# Treatment of the
# Rheumatic Diseases

SECOND EDITION

# Treatment of the Rheumatic Diseases

## Companion to *Kelley's Textbook of Rheumatology*

**Michael H. Weisman, M.D.**
Director
Division of Rheumatology
Cedars-Sinai Medical Center
Professor of Medicine
University of California at Los Angeles Medical Center
Los Angeles, California

**Michael E. Weinblatt, M.D.**
Professor of Medicine
Harvard Medical School
Co-Director of Clinical Rheumatology
Brigham and Women's Hospital
Boston, Massachusetts

**James S. Louie, M.D.**
Professor of Medicine
University of California at Los Angeles School of Medicine
Chief, Division of Rheumatology
Harbor–University of California at Los Angeles Medical Center
Torrance, California

**W.B. Saunders Company**
*A Harcourt Health Sciences Company*
Philadelphia London New York St. Louis Sydney Toronto

**W.B. SAUNDERS COMPANY**
*A Harcourt Health Sciences Company*

The Curtis Center
Independence Square West
Philadelphia, Pennsylvania 19106

**Library of Congress Cataloging-in-Publication Data**

Treatment of the rheumatic diseases : companion to Kelley's textbook of rheumatology/
[edited by] Michael H. Weisman, Michael E. Weinblatt, James S. Louie.—2nd ed.

p. ; cm.

ISBN 0–7216–8464–5

1. Rheumatism—Chemotherapy. 2. Arthritis—Chemotherapy. I. Weisman, Michael H.
II. Weinblatt, Michael E. III. Louie, James S.
 [DNLM: 1. Rheumatic Diseases—drug therapy. 2. Arthritis, Rheumatoid—drug therapy.

WE 544 D7938 2001]     RC927 .T74 2001
616.7′23061—dc21                                 99–051710

*Acquisitions Editor:* Richard Zorab
*Manuscript Editor:* Anne Ostroff
*Production Editor:* Natalie Ware
*Illustration Specialist:* Lisa Lambert
*Indexer:* Eleanor Kuljian

TREATMENT OF THE RHEUMATIC DISEASES:
Companion to Kelley's Textbook of Rheumatology          ISBN 0–7216–8464–5

Printed in the United States of America.

Last digit is the print number:     9     8     7     6     5     4     3     2     1

*To our patients and our families*
*who have inspired and have taught us*

# CONTRIBUTORS

**Jean-Jacques Abitbol, MD**
Associate Professor, Orthopedic Surgery, University of California, San Diego, California
*Neck Pain*

**Carlos A. Agudelo, MD**
Chief, Rheumatology Section, Emory University School of Medicine, Atlanta V.A. Medical Center, Decatur, Georgia
*Crystal Deposition Disease*

**Daniel A. Albert, MD**
Associate Professor of Medicine/Rheumatology, University of Pennsylvania; Attending Physician, Hospital of the University of Pennsylvania; Attending Physician, Children's Hospital of Philadelphia, Philadelphia, Pennsylvania
*Geriatric Rheumatology*

**Gene V. Ball, MD**
Professor of Medicine Emeritus, University of Alabama at Birmingham, Birmingham, Alabama
*Uncommon Rheumatic Diseases*

**Bonnie L. Bermas, MD**
Clinical Instructor in Medicine, Harvard Medical School; Associate Director of Clinical Affairs for Women's Health and Associate Rheumatologist, Brigham and Women's Hospital, Boston, Massachusetts
*The Treatment of Rheumatic Diseases During Pregnancy*

**Bram H. Bernstein, MD, CM**
Professor of Pediatrics, Keck School of Medicine, University of Southern California; Head, Division of Rheumatology, Children's Hospital of Los Angeles, Los Angeles, California
*The Rheumatic Diseases of Childhood*

**Robert S. Boretz, MD**
Chief Resident, Department of Orthopaedic Surgery, Long Island Jewish Medical Center, New Hyde Park, New York
*Neck Pain*

**Mark J. Borigini, MD**
Assistant Clinical Professor of Medicine, University of California, Irvine; Consulting Rheumatologist, Care More Medical Group, Downey, California
*Rheumatoid Arthritis*

**F. C. Breedveld, MD**
Professor of Rheumatology, Leiden University; Head, Department of Medicine, Leiden University Medical Center, Leiden, The Netherlands
*Novel Therapies for Rheumatoid Arthritis*

**Michael P. Brunelli, MD**
Resident in Orthopaedic Surgery, Mt. Sinai Hospital, New York, New York
*Shoulder Pain*

**Leonard H. Calabrese, DO**
R. J. Fasenmyer Chair of Clinical Immunology; Vice Chairman, Department of Rheumatic and Immunologic Disease, Cleveland Clinic Foundation, Cleveland, Ohio
*Vasculitis of the Central Nervous System*

**Jeffrey P. Callen, MD, FACP**
Professor of Medicine (Dermatology) and Chief, Division of Dermatology, University of Louisville, Louisville, Kentucky
*Treatment of Cutaneous Disease Associated with Rheumatic Disease*

**Loretta B. Chou, MD**
Assistant Professor of Orthopaedic Surgery, Stanford University, Stanford, California
*Foot and Ankle Pain*

**Daniel O. Clegg, MD**
Professor of Medicine and Chief, Division of Rheumatology, University of Utah School of Medicine, Salt Lake City, Utah
*The Seronegative Spondyloarthropathies (Ankylosing Spondylitis, Reactive Arthritis, Psoriatic Arthritis)*

**Doyt L. Conn, MD**
Professor of Medicine and Director of Allergy, Immunology and Rheumatology, Emory University School of Medicine; Professor of Medicine, Grady Hospital and Emory University Hospital, Atlanta, Georgia
*Extra-articular Manifestations of Rheumatoid Arthritis*

**Mary Patricia Corr, MD**
Assistant Professor in Residence, University of California, San Diego, La Jolla, California
*Differential Diagnosis of Acute and Chronic Polyarthritis*

**Miriam F. Delaney, MB, BCh, BAO, MRCPI**
Clinical Instructor in Medicine, Harvard Medical School; Associate Physician, Endocrine-Hypertension Division, Brigham and Women's Hospital, Boston, Massachusetts
*Osteoporosis and Rheumatic Disorders*

**Robin K. Dore, MD**
Associate Professor of Medicine, Division of Rheumatology, University of California, Los Angeles, School of Medicine, Los Angeles, California
*Developing Medical Documentation for Rheumatology Encounters*

**George F. Duna, MD**
Clinical Assistant Professor, Baylor College of Medicine; Chief of Rheumatology, Kelsey-Seybold Clinic and St. Luke's Episcopal Hospital, Houston, Texas
*Vasculitis of the Central Nervous System*

**Evan L. Flatow, MD**
Professor of Orthopaedic Surgery, Mt. Sinai School of Medicine; Chief of Shoulder Surgery, Mt. Sinai Hospital, New York, New York
*Shoulder Pain*

**Robert I. Fox, MD, PhD**
Member, Allergy and Rheumatology Clinic, Scripps Memorial Hospital and Research Foundation, La Jolla, California
*Approaches to the Treatment of Sjögren's Syndrome*

**Steven R. Garfin, MD**
Professor and Chair, Orthopaedics, and Professor of Orthopaedic Surgery, University of California, San Diego, Medical Center, San Diego, California
*Neck Pain*

**Ellen M. Ginzler, MD, MPH**
Professor of Medicine and Chief of Rheumatology, State University of New York–Health Science Center at Brooklyn, Brooklyn, New York
*Renal Disease in Systemic Lupus Erythematosus*

**Deirdre A. Gramas, MD, MPH**
Division Chair, Rheumatology, Penobscot Bay Medical Center, Rockport, Maine
*Osteoarthritis*

**Melanie A. Greenberg, PhD**
Associate Professor of Psychology, Health Psychology Programs, California School of Professional Psychology, San Diego, California
*The Effectiveness of Cognitive-Behavioral and Psychoeducational Interventions in the Management of Arthritis*

**Christopher G. Jackson, MD**
Associate Professor of Medicine, University of Utah School of Medicine, Salt Lake City, Utah
*The Seronegative Spondyloarthropathies (Ankylosing Spondylitis, Reactive Arthritis, Psoriatic Arthritis)*

**R. Kumar Kadiyala, MD, PhD**
Assistant Professor of Orthopaedic Surgery, University of Iowa Hospital, Department of Orthopaedic Surgery, Iowa City, Iowa
*Rheumatic Diseases of the Hand and Wrist*

**Jeffrey N. Katz, MD**
Associate Professor of Medicine, Harvard Medical School; Co-Director, Spine Center, Division of Rheumatology, Immunology and Allergy, Brigham and Women's Hospital, Boston, Massachusetts
*Lumbar Spine Disease*

**Nathaniel P. Katz, MD**
Assistant Professor of Anesthesia, Harvard Medical
School; Neurologist, Pain Management Center,
Brigham and Women's Hospital, Boston,
Massachusetts
*Lumbar Spine Disease*


**L. B. Klickstein, MD, PhD**
Assistant Professor of Medicine, Harvard Medical
School; Associate Physician, Brigham and Women's
Hospital, Boston, Massachusetts
*Rheumatologic Consultations in Organ Transplant
Recipients*


**Nancy E. Lane, MD**
Associate Professor of Medicine, University of
California, San Francisco; Co-Director,
Rheumatology Clinic, San Francisco General
Hospital, San Francisco, California
*Osteoarthritis*


**Carol A. Langford, MD, MHS**
Senior Investigator, National Institute of Allergy and
Infectious Diseases, National Institutes of Health,
Bethesda, Maryland
*Takayasu's Arteritis, Giant Cell Arteritis, and
Polymyalgia Rheumatica*


**Meryl S. LeBoff, MD**
Associate Professor of Medicine, Harvard Medical
School; Director, Skeletal Health and Osteoporosis
Program and Director, Bone Density Unit,
Endocrine-Hypertension Division, Brigham and
Women's Hospital, Boston, Massachusetts
*Osteoporosis and Rheumatic Disorders*


**Clifford D. Locks, JD**
Anaheim, California
*Developing Medical Documentation for Rheumatology
Encounters*


**Baron S. Lonner, MD**
Attending Surgeon, Albert Einstein College of
Medicine, Bronx; Montefiore Medical Center, Bronx;
The Hospital for Joint Diseases, Manhattan; and
Long Island Jewish Medical Center, Our Lady of
Mercy Hospital, Long Island, New York
*Neck Pain*


**James S. Louie, MD**
Professor of Medicine, University of California, Los
Angeles (UCLA); Chief, Division of Rheumatology,
Harbor–UCLA Medical Center, Torrance, California
*Monarticular Arthritis*
*Infectious Agent Arthritis*


**Milton H. Louie, MD**
Infectious Disease Consultants Medical Group,
Glendale, California
*Infectious Agent Arthritis*


**Roger A. Mann, MD**
Clinical Associate Professor of Orthopaedic Surgery,
University of California, San Francisco, San
Francisco, California
*Foot and Ankle Pain*


**Alan K. Matsumoto, MD**
Assistant Professor of Medicine, Johns Hopkins
University School of Medicine; Johns Hopkins
Bayview Medical Center, Johns Hopkins Hospital,
Baltimore, Maryland
*Scleroderma*


**Eric L. Matteson, MD, MPH**
Associate Professor of Medicine, Mayo Clinic and
Mayo Graduate School of Medicine; Consultant in
Rheumatology, Mayo Foundation, Rochester,
Minnesota
*Extra-articular Manifestations of Rheumatoid Arthritis*


**Paul Michelson, MD**
Division Chairman, Department of Ophthalmology,
Scripps Memorial Hospital, La Jolla, California
*Approaches to the Treatment of Sjögren's Syndrome*


**Perry M. Nicassio, PhD**
Professor of Psychology and Director of Health
Psychology Programs, California School of
Professional Psychology, San Diego; Associate
Adjunct Professor, Department of Psychiatry, School
of Medicine, University of California, San Diego,
La Jolla, California
*The Effectiveness of Cognitive-Behavioral and
Psychoeducational Interventions in the Management of
Arthritis*


**Ann L. Parke, MD**
Professor of Medicine, Division of Rheumatic
Diseases, University of Connecticut Health Center,
Farmington, Connecticut
*Antiphospholipid Syndrome*


**Harold E. Paulus, MD**
Professor of Medicine, University of California, Los
Angeles, School of Medicine, Los Angeles, California
*Rheumatoid Arthritis*

**Erik Peterson, MD**
Instructor, Department of Medicine, Abramson
Family Cancer Research Institute, University of
Pennsylvania, Philadelphia, Pennsylvania
*Reflex Sympathetic Dystrophy (Complex Regional Pain
Syndrome-I)*

**Michelle Petri, MD, MPH**
Associate Professor of Medicine and Director, Lupus
Center, Johns Hopkins University School of
Medicine, Baltimore, Maryland
*Systemic Lupus Erythematosus (Including Pregnancy
and Antiphospholipid Antibody Syndrome)*

**Boris Ratiner, MD**
Attending Physician, Northridge Hospital, and
private practice, Northridge, California
*Osteoarthritis*

**James T. Rosenbaum, MD**
Professor of Ophthalmology, Medicine, and Cell
Biology; Director, The Uveitis Clinic, Oregon Health
Sciences University, Portland, Oregon
*Inflammatory Eye Disease: Uveitis and Scleritis*

**Kenneth Saag, MD**
Associate Professor, Division of Clinical
Immunology and Rheumatology, Department of
Medicine, University of Alabama at Birmingham,
Birmingham, Alabama
*Reflex Sympathetic Dystrophy (Complex Regional Pain
Syndrome-I)*

**Edna P. Schwab, MD**
Assistant Professor of Medicine, Hospital of the
University of Pennsylvania and Philadelphia
Veterans Affairs Medical Center, Philadelphia,
Pennsylvania
*Geriatric Rheumatology*

**Nancy A. Shadick, MD, MPH**
Assistant Professor of Medicine, Harvard Medical
School; Rheumatologist, Robert B. Brigham Arthritis
Center, Brigham and Women's Hospital, Boston,
Massachusetts
*Lyme Disease*

**Bracha Shaham, MD**
Assistant Professor of Pediatrics, University of
Southern California Medical School; Attending
Physician, Division of Rheumatology, Children's
Hospital of Los Angeles, Los Angeles, California
*The Rheumatic Diseases of Childhood*

**Barry P. Simmons, MD**
Associate Professor of Orthopaedic Surgery,
Harvard Medical School; Chief, Hand and Upper
Extremity Service, Department of Orthopaedics,
Brigham and Women's Hospital, Boston,
Massachusetts
*Rheumatic Diseases of the Hand and Wrist*

**Robert W. Simms, MD**
Associate Professor of Medicine, Boston University
School of Medicine; Clinical Director, Rheumatology
Section, Boston Medical Center, Boston,
Massachusetts
*Fibromyalgia Syndrome*

**Bernhard H. Singsen, MD, MPH**
Head, Section of Pediatric Rheumatology,
Department of Rheumatology and Division
of Pediatrics, Cleveland Clinic Foundation,
Cleveland, Ohio
*Juvenile Rheumatoid Arthritis and the Pediatric
Spondyloarthropathies*

**Garth R. Smith, MD**
Co-Director, Hand Center, Anne Arundel
Orthopaedic Surgeons, Annapolis, Maryland
*Rheumatic Diseases of the Hand and Wrist*

**Gordon Starkebaum, MD**
Professor and Associate Dean, School of Medicine,
University of Washington, Seattle; Chief Medical
Officer, Veterans Affairs Puget Sound Health Care
System, Seattle, Washington
*Hematologic Disease*

**E. William St. Clair, MD**
Associate Professor of Medicine, Division of
Rheumatology, Allergy, and Clinical Immunology,
Duke University Medical Center, Durham, North
Carolina
*Vasculitis*

**Jryki Tornwall, MD, DDS, PhD**
Postdoctoral Fellow, The Scripps Research Institute,
La Jolla, California
*Approaches to the Treatment of Sjögren's Syndrome*

**Joan Marie Von Feldt, MD**
Assistant Professor of Medicine, Department of
Medicine—Rheumatology Division, University of
Pennsylvania; Attending Physician, Rheumatology,
Hospital of the University of Pennsylvania,
Philadelphia, Pennsylvania
*Treatment of Neuropsychiatric Systemic Lupus
Erythematosus*

**John Wade, MD, FRCP(C), FRCP(Rheum)**
Clinical Associate Professor, Department of
Medicine, Division of Rheumatology, University of
British Columbia; Clinical Associate Professor,
Vancouver General Hospital, Vancouver, British
Columbia, Canada
*Osteoporosis and Rheumatic Disorders*

**Michael H. Weisman, MD**
Director, Division of Rheumatology, Cedars-Sinai
Medical Center; Professor of Medicine, University of
California at Los Angeles Medical Center, Los
Angeles, California
*Differential Diagnosis of Acute and Chronic Polyarthritis*

**Sterling G. West, MD**
Professor of Medicine, University of Colorado
Health Sciences Center, Denver, Colorado
*Uncommon Rheumatic Diseases*

**Fredrick M. Wigley, MD**
Professor of Medicine, Johns Hopkins University
School of Medicine; Director, Division of
Rheumatology, Johns Hopkins University, Baltimore,
Maryland
*Scleroderma*
*Raynaud's Phenomenon*

**Christopher M. Wise, MD**
W. Robert Irby Associate Professor, Medical College
of Virginia, Virginia Commonwealth University,
Richmond, Virginia
*Crystal Deposition Disease*

**Robert L. Wortmann, MD**
Professor and Chair, Department of Internal
Medicine, The University of Oklahoma College of
Medicine–Tulsa, Tulsa, Oklahoma
*Idiopathic Inflammatory Diseases of Muscle*

# FOREWORD

The investment has paid off. Millions of dollars have been allocated for the study of the pathogenesis of rheumatic diseases. Research has involved the collegial interaction of investigators from many different fields, including clinical and humoral immunology, cell biology, molecular genetics, biochemistry, physical chemistry, and microbiology, to name a few. The central paradigm, that understanding the basic pathophysiology of disease will lead to effective therapy, has been validated. Consider, for example, the appreciation from studies done in many laboratories that tumor necrosis factor-alpha is an important driving factor in the development of proliferative and destructive synovitis. This led to development of antibodies to tumor necrosis factor-alpha as well as to recombinant production of the soluble receptor for this important cytokine. Both have been shown to be effective in breaking into the cycle of proliferation and inflammation that is rheumatoid synovitis and, in many cases, in causing the process to subside. Neither is a cure, but the logic of following the lead that these studies have given us has been given a basis in reality: Learn about the cellular processes that are activated in rheumatic diseases, and our modern biotechnology can exploit this new knowledge to generate products that can be used for alleviation, if not cure.

The 1990s were a time of new awareness of the subtleties of rheumatic disease and how, with close inspection, different syndromes could be separated out from what seemed initially to be the same basic disease. This knowledge has been useful in prognosis and therapy as well as classification. For example, it was realized that an acute febrile illness with small-joint arthritis and skin desquamation in young parents exposed to young children might be a viral disease, and the data linked these findings to infection with human parvovirus B19. It is both intriguing and disconcerting to realize that with each passing year, yet another "rheumatic" disease is determined to have an infectious cause.

A fascinating yet potentially complicated collaboration is that between academia and industry in clinical investigation. In its best form, the science of basic laboratories has given biotechnology companies the lead for development of new products that are useful in therapy. At its worst, dollars generated by investors poured into products with little or no scientific rationale for use have given false hope to practitioners as well as patients. The evidence is abundant: Careful studies of the pathophysiology of disease can lead to an occasional "eureka!" as a good therapy evolves from clinical investigation.

Michael Weisman, Michael Weinblatt, and James Louie have generated a second edition of *Treatment of the Rheumatic Diseases* that exploits the lessons learned in the years since the first edition and creates excitement about new treatments developed. A brief section on diagnosis of various phenotypes is followed by a section on management of syndromes before a definite diagnosis is made. After this is a section on management of the rheumatic diseases in those in whom a clear diagnosis has been made. Clear, logical algorithms for management using all the modalities available (e.g., physical, educational, and pharmacologic therapies) are presented in useful formats. It is both honest and useful that no attempt is made to promote untried or unproven treatment for any of these illnesses that we study and attempt to treat. It is a measure of the success of the links among basic laboratories, clinical investigation, and clinical trials that we can move in the same way toward amelioration and perhaps cure of the diseases that seem "untreatable" to us now.

This book will be an important resource for clinicians both in primary care and in rheumatology who see patients with the many syndromes that comprise the content of our specialty texts. This is a worthy companion to *Textbook of Rheumatology* and *Primary Care Rheumatology*.

EDWARD D. HARRIS, JR., MD

# PREFACE

The second edition of *Treatment of the Rheumatic Diseases: Companion to the Textbook of Rheumatology* is now worthy of the name "treatment." Since the first edition was published in 1995, advances in patient management for chronic rheumatic diseases have gone beyond what we ever dreamed or imagined. We now can target specific elements of the basic disease process in rheumatoid arthritis and systemic lupus erythematosus rather than rely on drugs borrowed from the fields of infectious disease or cancer. Furthermore, the emerging capability of identifying risk factors for disease severity before the disease is clinically manifest will help guide more aggressive management. Even with the slow-moving condition osteoarthritis, there are bright spots for disease control beyond symptomatic treatment. Nevertheless, as stated in the preface to the first edition, the most powerful aspect of chronic rheumatic disease management will continue to be the relationship of the doctor to the knowledgeable patient. In truth, newer drugs serve only to highlight that need.

The purpose of the second edition is to continue to provide accurate and up-to-date information for the specialist and generalist about the management of adults and children with rheumatic diseases. Accordingly, to accomplish that task, we have broadened and extended our definition of "information." Because you cannot treat it if you cannot diagnose it, we have added a section on the differential diagnosis of acute and chronic arthritis. Furthermore, we focus, in other new chapters, on the differential diagnosis and management of rheumatic syndromes such as shoulder pain, foot and ankle pain, and joint pain in the dialysis/transplant patient. In addition, we have added chapters on medical documentation, arthritis in the elderly, and pain/psychological management for the patient with chronic illness. All of the previous chapters have been rewritten, and we have added 18 new chapters overall, expanding into areas in which specific information is needed in order to manage the organ system complications of rheumatic diseases.

As in the first edition, we have asked our contributors not only to review available data upon which to base management questions but also to give specific recommendations that are personal and reflective of their own unique approach. Although the individual chapters have been organized internally as in the first edition, the editors have tried to maintain as much as possible the uniqueness and individuality represented by each author's contribution. Therefore, there may be some overlap of approach to the disease or drug use from chapter to chapter, and the reader will note that individual authors will view risk/benefit of drugs in a different manner. The editors feel that the "menu" provided by this volume should give multiple choices and different strategies from which to pick and choose. It is highly unlikely that any one person knows all the best answers.

We are most appreciative of the efforts of the W.B. Saunders staff under the direction and guidance of Richard Zorab. However, in the final analysis, the editors are enormously in debt to our contributors, who dropped everything to answer the call to write their chapters. We are very grateful and hope that this second edition is worthy of their commitment to *Treatment of the Rheumatic Diseases*.

MICHAEL H. WEISMAN, M.D.
MICHAEL E. WEINBLATT, M.D.
JAMES S. LOUIE, M.D.

# CONTENTS

## SECTION I

## Diagnosis    1

1  Monarticular Arthritis    1
   *James S. Louie*

2  Differential Diagnosis of Acute and
   Chronic Polyarthritis    4
   *Michael H. Weisman and Mary Patricia Corr*

   *Color plates follow page 12*

3  Geriatric Rheumatology    31
   *Daniel A. Albert and Edna P. Schwab*

## SECTION II

## Rheumatic Syndromes    45

4  Shoulder Pain    45
   *Michael P. Brunelli and Evan L. Flatow*

5  Neck Pain    51
   *Robert S. Boretz, Baron S. Lonner, Jean-Jacques Abitbol,
   and Steven R. Garfin*

6  Foot and Ankle Pain    65
   *Roger A. Mann and Loretta B. Chou*

7  Rheumatic Diseases of the Hand
   and Wrist    75
   *R. Kumar Kadiyala, Barry P. Simmons,
   and Garth R. Smith*

8  Lumbar Spine Disease    89
   *Jeffrey N. Katz and Nathaniel P. Katz*

9  Reflex Sympathetic Dystrophy (Complex
   Regional Pain Syndrome-I)    101
   *Erik Peterson and Kenneth Saag*

10  Rheumatologic Consultations in Organ
    Transplant Recipients    111
    *L. B. Klickstein*

11  Fibromyalgia Syndrome    120
    *Robert W. Simms*

12  Developing Medical Documentation for
    Rheumatology Encounters    132
    *Clifford D. Locks and Robin K. Dore*

13  The Effectiveness of Cognitive-Behavioral and
    Psychoeducational Interventions in the
    Management of Arthritis    147
    *Perry M. Nicassio and Melanie A. Greenberg*

## SECTION III

## Rheumatic Diseases    163

14  The Treatment of Rheumatic Diseases
    During Pregnancy    163
    *Bonnie L. Bermas*

15  Treatment of Cutaneous Disease Associated with
    Rheumatic Disease    175
    *Jeffrey P. Callen*

    *Color plates follow page 188*

16  Inflammatory Eye Disease:
    Uveitis and Scleritis    192
    *James T. Rosenbaum*

17  Hematologic Disease    198
    *Gordon Starkebaum*

18  Novel Therapies for
    Rheumatoid Arthritis    208
    *F. C. Breedveld*

19  Rheumatoid Arthritis    217
    *Mark J. Borigini and Harold E. Paulus*

20  Extra-articular Manifestations of
    Rheumatoid Arthritis    236
    *Eric L. Matteson and Doyt L. Conn*

21  Approaches to the Treatment of
    Sjögren's Syndrome    249
    *Robert I. Fox, Paul Michelson, and Jryki Tornwall*

**22**  The Seronegative Spondyloarthropathies (Ankylosing Spondylitis, Reactive Arthritis, Psoriatic Arthritis)    263
*Christopher G. Jackson and Daniel O. Clegg*

**23**  Systemic Lupus Erythematosus (Including Pregnancy and Antiphospholipid Antibody Syndrome)    274
*Michelle Petri*

**24**  Antiphospholipid Syndrome    289
*Ann L. Parke*

**25**  Renal Disease in Systemic Lupus Erythematosus    297
*Ellen M. Ginzler*

**26**  Treatment of Neuropsychiatric Systemic Lupus Erythematosus    313
*Joan Marie Von Feldt*

**27**  Vasculitis    323
*E. William St. Clair*

**28**  Vasculitis of the Central Nervous System    345
*Leonard H. Calabrese and George F. Duna*

**29**  Takayasu's Arteritis, Giant Cell Arteritis, and Polymyalgia Rheumatica    353
*Carol A. Langford*

**30**  Scleroderma    365
*Fredrick M. Wigley and Alan K. Matsumoto*

**31**  Raynaud's Phenomenon    382
*Fredrick M. Wigley*

**32**  Idiopathic Inflammatory Diseases of Muscle    390
*Robert L. Wortmann*

**33**  Juvenile Rheumatoid Arthritis and the Pediatric Spondyloarthropathies    403
*Bernhard H. Singsen*

**34**  The Rheumatic Diseases of Childhood    423
*Bracha Shaham and Bram H. Bernstein*

**35**  Crystal Deposition Disease    447
*Carlos A. Agudelo and Christopher M. Wise*

**36**  Osteoarthritis    461
*Boris Ratiner, Deirdre A. Gramas, and Nancy E. Lane*

**37**  Uncommon Rheumatic Diseases    487
*Sterling G. West and Gene V. Ball*

**38**  Infectious Agent Arthritis    503
*James S. Louie and Milton H. Louie*

**39**  Lyme Disease    515
*Nancy A. Shadick*

**40**  Osteoporosis and Rheumatic Disorders    528
*Miriam F. Delaney, John Wade, and Meryl S. LeBoff*

Index    547

# SECTION

# I Diagnosis

## CHAPTER

## 1 Monarticular Arthritis

*James S. Louie*

Monarticular arthritis, the manifestation of joint pain and swelling in a single joint, is the most important differential diagnosis in rheumatology. Within this differential diagnosis are the most treatable conditions in our specialty when the diagnosis and the therapies are effected quickly. Appropriately, the processes for early diagnosis require the basic skills taught in rheumatology. Thus, in an evaluation of 56 consecutive presentations of monarticular arthritis to a metropolitan emergency department, the history, physical examination, synovianalysis, and x-ray film elicited the diagnosis in 66% of patients.[1]

The differential diagnosis is best adapted to the following mnemonic: *"If I make the diagnosis, no more harm."* The following sections describe the elements of this mnemonic.

## INFECTION

It is rather curious that most infections present with pain and inflammation in a single joint, because infections are disseminated hematogenously. Perhaps the initial joints infected activate basic host defenses to control the infection in the other sites. Of course, polyarticular infections occur when the host defenses are immunocompromised by disease or drug or when a large number of microorganisms are disseminated.

Following the cues elicited from the history and physical examination, all patients presenting with a single inflamed joint should have synovial fluid aspirated and processed for bacterial identification by either culture or DNA hybridization molecular techniques such as the polymerase chain reaction (PCR). Gram staining of the cells identifies microorganisms in 60% of nongonococcal infections.[2] Once the synovial fluid is aspirated and submitted for culture, antibiotics should be prescribed empirically and then modified on identification of the specific microorganism. The discipline and care in processing the synovial fluid determine the effectiveness of identification. Thus, a careful and knowledgeable physician can identify by culture the fastidious gonococcus in 44% of cases, whereas the house staff at three major teaching institutions recover gonococcus in less than 10% of cases.[3, 4]

When monarticular arthritis persists with inflammatory signs, biopsy of the synovial tissue for culture or PCR and histologic examination identifies elusive organisms such as tuberculosis fungi, actinomycetes, or virus.[5-8] Biopsy is most effective under the direct viewing afforded by arthroscopy.

## INFLAMMATION

The three diseases that commonly present with monarticular arthritis are juvenile rheumatoid arthritis, rheumatoid arthritis, and acute reactive arthritis.

Monarticular juvenile rheumatoid arthritis occurs in 30% of children presenting with inflammatory arthritis. Girls are prone to acquire symptomatic iritis, particularly when identified as part of the subset of patients who display antinuclear antibody positivity. Iritis in boys is associated with the HLA-B27 spondyloarthropathy gene.

About a third of patients with rheumatoid arthritis, particularly males, present with inflammation in a single joint before displaying the usual symmetric small joint inflammatory pattern.

Acute reactive arthritis presents with a single inflamed joint, particularly in the lower extremity, often simulating acute gonococcal arthritis.[9] In 20% of cases, mucocutaneous lesions such as oral ulcers, circinate balanitis, or keratoderma blennorrhagicum on the soles differentiate the diagnosis of acute reactive arthritis from the erythematous macule, papule, and pustule of acute gonococcal arthritis.

## METABOLIC DISEASE

The crystalline-induced arthritides reflect changes of the metabolism of monosodium urate, calcium hydroxyapatite, calcium pyrophosphate, and other calcium molecules in the joint.

In gout, the crystals of urate deposit in the great toe (podagra), ankle, or knee in increasing order of frequency. Although calcium pyrophosphate was first described in the great toe (pseudogout), the usual presentations affect the knee, ankle, and great toe in decreasing order of frequency. Calcium hydroxyapatite can affect a single large joint such as a shoulder (see Chapter 35).

Again, diagnosis requires joint aspiration and processing the fluid for crystal identification. The most practicable method of crystal identification requires knowledge and experience in using a pair of polarizing filters and a third filter called a *first-order red compensator*. The polarizing filters are placed at right angles above and below the glass slide with the crystal-laden synovial fluid cells. The red compensator is placed with the slow plane of vibration directed vertically. Crystals that are vertical and yellow are negatively birefringent and are gout crystals. On occasion, after pricked with a needle or lancet, crystals can be expressed from a small tophus identified at the helix of the ear or from an olecranon nodule. Crystals that are vertical and blue are positively birefringent and are calcium pyrophosphate crystals. Because calcium pyrophosphate dihydrate crystals are weakly birefringent, it is useful to dim the overhead lights to view the crystals (see Chapter 35). Regrettably, current health care funding restricts identification of urate and calcium pyrophosphate dihydrate crystals to a Clinical Laboratories Improvement Act–approved laboratory for reimbursement, so these requirements have essentially removed the microscopes from the clinics and teaching institutions and thereby compromised the teaching of this skill to trainees. ◦

Calcium apatite crystals are 10 A and cannot be visualized with microscopy. The clinical method for tentative identification of these crystals requires staining of the synovial fluid cells with alizarin red S.[10]

## TRAUMA

External or internal trauma can lead to monarticular arthritis. Stress fractures can present with a monarticular presentation even in the setting of polyarticular disease.[11] Fractures that extend into the joint release marrow cells into the synovial fluid. These marrow cells glisten on gross inspection and layer over the serum and blood elements when sedimented in a vertical tube. Internal trauma includes the inadvertent introduction of foreign bodies such as sea urchin spines, rose thorns, and a variety of metallic, silicone, and cement particles.[12, 13]

## DEGENERATIVE DISEASE

Juvenile osteochondrosis, including true osteonecrosis of an apophyseal or epiphyseal center or a genetic or traumatic alteration of ossification, often leads to accel-erated degenerative changes in the affected joint.[14, 15] Thus, aseptic necrosis of the proximal femoral capital epiphysis of the hip (Legg-Calvé-Perthes disease) affecting boys aged 3 to 12 years and slipped capital femoral epiphysis affecting boys aged 16 to 19 years lead to accelerated degenerative hip disease.

In adults, degenerative changes in a single joint in the absence of prior trauma suggest a secondary form of osteoarthritis induced by calcium crystals. The marked destruction of a shoulder joint in elderly women associated with blood-tinged synovial fluid may demonstrate calcium apatite or pyrophosphate crystals (Milwaukee shoulder).[16] Anecdotes describe pain relief with closed needle drainage, colchicine, and magnesium-containing nonsteroidal anti-inflammatory drugs.[17]

## NEOPLASM

Benign neoplasms and tumoral conditions are the characteristic new growths in the joint. Pigmented villonodular synovitis is a locally invasive tumor-like growth of both A- and B-type synovial lining cells, histiocytes, giant cells, lipid-laden foam cells, lymphocytes, and hemosiderin deposits. The mononuclear and giant cells show the characteristics of osteoclasts.[18] Pigmented villonodular synovitis occurs in young adults who present with pain, swelling, and limitation of motion, particularly in the knee (80%); occasionally it presents in a localized form within tendon sheaths of the hands and feet. A bloody effusion alerts the clinician to this diagnosis. Radiographs may show irregular bony erosions, but radionuclide studies that show uptake of technetium but not gallium and magnetic resonance imaging (MRI) studies are more sensitive.[19] Surgical excision is the treatment of choice, but recurrences are common, particularly in the diffuse form, and are apparently related to incomplete removal. Other benign tumors include synovial chondromatosis of cartilage metaplasia that detaches from the synovium and presents as calcified loose bodies, lipoma arborescens of fatty synovial tissue, and hemangiomas. Each is diagnosed by radiography, MRI, and arthroscopy before surgical excision.[20]

Malignant tumors of the joint are rare. Primary sarcomas arise in the surrounding tissues, including the synovium, bone, cartilage, and fibrous tissue and extend into the joint by local extension. Metastatic carcinomas are rarely described in the knee and other joints.

## MISCELLANEOUS CONDITIONS

Several periodic syndromes present with a monarticular arthritis. Palindromic rheumatism and intermittent hydrarthrosis were described in the mid-1900s, with few substantive papers of new knowledge being written since then.[21] One suspects that these two syndromes were unusual presentations of infectious diseases or forme fruste of autoimmune diseases such as rheumatoid arthritis and systemic lupus erythematosus. Palindromic rheumatism was described as a recurring acute arthritis characterized by intense inflammation in one or two joints and adjoining tissues for several days interspersed with months of symptom-free periods. A retrospective study suggests that antimalarial drugs will delay and possibly reduce subsequent rheumatoid arthritis.[21a] Similarly, a report on intermittent hydrarthrosis or periodic benign synovitis described recurrent effusions in the knee or another large joint that recurred at regular intervals.[22] There have been no prospective reports of effective therapy.

## HEMATOLOGIC DISEASE

Hematologic diseases that present as monarticular arthritis include those that are heritable as well as those that are acquired. The hemophilias are sex-linked disorders that occur in 1 of every 10,000 males. The deficient clotting factors include factor VIII (hemophilia A), factor IX (hemophilia B or Christmas disease), and rarely factor V (von Willebrand's disease). Intra-articular hemorrhage produces tenderness, swelling, and warmth within the knee and other large joints. Repeated hemorrhage results in flexion contractures induced by hypertrophic, hemosiderin-laden synovium, and degenerative changes in the cartilage and bone.

The acute bleed is treated with intravenous replacement of the deficient clotting factor while the joint is placed at rest in extension with ice, analgesia, and nonsteroidal anti-inflammatory drugs. Arthrocentesis is indicated if infection is suspected. Intra-articular corticosteroids, yttrium 90, and arthroscopic synovectomy have been reported to be effective by some investigators.[23]

Acquired causes of intra-articular bleeds include heparin or warfarin administration in patients who suffer minor trauma to the joint.

## SUMMARY

Monarticular arthritis remains the most exciting differential diagnosis in rheumatology. Aspiration and examination of the fluid for infection and crystals is a skilled clinical pursuit that leads to early detection and offers cure or control of inflammatory processes that can lead to deformity or death. When the history, physical examination, radiographs, and synovianalysis do not reveal the diagnosis, arthroscopic or closed-needle biopsy for culture or PCR and histologic examination of the synovial tissue will identify the more elusive infections that are not easily cultured from the synovial fluid. *Chlamydia,* tuberculosis, and fungal infections are more efficiently identified from synovial tissue.

When monarticular arthritis persists, evaluation with an HLA-B27 gene protein and an MRI of the affected joint assists in the differential diagnosis. Thus, clinical skills and the use of emerging technologies will enhance our capabilities of diagnosing the causes of monarticular arthritis and effect appropriate therapies.

## REFERENCES

1. Freed JF, Nies KM, Boyer RS, et al: Acute monoarticular arthritis: A diagnostic approach. JAMA 1980; 243:2314–2316.
2. Goldenberg DL: Bacterial arthritis. *In* Kelley WN, Harris ED, Ruddy S, et al (eds): Textbook of Rheumatology, 5th ed. Philadelphia: WB Saunders, 1997.
3. Wise CM, Morris CR, Wasilauskas BL, et al: Gonococcal arthritis in an era of increasing penicillin resistance: Presentations and outcomes in 41 recent cases (1985–1991). Arch Intern Med 1994; 154:2690.
4. Liebling MR, Arkfeld DG, Michelini GA, et al: Identification of *Neisseria gonorrhoeae* in synovial fluid using the polymerase chain reaction. Arthritis Rheum 1994; 37:702.
5. Hunfeld KP, Rittmeister M, Wichelhaus TA, et al: Two cases of chronic arthritis of the forearm due to *Mycobacterium tuberculosis.* Eur J Clin Microbiol Infect Dis 1998; 17:344.
6. Stebbins S, Highton J, Croxson MC, et al: Chickenpox monoarthritis: Demonstration of varicella-zoster virus in joint fluid by polymerase chain reaction. Br J Rheumatol 1998; 37:311.
7. Matava MJ, Horgan M: Serial quantification of the human immunodeficiency virus in an arthroscopic effluent. Arthroscopy 1997; 13:739.
8. O'Duffy JD, Griffing WL, Li CY, et al: Whipple's arthritis—Direct detection of *Tropheryma whippelii* in synovial fluid and tissue. Arthritis Rheum 1999; 42:812.
9. McCord WC, Nies KM, Louie JS: Acute venereal arthritis. Comparative study of acute Reiter's syndrome and acute gonococcal arthritis. Arch Intern Med 1977; 137:858.
10. Paul H, Reginato AJ, Schumacher HR: Alizarin red S staining as a screening test to detect calcium components in synovial times. Arthritis Rheum 1983; 26:191–200.
11. Wei N: Stress fractures of the distal fibula presenting as monarticular flares in patients with rheumatoid arthritis. Arthritis Rheum 1994; 37:1555.
12. Cracchiolo A, Goldberg L: Local and systemic reactions to puncture injuries by the sea urchin spine and date palm thorn. Arthritis Rheum 1977; 20:1125.
13. Reginato AJ, Ferreiro JL, O'Connor CR, et al: Clinical and pathologic studies of twenty-six patients with penetrating foreign body injury to the joint, bursae, and tendon sheaths. Arthritis Rheum 1990; 33:1753.
14. Weinstein SL: Natural history and treatment outcomes of childhood hip diseases. Clin Orthop 1997; 314:227.
15. Wang L, Bowen JR, Puniak MA, et al: An evaluation of various methods of treatment for Legg-Calve-Perthes disease. Clin Orthop 1995; 314:225.
16. Fam AG: Calcium pyrophosphate deposition disease and other crystal deposition diseases. Curr Opin Rheumatol 1995; 7:364.
17. Patel KJ, Weidensaul D, Palma C, et al: A shoulder with massive bilateral cysts: Effective treatment for hydrops of the shoulder. J Rheumatol 1997; 24:2479.
18. Neale SD, Kristelly R, Gundle R, et al: Giant cells in pigmented villonodular synovitis express an osteoclast phenotype. J Clin Pathol 1997; 50:605.
19. Bravo SM, Winalski CS, Weissman BN: Pigmented villonodular synovitis. Radiol Clin North Am 1996; 34:311.
20. Martin S, Hernandez L, Romero J, et al: Diagnostic imaging of lipoma arborescens. Skeletal Radiol 1998; 27:325.
21. Hench PS, Rosenberg EF: Palindromic rheumatism: A "new" oft-recurring disease of joints (arthritis, peri-arthritis, para-arthritis) apparently producing no articular residues: Report of 34 cases; its relation to "angioneural arthrosis," "allergic rheumatism" and rheumatoid arthritis. Arch Intern Med 1944; 73:292.
21a. Gonzalez-Lopez L, Gamez-Nava JI, Jhangri G, et al: Decreased progression to rheumatoid arthritis or other connective diseases in patients with palindromic rheumatism treated with antimalarials. J Rheum 2000; 27:41.
22. Weiner AB, Ghormley RK: Periodic benign synovitis: Idiopathic hydrarthrosis. J Bone Joint Surg Am 1956; 38:1034.
23. Gilbert MS, Radomsli TE: Therapeutic options in the management of hemophilic synovitis. Clin Orthop 1997; 343:88.

# Differential Diagnosis of Acute and Chronic Polyarthritis*

*Michael H. Weisman and Mary Patricia Corr*

What is the purpose of a chapter on the differential diagnosis of acute and chronic polyarthritis in a book that deals with treatment? It is very simple: You cannot treat it if you cannot diagnose it.

It is important to remember that many of the patients who present to the physician with acute or short-duration inflammatory polyarthritis do not become chronically ill and do not need aggressive treatment. The conditions are often self-limited or resolve by themselves, even without a diagnosis. For example, Tunn and Bacon[1] described the natural history of patients with polyarthritis of short duration seen in an early arthritis clinic. Of the cohort, 50% displayed findings at 6 months, and only 25% continued to have polyarthritis at the end of a 1-year follow-up. Aggressive management with toxic medications in the majority of these patients at presentation would have been a mistake and, in fact, downright dangerous.

To accomplish this task, the current chapter is divided into two sections: differential diagnosis of chronic polyarthritis and differential diagnosis of acute polyarthritis. The distinction is somewhat arbitrary and based entirely on the authors' clinical experience and some observational data. For conditions or diseases that persist longer than 6 weeks, the term *chronic* is applied, and the first section of this chapter focuses on those diseases. A set of five fundamental rules is presented as a general guide for systematically narrowing and focusing the differential diagnosis on the basis of clinical presentation. The most common forms of chronic polyarticular arthritis are then examined with these rules in mind.

Much importance is attached to making an accurate and precise diagnosis among the many conditions with chronic polyarthritis. The prognosis and long-term outlook are dramatically different if the patient has rheumatoid arthritis (RA) versus osteoarthritis (OA). Furthermore, the distinction between RA and the diseases that resemble RA, such as psoriatic arthritis, has important implications for a patient's individual prognosis as well as for management decisions. Similarly, failing to make the diagnosis of chronic gouty arthritis would be a major mistake in the management of a patient with chronic joint complaints. Not recognizing

the possibility of calcium pyrophosphate dihydrate (CPPD) deposition disease in a patient with chronic joint complaints may prevent the clinician from diagnosing potentially treatable CPPD-associated conditions, such as hypothyroidism, hyperparathyroidism, or hemochromatosis. By approaching the patient with foreknowledge of the basic findings in relation to the pathologic processes of these diseases, common diagnostic pitfalls can be avoided.

The second part of this chapter addresses acute polyarthritis. The acute infectious diseases or postinfectious syndromes that are self-limited usually last 6 weeks or less. This appears to be true for most of the identifiable virus-induced syndromes (e.g., parvovirus, hepatitis B, and rubella) as well as for many of the conditions that resemble postviral syndromes but for which no viruses have as yet been isolated. Even rheumatic fever attacks generally do not last longer than 6 weeks. A differential diagnosis of patients potentially presenting with fever, rash, and arthritis is examined in detail through a series of case presentations. These cases highlight the distinguishing physical findings and pertinent laboratory data to rule out certain diseases and arrive at the most likely diagnosis.

## CHRONIC POLYARTHRITIS

### The Rules

The differential diagnosis of chronic polyarthritis remains a challenge to both the primary care and specialist physician as much today as it was in the mid-1970s. There is even some information that this situation has really not improved very much since then. Newly acquired data indicate that the "lag time," or the time from onset of symptoms to a final physician-made diagnosis of RA, is still quite long (18 weeks); the majority of this time delay takes place under the direct observation of the physician.[2]

It is also recognized that the expert specialist approach in evaluating a patient with chronic joint complaints can lead to a more timely diagnosis. The setting of the medical encounter (e.g., how much time was spent with this patient; the additional constraints of the visit) must certainly influence the ability to focus on the patient's articular findings. How to "download"

---

*\* All figures in this chapter except Figures 2–1 and 2–2 also appear in color following page 12.*

the expertise from the seasoned clinician to the primary care physician represents the greatest challenge for this chapter.

The initial approach for this section is to describe patients with textbook "full-blown" disease: that is, with completely classical physical findings. The cases presented in this way should be relatively easy to separate into different disease categories. However, it must be recognized that patients do not appear in textbook form, especially early in the course of their illness, when it may be difficult to separate their physical findings from "normal." In addition, many diseases evolve from one pattern into another or from the less specific into the more specific. In some cases, and just to add to the confusion, more than one disease may exist in the same patient at the same time (for instance, an attack of gout may occur in the fingers of a woman with OA). Therefore, the early forms of the disease are not "classical," but they are extremely important to recognize. Nevertheless, it is the knowledge of the full-blown classical disease pattern that permits the clinician to look and work backwards. Then it may be possible to identify the early forms, distinguish normal from abnormal, and increase the specificity of the diagnosis.

We present certain diseases in terms of how well they obey "rules," or domains for their behavior. These five rules, or domains, are listed in Table 2–1. For example, under rule 2 we describe conditions that are symmetric and diseases that involve only certain parts of the body. It is the knowledge of the rules that lets the expert clinician decide when certain diseases break the rules. In Table 2–2 we have listed the individual chronic rheumatic diseases that are discussed in this chapter and for which the rules are applied.

## Rule 1: Pathogenetic Aspects Predict Physical Findings

**RHEUMATOID ARTHRITIS.** An idealized joint is represented in Figure 2–1. The synovial membrane or synovium, a tiny structure normally only two cell layers

## TABLE 2–1
### The Five Rules for Understanding How Physical Findings Predict the Differential Diagnosis of Patients with Chronic Polyarthritis

1. Knowledge of the pathogenesis of the disease is of critical importance to predict physical findings.
2. The distribution of joint involvement around the body provides important clues to the differential diagnosis.
3. The unique involvement of the hand and foot (i.e., which joints or groups of joints are involved) refines the differential diagnosis into more specific diseases.
4. Extra-articular manifestations observed in the individual diseases often supply insight toward the diagnosis.
5. Certain conditions produce symptoms out of proportion to physical findings; awareness of this fact facilitates differential diagnosis.

## TABLE 2–2
### Conditions and Diseases To Be Recognized and Differentiated from One Another

Rheumatoid arthritis
The spondyloarthropathies
  Ankylosing spondylitis
  Reactive arthritis (formerly called Reiter's disease)
  Arthritis associated with inflammatory bowel disease
  Psoriatic arthritis
Crystal deposition diseases
  Gout
  Pseudogout (CPPD deposition disease)
Osteoarthritis
Connective tissue diseases
  Systemic lupus erythematosus
  Scleroderma
  Polymyositis
  Mixed connective tissue disease

CPPD = calcium pyrophosphate dihydrate.

thick, is the primary pathogenetic focus of the disease in RA. It is not known how or why the disease begins in this structure or what initiates the disease, but by the time RA is clinically evident, there appears to be a recognizable established inflammatory response in the synovium. As a result of this process, the cells of the synovium proliferate, the tissue hypertrophies and becomes thickened, and the physical findings reflect these processes. The joints become enlarged, warm, and tender and exude copious amounts of inflammatory fluid. The nickname for this inflammatory process is *synovitis*. What is important to recognize is the fact that this process takes place within the confines of the joint itself: that is, inside the boundaries formed by the thick fibrous band, connected to the periosteum, called the joint capsule (see Fig. 2–1).

**OSTEOARTHRITIS.** OA, a degenerative and typically not an inflammatory condition, probably does not have a single pathogenesis. However, the primary process

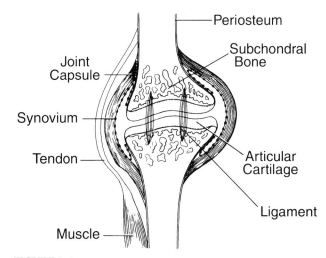

**FIGURE 2–1**
The sites of disease pathogenesis are illustrated in this drawing of an idealized joint.

probably begins either in the cartilage itself or in the bone just beneath the cartilage, called the subchondral bone (see Fig. 2–1). The joint itself can be thought of as behaving as a unit. This unit contains not only bone and cartilage but also tendons (attachments of muscles to bones), ligaments (attachments between bones), and muscles. In addition, fibrocartilage structures, called menisci, act as "spacers" within certain joints such as the knee.

Anything can and often does go wrong with the joint unit. Metabolic changes may occur within either the bone or cartilage, causing an inability of the joint to transmit normal biomechanical forces and to become less resistant to compression and mechanical stress. Injuries can affect the ligaments or menisci, and muscles may overwork, or in some cases even atrophy, producing abnormal effects on the joint unit. The net result in, for example, a weight-bearing joint is an aberrant transmission of normal forces, producing degeneration of cartilage and compaction of bone. This degeneration causes the joint to make attempts at repair; the repair takes the form of bony proliferation at the margins of the joint. These bony excrescences are called osteophytes and are palpable as well as often visible. Crepitation, or a grinding sensation that is felt by the examiner's hand placed on the joint, may occur when incongruous or damaged surfaces rub against each other as the joint is put through a range of motion. Small amounts of noninflammatory fluid are sometimes noted in osteoarthritic joints. Therefore, physical findings for an osteoarthritic joint often reveal bony enlargements (osteophytes) at the joint margins, crepitation on motion, deformities caused by joint incongruities, and small amounts of noninflammatory fluid.

SPONDYLOARTHROPATHIES. There are four diseases that are clearly distinguishable from RA by a variety of clinical findings; however, these conditions are often not easily distinguished one from another:

- ankylosing spondylitis
- reactive arthritis (formerly called Reiter's disease)
- arthritis associated with inflammatory bowel diseases (Crohn's disease and ulcerative colitis)
- psoriatic arthritis

In years past, they were lumped together and called the "rheumatoid variants" because they varied as a group from RA in a number of ways. They clearly have an existence of their own and have one important feature in common: They either exclusively or almost always involve the spine and sacroiliac joints. Therefore, they are most commonly called, collectively, the *spondyloarthropathies*. Unlike RA, which affects predominantly women, more men than women suffer from spondyloarthropathies; the reasons for these differences are not known.

Although the spondyloarthropathies do affect the synovial membrane and produce some of the physical findings described for RA, they more typically involve the supporting structures (see Fig. 2–1) around the joint. These structures are the joint capsule itself, the periosteum lining the surrounding bones, and even the attachments of tendons and ligaments to the bone.

Inflammation occurs separately in these sites, producing pain and swelling at a distance from and beyond the confines of the joint. Sometimes the inflammation and swelling in spondyloarthritic joints is so extensive that it reaches or extends from one joint to another. In a toe or finger, the descriptive term for this situation is a sausage digit. When inflammation occurs at remote sites of ligament and tendon attachments (called *entheses*), even where there is no joint, it is called *enthesitis*. This phenomenon is clearly in contrast to synovitis, which takes place in the synovial membrane within the confines of the joint.

CRYSTAL DEPOSITION DISEASES. There are two conditions that are caused by the deposition of crystalline material in the joint, and each has a recurrent acute form and a chronic form. The acute forms are called *gout* and *pseudogout*, and the chronic forms are called *tophaceous gout* and *CPPD deposition disease*. What makes these diseases unique and different from all others described in this chapter is the fact that there is a physical crystal that causes the acute inflammation. In the case of gout, the crystal is monosodium urate, and in the case of CPPD, the crystal is calcium pyrophosphate dihydrate.

In acute gout, the crystal-induced inflammation is thought by scientific investigators to begin in the fluid that is present in the joint space (see Fig. 2–1); however, the inflammation may become so intense that redness, swelling, and pain often extend well beyond the joint into the surrounding soft tissues. The physical findings are very dramatic: An attack of acute gout may even cause the skin to peel, and sometimes the attack is mistaken for bacterial cellulitis. In pseudogout, similar but generally less intense inflammation occurs. If both of these diseases continue (which they do not always do) into their chronic forms, joint destruction can occur. In the case of gout, collections of monosodium urate crystals coalesce and form hard, yellow masses in the surrounding joint tissues such as the synovium, periosteum, and bone. These "walled-off" crystal collections are called *tophi*. In the case of CPPD deposition disease, destruction of the joint most commonly takes the form of an aggressive, chronic type of OA, although the OA occurs in unusual locations (see later explanation). The physical findings in that situation are those of OA: palpable osteophytes, bony crepitus, and deformity.

## Rule 2: Distribution of Joint Involvement Around the Body Provides Clues to the Diagnosis

The pattern of articular involvement or joint distribution around the body provides very important information that points toward the diagnosis.

RA is a bilateral, symmetric (involving the same joint or groups of joints on each side of the body) polyarthritis; upper and lower extremities are equally affected. In addition, RA involves large joints (e.g., hip, knee, shoulder) as well as small joints (e.g., knuckles, fingers, toes). In contrast, the spondyloarthropathies are often unilateral, asymmetric diseases involving mostly large joints and concentrating more on the lower extremities than on the upper extremities. The descriptive term *oligoarthritis* refers to four or fewer joints that are commonly involved with this group of diseases.

The crystal deposition diseases do not have a unique pattern of involvement except that certain individual joints (knees, ankles, wrists, great toe joints) appear to be predominantly affected in most cases. OA takes several forms but most commonly involves the large weight-bearing joints of the lower extremities, such as the hips and knees. However, when OA involves the hand, it has a very special or unique distribution (to be illustrated). The connective tissue diseases do not have a unique body distribution or follow special rules to account for the arthritis that they produce.

### Rule 3: Distribution in the Hand and Foot ("Target Areas") Refines the Specificity of the Diagnosis

Recognizing the distribution of joint involvement in the hand and foot is extremely useful in the differential diagnosis of chronic rheumatic diseases. Figure 2–2 displays the relevant joint anatomy for reference; by convention, the joints are numbered beginning on the radial side (the thumb is "number 1"). It may be helpful to think of these unique distributions as "target areas" for the individual diseases, recognizing the fact that the rules apply in general but never 100%. RA almost always involves the metacarpophalangeal (MCP) joints and the wrist, in addition to the interphalangeal (IP) joints. However, OA almost never (with few exceptions, to be described) affects the MCP joints or the wrists. Osteoarthritis most commonly involves the IP joints, both proximal (PIP) and distal (DIP), and affects

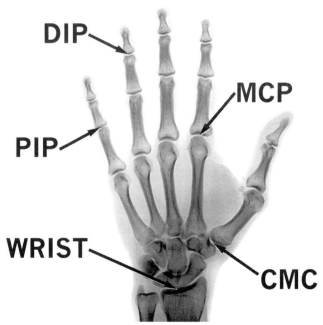

**FIGURE 2–2**
The joints in this hand diagram are the target areas for rheumatoid arthritis, osteoarthritis, calcium pyrophosphate dihydrate deposition disease, and the spondyloarthropathies.

as well a joint near the wrist at the base of the thumb called the first carpometacarpal (CMC) joint. Sometimes OA may affect the CMC alone, or it may do so in concert with the IP joints of the fingers. It is critically important for a proper differential diagnosis to distinguish, on physical examination, between RA involvement of the wrist and OA affecting the first CMC joint.

The spondyloarthropathies, as they affect the hand and foot, also have a unique joint distribution, in addition to their typical pathoanatomic findings such as sausage digits. They tend to involve the IP joints of the hand and foot out of proportion to the MCP joints in the hand and the metatarsophalangeal (MTP) joints of the feet. This is in great distinction to RA, in which arthritis in the MCP and MTP predominates. Furthermore, in the spondyloarthropathies, the involvement may be entirely asymmetric. For example, it is not unusual for a patient with psoriatic arthritis to have swelling and tenderness of a DIP on the index finger of one hand and the same manifestations in a PIP on the ring finger of the other hand as the only hand arthritis. The crystal deposition diseases, in either their acute or chronic forms, may affect any joint in the hand, wrist, foot, or ankle, and the distribution is not specific for either of the diseases. The connective tissue diseases, as well, do not have a unique joint distribution.

### Rule 4: Extra-articular Features Supply Additional Insight into the Diagnosis

Extra-articular features can be a clue to the differential diagnosis and should be looked for in every patient. In some cases (such as RA) they are not common, but in other situations they define the condition (e.g., psoriasis, in psoriatic arthritis) or dominate the illness (as in systemic lupus erythematosus). Examples are discussed in later sections dealing with the individual diseases.

### Rule 5: Symptoms Out of Proportion to Physical Findings Facilitate Differential Diagnosis

For purposes of this chapter, we consider the physical findings of four conditions that are often grouped together as connective tissue diseases: systemic lupus erythematosus (SLE), scleroderma, dermatomyositis, and mixed connective tissue disease. The skin, joints, and muscles are involved in all of these conditions, and some of the physical findings are unique to each individual disease, whereas other findings are common to all four conditions. Those examples are illustrated in the next section. However, the joint involvement has one feature common to these diseases: Symptoms are out of proportion to the physical findings. In other words, affected patients experience pain in a joint clearly beyond what might be expected or deduced from the visible signs of inflammation. The reason for this discrepancy is the hypothesis (there is really no proof for it) that the inflammation in the connective tissue diseases involves the soft tissues of the joint (e.g., the joint capsule, ligaments, and tendons). In this manner, the joint is only mildly swollen or red but extraordinarily tender to touch or painful with minimal movement. The term *periarticular inflammation* describes this phenomenon and characterizes the findings in the diseases referred to collectively as the connective tissue diseases.

## The Diseases

### Rheumatoid Arthritis

Figure 2–3 is an illustration of fully developed RA. There is clearly defined swelling of the target areas mentioned: the wrist, the MCP joint, and the PIP joints. The synovial swelling (synovitis) is anatomically contained within the confines of the joint and limited by the joint capsule. The swelling actually is visibly extensive, very soft in appearance, and obviously painful. However, recognizing RA at this fully developed stage of the disease is not what this chapter is about. It is much more important to recognize the patient in Figure 2–4 as having RA. In this particular patient, who has very early RA, there is a subtle but very important finding: In the second and third MCP joints in this figure, there is loss of the normal "valley," or indentation, between the heads of the metacarpals. In a normal hand, the "peaks" created by the metacarpal heads and the "valleys" represented by the spaces in between are visible. What fills the space from the patient in Figure 2–4 is inflammation contained in the synovial tissues of the MCP joints and probably the tendon sheaths as well. In addition, in a normal wrist, there is a normal "waist," or slight indentation at the end of the distal radius and ulna where the wrist is formed.

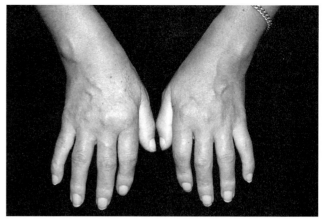

**FIGURE 2–4**
Early subtle synovitis with loss of the landmarks ("peaks" and "valleys") of the metacarpophalangeal joints and of the normal indentation ("waist") at the wrist.

Figure 2–4 illustrates the loss of this "waist," with flaring out on both sides at the wrist as a result of underlying wrist swelling. The top, or dorsum, of this patient's hand is also swollen at the wrist, with loss of the normal landmarks. The involvement of the MCP joints is diagnostic of RA and distinguishes it from other conditions, such as OA.

Figure 2–5 represents a later and more progressive stage of the disease. In this patient, the "peaks" and "valleys" between the metacarpal heads are filled in with inflammatory tissue, or synovitis. The wrist itself is completely involved, and a very characteristic finding is evident: On the ulnar side of the wrist, there

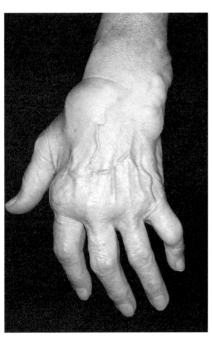

**FIGURE 2–3**
Fully developed rheumatoid arthritis with synovitis contained within the confines of the joint.

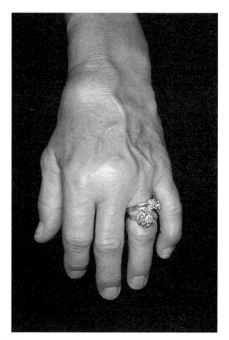

**FIGURE 2–5**
Clear-cut synovial hypertrophy in the wrist and metacarpophalangeal joints in a patient with established rheumatoid arthritis.

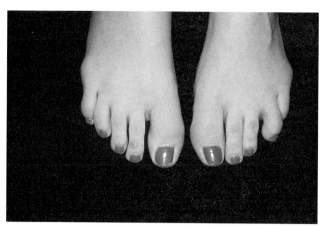

**FIGURE 2–6**
Spreading apart laterally of the metatarsal heads in rheumatoid arthritis produces space ("daylight") between the toes.

is a rubbery-feeling, thickened extensor carpi ulnaris tendon sheath, producing its typical ropy or knot-like appearance. Another finding is evident in this hand: lateral movement or displacement of the metacarpal heads, producing larger-than-normal spaces between the digits as a result of the marked swelling of the MCP joints. This type of physical finding is often quite dramatic in the rheumatoid foot. In a normal foot, all the toes are touching each other. When the MTP joints in the feet are swollen, the metatarsal heads are distracted laterally, and there are open spaces between the toes. The space between the toes is called the *daylight sign* of RA, affecting the MTP joints and forefoot (Fig. 2–6).

With further progression of the disease in the hand (Fig. 2–7), there appear additional characteristic findings, such as muscle atrophy of the intrinsic hand muscles, revealing very prominent swollen metacarpal heads.

Secondary changes then begin to take place; the wrist compartment is very vulnerable to loss of its integrity from this accumulated damage. The progressive rheu-

matoid synovitis erodes the supporting ligaments, producing a tetrad of destructive developments in the wrist: radial deviation, volar subluxation, ulnar translocation, and supination of the wrist at the end of the forearm. The outer (or ulnar) side of the wrist then "straightens out," producing a straight-line deformity along this side of the hand (Fig. 2–8), illustrating a late stage of irreversible bone, cartilage, tendon, and ligament damage. It is this picture that all physicians want to prevent through therapy. The wrists are now clearly rotated toward the radial side of the hand. Extensor tendons may slip down over the side of the PIP joints; instead of extending the joint, they produce flexion and the resultant "boutonnière" deformity of the PIP joint (not shown here). As illustrated in Figure 2–8, flexor tendons slip dorsally from underneath the PIP joints and actually extend the PIP joint while producing DIP flexion, causing the "swan-neck" hyperextension deformity of the PIP joint. At the MCP joints, there is such extensive damage that the ends of the bones making up the joint are no longer in congruity, and the base of the proximal phalanx slides under the metacarpal head, resulting in subluxation of the MCP joint. At the same time, largely because of the radial deviation at the wrist with pointing of the metacarpals into a radial direction, the extensor tendons pull the fingers toward the ulnar side of the hand. The entire, very destructive process results in the "Z," or zigzag-like, deformity of the end-stage rheumatoid hand, a well-recognized and regrettably all too common complication of late-stage RA.

As noted from Table 2–1 and rule 4, the extra-articular features of many chronic rheumatic diseases considered in this chapter may provide important clues to their diagnosis. However, in the particular case of RA, the prognosis or risk for a worse outcome is affected by the presence of extra-articular aspects of the disease. Recognizing these features during the course of managing a patient with RA should alert the clinician to a need for a change in therapy. The most com-

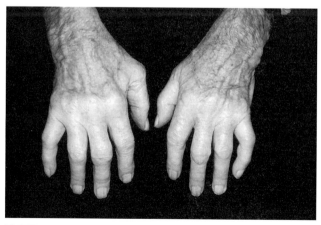

**FIGURE 2–7**
The later stages of rheumatoid arthritis produce hand intrinsic muscle atrophy and marked synovial thickening.

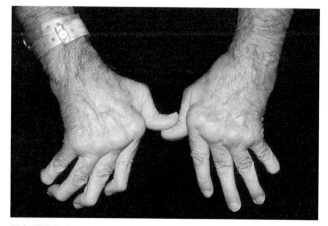

**FIGURE 2–8**
The end-stage rheumatoid arthritis–affected hand reveals radial deviation at the wrist, ulnar drift of the digits, and subluxation of the metacarpophalangeal joints along with "swan-neck" deformity of the proximal and distal interphalangeal joints.

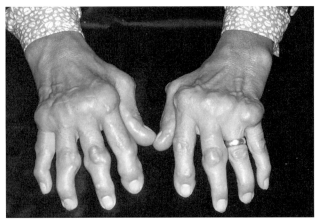

**FIGURE 2–9**
Rheumatoid nodules are illustrated; they typically occur over extensor surfaces or pressure joints.

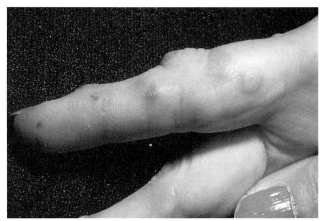

**FIGURE 2–11**
More extensive dermal nodules with skin infarctions caused by vasculitis.

monly noted feature is the rheumatoid nodule, a firm, gelatinous-feeling structure typically located in the subcutaneous tissues over pressure points or extensor surfaces of joints (Fig. 2–9). In some RA patients, a small blood vessel (usually a postcapillary venule) vasculitis produces a tiny skin infarction lesion, commonly located in the soft tissues at the distal nailbed; this is called a periungual infarct (Fig. 2–10). On occasion these skin infarctions accompany the nodules in the skin, producing a collection of dermal nodules and skin infarctions (Fig. 2–11). If the rheumatoid vasculitis affects larger blood vessels such as arteries of substantial size, there may be much more extensive destruction of tissue, as illustrated by Figure 2–12, which shows digital necrosis and gangrene.

Many patients with RA suffer from an accompanying condition called Sjögren's disease. This extra-articular process produces dryness of practically all of the moist mucous membranes in the body but is particularly troublesome in the mouth (xerostomia) and the eye (keratoconjunctivitis sicca). Sjögren's disease may exist alone (primary Sjögren's disease) or in

a secondary form accompanying RA (and other rheumatic diseases as well). The histologic feature that appears to define its pathogenesis is an infiltration of the glandular structures with lymphocytes, which in the case of the patient in Figure 2–13 produces a marked enlargement of the parotid gland.

## The Spondyloarthropathies

ANKYLOSING SPONDYLITIS. There is a marked contrast in physical examination findings between the patient with RA and the patient with ankylosing spondylitis. Although ankylosing spondylitis is defined on the basis of spinal involvement, the peripheral arthritis may be the presenting feature or may occur at any time during the course of the disease. For example, it is not uncommon for teenagers, usually males, to come to medical attention with a peripheral arthritis and for the correct diagnosis of ankylosing spondylitis to be made only after adulthood is reached. The peripheral arthritis can take the form of an asymmetric, large-joint, peripheral arthritis limited to the lower extremities (involving only a knee or an ankle, for example) or it can involve a limited number of small peripheral joints in the hand or foot. In the case of the patient in

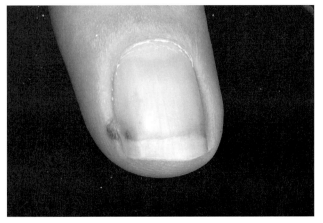

**FIGURE 2–10**
A periungual infarction caused by small-vessel vasculitis.

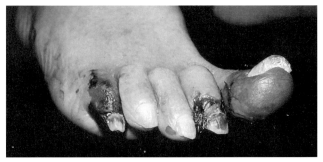

**FIGURE 2–12**
Large-vessel vasculitis has produced digital gangrene and necrosis, a rare occurrence.

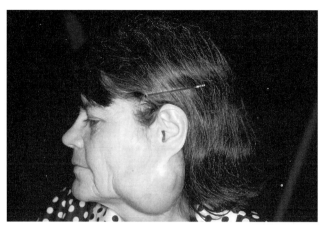

**FIGURE 2–13**
Sjögren's syndrome is illustrated in a patient with marked parotid enlargement.

Figure 2–14, the only joint involvement is an oligoarthritis and takes place in two areas: the PIP joint of the right hand and, more subtly, the fourth MCP joint of the opposite hand. Furthermore, the arthritis of the PIP joint extends beyond the confines of the joint capsule, which is consistent with the pathoanatomic features characteristic of the spondyloarthropathies.

ARTHRITIS ASSOCIATED WITH INFLAMMATORY BOWEL DISEASE (IBD). The peripheral arthritis associated with IBD is indistinguishable from the arthritis of ankylosing spondylitis. It is typically an asymmetric oligoarthritis, involving large joints, most commonly affecting the lower extremities. When it involves the hand or foot, it takes on the characteristic appearance of extending beyond the joint capsule, and it involves the IP joints more than the MCP or MTP joints. There appear to be two forms of IBD arthritis: The first is an acute process, quite inflammatory, often involving periarticular structures (producing a tenosynovitis), but paralleling the clinical course of the colitis or enteritis; when the bowel disease flares, so does the arthritis. The sec-

ond form is more indolent, persistent, and destructive; this type does not parallel the colitis or enteritis and is associated with spinal arthritis. Figure 2–15 is an excellent illustration of IBD arthritis: lower extremity, unilateral, asymmetric, and involving the midfoot, MTP joints, and a single toe digit in a dramatic way. Erythema nodosum (painful red bumps on the legs) often accompanies a flare of the arthritis of IBD. Microscopic evaluation shows this lesion to be a small vessel vasculitis in the septa of the subcutaneous fat. It is not known why these lesions occur.

REACTIVE ARTHRITIS. This condition, formerly known as Reiter's disease, comprises a tetrad of signs: arthritis, conjunctivitis, urethritis, and skin lesions. Not all of these manifestations occur in every patient, and they do not occur at the same time. Reactive arthritis typically affects young men more often than it does women; the reason for this difference is not known. It occurs after an infection of either the gastrointestinal or urinary tract in a genetically susceptible host. The triggering event is most commonly an acute infectious diarrheal illness, such as those caused by *Salmonella* or *Shigella* organisms. It less commonly occurs after genitourinary infection acquired through sexual contact; in these cases, it is a venereal disease, by definition. The term *reactive arthritis* refers to the clinical manifestations that appear to be a "reaction" to the triggering infectious insult. Although the genetics of susceptible individuals are increasingly well characterized and studied, exactly why the particular agent causes the remote effects in the body is still a mystery. In some patients the illness lasts a short time—a few months—without recurrences; in others, it is progressive and

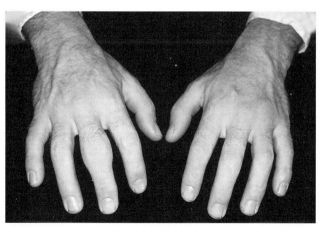

**FIGURE 2–14**
Patchy, asymmetric arthritis of the hands in a patient with ankylosing spondylitis involving the proximal interphalangeal joint of the right hand and the fourth metacarpophalangeal joint of the left hand.

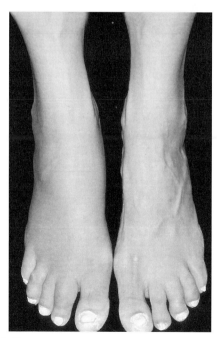

**FIGURE 2–15**
The arthritis associated with inflammatory bowel disease can be asymmetric, involving the lower extremities, with accentuation in a single toe joint.

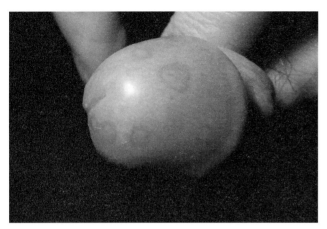

**FIGURE 2–16**
Circular, shallow, painless ulcers on the uncircumcised skin of the glans of the penis are called *circinate balanitis* in patients with reactive arthritis.

destructive and lasts a lifetime. Again, the reasons for these differences are not known.

The skin lesions of the disease are very distinctive and dramatic in appearance. On the uncircumcised skin of the glans penis (Fig. 2–16), the disease takes the form of circular shallow ulcers, called *circinate balanitis*. In spite of their angry appearance, they are entirely painless, quite in contrast to other types of ulcers that can occur on the penis, such as herpes simplex. These lesions, with a similar but not identical appearance, can take place on the moist surfaces inside the mouth on the buccal mucosa. When the lesion occurs on the keratinized skin surfaces exposed to ambient air, it takes on a different appearance (Fig. 2–17). In that case, the lesion becomes hyperkeratotic and scaling, resembling a psoriatic plaque, and is called *keratoderma blennorrhagicum*. The conjunctivitis can be transient and almost inapparent in many patients and sometimes hemorrhagic in other patients. The arthritis of reactive arthritis is an asymmetric, large-joint condition predominantly of the lower extremities. Like the other spondyloarthropathies, it may involve only a single digit in the hand or foot. Figure 2–18 illustrates the single swollen toe, often called a sausage digit, that may be a prominent finding in a patient with acute reactive arthritis. In the later stages of the chronic and persistent form of the disease, a patient may exhibit very destructive arthritis of several toes, which often leaves other toes in the foot relatively unaffected.

**PSORIATIC ARTHRITIS.** Psoriatic arthritis, or the arthritis associated with the skin disease psoriasis, shares many features in common with the other spondyloarthropathies such as asymmetry, sausage digits, and large-joint predominance. However, it differs importantly in two ways; it tends to affect the upper extremities as often as the lower ones and affects equal numbers of women and men. It is probably the most commonly encountered condition among the spondyloarthropathies. Psoriatic arthritis can take an oligoarthritic form (just a few joints) or affect multiple joints of the hands and feet, even resembling classical RA. In general, the skin disease bears no relationship to the arthritis in terms of location or extent; some patients have extensive joint disease with tiny amounts of skin psoriasis, and the opposite (widespread psoriasis and a single joint involvement) also occurs.

Figure 2–19 displays hands of a typical patient with psoriatic arthritis, with involvement of the joints in a patchy asymmetric way, affecting some (the thumb IP and MCP on one side, the PIP on the fourth finger of the opposite hand) and sparing others. In addition, there is extensive swelling beyond the confines of the joint capsule, producing the circumferential swelling of the joint characteristic of psoriatic arthritis. Figure 2–20 illustrates the sausage toe in a foot of a man with psoriatic arthritis.

In order to make an accurate diagnosis, it is important to look for subtle signs of psoriasis in a patient with a pattern of arthritis that is indicative of psoriatic arthritis. Two typical areas where psoriasis may be hidden, even from the patient, are the umbilicus and the natal cleft. Another area to find subtle psoriasis,

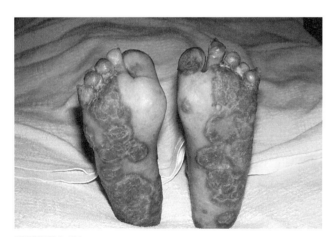

**FIGURE 2–17**
Scaling, hyperkeratotic plaques, typically located on the hands and feet of patients with reactive arthritis, are called *keratoderma blennorrhagicum.*

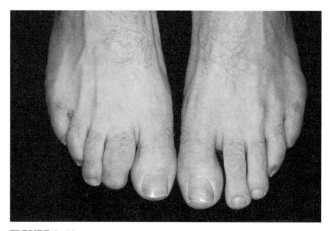

**FIGURE 2–18**
The single swollen toe is called a *sausage digit* in the spondyloarthropathies because the swelling extends throughout the digit well beyond the confines of the joints.

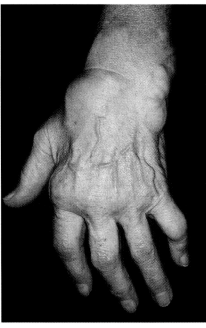

**FIGURE 2–3**
Fully developed rheumatoid arthritis with synovitis contained within the confines of the joint.

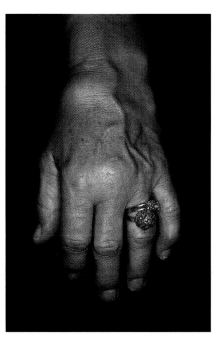

**FIGURE 2–5**
Clear-cut synovial hypertrophy in the wrist and metacarpophalangeal joints in a patient with established rheumatoid arthritis.

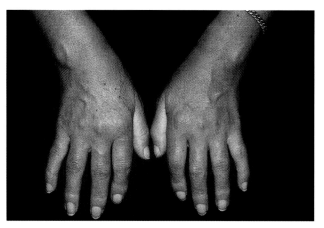

**FIGURE 2–4**
Early subtle synovitis with loss of the landmarks ("peaks" and "valleys") of the metacarpophalangeal joints and of the normal indentation ("waist") at the wrist.

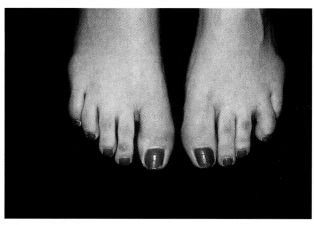

**FIGURE 2–6**
Spreading apart laterally of the metatarsal heads in rheumatoid arthritis produces space ("daylight") between the toes.

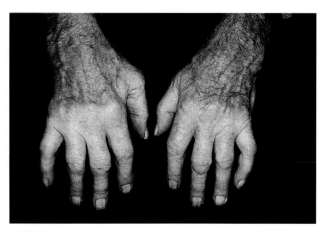

**FIGURE 2–7**
The later stages of rheumatoid arthritis produce hand intrinsic muscle atrophy and marked synovial thickening.

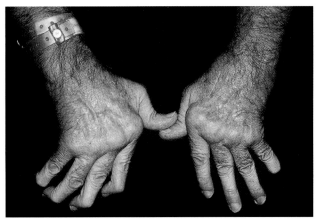

**FIGURE 2–8**
The end-stage rheumatoid arthritis–affected hand reveals radial deviation at the wrist, ulnar drift of the digits, and subluxation of the metacarpophalangeal joints along with "swan-neck" deformity of the proximal and distal interphalangeal joints.

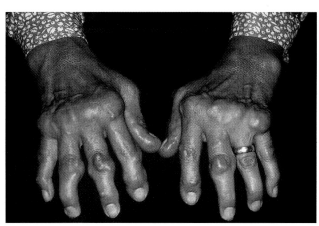

**FIGURE 2–9**
Rheumatoid nodules are illustrated; they typically occur over extensor surfaces or pressure joints.

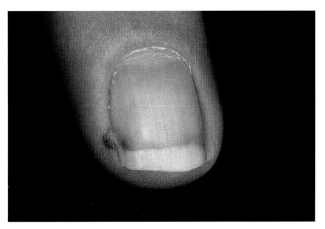

**FIGURE 2–10**
A periungual infarction caused by small-vessel vasculitis.

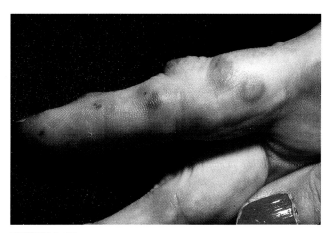

**FIGURE 2–11**
More extensive dermal nodules with skin infarctions caused by vasculitis.

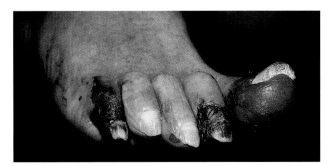

**FIGURE 2–12**
Large-vessel vasculitis has produced digital gangrene and necrosis, a rare occurrence.

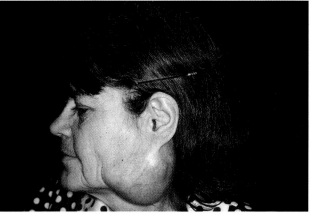

**FIGURE 2–13**
Sjögren's syndrome is illustrated in a patient with marked parotid enlargement.

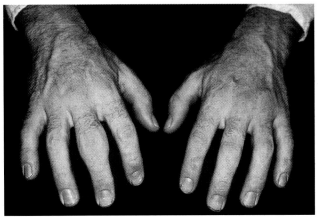

**FIGURE 2–14**
Patchy, asymmetric arthritis of the hands in a patient with ankylosing spondylitis involving the proximal interphalangeal joint of the right hand and the fourth metacarpophalangeal joint of the left hand.

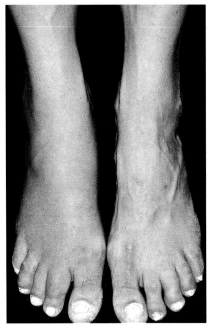

**FIGURE 2–15**
The arthritis associated with inflammatory bowel disease can be asymmetric, involving the lower extremities, with accentuation in a single toe joint.

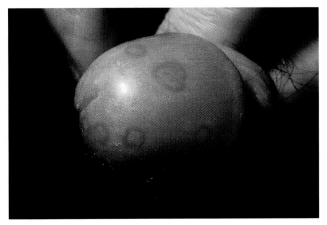

**FIGURE 2–16**
Circular, shallow, painless ulcers on the uncircumcised skin of the glans of the penis are called *circinate balanitis* in patients with reactive arthritis.

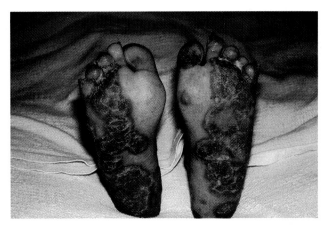

**FIGURE 2–17**
Scaling, hyperkeratotic plaques, typically located on the hands and feet of patients with reactive arthritis, are called *keratoderma blennorrhagicum.*

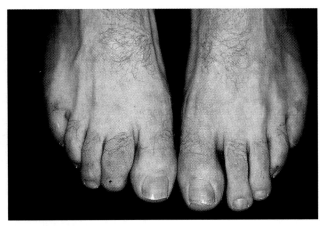

**FIGURE 2–18**
The single swollen toe is called a *sausage digit* in the spondyloarthropathies because the swelling extends throughout the digit well beyond the confines of the joints.

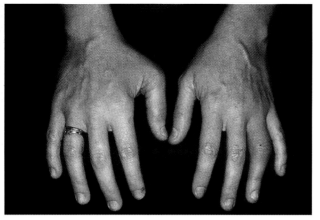

**FIGURE 2–19**
Psoriatic arthritis in the hands takes the form of a patchy asymmetric arthritis with circumferential swelling around a single digit.

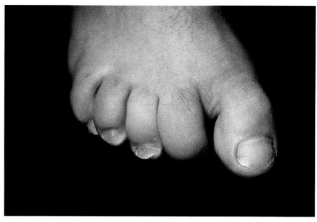

**FIGURE 2–20**
A sausage toe in a patient with psoriatic arthritis; this is often the only involved joint in an individual case.

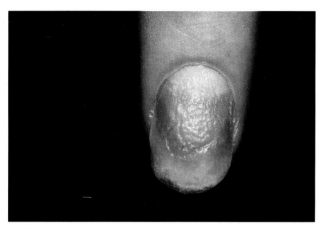

**FIGURE 2–21**
Nail pitting of psoriasis should be sought as a clue to the diagnosis for a patient with asymmetric arthritis.

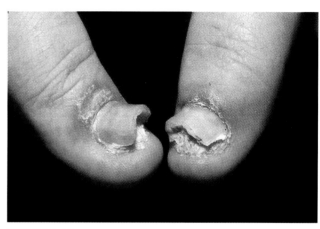

**FIGURE 2–22**
Extensive distal nail hypertrophy with chipping and cracking produces onycholysis in a patient with psoriatic arthritis.

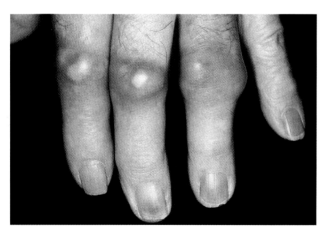

**FIGURE 2–23**
Acute gouty arthritis in multiple finger joints.

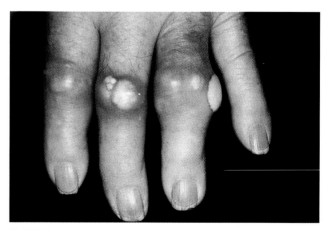

**FIGURE 2–24**
The build-up of monosodium urate crystals 3 weeks later in and around the joints, from the same patient as in Figure 2–23, has caused tophaceous gout.

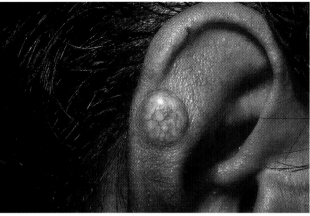

**FIGURE 2–25**
Tophaceous deposits, or tophi, are the accumulation of monosodium urate crystals; this may take place where there are no joints, such as the helix of the ear.

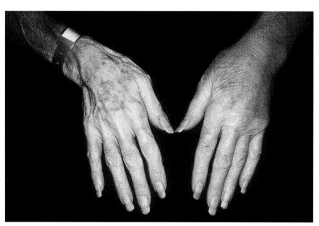

**FIGURE 2–26**
Acute pseudogout, as in this case, is clinically identical to urate gout; the inflammation typically extends beyond the confines of the joint.

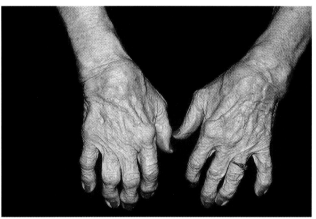

**FIGURE 2–27**
Calcium pyrophosphate dihydrate deposition disease produces osteoarthritis in areas not usually involved with garden-variety osteoarthritis, as in the wrists of this patient; this is called the pseudo-osteoarthritis form of the disease.

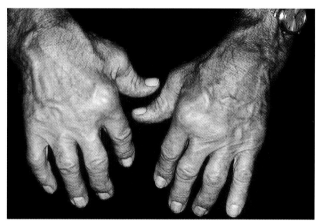

**FIGURE 2–28**
On occasion, calcium pyrophosphate dihydrate deposition disease produces synovial hypertrophy and resembles rheumatoid arthritis (RA); this is called the pseudo-RA form of the disease.

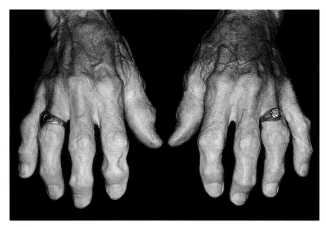

**FIGURE 2–29**
Osteoarthritis of the hands causes bony enlargement of the interphalangeal joints and first carpometacarpal joint, sparing the wrist and metacarpophalangeal joints.

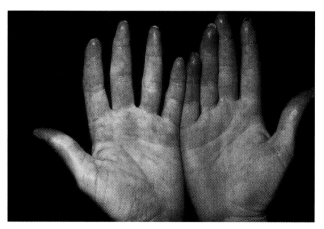

**FIGURE 2–30**
Raynaud's phenomenon, also called digital vasospasm, manifests with color changes that are typically limited to the digits and not involving the whole hand.

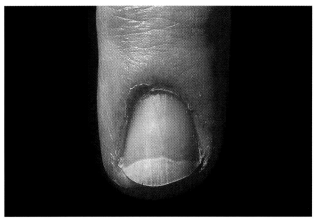

**FIGURE 2–31**
Periungual telangiectasia is a result of dilated and distorted capillary loops, as seen in a patient with dermatomyositis.

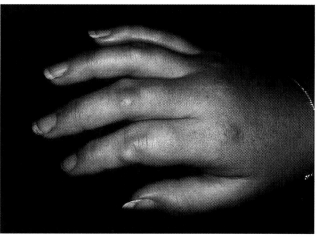

**FIGURE 2–32**
The swollen hand of a patient with a connective tissue disease is caused by periarticular inflammation, as in this case of a patient with systemic lupus erythematosus.

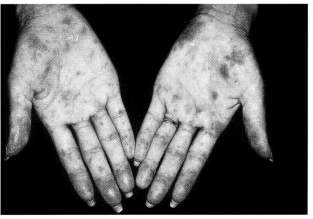

**FIGURE 2–33**
Vasculitis of the palms and soles has a limited differential diagnosis; systemic lupus erythematosus should be strongly suspected.

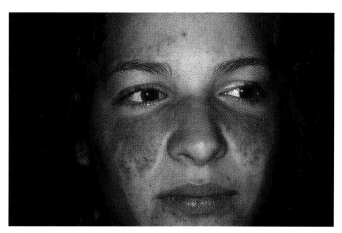

**FIGURE 2–34**
The butterfly rash of systemic lupus erythematosus is an uncommon finding; it is typically seen in teenagers, as in this case.

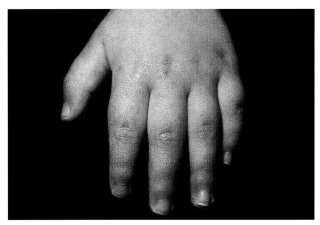

**FIGURE 2–35**
Gottron's papules are considered pathognomonic of dermatomyositis; they consist of pink raised scaling lesions, symmetrically distributed, on extensor surfaces over joints.

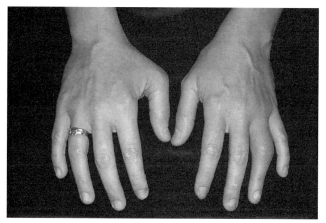

**FIGURE 2–19**
Psoriatic arthritis in the hands takes the form of a patchy asymmetric arthritis with circumferential swelling around a single digit.

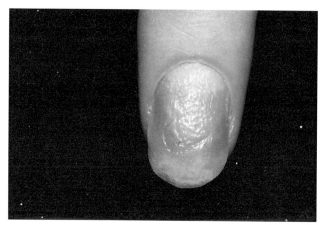

**FIGURE 2–21**
Nail pitting of psoriasis should be sought as a clue to the diagnosis for a patient with asymmetric arthritis.

and much more accessible to the examination, is the nail. Psoriatic nails may take the form of pitting (Fig. 2–21), undermining of the distal nail with chipping and cracking, or even extensive onycholysis and hyperkeratotic changes (Fig. 2–22). As with skin psoriasis and arthritis elsewhere in the body, there is no correlation between the extent of contiguous nail and DIP joint disease in any individual patient, in spite of the fact that DIP joint involvement by itself is very common in psoriatic arthritis.

### The Crystal Deposition Diseases

GOUT. An attack of gout is caused by a physical crystal that forms because our bodies are supersaturated with uric acid. In addition, physicians often administer drugs to patients that aggravate this state by blocking even further the normal excretion mechanisms for uric acid. The use of these drugs is not arbitrary or capricious; it is necessary for life in certain cases (such as cyclosporine administration for transplant recipients).

Why a particular joint is susceptible to a gout attack is not known, but local changes in temperature and blood flow, prior trauma, and even degenerative arthritis in that joint are suspected to play a role. Attacks of gout can occur in a single joint or in multiple joints simultaneously. The erythema and swelling of a gout attack are dramatic and unmistakable to the clinician; an attack of gout is thought to be one of the most painful experiences a human being can endure. Gouty inflammation is so intense that it can spread across soft tissues beyond the confines of the joint and can cause the skin to peel. Usually an attack lasts, at most, 10 days to 2 weeks until the crystals are cleared or are coated with materials that reduce or eliminate their inflammatory potential.

If the conditions that cause the attack are not managed properly and the patient suffers repeated attacks, the build-up of monosodium urate crystals probably continues unabated. This situation is called *chronic to-*

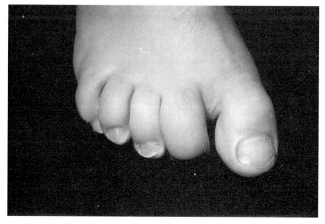

**FIGURE 2–20**
A sausage toe in a patient with psoriatic arthritis; this is often the only involved joint in an individual case.

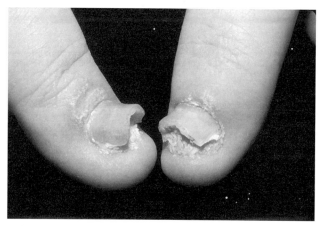

**FIGURE 2–22**
Extensive distal nail hypertrophy with chipping and cracking produces onycholysis in a patient with psoriatic arthritis.

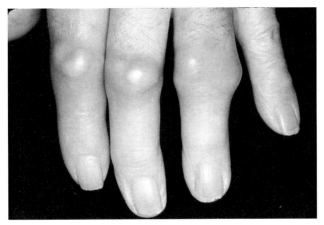

**FIGURE 2–23**
Acute gouty arthritis in multiple finger joints.

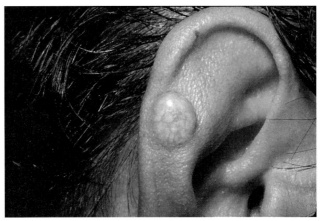

**FIGURE 2–25**
Tophaceous deposits, or tophi, are the accumulation of monosodium urate crystals; this may take place where there are no joints, such as the helix of the ear.

*phaceous gout*. The patient in Figures 2–23 and 2–24 was having repeated attacks of gout in his fingers, and within a few weeks (Fig. 2–24 is taken 3 weeks after Fig. 2–23), monosodium urate crystal deposits formed into yellow masses called *tophi* in and around the joints. It may take years for these tophi to be resorbed with proper treatment. For reasons that are not known, some tophi actually appear and grow in places where there is no joint at all, such as in the helix of the ear (Fig. 2–25). Looking for the presence of a tophus in the ear of a patient with chronic arthritis should be part of the rheumatologic examination of the patient.

PSEUDOGOUT AND CPPD DEPOSITION DISEASE. An attack of pseudogout was first identified when a patient's joint fluids were examined for crystals in an otherwise clinically typical gout attack. Instead of the finding of monosodium urate, CPPD crystals were observed being engulfed by inflammatory cells.[3] At the same time, calcification of cartilage was noted in the plain radiographs of the joints in many of these same patients, along with other distinctive radiogaphic features suggesting a syndrome. Subsequently, more so-

phisticated x-ray crystallography studies performed on patients' specimens identified the material observed on radiographs and in the joint fluid examination as CPPD.[4]

Figure 2–26 displays an attack of pseudogout in the wrist of a hospitalized woman; it is not uncommon for patients already in the hospital for another reason to have an attack of either gout or pseudogout, a clinical finding that remains unexplained. The inflammation is intense and extends beyond the joint itself, a finding in common with both gout and pseudogout.

If the disease becomes chronic, and in most cases it does, additional clinical variants of CPPD deposition disease that resemble and can be confused with other chronic rheumatic diseases may emerge. CPPD deposition disease commonly produces cartilage and bone degeneration very similar to that produced by OA, but the location of this degeneration is not in areas where OA is usually seen. The OA caused by CPPD deposition disease may occur in the MCP joints, the wrist, the shoulder, or the ankle, which are joints not at all

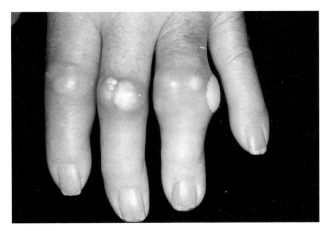

**FIGURE 2–24**
The build-up of monosodium urate crystals 3 weeks later in and around the joints, from the same patient as in Figure 2–23, has caused tophaceous gout.

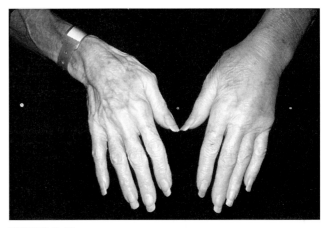

**FIGURE 2–26**
Acute pseudogout, as in this case, is clinically identical to urate gout; the inflammation typically extends beyond the confines of the joint.

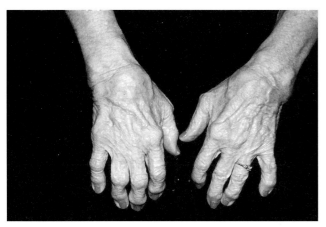

**FIGURE 2–27**
Calcium pyrophosphate dihydrate deposition disease produces osteoarthritis in areas not usually involved with garden-variety osteoarthritis, as in the wrists of this patient; this is called the pseudo-osteoarthritis form of the disease.

typically affected by garden-variety or usual OA. This particular form of CPPD deposition disease is called the *pseudoosteoarthritis* form of the disease, as illustrated by Figure 2–27, which displays OA of the wrist caused by CPPD deposition disease.

For reasons that are not known, CPPD deposition disease can produce synovial hypertrophy, or synovitis, along with the degenerative changes in the underlying cartilage and bone. This synovial hypertrophy, not only because of its tactile features but also because of its location, superficially resembles RA. This particular variant is called the *pseudo-rheumatoid* form of the disease and is illustrated by Figure 2–28. The patient in the photograph has thickened synovium in the MCP joints with spreading apart of the digits, a physical finding identical to that in RA. The only way to tell the difference between CPPD deposition disease and RA in this case is either to perform x-ray studies and look for cartilage calcification and degenerative instead

of erosive changes or to aspirate joint fluid in order to find CPPD crystals.

Why is it necessary to make a diagnosis of CPPD? The most important reason concerns the proven clinical association of certain underlying and potentially reversible metabolic abnormalities (hyperparathyroidism, hemochromatosis, and hypothyroidism) with the disease. A patient with one of these metabolic conditions can present with CPPD manifestations and thus enable the underlying diagnosis to be made. The second reason is that the natural history of the disease, prognosis, and treatment plan are different if the patient has RA as opposed to the pseudo-rheumatoid form of CPPD deposition disease. The third reason is that there are safe and effective ways of treating and preventing attacks of pseudogout.

**OSTEOARTHRITIS.** The patient's hands in Figure 2–29 show the most common form of arthritis: OA. The abnormalities reveal bony enlargement of the PIP and DIP joints; the MCP joints and the wrist are spared. The deformities of the fingers take on their characteristic "random" appearance, in which some joints display an ulnar angulation, whereas others have a radial angulation. This deformity gives the hand a crooked or knotted appearance and is particularly unsightly or embarrassing for some patients. On the patient's left hand, the deformity of the first CMC joint is demonstrated with prominent bony enlargement at the base of the thumb. If this deformity is particularly dramatic with subluxation of the joint, the appearance of the hand resembles a square, often termed the *square hand* of a patient with OA.

**THE CONNECTIVE TISSUE DISEASES.** SLE, scleroderma, dermatomyositis, and mixed connective tissue disease may produce very characteristic appearances of the hand, and these appearances can be helpful in the diagnosis. However, there are certain features in common among all four of these diseases that cannot be used to separate one from another but can point to the entire group as a whole in distinction from, for example, RA or OA. One of those features that is com-

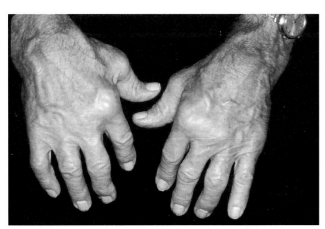

**FIGURE 2–28**
On occasion calcium pyrophosphate dihydrate deposition disease produces synovial hypertrophy and resembles rheumatoid arthritis (RA); this is called the pseudo-RA form of the disease.

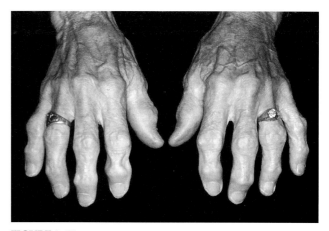

**FIGURE 2–29**
Osteoarthritis of the hands causes bony enlargement of the interphalangeal joints and first carpometacarpal joint, sparing the wrist and metacarpophalangeal joints.

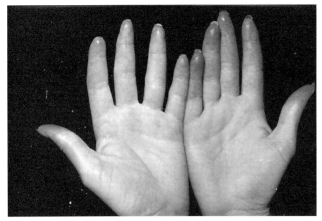

**FIGURE 2–30**
Raynaud's phenomenon, also called digital vasospasm, manifests with color changes that are typically limited to the digits and not involving the whole hand.

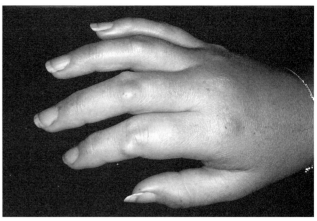

**FIGURE 2–32**
The swollen hand of a patient with a connective tissue disease is caused by periarticular inflammation, as in this case of a patient with systemic lupus erythematosus.

mon to all four of the connective tissue diseases is Raynaud's phenomenon, or digital vasospasm (Fig. 2–30). This condition, brought on by cold exposure or emotions, produces pain and color changes in the digits. The color can change from white to red to blue, or any combination of these colors may exist. The important and diagnostic clinical feature of Raynaud's phenomenon that distinguishes it from other conditions that cause color changes in the hand, such as acrocyanosis, is that the color changes are limited to the digits and typically do not involve the whole hand. In fact, it is not uncommon, as illustrated in Figure 2–30, for the color changes to involve just a partial digit, a single digit, or a few digits.

Another feature shared by all four diseases is periungual telangiectasia. These dilated and distorted blood vessels in the skin surrounding the nailbed, if dramatic, can sometimes be seen with the naked eye (Fig. 2–31). However, the findings are usually more subtle and appreciated only with the aid of a dissecting microscope or the use of an ophthalmoscope at high power

with a drop of oil placed on the nailbed. The final aspect that unites these diseases is the very early finding, in all four conditions, of a "swollen hand" (Fig. 2–32), which is often accompanied by pain, sometimes quite intense, that appears to be out of proportion to the degree of inflammation observed in the hand. This feature of disproportionate pain is quite common in the connective tissue diseases, especially in SLE.

In addition to the aspects in common among the four diseases, there are individual features of the hands and skin that can distinguish one disease from another. SLE produces painful, sometimes necrotic-appearing skin lesions, typically on the palms of the hand (Fig. 2–33). The "butterfly rash" (Fig. 2–34), sparing the nasolabial folds, is a finding observed usually among teenagers with the disease and is not very commonly encountered in spite of its notoriety as a diagnostic hallmark of the condition. For patients with scleroderma, subcutaneous calcinosis is a characteristic finding. It is also seen in some patients with dermatomyo-

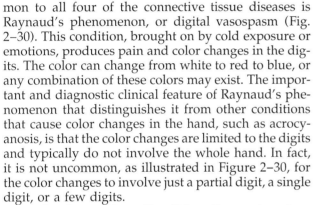

**FIGURE 2–31**
Periungual telangiectasia is a result of dilated and distorted capillary loops, as seen in a patient with dermatomyositis.

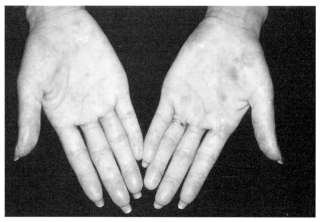

**FIGURE 2–33**
Vasculitis of the palms and soles has a limited differential diagnosis; systemic lupus erythematosus should be strongly suspected.

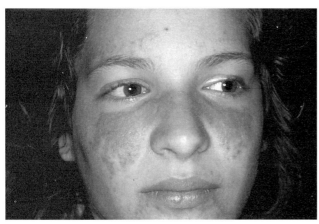

**FIGURE 2–34**
The butterfly rash of systemic lupus erythematosus is an uncommon finding; it is typically seen in teenagers, as in this case.

sitis or mixed connective tissue disease. Patients with dermatomyositis often display the very specific skin finding called Gottron's papules, a hypertrophic scaling skin lesion located over extensor surfaces of the joints, as illustrated in a 2-year-old child with the disease (Fig. 2–35).

The fourth condition is termed *mixed connective tissue disease* because it contains mixtures of the individual features seen typically with RA, scleroderma, and dermatomyositis. All of the physical and clinical findings described earlier, including swollen hands, Raynaud's phenomenon, calcinosis, periungual telangiectasia, and symptoms of pain out of proportion to the physical findings, may be seen with this condition. Patients with mixed connective tissue disease, when identified, appear to have a mild course and share a good outcome with patients who have mild, non–organ-threatening SLE.

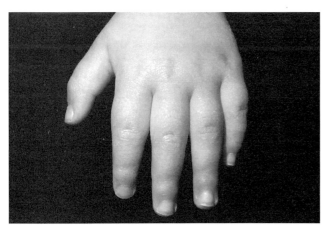

**FIGURE 2–35**
Gottron's papules are considered pathognomonic of dermatomyositis; they consist of pink raised scaling lesions, symmetrically distributed, on extensor surfaces over joints.

## ACUTE POLYARTHRITIS

### Fever, Rash, and Arthritis

Acute polyarthritis is probably fairly common in the population, but in truth, no one really knows exactly how prevalent it is. A sense of how often acute polyarthritis occurs can be estimated from information contained in a few population-based studies and compared to what we know about RA. For example, as noted by Tunn and Bacon[1] in the early arthritis clinic population followed prospectively, for every four patients with acute arthritis, three have a self-limited polyarthritis or some other recognizable syndrome that disappears over the course of that year. Similarly, in the large population-based study from Sudbury, Massachusetts, of 118 patients in the cohort who were observed to have polyarthritis, only 27.5% actually ended up with RA at follow-up 3 to 5 years later.[5] The figure of three self-limited cases for every one that ends up with RA appears consistent across population-based and early arthritis clinic studies.[6]

Furthermore, acute polyarthritis appears to be very common to the authors of this chapter because in the health care system in which the authors work, patients with joint complaints have immediate access to a specialist. In medical care delivery systems in which there may be limited access to a specialist who will recognize the arthritis, the problem may not appear to be very common.

Nevertheless, when a patient does arrive in a physician's office with acute polyarthritis, the clinical problem should be framed as the differential diagnosis of fever, rash, and arthritis. Most of the patients who seek medical attention in this way exhibit these individual components, in one manner or another. The search for the specific characteristics or distinguishing features of the fever, rash, and arthritis forms the backbone of the differential diagnosis. That concept is developed further in this chapter.

Because most of the patients who present with acute polyarthritis have a self-limited illness, the clinical problem is mostly an exercise in self-control for the physician and extreme anxiety for the patient. There is always the urge to make a specific diagnosis of an illness if only to avoid the uncertainty of the current situation. However, the watchwords are *patience* and, of course, *restraint*. Nevertheless, a few cases presented in this way do represent an acute exacerbation of an unrecognized chronic illness or the beginning of something lifelong and chronic. The truth, of course, is that even if the patient is displaying the initial signs and symptoms of a connective tissue disease, there is nothing that can be done to prevent the problem from becoming chronic or persistent. Therefore, it makes sense to anticipate that the situation will have a favorable outcome for all concerned.

Even if the process is self-limited, the actual diagnosis may be important for the future because many of the diseases that manifest with fever, rash, and arthritis have a relationship to either a known or suspected prior infectious process. The diagnosis of an acute infection with the human immunodeficiency virus (HIV), hepatitis B or C, or acute rheumatic fever has major implications for future health beyond the single episode of fever, rash, and arthritis, which in fact may never recur. Furthermore, and it should be emphasized, for most of these self-limited episodes it will not be known which infectious agents were involved; physicians' current ability to diagnose all of these suspected infections has not been fully realized.

Clearly, knowledge about the pathogenesis of the arthritis that derives from known viral infections is insufficient.[7] For example, even though the spectra of clinical events that result from parvovirus B19 and hepatitis C infections have been broadened, the link between the virus and the clinical manifestations has not yet been elucidated.[8] All these issues become even more important in the fundamental and perhaps more important search for the possible relationship between a viral infectious agent and the onset of a chronic rheumatic disease.[9]

In direct contrast to the differential diagnosis of chronic polyarthritis, the laboratory tests *are* helpful in the differential diagnosis of acute polyarthritis. Often, however, the clinical manifestations typically do *not* provide a clear or distinct separation of one disease from another. It is fair to state that many of the clinical features of the individual syndromes are not very different from each other. Knowledge of when to order the specific serologic assay and how to interpret the results is critical in the diagnosis and subsequent management of a patient with fever, rash, and arthritis.

## The Cases

The authors of this chapter believe that the best way of teaching how to accurately diagnose cases of acute polyarthritis is through illustrative patient presentations. The following have been constructed from real-life cases in the authors' experiences; such patients can be found either in the outpatient or the inpatient setting. Just as in chronic polyarthritis, it is necessary to go through an exercise of identifying domains or areas of inquiry that contain the critical information necessary to make the differential diagnosis. Each of these domains, listed in Table 2–3, should be addressed and the characteristics identified when a patient is seen with fever, rash, and arthritis.

For purposes of this teaching exercise, we consider a short list (Table 2–4) containing 14 entities—7 infectious or postinfectious diseases and 7 chronic rheumatic diseases—as part of the differential diagnosis for each of the cases below. Most certainly there are many more entities that could be responsible for fever, rash, and arthritis. However, if the reader can learn the key characteristics about the following diseases, the differential diagnosis can easily be extended to other, less commonly encountered conditions.

Also, it must be recognized that we are using examples of only four viral illnesses (hepatitis B, hepatitis C, parvovirus, and rubella) in the differential diagnosis. There certainly must be many more viruses that can

## TABLE 2–3
### Domains of Inquiry to Characterize Disease and Establish Specific Diagnosis of Fever, Rash, and Arthritis

> Arthritis
> Rash
> Fever curve
> Sore throat
> Pulmonary involvement
> Renal involvement
> Liver function tests
> ESR/CRP
> WBC count, platelet count
> Serologic tests (ANA, rheumatoid factor, viral studies)

ANA = antinuclear antibodies; CRP = C-reactive protein; ESR = erythrocyte sedimentation rate; WBC = white blood cell.

cause fever, rash, and arthritis, inasmuch as we are unable to identify the virus in the majority of patients who present in this way. Furthermore, HIV has been recognized to cause an acute viral illness syndrome when the patient is acutely infected, and there are a variety of chronic arthritic and musculoskeletal manifestations attributed to HIV. The HIV-related issues are not addressed in this chapter. Finally, for each of the patient cases presented, we consider a portion of the diagnoses from Table 2–4.

### Case 1: The 28-Year-Old Female First-Year Pediatric Resident

#### HISTORY
The patient has a 6-day history of pain and swelling in her hands and feet. She has observed daily fevers as high as 101° F but no chills. There is no complaint of a sore throat, and no rash has been noted.

## TABLE 2–4
### Fourteen Diagnoses with the Potential for Fever, Rash, and Arthritis

**Infectious or Postinfectious Diseases**
Hepatitis B
Hepatitis C
Parvovirus
Rubella
Subacute bacterial endocarditis
Acute rheumatic fever
Lyme disease

**Chronic Rheumatic Diseases**
Adult-onset Still's disease
Rheumatoid arthritis
Systemic lupus erythematosus
Wegener's granulomatosis
Giant cell arteritis
Mixed cryoglobulinemia
Sjögren's syndrome (benign hypergammaglobulinemic purpura of Waldenström)

The patient was married recently, and all premarital blood test results were either normal or negative. She has never been pregnant, and she has been using birth control pills for the past 3 years without incident. There is no history of recent travel outside of the country or camping trips into the local mountains. There have been no prior blood transfusions or needlesticks. She has never had a serious medical or surgical illness, and she and her husband recently passed a physical examination for life and disability insurance, including blood testing for HIV. She has been vaccinated with hepatitis B and rubella vaccines as a condition of employment.

For the past month and a half, she has worked in the pediatric intensive care unit, taking care of very sick children with the acquired immunodeficiency syndrome, hematologic and other malignancies, sickle cell disease, and cystic fibrosis.

### PHYSICAL AND LABORATORY EXAMINATIONS

- Arthritis: Hands and feet were diffusely swollen and tender, with accentuation of the swelling and tenderness in the joints. The joints that appeared to be involved were the PIPs, MCPs, and wrists, along with the ankles and MTPs.
- Rash: None.
- Fever curve: Persistent low-grade fever, the highest being 101° F, going down to 99.6° F in the evening.
- Sore throat: None.
- Pulmonary involvement: None.
- Renal involvement: None.
- Liver function tests: Alanine aminotransferase (ALT) = 47 U/L; aspartate aminotransferase (AST) = 30 U/L; alkaline phosphatase = 144 U/L; bilirubin = 0.1/0.4 mg/dL.
- Erythrocyte sedimentation rate (ESR)/C-reactive protein (CRP): ESR = 36 mm/hr (Westergren); CRP = 1.2 mg/dL.
- White blood cell (WBC)/platelet count: Both normal.
- Serologic tests: Results for antinuclear antibodies (ANA) and rheumatoid factor (RF) were negative; viral studies are pending.

### WHAT IS THE DIFFERENTIAL DIAGNOSIS?

The differential diagnosis of an acute polyarthritis without renal or pulmonary involvement and without a rash should be initially considered to include an infectious process, either directly or indirectly. Alternatively, this could be the beginning of a chronic rheumatic disease such as RA or SLE. However, there is little to be accomplished by making the diagnosis of a chronic rheumatic condition at the present time. On the other hand, there is quite a bit to be gained by making a precise diagnosis of an infectious process because in certain situations the patient can be treated and complications prevented (as in Lyme disease, subacute bacterial endocarditis, or acute rheumatic fever). Furthermore, the identification of a self-limited postinfectious process can be reassuring to the patient, who is obviously going to fear the beginning of a chronic rheumatic disease. In addition, the fact that the process is self-limited can be used to avoid the institution of potentially toxic therapy.

What should be considered at this time? From our original list, there are seven infectious or postinfectious syndromes. We now consider each of these conditions.

*HEPATITIS B.* Although not seen as frequently today as in the mid-1970s, largely because of effective viral testing and adherence to safety precautions, accidental exposure to this virus still takes place. Typically 10 to 14 days after inoculation, the patient experiences fever, rash, and arthritis. During this period the test for hepatitis B surface antigen yields positive results, and the liver function test results are normal. Later, usually after regression of the acute symptoms, liver function becomes abnormal, and antibodies to virus are detected. This syndrome is self-limited and is associated with permanent immunity to the virus. It has been described as a "serum sickness" reaction because it resembles the classical syndrome, described many years ago, that resulted when horse serum products were employed to treat infectious diseases.

A rash (described as ranging from urticaria to vasculitis) may be observed after acute infection with this virus, although it may not always occur. Sore throat and pulmonary and renal involvement are not features of this condition. Liver function tests yield abnormal results later in the course, and ESR and CRP may actually be normal or at least much lower than predicted by the amount of inflammation observed in the patient. WBC and platelet count are unremarkable, and serologic tests yield normal results except for the positive finding for hepatitis surface antigen. This patient had a prior vaccination for hepatitis B.

*HEPATITIS C.* An acute syndrome is said to follow exposure to hepatitis C infection, but descriptions of its clinical course are lacking. It is entirely likely that a serum sickness reaction, similar to that of hepatitis B, occurs in some patients, but hepatitis C is associated mostly with chronic extrahepatic conditions such as cutaneous vasculitis, mixed cryoglobulinemia and vasculitis, and polyarteritis nodosa. This patient's antibody to hepatitis C was negative.

*RUBELLA.* After infection with the native virus or immunization with the killed virus vaccine, a syndrome of self-limited fever and arthritis can occur. The arthritis is a symmetric polyarthritis of the hands and feet, and it resembles RA in its distribution and its clinical features. Findings for all the other domains listed in Table 2–3 are essentially negative or normal. This patient was vaccinated for rubella 3 years ago.

*SUBACUTE BACTERIAL ENDOCARDITIS.* Fever, rash, and arthritis can occur with this condition; however, the clinical features are usually quite different. The arthritis typically involves the proximal large joints (shoulders, hips), resembling polymyalgia rheumatica, although hands may also be swollen. Vasculitis (causing a rash) can occur in subacute bacterial endocarditis, but the clinical setting is more of a chronic illness typically seen with long-standing infection of a prosthetic valve; immune complex deposition is thought to be the mechanism. Subacute bacterial endocarditis should always be considered in the setting of fever, rash, and arthritis, because of the danger to the patient of missing the diagnosis. Echocardiography and blood cultures should be obtained, but the possibility of subacute bacterial endocarditis with this patient's clinical findings is very remote.

*ACUTE RHEUMATIC FEVER (ARF).* Fever, rash, and arthritis certainly occur with ARF, but the characteristics are decidedly different from those in this case. The rash of ARF is almost always associated with carditis, and carditis is almost never seen in adults with ARF. The arthritis of ARF is an additive large-joint polyarthritis, with symptoms out of proportion to physical findings. Swollen hands and feet as the lone manifestation of ARF arthritis would be distinctly unusual.

*LYME DISEASE.* Lyme disease, caused by the infectious agent *Borrelia burgdorferi*, should always be considered in the circumstance of fever, rash, and arthritis because of the reversibility of the disease with antibiotic treatment. However, the rash (erythema chronicum migrans) of Lyme disease is associated with the tick bite and occurs months before the arthritis. Although fever and muscle aches (myalgias) may accompany the acute infection, the actual arthritis involves large joints, resembling the chronic oligoarthritis of juvenile rheumatoid arthritis. It is easy to recall the characteristics of Lyme arthritis if it is remembered that the disease was first identified because there was an unusual cluster of children with juvenile rheumatoid arthritis living in the area around Old Lyme, Connecticut. However, this patient's findings are not at all consistent with Lyme disease.

*PARVOVIRUS.* This case is of a typical patient with human parvovirus (HPV B19) arthritis. Two thirds of the adult patients with arthritis are young women, and the reason for this is not known, although it may be explained in part by the exposure risks in this group. The virus is responsible for erythema infectiosum, the "slapped cheek" or fifth disease in childhood. Women who are frequently around small children are at risk. In addition, the effects of this small single-stranded DNA virus may be seen in the hospital setting, where it has been known to be responsible for a syndrome of transient aplastic crisis observed in chronic hemolytic anemia states. A pediatric house officer would be particularly vulnerable to exposure under these circumstances.

The arthritis of parvovirus infection is described with swollen hands and feet as the typical manifestations as in this patient. There are no renal, cardiovascular, respiratory, or gastrointestinal manifestations. The slapped-cheek appearance in adults is usually absent; instead there may be a reticular rash on the trunk and extremities. General laboratory testing is usually not specific, but the parvovirus titer indicating an immunoglobulin M (IgM) response is positive in this syndrome, and this result is diagnostic. The immunoglobulin G response to the virus occurs later on and indicates a past infection. The actual pathogenesis of the arthritis is not yet known, but because some of the cases have become chronic (although most are self-limited), investigators have always been fascinated with the hypothesis that a parvovirus-like trigger is responsible for initiating RA in susceptible hosts.

## Case 2: The 54-Year-Old Male Lawyer

### HISTORY

The patient was referred to the physician by his neighbor, a radiologist. The neighbor observed that the patient was not doing his usual gardening on the weekend and asked why. The answer was that the attorney's hands were painful and swollen. The patient comes to the physician's office for an evaluation. He has had fevers for the past 4 to 6 weeks, but only intermittently and occasionally up to 102° F. His hands have been swollen and painful for the past 2 to 3 weeks. There has been no rash or sore throat.

A year and a half ago, the patient was admitted to a local hospital for a respiratory illness characterized as bilateral pneumonia that did not respond to outpatient antibiotic therapy. During that hospitalization, both bronchoscopy and an open lung biopsy were performed; neither tumor nor tuberculosis was demonstrated. The illness ultimately resolved after 6 months, with spontaneous regression of the chest findings.

Six months ago the patient experienced a severe nosebleed while on an airplane descending for a landing. He was taken to an emergency room and treated with antibiotics and an anterior nasal pack. This problem has not recurred. The patient brings records from his internist, who has been performing yearly physical examinations. He always has measurements of 1+ to 2+ protein in the urine, 2 to 5 WBCs per high-power field (hpf), and 6 to 10 red blood cells (RBCs)/hpf. His prostate is checked regularly for this problem, and he has undergone a cystoscopy, with negative findings. The urine abnormality remains undiagnosed.

### PHYSICAL AND LABORATORY EXAMINATIONS

- Arthritis: Swelling and tenderness was noted in the PIPs, MCPs, wrists, knees, and ankles.
- Rash: None.
- Fever curve: There is a consistent elevation of temperature over the past 4 to 6 weeks, but not every single day; on occasions it has been measured as high as 102° F.
- Sore throat: None.
- Pulmonary involvement: Chest examination was clear, but the chest radiograph revealed some scarring at both lung bases and some streaking in the right mid lung field that was interpreted as "old."
- Renal involvement: Urine analysis revealed 3+ protein, 10 to 20 WBCs/hpf, 20 to 50 RBCs/hpf, and granular casts. Blood urea nitrogen (BUN) = 36 mg/dL, creatinine = 2.9 mg/dL.
- Liver function tests: AST = 59 U/L, ALT = 62 U/L, serum albumin = 2.3 g/dL, and total protein level = 6.5 g/dL.
- ESR/CRP: ESR = 92 mm/hr, CRP = 4.6 mg/dL.
- WBC, platelet count: WBC count = 11,500/mm³, platelet count = 560,000/mm³.
- Serologic studies: All test results were negative except an ANA of 1:40 and RF positive at 1:80.

### WHAT IS THE DIFFERENTIAL DIAGNOSIS?

This patient has findings of arthritis and fever. However, clearly he is systemically ill with pulmonary and renal involvement. The first order of business is to determine whether he has an acute self-limited infectious/postinfectious illness or a chronic rheumatic disease (with an acute exacerbation). His serum albumin level is low, which suggests a chronic condition or at least an illness that has been present for several months, perhaps longer. The findings of significant renal impairment, with an active-appearing urinary sediment, suggest acute glomerulonephritis. This finding should be coupled with the background presence of a prior episode of self-limited pulmonary disease and a persistent abnormal urinary sediment, which are consistent with chronic glomerular inflammation. The entire picture strongly suggests an acute exacerbation of a chronic rheumatic disease that affects not only the joints but also the kidneys and lungs.

From the original list of 14 possible diagnoses, the second 7 are chronic illnesses and potential diagnoses for this patient. We describe and consider each of these illnesses; of importance in this specific case is the presence of renal insufficiency with the assumption that it could be potentially reversible.

*ADULT-ONSET STILL'S DISEASE (AOS)*. The arthritis of this particular patient could be seen in AOS, but the fever pattern is not consistent. No rash is noted, and sore throat is absent; both rash and fever are features of AOS. Although transient pulmonary infiltrates and effusions are described in AOS, they are usually not this extensive and do not occur in the absence of other systemic findings, as happened in this patient. Liver function test results, ESR, and CRP are elevated in AOS, as in this case, but AOS does not produce serologic abnormalities. However, the major differentiating feature from AOS is the presence of acute and chronic renal disease in this patient.

*RHEUMATOID ARTHRITIS*. Although the arthritis as described in this case can occur in RA, as can slightly elevated liver function test results, ESR, and CRP, the presence of renal disease would be sufficient to rule out this diagnosis. Pulmonary manifestations do take place in RA, but their occurrence in the absence of joint disease (as in this patient) would be distinctly unusual. The serologic findings are consistent with RA, but the overall clinical picture is not.

*SYSTEMIC LUPUS ERYTHEMATOSUS*. Many, if not all, of the features of this case are consistent with SLE, including the arthritis, fever, pulmonary and renal involvement, and elevated liver function test results, CRP, and ESR. However, the absence of a rash makes the diagnosis of SLE quite unlikely. A rash would be expected in SLE because it is the most commonly encountered clinical feature of the disease (in over 90% of cases); its absence in this patient with a chronic illness contradicts the diagnosis of SLE. In addition, in a very sick SLE patient with renal disease, as described in this case, leukopenia and thrombocytopenia might be expected. However, the very low ANA titer in this patient further contradicts the diagnosis of SLE.

*GIANT CELL ARTERITIS (GCA)*. Patients with GCA can present to the physician with fever and nonspecific signs of a chronic illness (low serum albumin, anemia, and so forth). However, it is distinctly unusual to find evidence of painful objective arthritis, signs of glomerulonephritis, and significant pulmonary involvement. These latter features are prominent in this patient and effectively rule out GCA in this case.

*MIXED CRYOGLOBULINEMIA (MCG)*. Although arthritis, fever, and pulmonary, hepatic, and renal involvement can occur in this disease, the absence of a vasculitic rash in the course of this patient's illness would distinctly contradict the diagnosis of MCG. The serologic study results are compatible with MCG; viral studies for hepatitis B and C should be performed. However, without cutaneous vasculitis in the history or on examination, this diagnosis is suspect.

*SJÖGREN'S SYNDROME*. This disease can have widespread systemic manifestations beyond keratoconjunctivitis sicca symptoms in the eyes and xerostomia in the mouth. Arthritis, fever, pulmonary involvement, elevated liver function test results, and elevated ESR and CRP occur in Sjögren's syndrome, but renal disease to this magnitude is distinctly unusual and effectively rules out Sjögren's syndrome in this patient. In addition, a vasculitic rash is typically seen in the systemic form of Sjögren's syndrome; it is absent in this patient.

*WEGENER'S GRANULOMATOSIS (WG)*. This patient demonstrates the classical clinical features and time course of an acute exacerbation of WG. What appears to distinguish WG from RA or SLE is its tendency to produce different clinical manifestations over time, often with long disease-free periods in between. This patient, for example, developed pulmonary disease, then upper airway disease, and then renal disease over a period of years. This intermittent course of disease activity is probably why the diagnosis of WG is often delayed and sometimes missed until a collection of different manifestations have occurred over time. In fact, there is little to distinguish the clinical features of WG (fever, rash, and involvement of the lungs, kidneys, skin, joints, upper airway) from other rheumatic diseases until a biopsy reveals the specific findings of granulomatous vasculitis. However, the on-and-off clinical course in this patient, with additive clinical features over time, is certainly typical of WG. Sometimes a high-titer positive antineutrophil cytoplasmic antibody result will confirm the diagnosis.

## Case 3: The 32-Year-Old Registered Nurse

### HISTORY

This female patient was referred by her primary care physician for pain in her shoulders, elbows, knees, and wrists. These symptoms have been present for 2 to 3 months; no joint swelling has been noted. She has complained of a feverish feeling, but no temperature has been taken. There has been moderate fatigue and some weight loss, estimated to be 5 to 10 lbs (3 to 5 kg). She has experienced a sore throat, back pain, and some anterior chest pain in the last 1 to 2 weeks. She has also had a rash with itching present on her face, forehead, and shoulders, along with some hair loss in a patchy distribution. In the last few weeks she has noticed much more hair loss in her comb and in the shower. She is unmarried and has never been pregnant. She works the night shift in an oncology ward at a local hospital.

Her mother died in a rural area in the Philippines 8 years ago from a fulminant multisystem illness characterized at the end by rapidly progressive renal failure. No specific diagnosis was made, according to the patient, but her mother did experience pain all over and a rash. At age 14 the patient experienced an episode of idiopathic thrombocytopenic purpura (ITP) that was unresponsive to glucocorticoids, and she ultimately required a splenectomy. There has been no recurrence of the ITP.

#### PHYSICAL AND LABORATORY EXAMINATIONS

- Arthritis: Marked tenderness to palpation was noted over the wrists, knees, and elbows. Pain was experienced on full abduction of both shoulders and on hyperextension of the knees and elbows. No joint swelling was appreciated; however, the hands appeared "puffy" on inspection.
- Rash: A maculopapular rash was noted, with raised edges, on the shoulders, neck, forehead, and calf. Several areas of patchy alopecia were noted in the scalp, and the patient's hair at the forehead hairline appeared lanugo-like, soft, and curly. There was a small (2- to 3-mm) shallow ulcer at the apex of the hard palate.
- Fever curve: Temperature was noted to be 99° F.
- Sore throat: This has been present for the past 1 to 2 weeks.
- Pulmonary involvement: None. Normal chest radiograph.
- Renal involvement: BUN and creatinine = 18 mg/dL and 1.0 mg/dL, respectively; urine analysis revealed 1+ protein, 2 to 5 RBCs/hpf, 6 to 10 WBCs/hpf.
- Liver function tests: ALT = 64 U/L, AST = 86 U/L, albumin = 3.0 g/dL, total protein level = 7.2 g/dL.
- ESR/CRP: ESR = 48 mm/hr, CRP = <0.8 mg/dL.
- WBC count, platelet count: WBC count = 2800/mm³, platelet count = 420,000/mm³.
- Serologic tests: ANA > 1:1280, RF = 1:80. Viral studies all yielded negative results.

#### WHAT IS THE DIFFERENTIAL DIAGNOSIS?

The patient has a multisystem illness characterized by fever, rash, and arthritis; additional features include chest and back pain, sore throat, and oral ulcers. Furthermore, there is a strong suggestion that the illness is familial (the patient's mother died of a fulminant multisystem illness ending with renal failure), and the patient's illness likely began when she was a teenager, with an episode of ITP at age 14. Chronicity is documented by the low serum albumin level, and mild renal glomerular inflammation is suggested by the findings on urine analysis. The patient has leukopenia, a high ANA-positive titer, and an elevated platelet count associated with a prior splenectomy.

Therefore, the clinical picture is one of a progressive, systemic rheumatic disease going back at least several months, perhaps longer. The differential diagnosis is very likely beyond the self-limited syndromes (infectious, postinfectious, viral) and should focus on chronic rheumatic diseases, such as the second list of 7 conditions referred to earlier.

***ADULT-ONSET STILL'S DISEASE.*** Although fever, rash, and arthritis as well as sore throat are present, the other characteristics in this patient are quite different from those seen in AOS. In patients with AOS, the fever is high, spiking up to 104° or 105° F, and returns to normal daily, and the rash is transient, almost evanescent, nonpruritic, and without raised borders. The renal involvement, leukopenia, and serologic abnormalities are quite in contradiction to AOS, along with the patient's history of familial illness and ITP.

***RHEUMATOID ARTHRITIS.*** The specific characteristics of the fever, rash, and arthritis in this patient all contradict the diagnosis of typical adult RA, whether seropositive or seronegative. RA patients may on rare occasions experience a vasculitic rash, although not the one described in this patient, and fever is typically absent. This patient's arthritis is not consistent with the typical features of objective synovitis seen in RA. Furthermore, renal involvement is absent in RA except for instances of drug toxicity or, very rarely, severe vasculitis. The systemic nature of this patient's findings, including the rash, the family history of a multisystem illness, and the personal history of ITP, is inconsistent with the diagnosis of RA and suggests another diagnosis.

***GIANT CELL ARTERITIS.*** None of the fever, rash, and arthritis characteristics of this patient are part of the typical manifestations of GCA. The history of past familial multisystem illness, the findings of leukopenia, high ANA titer, and glomerular inflammation all contradict the diagnosis of GCA.

***MIXED CRYOGLOBULINEMIA.*** There is no doubt that MCG could be confused with the picture presented by this patient, especially the multisystem nature of the illness. However, the rash of MCG is typically vasculitis, not seen in this patient. A laboratory test for cryoglobulins should be performed in this case; it may even yield a positive result in other diseases (such as RA or SLE), but the titers or amounts of cryoglobulins in MCG would be expected to be much higher. Laboratory tests for viral pathogens (hepatitis B or C) might be positive in MCG; they were negative in this patient.

***SJÖGREN'S SYNDROME.*** The specifically described rash, arthritis, and fever in this patient do not resemble the characteristic features of Sjögren's syndrome. In that condition, vasculitis of the lower extremities predominates. Renal disease, the history of past familial multisystem disease, and a prior splenectomy for ITP in this patient would contradict the diagnosis of Sjögren's syndrome.

***WEGENER'S GRANULOMATOSIS.*** Many of the findings in this patient could be found in WG. However, there are important, if subtle, differences. The rash of WG is typically a vasculitis and papular/nodular, sometimes with ulceration; this patient has quite different findings. The presence of leukopenia and the absence of upper and lower airway disease in this patient contradict the diagnosis of WG. In addition, the patient's history of ITP is clearly inconsistent with the diagnosis of WG.

SYSTEMIC LUPUS ERYTHEMATOSUS. All the features of this patient's illness are totally consistent with SLE. The arthritis causes pain out of proportion to the physical findings of inflammation; the joints only appear slightly "puffy," but the pain on motion is intense. The rash is maculopapular and located in areas with the greatest exposure to ultraviolet light. A sore throat and fever are present, and the patient has lost hair, experienced fatigue and weight loss, and noted anterior chest pain and back pain; these clinical findings are consistent with active SLE. Oral ulceration on physical examination typically denotes active SLE.

The patient's family history of her mother with a multisystem illness ending in renal failure is consistent with familial SLE, and of course the past history of an ITP-like illness, necessitating a splenectomy, may be found in an SLE patient's background. The laboratory studies are typical for SLE patients, including findings of mild glomerulonephritis, elevated transaminase levels, low serum albumin level with a high globulin concentration, leukopenia, and a high ANA-positive titer.

## Case 4: The 28-Year-Old Computer Scientist

### HISTORY
The patient is a woman with a 4- to 6-week history of high fevers (when taken, up to 104° F), chills, and sweats, occurring almost every day. Because of an accompanying severely sore throat at the beginning of the illness, the patient was given a 7-day course of antibiotics; no effect on the fever or sore throat was observed. Anorexia, weight loss, and marked fatigue ensued, and the patient went to another physician, who took a chest radiograph and noted a right-sided pulmonary infiltrate, dehydration (postural hypotension), lymphadenopathy, and an enlarged spleen. The patient was subsequently hospitalized with the initial diagnosis of fever of unknown origin.

This patient had no history of a previous similar illness, undiagnosed illness in childhood, or any other major medical or surgical condition. She has been married for the past 4 years, has taken oral contraceptives, and has no exposure or travel history. For the past several weeks she had been complaining to her husband that her elbows and knees hurt, but there was no sign of swelling.

### PHYSICAL AND LABORATORY EXAMINATIONS

- Arthritis: There was pain on full extension of both elbows and a moderate-sized effusion in the right knee, which was minimally tender to palpation.
- Rash: None.
- Fever curve: Temperature was 103.8° F at 4 p.m. the day of admission.
- Sore throat: The patient's throat was so severely sore that she had difficulty swallowing; the examination revealed only erythema.
- Pulmonary involvement: On chest radiograph, a hazy infiltrate was noted at the right lung base along with a small pleural effusion on the right side.
- Renal involvement: None.

- Liver function tests: ALT = 80 U/L, AST = 90 U/L, albumin/globulin ratio = 2.9/4.6, alkaline phosphatase = 360 U/L.
- ESR/CRP: ESR = 117 mm/hr, CRP = 4.8 mg/dL.
- WBC/platelet count: WBC = 36,000/mm$^3$, platelets = 760,000/mm$^3$.
- Serologic tests: All negative.

### HOSPITAL COURSE
Further physical examination in the hospital revealed moderate lymphadenopathy in all locations, and the patient's liver and spleen were easily palpated. After cultures were taken, the patient was given broad-spectrum antibiotics for the possibility of a community-acquired pneumonia. Fevers persisted in the afternoon, sometimes up to 104° F, but the temperature was typically normal in the early morning. There was no apparent response to antibiotics. All cultures of the throat, blood, urine, sputum, and stool were negative. Echocardiography yielded negative findings. Serologic studies yielded negative results for HIV, other retroviruses, hepatitis viruses, Lyme disease, antistreptolysin O and other streptococcal antigens, Brucella, and febrile agglutinins. A faint, nonpruritic maculopapular rash was observed on the patient's back and neck 2 days after antibiotics were stopped; the rash was attributed to a drug reaction. The patient was hospitalized for a total of 14 days and left without a diagnosis, still moderately symptomatic.

### WHAT IS THE DIFFERENTIAL DIAGNOSIS?
The patient's entire illness, from beginning of symptoms to the end of hospitalization, was at least 2 months in duration. All serologic studies for an acute infectious or postinfectious syndrome yielded negative findings, and all cultures for pathogens were negative. Therefore, the differential diagnosis must focus on the possibility that this case of fever, rash, and arthritis represents the beginning of a chronic rheumatic disease.

RHEUMATOID ARTHRITIS. Although systemic features may be present in an occasional RA patient, they will not persist out of proportion to the arthritis, as seen in this patient. Conventional, garden-variety RA is highly unlikely in this case without more obvious physical findings of arthritis, which were present but minimal in this patient.

SYSTEMIC LUPUS ERYTHEMATOSUS. Although the multisystem nature of this illness suggests SLE, many features contradict this diagnosis: for example, the very high WBC and platelet counts and, of course, the negative ANA titer. Although ANA-negative SLE does occur, it is very rare and is typically associated with obvious cutaneous manifestations, which are absent in this case.

WEGENER'S GRANULOMATOSIS. Without significant pulmonary, renal, or upper airway involvement in this very sick, chronically ill patient, the diagnosis of WG is very remote.

GIANT CELL ARTERITIS. The widespread systemic findings in this case, which included lymphadenopathy and hepatosplenomegaly, make this diagnosis quite unlikely. In spite of the fact that fever and anemia with a high sedimentation rate are the hallmarks of

GCA, the fever curve presented by this patient (high spiking, returning to normal daily) is not typical of GCA.

*MIXED CRYOGLOBULINEMIA.* The absence of a vasculitic rash, renal involvement, and positive hepatitis serologies in this patient makes the diagnosis of MCG highly unlikely.

*SJÖGREN'S SYNDROME.* Although systemic features may occur in Sjögren's syndrome, they are much less dramatic and more chronic than in this case. In addition, positive RF activity associated with other autoantibodies and cutaneous vasculitis almost always occurs in the setting of systemic Sjögren's syndrome. None of these are evident in this patient.

*ADULT-ONSET STILL'S DISEASE.* This patient's illness is a classical case of AOS. This syndrome is a tetrad of findings: fever, rash, polyarthritis, and sore throat. Each may predominate at the onset of the illness, and sometimes they do not occur simultaneously, a scenario that often delays the diagnosis. The AOS fever is widely fluctuating, extraordinarily high especially in the afternoon but always coming down to normal at least once during each 24-hour cycle. The arthritis may be subtle, overshadowed by the marked systemic features, and not easily detected unless specifically sought. The rash is evanescent and may occur only when the fever is the highest in the midafternoon, when the hospitalized patient is least likely to be observed by a physician.

Extensive malignancy and infectious disease workups are typically negative and often repeated in spite of their negativity in these cases, and the lymphadenopathy and organomegaly may be very dramatic to the point of provoking the physician to order a biopsy. Biopsies and bone marrow examinations are uniformly nondiagnostic. Levels of acute-phase proteins are impressively elevated. The peripheral WBC count may suggest a "leukemoid" reaction, often between 25,000 and 50,000 cells/mm$^3$, and the platelet count may exceed 1,000,000. A ferritin level, if measured, is in the thousands, which is strongly suggestive of the diagnosis.

The sore throat that occurs with AOS can be so severe as to provoke empiric therapy for the presumptive diagnosis of ARF. However, the sore throat is a typical systemic feature of the disease, occurring as often as the rash in large series of patients. Finally, it is important to point out that the presence of arthritis is probably the best way to distinguish AOS from infectious diseases and malignancies, although it does not help to distinguish the different rheumatic diseases from each other.

## Case 5: The 19-Year-Old Male Migrant Farm Worker

### HISTORY

The patient comes to the emergency room with a 7-day history of severe joint pains in his back, knees, and hips. He has been feverish for 2 to 3 days, and he has complained of a sore throat for several weeks. He denies all other symptoms referable to other organ systems, but he appears frightened and unwilling to talk. He is brought into the emergency room by a fellow worker who claimed to know nothing else about the patient; therefore, the patient was admitted to the hospital.

### PHYSICAL AND LABORATORY EXAMINATIONS

- Arthritis: Marked pain throughout range of motion of the shoulders and hips was noted. The right knee was exquisitely tender to touch, was swollen, and contained a moderate effusion. The left knee was mildly swollen, was less tender, and contained a minimal effusion.
- Rash: None.
- Fever curve: Temperature in the emergency room was 102.6° F.
- Sore throat: The patient's throat was red without an exudate, and cervical lymphadenopathy was observed.
- Pulmonary involvement: None.
- Renal involvement: None.
- Liver function tests: Normal.
- ESR/CRP: ESR = 88 mm/hr, CRP = 4.8 mg/dL.
- WBC/platelet count: Normal.
- Serologic tests: All normal.

### HOSPITAL COURSE

On admission the patient appeared acutely ill. The general physical examination yielded normal findings; there was no heart murmur, and echocardiography yielded negative results. Cultures of urine, blood, and stool were negative. Throat culture revealed β-hemolytic streptococci; the antistreptolysin O titer was reported as positive. Lyme disease, parvovirus, and all hepatitis serologic results were negative. Arthrocentesis of the right knee produced 20 mL of cloudy fluid; the total cell count was 50,000/mm$^3$, all were polymorphonuclear cells, and the culture was negative. While culture results were pending, broad-spectrum antibiotics were administered for 48 hours; the patient did not respond clinically, and antibiotics were discontinued.

The patient's family members visited in the hospital and were able to give additional details for the history. In the past year, the patient has had at least two similar episodes of sore throat, fever, and arthritis, each lasting about 2 to 4 weeks. He had been given antibiotics in the past; for this episode, he took some leftover drug at home. All of these family members, including the patient, suffered repeated sore throats; they lived in close quarters in a migrant field worker camp outside of town. Subsequently, the patient was given indomethacin and was discharged when his fever curve was normal for 24 hours.

### WHAT IS THE DIFFERENTIAL DIAGNOSIS?

The patient presents with an acute febrile illness and arthritis. However, additional history from the family indicates that it was a recurrent problem over the past year, each episode lasting less than 30 days. Nevertheless, the differential diagnosis must focus on what may be treatable or reversible disease: that is, the infectious or postinfectious syndromes. The clinical characteristics of this patient's fever, rash, and arthritis, as well as the serologic findings, when carefully examined, indicate a specific diagnosis.

*HEPATITIS B AND HEPATITIS C.* The absence of rash and exposure history, and the negative serologic findings, are strong evidence against these diagnoses. The multisystem involvement caused by hepatitis C is not present in this patient. An acute self-limited polyarthritis of the hands and feet is typical for hepatitis B; this patient's recurrent disease in large joints contradicts that diagnosis.

*PARVOVIRUS AND RUBELLA.* An acute polyarthritis of the hands and feet is the rule in these postviral syndromes; this patient's physical and clinical findings are those of a large-joint oligoarthritis, making these diagnoses less likely. In addition, the negative viral study findings are strong evidence against these postviral conditions.

*SUBACUTE BACTERIAL ENDOCARDITIS.* This diagnosis is always possible in a young person with the acute onset of fever and a large-joint oligoarthritis. However, results of cardiac examination, echocardiography, and blood cultures were all negative, ruling out this diagnosis.

*LYME DISEASE.* This diagnosis should always be a consideration for a patient with recurrent large-joint oligoarthritis and potential exposure history. However, the negative serologic results rule out this diagnosis, especially because the arthritis is recurrent and the Lyme serologic result would be expected to be positive in that setting.

*ACUTE RHEUMATIC FEVER.* This patient's presentation is a classical case of ARF in a young adult. A large-joint, additive oligoarthritis is characteristic for adults with this condition. Severe pain, sometimes out of proportion to physical findings of inflammation, is the rule, especially in the proximal limb girdles. Rheumatic fever in adults manifests almost exclusively as arthritis; cardiac involvement is extremely rare after childhood. As a result, in these adult cases, the usual accompaniments of carditis, such as erythema marginatum or chorea, are not seen. Attacks usually last less than 6 weeks, as in this case, and may be recurrent, depending on the frequency and severity of the antecedent streptococcal throat infections.

The antistreptolysin O titer should be high in this case, reflecting the severity of the pharyngitis and the risk of rheumatic fever resulting from the infection. Rheumatic fever still exists in all parts of the world as long as there are socioeconomic conditions that allow for recurrent streptococcal pharyngitis. With regard to the articular findings of ARF, a response to aspirin or nonsteroidal anti-inflammatory agents should be relatively dramatic and complete, providing more definitive evidence for the diagnosis.

## Case 6: The 78-Year-Old Retired Engineer

### HISTORY

The patient is brought to the physician's office by a colleague. The physician is told that the patient is the colleague's father, who is visiting from Minnesota and has been complaining of an illness going back over

several months. The characteristics of this illness are that the patient has lost weight and complained of stiffness in his muscles, especially in the morning. His shoulders have been particularly painful. More recently the patient has been unable to perform his hobbies, such as repairing children's toys for charity resale; he has always been the local handyman for the neighbors, and he has been unable to work in this capacity in recent weeks. When he had a persistent "low-grade" fever, he went to his primary care physician, who performed a series of examinations and tests; no diagnosis was made except for a flu-like illness. He was told he was "slightly anemic" and given iron and multivitamin pills to take.

The patient has not experienced the onset of a new headache, rash, or cardiopulmonary, genitourinary, or gastrointestinal symptoms. There is no recent change in his bowel habits. He does not complain of dry eyes or dry mouth. His history is negative for any past serious medical or surgical illnesses. He retired 6 years ago, and until recently, he was completely fit.

### PHYSICAL AND LABORATORY EXAMINATIONS

- Arthritis: The patient's hands were slightly swollen with a positive Tinel's sign; tenderness was localized over the MCP and PIP joints. Pain was exhibited on dorsiflexion of both wrists. There was moderately diminished range of motion of both shoulders, each limited by moderate pain to only 60 to 70 degrees of abduction bilaterally. Both knees displayed some bone crepitus without effusions. The rest of the joint examination was normal.
- Rash: None.
- Fever curve: Temperature in the office was 99.7° F.
- Sore throat: None.
- Pulmonary involvement: None.
- Renal involvement: None.
- Liver function tests: ALT = 47 U/L, AST = 39 U/L, alkaline phosphatase = 140 U/L.
- ESR/CRP: ESR = 98 mm/hr, CRP = 2.0.
- WBC/platelet count: Both were normal.
- Serologic tests: All normal, including viral studies, except for a positive ANA titer of 1:40.

### WHAT IS THE DIFFERENTIAL DIAGNOSIS?

This gentleman in his late 70s presents with the insidious onset, over many months, of low-grade fever, muscle aches, shoulder pain, and difficulty in using his hands. Examination reveals swollen hands, findings of carpal tunnel syndrome, and moderate to marked limitation of mobility of both shoulders in association with pain. The laboratory test results indicate an anemia and a markedly elevated sedimentation rate; serologic studies yield normal results. The process has been going on for at least 6 months, perhaps longer in this stoic gentleman. The differential diagnosis is among the chronic rheumatic diseases listed in Table 2–4, and the clinical findings along with the laboratory testing will lead to the correct diagnosis.

*ADULT-ONSET STILL'S DISEASE.* Although AOS has been described in this age group, it is nonetheless distinctly unusual. The clinical absence in this patient of all three elements—sore throat, a typical fever pattern, and a rash—firmly contradict the diagnosis of AOS.

*RHEUMATOID ARTHRITIS.* RA in the elderly can manifest exactly in the same manner as in this patient. The presence of low-grade fever, an inflammatory arthritis involving the shoulders, and swollen hands may be entirely consistent with RA in this subpopulation of patients. In addition, these RA patients are typically seronegative, as in this case. It may not be possible to distinguish this diagnosis from the one suggested later for this patient.

*SYSTEMIC LUPUS ERYTHEMATOSUS.* The articular findings in this patient and the presence of a low-grade fever are consistent with SLE. However, the absence of a rash and lack of multisystem (pulmonary, renal) involvement make this diagnosis much less likely. The ANA titer is barely positive and can be considered falsely positive in this elderly gentleman; therefore, SLE is effectively ruled out.

*WEGENER'S GRANULOMATOSIS.* Although the articular findings and presence of fever in this patient could be found in WG, the absence of upper airway disease, pulmonary, or renal involvement makes this diagnosis extremely unlikely.

*MIXED CRYOGLOBULINEMIA.* The hallmarks of MCG (vasculitis, glomerulonephritis, and serologic abnormalities) are absent in this patient. In addition, viral serologic results are negative, making this diagnosis implausible.

*SJÖGREN'S SYNDROME.* This patient's fever and articular findings could be explained by Sjögren's syndrome. However, the absence of vasculitis, of symptoms of xerostomia (dry mouth) and keratoconjunctivitis sicca (dry eyes), and of serologic abnormalities makes this diagnosis very unlikely.

*GIANT CELL ARTERITIS.* Patients with the syndrome of GCA may have typical symptoms as in this case, and GCA is the most likely diagnosis for this patient, who displays fever, weight loss, anemia, a high sedimentation rate, proximal limb girdle pain, swollen hands, and carpal tunnel syndrome. However, it is important to remember that there are several other unique syndromes considered subsets of GCA: temporal arteritis (localized or unilateral head and neck symptoms) and polymyalgia rheumatica (abrupt onset of proximal muscle pain). The histologic features of GCA may occur in arteries throughout the body, both above and below the diaphragm, and in the great vessels in the head and neck.

GCA, in its many forms, does not commonly involve internal organs (kidneys, lungs, heart, peripheral nervous system), but on very rare occasions patients may have ischemia from arteritis in mesenteric vessels. The most feared complication of GCA is sudden unilateral blindness, resulting from arteritis of the posterior ciliary branch of the ophthalmic artery, which causes nonreversible ischemic optic atrophy.

Strictly from a clinical perspective, it is not possible to make a clear distinction between the polymyalgia rheumatica subset of GCA and seronegative RA manifesting in the elderly. The prognosis and treatment plan are fundamentally the same, regardless of which

diagnosis is entertained, and the results of a temporal artery biopsy would not influence the patient's management. At best, a temporal artery biopsy would yield a positive result in one third to half of suspected cases. In the future, the use of combined magnetic resonance angiography and magnetic resonance imaging may lead to less invasive diagnostic testing with higher sensitivity and specificity.

## Case 7: The 27-Year-Old Female Mortgage Broker

### HISTORY

This patient was referred by a dermatologist for evaluation of systemic disease with a biopsy-proven diagnosis of cutaneous vasculitis. For the past several months, the patient has experienced raised, red, painful, "burning" skin lesions on her lower extremities. The pain in these lesions is worsened with standing or at the end of a working day and often regresses with elevation of her legs, especially after lying down overnight, or on weekends when she reclines at home. Tight constricting bands on her stockings will accentuate the rash. The highest point of the rash has been her upper thighs; it has not appeared on her trunk or arms. The patient has noted new lesions appearing as the old ones fade; the fading lesions turn a golden yellow color as they disappear.

The dermatologist has performed a punch biopsy on a fresh lesion; the pathology report brought by the patient reveals a description of leukocytoclastic vasculitis. There are a variety of laboratory reports that come with the patient as well, suggesting a systemic illness.

The patient's history is negative for prior episodes similar to this one, and she denies arthritis, cardiopulmonary symptoms, fatigue, fever, weight loss, and change in bowel habits. There is no history of exposure to blood or blood products, needlesticks, or people with hepatitis. Approximately 1 year ago the patient noted swelling of her parotid gland on the right side; work-up at that time yielded results negative for tumor or stones, and the swelling regressed. She has noted dryness of her eyes in recent months, and her contact lenses have become difficult to wear; she is currently unable to wear them at all.

### PHYSICAL AND LABORATORY EXAMINATIONS

- Arthritis: None.
- Rash: There was a punctate as well as a confluent red/purple macular rash on the lower extremities, several areas of which were raised and palpable. The highest point of the rash was the upper thigh. The areas of confluence occurred around the ankles and tops of the feet. There were fresh-appearing red lesions alongside brown and golden areas of hyperpigmentation on the calf.
- Fever curve: None.
- Pulmonary involvement: None.
- Renal involvement: None.
- Liver function tests: AST = 67 U/L, ALT = 42 U/L, albumin = 3.5 g/L, total protein = 8.7 g/L, alkaline phosphatase = 175 U/L.

- ESR/CRP: ESR = 56 mm/hr, CRP < 0.8 mg/dL.
- WBC/platelet count: Normal.
- Serologic tests: ANA = 1:640, RF = 1:1280, anti–Sjögren's syndrome antigen A (anti–SS-A+) = 1:320, anti–Sjögren's syndrome antigen B (anti–SS-B+) = 1:40; anti-DNA results were negative; results of viral studies (including hepatitis serologic results) were negative. Cryoglobulins were not present.

#### WHAT IS THE DIFFERENTIAL DIAGNOSIS?

The patient has cutaneous vasculitis, waxing and waning over several months, and laboratory studies strongly suggest a systemic rheumatic disease. A variety of autoantibodies are positive, and the patient has markedly elevated serum globulin values on routine chemistry testing. Therefore, the differential diagnosis is to include one of the causes of cutaneous vasculitis in this clinical setting. There are several distinct possibilities among the seven causes of fever, rash, and arthritis to be considered below.

*ADULT-ONSET STILL'S DISEASE.* The classical features of AOS, such as high spiking fevers, evanescent rash, arthritis, and sore throat, are absent in this patient. In addition, the finding of cutaneous vasculitis with marked serologic abnormalities in this case firmly contradicts the diagnostic possibility of AOS.

*RHEUMATOID ARTHRITIS.* A symmetric polyarthritis is absent in this patient in spite of months of widespread lower extremity cutaneous vasculitis; this renders the diagnosis of RA very implausible in this case.

*SYSTEMIC LUPUS ERYTHEMATOSUS.* The lack of fever, photosensitive rash, and arthritis in this patient is inconsistent with SLE as a diagnosis. Furthermore, this patient does not display the widespread internal organ involvement (renal, cardiopulmonary, nervous system) seen frequently in SLE cases.

*WEGENER'S GRANULOMATOSIS.* The key diagnostic feature of WG—involvement of the upper and lower airways and the kidneys—is not found in this patient, making this diagnosis very unlikely. Although cutaneous vasculitis may occur in WG, as a single feature alone it is insufficient to establish that diagnosis.

*GIANT CELL ARTERITIS.* The important clinical aspects of GCA, such as the systemic findings of fever, weight loss, anemia, and proximal limb girdle pain, are absent in this patient. Furthermore, the autoantibodies present in high titers in this case are not typical of GCA. Therefore, this diagnosis is very unlikely.

*MIXED CRYOGLOBULINEMIA.* Patients with MCG may present exactly as in this case, with lower extremity vasculitis, and the condition can be difficult to distinguish from Sjögren's syndrome and other causes of cutaneous vasculitis. However, patients with MCG may have internal organ involvement such as glomerulonephritis or mononeuritis multiplex; these are absent in this case. Nevertheless, the absence of cryoglobulins and the presence of negative serologic results indicating a concomitant hepatitis B or C infection make MCG unlikely.

*SJÖGREN'S SYNDROME.* This patient presents with classical signs and symptoms of hypergammaglobulinemic purpura associated with Sjögren's syndrome.

In some patients the symptoms of xerostomia and keratoconjunctivitis sicca predominate; in other cases, vasculitis is the main clinical feature. Because so many of the features are shared, it is useful to consider Sjögren's syndrome and hyperglobulinemic purpura to be subsets of the same condition. The lower extremity vasculitis, as in this patient, is typically effected by factors that promote deposition of immune complexes (the proposed mechanism), such as increased hydrostatic pressure or local trauma to blood vessels. That proposed pathophysiologic mechanism appears to explain why the patients experience a marked increase in signs and symptoms with weight bearing and amelioration of these manifestations with a recumbent position or just elevating the legs.

The hyperglobulinemia represents an elevation of gamma globulins, almost always polyclonal, as in this case. Autoantibodies, such as antinuclear antibodies and rheumatoid factors, are typically present along with other antibodies more commonly associated with Sjögren's syndrome, such as anti–SS-A and anti–SS-B. Hepatitis C and HIV infections are associated with Sjögren's syndrome and sicca syndrome; hence virus-associated antibodies may be present. Additional features of Sjögren's syndrome, such as intermittent parotid swelling, lymphadenopathy, and dryness of the eyes and mouth, probably appear in many of these patients over time. This patient has had one prior episode of parotid swelling. The course in this subset of patients with cutaneous vasculitis is chronic, remitting and relapsing, very much affected by the ability of the patient to avoid conditions that aggravate the rash. It is often referred to as *palpable purpura* because of its visible resemblance to thrombocytopenic purpura, and the inflammation and necrosis caused by the vasculitis produce a palpable lesion.

### Case 8: The 38-Year-Old Occupational Therapist

#### HISTORY

The patient is admitted to the hospital with a 4- to 6-week history of a rash on her trunk and lower extremities; initially the rash had the appearance of hives, but lately she has noted purple blotches on her legs, some of which have become ulcerated. She has experienced a mild fever on one or two occasions, up to 100° F, and has noted joint pains in her hands and elbows. The skin lesions are becoming painful, especially the ulcerated ones. In the past 2 weeks she has experienced weakness in her legs and marked overall fatigue. There is numbness on the bottom of her feet; she reports that when she is barefoot, she feels as if she is wearing socks. On her own she took a course of oral antibiotics during the past week, with no effect. Her husband reports that the patient told him she had a similar but much less extensive rash on her lower legs and feet 6 months ago; it lasted about a week and disappeared. She denies a history of dry eyes or dry mouth.

Her personal history is fairly unremarkable for any other serious medical or surgical illnesses. However, she was hospitalized about 15 years ago for a postpartum hemorrhage that necessitated multiple transfusions. At the time she was told that the blood was safe from HIV transmission; she has not had any blood tests to check for this since.

The findings of the general examination were very remarkable and included cervical lymphadenopathy, hepatosplenomegaly, and a blood pressure of 160/100. Results of cardiac examination and echocardiography were negative. Neurologic examination revealed diminished sensation in both lower legs and feet in a stocking-glove distribution. There was weakness of dorsiflexion and eversion in the right foot.

### PHYSICAL AND LABORATORY EXAMINATIONS

- Arthritis: The patient's hands were generally swollen and tender; the swelling and tenderness were accentuated at the wrists and MCP joints. The elbows were painful on full extension.
- Rash: There was a bilateral and extensive maculopapular eruption from her waist to her toes, accentuated on the lower legs and feet, with confluent areas on the calf. The color was red/purple, and the lesions ranged in size from 1 to 2 mm to 5 to 6 mm; on the confluent areas, there were several small ulcerations with serous drainage. The lesions were palpable.
- Fever curve: The temperature during the examination was 99.6° F.
- Sore throat: None.
- Pulmonary involvement: None.
- Renal involvement: Urinalysis revealed 2+ protein, 5 to 10 WBCs/hpf, 30 to 40 RBCs/hpf, and both hyaline and red blood cell casts. BUN and creatinine levels were 24 and 1.6 mg/dL, respectively.
- Liver function tests: AST = 87 U/L, ALT = 122 U/L, albumin = 2.8 g/L, globulin = 4.7 g/L, alkaline phosphatase = 245 U/L.
- ESR/CRP: ESR = 87 mm/hr, CRP = 4.0 mg/dL.
- WBC/platelet count: WBC count = 3600/mm$^3$, platelet count = 110,000/mm$^3$.
- Serologic tests: ANA = 1:40, RF = 1:2560; anti–SS-A and anti–SS-B results were negative, anti-DNA was not detected; complement components: C3 = 24 mg/dL, C4 = 14 mg/dL; hepatitis B surface antigen results were negative, HIV results were negative, anti–hepatitis C results were positive, and cryoglobulin levels were markedly positive.

### WHAT IS THE DIFFERENTIAL DIAGNOSIS?

This patient has widespread palpable vasculitic lesions of her trunk and lower extremities, some of which have ulcerated. She has marked systemic manifestations, including symptoms of joint pain (arthralgias), weakness, and paresthesias, in addition to physical findings of hypertension, arthritis, neuropathy, lymphadenopathy, and abdominal organomegaly. The laboratory examination reveals low serum albumin levels, elevated globulin levels, and abnormal transaminase levels; she has positive levels of RF and cryoglobulins, and antibodies to hepatitis C are present. There are very mild leukopenia and thrombocytopenia. The blood pressure is elevated, and the urinalysis reveals an active urinary sediment suggestive of glomerular inflammation.

This entire picture is consistent with the onset of a serious chronic systemic illness affecting blood vessels not only in the skin but throughout the body, including the liver, kidneys, and bone marrow. Clinically the rash has the appearance of vasculitis. From our list of 14 possible diagnoses, we consider the second group of 7 chronic rheumatic diseases.

*ADULT-ONSET STILL'S DISEASE.* The presence of arthritis, fever, organomegaly, lymphadenopathy, and liver function abnormalities is consistent with AOS, but everything else is not. Sore throat is not present, and the rash of AOS is a transient evanescent process, which is quite different from that in this patient. The presence of a widespread vasculitic rash, neuropathy, glomerulonephritis, and hypertension is inconsistent with AOS. In addition, laboratory studies revealing positive RF activity, low complement values, mild leukopenia and thrombocytopenia, and the presence of cryoglobulins contradict the diagnosis of AOS.

*RHEUMATOID ARTHRITIS.* Some of the findings of widespread vasculitis seen in this patient are rarely noted in RA subjects; usually they appear only in patients with long-standing joint disease. These include, in addition to arthritis, the findings of cutaneous vasculitis, neuropathy, elevated globulin levels and liver function findings, organomegaly, and the laboratory abnormalities (positive RF activity, low levels of complement components, mild leukopenia, and mild thrombocytopenia). Even cryoglobulins may be positive in these patients, but always in amounts much smaller than seen here. However, findings consistent with glomerulonephritis are not commonly seen in this subset of RA patients, and the presence of antibodies to hepatitis C would not be expected to occur except by chance association. On purely clinical grounds, the diagnosis of RA with systemic features of vasculitis would closely resemble the condition of this patient. However, widespread vasculitis in RA is seen in much later stages with deforming joint disease; that is not the case with this patient.

*SYSTEMIC LUPUS ERYTHEMATOSUS.* In a manner similar to RA, many of the features of a systemic vasculitis may be seen in and are a part of SLE. These findings include this patient's hypertension, arthritis, vasculitic rash, neuropathy, organomegaly, and lymphadenopathy, as well as laboratory findings of mild cytopenias, glomerular inflammation, positive RF activity, low complement components, and abnormal liver function findings. However, the ANA titer in a systemically ill SLE patient would be expected to be very high; the borderline elevated ANA titer in this case firmly contradicts the diagnosis of SLE. Furthermore, in the presence of SLE-related glomerulonephritis, a patient with SLE would be expected to have antibodies to native DNA. This test yielded negative results in this patient. In addition, the absences of a photosensitive rash and Raynaud's phenomenon contradict the diagnosis of SLE in this case.

*GIANT CELL ARTERITIS.* The presence of a widespread vasculitic rash is extremely unusual in cases of GCA, but they have been known to occur. However, the systemic features of this patient's vasculitic illness in different organ systems (hepatosplenomegaly, glomerulonephritis, neuropathy) are not seen in GCA, and the marked serologic abnormalities observed in this case (including cryoglobulin levels) are always absent in GCA.

*SJÖGREN'S SYNDROME.* A widespread vasculitic rash and the type of arthritis seen in this patient may be typical features of Sjögren's syndrome. In addition, patients with Sjögren's syndrome display neuropathy, organomegaly, and lymphadenopathy, as well as the laboratory abnormalities of cytopenias, abnormal liver function findings, and high positive RF activity. Certainly there is the possibility of a clinical overlap between Sjögren's syndrome and this patient's diagnosis. However, glomerulonephritis is not a feature of Sjögren's syndrome, and if cryoglobulins are present in Sjögren's syndrome, they are observed in much smaller amounts. This patient does not have any features of dry eyes and dry mouth, which rules out the diagnosis of Sjögren's syndrome.

*WEGENER'S GRANULOMATOSIS.* Some of this patient's clinical and laboratory features, such as neuropathy, glomerulonephritis, vasculitic rash, elevated levels of acute-phase proteins, and arthritis, are seen in WG; however, the absence of sinus and upper airway disease and the absence of pulmonary involvement make this diagnosis distinctly unlikely.

*MIXED CRYOGLOBULINEMIA.* Mixed cryoglobulinemia is characterized by recurrent purpura, weakness, peripheral neuropathy, arthralgias/arthritis, organomegaly, and glomerulonephritis. This condition was formerly called *essential cryoglobulinemia* because it was idiopathic and not associated with a hematologic malignancy. This patient's illness is a textbook example of that condition. The laboratory abnormalities seen in this case (cytopenias, abnormal liver functions, elevated levels of acute-phase proteins, very high serum RF activity, low levels of complement components) are classical for patients with MCG.

Cryoglobulin simply means "cold protein," or proteins that precipitate when serum is placed in the cold environment of a refrigerator at 4° C after 48 to 72 hours of incubation. The composition of this cold-precipitated protein, or cryoglobulin, is a mixture (hence the name) of IgM and immunoglobulin G, wherein the IgM has RF activity. Sometimes the IgM is monoclonal, but not always. Why some proteins precipitate in the cold is not totally understood, but the observation has been made that antigen-antibody complexes of any sort or type are physically vulnerable to cold precipitation.

As stated elsewhere in this book (see Chapter 27, Vasculitis), hepatitis C appears to play an important role in the pathogenesis of MCG. This patient gives a history of hepatitis C exposure. The skin lesions reveal both vasculitis and perivascular inflammation, and hepatitis C virus has been identified in the vessel wall of some of these lesions. The cryoglobulin itself is thought to represent aggregates of antigen-antibody complexes. The other organ systems involved in MCG reveal histologic evidence of small-vessel vasculitis. MCG is a chronic, remitting and relapsing condition; in some patients, the disease converts to a lymphoid malignancy.

# REFERENCES

1. Tunn EJ, Bacon PA: Differentiating persistent from self-limiting symmetrical synovitis in an early arthritis clinic. Br J Rheumatol 1993; 32(2):97–103.
2. Chan KW, Felson D, Yood RA, et al: The time lag between onset of symptoms and diagnosis of rheumatoid arthritis. Arthritis Rheum 1994; 37(6):814–820.
3. McCarty DJ, Kohn NN, Faires JS: The significance of calcium phosphate crystals in the synovial fluid of arthritis patients: The "pseudogout syndrome." I. Clinical aspects. Ann Intern Med 1962; 56:711–737.
4. Ryan LM, McCarty DJ: Calcium pyrophosphate crystal deposition disease, pseudogout, and articulor chondrocalcinosis. *In* Koopman WD (ed): Arthritis and Allied Conditions, 13th ed. Baltimore: Williams & Wilkins, 1997: 2103–2125.
5. O'Sullivan JB, Cathcart ES: The prevalence of rheumatoid arthritis: Follow-up evaluation of the effect of criteria on rates in Sudbury, Massachusetts. Ann Intern Med 1972; 76(4):573–577.
6. Kim JM, Weisman MH: When does rheumatoid arthritis begin and why do we need to know. Arthritis Rheum, 2000; 43(3):473–484.
7. Schnitzer TJ, Penmetcha M: Viral arthritis. Curr Opin Rheumatol 1996; 8(4):341–345.
8. Phillips PE: Viral arthritis. Curr Opin Rheumatol 1997; 9(4): 337–344.
9. Naides SJ: Viral arthritis including HIV. Curr Opin Rheumatol 1995; 7(4):337–342.

CHAPTER

# 3 | Geriatric Rheumatology

*Daniel A. Albert and Edna P. Schwab*

## RHEUMATIC DISEASE IN THE ELDERLY

### Epidemiology

The treatment of rheumatologic disorders in the elderly can be extremely challenging. As the percentage of elderly in the population increases, the prevalence of chronic diseases will also rise. The proportion of elderly in the population is expected to rise from its present rate of 13% to 20% as we enter the 21st century.[1] In 1995, 40 million persons in the United States were affected by arthritis (using the 1990 prevalence rate of 15%). By the year 2020, 59.4 million persons, or 18.2% of the population, will be affected.[2] Arthritis is the most common chronic condition among noninstitutionalized adults over the age of 65 years.[3] Although arthritis affects 5.1% of persons under the age of 44 years,[4] the National Arthritis Data Work Group demonstrated that the incidence rises to 36.5% for persons between the ages of 55 and 64 years, to 45% among 65- to 74-year-olds, to 55.2% among 75- to 82-year-olds, and to 57.1% among those older than the age of 85 years.[2] Arthritis is also the most frequent cause of physical disability in older adults and the leading cause of work-related disability among Americans older than the age of 65 years.[2, 4, 5] Yelin and Callahan reviewed the profound economic impact of musculoskeletal and associated disorders in terms of lost wages, disability benefits, and hospital, nursing home, and home care expenses in addition to physician and other professional and medication costs. Using 1992 dollars, the total cost of care for all age groups amounted to $149.4 billion, or 2.5% of the 1992 gross national product. The elderly were found to incur the largest proportion of direct costs associated with medical care and $13.5 billion in indirect costs related to lost wages. Expenses such as those related to care of the elderly and to the inability to perform avocational activities were more difficult to quantify.[6]

The prevalence of limited activity as a consequence of arthritis is expected to rise as the proportion of elderly in the population grows.[2, 5] In 1990, 2.8% of the population experienced a limitation of activity as a result of arthritis and other musculoskeletal disorders. This figure is expected to increase to 3.6% by the year 2020, affecting 11.6 million persons.[2]

Among the 55% of the elderly who report having arthritis, 78% report limitation in a physical activity,

34% are limited in five or more activities, and 36% are limited in activities of daily living (ADLs).[7] The National Arthritis Data Work Group found that arthritis and its limitations were more prevalent among women than among men, perhaps as a result of a predominance of women in the older population.[2, 8]

Musculoskeletal conditions have a significant impact on a person's psychological and social well-being. Psychological distress, depression, and anxiety have been associated with the presence of arthritis,[6] and these conditions result in an increased utilization of health services. The consequences of pain and limitation in function from arthritis and other comorbid conditions include impaired mobility, diminished quality of life, mood disorders, and ultimately limited independence.[9] Hughes and Dunlop reported that arthritis was the most prevalent chronic condition in older homebound patients. Analysis of Health Care Financing Administration data on home care use revealed that musculoskeletal disorders were the second most commonly ranked diagnoses,[10] whereas the National Long Term Care Survey, a national survey of persons older than 65 years of age with ADL disability or with impairment of instrumental activities of daily living (IADLs), found that arthritis, dementia, and atherosclerosis accounted for the greatest amount of disability. The Longitudinal Study on Aging, a prospective study of community-dwelling elderly, and a longitudinal study of elderly patients in metropolitan Chicago both demonstrated that arthritis in combination with comorbid conditions increased the risk for the development of disability.[10, 11] Yelin's review of these data also demonstrated that individuals who had arthritis along with other comorbid conditions had greater limitations in their ADLs and IADLs: 41% and 82%, respectively. Persons with baseline disability, arthritis, and ADL impairment were found to be twice as likely to die or five times more likely to require nursing home placement in comparison with elderly without limitations.[7]

### Evaluation and Treatment of the Geriatric Patient

Pain may be the primary presenting symptom of a musculoskeletal disorder in the older person. It may present as increased confusion or functional decline. Among nursing home residents, pain as a consequence of a rheumatic condition has been reported in more than 40% of residents surveyed.[12] However, it is seldom the reason for nursing home placement.[13] Symptoms of arthritis may not be as apparent in the elderly as in younger persons because of the difficulty eliciting information from patients with impaired cognition as well as an under-reporting of symptoms.[14] Atypical disease presentations, false-positive serologic test results, and multiple coexisting conditions may delay an accurate diagnosis.[15] Often a musculoskeletal disorder can present as a subtle decline in functional status, mood, or behavioral disturbance that may not be perceived by the patient, family, or medical professional until the impairment or disability interferes with ADLs or IADLs.[12]

In any patient with a musculoskeletal complaint, a thorough history and physical examination are key elements in establishing an early and accurate diagnosis. Radiographs of affected areas and laboratory studies may provide important information when conservative measures fail or in patients with a suspected inflammatory condition.[16] In the geriatric patient, the inclusion of a complete geriatric assessment that encompasses functional assessments (ADLs and IADLs); visual, dental, and audiologic evaluations; and nutritional status, cognitive status, and psychosocial evaluations helps provide a more comprehensive picture of the individual's clinical as well as social situation. It allows the practitioner to individualize an intervention based on the patient's needs and social support. Depending on the medical diagnosis and other comorbid conditions, the safest and most effective therapeutic interventions can be implemented. They often consist of physical therapy with the prescription of assistive devices to maximize independence and safety, localized joint and soft tissue injections to avoid systemic therapy and associated toxicities, and, if needed, prescriptions of medications with the safest side effect profiles. Continuous assessment of functional status on return visits can often provide a good measure of an individual's response to therapy. A multidisciplinary team approach to assessment and treatment becomes necessary because many frail elderly patients have multiple medical and psychosocial problems that require simultaneous attention and treatment. Many elderly are unable to undergo requested studies or return for repeated visits because of physical limitations from arthritis or other chronic disease states, an inability to access transportation, or a lack of social and familial support.

Team approaches can be provided in various settings. Team members may include physician, nurse, nurse practitioner, social worker, and physical and occupational therapists. Ideally, as in our geriatric-rheumatology practice, treatment is provided in the traditional office setting with the support of a social worker and a nurse practitioner, who assist in complete geriatric, cognitive, psychosocial, and functional assessments. In the alternative setting of the day hospital, which is most commonly found in the United Kingdom, evaluation and treatment are provided with the support of a physician, a nurse practitioner, physical therapists, occupational therapists, a psychological counselor, and a social worker on the premises. Medical, nutritional, psychosocial, and functional evaluations are performed and treatment plans are implemented that consider the specific medical and psychosocial constraints of the patient. In addition to physical therapy and occupational therapy, safety evaluations in the home are performed to prevent falls and injuries. The team also monitors for adverse drug reactions, symptoms of depression, and exacerbation of any comorbid condition. Drug regimens are simplified if possible and patient education about exercise, drug compliance, and medication safety is reviewed. The medical director oversees the care delivered by these professionals. The referring physicians communicate with these providers on a continuous basis and approve the plan of care for the individual patient.

Patients enrolled in home care also have the benefit of having their care delivered by a team of providers that includes a physician, a nurse practitioner or nurse, physical and occupational therapists, and a home health aide. Patients who are homebound often opt for having this type of care because of their physical inability to leave home. As with the day hospital, the referring physician oversees the care delivered by various team members. Necessary radiographs and laboratory studies can be obtained by mobile units. The treatment of rheumatic conditions in the nursing home is also ideally delivered by a multidisciplinary team that includes a physician; a nurse practitioner; physical, occupational, and recreational therapists; and a social worker. Psychiatrists as well as psychological counselors are also available to provide ongoing treatment, whereas the pharmacist on the premises supports the physician in monitoring the patient for adverse drug reactions, commonly found in this frail elderly population. Certainly care delivered in these settings with a team of qualified individuals is always limited by financial constraints.

## Pharmacokinetics of Drugs

Medications prescribed for the elderly should be those with the safest side effect profile. The older person requires close drug surveillance for several reasons: The numerous coexisting diseases found in this population commonly result in polypharmacy, and the increased complexities of medical regimens create significant problems with medication noncompliance, drug interactions, and adverse drug reactions.

Normal aging is associated with several changes in drug distribution, metabolism, excretion, and drug half-life. Drug distribution is altered with changes in body composition. As total body water is reduced, total body fat increases, thereby increasing the plasma concentration of water-soluble drugs and lowering plasma concentration of lipid-soluble drugs. As serum albumin levels fall, even in well elderly persons, it increases the availability of the free fraction of medication that is normally protein bound.[17, 18] Hepatic metabolism falls with aging, secondary to decreased hepatic blood flow and decreased liver mass.[19] There are conflicting studies regarding alterations in phase I enzyme reactions. Renal clearance is often impaired with aging, secondary to alterations in renal blood flow, glomerular filtration, and active tubular secretion and reabsorption. The impairment in renal function may not be reflected in elevated blood urea nitrogen or serum creatinine levels because muscle mass found in many elderly individuals is decreased. Drug absorption does not appear to be significantly altered with normal aging.[17, 19] At any given plasma level, the elderly have increased receptor sensitivity to many agents, particularly psychoactive and analgesic drugs. Therefore, when prescribing medication for any rheumatic condition, the physician must take into consideration these alterations and monitor for adverse drug effects even at low or therapeutic doses.[18]

## Overview

In this chapter we describe common rheumatologic conditions diagnosed in the senior population and discuss both diagnostic and therapeutic approaches. Conditions that are more prevalent in adults older than 50 years are reviewed and include osteoarthritis (OA), gout, calcium pyrophosphate deposition disease (CPDD), hydroxyapatite deposition disease, elder-onset rheumatoid arthritis, polymyalgia rheumatica (PMR), and fibromyalgia. As the proportion of elderly patients in the population grows, there will be greater necessity for rheumatologists and primary care physicians to identify risk factors that precede the development of these musculoskeletal disorders so that the magnitude of their effects on the senior adult can be diminished.[20] Early recognition and implementation of effective therapeutic interventions help prevent or retard disability and maintain an older individual's independence and quality of life. The goal of therapy is to diminish pain and enhance functional status, mobility, and independence. Given the complexities often found in this age group, these interventions are best delivered by a coordinated, multidisciplinary approach provided by a team of health care professionals.

## OSTEOARTHRITIS

OA is by far the most common and disabling rheumatic disorder in patients older than 55 years of age and was associated with increased mortality rates (independent of age, history of diabetes, body mass index, smoking, and alcohol use) when reviewed by Callahan and Pincus.[21] It affects 12% of the population[2] and more than 65% of the senior population.[22] Oliveria and colleagues observed an incidence of 88/100,000 person-years for hip OA and 240/100,000 person-years for knee OA among a large population of patients enrolled in a health maintenance organization. The incidence increased with age and affected women at higher rates than for men, especially after the age of 50 years, and plateaued after the ages of 80 to 89 years.[23]

It is the leading cause of disability and pain in the senior population and the second most common diagnosis found among adults receiving Social Security benefits.[2] It contributes to the growing economic burden in terms of lost income, disability costs, hospital costs (related to the increasing numbers of persons undergoing joint replacements),[24] nursing home care, home care to elderly, medical expenditures (physicians and other health care practitioners), and drug expenditures.[6, 25] The number of persons affected with arthritis and its resultant economic impact are expected to grow as the population ages.[6]

The functional impact of OA is specific to the joints affected and the performance of required tasks. OA of the knee affects ambulation, stair climbing, and transfers, whereas OA affecting the hands and shoulders may have an impact on basic ADL abilities.[26] Predictors of disability have been found to include the severity of other coexisting diseases, functional capacity, social support, education level, income, and availability of social and home care services.[27] Anxiety, depression, and coping styles have also been associated with the development and severity of disability.[26]

## Clinical Features

Generalized OA is the most prevalent form of the disorder found in elderly women and may be related to menopause. It primarily involves the distal interphalangeal joints (Heberden's nodes), proximal interphalangeal joints (Bouchard's nodes), first carpometacarpal joints, knees, cervical and lumbar spine, first metatarsophalangeal joints, and possibly the hip.[13, 14, 28] The prevalence of OA affecting weight-bearing areas such as the knees, hips, and spine increases in both sexes with age. OA involving the hands, feet, knees, and possibly the hip appears to be more prevalent in women, whereas involvement of the cervical and lumbar spine is more prevalent in men.[2, 8, 9]

An unusual presentation of OA is erosive OA found among the elderly. It most often involves the distal and proximal interphalangeal joints and is associated with synovitis and joint erosions.[13, 14] Verbrugge and Veys found that erosive changes affected 50% of their study population and suggest that this may be a stage in the evolution of the disease resulting in Heberden's and Bouchard's nodes.[13] A unilateral destructive arthropathy involving the hip has been reported in elderly women; it is characterized by femoral head collapse followed by bony resorption. Synovial fluid analysis demonstrates the presence of basic calcium phosphate (apatite) crystals. Similarly, in the destructive arthropathy of the shoulder referred to as "Milwaukee shoulder" (commonly reported in association with rotator cuff tears),[14] hemorrhagic effusions and calcium crystals are almost always identified.[29]

In any age group, OA is diagnosed by symptoms, clinical examination findings, and radiographic features. Characteristic symptoms of OA include early morning stiffness lasting 20 to 30 minutes. Patients may complain of stiffness and pain associated with activity and relieved by rest, joint buckling or instability, or loss of function. If joint destruction is severe, pain may be present with rest as well. Physical findings may include joint swelling, tenderness with palpation, pain on motion, decreased range of motion, crepitus, and deformity or malalignment of the affected joint. OA may also be found to coexist with inflammatory conditions such as end-stage rheumatoid arthritis or polymyalgia rheumatica, as well as in patients with fibromyalgia and regional pain syndromes. The presence of symptomatic OA often makes the diagnosis of these other entities more difficult.

## Treatment

### Nonpharmacologic Therapy

There is no agent that cures or retards the progression of OA. By the time an older patient presents with symptoms consistent with OA, prevention may no longer be an option. The emphasis of treatment is on the alleviation of pain and disability in addition to maximizing function. Preventive techniques such as behavioral modification for weight loss and preventing injury during exercise may be implemented for healthy elderly persons as well as frail community-dwelling and institutionalized elders.[14, 24, 30–32] Interventions should include patient education, joint protection, relaxation techniques, psychological counseling, bracing, and using proper foot wear.[24, 31, 33] These modalities are readily accepted by patients and may be preferred to avoid pharmacologic therapies and their associated toxicities.

Physical therapy aimed at strengthening the muscles surrounding the joint in addition to the use of assistive devices provides patients with stability, enables mobility, and decreases joint load. Several clinical trials have demonstrated the efficacy of routine aerobic exercise and aquatic therapy in improved function and pain control.[24] Aerobic and resistance exercises have been shown to improve joint pain and disability in these patients.[34] Quadriceps strengthening in the elderly may retard the rate of muscle loss, diminish pain, improve gait and knee strength, and decrease joint trauma.[35–37] Many patients acquire more confidence with ambulation after going through a prescribed physical therapy program.

Although controlled studies have not demonstrated clinically significant improvement with acupuncture, many patients do seek such alternative therapies when pain has not responded to either pharmacologic or other traditional nonpharmacologic modalities. This may be an option for elderly patients who are intolerant of medications because of side effects or drug interactions. The application of heat or cold has also been used to control pain.[24, 38] Acute pain often responds to the application of cold, whereas chronic pain improves with heat. Patient preference determines the mode of therapy. Other forms of nonpharmacologic treatment that may be used include transcutaneous electrical nerve stimulation, low-power laser treatment, and pulsed electric and electromagnetic field therapy. Unfortunately none of these treatment regimens has been as extensively studied as pharmacologic therapies, especially in the elderly.[38]

## Pharmacologic Therapy

Pharmacologic therapy frequently supplements nonpharmacologic modalities when pain from OA persists. In any patient, but especially in frail elderly persons, one has to consider the side effect profile of the drug, comorbidities present in the patient, alterations in drug metabolism that occur with aging, and potential drug interactions when prescribing a particular agent. The general dictum among physicians who care for the elderly is "start low and go slow."

### Non-narcotic Analgesics

Non-narcotic analgesics are the drugs of choice for the initial pharmacologic treatment of OA in the elderly. Acetaminophen in therapeutic doses of 4 g/day is the first line of therapy and has been found to be as effective an agent in the short term for pain relief as naproxen or ibuprofen in OA of the knee, with fewer side effects than those seen with the use of most nonsteroidal anti-inflammatory drugs (NSAIDs).[39–41]

### Narcotic Analgesics

Opioids such as codeine and oxycodone may be used when conservative therapies are ineffective or when contraindications exist to the use of traditional NSAIDs. Patients with end-stage OA involving the hip, knee, or spinal canal (spinal stenosis) who are not surgical candidates may obtain pain relief with these agents. Other centrally acting analgesics such as tramadol have been found to be effective in controlling symptoms.[42] Common side effects to watch for include delirium, dizziness, somnolence, and constipation. When a patient is using other agents with central nervous system (CNS) effects such as antidepressants, an adverse CNS drug reaction may be potentiated, such as seizures.[24, 43] Just as with any other drug, doses of opioid analgesics should be adjusted in the elderly because of altered distribution and clearance and enhanced sensitivity.[42] Many elderly may be reluctant to use narcotics because of their concern about dependence or addiction. The physician treating these patients should reassure them that although addiction occasionally occurs, relief of pain and maximizing function are the goals of treatment.

### Topical Agents

Other useful forms of treatment in the elderly include the use of topical analgesic creams such as methylsalicylate or capsaicin, an inhibitor of the release of substance P from nerve terminals. These creams have been helpful in alleviating the symptoms of pain from OA of the knee.[38, 44]

### Nonsteroidal Anti-inflammatory Agents

NSAIDs are the most commonly prescribed agents used to treat OA in all age groups. When analgesics such as acetaminophen fail to alleviate pain, NSAIDs are often initiated and titrated to the lowest dose that provides analgesia.[45] Since response to various NSAIDs is variable, a trial of nonacetylated salicylates should initially be attempted, followed by more potent NSAIDs if treatment fails.[14, 46] Low doses of these agents are commonly purchased by patients as over-the-counter drugs. Physicians should routinely review the patient's drug regimen so that multiple NSAIDs are not erroneously used simultaneously.

The elderly are more likely to experience toxicities related to NSAIDs, including gastrointestinal toxicity such as inflammation, ulceration (reported in both small and large bowel),[47] bleeding, and perforation; nephrotoxicity; hepatotoxicity;[46] cardiovascular effects such as volume overload; CNS effects including dizziness, confusion, cognitive impairment, and memory loss; and hematologic abnormalities such as thrombocytopenia, neutropenia, and hemolytic anemia.[14, 19, 45] Risk factors identified for the development of gastrointestinal complications include increasing age, history of peptic ulcer disease, concomitant use of corticosteroids or anticoagulants, cigarette smoking or alcohol use, and ingestion of multiple NSAIDs.[14, 19, 24] Misoprostol, a prostaglandin $E_2$ inhibitor, or histamine-2 ($H_2$) blockers may be prescribed in these patients[24, 45]; however, we find their side effects to be unacceptable to many patients, and cost may be prohibitive. Agents with cyclooxygenase-2 (COX-2) inhibition may provide protection from more serious gastrointestinal side effects; however, further clinical trials must be conducted to assess their safety in the elderly.[48, 49]

Risk factors for hepatoxicity due to NSAIDs include increasing age, poor renal function, multiple drug therapies, high dosage, and long duration of therapy. Patients placed on NSAID therapy should have blood counts and renal and liver function monitored at baseline, 1 month after initiating therapy, and then routinely.[14]

### Intra-articular Injections

When pain from OA affects one or two joints, intra-articular injections of the steroid triamcinolone hexacetonide should be used to avoid potential systemic toxicity with pharmacologic agents. Intra-articular injections frequently provide short-term pain relief from arthritis.[24, 46, 50, 51] The concern for deleterious effects of steroids on joint cartilage limits their usefulness in long-term management[50]; however, in patients with severe disease that has not improved with other modalities we often accommodate their request for more frequent injections. Viscosupplementation with hyaluronic acid derivatives is useful in relieving pain and improving mobility in geriatric patients with OA of the knee and is favorable to systemic treatment with analgesics, narcotics, or anti-inflammatory agents.[46, 52, 53] One intra-articular injection weekly for 3 weeks has provided superior relief when compared with intra-articular corticosteroids and some NSAIDs.[53] The principal side effect of injection is a local reaction, noted

in 10% of patients.[24] The major limitation to this treatment is cost (especially for elderly on fixed incomes) as well as the need for weekly office visits.

### Alternative Agents

The use of alternative remedies has become extremely popular among older patients with OA. Glucosamine sulfate and chondroitin sulfate, available in nutritional stores, have been advertised as "cures for arthritis."[52] Although there are a few European studies demonstrating that these agents may ameliorate symptoms from OA, there are no double-blind placebo-controlled trials revealing altered cartilage structure. Despite this information, many patients prefer trying this form of therapy when other treatment regimens have failed or when wishing to avoid other systemic therapies.[54] The role of antioxidants such as vitamin C, beta carotene, and vitamin E in protecting against progression of OA still has to be established.[24] They may be useful as long as toxicities are limited.

### Invasive Therapies

Joint lavage and arthroscopic débridement appear to have limited usefulness. The efficacy of lavage results from the removal of debris and inflammatory mediators.[32, 40] When mobility and function are limited by pain, joint replacement is indicated. This often occurs when pharmacologic and nonpharmacologic remedies have failed to provide adequate pain relief. Although a study of 80-year-olds undergoing total hip arthroplasty showed beneficial results, the complication rate in this age group was 2.5 to 3.5 times higher than in younger patients. Thirty percent of patients older than 80 years had a prolonged course of rehabilitation, primarily owing to cognitive impairment.[14] Patients undergoing replacement should be monitored closely by a geriatrician for delirium and other postoperative complications. The patient should receive adequate pain relief, and physical therapy should be initiated within 48 hours. In order to decrease the incidence of postoperative complications, unnecessary catheters should be removed, incentive spirometry started, and prophylaxis against deep venous thrombosis with anticoagulants initiated.

## CRYSTAL DEPOSITION DISEASES

Crystal deposition diseases are common in the elderly[55] and increase in prevalence with increasing age. This increase is the result of increasing prevalence of each of the major crystal deposition diseases: gout, CPDD, and hydroxyapatite deposition disease.

### Gout

Gout classically presents in men in early adulthood with podagra or acute monoarthritis of the midfoot or ankle. Less commonly it presents with knee or upper extremity arthritis. It is prevalent in the elderly. Up to 4% of patients aged 50 to 74 have gout. The presentation is, however, sufficiently different from that in the younger patient to make diagnosis difficult in certain cases.[14] The primary problem is the presentation of chronic tophaceous gout in elderly women with OA.[56] Even radiographically it can be difficult to distinguish erosive OA from gout complicating Heberden's and Bouchard's nodes. It is important to aspirate these joints if the diagnosis of gout is in question either on radiographs or because of hyperuricemia or if the patient is taking diuretics.[22] Another unusual presentation in the elderly is a polyarticular attack with fever and delirium. Both monoarticular and polyarticular attacks are sometimes complicated by coexisting CPDD.

The treatment of an acute gouty monoarticular arthritis is similar in younger and elderly patients. These patients are frequently treated with NSAIDs, which are uniformly effective if given in high enough doses for long enough. Unfortunately, their use is often limited by toxicity or anticipated toxicity. These problems are greater in the elderly population because of baseline renal insufficiency, comorbid conditions of congestive heart failure and hypertension, and the sensitivity of the elderly to the gastrotoxic and the CNS side effects of these drugs. The alternative therapies are also occasionally troublesome. Colchicine is suppressive of the hematologic system in the elderly and must be used with caution. Its inherent low margin between an effective dose and a gastrotoxic dose is especially problematic in the frail elderly patient. Lastly, corticosteroids are frequently used either in a short course of oral steroids or the equivalent given parenterally in the postoperative patient or by intra-articular administration. Parenteral intramuscular adrenocorticotropic hormone is frequently followed 72 to 96 hours later by a rebound; a second injection can be given, or the first injection can be followed by a daily maintenance dose of colchicine or an NSAID. The (Medrol) Dosepak (methylprednisolone), which gives a tapering dose over 6 days, is usually sufficient for an acute attack. The problem with intra-articular steroids is the difficulty of administration when the involved structure is not a large joint and the tendency of gout to involve periarticular structures. Intra-articular steroids are not an attractive choice in a polyarticular attack. The role of the new COX-2 inhibitors is unknown, but they may become the drugs of choice for the treatment of acute gout.

Like younger patients, most older patients have an idiopathic defect in the excretion of uric acid by the kidney, and an increasing frequency of attacks develops as does an increasing frequency of polyarticular attacks unless the defect is corrected by administration of a uricosuric agent or bypassed by the xanthine oxidase inhibitor allopurinol. The rare patient with a genetic defect in the production of uric acid such as Lesch-Nyhan disease or phosphoribosylpyrophosphate disease usually comes to medical attention earlier in life. In contrast, the prevalence of drug-related gout increases in elderly patients as the need for thiazide-type diuretics and other agents that increase serum uric acid increases with age. Patients taking thiazides can pose a therapeutic dilemma because they often need a diuretic that increases serum uric acid. Furosemide is less of a stimulus than thiazides, but it is preferable if the patient can be maintained without diuretics, perhaps with the use of angiotensin-converting enzyme inhibitors and calcium channel blockers. Patients taking diuretics do not respond well to uricosuric agents in part because thiazide site of action is proximal to the site of uricosuric agent action in the renal tubule and in part because there is a variable amount of renal insufficiency in these persons. These patients respond appropriately to allopurinol with several caveats. First, there is a clinical observation that many individuals in whom allopurinol hypersensitivity develops have hyperuricemia induced by thiazide diuretics. Second, allopurinol is a potential marrow-suppressing agent and should be introduced in an escalating-dose fashion starting at 50 mg or 100 mg/day and gradually building up to a dose necessary to reduce the serum uric acid to less than 6 mg/dL. At this dose or less, the patient's total body burden of sodium urate should gradually be reduced, including tophaceous deposits. Other causes of drug-induced gout such as cyclosporine and pyrazinamide administration are beyond the scope of this chapter, as is gout in the transplant patient. If the patient is an underexcretor (<400 mg of urate excreted in 24 hours) and has a creatinine clearance rate greater than 40 mL/minute, uricosuric drugs such as probenecid or sulfinpyrazone can be tried.

## Calcium Pyrophosphate Dihydrate Deposition Disease

CPDD is a disease almost exclusively of the elderly. Approximately 15% of patients older than age 65 have CPDD. It presents in a variety of forms. The most common form is the asymptomatic calcification of articular cartilage primarily in the menisci of the knee and the triangular cartilage of the wrist but also in hyaline cartilage in the humeral and femoral heads and in the symphysis pubis. There is some association of this radiographic finding with OA, but the significance is unclear. The prevalence of this finding is as high as 25% in patients aged 75 years. These patients occasionally have attacks of pseudogout primarily in the knee and wrist but also in the elbow, ankle, and feet. Acute pseudogout, like acute gout, is frequently observed in postoperative patients. In these cases, it is critical to exclude infection because bacterial arthritis and CPDD occasionally coexist, unlike urate gout and bacterial infection, which rarely are seen together. Infrequently, a patient presents with a chronic polyarthritis of the small joints of the hands and feet. These patients have characteristic radiographs, and blood test results are rheumatoid factor–negative.

The treatment of asymptomatic chondrocalcinosis is unknown because no specific therapy reduces the rate of progression. Patients should have any underlying metabolic condition examined, especially hyperparathyroidism and hemochromatosis, although such conditions account for less than 5% of cases. It is, however, unclear whether effective treatment of these conditions arrests or ameliorates the articular disease. Acute pseudogout is treated in similar fashion to that for acute gout but it is somewhat less likely to respond to colchicine. Gout is rarely found in conjunction with septic arthritis; thus, corticosteroids may be given with confidence when negatively birefringent crystals of sodium urate are observed in joint fluid. However, the same cannot be said for pseudogout, which can coexist with infection. Chronic CPDD polyarthritis is a difficult management problem, but some rheumatologists use hydroxychloroquine.

## Hydroxyapatite Deposition Disease

A third crystal, hydroxyapatite, is associated with several syndromes found in elderly patients. Occasionally, it is found in a rapidly destructive lytic articular disorder best known in the shoulder as the *Milwaukee shoulder*. The pathogenesis and treatment are unknown, but it is commonly treated with NSAIDs and intra-articular steroids. In rare instances, this syndrome is seen in other, usually large, joints.

## RHEUMATOID ARTHRITIS

The diagnosis, therapy, and management of elderly patients with rheumatoid arthritis are largely the same as for younger patients, with some important caveats.[57] Although the peak incidence of the disease is between the third and the fifth decades of life, the peak prevalence is in the elderly, and this is rising.[58] Interestingly, the gender discordance found in younger age groups is thought to be less prominent in the elderly, and the male to female ratio is thought to approach unity. In addition, although a proportion of younger patients have a palindromic presentation, this is seen less frequently in the elderly. Younger patients occasionally have asymmetric involvement, often without rheumatoid factor. By contrast, elderly patients have unique presentations: a polymyalgia rheumatica syndrome and remitting seronegative symmetric synovitis with pitting edema (RS3PE). The management of these two conditions is discussed at the end of this section.

### Diagnosis

The diagnosis of rheumatoid arthritis in the elderly is largely the same as in younger patients. Persistent synovitis is present in more than one joint and is usually symmetrically distributed and accompanied by constitutional symptoms that include morning stiffness, and there is laboratory evidence of acute inflammation. More specific attributes such as nodules, radiographic erosions, and rheumatoid factor assist in confirming the diagnosis but are often late manifestations, and specific treatment should not await these features. The American College of Rheumatology criteria for the diagnosis of rheumatoid arthritis are used in the elderly, and there is no evidence that they lose their operating characteristics in this population. Patients fulfilling these criteria are likely to have rheumatoid arthritis, and spontaneous remissions in these patients are rare. There are no special diagnostic procedures necessary or indicated for elderly patients suspected of having rheumatoid arthritis. In addition to a complete history and physical examination, patients should have a detailed musculoskeletal examination and a joint count that assesses the swelling and tenderness of at least the typical target joints in rheumatoid arthritis—the proximal interphalangeal and metacarpophalangeal joints, wrists, elbows, shoulders, hips, knees, ankles, and metatarsophalangeal joints. Blood count and chemistry panels that include liver and renal function tests, erythrocyte sedimentation rate, and C-reactive protein should be performed. Synovial fluid analysis is especially useful in the elderly to exclude CPDD, which can mimic rheumatoid arthritis (see further on). Radiographs of at least the hands, as well as other target joints as indicated by the joint examination, are also useful to implicate rheumatoid arthritis if the characteristic periarticular osteopenia and marginal erosions are seen and to exclude clinically similar diseases such as CPDD with the finding of chondrocalcinosis. When indicated, additional serologic studies may be helpful in excluding systemic lupus erythematosus, drug-induced lupus, Sjögren's syndrome, and, in rare circumstances, Lyme disease, parvovirus, and rheumatoid variants. Rheumatoid factor positivity increases with age, and therefore the positive predictive value of the test diminishes because of an increase in false-positive values. Up to 15% of healthy patients aged 65 and older test positive for rheumatoid factor.[57] The positive predictive value rises with the titer, and very high titers are found predominantly in patients with rheumatoid arthritis. Seronegative patients with severe constitutional symptoms should undergo a thorough investigation for malignancy, especially hematologic disorders, but the typical elderly patient with polyarthritis does not warrant a malignancy work-up. In rare cases, elderly patients with synovial thickening and carpal tunnel syndrome have amyloidosis, the diagnosis of which almost always requires a synovial biopsy.

### Drug Therapy

As with other age groups, the primary controversy is in the drug management of elderly patients with rheumatoid arthritis. Traditional approaches have focused on the nonfatal, slowly progressive, spontaneously remitting aspects of the disease as well as the significant toxicity of the medications used to treat it. These arguments are strengthened by reports that overall the disease is milder in older individuals,[59] with up to 50% of patients being rheumatoid factor–negative, and the drugs are more toxic in this age group,[60] in part because of polypharmacy, which results in adverse reactions from drug interactions. This is most significant with the increased gastrointestinal morbidity of NSAIDs.[61, 62] Increased hematologic suppression by methotrexate in the elderly is not supported by careful analysis.[63] More recent data suggest that the disease in the elderly may not be milder,[64] but the loss of functional capacity is greater in these patients[65] and a more aggressive approach may be indicated to maintain independent living, especially in the elderly living alone or with a functionally impaired spouse. None of the medications available to treat rheumatoid arthritis in younger patients is proscribed in the elderly, but caution must be exercised in their use. There are no data to suggest differential efficacy of antirheumatic drugs in the elderly as opposed to younger patients with rheumatoid arthritis, although some authors suggest the use of corticosteroids in lieu of second-line agents.[66] Overall, the effect of age on outcome in rheumatoid arthritis is controversial.[57, 66, 67] Likewise, age itself is not a strong predictor of adverse drug reactions.[68]

NSAIDs are effective in the elderly to roughly the same extent that they are in younger patients; however, their toxicity is greater, at least in part because of the increased prevalence of comorbid diseases such as hypertension, congestive heart failure, and renal insufficiency, which result in adverse reactions.[69] In general, it is wise to avoid the more gastrotoxic nonsteroidal agents in this population and to use nabumetone, etodolac, or one of the COX-2 inhibitors. It is important to realize that elderly patients with normal serum creatinine levels may have significant renal insufficiency, especially if they have small muscle mass. These patients are at increased risk for all the complications of nonsteroidal agents, including renal insufficiency, which is usually dose related, and gastrointestinal complications. One nonsteroidal agent that should probably be avoided in the elderly is piroxicam, which has a long half-life and high gastrointestinal toxicity in this age group. Our experience is that elderly patients have a far higher incidence of cognitive, affective, and dysphoric reactions to nonsteroidal agents than do younger patients. Great caution should be exercised with use of these drugs in combination with corticosteroids because they have additive or synergistic gastrointestinal toxicity. As in other age groups, the gastrointestinal toxicity of nonsteroidal agents is increased in older patients with a history of peptic ulcer disease and in those who smoke.

Hydroxychloroquine is well tolerated in the elderly,[70] but attention must be paid to the guidelines for dosing. There is general agreement that the daily dose of hydroxychloroquine should not exceed 6.5 mg/kg/day with the caveat that higher loading doses may be given in the first 6 weeks. This daily dose should be reduced in individuals with renal insufficiency because the drug is partially cleared through the kidney. A dose reduction is not agreed on, but as a rough guide half the dose is given to patients receiving dialysis. Our experience is that elderly patients have a somewhat increased frequency of blurred vision and gastrointestinal side effects from the drug. Occasionally, elderly patients have gastrointestinal side effects with generic hydroxychloroquine but not with the Sanofi-Winthrop brand Plaquenil. The frequency of

rash and photosensitivity does not seem to be increased. Late retinal toxicity is rare in all age groups, and there is no consensus about maximal total dose. Because there is a high incidence of unrelated ocular disease in the elderly, such as cataracts, macular degeneration, and glaucoma, we advocate yearly ophthalmologic examinations.

Methotrexate is also well tolerated in the elderly if care is given to gradual dose escalation. As with hydroxychloroquine, the clearance of methotrexate is partially through the kidney and reduced renal function can lead to excessive toxicity.[71] The primary toxic effect that is overrepresented in the elderly is hematologic. We introduce the drug in the elderly, increasing from one tablet (2.5 mg) a week to an additional tablet every 2 weeks, checking blood counts before the increase. We maintain a dose of 7.5 mg/week for several months to determine its efficacy before we contemplate further increases. We supplement with folic acid, 1 mg/day. We have not been impressed by the finding that gastrointestinal or pulmonary toxicity is increased in the elderly. Although there are a few cases of methotrexate-dependent lymphoma, this sequela is rare and not apparently disproportionately greater in frequency in the elderly.

Cyclosporine is a difficult drug to use in rheumatoid arthritis. It is not effective for use as monotherapy unless the dose approaches toxicity (5 mg/kg/day), and we do not recommend it. As an adjunct to methotrexate given in doses as low as 25 mg BID, cyclosporine is partially effective in the 50% of patients who get a partial response to methotrexate in these doses. At such doses, there is no reason to measure drug levels and there is little risk of hypertension or renal insufficiency.

Sulfasalazine is well tolerated in the elderly with gradual dose escalation, but gastrointestinal problems are common. Side effects are minimized with use of the enteric-coated preparation, but headaches, occasional abnormal liver function test results, and rare hematologic toxicity are not diminished by this formulation. Sulfasalazine in combination with hydroxychloroquine is a safe, well-tolerated combination that appears to have superior efficacy to that of each drug alone.

Azathioprine is somewhat less effective than methotrexate but is an option for individuals who do not tolerate methotrexate. The dose should be escalated from 50 mg/day to between 2 and 3 mg/kg/day, with an upper limit of 150 mg/day. It is essential to monitor blood count and liver function on a periodic basis.

Penicillamine and gold therapy are less popular at present. Although use of these agents is associated with serious toxicity in up to 50% of cases, there are no special precautions that need to be made for the elderly. In general, these drugs are given in escalating doses. We give penicillamine starting at 125 mg/day, increasing the dose by 125-mg increments every month. We monitor hematologic, dermatologic, and renal function for toxicity. Gold is given in weekly injections starting with a test dose of 1 or 10 mg and increasing to 25 mg and then to 50 mg. After approximately 6 months, the maximal effect of the drug is achieved, but most patients who will improve notice improvement after 3 months. Oral gold may be well suited to elderly patients with mild disease.[72]

The newer agents leflunomide and etanercept are approved for treatment of rheumatoid arthritis without an age limitation. There is no current evidence that elderly patients have an unusual toxicity profile with either of these agents. Etanercept is particularly well tolerated and can be used in conjunction with methotrexate for patients in whom control is not achieved with a single agent. Leflunomide is associated with some gastrointestinal toxicity during the 3-day loading phase with doses of 100 mg/day but is extremely well tolerated on the daily dose of 20 mg. The major issue is the elevation of liver function test values, which occurs in about 10% of patients. There are few data on minocycline or Prosorba column specifically targeted to the elderly.

The most controversial therapeutic decision concerns the use of corticosteroids. There are data that corticosteroids are effective in reducing disability and even radiographic destruction (perhaps by inhibiting metalloproteinases) at least in the short term. Conversely, there is excessive morbidity and mortality specifically attributable to corticosteroids, and the elderly are especially prone to the complications of cataracts, osteoporosis, accelerated atherosclerotic disease, and glaucoma. In a sense, the rationale, both pro and con, is especially salient in the elderly, making the decision much more difficult. If corticosteroids are employed, the lowest dose possible should be used, preferably less than 7.5 mg/day and if possible without the concurrent use of nonsteroidal agents. Patients should automatically get antiresorptive therapy to forestall steroid-induced osteoporosis.

## Differential Diagnosis

PMR is a common disorder of the elderly that is covered in detail further on. There is a genuine difficulty in distinguishing PMR from rheumatoid arthritis in some patients; however, there are features that are useful in distinguishing one from the other. At one extreme an elderly patient with the abrupt onset of proximal hip and shoulder girdle pain with constitutional symptoms and little or no synovitis is likely to have PMR; in contrast, a patient with the subacute or insidious onset of significant synovitis of the hands and feet with morning stiffness is more likely to have rheumatoid arthritis. Either disorder can have constitutional features such as weight loss, fever, anemia, or seropositivity for acute-phase reactants. Distinguishing features of PMR are rapid and complete response to low doses of corticosteroids, extreme elevations of the erythrocyte sedimentation rate (ESR >100 mm/hour), prominent shoulder symptoms, and abrupt onset. If the patient has features consistent with giant cell arteritis, rheumatoid arthritis is effectively ruled out. Distinguishing features of rheumatoid arthritis are proliferative synovitis in the hands or feet, especially with radiographic changes and significant titers of rheumatoid factor. A significant proportion of patients do not possess enough features to categorize them initially but over time, usually less than a year, most patients are appropriately categorized.

A frequently troublesome consideration in the differential diagnosis is Sjögren's syndrome. Primary Sjögren's syndrome in the elderly is a common[73] disease with a female predominance and characterized by salivary and lacrimal glandular hyperplasia caused by lymphoid cell infiltration. Most patients have keratoconjunctivitis sicca and xerostomia. Many patients have the autoantibody SSA or SSB, or both. About 20% of these patients have synovitis of the small joints of the hands or feet, or both, in the same distribution as for rheumatoid arthritis. Further confusion arises because many of these patients have a positive rheumatoid factor test result; however, they lack some of the radiologic hallmarks of rheumatoid arthritis, especially erosive destructive disease. Because about 20% of patients with rheumatoid arthritis have secondary Sjögren's syndrome, it is sometimes difficult to distinguish these two disorders. Fortunately, in general the diseases are treated similarly; however, the risk of lymphoma is much greater in patients with primary Sjögren's syndrome than in those with rheumatoid arthritis and secondary Sjögren's syndrome.

Another disorder that occasionally poses a difficulty in the differential diagnosis in the elderly is fibromyalgia. This syndrome of generalized aching is more commonly a problem in the evaluation for possible PMR but occasionally leads to confusion with rheumatoid arthritis. In this case, the key distinguishing feature is the invariable presence of inflammatory parameters in rheumatoid arthritis and their complete absence in fibromyalgia. Unfortunately, sometimes that is easier stated than observed. The inflammatory feature of rheumatoid arthritis may be subtle in presentation, such as morning stiffness, or weight loss or anemia could be attributed incorrectly to other causes.

Systemic lupus erythematosus presenting in the elderly is often predominantly a symmetric small joint polyarthritis. These patients have fewer double-stranded DNA antibodies, less hypocomplementemia, and less renal disease[74] than do younger patients. Despite the lessened frequency of renal disease, elderly patients with lupus do poorly.[75] These patients may have rheumatoid factor but do not show typical juxta-articular (marginal) erosions on radiographs. The evaluation of a patient with symmetric small joint polyarthritis should include an antinuclear antibody test; if results are positive, further determinations of antibodies to double-stranded DNA and serum complement levels are indicated. These patients often have subtle or even clinically silent visceral disease, making the serologic evaluation even more crucial.

A rare disorder that has some of the features of rheumatoid arthritis and some features of PMR is the disorder *RS3PE* described by McCarty and colleagues.[76] These individuals are elderly, with a male predominance. There is an abrupt onset of pitting edema of the hands and to a lesser extent the feet, with pain, moderate tenderness, and functional limitation resulting from both the edema and the mechanical limitation imposed by the swelling itself. These patients often respond dramatically to corticosteroids; however, some acquire typical rheumatoid arthritis and others may acquire features of a spondyloarthropathy.[77] In general the outcome is good.[78] The key feature in *RS3PE* is the presence of pitting edema beyond the confines of the synovial cavity in a glovelike distribution.

## POLYMYALGIA RHEUMATICA

PMR is a systemic inflammatory disease that occurs most commonly in middle-aged and elderly women. It frequently manifests with aching and morning stiffness involving the shoulder and hip girdle as well as an elevated ESR. In a large population-based epidemiologic investigation of PMR among the residents of Olmsted County, Minnesota, from 1970 to 1991, the annual incidence of PMR was found to be 52.5/100,000 population among those older than 50 years. The incidence appeared to rise with each decade past 50 years, and the highest rate was reported among women in their eighth decade of life (167.7/100,000).[79] Although it often occurs in the absence of giant cell arteritis, we always screen patients for symptoms and clinical findings suggestive of vasculitis to prevent the dreaded complications of blindness and stroke.[80] In patients diagnosed with PMR with negative temporal artery biopsy results, Weyand and colleagues demonstrated the presence of proinflammatory cytokines in a pattern resembling that seen in giant cell arteritis and suggested that PMR is a forme fruste of arteritis even in the absence of typical vascular lesions.[81, 82]

### Diagnosis

PMR is diagnosed when symptoms of pain and morning stiffness are present for at least 1 month and other diagnostic possibilities have been excluded. PMR is most frequently found in white women.[83, 84] Patients are often older than 50 years of age, and pain and stiffness are present in two of the three following regions: the neck and torso, shoulder girdle and upper arms, and hip girdle and thighs. Morning stiffness often persists for more than an hour. The ESR is frequently greater than 40 mm/hour and may be as high as 80 to 100 mm/hour.[83, 85] Normal ESRs have been reported in up to 20% of patients.[86] Other laboratory abnormalities include increased serum concentrations of C-reactive protein and interleukin 6 (IL-6).[81] It may be difficult to make the diagnosis in patients who also have pain secondary to generalized OA involving the cervical spine, lumbar spine, or hips or when myalgias may be secondary to fibromyalgia or regional pain syndromes. The presence of constitutional symptoms and physical examination findings of muscle tenderness, synovitis, limited range of motion, and absence of tender points in addition to laboratory studies indicative of systemic inflammation help differentiate PMR from other noninflammatory conditions such as OA and fibromyalgia. However, the presence of these features makes it more difficult to distinguish PMR from other inflammatory disorders such as elder-onset seronegative rheumatoid arthritis. The more difficult scenario arises when the older person has no evidence of inflammation, but pain and constitutional symptoms are present in the setting of other diseases such as depression and generalized OA. Sometimes a therapeutic trial of low-dose corticosteroids helps confirm the diagnosis.

An older person who presents with constitutional symptoms such as fatigue, malaise, anorexia, weight loss, and depression should have a thorough evaluation for other systemic inflammatory disorders before the diagnosis of PMR is established. Disorders that may be considered include viral and bacterial infections (i.e., subacute bacterial endocarditis), hypothyroidism or hyperthyroidism, metabolic bone disorders, elder-onset rheumatoid arthritis, inflammatory myopathy, and malignancy.[14, 16, 85] Infrequently, paraneoplastic syndromes have been manifested as PMR-like symptoms, usually from humoral factors produced by the malignancy.[85]

PMR with involvement of distal extremities has been described in approximately 8% of patients, confusing the diagnosis with the entity referred to as *RS3PE*.[84, 87, 88] Symptoms are usually less severe than in the proximal muscles but may also include aching, stiffness, synovitis in more than one joint, tenosynovitis, and carpal tunnel syndrome.[87, 88] It is not uncommon to have an older person who presents with synovitis of the wrists and knees. This may occur in 15 to 30% of patients, confusing the diagnosis with seronegative rheumatoid arthritis. There are descriptions of seronegative rheumatoid arthritis developing after the onset of PMR, and some investigators have suggested that they could be different presentations of the same disease.[14, 83, 85]

### Treatment

PMR frequently is not responsive to NSAIDs but requires treatment with corticosteroids. Both agents are associated with their own significant toxicities especially in the elderly. We have not found NSAIDs to be effective. These agents are associated with numerous toxicities, including the gastric ulceration and bleeding, hepatotoxicity, nephrotoxicity, cardiovascular effects, hematologic effects, and CNS abnormalities, as described previously.[19, 45] Corticosteroids are most often used to treat PMR.[14, 85] A rapid response to low-dose corticosteroids, 10 to 15 mg/day of prednisone, is often diagnostic of the disease. There appears to be no clear consensus, however, regarding appropriate initial doses. Some studies report starting doses as high as 20 to 30 mg/day of prednisone.[83] Weyand and colleagues tried to stratify patients according to ESR and IL-6 values. Elevated IL-6 concentrations following a single 20-mg dose of prednisone appeared to identify patients who required higher doses of corticosteroids and experienced frequent relapses.[81] The goal of therapy is to relieve pain and stiffness and suppress systemic symptoms with the lowest effective dose. Once symptoms have resolved and the ESR has normalized, corticosteroids are tapered by 10%/week until a prednisone dosage of 10 mg/day is achieved, followed by dose reductions of 1 mg/month, depending on the patient's clinical response. Disease relapse may occur when reductions are instituted too rapidly. Clinical improvement and ESR change are the most reliable parameters of therapeutic response. Unfortunately, response and the duration of treatment are variable and are reported to range from 2 years to longer than 5 years.[83, 81] This exposes the elderly patient to the multiple side effects of steroids, which include diabetes, osteoporosis and painful compression fractures, cataracts, and anxiety as well as delirium.[14, 85] Measures should be taken to retard the progression of some of these side effects such as increasing calcium intake, prescribing vitamin D, and initiating antiresorptive therapy with either an estrogen-progesterone combination or other antiresorptive agents approved for prevention and treatment of osteoporosis. Physical therapy and a weight-bearing exercise program should also be started so that patients can maintain strength and function. Steroid-sparing agents such as methotrexate and azathioprine have not been uniformly useful in the treatment of this disease. Studies on tumor necrosis factor blockade are in progress.

## FIBROMYALGIA

Fibromyalgia is a noninflammatory musculoskeletal syndrome manifested by the presence of widespread pain both above and below the waist, on the left and right sides of the body, and in the axial skeleton[2] as well as dysregulation of neuroendocrine function and sleep.[89] It has not been well studied in the elderly, although recently it has received more attention. The prevalence of fibromyalgia syndrome in the population has been estimated to be 2% for both sexes: 3.4% for women and 0.5% for men.[90] In a survey conducted over 10 years by Kennedy and Felson, women were found to be affected more frequently than men, with a mean age at presentation of 43.5 years.[91] It has also been observed that its prevalence increases with increasing age.[92] Yunus and associates reported that 45% of their elderly cohort of patients with fibromyalgia acquired symptoms after age 60 years, whereas 65% presented with symptoms at age 65 years or older.[93] A prevalence study conducted by Wolfe and colleagues demonstrated that the prevalence of fibromyalgia among women rose from 2% in 30- to 39-year-olds to 5.6% in 50- to 59-year-olds, and 7.4% in those older than 70 years. Among men, the prevalence rose from 0.2 to 0.8% and 1.2% in each age group, respectively. Fibromyalgia was found to be six times more prevalent in women older than 50 years of age than in men. It has been suggested that the presence of other musculoskeletal pain disorders may contribute to the development of fibromyalgia.[90]

As in younger patients, characteristic symptoms include widespread pain and tenderness, stiffness, fatigue, memory and concentration difficulties, and disrupted sleep, which often becomes chronic.[16, 90, 91, 94, 95]

Other associated signs and symptoms may include Raynaud's phenomenon, subjective hand puffiness, dizziness, paresthesias, sicca symptoms, irritable bowel syndrome, irritable bladder syndrome, and temporomandibular joint dysfunction.[96–98] Psychological distress manifested as tension, anxiety, and chronic functional headaches have been reported less frequently in the elderly, whereas other associated symptoms such as subjective hand puffiness, paresthesias, and irritable bowel syndrome have been reported as frequently as in younger patients.[93] Pain in the axial skeleton is found in both age groups and may affect the scapular region; shoulders; trapezius muscles; cervical, thoracic, and lumbar spine; posterior iliac crest; gluteal area; and trochanteric region. In both age groups, fatigue (felt to be secondary to sleep disruption) appears to be a prominent feature and has been reported in more than 50% of patients in Kennedy and colleagues' survey.[91] The achiness and stiffness seen in fibromyalgia often wax and wane. When compared with younger patients, the elderly were less frequently affected by fatigue, inactivity, psychological stress, poor sleep, and adverse weather conditions (cold or humid weather).[93] Fibromyalgia may coexist with other rheumatic disorders commonly found in the elderly such as OA, rheumatoid arthritis, systemic lupus erythematosus, Sjögren's syndrome, and psoriatic arthritis.[94] In the elderly it may present with symptoms consistent with degenerative disc disease, nerve entrapment, and OA, making the diagnosis more difficult. It has frequently been misdiagnosed as OA.[92]

## Diagnosis

Criteria for the diagnosis of fibromyalgia have been established by the American College of Rheumatology and also apply to the elderly. They include widespread pain present for at least 3 months and the presence of pain on digital palpation with a pressure of 4 kg in 11 of 18 tender point sites.[99] Other than less frequent tenderness involving the medial aspects of the elbows, no differences were detected in the number or sites of tender points found among elderly patients when compared with younger patients.[93]

Laboratory and radiographic studies are often unremarkable in patients with fibromyalgia. However, in the older adult with new onset of symptoms, other causes such as infection, PMR, hypothyroidism, systemic lupus erythematosus, and malignancies should be considered.[100] Patients with fibromyalgia may have elevated levels of antibodies including antinuclear antibodies and immune complexes as a result of immune changes seen with chronic stress.[94] Healthy elderly persons may also have rheumatoid factor and antinuclear antibodies in low (but sometimes high) titers as well as a mildly elevated ESR.[93]

Patients with fibromyalgia report poor sleep quality and exhibit more psychological distress. Certainly, poor sleep and insomnia are frequent complaints among the elderly and have been associated with symptoms of myalgias and fatigue.[89, 96, 101] Fibromyalgia is also strongly associated with a current or past history of depression as well as a family history of depression and alcoholism.[92, 98] These two disorders are prevalent among the elderly. In a survey of patients with fibromyalgia, Wolfe and colleagues found that somatization, anxiety, and depression were significantly associated with symptoms of fibromyalgia. Many patients report severe disability preventing meaningful employment secondary to fatigue, weakness, and difficulties with memory and concentration. In contrast to the case in younger patients, work-related disability does not appear to be prevalent among those older than 65 years.[90] When the diagnosis of fibromyalgia is entertained, patients should also be screened for symptoms of depression, and treatment should be initiated when indicated.[91, 96, 97]

## Treatment

The elderly who present with fibromyalgia are often misdiagnosed and inappropriately treated. In his cohort of patients, Yunus found that 55% were diagnosed initially with rheumatoid arthritis, PMR, or OA. Forty percent inappropriately received corticosteroids, thereby subjecting older patients to the potential toxicities of corticosteroids, including osteoporosis with compression fractures, diabetes mellitus, cataracts, anxiety, and delirium.[93] Treatment efforts should concentrate on addressing the psychosocial aspects of having a chronic disease in addition to preserving function and restoring sleep. Reassurance that the condition is not deforming or fatal should be provided.[103] Patient education, rehabilitation, and low-impact aerobic exercise have been found to be effective forms of therapy.[91, 97] In patients who also require medication for analgesia, low doses of tricyclic antidepressants may be initiated and titrated until restorative sleep is obtained. In younger patients, blinded randomized trials using the tricyclic agent amitriptyline or the pharmacologically related drug cyclobenzaprine, as well as the serotonin reuptake inhibitor fluoxetine, have shown modest responses in sleep quality and pain control.[94, 97, 103, 104] Unlike younger patients, older patients are more likely to experience adverse effects from tricyclic antidepressants, including anticholinergic effects and orthostasis, frequently described with amitriptyline, a potent tricyclic agent. We avoid amitriptyline in the elderly because of these potential toxicities. If an agent with sedating properties is desired, low doses of nortriptyline or trazodone may be initiated and titrated to the lowest effective dose; however, sedation, anticholinergic effects, and orthostasis still must be monitored for.[14] We do not recommend using combinations of antidepressants such as amitriptyline and fluoxetine[104] because of potentiating the risk of side effects in the elderly. Zolpidem has been reported to increase sleep time and improve energy in younger patients.[96, 97] In older patients, low doses should be initiated. We have not found trigger point injections with a local anesthetic to be that effective, but others have reported improvement in range of motion and pain intensity.[96] NSAIDs are also commonly prescribed but may not be beneficial. As discussed previously, they are associated with numerous toxicities in the elderly,[105] including gastrointestinal toxicity; nephrotoxicity; hepatotoxicity; cardiovascular effects such as volume overload, CNS effects including dizziness, confusion, cognitive impirment, and memory loss; and hematologic abnormalities such as thrombocytopenia, neutropenia, and hemolytic anemia.[14, 19, 45] Tramadol, a centrally acting analgesic, has been shown to be effective in low doses. This agent should be used judiciously because toxicities are experienced more frequently by the elderly. Dose adjustments are recommended for patients older than 75 years of age and for patients with renal or hepatic impairment. The elderly are more vulnerable to side effects secondary to altered drug distribution, reduced clearance, and enhanced sensitivity to opioid analgesics.[42] Although studies have demonstrated the usefulness of narcotic analgesics in these patients, this class of agent is seldom the first choice for treatment in any age group.[98, 106]

We often encourage the use of alternative therapies such as massage, relaxation therapy, acupuncture, psychological counseling, physical therapy with ultrasound, and water exercises in addition to a routine exercise regimen. These therapies have frequently been reported to be effective. Heat and whirlpool baths may also provide temporary relief.[91, 96, 97]

*Acknowledgment*

*The authors acknowledge the assistance of Agnes R. Robideaux in the preparation of this chapter.*

## REFERENCES

1. Hamerman D (ed): Osteoarthritis: Public Health Implications for an Aging Population. Baltimore: Johns Hopkins University Press, 1997.
2. Lawrence RC, Helmick CG, Arnett FC, et al: Estimates of the prevalence of arthritis and selected musculoskeletal disorders in the United States. Arthritis Rheum 1998; 41:778–799.
3. Olshansky SJ, Casel CK: *In* Hamerman D (ed): Osteoarthritis: Public Health Implications for an Aging Population. Baltimore: Johns Hopkins University Press, 1997: 15–29.
4. Helmick CG, Lawrence RC, Pollard RA, et al: Arthritis and other conditions: Who is affected now, who will be affected later? Arthritis Care Res 1995; 8:203–211.
5. Badley EM, Wang PP: Arthritis and the aging population: Projections of arthritis prevalence in Canada 1991 to 2031. J Rheumatol 1998; 25:138–144.
6. Yelin E, Callahan LF: The economic cost and social and psychological impact of musculoskeletal disorders. Arthritis Rheum 1995; 38:1351–1362.
7. Yelin E: The cumulative impact of a common chronic condition. Arthritis Rheum 1992; 35:489–497.
8. Verbrugge LM: Women, men and osteoarthritis. Arthritis Care Res 1995; 8:212–220.
9. Abyad A, Boyer JT : Arthritis and aging. Curr Opin Rheumatol 1992; 4:153–159.
10. Hughes SL, Dunlop D. The prevalence and impact of arthritis in older persons. Arthritis Care Res 1995; 8:257–264.
11. Hughes SL, Dunlop D, Edelman P, et al: Impact of joint impairment on longitudinal disability in elderly persons. J Gerontol 1994; 49:291–300.
12. Ferrell BA: Pain evaluation and management in the nursing home. Ann Intern Med 1995; 123:681–687.

13. Verbrugge G, Veys EM: Numerical scoring systems for the anatomic evolution of osteoarthritis of the finger joints. Arthritis Rheum 1996; 39:308–320.

14. Michet CJ Jr, Evans JM, Fleming KC, et al: Common rheumatologic diseases in elderly patients. Mayo Clin Proc 1995; 70:1205–1214.

15. Loeser RF: Evaluation of musculoskeletal complaints in the older adult. Clinics Geriatr Med 1998; 14:401–415.

16. American College of Rheumatology Ad Hoc Committee on Clinical Guidelines: Guidelines for the initial evaluation of the adult patient with acute musculoskeletal symptoms. Arthritis Rheum 1996; 39:1–8.

17. Woodhouse KW: Pharmacokinetics of drugs in the elderly. J R Soc Med 1994; 87(suppl 23):2–4.

18. Everitt DE, Avorn J: Drug prescribing for the elderly. Arch Intern Med 1986; 146:2393–2396.

19. Fleming A: Drug management of arthritis in the elderly. J R Soc Med 1994; 87(suppl 23):22–25.

20. Fries JF, Singh G, Morfeld D, et al: Relationship of running to musculoskeletal pain with age. Arthritis Rheum 1996; 39:64–72.

21. Callahan LF, Pincus T: Mortality in the rheumatic diseases. Arthritis Care Res 1995; 8:229–241.

22. Cicuttini FM, Spector TD: In Hamerman D (ed): Osteoarthritis: Public Health Implications for an Aging Population. Baltimore, Johns Hopkins University Press: 1997.

23. Oliveria SA, Felson DT, Reed JI, et al: Incidence of symptomatic hand, hip and knee osteoarthritis among patients in a health maintenance organization. Arthritis Rheum 1995; 38:1134–1141.

24. Creamer P, Flores R, Hochberg M: Management of osteoarthritis in older adults. Clin Geriatr Med 1998; 14:435–454.

25. Coyte PC, Asche CV, Croxford R, et al: The economic costs of musculoskeletal disorder in Canada. Arthritis Care Res 1998; 11:315–325.

26. Guccione AA: In Hamerman D (ed): Osteoarthritis: Public Health Implications for an Aging Population. Baltimore: Johns Hopkins University Press, 1997: 84–98.

27. Swedburg JA, Steinbaur JR: Osteoarthritis. Am Fam Phys 1992; 45:557–567.

28. Felson DT, Zhang Y, Hannan MT, et al: The incidence and natural history of knee osteoarthritis in the elderly. The Framingham Osteoarthritis Study. Arthritis Rheum 1995; 38:1500–1505.

29. Schumacher HR: Osteoarthritis and crystal deposition diseases. Curr Opin Rheumatol 1998; 10:244–245.

30. Felson DT, Zhang Y: An update on the epidemiology of knee and hip osteoarthritis with a view to prevention. Arthritis Rheum 1998; 41:1343–1355.

31. Felson DT: Preventing knee and hip osteoarthritis. Bull Rheum Dis 1998; 47:1–4.

32. Creamer P, Hochberg MC: Osteoarthritis. Lancet 1997; 350:503–509.

33. Hampson SE, Glasgow RE, Zeiss AM: Coping with osteoarthritis by older adults. Arthritis Care Res 1996; 9:133–141.

34. Ettinger WH, Burns RB, Messier SO, et al: A randomized trial comparing aerobic exercise and resistance exercise with a health education program in older adults with knee osteoarthritis. The Fitness Arthritis and Seniors Trial. JAMA 1997; 227:25–31.

35. Hamerman D: Aging and the musculoskeletal system. Ann Rheum Dis 1997; 56:578–585.

36. O'Reilly S, Jones A, Doherty M: Muscle weakness in osteoarthritis. Curr Opin Rheumatol 1997; 9:259–262.

37. Slemenda C, Brandt K, Heiman D, et al: Quadriceps weakness and osteoarthritis of the knee. Ann Intern Med 1997; 127:97–104.

38. Puett DW, Griffin MR: Published trials of nonmedicinal and noninvasive therapies for hip and knee osteoarthritis. Ann Intern Med 1994; 121:133–140.

39. Bradley JD, Brandt KD, Katz BP, et al: Comparison of an antiinflammatory doses of ibuprofen, an analgesic dose of ibuprofen, and acetaminophen in the treatment of patients with osteoarthritis of the knee. N Engl J Med 1991; 325:87–91.

40. Hochberg JC, Altman RD, Brandt KD, et al: Guidelines for the medical management of osteoarthritis. Part I. Osteoarthritis of the knee. American College of Rheumatology. Arthritis Rheum 1995; 38:1535–1540.

41. Hochberg JC, Altman RD, Brandt KD, et al: Guidelines for the medical management and treatment of osteoarthritis: Part II. Osteoarthritis of the hip. American College of Rheumatology. Arthritis Rheum 1995; 38:1541–1546.

42. Gibson TP: Pharmacokinetics, efficacy and safety of analgesia with a focus on tramadol HCl. Am J Med 1996; 101:47S–53S.

43. Ytterberg SR, Maowald ML, Woods SR: Codeine and oxycodeine use in patients with chronic rheumatic disease pain. Arthritis Rheum 1998; 41:1603–1612.

44. Herst EV, Pertes RA, Ochs HA: Topical capsaicin: Pharmacology and potential role in the treatment of temporomandubular pain. J Clin Dent 1994; 5:54–59.

45. Simon LS: Biology and toxic effects of nonsteroidal anti-inflammatory drugs. Curr Opin Rheumatol 1998; 10:153–158.

46. Furst DE: Update on clinical trials in the rheumatic diseases. Curr Opin Rheumatol 1998; 10:123–128.

47. Davies NM, Jamali F, Skeith KJ: Nonsteroidal anti-inflammatory drug-induced enteropathy and severe chronic anemia in a patient with rheumatoid arthritis. Arthritis Rheum 1996; 39:321–324.

48. Simon LE, Lanza FL, Lipsky PE, et al: Preliminary study of the safety and efficacy of SC-58635, a novel cyclooxygenase 2 inhibitor: Efficacy and safety in two placebo-controlled trials in osteoarthritis and rheumatoid arthritis, and studies of gastrointestinal and platelet effects. Arthritis Rheum 1998; 41:1591–1602.

49. McAdam BF, Catella-Lawson F, Mardini IA, et al: Systemic biosynthesis of prostacyclin by cyclooxygenase (COX)-2: The human pharmacology of a selective inhibitor of COX-2. Proc Natl Acad Sci U S A 1999; 96:272–277.

50. Towheed TE, Hochberg MC: A systematic review of randomized controlled trials of pharmacological therapy in osteoarthritis of the knee, with an emphasis on trial methodology. Semin Arthritis Rheum 1997; 26:755–770.

51. Jones A, Doherty M: Intra-articular corticosteroids are effective in osteoarthritis but there are no clinical predictors of response. Ann Rheum Dis 1996; 55:829–832.

52. Lozada CL, Altman RD: Chondroprotection in osteoarthritis. Bull Rheum Dis 1997; 46:5–7.

53. Cohen MC: Hyaluronic acid treatment (viscosupplementation) for OA of the knee. Bull Rheum Dis 1998; 47:4–7.

54. Constantz RB: Hyaluronan, glucosamine, and chondroitin sulfate: Roles for therapy in arthritis. In Kelley WN, Harris ED Jr, Ruddy S, et al (eds): Textbook of Rheumatology Update 27. Philadelphia: WB Saunders, 1998: 1–6.

55. Bomalaski JS: Acute rheumatic disorders in the elderly. Emerg Med Clin North Am 1990; 8:341–359.

56. Campbell SM: Gout: How presentation, diagnosis, and treatment differ in the elderly. Geriatrics 1988; 43:71–77.

57. Kavanaugh A: Rheumatoid arthritis in the elderly: Is it a different disease? Am J Med 1997; 103:40S–48S.

58. Kaipiainen-Seppanen O, Aho K, Isomaki H, et al: Shift in the incidence of rheumatoid arthritis toward elderly patients in Finland during 1975–1990. Clin Exp Rheumatol 1996; 14: 537–542.

59. Deal C, Meenan RF, Goldenberg DL, et al: The clinical features of elderly-onset rheumatoid arthritis. Arthritis Rheum 1985; 28:987–994.

60. Montamat SC, Cusack B, Vestal RE: Management of drug therapy in the elderly. N Engl J Med 1998; 321:303–309.

61. Llewellyn JG, Pritchard MH: Influence of age and disease state in nonsteroidal antiinflammatory drug associated gastric bleeding. J Rheumatol 1988; 154:691–694.

62. Griffin MR, Piper JM, Daugherty JR, et al: Nonsteroidal anti-inflammatory drug use and increased risk for peptic ulcer disease in elderly persons. Ann Intern Med 1991; 114:257–263.

63. Wolfe F, Cathey MA: The effect of age on methotrexate efficacy and toxicity. J Rheumatol 1991; 18:973–977.

64. van der Heijde DM, van Reil PL, van Leeuwen MA, et al: Older versus younger onset rheumatoid arthritis: Results at onset and after 2 years of a prospective followup study of early rheumatoid arthritis. J Rheumatol 1991; 18:1285–1289.

65. Sherrer YS, Bloch DA, Mitchell DM, et al: The development of disability in rheumatoid arthritis. Arthritis Rheum 1986; 29:494–500.

66. van der Heijde DM, van Riel PL, van Rijswik MH, et al: Influence of prognostic features on the final outcome in rheumatoid arthritis: A review of the literature. Semin Arthritis Rheum 1988; 17:284–292.

67. Anderson ST: Mortality in rheumatoid arthritis: Do age and gender make a difference? Semin Arthritis Rheum 1996; 25:291–296.

68. Gurwitz JH, Avorn J: The ambiguous relation between aging and adverse drug reaction. Ann Intern Med 1991; 114:956–966.

69. Ailabouni W, Eknoyan G: Nonsteroidal anti-inflammatory drugs and acute renal failure in the elderly. A risk-benefit assessment. Drugs Aging 1996; 9:341–351.

70. Gardner G, Furst DE: Disease-modifying antirheumatic drugs. Potential effects in older patients. Drugs Aging 1995; 7:420–437.

71. Bressolle F, Bologna C, Kinowski JM, et al: Total and free methotrexate pharmacokinetics in elderly patients with rheumatoid arthritis. A comparison with young patients. J Rheumatol 1997; 24:1903–1909.

72. Glennas A, Kvien TK, Andrup O, et al: Auranofin is safe and superior to placebo in elderly-onset rheumatoid arthritis. Br J Rheumatol 1997; 36:870–877.

73. Strickland RW, Tesar JT, Berne BH, et al: The frequency of sicca syndrome in an elderly female population. J Rheumatol 1987: 14;766–771.

74. Ward MM, Studenski S: Age-associated clinical manifestations of systemic lupus erythematosus: A multivariate regression analysis. J Rheumatol 1990; 17:476–481.

75. Reveille JD, Bartolucci A, Alarcon GS: Prognosis in systemic lupus erythematosus. Arthritis Rheum 1990; 33:37–48.

76. McCarty DJ, O'Duffy JD, Pearson L, et al: Remitting seronegative symmetrical synovitis with pitting edema. JAMA 1985; 254:2763–2767.

77. Schaeverbeke T, Fatout E, Marce S, et al: Remitting seronegative symmetrical synovitis pitting oedema: Disease or syndrome? Ann Rheum Dis 1995; 54:681–684.

78. Roblot P, Zaim A, Azais I, et al: RS3PE: A clinical diagnosis, a prognosis more simple than its name [In French]. Rev Med Interne 1998; 19:542–547.

79. Salvarani C, Gariel S, O'Fallon WM, et al: Epidemiology of polymyalgia rheumatica in Olmsted County, Minnesota, 1970–1991. Arthritis Rheum 1995; 38:369–373.

80. Gonzalez-Gay MA, Blanco R, Rodriguez-Valverdem V, et al: Permanent visual loss and cerebrovascular accidents in giant cell arteritis. Arthritis Rheum 1998; 41:1497–1504.

81. Weyand CM, Fulbright JW, Evans JM, et al: Corticosteroid requirements in polymyalgia rheumatica. Arch Intern Med 1999; 159:577–584.

82. Weyand CM, Hicock KC, Hunder GG, et al: Tissue cytokine patterns in patients with polymyalgia rheumatica and giant cell arteritis. Ann Intern Med 1994; 121:484–491.

83. Balas S, Ramos-Remus C, Davis P: Clinical outcome of 149 patients with polymyalgia rheumatica and giant cell arteritis. J Rheumatol 1998; 25:99–106.

84. Healey LA: What's in a name? J Rheumatol 1998; 25:5.

85. Evans JM, Hunder GG: Polymyalgia rheumatica and giant cell arteritis. Clin Geriatr Med 1998; 14:455–473.

86. Helfgott SM, Kieval RI: Polymyalgia rheumatica in patients with a normal erythrocyte sedimentation rate. Arthritis Rheum 1996; 39:304–307.

87. Salvarani C, Gabriel S, Hunder GG: Distal extremity swelling with pitting edema in polymyalgia rheumatica. Arthritis Rheum 1996; 39:73–80.

88. Salvarani C, Cantini F, Macchioni P, et al: Distal musculoskeletal manifestations in polymyalgia rheumatica. Arthritis Rheum 1998; 41:1221–1226.

89. Pillemer SR (ed): The Neuroscience and Endocrinology of Fibromyalgia. Binghamton, NY: Haworth Medical, 1998.

90. Wolfe F, Ross K, Anderson J, et al: The prevalance and characteristics of fibromyalgia in the general population. Arthritis Rheum 1995; 38:19–28.

91. Kennedy M, Felson DT: A prospective long-term study of fibromyalgia syndrome. Arthritis Rheum 1996; 39:682–685.

92. Goldenberg DL: Fibromyalgia syndrome a decade later. What have we learned? Arch Intern Med 1999; 159:777–785.

93. Yunus MB, Holt GS, Masi AT, et al: Fibromyalgia syndrome among the elderly: Comparison with younger patients. J Am Geriatr Soc 1988; 36:987–995.

94. Clauw DJ, Katz P: The overlap between fibromyalgia and inflammatory rheumatic disease: When and why does it occur? J Clin Rheumatol 1995; 1:335–341.

95. Hsu V, Patella S, Sigal LH: "Chronic Lyme disease" as the incorrect diagnosis in patients with fibromyalgia. Arthritis Rheum 1993; 36:1493–1500.

96. Bennett R: Fibromyalgia, chronic fatigue syndrome and myofascial pain. Curr Opin Rheumatol 1998; 10:95–103.

97. Goldenberg DL: Fibromyalgia, chronic fatigue syndrome and myofascial pain syndrome. Curr Opin Rheumatol 1997; 9:135–143.

98. Bennett RM: Emerging concepts in the neurobiology of chronic pain: Evidence of abnormal sensory processing in fibromyalgia. Mayo Clin Proc 1999; 74:385–398.

99. Wolfe F, Smythe HA, Yunus MB, et al: The American College of Rheumatology 1990 Criteria for Classification of Fibromyalgia. Report of the Multicenter Criteria Committee. Arthritis Rheum 1990; 33:160–172.

100. Holland NW, Gonzalez EB: Soft tissue problems in older adults. Clin Geriatr Med 1998; 14:601–611.

101. Moldofsky H: Sleep influences on regional and diffuse pain syndromes associated with osteoarthritis. Semin Arthritis Rheum 1989; 18(4, suppl 2):18–21.

102. White KP, Speechley M: Comparing self-reported function and work disability in 100 community cases of fibromyalgia syndrome versus controls in London, Ontario: The London Fibromyalgia Epidemiology Study. Arthritis Rheum 1999; 42:76–83.

103. Block SR: What to say to the patient who has just been diagnosed as having generalized rheumatism (fibromyalgia). J Clin Rheumatol 1995; 1:343–346.

104. Goldenberg D, Mayskiy M, Mossey C, et al: A randomized, double-blind crossover trial of fluoxetine and amitriptyline in the treatment of fibromyalgia. Arthritis Rheum 1996; 39:1852–1859.

105. Wolfe F, Anderson J, Harkness D, et al: A prospective, longitudinal, multicenter study of service utilization and cost in fibromyalgia. Arthritis Rheum 1997; 40:1560–1570.

106. Russell IJ: Fibromyalgia syndrome: Formulating a strategy for relief. J Musculoskeletal Med 1998; (November), pp 4–21.

# SECTION

## II Rheumatic Syndromes

## CHAPTER

## 4 | Shoulder Pain

*Michael P. Brunelli and Evan L. Flatow*

Rheumatoid arthritis (RA) is a potentially devastating disease, ranging from mild discomfort to inexorable crippling and destruction of multiple joints. The pathophysiology and genetic predisposition of this disease process have been well described and are not discussed here. Instead, this chapter focuses on all aspects of RA as they pertain to the shoulder joint, as well as those of other shoulder conditions that need to be considered in the differential diagnosis.

## EPIDEMIOLOGY

The prevalence rate of RA is difficult to specify because multiple studies have yielded many different rates for both men and women with a wide range of ages.[1, 2] This topic is discussed in other chapters. With regard to the shoulder, two separate groups of RA patients have been distinguished: Elderly-onset rheumatoid arthritis (EORA) by definition occurs after the age of 60; younger-onset rheumatoid arthritis (YORA) occurs before age 60. EORA is further distinguished by an equal age distribution between sexes, more acute onset with higher disease activity, lower frequency of seropositivity for rheumatoid factor, and higher incidence of involvement of the large joints, particularly the shoulder.[1] It has been shown that the shoulder is the first problematic joint in 21% of EORA patients.[3] Other investigators have shown EORA patients to have higher incidence of shoulder involvement than do YORA patients at diagnosis.[4, 5] Understanding these differences within the rheumatoid population may better serve the physician in the decision-making process, diagnosis, and treatment.

## CLINICAL PRESENTATION

Shoulder involvement is usually seen with polyarticular disease,[6] but monoarticular involvement of the shoulder (or at least manifestations in the shoulder as the first affected joint) does occur. Pain is the major complaint and is aggravated by movement, followed by decreased range of motion and functional capacity. There may be concomitant gross swelling about the shoulder as a result of synovial inflammation, and/or there may be subdeltoid bursitis with associated warmth. Erythema is an uncommon manifestation of the rheumatoid shoulder and suggests infectious etiologies as a cause of the shoulder pain. During acute episodes of inflammation, patients may prefer flexion of the shoulder to relieve capsular distention.[7]

Further visual inspection may show prominence of the clavicle and the acromion secondary to muscle wasting and medialization of the humeral head. This may result in cosmetic complaints, usually of loss of the "roundness" of the shoulder. Fluid in the subdeltoid bursa can be either caused by primary involvement or joint fluid extravasation secondary to a rotator cuff tear. In the latter case, the examiner may expect to find anterosuperior subluxation of the humeral head that results from unopposed pull of the deltoid muscle.[8]

Any of the joints about the shoulder, including the sternoclavicular joint, may be involved. This is also true of the many bursae about the shoulder, including the scapulothoracic bursa. These areas contain synovium, which may become involved in the disease process, causing pain and swelling. Direct palpation can be helpful in revealing joint line tenderness.

## USE OF IMAGING

Plain films are usually the first studies obtained and are the most helpful in preoperative planning. This series should contain four views: An anteroposterior view of the shoulder joint in internal rotation, one in external rotation, an axillary view, and a projection in the scapular Y plane. These changes might be seen on the anteroposterior radiographs alone, but the additional views can give important information. The axillary view shows any glenoid destruction or loss of bone stock, which will help in planning for implantation of a prosthesis. The Y view is useful for detecting any acromial disease or may suggest impingement of a high-riding humeral head. A full assessment should characterize bone destruction, the presence of erosions or infection, the position of the humeral head, and associated AC joint involvement.[9]

Cuomo and associates[6] summarized the radiographic changes, which occur in RA of the shoulder. Osteopenia is first noted, followed by marginal erosions at the junction of the humeral head and anatomic neck. These marginal erosions usually represent enthesopathies: erosions at the sites of tendon and capsular attachments. Symmetric cartilage narrowing occurs and, in advanced disease, leads to bone loss and medialization of the humeral head as results of erosions of the glenoid. In general, sclerosis and osteophytes are seen far less frequently in RA than in osteoarthritis, but they can occur in some patients and do not rule out a rheumatologic diagnosis. As the osseous destruction continues, there may be loss of the greater tuberosity and anatomic neck of the humerus. As soft tissue succumbs to synovial inflammation, elevation of the humeral head can be seen.[6]

Synovial inflammation of the acromioclavicular joint can lead to osseous destruction on both sides of the joint, but it is worse at the distal third of the clavicle.[10] This has been noted commonly in rheumatoid patients, with the progression of subchondral erosion, tapering, and osteolysis of the lateral aspect of the clavicle worsening with time.

It must be realized that long before any changes may be detected by plain film, the disease process may be present for some time. Magnetic resonance imaging (MRI) allows visualization of the inflammatory synovitis and pannus before it begins to erode cartilage and bone[11] and therefore may be of greater advantage at an earlier stage of the disease by allowing the physician to modify the course of the disease.

Studies comparing MRI with radiography have shown MRI to be more sensitive than radiography for detecting erosions and subchondral cysts of large joints.[12, 13] In general, MRI is useful for all soft tissue planes, bursae, tendons, and ligaments about the shoulder. It shows evidence of synovitis and presence of pannus. In particular, it may detect a rotator cuff tear before the tear is clinically significant. One study in a rheumatoid population suggested that injection of gadolinium further improves the ability to detect tears of the supraspinatus and may be useful for early intervention in a younger, more active population before the tear can propagate.[14] In patients requiring MRI but who are unable to undergo the procedure (pacemaker, claustrophobia), a computed tomographic (CT) arthrogram may be considered in order to rule out the presence of a rotator cuff tear.

In the treatment and evaluation of the rheumatoid shoulder, further studies are rarely used. However, to visualize bony anatomy most accurately, a CT scan of the shoulder may be obtained. This might be of particular use in the case of severe glenoid erosion, which can be suggested on the axillary radiograph. The information would be valuable in the case of preoperative planning for a prosthesis.

Ultrasonography, like MRI, has been reported to show bursitis, synovitis, rotator cuff tears, and biceps tendonitis quite early in the course of disease.[15] This imaging method has rarely been used by our office.

## DIFFERENTIAL DIAGNOSIS

Glenohumeral osteoarthritis, or secondary arthritis (e.g., occurring after trauma), is usually distinguished by lack of a systemic diagnosis and a history of fewer crescendo episodes (flares) than occur in RA patients. Radiographs show sclerosis, osteophytes, posterior glenoid wear, lack of superior head migration, and small subchondral cysts. Osteopenia, central glenoid erosion, superior head migration, and large resorptive cysts are seen in rheumatoid disease by way of contrast.

Rotator cuff disease is an extremely common condition and is an important part of the differential diagnosis to be considered in the evaluation of shoulder pain. Pain from bursal and rotator cuff conditions tends to refer to the anterior upper arm (deltoid area) between the shoulder and the elbow, and patients often deny they have "shoulder pain" but rather insist they have "arm pain." Cuff disease usually occurs after age 40. Physical examination usually reveals full passive motion but pain with overhead use or resisted elevation. With large cuff tears, there may be weakness of elevation and external rotation, and the bursa may be distended as a result of joint fluid leakage through the tear. Loss of shoulder contour is rare, however. Radiographs usually show a normal glenohumeral joint, sometimes with cysts and sclerosis at the head-tuberosity junction and anterior acromial spurs. MRI shows tendon abnormalities of the supraspinatus or even tears and frank defects. Usually the glenohumeral joint is fully intact. Two groups of patients present difficulties in assessment. First, even patients with diagnosed polyarticular rheumatoid disease may have typical degenerative rotator cuff disease. Because cadaver studies have shown that up to 50% of persons develop rotator cuff degeneration by the seventh and eighth decades, it seems unsurprising that RA does not "protect" against noninflammatory cuff disease. The other group with difficulties has been described as having "cuff-tear arthropathy" by orthopedic surgeons and crystalline arthropathy or "Milwaukee shoulder" by rheumatologists. In this condition there are a massive rotator cuff tear, extreme superior humeral migration, and extensive loss of the glenohumeral joint. There is usually more sclerosis and less erosion than in RA. Although the surgical treatment is the same (arthroplasty), it is important to avoid a mistaken diagnosis of rheumatoid disease with monarticular involvement.

Fractures are usually easily diagnosed, but a tuberosity fracture in a patient with rheumatoid disease may be mistaken for a flare of the disease if a history of trauma, however slight, does not lead to careful radiographic assessment. Any time a fracture is suspected, radiographs in three planes should be obtained: a true anteroposterior view and a lateral view of the scapula and an axillary view.

Infection must always be considered, especially in the patient with rheumatoid disease that has already been treated with cortisone injections. Warmth over the shoulder, fever, malaise, and sudden severe increase in pain should be investigated by arthrocentesis for cell count and culture. When the results are unclear (e.g., an intermediate cell count and a culture suspected of being contaminated), an arthroscopic clean-out and synovial biopsy for culture should be considered; the rate of morbidity from this procedure is very low.

## CONSERVATIVE TREATMENT

The systemic treatment of RA, a complex, multisystem disease, is discussed in Chapter 19. Medical management is, of course, the mainstay.[16, 17] When shoulder involvement develops, patients must be counseled as to activity modification, especially in the use of wheeled luggage or porters and avoidance of activities that lead to flares of pain.

Physical therapy, if gentle, may be of help early in shoulder involvement. Deterioration of shoulder biomechanics is a chronically progressive course with formation of adhesions leading to stiffness. Cuff muscles become weak and atrophic from periods of disuse. Therapy can help loosen stiff shoulders, strengthen muscles, and help return some function early in the course of disease. As the articular surface destruction progresses, such therapy becomes less valuable. Aggressive stretching or manipulations can fracture osteoporotic bone or tear frail cuff tissue. Rest and physical therapy modalities may also help ameliorate some symptoms. Isometric exercises may be useful during periods of inflammation.

## INVASIVE TREATMENT

The discussion of bursal and intra-articular injection technically concerns nonoperative treatment and might be included under the heading of conservative treatment. It is our opinion, however, that this procedure is not without risk and should be considered invasive treatment. The literature on local injection about the shoulder is scarce but indicates a higher rate of tendon damage and rupture after injection of steroid about the hand.[18] Also, we believe that injection in a potentially immunosuppressed population may lead to a higher chance of infection. The literature on the subject of steroid injection is dated and clearly is an area open for reexploration.

One author discussed the use of bursal injection for the treatment of subdeltoid bursitis, a common problem in this population.[19] Affected patients have pain, swelling, and restricted range of motion. The symptoms are best alleviated with one or multiple intra-bursal injections of hydrocortisone. Over time, the repeated inflammatory cycle leads to fibrosis and obliteration of this bursa. In rare instances, it becomes chronically distended, filled with synovial fluid and necessitating open bursectomy. The same article also described the use of injection for rotator cuff tendonitis in RA of the shoulder. The author stated that 5 mL of 1% procaine and 25 mg of hydrocortisone would give both immediate and long-lasting relief.[19]

At least one group of authors has stated that medication, except for local injection, is not helpful in the rheumatoid shoulder. Weiss and colleagues[20] found that systemic treatment, including nonsteroidal anti-inflammatory agents and other disease-modifying drugs, had little effect on a patient's pain and loss of function. They recommended a regimen of heat, rest, range-of-motion exercises, and repeated intra-articular injections, which they found useful in decreasing pain and increasing functional capacity. There was no description of technique or dosage of steroid used.

Yet another group of authors believed local injection to be of no value at all. Rylance and Chalmers,[21] in a blind clinical trial, compared the intra-articular injection of hydrocortisone acetate, acetylsalicylic acid, and normal saline in a population with rheumatoid shoulder. They found no difference in results between groups. Each group showed the same amount of improvement in range of motion and relief of pain. They therefore questioned the use of steroid injection at all.

It is our belief that the careful use, once or at most twice, of bursal and intra-articular steroid injections can be useful in the early treatment of the rheumatoid shoulder. Because the goal is to break the inflammatory cycle of synovitis, local steroid at the appropriate point is critical. Rarely is an injection given on a patient's first visit, regardless of symptoms. No more than two doses are ever recommended, because of possible tendon side effects.

Our steroid of choice is dexamethasone acetate, 16 mg in 1 mL, mixed with 3 mL of 1% lidocaine, 3 mL of 0.5% bupivacaine, and 0.5 mL of bicarbonate (1 mEq/mL). For subdeltoid or subacromial bursitis, the mixture is introduced with a 22-gauge needle. Under sterile conditions, the needle is introduced just anterior and lateral to the anterolateral corner of the acromion through the deltoid and bursa until bone (the greater tuberosity) is felt. With light pressure on the syringe, the needle is slowly withdrawn until suddenly the plunger of the syringe moves easily. This represents the subdeltoid space, which is continuous with the subacromial space. A similar injection may be directed into the glenohumeral joint if intra-articular synovitis is suspected. The most useful site for this injection is the posterior arthroscopic portal site.

Certain patients do not respond to local injection and go on to form a chronic synovitis about the shoulder. On physical examination, these patients have a painful, boggy shoulder with decreased range of motion. This scenario may represent bursal hypertrophy or a rotator cuff tear with extension of fluid and synovial tissue into the subdeltoid bursa. The situation may be deciphered best through an MRI. Synovectomy is a controversial procedure with little evidence of its value in the shoulder. Arthroscopic synovectomy has largely replaced open procedures and should be reserved for patients with articular cartilage of at least half of its normal thickness. Additional benefits of arthroscopy include removal of loose bodies, débridement, and obtaining synovium for study.[22]

Open synovectomy has nevertheless been described. Matsen and coworkers[22] reported on open-shoulder synovectomy through the deltopectoral approach. The subdeltoid tissue is excised during the procedure, with care not to damage the circumflex branch of the axillary nerve on the undersurface of the deltoid. The joint is approached through the subscapularis tendon, and the shoulder capsule is then released from the inferior aspect on the humerus (6-o'clock position) up to the articular margin and along the long head of the biceps to the articular margin. Synovium is removed from the anterior aspect of the joint, with care to protect the axillary nerve. The surgeon must work around the joint to the posterior aspect, for which dislocation of the joint might be helpful. Drains are important, as is physical therapy after 2 to 3 days.

Pahle and Kvarnes[23] reported their experience with open synovectomy. In addition to removing all signs of synovitis, they smoothed and débrided any osteophytes or imperfections of the joint surface. The results revealed a decrease in pain in 44 of 54 shoulders. Motion, however, was found to improve only slightly.

Wakitani et al[24] studied 47 rheumatoid shoulders, which were divided into groups on the basis of five different destruction patterns. Using arthroscopic techniques, they produced pain relief and increased range of motion in the nonprogressive pattern and produced only pain relief in the shoulders with erosive disease.

Some authors[25, 26] have recommended glenoidectomy at the time of synovectomy. This procedure theoretically removes the diseased articular cartilage and pannus, which may be of benefit in decreasing pain and recurrence. However, this remains controversial as no clear advantage over simple synovectomy has been demonstrated.

As the disease severity increases and symptoms become more severe, none of the aforementioned techniques may be useful. At this point, the next option is arthroplasty, regardless of patient's age. Arthrodesis and resection arthroplasty should be used only as salvage procedures. Arthrodesis is indicated in cases of severe bone/muscle loss with paralysis of all shoulder muscles or if a history of infection precludes arthroplasty. Although this allows the elbow to present the hand to the face, it increases stresses at the elbow, which may be involved with the disease. Control of pain is less predictable with resection arthroplasty than with total shoulder replacement. These joints are usually unstable early with poor motion and progression to stiffness and weakness, rendering the upper extremity useless, especially when other joints are involved.[27]

If the decision is made to use a prosthesis, the physician must first consider the patient's overall health, the state of the ipsilateral joints, the possibility of septic shoulder, and the stability of the cervical spine. The

results of shoulder replacement are far better before severe bone and cuff tendon loss have occurred. For this reason, we advocate early replacement once it is clear that the joint is unsalvageable and replacement will eventually be required. It is unfortunate for a patient to undergo surgery on the knees, hips, hands, and feet only to end up with totally eroded shoulders because the patient was told to "live with it as long as possible."

As in all of our shoulder procedures, we prefer to use an interscalene block with long-acting local agents. This provides excellent intraoperative pain control and decreased postoperative pain and morbidity for the patient. The surgeon must know the status of the cervical spine in case of unforeseen problems, which may necessitate endotracheal intubation.

These considerations aside, the decision of hemiarthroplasty versus total shoulder arthroplasty must be considered. The ultimate decision usually cannot be made until the joint has been opened and the tissues and bone have been inspected; however, some idea might be gained preoperatively from radiographs, CT scan, or MRI. We rarely obtain the latter two studies, however. In the rheumatoid shoulder, it is generally better to perform a total shoulder arthroplasty whenever possible because of more predictable pain control and better postoperative range of motion. For these reasons, it is important to resort to total shoulder arthroplasty before advanced disease can lead to anatomic deficiency that might preclude its use.[28] Leaving behind any articular surface might allow the synovitis and pannus formation to continue.[29] In cases with severe loss of glenoid bone or massive rotator cuff tear, a hemiarthroplasty is appropriate. The basic decision hinges on two factors: (1) Is there enough rotator cuff function to center the head in the glenoid, or has the head migrated up under the acromion? If the latter, then a hemiarthroplasty without glenoid replacement is used. (2) Is there adequate bone for glenoid component implantation? If there is not, then again a humeral head replacement alone is employed.

There is a growing number of articles in the literature that suggest that if repair of the rotator cuff is possible, a total shoulder prosthesis may be used.[30–32] In general, the results reported are better than those of hemiarthroplasty, but the actual groups of pure rheumatoid shoulders included in these studies are small. The cuff tissue of the rheumatoid is thin and friable, and it is difficult to obtain a dependable repair. The cuff should be in good condition or have a reasonable repair to prevent early glenoid loosening as a result of the "rocking horse effect," or eccentric superior loading of the glenoid component.[33] For irreparable tears of the rotator cuff, the hemiarthroplasty is a better choice than resection or constrained arthroplasty.[34] Sneppen and associates[35] suggested stricter indications for arthroplasty and cemented hemiarthroplasty for all advanced disease, to avoid the long-term complications of proximal migration and glenoid loosening.

Final considerations for implantation include the constrained prosthesis. This is not an appropriate choice in the rheumatoid population because undue stress may be transmitted to the osteoporotic bone, leading to periprosthetic fracture. The bipolar prosthesis advocated by Worland and Arredondo[36] is an attempt to deal with the specific concern of the high rate of glenoid complications and therefore is designed to function without a glenoid component. Although their results are promising, the study population contained only two rheumatoid cases, and the follow-up period was only 2.9 years. Our experience with the bipolar prosthesis is limited.

Finally, before beginning surgery, it is necessary to have the long-stem revision–type prosthesis available. This would be needed if the combination of joint contracture and osteoporotic bone leads to fracture of the humeral shaft. The surgeon must be prepared to cement the prosthesis because bone loss may obviate a good interference fit.

The deltopectoral approach is used for implantation of the prosthesis. During dissection, great care and consideration is given to the tissues. Periodically, all retractors are removed to allow tissue to reperfuse. The rotator interval is located exactly so as not to split into the substance of either muscle. The cephalic vein is unroofed and retracted medially with the pectoralis major. The deltoid is elevated from the humerus distally from its tendon insertion to proximally where the circumflex branch of the axillary nerve can be palpated. At this point, the subdeltoid and subacromial bursae can be débrided. The biceps tendon can be inspected, débrided, or, if severely diseased, resected. A tenodesis is performed at the most proximal aspect of the remaining tendon at the level of the pectoralis major tendon insertion.

The rotator cuff integrity can now be inspected for any bear spots. Better visualization is possible after disarticulation and resection of the head. The subscapularis is incised in one cut approximately 1 cm from its insertion with the capsule after the circumflex vessels are located and tied anteroinferiorly. The rotator interval is separated, and after the axillary nerve is located and protected inferomedially, the subscapularis can be completely mobilized. With retraction sutures in the tendinous substance, the capsule can be separated and excised down to the anterior glenoid. If the tissues are thin, the capsule is not excised but left with the subscapularis tendon. The subscapularis can then move as the surgeon pulls on the sutures. This release usually is enough so that a lengthening of the subscapularis tendon is not necessary.

If osteophytes are visible on the now-dislocated humerus, they are removed at their base with a curved osteotome. The presence of osteophytes, especially inferomedial osteophytes, can make the osteotomy cut of the head in too much varus. After the anatomic head is excised, the glenoid and rotator cuff can be completely inspected, and decisions about cuff repair and/or glenoid placement can be made.

Next, the proximal humerus is reamed progressively to find the appropriate stem size to be cemented in place. A stem is then trialed in about 20 to 30 degrees of retroversion. If a glenoid is to be placed, attention is now aimed at its preparation. The coracoacromial arch must be preserved as a buffer against superior humeral migration.

The glenoid may require reaming to smooth its surface to match the back of the glenoid trial. A burr is used to create a channel for the keel of the glenoid component. Its entry into the subchondral bone is slender, just permitting the keel, but an undercut is made slightly in all directions to allow the cement to grip the glenoid under surface. The direction of the keel entrance is important, because the glenoid is retroverted 4 to 12 degrees. Care must be taken not to perforate the glenoid. When this maneuver is complete, the canal is packed with a thrombin-soaked sponge and then peroxide-soaked sponge while cement is being mixed. The cement is packed into the glenoid with a lap sponge, and finally the all polyethylene glenoid is introduced and held until the cement is hardened.

Once this is complete, the prosthesis can be tested for stem and head size. A cement plug is inserted beyond the tip of the prosthesis. The canal is irrigated and prepared, as was the glenoid. Nonabsorbable sutures are placed through the edge of the prepared tuberosity for later approximation of the subscapularis tendon. Cement is mixed to a loose consistency and introduced over a suction tube with a 60-mL syringe. The prosthesis is introduced with the appropriate retroversion. Once the cement has hardened, the head is placed and the shoulder tested. It should have about 50% anteroposterior and superoinferior translation.

The subscapularis is secured anatomically with the preplaced sutures in a series of Mason-Allen and simple sutures. The lateral part of the rotator interval is reapproximated with absorbable sutures. The wound is irrigated and closed in layers over a drain with absorbable sutures.

The following day, physical therapy, consisting of all passive exercises, is begun. These exercises include pendulum, elevation in the scapular plane, external rotation with a stick, and hand and elbow range of motion. Physical therapy is continued on an outpatient basis, and active exercising is gently progressed to resistive exercising over several months. The results have been more durable than those of hip and knee replacement, and they are extremely gratifying as to pain relief. Function has depended on the status of the muscles (especially the rotator cuff) at the time of arthroplasty.

## CONCLUSIONS

Shoulder involvement in RA generally leads to replacement arthroplasty. The results are far better if performed before irreversible loss of bone and tendons preclude a complete reconstruction.

## REFERENCES

1. Schaardenburg van D, Breedveld FC: Elderly-onset rheumatoid arthritis. Semin Arthritis Rheum 1994; 23:367–378.

2. Ward RH, Hasstedt SJ, Clegg DO: Population prevalence of rheumatoid arthritis is lower than formerly supposed. Arthritis Rheum 1992; 35:S126.
3. Dordick JR: Rheumatoid arthritis in the elderly. J Am Geriatr Soc 1956; 4:588–591.
4. Deal CL, Meenan RF, Goldenberg DL, et al: The clinical features of elderly-onset rheumatoid arthritis. Arthritis Rheum 1985; 28:987–994.
5. Inoue K, Shichikawa K, Nishioka J, et al: Older age onset rheumatoid arthritis with or without osteoarthritis. Ann Rheum Dis 1987; 46:908–911.
6. Cuomo F, Greller MJ, Zuckerman JD: The rheumatoid shoulder. Rheum Dis Clin North Am 1998; 24:67–82.
7. Lipsky PE: Rheumatoid arthritis. *In* Wilson JD, Braunwald E, Isselbacher KJ (eds): Harrison's Principles of Internal Medicine, 12th ed. New York: McGraw-Hill, 1991:1437–1442.
8. Cofield RH: Degenerative and arthritic problems of the glenohumeral joint. *In* Rockwood CA, Matsen FA (eds): The Shoulder. Philadelphia, WB Saunders, 1990:678–749.
9. Slawson SH, Everson LI, Craig EV: The Radiology of Total Shoulder Replacement. Radiol Clin North Am 1995; 33:305–318.
10. Petersson CJ: The acromioclavicular joint in rheumatoid arthritis. Clin Orthop 1987; 223:86–93.
11. Winalski CS, Palmer WE, Rosenthal DI, et al: Magnetic resonance imaging of rheumatoid arthritis. Radiol Clin North Am 1996; 34:243–258.
12. Poleksic L, Zdravkovic D, Jablanovic D, et al: Magnetic resonance imaging of bone destruction in rheumatoid arthritis: Comparison with radiography. Skeletal Radiol 1993; 22:577.
13. Gubler FM, Algra PR, Maas M, et al: Gadolineum-DTPA–enhanced magnetic resonance imaging of bone cysts in patients with rheumatoid arthritis. Ann Rheum Dis 1993; 62:716.
14. Munk PL, Vellet AD, Levin MF, et al: Intravenous administration of gadolinium in the evaluation of rheumatoid arthritis of the shoulder. Can Assoc Radiol J 1993; 44:99.
15. Behrend R: Ultrasonographic diagnosis of inflammatory-rheumatic changes of the shoulder. Orthopedics 1993; 22:301–306.
16. O'Callaghan JW, Brooks PM: Disease-modifying agents and immunosuppressive drugs in the elderly. Clin Rheum Dis 1986; 12:275–289.
17. Lamy PP: Drug prescribing in the elderly. *In* Reichel W (ed): Clinical Aspects of Aging. Baltimore: Williams & Wilkins, 1983:21–71.
18. Karpman RR, McComb JE, Volz RG: Tendon rupture following local steroid injection: Report of four cases. Postgrad Med 1980; 68(1):169–174.
19. Sbarbaro JL Jr: The rheumatoid shoulder. Orthop Clin North Am 1975; 6(2):593–596.
20. Weiss JJ, Thompson GR, Doust V, et al: Rotator cuff tears in rheumatoid arthritis. Arch Intern Med 1975; 135:521–525.
21. Rylance HJ, Chalmers TM: Clinical trials of intra-articular aspirin in rheumatoid arthritis. Lancet 1980; 81:1099–1102.
22. Matsen FA, Rockwood CA, Wirth MA, et al: Glenohumeral arthritis and its management. *In* Rockwood CA, Matsen FA, Wirth MA, et al (eds): The Shoulder, 2nd ed. Philadelphia: WB Saunders, 1998:840–964.
23. Pahle JA, Kvarnes L: Shoulder synovectomy. Ann Chirurg Gynaecol 1985; 198(suppl 75):37–39.
24. Wakitani S, Imoto K, Saito M, et al: Evaluation of surgeries for rheumatoid shoulder based on the destructive pattern. J Rheumatol 1999; 26:41–6.
25. Gariepy R: Glenoidectomy in the repair of the rheumatoid shoulder. J Bone Joint Surg Br 1977; 59:122.
26. Wainwright D: Glenoidectomy in the treatment of the painful arthritic shoulder [Abstract]. J Bone Joint Surg Br 1976; 58:377.
27. Waldman BJ, Figgie MP: Indications, technique, and results of total shoulder arthroplasty in rheumatoid arthritis. Orthop Clin North Am 1998; 29:435–444.
28. Shon FG, Connor PM, Arroyo JS, et al: Shoulder arthroplasty for rheumatoid arthritis. Orthop Trans 1997; 21:17.
29. Boyd AD, Thomas WH, Scott RD, et al: Total shoulder arthroplasty versus hemiarthroplasty. J Arthroplasty 1990; 5:329–336.
30. Levine WN, Pollock RG: Prosthetic replacement in the rotator cuff-deficient patient. Semin Arthroplasty 1997; 8:321–327.
31. Rozing PM, Brand R: Rotator cuff repair during shoulder arthroplasty in rheumatoid arthritis. J Arthroplasty 1998; 13:311–319.
32. Zeman CA, Arcand MA, Cantrell JS, et al: The rotator cuff-deficient arthritic shoulder: Diagnosis and surgical management. J Am Acad Orthop Surg 1998; 6:337–348.
33. Franklin JL, Barrett WP, Jackins SE, et al: Glenoid loosening in total shoulder arthroplasty. Association with rotator cuff deficiency. J Arthroplasty 1988; 3:39–46.
34. Williams GR, Rockwood CA: Hemiarthroplasty in rotator cuff-deficient shoulders. J Shoulder Elbow Surg 1996; 5:362–367.
35. Sneppen O, Fruensgaard S, Johannsen HV, et al: Total shoulder replacement in rheumatoid arthritis: Proximal migration and loosening. J Shoulder Elbow Surg 1996; 5:47–52.
36. Worland RL, Arredondo J: Bipolar arthroplasty for painful conditions of the shoulder. J Arthroplasty 1998; 13:631–637.

# 5 | Neck Pain

*Robert S. Boretz, Baron S. Lonner, Jean-Jacques Abitbol, and Steven R. Garfin*

Neck pain is one of the most common complaints confronting the health care provider.[1] The source of discomfort is usually related to cervical spine pathology, but neck pain can be referred from adjacent structures or be related to systemic diseases.

Cervical pain is a subjective complaint that can be defined as pain perceived between the occiput and midscapular region. Although neck pain is often an isolated complaint, it may occur in association with headache, radiculopathy, or myelopathy.

The physician must seek a pathologic basis for a patient's symptoms in order to coordinate a treatment plan and to determine prognosis. A thorough understanding of cervical spine anatomy, available diagnostic modalities, and differential diagnosis enables the physician to formulate a treatment plan aimed at a specific pathology or group of organic causes of pain.

This chapter provides an overview of cervical spine anatomy, pain generators, and the multiple conditions that cause neck discomfort, with an emphasis on diagnosis and treatment.

## ANATOMY

The neck comprises the region between the base of the skull and the thoracic inlet. The cervical spine functions to support the head in space, to allow a wide range of motion (ROM), and to protect the spinal cord and other vital structures. Knowledge of cervical spine anatomy is important to understanding its role in painful conditions.

## Functional Anatomy

The cervical spine is composed of seven cervical vertebrae, which articulate with the occiput cranially and the thoracic spine caudally. The atlas (C1) is a ringlike structure that articulates with the occipital condyles to form a diarthrodial joint that allows for flexion, extension, and lateral bending. The second cervical vertebra or axis (C2) serves as a pivot for C1, allowing approximately 50% of cervical spine rotational motion.[2] The subaxial spine articulates posteriorly through the zygapophyseal joints that contain hyaline cartilage. The facet joints are synovial-lined, diarthrodial joints that are oriented approximately 45 degrees

to the horizontal and become more vertically oriented caudally. Mechanical and nociceptive nerve endings have been located in the facet capsules.[3] Furthermore, the vertebral bodies of C2 through C7 articulate at the synovial-lined uncovertebral joints (joints of Luschka), which are formed at the posterolateral aspects of the vertebral bodies. The intervertebral discs are composed of the outer annulus fibrosis surrounding the centrally located nucleus pulposus. The main ligamentous structures of the cervical spine include the anterior longitudinal ligament, posterior longitudinal ligament (PLL), ligamentum flavum, interspinous ligaments, supraspinous ligaments, and facet joint capsules (Fig. 5–1). The transverse ligament is an important restraint to anterior translation at the atlantodental articulation, which is itself synovial-lined. This joint is often involved early in rheumatoid disease, resulting in attenuation and, at times, complete disruption of the transverse ligament. The apical and alar ligaments are secondary restraints to occipitocervical motion.

## Neuroanatomy and Pain Generators

The spinal canal contains the spinal cord, which is encased by the thecal sac. Dorsal (sensory) and ventral (motor) roots exit the spinal cord to give rise to the spinal nerves. The ventral nerve root lies adjacent to the uncovertebral joint, and the dorsal nerve root lies adjacent to the facet joint. This has implications with respect to radicular pain in degenerative cervical spine disease. Just proximal to the formation of the spinal nerve, the dorsal nerve root enlarges to become the dorsal root ganglion (DRG) within the intervertebral foramina. The DRG appears to be sensitive to mechanical stresses and pressure increases caused by edema and direct compression and is at least partially responsible for the onset of radicular pain.[4, 5] Just distal to the DRG, the sinuvertebral nerve originates from a somatic root (ventral ramus) and an autonomic root (vertebral nerve). This nerve innervates the PLL, the outer third of the annulus fibrosus, the dura mater, epidural veins, and the nerve root sleeves[6–8] (Fig. 5–2).

Medial branches of the cervical dorsal rami richly innervate the facet joints.[9–11] Trauma and degeneration of the facet joints may lead to neck pain. In one study, 26% of patients in a group of 318 had facet joint pain

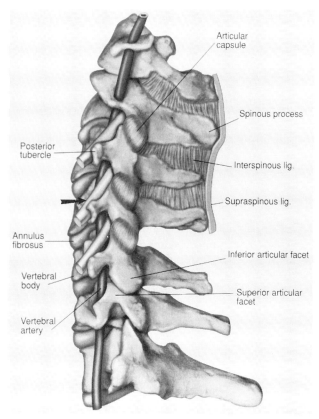

**FIGURE 5–1**
Lateral drawing of cervical spine. The *arrow* indicates a spinal nerve. (From Clark CR [ed]: The Cervical Spine, 3rd ed. Philadelphia: Lippincott-Raven, 1998:11.)

alone or in combination with discogenic pain after facet joint injection.[12] Furthermore, the proximity of the dorsal nerve root to the facet joint implicates hypertrophic degenerative changes in the cause of radicular pain.

The uncovertebral joints are not thought to play a major role in axial pain generation. However, degenerative changes of the uncovertebral joints may contribute to neuroforaminal narrowing and subsequent radicular pain.

The intervertebral discs receive a rich nerve supply, and annular tears have been implicated as a cause of neck pain.[6] Also, disc herniation can cause pain by direct pressure on the cervical nerve roots, spinal cord, or PLL.

The nociceptive response from nerve root compression is not solely a result of mechanical compression of nerve elements. In fact, persistent nerve root compression has been demonstrated on imaging studies despite resolution of pain.[13] Chemical mediators most probably play a role in pain pathways. Neurotransmitters such as substance P and somatostatin, along with chemicals such as bradykinin, serotonin, and histamine from non-neural tissues, modulate pain responses.[14, 15]

## EPIDEMIOLOGY

There has been a paucity of literature on the prevalence of neck pain in the general population, as compared with low back pain studies. This may in part reflect the fact that the economic impact of neck pain does not parallel that of low back pain.[16] Work absence is less commonly associated with neck pain than with back pain.

In a study from Norway, 34% of 9918 patients responded in a questionnaire that they had had an episode of significant neck pain within the past year.[17] Fourteen percent reported chronic pain (lasting longer than 6 months); this finding is comparable to the results of a Finnish questionnaire study of 8000 adults.[18] Chronic neck pain increased in frequency with age and was more common in women than in men.[17]

## DIAGNOSTIC EVALUATION

### History

A comprehensive history is invaluable toward making a diagnosis in a patient with neck pain. Often the diagnosis can be made solely from a detailed history, with the physical examination and imaging studies used for confirmation.

The history should elicit the nature of the pain, its location, its duration, and its intensity. The time of onset should be determined. Insidious onset might imply a degenerative condition, a tumor, or even an indolent infection. Acute onset may be associated with disc

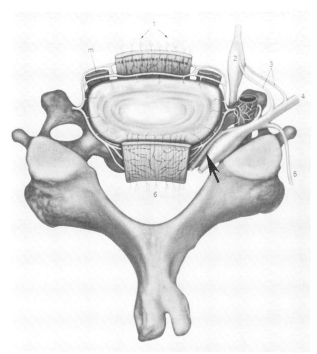

**FIGURE 5–2**
Schematic diagram of nerve plexus of the cervical spine.
(1) Anterior longitudinal ligament, (2) sympathetic trunk, (3) rami communicans, (4) ventral ramus of spinal nerve, (5) dorsal ramus of spinal nerve, (6) posterior longitudinal ligament. The *arrow* indicates a sinuvertebral nerve; m = longus coli muscle. (From Clark CR [ed]: The Cervical Spine, 3rd ed. Philadelphia: Lippincott-Raven, 1998:18.)

herniation or trauma. A helpful way to quantify a patient's perception of pain is to ask the patient to rate the pain on a scale from 1 to 10, with 1 as minimal and 10 as maximal, or on a pain analog diagram. Severe pain is more likely to be related to disc herniation or fracture. Pain worsening with a Valsalva maneuver may imply a space-occupying lesion such as a herniated disc. A history of radiating arm pain indicates nerve root impingement.

It is important to inquire about neurologic complaints. The presence of myelopathic symptoms such as poor balance, difficulty with ambulation, bowel and bladder dysfunction, and spasticity indicates spinal cord compression and adds urgency to diagnosis and treatment so as to prevent neurologic deterioration.

A thorough past medical history should include questions about malignancies, arthritis, and systemic disorders affecting bone. For example, a patient who has a history of inflammatory bowel disease may have an associated spondyloarthropathy that involves the cervical spine. Rheumatoid arthritis (RA) has a high predilection for involving the cervical spine.[19] Finally, a patient's employment status should be sought, as well as whether the pain is work related or associated with a worker's compensation claim. A history of ongoing litigation or other factors that might affect outcome should be sought. Psychosocioeconomic factors have been clearly shown to influence a patient's prognosis.[20]

## Physical Examination

A thorough general physical examination and evaluation of the neck, combined with a neurologic examination, is essential toward establishing a diagnosis for a patient with neck pain. The examination begins when the patient enters the room by inspecting how he or she holds the head. Splinting towards one side or torticollis may point to muscle spasm related to sprain, strain, fracture, or subluxation.

Next, the midline spinous processes of the cervical spine are palpated to assess for tenderness that would be consistent with fracture or ligamentous disruption. Muscle palpation is performed to assess for spasm. Anterior neck palpation is performed to assess for cervical lymph nodes, thyroid enlargement, or other masses that may represent benign or malignant tumors.

ROM should be assessed in flexion-extension, lateral rotation, and lateral bending. Passive ROM in which the examiner moves the spine through an arc of motion should be avoided, especially in the setting of trauma, to avoid possible fracture displacement and neurologic deterioration. In cases of trauma, radiographs should be evaluated before assessment of ROM. Limited motion may occur secondary to muscle spasm, pain, or congenital vertebral anomalies such as with a Klippel-Feil deformity, in which vertebrae are fused (Fig. 5–3).

The importance of the neurologic examination cannot be overstated. Cervical spine pathology often manifests with nerve root and/or spinal cord involvement. A detailed examination of nerve root function by evaluation of specific muscles, dermatomes, and reflexes indicates the level of pathology as well as degree of

severity (Table 5–1). For example, a C5–6 herniated intervertebral disc most commonly manifests with C6 radicular findings (i.e., weakness of wrist dorsiflexion; diminished sensation in the radial aspect of the forearm, thumb, and index finger; and absence of the brachioradialis reflex). Upper motor neuron signs may be indicative of spinal cord compression and should be tested. These include hyperreflexia of deep tendon reflexes caudal to the level of spinal cord involvement, Hoffman's sign, ankle clonus, Babinski reflexes, and spasticity. Lhermitte's sign is a shocklike sensation experienced when the patient's head is flexed or extended; it is associated with myelopathy caused by spinal cord compression. Because a number of lesions and diseases other than degenerative disc disease can manifest with these findings, a careful evaluation is essential. These other entities include but are not limited to syringomyelia, hydrocephalus, space-occupying lesions in the calvarium and spinal canal, multiple sclerosis, Friedreich's ataxia, and tabes dorsalis.

There are several specialized tests that are helpful in assessing cervical spine pathology. The distraction and compression tests may relieve or exacerbate pain related to degenerative narrowing of the neuroforamina.[21, 22] These tests are performed by gently distracting and compressing the patient's head axially and assessing for a change in radicular symptoms indicating nerve root compression in degenerative disc disease. Spurling's test is performed by having the patient turn the head toward the side of arm pain and applying compression to the head (Fig. 5–4). This test is also specific for reproducing nerve root symptoms. Neck or radicular pain with a Valsalva maneuver that worsens may suggest a space-occupying lesion such as a disc herniation or tumor.

Finally, the physical examination should include related areas that can cause referred neck pain. The temporomandibular joint is a common site for pain, which may occur concomitantly with cervical injury after a so-called whiplash injury. The shoulder should also be examined carefully. Rotator cuff pathology and glenohumeral arthritis can produce symptoms similar to those of referred neck pain or radiculopathy.

## Diagnostic Modalities

Imaging, electrodiagnostic studies, and laboratory studies can all provide useful information in the evaluation of a patient with neck pain. Imaging studies are essential to determine the exact site of pathology and confirm a clinical diagnosis. Importantly, radiographic findings do not always correspond to clinically relevant pathology; the physician must always correlate imaging findings with the patient's presentation. Boden et al. demonstrated a major abnormality on cervical spine magnetic resonance imaging (MRI) in 19% of asymptomatic subjects.[23]

A plain radiograph should be the first imaging study obtained. It is a good screening tool for assessing for fractures, degenerative disease, destructive lesions, and congenital anomalies. Recommended standard

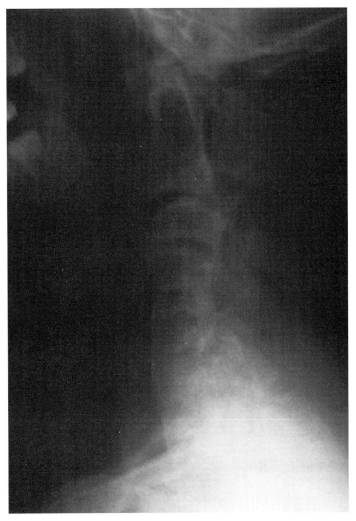

**FIGURE 5–3**
Lateral radiograph of congenitally fused cervical vertebrae in a patient with Klippel-Feil syndrome.

cervical spine views include an open-mouth antero-posterior view, an anteroposterior view of the lower cervical spine, and a lateral view. Specialized views of the cervical spine may provide additional detail. These include a Fuchs (odontoid) view, oblique views, swimmer's view, and pillar view. A Fuchs view is useful to assess injuries to the dens. Oblique views demonstrate the patency of the neural foramina for patients with radicular findings. In the setting of trauma, the cervical spine cannot be cleared radiographically without visualizing the cervicothoracic junction. A swimmer's view demonstrates this area when downward traction of the shoulders on a lateral view fails to do so. After fractures and dislocations have been ruled out, flexion-extension views can be performed in an alert patient to rule out instability caused by ligamentous injuries.[24] This study

## TABLE 5–1
### Cervical Nerve Root Innervation

| NERVE ROOT | MUSCLES | REFLEX | SENSATION |
| --- | --- | --- | --- |
| C5 | Deltoid, biceps | Biceps | Lateral arm |
| C6 | Biceps, wrist extensors | Brachioradialis | Lateral forearm |
| C7 | Triceps, wrist flexors, finger extensors | Triceps | Middle finger |
| C8 | Hand intrinsics, finger flexors | None | Medial forearm |
| T1 | Hand intrinsics | None | Medial arm |

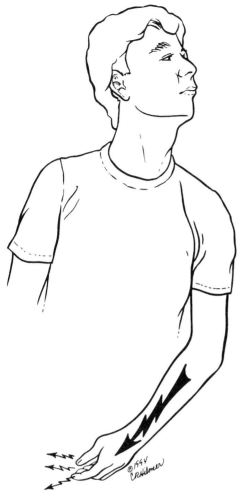

**FIGURE 5–4**
Spurling's sign. Extension and rotation toward the symptomatic side reproduces the radiculopathy. (From Clark CR [ed]: The Cervical Spine, 3rd ed. Philadelphia: Lippincott-Raven, 1998:759.)

must be done actively. Passive ROM should not be performed, because it may result in displacement of a fracture or dislocation. When the maneuver is performed actively by the patient, guarding prevent this from occurring. The utility of flexion-extension views in the acute setting is limited because muscle spasm may mask subtle instability. If a high degree of suspicion exists for instability, flexion-extension views should be obtained several days later.

Computed tomography (CT) of the cervical spine is indicated to evaluate fractures, spinal stenosis, congenital anomalies, ossification of the PLL, and bone tumors. CT affords excellent bone detail and is useful to characterize fractures as well as to detect occult fractures.[25] MRI is preferred to CT for detection of disc herniation and soft tissue lesions; however, one study found contrast-enhanced CT to be equal to MRI in detecting central herniations and more sensitive for lateral herniations.[26] When combined with myelography, CT is highly effective in delineating the extent and causes of neural compression. Myelography is an invasive test that can result in spinal headache, nau-

sea/vomiting, and back pain. It is usually reserved for cases requiring surgical intervention to provide additional detail and when MRI is contraindicated.

MRI is unparalleled in its resolution of the central nervous system and associated soft tissue. Myelopathy caused by intrinsic spinal cord abnormalities or by compression from herniated disc material, tumor, infection, or hematoma is best diagnosed with MRI. Also, MRI can detect changes in vertebral marrow signal that may represent infection, tumor, or fracture. Intravenous gadolinium enhancement can help differentiate granulation tissue from recurrent disc herniation in a patient who has had surgery, and it is also useful in assessing the vascularity of a neoplasm.

Discography involves direct injection of the cervical discs percutaneously with contrast under fluoroscopy. The modality is used to assess disc morphology as well as symptom production. The test is considered positive when concordant symptoms are produced (i.e., the patient experiences pain similar to that experienced clinically). The injection of a local anesthetic with resolution of pain has also been deemed a positive test. Discography may be indicated in patients with chronic discogenic neck pain when imaging results are nonspecific and to evaluate the main pain generators when imaging shows multilevel disease.[27] The clinical utility of this modality is controversial.[28, 29] Furthermore, in one study 13% of patients suffered a major complication, including one who developed quadriplegia.[29]

Scintigraphy plays a limited role in the evaluation of neck pain. Technetium bone scanning is a useful adjunct for detection of radiographically occult fractures, metabolically active tumors, and infection and for screening for distant lesions in metastatic disease. Single photon emission computed tomography (SPECT) provides an axial image of the cervical spine and can detect occult fractures and periostitis after trauma.[30]

Electromyography and nerve conduction studies provide further confirmation and clarification of clinically significant nerve compression. They can be used to distinguish between lesions at the level of the nerve root, brachial plexus, or peripheral nerve. Cervical nerve root compression may occur in combination with a peripheral nerve lesion; this has been termed the "double crush" syndrome.[31] It can present a diagnostic and treatment dilemma that may be further evaluated with use of this diagnostic modality.

Laboratory studies can be useful in diagnosing a patient with neck pain related to systemic disease such as hyperparathyroidism, RA, multiple myeloma, human immunodeficiency virus myelopathy or infection. An elevated white blood cell count, erythrocyte sedimentation rate, and C-reactive protein concentration are suggestive of infection. Serum protein electrophoresis and urine testing for Bence Jones proteins make the diagnosis of multiple myeloma. Serum calcium, phosphate, and parathyroid hormone levels are evaluated to rule out hyperparathyroidism. In a patient with suspected meningitis, cerebrospinal fluid testing is mandatory.

# SPECIFIC CAUSES OF NECK PAIN

The causes of neck pain are multiple and encompass a wide spectrum of pathology. General categories include cervical degenerative disc disease, traumatic causes, inflammatory, infectious, neoplastic, congenital, nonspinal, and psychological etiologies (Table 5–2). Specific entities and their treatment are discussed in this section.

## Cervical Degenerative Disc Disease

Degenerative disc disease can be divided into two types of clinical presentation. Soft disc herniations tend to occur in middle-aged patients who present with acute neck pain, radiculopathy, and/or myelopathy. Pain may be related to the annular tear, tension in the bulging disc, or neural compression.[32]

Spondylosis is the normal result of aging and is seen in a majority of patients over 70 years of age. With age, the intervertebral disc desiccates, with resultant narrowing, increased motion, disc bulging, and endplate osteophyte formation.[33–35] Also, increased motion results in facet joint degeneration, with osteophyte formation and ligamentum flavum hypertrophy resulting in spinal stenosis. Axial neck pain, radicular pain, and/or myelopathy may ensue.

Nonoperative treatment consists of nonsteroidal anti-inflammatory drugs (NSAIDs) and early gentle passive ROM exercises. Narcotics may be used acutely for severe pain, but prolonged use is discouraged, particularly in the elderly. Active modalities may begin when pain improves.

Surgical treatment is reserved for patients with persistent radicular symptoms unresponsive to nonopera-

## TABLE 5–2
## Causes of Neck Pain

Degenerative cervical disc disease
    Disc herniation
    Cervical spondylosis
    Cervical stenosis
Trauma
    Soft tissue injuries (strain, sprain, whiplash syndrome)
    Fractures and dislocations
Inflammatory causes
    Rheumatoid arthritis
    Seronegative spondyloarthopathies (ankylosing spondylitis,
        psoriatic arthritis, reactive arthritis, inflammatory bowel
        disease)
Infectious causes
    Discitis
    Vertebral osteomyelitis
    Grisel's syndrome
Neoplastic causes
    Primary bone, soft tissue, and neural tumors
    Metastatic disease
Congenital causes
    Klippel-Feil (congenital fusion)
    Arnold-Chiari malformations (syringomyelia)
Nonspinal causes
    Esophagitis, lymphandenitis, TMJ pathology, other
Psychogenic causes

tive treatment for 6 weeks, progressive neurologic deficit, or static neurologic deficits with significant radicular pain.[36] In addition, there must be confirmatory imaging that correlates with the patient's symptoms. The mainstay of surgical treatment has been an anterior discectomy with fusion for one- or two-level degenerative disease or disc herniation.[37, 38] In cases in which myelopathy is present in association with large osteophytes, vertebrectomy with strut grafting is indicated (Fig. 5–5). At times a more extensive anterior and posterior approach is required. A posterior decompression via a multilevel laminectomy may be indicated for patients with multilevel stenosis when cervical lordosis is preserved.

Surgical treatment for neck pain alone is generally discouraged because results have not improved upon the natural history of the problem.[36] If there is no clearly identifiable lesion on imaging studies, discography and/or facet joint injections may be indicated to localize the pain generator.[39, 40]

## Traumatic Causes

The spectrum of injury that can cause neck pain ranges from a sudden twisting injury to fracture-dislocations resulting from high-energy trauma. The most frequently identifiable causes of fracture in adults are motor vehicle accident (38%), falls (26%), diving accidents (11%), and gunshot wounds (4%).[41]

Soft tissue injuries of the cervical spine usually result from an acceleration injury of the head on the thorax. It is usually the result of a rear-end motor vehicle accident and has been termed *whiplash, acceleration injury, cervical sprain-strain syndrome,* or *hyperextension injury.* The patient usually presents with nonradiating neck pain and occipital headache. Diagnostic imaging studies are usually inconclusive. If a patient's symptoms persist, flexion-extension views, facet joint injections, or discography may assist to identify the pain generator. The majority of patients fully recover within 3 months; however, up to 40% of patients develop chronic pain.[42] Poor prognostic indicators include increased severity and prolonged duration of symptoms, age older than 50 years, ongoing litigation, pain radiation into the upper extremities, and associated thoracic and lumbar pain.[42]

Although traditional treatment of whiplash has been immobilization and rest, more recent studies have documented no difference in outcome with early treatment with immobilization and traction versus uncontrolled ROM.[43–45] In general, recommended treatment consists of minimal immobilization with a soft collar, NSAIDs, and early return to normal activities.[46, 47]

A patient who presents with neck pain after significant trauma should be immobilized and a cervical spine fracture should be suspected until proven otherwise. The consequences of a missed fracture include neurologic deficit, paralysis, and death. The history should elicit the mechanism of injury and the amount of energy involved. A cross-table lateral cervical spine radiograph demonstrates the majority of fractures. Additional views increase the diagnostic yield, but CT is

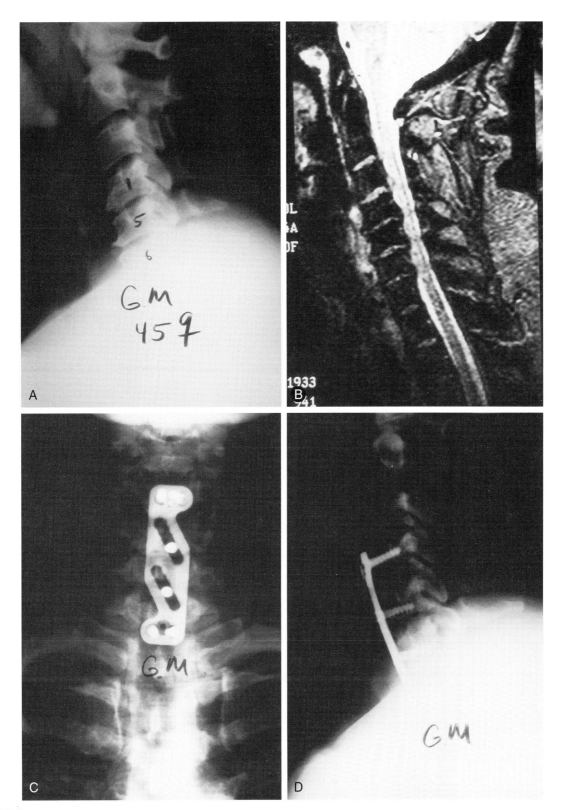

**FIGURE 5–5**
Preoperative and postoperative radiographs and magnetic resonance images (MRI) of three-level discectomy and fusion with instrumentation for multilevel degenerative disc disease. *A,* Preoperative lateral radiograph. *B,* Preoperative sagittal T2-weighted MRI. *C,* Postoperative anteroposterior radiograph. *D,* Postoperative lateral radiograph.

superior to identify occult fractures and to better define known fractures.

Fractures and dislocations of the cervical spine are divided into those occurring in the upper cervical spine and those in the subaxial spine. Upper cervical spine injuries include occipital condyle fractures, occipito-atlantal dislocations, atlas fractures, odontoid fractures, traumatic spondylolisthesis of the axis, and atlantoaxial rotatory instability. Allen and coworkers classified injuries to the subaxial spine into six groups and subdivided them by severity.[48] These groups are classified by mechanism of injury and include compression-flexion, distraction-flexion, vertical compression, compression-extension, distraction-extension, and lateral bending. White and colleagues classified cervical spine stability on the basis of radiographic alignment, degree of anatomic disruption, and functional neurologic deficit.[49] Angulation of more than 11 degrees, angular motion of more than 22 degrees, or translation of more than 3.5 mm at a spinal segment is considered unstable (Fig. 5–6).

It is beyond the scope of this chapter to discuss particular injuries and their respective treatment. In general, stable injuries are treated with a period of immobilization in a cervical collar or cervicothoracic orthosis. Unstable injuries may require surgical treatment. Management decisions depend on the degree of instability and neurologic injury, concomitant injuries, and available resources. In general, spinal alignment is restored, decompression of neural elements is performed, and the spine is stabilized via arthrodesis.

## Inflammatory Causes

The cervical spine is involved in the majority of patients with RA, with 43% to 86% developing subluxations and 7% to 34% developing a neurologic deficit.[50] The most common type of cervical subluxation is atlantoaxial instability, followed by basilar invagination and subaxial subluxations.

Routine evaluation of patients with RA must include a thorough neurologic examination and baseline radiographs to rule out cervical instability patterns. Objective neurologic motor grading is often made difficult by the generalized weakness and severe deformity of the extremities associated with the disease. Atlantoaxial subluxation can be assessed on the lateral radiograph by measuring the anterior atlantodental interval (AADI) and the posterior atlantodental interval (PADI) (Fig. 5–7). The normal AADI is 3 mm or less in adults and 4 mm or less in children. Flexion-extension views may demonstrate dynamic instability. MRI is more sensitive in establishing spinal cord compression because the cord can be directly visualized. The presence of a soft tissue pannus at the atlantoaxial articulation which limits the space available for the spinal cord is also best demonstrated on MRI.[51] Many radiographic lines and measurements have been described to assess for basilar invagination or atlantoaxial impaction.[52, 53] Finally, subaxial instability is best assessed on lateral radiographic dynamic views and MRI. Flexion-extension MRI studies provide additional information on the dynamic nature of instability and neural com-

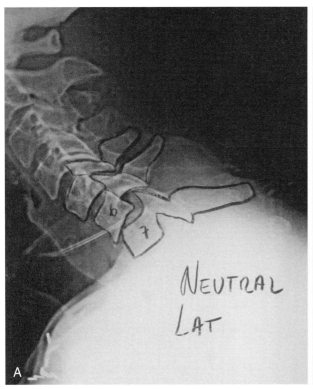
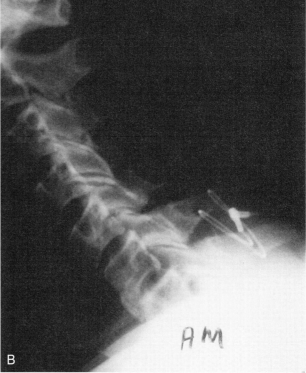

**FIGURE 5–6**
Lateral radiograph demonstrating late post-traumatic instability and kyphosis at C6–7 treated with posterior wiring. *A,* Preoperative lateral radiograph. *B,* Postoperative lateral radiograph.

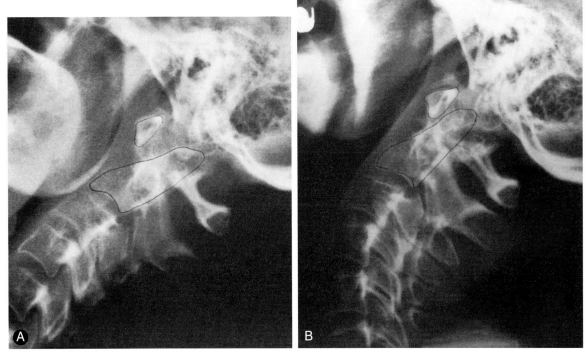

**FIGURE 5–7**
Lateral flexion-extension views of the cervical spine in a patient with rheumatoid arthritis, demonstrating dynamic instability at C1–2 with increase in the anterior atlantodental interval (AADI) with flexion. *A*, Flexion lateral radiograph. *B*, Extension lateral radiograph.

pression.[54] Any patient with RA who is scheduled to undergo general anesthesia must be evaluated with lateral flexion-extension radiographs to rule out instability that may result in intraoperative quadriplegia.

The goals of management for the patient with RA and neck pain are to prevent irreversible neurologic deficit and maintain comfort. Indications for fusion include intractable neck pain, neurologic deficits, or both in association with cervical instability. Any patient with radiographic instability should be referred for surgical evaluation.

The seronegative spondyloarthropathies may also manifest with neck pain secondary to inflammation or ossification of ligamentous and tendinous structures. They include ankylosing spondylitis (AS), psoriatic arthritis, reactive arthritis (formerly known as Reiter's syndrome), and inflammatory bowel arthropathy. The mainstay of treatment for these patients is NSAIDs, especially indomethacin, as well as physical therapy.[55] Of particular significance, patients with AS develop a rigid (fused) neck. These patients may develop unrecognized fractures in response to minimal trauma or expanding epidural hematomas that can result in catastrophic neurologic injury if not addressed immediately.[55, 56] Therefore, after trauma any patient with AS should be immobilized and evaluated with radiographs. MRI is useful to detect occult fractures and to evaluate for spinal cord compression caused by epidural hematoma or by translocation of the fractured spinal column. There is a high incidence of neurologic complications in patients with AS, so immediate immobilization and, in some instances, surgical stabilization are indicated.[55]

## Infectious Causes

Infections do not involve the cervical spine as frequently as they involve the thoracic or lumbar spine. However, there is a greater potential for severe neurologic sequelae and disability because of the relatively small diameter of the spinal canal in this region. Prompt diagnosis is necessary to minimize morbidity.

Infections often originate in the intervertebral disc (discitis) or endplate and then commonly spread to the vertebrae, resulting in osteomyelitis. Epidural abscess may occur primarily or secondary to osteomyelitis or prior surgery. Infection may occur as a result of hematogenous spread, iatrogenic seeding from surgery, or locally from penetrating trauma. Hematogenous vertebral osteomyelitis, discitis, and epidural infections have been increasing in frequency, owing in part to an increase in intravenous drug use, an increase in the elderly population, and an increase in the number of immunocompromised individuals. Responsible organisms include staphylococci, streptococci, and *Mycobacterium tuberculosis*. In immunosuppressed patients, atypical mycobacteria and fungi must be considered.

If the diagnosis is suspected by history, physical examination, and laboratory studies, an MRI should be performed. MRI is 96% sensitive and 93% specific in detecting vertebral infection.[57] The addition of gadolinium can further increase sensitivity, especially for abscess formation. However, biopsy is necessary to make an absolute diagnosis and to determine the specific organism involved. CT-guided aspiration may prove useful, although false-negative aspirations are not uncommon. The mainstay of treatment is immobilization and intravenous antibiotic therapy. Surgery is indicated for abscess formation, for failure of the infection to respond to nonoperative management, to decompress neural elements in the presence of neurologic deficits, and to correct deformity (Fig. 5–8). Tuberculous spondylitis is most commonly treated with a 9-month course of rifampin and isoniazid.[58] Drug resistance is becoming more prevalent; therefore, when possible drug sensitivities should be determined. Surgical indications are the same as for pyogenic infection.

Grisel's syndrome usually occurs in patients less than 30 years of age, who present with neck pain and torticollis as a result of atlantoaxial rotatory subluxation. This occurs as a result of ligamentous laxity from parapharyngeal inflammation. Treatment is directed at the underlying infection. Neck immobilization is provided for comfort. If rotatory subluxation does not resolve, traction may be used. In rare instances, surgical reduction and stabilization are required.

## Neoplastic Causes

Neck pain is often a presenting complaint in patients with a cervical spine tumor. Primary tumors occurring in the cervical spine can be classified as extradural, intradural extramedullary, and intramedullary. The site of the tumor determines the exact clinical presentation.

Extramedullary tumors are the most common. They arise outside the dura in vertebral bodies and epidural tissue. Benign extradural tumors involve the cervical spine less commonly than do malignant tumors.[59] Benign tumors include osteoid osteoma, aneurysmal bone cyst, giant cell tumor, neurofibroma, osteoblastoma, and eosinophilic granuloma. Malignant tumors and metastatic disease occur in an older population. Primary malignant tumors include multiple myeloma, osteosarcoma, chondrosarcoma, Ewing's sarcoma, and chordoma. When a patient with a known history of malignancy presents with neck pain, a diagnosis of metastatic disease should be sought, because the spine is the most common site for osseous metastases.[60, 61] An MRI and technetium bone scan should be performed.

The majority of benign bone tumors can be treated nonoperatively or with simple excision. Specifically, osteoid osteomas can be managed with aspirin or NSAIDs alone.[62] Simple excision is indicated if medical treatment fails. Treatment of primary malignant extradural spine tumors usually involves wide excision with adjuvant therapy if the tumor is sensitive. The prognosis for these tumors is generally poor because of the difficulty in achieving complete resection with negative margins at their particular locations. Finally, treatment of metastatic disease is dependent on many variables, including the patient's life expectancy, tumor type, neurologic compromise, stability of the spine, and radiosensitivity of the tumor. If there is no deformity, instability, or neurologic involvement without bone destruction, prophylactic immobilization with a rigid orthosis, radiation, and chemotherapy is indicated. Surgical decompression, spinal reconstruction, and stabilization are indicated for progressive neurologic deficit, deformity, and instability[60] (Fig. 5–9).

Intradural extramedullary tumors occur in the leptomeninges or nerve roots. The most common tumors

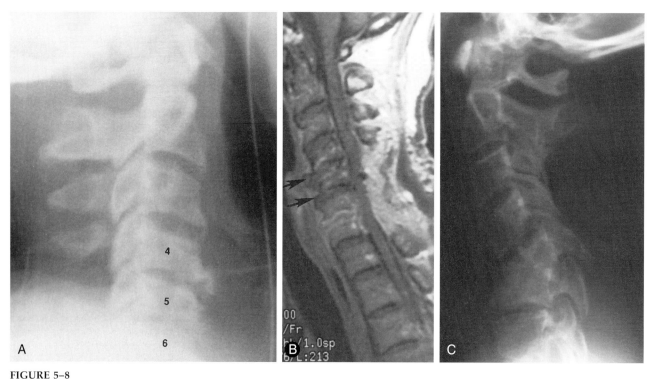

**FIGURE 5–8**
Lateral cervical spine radiographs and magnetic resonance image (MRI) demonstrating disc space narrowing and endplate destruction at C4–5 and C5–6 secondary to pyogenic infection. *A*, Lateral radiograph. *B*, Sagittal T2-weighted MRI. *C*, Lateral radiograph.

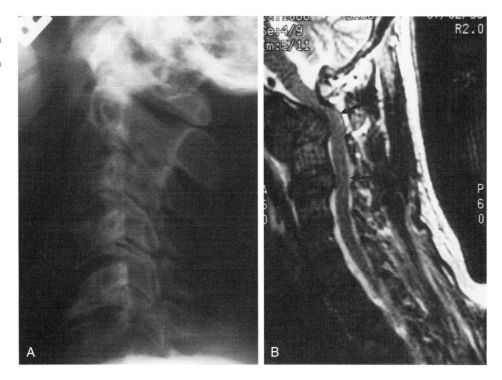

**FIGURE 5–9**
Lateral cervical spine radiograph and magnetic resonance image (MRI) demonstrating destruction of C3 and C5 with collapse, kyphosis, and spinal cord compression secondary to metastatic disease. *A*, Lateral radiograph. *B*, Sagittal T2-weighted MRI. The arrow indicates spinal cord compression.

are meningiomas and neurofibromas. Less commonly, sarcomas and metastases occur in this location. Treatment involves excision and is often curative, because the majority of intradural extramedullary tumors are benign.

Intramedullary tumors occur within the substance of the spinal cord and are uncommon. The majority are benign glial tumors, including astrocytoma and ependymoma. Cervical hemangioblastomas are seen frequently in patients with von Hippel–Lindau syndrome, an autosomal dominant inherited disorder characterized by retinal and cerebellar hemangioblastomas. Less common tumor types include lipomas, dermoids, epidermoids, teratomas, and neuroblastomas. Long-term control or cure can be achieved with microsurgical resection.

## Congenital Causes

Congenital cervical spine anomalies are an uncommon cause of neck pain. Klippel-Feil syndrome refers to any patient with congenitally fused cervical vertebrae (see Fig. 5–3). Classically, the patient with Klippel-Feil syndrome has a short webbed neck, low posterior hairline, and limited neck motion. These patients are prone to develop neck pain from degenerative disc disease at levels adjacent to fused vertebrae. Treatment is the same as for degenerative disc disease; however, these patients often require arthrodesis.

Arnold-Chiari malformation consists of herniation of a portion of the hindbrain into the cervical canal. There is a high association of syringomyelia in patients with Arnold-Chiari malformations. A syringomyelia is a fluid-filled cyst within the spinal cord that may cause neck pain and neurologic deficits. Also, syringo-

myelia occurs with other craniocervical junction malformations, congenital spinal malformations, intramedullary tumors, trauma, and infection. The natural history for syrinxes often involves progression of neurologic deficits, in which case surgical intervention is recommended. Treatment options include posterior fossa decompression, shunting procedures, and opening the cyst into the subarachnoid space.

## Nonspinal Causes

There are many conditions causing neck pain that are nonspinal in origin. Neck conditions that can mimic cervical pathology are esophagitis, lymphadenitis, and temporomandibular joint pathology. These can usually be diagnosed with an adequate history and physical examination.

Neck pain can be referred from structures with cervical innervation. The diaphragm is innervated by the third, fourth, and fifth cervical nerves. Subphrenic abscesses, hiatal hernias, and lower lung infiltrates can cause referred neck pain. Furthermore, a Pancoast tumor, which occurs in the apex of the lung, can manifest with neck pain. Inflammation involving the shoulder can cause deltotrapezial pain, which may be perceived as neck pain by the patient.

## Psychological Causes

The experience of neck pain is subjective. The emotional response to pain can be influenced by psychological and socioeconomic factors. Appreciating these factors enables the treating physician to screen for these barriers to recovery. Depression, personality disorders, alcoholism, and substance abuse can all contribute to the chronicity of a patient's condition. Also, monetary compensation has been shown to increase reports of pain and to have an adverse effect on prognosis.[20]

## APPROACH TO THE PATIENT WITH NECK PAIN

### Acute Neck Pain

The evaluation of the patient with acute neck pain begins with a careful history. Traumatic and nontraumatic causes of pain must be differentiated. If a patient has suffered trauma, the mechanism of injury and the energy involved in the impact must be determined. High-energy injuries that occur as a result of motor vehicle accidents or falls from heights may be associated with fractures or ligamentous disruption, which can lead to acute instability and neurologic deficits. In patients who are victims of trauma, the cervical spine must be immobilized immediately.

Physical examination consists of (1) palpation of the neck for areas of tenderness and/or step-offs that may indicate subluxation or dislocation of the spine and (2) a thorough neurologic examination. This is followed by radiographic assessment of the cervical spine. If there is evidence of fracture or ligamentous disruption, orthotic immobilization, halo vest immobilization, and/or surgical intervention may be indicated. The treatment of specific injuries is beyond the scope of this chapter. If fracture or dislocation has not occurred, the patient probably has a cervical sprain/strain syndrome, which often is ameliorated by periods of soft collar immobilization, nonsteroidal anti-inflammatory medication, ice and heat applications, physical therapy, and, in some cases, narcotic administration early on. Cervical sprain/strain (whiplash) is often characterized by relatively long symptomatic periods and may be refractory to the aforementioned interventions. In these cases, referral to a pain management service for injection therapy and other modalities may be indicated. Cineradiography and other imaging modalities should be used as needed to check for subtle instability injuries.

Even relatively low-energy impact may result in significant injuries. One of the authors treated a patient with previously undiagnosed ankylosing spondylitis who had been in a motor vehicle accident at approximately 20 miles per hour that resulted in an unstable fracture through the lower cervical spine. Patients with ankylosing spondylitis are prone to fracture even with minor injuries and are at risk for severe neurologic compromise and/or death as a result of epidural hematoma formation.

Other causes of acute neck pain include cervical disc herniation, pathologic fractures caused by neoplasm, and acute pyogenic disc space infection and secondary osteomyelitis.

Acute neck pain with or without radiculopathy should be assessed with a screening radiograph. If radiographs are normal and objective neurologic findings are minimal, the patient may be treated effectively with a nonsteroidal anti-inflammatory medication, brief periods of immobilization with a soft cervical collar, outpatient cervical traction, and physical therapy. If the patient fails to respond to a course of this conservative therapy, MRI of the cervical spine should be performed. Imaging should be performed immediately in patients who have significant objective neurologic findings.

### Chronic Neck Pain

The patient with chronic neck pain is also evaluated with a careful history, physical examination, and imaging studies. Information about the onset of pain, nature of symptoms, presence of constitutional or neurologic symptoms, and history of malignancy is elicited.

A very common presentation is that of a patient with neck pain and stiffness and diminished ROM accompanied by crepitus, in whom radiographs reveal diffuse osteoarthritis and degenerative disc disease. Such patients are best managed with a nonsteroidal anti-inflammatory medication or acetaminophen in combination with ROM and isometric strengthening exercises. Brief periods of soft collar immobilization may provide symptom relief. Physical therapy with a variety of modalities may also be of some benefit. Patients with neurologic deficits are evaluated with three-dimensional imaging studies such as MRI or CT myelography. Radicular symptoms associated with foraminal stenosis and disc herniation in the absence of profound neurologic deficit may be ameliorated by a trial of cervical epidural steroid injections. Myelopathy secondary to central stenosis necessitates operative decompression.

High-risk patients with rheumatoid arthritis should be evaluated and monitored annually with radiographs, including lateral flexion/extension views, to rule out instability. In patients with a history of malignancy, metastatic disease to the cervical spine can manifest as insidious neck pain. Similarly, nonvirulent bacterial organisms or mycobacteria may have an insidious onset and must be considered in the appropriate clinical setting. Disease metastatic to the spine in the absence of neurologic deficits, acute structural collapse, and progressive deformity is often treated effectively with a combination of local radiation therapy and halo or rigid collar immobilization. Infection can often be effectively managed with a combination of orthotic immobilization and chemotherapy.

## SUMMARY

There are a multitude of causes of neck pain, most of which result from cervical spine pathology. A thorough understanding of the conditions that afflict the cervical spine and the structures that cause pain enables the treating physician to formulate a diagnosis and treatment plan. A careful history and physical examination supplemented with diagnostic modalities lead to a timely diagnosis and treatment plan in the majority of patients. Early referral to a spine surgeon may be indicated to assist in management and to prevent neurologic deterioration.

# REFERENCES

1. Gore DR, Sepic SB, Gardner GM, et al: Neck pain: A long-term follow up of 205 patients. Spine 1987; 12:1–5.
2. Pennig L, Wilmink JT: Rotation of the cervical spine: A CT study on normal subjects. Spine 1987; 12:732–738.
3. McLain R: Mechanoreceptor endings in human cervical facet joints. Spine 1994; 19:495–502.
4. Rydevik D, Myer RR, Powel HC: Pressure increase in the dorsal root ganglion following mechanical compression: Closed compartment syndrome in nerve roots. Spine 1989; 14:574–576.
5. Vanderlinden RG: Subarticular entrapment of the dorsal root ganglion as a cause of sciatic pain. Spine 1984; 9:19–22.
6. Bogduk N, Windsor M, Inglis A: The innervation of the cervical intervertebral discs. Spine 1988; 13:2–8.
7. Groen G, Baljet B, Drukker J: Nerves and nerve plexuses of the human vertebral column. Am J Anat 1980; 188:282–296.
8. Groen G, Baljet B, Drukker J: The innervation of the spinal dura mater: Anatomy and clinical implications. Acta Neurochir 1988; 92:39–46.
9. Bogduk N, Aprill C: On the nature of neck pain, discography and cervical zygapophyseal joint block. Pain 1993; 54:213–217.
10. Bogduk N, Marslan A: The cervical zygapophyseal joints as a source of neck pain. Spine 1988; 13:610–617.
11. Bogduk N: The clinical anatomy of the cervical dorsal rami. Spine 1982; 7:319–330.
12. Aprill C, Bogduk N: The prevalence of cervical zygapophyseal joint pain. Spine 1991; 17:744–747.
13. Garfin SR, Rydevik BL, Brown RA: Compressive neuropathy of spinal nerve roots: A mechanical or biological problem? Spine 1991; 16:162–166.
14. Aimone LD: Neurochemistry and modulation of pain. In Sinatra RS (ed): Acute Pain: Mechanism and Management. St. Louis: Mosby–Year Book, 1992:29–43.
15. Marx JL: Brain peptides: Is substance P a transmitter of pain signals? Science 1979; 205:886–889.
16. Cats-Baril WL, Frymoyer JW: The Economics of Spinal Disorders. In Frymoyer JW (ed): The Adult Spine. New York: Raven Press, 1991:85–105.
17. Bovim G, Schrader H, Sand T: Neck pain in the general population. Spine 1993; 19:1307–1309.
18. Makela M, Heiovaasa M, Sievers K, et al: Prevalence, determinants, and consequences of chronic neck pain in Finland. Am J Epidemiol 1991; 134:1356–1367.
19. Lonner BS, Cammisa FP Jr, Ranawat CS: Rheumatoid arthritis of the cervical spine. Semin Arthrop 1995; 6:193–210.
20. Rohling MC, Binder LM, Langhinrichsen-Rohling J: Money matters: meta-analytic review of the association between financial compensation and the experience and treatment of chronic pain. Health Psychol 1995; 14:537–547.
21. Hoppenfeld S: Evaluation of nerve root lesions involving the upper extremity. In Hoppenfeld S (ed): Orthopaedic Neurology. Philadelphia: Lippincott, 1977:7–42.
22. Hoppenfeld S: Physical examination of the cervical spine and temporomandibular joint. In Hoppenfeld S (ed): Physical Examination of the Spine and Extremities. Norwalk, CT: Appleton-Century-Crofts, 1976:105–132.
23. Boden SD, McCowin PR, Davis DO, et al: Abnormal magnetic-resonance scans of the cervical spine in asymptomatic subjects: A prospective investigation. J Bone Joint Surg Am 1990; 72: 1178–1184.
24. Davidorf J, Hoyt D, Rosen P: Distal cervical spine evaluation using swimmer's flexion-extension radiographs. J Emerg Med 1993; 11:55–59.
25. Acheson MB, Livingstone RR, Richardson ML, et al: High resolution CT scanning in the evaluation of cervical spine fractures: Comparison with plain film examinations. AJR Am J Roentgenol 1987; 148:1179–1185.
26. Yousem DM, Ata SW, Hackney DB: Cervical spine disk herniation: Comparison of CT and 3DFT gradient echo MR scans. J Comput Assist Tomog 1992; 16:345.
27. Zeidman SM, Thompson K: Cervical discography. In Clark CR (ed): The Cervical Spine, 3rd ed. Philadelphia: Lippincott-Raven, 1998:205–218.
28. Cloward R: Cervical discography defended. JAMA 1975; 233:862.
29. Connor PM, Darden BV 2nd: Cervical discography complications and clinical efficacy. Spine 1993; 18:2035–2038.
30. Seitz JP, Unguez CE, Wooten WW: SPECT of the cervical spine in the evaluation of neck pain after trauma. Clin Nucl Med 1995; 20:667–673.
31. Upton ARM, McComar AJ: The double crush in nerve entrapment syndromes. Lancet 1973; 2:359–362.
32. Rhoton AL Jr, Henderson ED: Cervical disc disease with neural compression: Anterior surgical approach. Minn Med 1972; 55:998–1002.
33. Lestini WF, Wiesel SW: The pathogenesis of cervical spondylosis. Clin Orthop 1989; 239:69–93.
34. Levine MJ, Albert TJ, Smith MD: Cervical radiculopathy: Diagnosis and nonoperative management. J Am Acad Orthop Surg 1996; 4:305–316.
35. Zeidman SM, Ducker TB: Evaluation of patients with cervical spine lesions. In Clark CR (ed): The Cervical Spine, 3rd ed. Philadelphia: Lippincott-Raven, 1998:143–162.
36. Fischgrund FS, Herkowitz HN: Cervical degenerative disc disorders. In Kasser JR (ed): Orthopaedic Knowledge Update 5. Rosemont, IL: AAOS, 1996:593–602.
37. Herkowitz HN, Kurz LT, Overholt DP: Surgical management of cervical soft disc herniation: A comparison between anterior and posterior approach. Spine 1990; 1:1026–1030.
38. Herkowitz HN: A comparison of anterior cervical fusion, cervical laminectomy, and cervical laminoplasty for the surgical management of multiple level spondylitic radiculopathy. Spine 1988; 8:693–699.
39. Parfenchuck TA, Janssen ME: A correlation of cervical magnetic resonance imaging and discography and discography/computed tomographic discograms. Spine 1994; 19:2819–2825.
40. Schellhas KP, Smith MD, Gundy CR, et al: Cervical disc pain: Prospective correlation of magnetic resonance imaging and discography in asymptomatic subjects and pain sufferers. Spine 1996; 21:300–311.
41. Meyer PR Jr: Cervical spine fractures: Changing management concepts. In Bridwell KH (ed): The Textbook of Spinal Surgery, 2nd ed. Philadelphia: Lippincott-Raven, 1997:1679–1741.
42. Barnsley L, Lord S, Bogduk N: Whiplash injury. Pain 1994; 58:283–307.
43. Borchgrevink GE, Kaasa A, McDonagh D, et al: Acute treatment of whiplash neck sprain injuries: A randomized trial of treatment during the first 14 days after a car accident. Spine 1998; 23:25–31.
44. McKiney LA, Dornan JD, Ryan M: The role of physiotherapy in the management of acute neck sprains following road-traffic accidents. Arch Emerg Med 1989; 6:27–33.
45. Pennie BH, Agambar LJ: Whiplash injuries: A trial of early management. J Bone Joint Surg Br 1990; 72:277–279.
46. Spitzer WD, Skovron ML, Salmi LR, et al: Scientific monograph of the Quebec task force on whiplash-associated disorders: Redefining "whiplash" and its management. Spine 1995; 20(suppl 8):S1–73.
47. Suissa S, Harder S, Veilleux M: The Quebec whiplash-associated disorder cohort study. Spine 1995; 20:12–39.
48. Allen BL Jr, Ferguson RL, Lehmann TR, et al: A mechanistic classification of closed, indirect fractures and dislocations of the lower cervical spine. Spine 1982; 7:1–27.
49. White AA, Southwick WO, Panjabai MM: Clinical instability in the lower cervical spine: A review of past and current concepts. Spine 1976; 1:15–17.
50. Pellici PM, Ranawat CS, Tsaisis P, et al: A prospective study of the progression of rheumatoid arthritis of the cervical spine. J Bone Joint Surg Am 1981; 68:342–350.
51. Kawaida H, Sakou T, Morizono Y, et al: Magnetic resonance imaging of upper cervical disorders in rheumatoid arthritis. Spine 1989; 14:1144–1148.
52. Ranawat CS, O'Leary P, Pellici P, et al: Cervical spine fusion in rheumatoid arthritis. J Bone Joint Surg Am 1979; 61:1003–1010.

53. Redlund-Johnell I, Pettersson H: Radiographic measurement of the craniovertebral region: Designed for evaluation of abnormalities in rheumatoid arthritis. Acta Radiol 1984; 25:23–28.

54. Dvorak J, Gob D, Baumgartner J, et al: Functional evaluation of the spinal cord by magnetic resonance imaging in patients with rheumatoid arthritis and instability in the upper cervical spine. Spine 1989; 14:1057–1064.

55. Brigham CD: Ankylosing spondylitis and seronegative spondyloarthopathy. *In* Clark CR (ed): The Cervical Spine, 3rd ed. Philadelphia: Lippincott-Raven, 1998:715–719.

56. Bohlman HH: Acute fractures and dislocations of the cervical spine. J Bone Joint Surg Am 1979; 61:1119–1142.

57. Modic MT, Feiglin DH, Piraino DW: Vertebral osteomyelitis: Assessment using MR. Radiology 1985; 157:157–166.

58. Medical Research Council Working Party on Tuberculosis of the Spine: A comparison of 6 or 9 month course regimen of chemotherapy in patients receiving ambulatory treatment or undergoing radical surgery for tuberculosis of the spine. Int J Tuberc Lung Dis 1989; 36 (suppl):1.

59. Levine AM, Boriani S, Donati D, et al: Benign tumors of the cervical spine. Spine 1992; 17:5399–5406.

60. Harrington KD: Current concept review: Metastatic disease of the spine. J Bone Joint Surg Am 1986; 68:1110–1115.

61. Schaberg J, Gainor BJ: A profile of metastatic carcinoma of the spine. Spine 1985; 10:19–20.

62. Kneisl JS, Simon MA: Medical management compared with operative treatment for osteoid osteoma. J Bone Joint Surg Am 1992; 74:179–185.

# 6 | Foot and Ankle Pain

*Roger A. Mann and Loretta B. Chou*

## BIOMECHANICS

The biomechanics of the foot and ankle are very complex, but a general understanding of the functional biomechanics enables the clinician to have a better appreciation of what occurs in the foot and ankle during normal gait. The foot provides contact with the environment and needs to be able to adapt to it. The adaptation may be in terms of walking up or down a hill, on a side slope, or on rough terrain. With normal function of the joints about the foot and ankle, this task is very simple. However, when an abnormality exists in a joint, it may prevent normal function from occurring, thereby creating a disability.

At the time of initial ground contact, when the heel strikes the ground, the foot is flexible in order to absorb the impact of the body hitting the ground. The absorption occurs through the plantar flexion of the ankle joint and the pronation or collapse of the medial arch, which is a normal event at ground contact. As the center of gravity of the body passes over the foot that is on the ground, the heel rises and weight is transferred onto the ball of the foot, biomechanically converting the foot into a rigid structure in preparation for toe-off. Therefore, at initial ground contact, the foot is flexible to absorb impact; at the time of toe-off, the foot is rigid. The former mechanism is passive, whereas the latter mechanism is active, requiring the coordinated function of the ankle, subtalar, and transverse tarsal and metatarsophalangeal (MTP) joints, as well as the muscles controlling these joints.

The magnitude of the force that is dissipated by the foot can be illustrated as follows: If a 150-pound person walks 1 mile, each foot dissipates approximately 63 tons of force. Therefore, if there is some type of dysfunction about the foot and ankle and this mechanism to absorb impact is lost, a significant disability may result.

Evaluation of the patient with a foot and ankle disorder begins with a history of the problem, as well as the relevant past history such as trauma and systemic disorder. The degree of disability in the patient's activities of daily living, work, and recreational activities needs to be explored. The area of maximal pain and its characteristics should be defined as precisely as possible. Determining aggravating factors is often helpful in defining the problem. What the patient has done to treat the problem (e.g., change shoes; use a pad, brace, or orthosis) should be determined.

Next, a physical examination is undertaken. It starts with the patient standing so that the alignment of the knees, ankles, feet, and toes is noted, first for symmetry and then for specific abnormalities. The basic knee abnormalities are bowing (genu varum), knock-knee (genu valgum), the presence of a back-knee deformity, and swelling of the knees.

The alignment of the ankle and hindfoot with the tibia is then observed. In this situation, the examiner is trying to define whether the calcaneus (heel) is in neutral position (in line with the tibia), in varus (tilted towards the midline), or in valgus (tipped away from the midline).

Next, the alignment of the foot is noted. It is very important to look for any asymmetry between the longitudinal arches of the two feet. An acquired flatfoot deformity, often caused by posterior tibial tendon dysfunction or arthrosis of the tarsometatarsal joints, may be present. In the alignment of the forefoot with the hindfoot, the front part of the foot is adducted (angled toward the midline) or abducted (angled away from the midline).

The alignment of the tarsometatarsal joints is next observed. An abduction deformity associated with thickening through this area would indicate arthrosis of these joints.

The alignment of the great toe is observed for a possible hallux valgus deformity, cock-up deformity (extension of the hallux), or occasionally a hallux varus (hallux pointing medially).

The lesser toes are assessed observing whether they lie flat on the floor or are cocked up secondary to contracture of the MTP joints. The toes themselves should be noted for hammer toe formation with associated calluses.

The patient is then asked to walk; this gives the clinician the opportunity to observe the patient's balance and ability to ambulate with a symmetric gait and to assess the degree of disability. The patient is then asked to stand on the toes, which requires a coordinated function of both the muscles and joints about the foot and ankle. When performing this task, the patient should be permitted to touch the wall for balance.

The patient is then seated on the examining table, and the range of motion of the joints about the foot and ankle is observed.

ANKLE JOINT. The ankle joint range of motion consists of dorsiflexion of about 20 degrees and plantar flexion of about 50 degrees. The ankle joint is then palpated for the presence of thickened synovial tissue and areas of pain. The lateral ankle ligament is assessed by gently pulling the foot in a forward and slightly internally rotated direction; the examiner notes whether there is any give in the anterior talofibular ligament structure.

SUBTALAR JOINT. The subtalar joint is the joint between the talus and calcaneus. Motion of this joint is called inversion (moving inward) and eversion (moving outward). Normally there are 25 degrees of inversion and 10 degrees of eversion.

TRANSVERSE TARSAL JOINT. Transverse tarsal joint motion occurs between the talonavicular and calcaneocuboid joints. It is assessed by moving the foot into adduction (medial deviation) and abduction (lateral deviation) of the forefoot in relation to the hindfoot. Normally there are approximately 20 degrees of adduction and 10 degrees of abduction.

TARSOMETATARSAL JOINTS. Tarsometatarsal motion is tested by grabbing the tarsal bones and the metatarsal bones and observing what type of motion is present. Usually only a trace amount of dorsiflexion and plantar flexion is present in this joint.

METATARSOPHALANGEAL JOINTS. MTP joint motion consists of dorsiflexion and plantar flexion. This motion can be quite variable from patient to patient, but there are usually about 60 degrees of dorsiflexion and 20 degrees of plantar flexion.

Once the range of motion of the joints about the foot and ankle has been determined, the plantar aspect of the foot needs to be assessed. The area beneath the metatarsal heads, where normally the fat pad is present, is observed for possible atrophy or callus formation. A callus beneath a metatarsal head may be a diffuse type of callus or a localized callus. A localized callus has a central core when it is trimmed, as opposed to a diffuse callus, which is just a generalized thickening of the skin. Normally there is a certain amount of thickening of the skin beneath the metatarsal heads.

The lesser toes are examined for a contracture of the proximal interphalangeal joint (hammer toe) or of the distal interphalangeal joint (mallet toe). Callus formation over the joint should also be observed. A toe that is dorsiflexed at the MTP joint and in which a hammer toe deformity is also present is known as a claw toe deformity.

## FOOT POSTURE

A foot should be in contact with the ground in such a way that weight is equally distributed on the bottom of the foot. This is known as a plantigrade foot, in which the calcaneus is perpendicular to the forefoot: namely, the metatarsal head region. This is assessed with the patient sitting on an examination table. The calcaneus is placed in line with the tibia; then the medial aspect of the head of the talus is covered by the navicular bone. The forefoot should be at a 90-degree angle to the hindfoot. When this anatomic alignment is present, the foot is considered to be a neutral foot, which is a plantigrade foot. If the lateral border of the

foot is more plantar flexed than the medial border, it is a *forefoot varus* deformity and is often associated with a flatfoot deformity. If the medial border of the foot is more plantar flexed than the lateral border of the foot, it is a *forefoot valgus* deformity, and this is often associated with a cavus, or high-arch, foot. Frequently in patients with rheumatoid arthritis, with posterior tibial tendon dysfunction, or after trauma, the relationship of the hindfoot and forefoot is altered so that the patient cannot walk with a plantigrade foot. When this occurs, excessive stress is placed on various portions of the foot and ankle, which results in varying degrees of disability. If a patient has a nonplantigrade foot, the clinician needs to determine why this abnormality is present.

## HINDFOOT PAIN: DIFFERENTIAL DIAGNOSIS

The hindfoot consists of the following anatomic structures: the calcaneus, talus, Achilles tendon, and plantar fascia. There are many causes of hindfoot pain, and the most common are disorders of the Achilles tendon, heel pain syndrome, subtalar joint pain, and transverse tarsal (talonavicular-calcaneocuboid) joint pain.

### Disorders of the Achilles Tendon

The Achilles tendon is the largest and strongest tendon in the leg and is made of contributions from the gastrocnemius and soleus muscles. The gastrocnemius and soleus muscles function in stance and undergoes eccentric (lengthening) and concentric (shortening) contractions with walking and running. It has unique anatomic features that make it susceptible to injury and disease. Vascular studies demonstrate that the blood supply to the tendon is deficient 4 to 5 cm above its insertion,[1, 2] which is the area most commonly ruptured. The Achilles tendon rotates 90 degrees, 2 to 6 cm proximal to the insertion, which can cause further stress forces in the tendon.[3]

There are many disorders involving the Achilles tendon. Noninsertional disorders occur proximal to its insertion and above the level of the retrocalcaneal bursa. These disorders include Achilles tendinitis, tendinosis, and rupture. Achilles tendinitis is inflammation of the tendon sheath. Achilles tendinosis is an intrasubstance process, caused by aging, microtears, and degeneration, and there may be an associated tendinitis.

Insertional disorders begin in the area posterior to the retrocalcaneal bursa to the insertion. These include Achilles calcification at the insertion, tendinosis, and Haglund's deformity. Calcification at its insertion into the calcaneus may exist without tendinosis. Achilles tendinosis can occur at its insertion with or without associated calcification. Haglund's deformity is caused by an increase in the size of the posterosuperior prominence of the calcaneal tuberosity that may be associated with Achilles tendinitis and retrocalcaneal bursitis.

Achilles tendinitis is one of the most common ailments of athletes, and the usual cause is overuse or training errors. Other causes are an equinus contracture, ill-fitting shoes, and hyperpronation of the foot. In contrast, Achilles tendinosis is a degenerative process of the tendon, and Achilles tendon ruptures are associated with tendinosis.[4, 5]

A careful history includes identifying the point of maximal pain, type of pain, associated swelling and increased warmth, and the time of onset of the symptoms. The patient's age, sex, occupation, type of shoewear, sports activities, and previous occurrences and treatment are documented. The symptoms usually begin with prolonged weight-bearing activities or exercise. In chronic cases, a patient may complain of pain and swelling with daily activities or even at rest. The physical examination begins by observing the patient's gait and observing the patient while he or she stands and sits. The posture of the foot, swelling, redness, and masses should be noted. The patient is instructed to rise on all the toes on one foot (perform a single toe rise) several times. This test helps distinguish a tendinosis from a tendinitis; a patient with a tendinosis usually cannot perform a single toe rise, whereas those with tendinitis usually can. The tendon is palpated for swelling, tenderness, localized or diffuse thickening, increased warmth, and crepitation.

In Achilles tendinitis, the peritenon is inflamed. Therefore, findings are tenderness, swelling, increased warmth, and crepitation. Nodules are not usually palpated in the tendon while the ankle is ranged. With tendinosis, the tendon is thickened over a length of 2 to 5 cm. There is tenderness with deep palpation or squeezing the involved area. The involved area moves when the ankle is placed through a range of motion.

In the patient with an inflamed retrocalcaneal bursa, the pain is usually well localized between the tendon and the calcaneus and proximal to the insertion of the tendon. The swollen bursa can be palpated, and there may be tenderness over the bursal area anterior to the Achilles tendon. The Achilles tendon is not tender, and there is usually no thickening of the tendon.

The insertional disorders of the Achilles tendon manifest in two forms. One involves a well-localized area of pain at the insertion of the Achilles tendon. The tendon is not thickened except in the localized area of the pain. Affected patients usually can perform a single toe rise without difficulty. Such patients usually have pain secondary to a bone spur at the insertion of the tendon. The other form of insertional disorders involve thickening of the tendon at its insertion. Tenderness to palpation, increased warmth, and a palpable bony prominence are present. Affected patients have difficulty with a single toe rise and have tendinosis.

Plain radiographs can show calcification at the insertion site. Calcifications can also be seen on computed tomography, and the focal area of calcification is usually correlated with tenderness at the insertion. Magnetic resonance imaging (MRI) may be used to show abnormalities associated with tendinosis. The Achilles tendon may be thickened and may have intrasubstance

cysts. The amount of thickening and intrasubstance inhomogeneity varies, depending on the degree of degeneration.

Nonoperative measures are generally successful in treatment of Achilles tendon disorders. The initial treatment is determined by the severity of the pain and disability. In acute conditions, rest and the use of nonsteroidal anti-inflammatory drugs (NSAIDs) often ameliorate symptoms. Also, the use of ice and elevation can be helpful in decreasing inflammation and swelling. Once the patient is more comfortable, he or she may begin gentle stretching exercises of the Achilles tendon. Some patients find physical therapy modalities, such as ultrasound therapy and massage, helpful for their symptoms.

Patients active in sports may require modification of shoewear or of the training program. The shoewear should have a high, soft cushion heel. A viscoelastic heel insert may be used in all shoes, including athletic shoewear. The insert provides absorption of static and dynamic loading. Also, a softer heel-counter decreases pressure and irritation in the area of the Achilles tendon. If indicated, an orthotic device with a medial sole and heel wedge diminishes severe pronation. Most patients find amelioration of their symptoms with these measures, but for symptoms that persist, a short period of cast immobilization has a good success rate. A removable cast is preferable to a fiberglass cast because it allows the patient to continue stretching exercises and physical therapy. Immobilization is especially useful for patients with insertional tendinosis. In chronic recurring cases, a polypropylene ankle-foot orthosis with no motion of the ankle joint has the same effect as a walking cast. Steroid injections about the Achilles tendon are not recommended because of the risk of tendon rupture caused by the steroids.

If a 6-month course of nonoperative treatment fails, operative treatment may be considered. The most successful outcome occurs in patients with a well-localized area of tenderness and corresponding calcification at the insertion. Through a small incision, the calcified area is shelled out and the defect in the Achilles tendon is repaired. When the area of involvement is extensive with concurrent tendinosis, the success rate is not as reliable.

Achilles tendinitis almost always responds to conservative management. For cases in which the symptoms persist, release and débridement of the peritenon has been reported to be successful.[6] In chronic cases of tendinosis, the tendon is explored. There is usually an area of thickening of the tendon, but rarely is a distinct cyst observed. The repair involves use of the plantaris tendon woven into the Achilles tendon to stimulate an inflammatory healing response. The reconstruction is protected postoperatively in a non–weight-bearing cast for 4 weeks, followed by a walking cast for an additional 4 weeks. During the second month, a removable cast allows for range-of-motion and gentle strengthening exercises.

After cast immobilization, the activities may be progressed gradually. Six to 12 months may be necessary for the Achilles tendon to reach maximal strength.

Some thickening of the tendon persists, but the pain usually diminishes.

In a patient with chronic retrocalcaneal bursitis without tendinosis, an operative procedure to excise Haglund's deformity—the superior aspect of the calcaneus adjacent to the Achilles tendon—decompresses the bursa.[6] The Achilles tendon can be adherent to the calcaneus, and with the excision, the symptoms diminish.

## Heel Pain Syndrome

Heel pain syndrome is pain in the subcalcaneal area and is commonly known as plantar fasciitis. It is a common problem, and affected patients usually seek medical attention from the primary care physician. Because there are multiple causes, a precise diagnosis is important for properly treating this condition. Other causes, such as infection, tumor, inflammatory arthritis, Achilles tendon disorders, nerve entrapment, and stress fracture of the calcaneus, should be considered when heel pain is evaluated.

The anatomic structures involved are the calcaneus, plantar fascia, plantar fat pad, medial and lateral plantar nerves, and medial calcaneal nerves. The plantar fascia is an aponeurosis between the subcutaneous fat and intrinsic structures. It originates from the calcaneal tubercle and inserts into the plantar aspect of the bases of the toes. Its role is to stabilize the arch of the foot during the toe-off phase of gait. It is also one of the important static supporting structures for the arch of the foot. With chronic overuse, degeneration of the fascia can result. There may be a component of nerve entrapment involving the first branch of the lateral plantar nerve or a tarsal tunnel syndrome.

This entity is more commonly seen in athletes, obese persons, and middle-aged persons.[7] Abnormal biomechanics associated with this condition include a tight Achilles tendon and pes cavus or pes planus deformities.

This clinical syndrome has very characteristic signs and symptoms; the diagnosis can generally be made on the basis of the history and physical examination. The pain is worse with the first steps in the morning, generally improves, but can return with prolonged weight-bearing activities. The pain is described as a dull ache, throbbing, and burning or sharp pain and is commonly localized to the medial tubercle of the calcaneus. There may be atrophy of the plantar fat pad. Rest helps symptoms diminish, although many patients complain of recurrent or chronic pain. Radiographic examination helps rule out a stress fracture, tumor, and infection. A bone spur is frequently seen and is thought to be a coincidental finding. A bone scan may show increased uptake at the attachment of the plantar fascia, and MRI may show edema of the plantar fascia with or without involvement of the calcaneus.

Because the pathoanatomy has not been definitively identified, there are many treatment modalities. Eighty-five percent of patients improve with nonsurgical modalities.[8] The initial treatment involves a combination of activity modification, heel cord Achilles tendon stretching, shoewear modification, and NSAIDs. Other treatment options include physical therapy, nighttime splinting, cortisone injections, and casting. Cast immobilization in a fiberglass walking cast has been found to be the most effective treatment.[7]

Wolgin and associates[9] found that heel pads were the most successful treatment in 83 of 100 patients. Pfeffer and colleagues[8] reported results of 236 patients, from 15 centers, who were treated nonoperatively for heel pain syndrome and found that a prefabricated shoe insert with a stretching program was more effective than a custom polypropylene orthotic device. In patients in whom the pain is resistant to treatment, a work-up should be performed to detect a seronegative arthropathy.

## Subtalar Joint Pain

The subtalar joint is between the talus and calcaneus. Inversion and eversion occur at this joint. The most common cause of subtalar joint pain is arthrosis. Trauma is the usual cause of subtalar arthritis, as the result of an intra-articular talus or calcaneus fracture or avascular necrosis of the talus. Other causes of arthrosis of the subtalar joint include primary osteoarthritis, rheumatoid arthritis, psoriatic arthritis, ankylosing spondylitis, and tarsal coalition involving the talocalcaneal joint. Posterior tibial tendon dysfunction is associated with a hindfoot valgus deformity that can become fixed and painful.

Affected patients complain of pain localized to the subtalar joint region, and sometimes there is associated pain in the ankle. Weight-bearing activities, particularly ambulating on uneven surfaces, worsen the symptoms.

Treatment for subtalar joint arthritis is initially symptomatic with rest, NSAIDs, and possibly a short course of immobilization. Moderate to severe involvement may necessitate support, such as an ankle-foot orthosis. For pain that persists, a subtalar arthrodesis yields reliable pain relief.[10]

## Transverse Tarsal Joint Pain

The transverse tarsal joint, also known as Chopart's joint, is made up of the talonavicular and calcaneocuboid joints. Adduction and abduction of the foot occurs in this joint. Pain and deformity involving the transverse tarsal joint can occur with posterior tibial tendon dysfunction, inflammatory arthritis, post-traumatic arthritis, and Charcot joint. When arthrosis is present, it usually involves the talonavicular joint.

Patients complain of pain about the midfoot and arch with weight-bearing activities, especially on uneven surfaces. The physical examination demonstrates localized tenderness and swelling to the transverse tarsal joint. The most common deformity seen with transverse tarsal joint arthritis is pes planovalgus.

Treatment of symptomatic transverse tarsal joint disease begins with rest, immobilization, and NSAIDs. Some patients benefit from a brace such as an ankle-foot orthosis. Talonavicular arthritis can be treated operatively with arthrodesis. Involvement of the calcaneocuboid and subtalar joints must be ruled out because residual pain may persist if these joints are not treated. Talonavicular fusion can be used to successfully treat isolated rheumatoid arthritis of that joint. Arthrodesis of the talonavicular joint eliminates subtalar and calcaneocuboid joint motion. Therefore, with a double arthrodesis (fusion of the talonavicular and calcaneocuboid joints), further motion is not lost, and the fusion is more stable than an isolated talonavicular arthrodesis.

## DIFFERENTIAL DIAGNOSIS OF THE ACQUIRED FLATFOOT

The most common origin of adult acquired flatfoot deformity is posterior tibial tendon dysfunction. Other causes are Charcot joint, arthrosis of the tarsometatarsal joints, crush injury, and rheumatoid arthritis.

The midfoot is made up of the tarsometatarsal (TMT), cuneiform, metatarsocuboid, and cuneiform cuboid joints. The transverse and longitudinal arch of the foot is composed of these joints and their interosseous ligaments. The second to fifth tarsometatarsal joints are connected with interosseous ligaments, and there is no connection between the first and second metatarsal joints. There is, however, a strong ligament between the medial cuneiform and second metatarsal base, known as Lisfranc's ligament. There is a ligament between the first metatarsal and medial cuneiform. Disruption of these ligaments or disease of these joints can result in loss of the arch of the foot because of dorsiflexion and abduction of the metatarsals.

### Posterior Tibial Tendon Dysfunction

Posterior tibial tendon dysfunction can result in an acquired flatfoot deformity. It is progressive, and in severe forms there is associated arthritis. Early reports by Fowler[11] and Williams[12] describe this disease and the treatment.

The role of the posterior tibial tendon is to invert and plantar-flex the foot and ankle. The posterior tibial muscle is important during the gait cycle: It initiates inversion of the hindfoot, to allow for push-off. If the posterior tibial tendon does not function normally, the peroneus brevis muscle is unopposed, thus flattening the arch. Other important structures involved with the deformity are the deltoid and spring ligaments. The natural history of dysfunction of the posterior tibial tendon is loss of the medial longitudinal arch, progressing to development of hindfoot valgus and forefoot abduction. The deformity is initially flexible; however, it becomes fixed with chronic disease.

Although the cause of posterior tibial tendon insufficiency is unknown, the vascular supply to the area of tendon involvement has been shown to be decreased.[13] Holmes and Mann[14] noted an association of this disease with obesity, hypertension, and the use of steroids. The majority of surgical specimens show intrasubstance abnormality, with longitudinal tears, discoloration, swelling, and elongation of the tendon.

Affected patients exhibit pain and swelling of the posterior medial aspect of the foot. With time they observe that the arch is flattening and the foot turns outward. Approximately one third to one half of patients have a history of injury or trauma, usually a twisting injury to the foot and ankle. Patients can have associated swelling and experience limitation of walking and other weight-bearing activities, such as playing tennis and hiking. Examination with a patient standing demonstrates swelling along the posterior tibial tendon, loss of the medial longitudinal arch, the "too many toes" sign (forefoot abduction), and increased hindfoot valgus, in comparison to the unaffected side. Most affected patients cannot perform a single heel rise on the affected limb, and if he or she can accomplish this, the examiner can see that the patient does not invert the hindfoot. The most accurate test is resisted inversion; with the patient sitting, the foot is placed in equinus and abduction, and the patient is instructed to adduct against the examiner's hand. This maneuver isolates the posterior tibial tendon from the tibialis anterior tendon and shows abnormal posterior tibial tendon function. Weight-bearing radiographs of the foot and ankle are obtained to evaluate bone anatomy. Depending on the severity of the deformity, the lateral radiograph can show sagging of the talonavicular joint, in comparison to the unaffected side, and the anteroposterior radiograph shows lateral subluxation of the navicular (also known as uncovering of the talar head). The joints are evaluated for the presence of arthrosis, which can influence the treatment. Other imaging studies are usually unnecessary after a thorough history and physical examination by an experienced examiner. An MRI study can help confirm the abnormality of the posterior tibial tendon and fluid in the tendon sheath.

Posterior tibial tendon insufficiency constitutes a spectrum of pathoanatomy. Johnson and Strom[15] provided a classification to describe the stage of the disease and associated treatment: Stage I is tenosynovitis causing pain and swelling; there is no deformity of the foot and ankle. Stage II shows further progression of the disease; in addition to pain and swelling, patients note some loss of the arch and turning out to the foot, and on examination, the foot and ankle remain supple, but the hindfoot has increased valgus with the presence of the "too many toes" sign. Stage III disease involves a fixed pes planovalgus deformity with associated radiographic findings of arthrosis.

Treatment of posterior tibial tendon insufficiency can be nonoperative or operative. Stage I disease is treated with rest, cast immobilization, and NSAIDs. Steroid injections of the tendon are not recommended because of the association with tendon rupture. Once the tenosynovitis improves, an orthotic device with a medial arch can provide support. With stage II involvement, the deformity is more difficult to treat; therefore, an ankle-foot orthosis or University of California Biomechanical Laboratory (UCBL) insert is required for adequate support of the deformity.

Patients in whom a course of nonoperative treatment fails can be candidates for operative treatment. Stage I disease can be treated with a synovectomy. With early débridement, this procedure has been reported to yield good results.[15] More severe deformity necessitates more extensive reconstruction. One of the most common procedures is posterior tibial tendon reconstruction with transfer of the flexor digitorum longus tendon. A medial displacement calcaneal osteotomy can be added to the reconstruction if there is increased hindfoot valgus. Early reports show greater patient satisfaction and more improvement of the longitudinal arch by radiograph than with tendon reconstruction alone. Stage III disease is treated with arthrodesis of the involved joints. Which arthrodesis is used is dependent on the severity of the deformity. Therefore, subtalar, double, or triple arthrodesis may be indicated. Most of the deformity can be corrected with these fusions. A tendo Achilles lengthening can be added to correct an associated equinus deformity.

## Diabetes with a Charcot Joint

A Charcot joint is caused by a neuropathic process, such as syringomyelia, syphilis, leprosy, and diabetes. Whereas the first three diseases are uncommon, diabetes affects 10 million people in the United States[16] and is the leading cause of Charcot joints. The origin of the neuroarthropathy has been attributed to repetitive microtrauma because of diminished protective sensation.

The most common areas of neuroarthropathy are the midfoot and hindfoot.[16] With destruction of one or more joints in the midfoot, instability of the arch results, with eventual collapse of the midfoot. With abnormal bony prominences, ulceration and infection can develop. There is often a delay in the diagnosis of a Charcot joint because other diseases, such as osteomyelitis, posterior tibial tendon insufficiency, and arthritis, can manifest with similar findings.

Some patients relate a history of injury or trauma, such as a twisting injury to the foot or ankle. They can have a variable amount of pain, swelling, loss of the arch, and turning out of the foot. The examination demonstrates swelling, loss of the medial longitudinal arch, erythema, and increased warmth. The peripheral neuropathy is manifested by loss of deep tendon reflexes and sense of vibration. Severe deformities may by accompanied by associated skin breakdown or ulcers in areas of increased pressure. Weight-bearing radiographs of the foot and ankle show diffuse destruction of the joint, with collapse, bony fragmentation, subluxation, or frank dislocation.

The Charcot joint can be described according to Eichenholtz's classification.[17] Stage I is the acute phase, in which the patient is found to have edema, erythema, increased warmth, and radiographic changes that include bone fragmentation. Stage II, which also manifests with swelling, erythema, and increased warmth, is the reparative phase; radiographs show healing with the presence of new bone

formation. Stage III is the resolution phase, with decreasing inflammatory signs and radiographic consolidation of the involved joint.

Treatment of Charcot joint depends on the stage. Eichenholtz's stage I is treated with a total-contact cast, non–weight-bearing, and elevation to decrease swelling. Once the inflammation resolves, which may take several months, the patient can be placed in a custom ankle-foot orthosis to support the foot.

Surgical treatment is reserved for patients in whom nonoperative treatment fails. The fusion rate is only 50% to 60% successful, and other complications include wound healing problems. A bony prominence that is the cause of a recurrent or nonhealing ulcer can be treated with a simple excision. Because the joints are unstable, the deformity can progress, and the bony prominence can recur. Thus, open reduction and arthrodesis or in situ fusion is advocated by some authors to correct the instability and prominence of the involved joints. Myerson and associates[16] reported on 68 patients with diabetes and neuroarthropathy of the midfoot. Thirty-seven feet were treated surgically, and arthrodesis was the most common procedure. Overall, the treatment was successful in 95% of cases. Patients with severe deformity, ulceration, infection, or ischemia may require amputation.

The postoperative course requires prolonged cast immobilization and limited weight-bearing. Even after successful fusion, a brace should be used to provide support to the fusion site and surrounding joints.

## Lisfranc Joint Arthrosis

A Lisfranc fracture is a fracture-dislocation of the TMT joint. One of the devastating consequences of this injury is post-traumatic arthritis associated with a dorsiflexion-abduction deformity. Primary arthrosis of the TMT joints can also cause equally severe deformity.

Affected patients have pain and swelling at the Lisfranc joint related to weight-bearing activities. The joint may be tender with palpation of the osteophytes. The symptoms can be reproduced with attempted stress of the affected joints. Usually, such patients cannot perform a single toe rise. Radiographic findings of post-traumatic Lisfranc joint arthritis include loss of joint space, osteophytes, and a variable degree of loss of the longitudinal arch manifested by dorsiflexion and abduction at the TMT joints.

This disorder can be treated with a total-contact orthosis to provide support of the arch. The patient with a severe fixed deformity may not be able to tolerate an arch support. The surgical treatment involves an arthrodesis of the TMT joints, often with an osteotomy to correct the deformity.

## Crush Injury of the Foot

The foot can be subject to traumatic injuries, and one of the most potentially devastating is a crush injury. This injury can occur in many different settings, such as in the workplace, in a motor vehicle accident, or at home. The mechanism and the amount of weight involved are important to ascertain during the initial evaluation.

An open wound is commonly associated with the injury and necessitates débridement and antibiotic prophylaxis. A crush injury can cause a compartment syndrome of the foot. If left untreated, the foot becomes stiff and deformed. The intrinsic muscles are atrophied, and there is an imbalance of the intrinsic and extrinsic musculature, leading to claw toe deformities.

Crush injuries to the midfoot should be treated with closed reduction and pinning. An open reduction may be required if anatomic reduction cannot be achieved because of interposition of soft tissue or severe comminution. The foot should be protected with a splint, and once the swelling subsides, a short leg cast with non–weight-bearing is used for 6 weeks, depending on the severity of the injury. After the cast is removed, the patient begins range-of-motion exercises and returns to usual activities. Also, a total-contact orthosis with a medial arch support may be necessary.

## Rheumatoid Arthritis

Rheumatoid arthritis is the most common inflammatory arthritis and affects the foot and ankle in 40% to 89% of cases.[18] The forefoot is most commonly involved, followed by the hindfoot and the ankle. As with the hands, both feet are affected but not necessarily symmetrically. The initial synovitis can involve the hindfoot and midfoot, which can result in collapse of the arch.

Patients complain of pain with weight-bearing and may have difficulty with shoewear. The examination shows loss of the arch, forefoot abduction, and increased hindfoot valgus. There can be associated tenderness and swelling. Radiographic examination shows typical rheumatoid findings with loss of joint space, periarticular erosions, and osteopenia. The longitudinal arch may be flattened.

Many patients can be treated conservatively. The goals of treatment are relief of pain, prevention of deformity, and improvement of function. Physical therapy involves range-of-motion and strengthening exercises. Injections with steroids, although commonly used in other joints, are difficult to administer to joints of the midfoot because of the small joint space. NSAIDs and an ambulatory aid can be helpful in decreasing symptoms. The most common nonoperative treatment involves shoewear modification. An orthotic device can provide arch support and relieve pressure under the metatarsal heads. Often, an extra-depth shoe is necessary to accommodate the deformity and orthotic device.

Surgical treatment is reserved for patients in whom nonoperative treatment has failed. A synovectomy helps decrease pain and swelling and may delay worsening of the deformity. However, severe disease may necessitate arthrodesis of the affected joints to produce a painless plantigrade foot.

## LESSER TOE PROBLEMS

The lesser toes are the second through fifth toes. The most common deformities are hammer toe, mallet toe, and claw toe. The anatomic structures involved are the extensor tendon, flexor tendon, interosseous muscle, lumbrical muscle, joint capsule, and collateral ligaments. Deformities are the result of an imbalance of the intrinsic and extrinsic muscle forces. The imbalance may be caused by trauma, arthritis, neurologic disease, or environmental factors (e.g., ill-fitting shoes). Rheumatoid arthritis begins in the forefoot in 17% of cases.[18] The most common deformities are hallux valgus and associated claw toe deformities of the lesser toes. The MTP joints are destroyed by the synovitis and then dorsal subluxation or dislocation of the MTP joint results.

A mallet toe is a flexion contracture of the distal interphalangeal (DIP) joint. A hammer toe is a flexion contracture of the proximal interphalangeal (PIP) joint. A claw toe is hyperextension of the MTP joint with a flexion contracture of the PIP joint.

Patients complain of pain over the involved joint; for example, there are usually a corn on the dorsum of the DIP joint with a mallet toe and a corn on the dorsum of the PIP joint with a hammer and claw toe deformity. The physical examination demonstrates a flexion deformity of the PIP joint in a hammer toe deformity and of the DIP joint in a mallet toe deformity. It should be determined whether the deformity is flexible or fixed. A flexible deformity can be corrected by placing dorsal pressure on the metatarsal heads.

The claw toe deformity has the lesser toe deformity, as noted, plus varying degrees of dorsiflexion of the MTP joint. The patient with rheumatoid arthritis has the most severe deformities, which lead to dislocations of the MTP joints. This forces the metatarsal heads into the plantar skin, resulting in severe atrophy of the fat pad and in callus.

Treatment for these deformities includes shoewear modification to help alleviate a majority of the symptoms. An extra-depth shoe with a soft upper part helps decrease pressure on the dorsum of the lesser toes. The affected toes can be padded with foam or silicone sleeves. Metatarsal pads or bars, toe slings, or tape can help correct a flexible deformity and decrease the weight-bearing pressure under the metatarsal heads. If the cause is an inflammatory arthritis, medical treatment of the systemic disease should be initiated.

If nonoperative modalities of treatment fail, an operative repair can be considered. The procedure is determined by the flexibility of the deformity as well as by the severity. A flexible hammer toe can be treated with a flexor tendon transfer to the extensor mechanism (a Girdlestone-Taylor procedure). A fixed hammer toe, however, necessitates a bone procedure to fully correct the deformity. This is best accomplished with a PIP joint arthroplasty with a flexor tenotomy. A mallet toe is treated with a flexor tenotomy and arthroplasty of the joint. A claw toe repair is similar to the hammer toe procedure, but the MTP joint is corrected by an extensor tenotomy and by capsulotomy to include the collateral ligaments. If there is a severe deformity, as in rheumatoid arthritis, a resection arthroplasty of the metatarsal head may be necessary to decompress the joint. Temporary fixation is accomplished with a Kirschner wire placed in the intramedullary canal of the toe and, in treating a severe deformity, into the metatarsal.

The fifth toe can have unique abnormalities because it lies on the lateral border of the foot and has direct pressure from the shoe. These deformities may be congenital or acquired, and they include overlapping, underlapping, and cock-up deformities. A common variant is the two-bone fifth toe, which is associated with a higher rate of problems.

Fifth toe problems can be treated nonoperatively as outlined for lesser toe problems. Operative treatment for a cock-up fifth toe is similar to that of deformities of the other lesser toes. An overlapping or underlapping toe is treated with release of the contracted tissue and may necessitate a Z-plasty of the contracted skin. A severe claw toe deformity of the fifth toe may necessitate resection of the proximal phalanx, a Ruiz-Mora procedure.

METATARSALGIA. Metatarsalgia means pain on the plantar aspect of the foot beneath the metatarsal heads. It does not define the specific problem; it is analogous to saying someone has heart disease, which encompasses many diagnoses. As with anything else in orthopedics and medicine in general, a specific diagnosis needs to be made. There are various causes of metatarsalgia and these are outlined as follows:

A. Skeletal causes
   1. Enlarged fibular condyle
   2. Long metatarsal
   3. Morton's foot
   4. Hypomobile first MTP joint
   5. Bony abnormality secondary to trauma
   6. Bony abnormality following surgery
B. Dermatologic causes
   1. Wart
   2. Callus
   3. Seed corn
   4. Hyperkeratotic skin
   5. Atrophy of the plantar fat pad
   6. Plantar scar
C. Iatrogenic causes
   1. Plantar incision
   2. Metatarsal surgery
D. MTP joint disorders
   1. Freiberg's infarction
   2. Nonspecific synovitis
   3. Plantar plate degeneration
   4. Infection
E. Neurologic causes
   1. Interdigital neuroma
   2. Tarsal tunnel syndrome
   3. Peripheral neuropathy
   4. Recurrent interdigital neuroma
   5. Discogenic disease
F. Soft tissue causes
   1. Atrophy of the plantar fat pad
   2. Crush injury: sequelae
   3. Plantar scar
   4. Neuroma
G. Systemic disease
   1. Rheumatoid arthritis
   2. Psoriatic arthritis
   3. Gout

After making a specific diagnosis of the cause of the metatarsalgia, the physician should undertake conservative management of the problem. The initial treatment consists of explaining the nature of the problem to the patient and the need to obtain a wide, soft, laced shoe. It is not possible to treat metatarsalgia with a fashionable woman's shoe. Many sports shoes and walking oxfords are available to satisfy almost any patient's needs. If regular shoes are not adequate, the patient should try orthopedic shoes. Very rarely does a patient require a custom-made shoe. Sometimes it is necessary to have a shoemaker relieve pressure points over bony prominences such as over the medial eminence of a bunion or hammer toes. Once a shoe of adequate size has been obtained, some type of metatarsal support within the shoe can be used to relieve pressure on the metatarsal head area. It must always be kept in mind that whenever something is added inside the shoe, it consumes space; therefore, if the shoe is not of adequate size, more pressure is placed upon the foot, making it uncomfortable.

The initial type of support should be a soft pad, which will relieve pressure underneath several metatarsal heads. This simple method is very useful in relieving pressure points. The pad should be placed under the longitudinal arch and should end just proximal to the metatarsal head or heads that are involved. The only disadvantage of this type of support is that a separate pad is required for each shoe. If the patient is comfortable with the support, he or she can obtain a customized orthotic device if desired. It is important that the top material of the orthotic device be soft, because hard acrylic or carbon fiber only adds to the patient's level of discomfort. If these basic conservative measures fail, the patient should be referred to an orthopedic surgeon for further evaluation, shoe modification, and, if necessary, corrective surgery.

# REFERENCES

1. Inglis AE, Scott WN, Sculco TP, et al: Rupture of the tendo Achilles. An objective assessment of surgical and non-surgical treatment. J Bone Joint Surg Am 1976; 58:990–993.
2. Lagergren C, Lindholm A: Vascular distribution in the Achilles tendon. An angiographic and microangiographic study. Acta Chir Scand 1958–1959; 116:491–496.
3. Inman VT: Applications to orthopaedics and areas for further clinical research. *In* Joints of the Ankle. Baltimore: Waverly Press, 1976:75–80.
4. Arner O, Lindholm A: Subcutaneous rupture of the Achilles tendon. A study of 92 cases. Acta Chir Scand 1959; Supplementum 239.

5. Clancy WG Jr, Neidhart D, Brand RL: Achilles tendinitis in runners: A report of 5 cases. Am J Sports Med 1976; 4:46–57.

6. Schepsis AA, Leach RE: Surgical management of Achilles tendinitis. Am J Sports Med 1987; 15:308–315.

7. Gill LH: Plantar fasciitis: Diagnosis and conservative management. J Am Acad Orthop Surg 1997; 5:109–117.

8. Pfeffer G, Bacchetti P, Deland J, et al: Comparison of custom and prefabricated orthoses in the initial treatment of proximal plantar fasciitis. Foot Ankle Int 1999; 20:214–221.

9. Wolgin M, Cook C, Graham C, et al: Conservative treatment of plantar heel pain: Long-term follow-up. Foot Ankle Int 1994; 15:97–102.

10. Mann RA, Beaman DN, Horton GA: Isolated subtalar arthrodesis. Foot Ankle Int 1998; 19:511–519.

11. Fowler AW: Tibialis posterior syndrome [Abstract]. J Bone Joint Surg Br 1955; 37:520.

12. Williams R: Chronic non-specific tendovaginitis of tibialis posterior. J Bone Joint Surg Br 1963; 45:542–545.

13. Frey C, Shereff M, Greenidge N: Vascularity of the posterior tibial tendon. J Bone Joint Surg Am 1990; 72:884–888.

14. Holmes GB Jr, Mann RA: Possible epidemiological factors associated with rupture of the posterior tibial tendon. Foot Ankle 1992; 13:70–79.

15. Johnson KA, Strom DE: Tibialis posterior tendon dysfunction. Clin Orthop 1989; 239:196–206.

16. Myerson MS, Henderson MR, Saxby T, et al: Management of midfoot diabetic neuroarthropathy. Foot Ankle Int 1994; 15:233–241.

17. Eichenholtz SN: Charcot Joints. Springfield, IL: Charles C Thomas, 1966:220–223.

18. Abdo RV, Iorio LJ: Rheumatoid arthritis of the foot and ankle. J Am Acad Orthop Surg 1994; 2:326–332.

# 7 | Rheumatic Diseases of the Hand and Wrist

*R. Kumar Kadiyala, Barry P. Simmons, and Garth R. Smith*

The hand and wrist are commonly affected in many rheumatic conditions. A thorough understanding of potential deformities and their history is important when caring for patients with these afflictions. In addition, a cooperative relationship among the primary care physician, the rheumatologist, the hand surgeon, the hand therapist, and others is critical to address the many needs of these patients adequately.

## PATIENT EVALUATION

As with any anatomic system, a thorough history and physical examination are paramount. The wrist should be evaluated for localized areas of pain as well as for swelling indicative of synovitis. Range of motion evaluated and compared over time is important when disease progression is sought. The carpometacarpal (CMC), metacarpophalangeal (MCP), and interphalangeal (IP) joints should be evaluated separately for swelling, deformity, and pain. Tendon function of the various wrist and digit flexors and extensors should be evaluated for integrity. Finally, sensation and strength should be assessed and recorded.

## RHEUMATOID ARTHRITIS

Patients with rheumatoid arthritis commonly experience problems with the hand and wrist and benefit from medical as well as surgical interventions.

### Nonsurgical Treatment

Rest, exercise, splinting, and injections play a critical role not only initially but also during all stages of the disease.[1, 2]

### Rest and Exercise

The patient with rheumatoid arthritis should understand the principles of rest and exercise and their practical application. When a joint is abnormally warm, painful, and inflamed, exercise must be reduced and rest increased. As the inflammatory process subsides, exercise can be resumed. Short, frequent periods of exercise are more beneficial than long, vigorous ones, which can aggravate synovial inflammation. A hand therapist is invaluable for working with patients and teaching them to decide how much exercise and activity they can carry out. If after a particular activity, hands become swollen, painful, or stiff, the activity has been too strenuous and should be modified.

### Splinting

Resting and dynamic splints alleviate pain, may decrease the progression of deformity during the active stages of the disease, and aid in postoperative management. Resting splints are especially effective for wrist pain and allow patients to use the hand while wearing the splint.[2] Various types of dynamic splints are used to stretch out fixed deformities, such as boutonnière deformities. However, dynamic splinting is used mainly after reconstructive surgery, especially after MCP joint arthroplasty.[3]

### Steroid Injections

The judicious use of local injections of steroids often lessens active synovitis and tenosynovitis. Steroids can be used for symptomatic carpal tunnel syndrome, flexor and dorsal tenosynovitis, and any joint that does not respond to medical treatment. Frequent and repeated administration to the same area may cause tendon ruptures, steroid-induced arthropathies, or subdermal skin atrophy. One joint or tendon sheath should probably not receive injections more than two or three times a year.[2] If the local disease persists or increases after this time, surgical intervention is indicated.[4]

### Preventive and Therapeutic Surgery

#### Tenosynovitis

Tenosynovitis is a frequent manifestation of rheumatoid hand disease resulting from a proliferation of the tenosynovium that surrounds the extensor or flexor tendons of the wrist and hand.[4-16] Early recognition of dorsal tenosynovitis affecting extensor tendons or flexor tenosynovitis is key to ensure a good outcome.

## Extensor Tendon Rupture

If dorsal tenosynovitis is ignored or inadequately controlled medically, extensor tendons may rupture from either direct infiltration or attrition (as in extensor pollicis longus rupture around Lister's tubercle).[11, 12] A soft, nonpainful mass located along any or all the extensor compartments is typically present initially. Any accompanying pain should alert the physician to underlying radiocarpal or radioulnar involvement.[4, 6] The most frequent tendons to rupture are the extensors to the small and ring fingers (the so-called Vaughan-Jackson lesion)[13] (Fig. 7–1) and the extensor pollicis longus. In severe destructive disease, multiple digital extensor tendons rupture. Even the wrist extensor tendons can

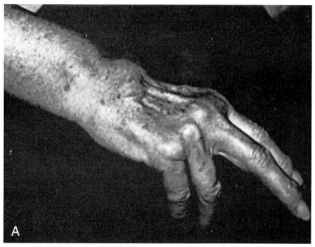

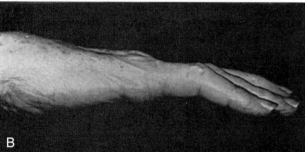

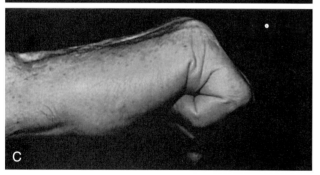

**FIGURE 7–1**
Example of a patient with dorsal tenosynovitis and tendon rupture. *A,* Dorsal tenosynovitis and double tendon rupture. *B and C,* Range of motion demonstrated 3 months postoperatively. (From Kelley WN, Harris ED Jr, Ruddy S, et al [eds]: Textbook of Rheumatology. vol II. 5th ed. Philadelphia: WB Saunders, 1997:1648–1649.)

rupture, with resulting severe flexion deformity of the wrist.[14] Diagnosis and early surgical treatment are important: first, to repair the tendons or perform tendon transfers and, second, to perform a tenosynovectomy to prevent further tendon rupture. There is little doubt about the benefit of prompt surgical intervention, even with a single extensor tendon rupture.[4, 15]

The patient with extensor tendon rupture experiences a loss of active MCP extension and loses the tenodesis effect when flexing and extending the wrist. As the wrist is passively flexed, the tenodesis effect causes MCP and proximal interphalangeal (PIP) joint extension. Conversely, as the wrist is passively extended, the PIP and MP joints are flexed via the tenodesis effect. Other conditions may mimic extensor tendon rupture, namely (1) ulnarly subluxated tendons with extensor hood attenuation secondary to MCP synovitis, (2) posterior interosseous nerve palsy usually secondary to elbow synovitis, and (3) MCP joint destruction and contracture.

With ulnarly subluxated tendons, the patient should be able to hold the MCPs in full extension if they are first positioned passively in extension. Also, the tendons can often be visualized through the thin dorsal skin and seem to subluxate with MCP flexion. Regarding the rare posterior interosseous nerve palsy, the patients usually have elbow complaints, and there is often more diffuse involvement of the posterior interosseous innervated muscles than of isolated finger extensor tendons. This problem can be evaluated further with electrodiagnostic studies. If there is elbow synovitis, a corticosteroid injection may lessen the synovitis and decompress the nerve. MCP joint destruction and dislocation are common in advanced disease and can make diagnosis difficult. It is, therefore, important to have high clinical suspicion for extensor tendon ruptures in advanced disease.

The morbidity and results are directly proportional to the number of tendons ruptured plus the status of the adjacent joints. Because much of the hand must be immobilized for 4 weeks after surgery to allow tendon healing, joint stiffness may develop, and therefore rehabilitation requires more time. Because of this, both patients and physicians should be alerted to the complications of dorsal tenosynovitis. Ideally, early tenosynovectomy should be carried out before tendon rupture occurs. Recurrence after dorsal tenosynovectomy is low at 5% to 6%,[9, 19] and future tendon rupture is effectively prevented.

FLEXOR TENOSYNOVITIS. Flexor tenosynovitis is a result of proliferation of tenosynovium that normally lies in flexor tendons. It can be categorized as wrist, palmar, and digital flexor tenosynovitis. As with dorsal tenosynovitis, early diagnosis and prompt treatment of flexor tenosynovitis prevent the complications of tendon rupture and permanent damage from prolonged median nerve compression.[4, 7, 17]

WRIST FLEXOR TENOSYNOVITIS. This condition may manifest with signs and symptoms of carpal tunnel syndrome because of tenosynovitis within the carpal tunnel causing compression at the median nerve. Some patients may have limited active digital flexion because of impaired flexor tendon excursion. The signs are minimal on physical examination unless there is limited active range of motion. Because the flexor tendons are covered by thick fascia, wrist flexor tenosynovitis does not bulge much. In contrast to dorsal tenosynovitis, it is much less apparent on examination. If the volar surface of the skin is observed carefully, loss of skin wrinkles and lack of venous markings can sometimes be observed. In addition, evidence of thenar muscle atrophy may be noted, especially with long-standing median nerve compression. The treatment for early wrist flexor tenosynovitis is steroid injection, wrist splinting, and medical management. For persistent wrist flexor tenosynovitis or prolonged median nerve symptoms, carpal tunnel release and tenosynovectomy should be carried out to prevent permanent median nerve damage, restore active digital flexion, and prevent tendon rupture (Fig. 7–2).[4, 7]

PALMAR (STENOSING) TENOSYNOVITIS. Palmar stenosing tenosynovitis (trigger finger) occurs when proliferating tenosynovium in the palm causes snapping and locking as the tendon glides within the flexor tendon sheath. Patients can usually flex the digit fully, but as the digit extends, a hypertrophied nodule of synovium catches on the proximal edge of the tendon sheath (the A1 pulley, just proximal to the MCP joint), and the digit snaps into extension. Sometimes the digit becomes locked acutely in flexion and cannot be extended actively. A painful snap occurs as the digit is passively extended. On examination, the flexor tendon nodule can be palpated, and the examiner can feel crepitation as the patient actively flexes and extends the digit.[4, 7]

The initial treatment is steroid injection into the flexor sheath. If the condition does not improve after two injections, flexor tenosynovectomy with or without release of the A1 pulley should be performed.

DIGITAL FLEXOR TENOSYNOVITIS. In contrast to stenosing tenosynovitis, digital flexor tenosynovitis is caused by proliferation of tenosynovium within the digit. The most common finding in this condition is loss of active digital flexion with preserved passive digital flexion.

This is a result of impairment of tendon excursion within the narrow tendon sheath. In addition, crepitation and locking can be seen as the nodule slides within the sheath, and the fullness can sometimes be felt and observed on the volar surface of the digit.[4, 7] A less common, but important, manifestation of digital flexor tenosynovitis is stiffness of the PIP joints. This occurs because the patient is unable to flex the digits actively. This, plus the associated PIP joint synovitis and pain, leads to joint stiffness. Initial treatment is flexor sheath injections; if there is no response, digital flexor tenosynovectomy is indicated. If the patient has associated PIP stiffness, and preservation of the joint space is seen on the radiograph, joint manipulation or release followed by vigorous postoperative hand therapy can restore considerable range of motion.[4, 7]

### Flexor Tendon Rupture

Flexor tendon rupture most commonly occurs at the wrist within the carpal tunnel. On rare occasions, it occurs in the palm or digit. Fortunately, it is not common. Results of treatment for multiple palmar and digital flexor tendon ruptures are not as good as those for their extensor counterparts.

At the wrist, attritional ruptures of the flexor pollicis longus or the flexors of the index finger are caused by a bony spur of the scaphoid that protrudes volarly (Mannerfelt and Norman's lesion).[18] In addition, flexor tendon rupture within the carpal tunnel can occur from infiltrative flexor tenosynovitis.[4–7] As in the case of extensor tendon rupture, early diagnosis and treatment are key to maximize results. This is outlined in detail elsewhere.[19]

## Synovectomy

There are limited data to show that synovectomy appreciably alters the natural course of the disease. Even though long-term results of synovectomy cannot be predicted, the procedure does have some definite, al-

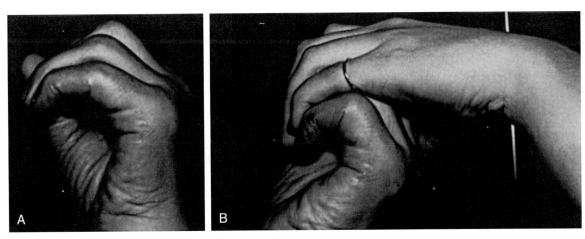

**FIGURE 7–2**
Patient with flexor tenosynovitis. *A*, Patient presents with symptoms of carpal tunnel syndrome. Note limited active digital flexion. *B*, Passive digital flexion preserved. (From Kelley WN, Harris ED Jr, Ruddy S, et al [eds]: Textbook of Rheumatology, 5th ed. Philadelphia: WB Saunders, 1997:1648–1649.)

though narrow, indications in the hand.[2, 6] The primary indications for synovectomy of the wrist or digital joint are for a small group of patients with smoldering, slowly progressive disease, who are responding to systemic medication but continue to show synovitis in one or more of the joints. Typically these patients have responded to three steroid injections over a 6- to 12-month period but continued to have recurrent synovitis, sometimes with pain. Radiographs show minimal joint involvement with little evidence of progression. Synovectomy can alleviate pain and, ideally, delay or prevent further joint destruction.

## Reconstructive and Salvage Surgery

Despite early recognition, splinting, and prophylactic surgery, the natural progression of rheumatoid arthritis often leads to destructive changes in the joints of the hand and wrist. The surgeon must then resort to either reconstructive surgery or salvage surgery to relieve pain and provide joint stability. The surgeon has one of two choices in the management of destroyed joints: arthrodesis or arthroplasty. Each of these procedures has benefits and drawbacks and, therefore, represents a compromise of full function. Choosing between these two operations takes judgment and experience.

### Wrist

The wrist is a foundation on which hand function is built. A painful, unstable wrist reduces hand function even without digital involvement. In fact, it may be a primary factor in producing digital deformities. In advanced cases, surgical attempts to realign the wrist and alleviate pain include total or partial fusion or arthroplasty.[20] The choice between these procedures depends on many factors, including the condition of the wrist extensors, the amount of bone resorbed in the carpus, and the status of the hand, the opposite wrist, and even the lower extremities.

WRIST ARTHRODESIS. Total wrist arthrodesis eliminates pain, provides stability for hand function, corrects alignment, and is still the gold standard of treatment.[21-23] Although the patient gives up flexion and extension motions, forearm supination and pronation are preserved. The advantages of a solid wrist fusion are stability and dependability. Disease is arrested at this site and is no longer a source of pain. Progression or recurrence of the deformity is now halted. If the patient has lower extremity problems that require the use of a cane or crutches, a fused wrist provides the necessary support. The benefits of a single fused wrist far outweigh the disadvantages of loss of flexion and extension; even in young, vigorous patients, this is a reliable solution to the problem of a destroyed wrist joint.

Although the total wrist fusion has been an accepted treatment for the severely involved wrist, there are many patients in whom the major changes are limited to the radiocarpal joints, whereas the midcarpal area is preserved. In these patients, limited arthrodesis may

be indicated. The radiolunate fusion restores the anatomy to a more normal situation and can preserve up to 50% of normal wrist motion.[24] If the radioscapholunate joint is destroyed, it can be fused, but there is a greater loss of motion, leaving only between 40 and 50 degrees.[25] The theoretical benefit of these limited arthrodesis procedures is that by restoring the wrist to a more normal anatomic position, the midcarpal joints are protected. However, one report indicates that prevention may not be possible and that in certain patients progression may be inevitable.[26]

WRIST ARTHROPLASTY. Because wrist arthropathy is usually symmetric in its distribution, the loss of bilateral wrist motion can create functional loss for the patient. Bilateral wrist arthrodesis is often preferred; however, in patients whose major difficulty with the wrist is pain with retention of significant motion, an alternative treatment, arthroplasty, is available.

A flexible wrist implant shaped like the digital implant was introduced in the late 1960s.[3] Early results with this type of implant were encouraging; however, long-term studies revealed a high incidence of implant problems.[27-31] This type of implant is mainly indicated for the extremely low-demand patient with bilateral wrist disease and no dependence on crutches.

The success of metal-to-plastic prostheses in the hip, knee, and shoulder has led to similar devices for the wrist.[32-37] Their early development was marked by problems with imbalance. Good results for up to 10 years can be achieved with newer generation designs.[28, 38, 39] In properly selected patients, wrist arthroplasty has a definite role. Arthrodesis, however, is still the mainstay of treatment.

### Distal Radioulnar Joint

Mention should be made of the distal radioulnar joint or, more appropriately, the distal ulna, in rheumatoid arthritis. As the disease progresses, instability of the distal ulna is noted. In particular, dorsal dislocation can cause extensor tendon rupture through attritional wear. Resection of the distal ulna with or without soft tissue reconstruction is the procedure of choice.[40] If adequate soft tissues are preserved, the remaining ulna, although mobile, does not cause symptoms, and the risk of extensor tendon rupture is minimized. On rare occasion, only the articular surface of the distal ulna is resected, that is, a distal radioulnar joint hemiarthroplasty.

### Thumb

The thumb of the rheumatoid arthritis patient deserves special comment. Its importance to hand function is well recognized. Unfortunately, it is frequently involved with rheumatoid arthritis and can, as a result of muscular imbalance or joint destruction, assume bizarre deformities.[41] The most common deformity seen is the boutonnière deformity (MCP flexion and IP hyperextension). This thumb deformity is made worse with pinch force on the thumb against other digits. The reverse deformity (swan-neck), with MCP hyperextension and IP flexion, is usually secondary to changes at the CMC joint from synovitis. Other deformities can occur as a result of collateral ligament or tendon ruptures occurring in combination with joint changes.

With regard to the specific thumb deformities, a systematic, joint-oriented approach is best. Early reconstruction is generally more satisfying than late salvage procedures. The distal joint of the thumb (IP) is treated in a manner similar to that for the distal joints of the other digits: by fusion. It is usually fused in the straight or slightly flexed position to restore a stable pinch (Fig. 7–3).

At the thumb MCP joint level, the choice is between fusion and arthroplasty. With isolated MCP joint disease, a fusion in 15 degrees of flexion gives excellent results with little functional loss. With associated IP joint disease, however, arthroplasty is preferred at the MCP level to avoid fusion in adjacent joints. The silicone implant gives excellent results, with good pain relief, about 25 degrees of motion, and good stability.[42]

At the CMC joint level, it is important to maintain motion. Fusion here could become disabling if subsequent instability developed and the patient required fusion distally. In general, resection arthroplasty of the CMC joint has been preferred over implants in patients with rheumatoid arthritis.[43]

## Metacarpophalangeal Joints

The MCP joints of the hand are single condylar joints allowing 80 to 90 degrees of flexion as well as rotary and lateral motions. They play an important role in positioning the fingers. If they are fixed in poor position, hand function is greatly reduced. Unfortunately, MCP joint involvement is common in rheumatoid arthritis. The capsular laxity, which gives the joint varied mobility, makes MCP joint subluxation and dislocation common late sequelae of synovitis.

Soft tissue reconstruction for MCP joint deformity might be considered.[44] However, this mandates a good joint space, and there is a tendency for recurrence. To

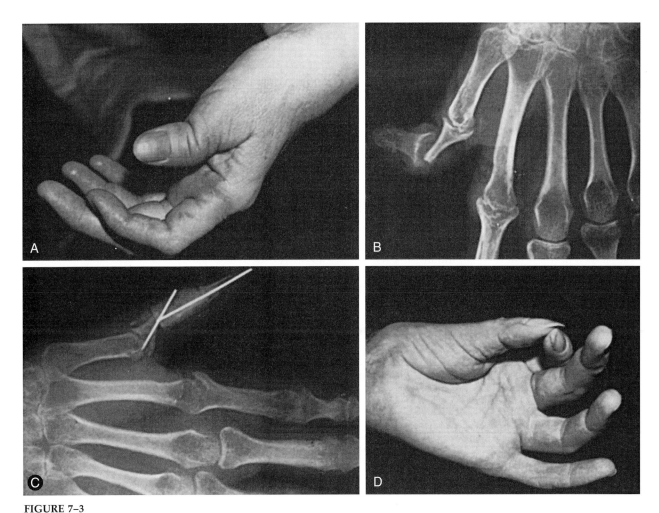

**FIGURE 7–3**
Unstable distal joint treated by fusion and bone graft.
*A,* Clinical appearance of the thumb with collapse of the interphalangeal joint. *B,* Radiograph shows significant absorption of the distal end of the proximal phalanx. *C,* Postoperative radiograph shows use of one graft to restore length and facilitate joint fusion. *D,* Note stable pinch between lengthened thumb and index finger. Distal joint fused in slight flexion. (From Kelley WN, Harris ED Jr, Ruddy S, et al [eds]: Textbook of Rheumatology, 5th ed. Philadelphia: VB Saunders, 1997:1656.)

restore function, arthroplasty is a treatment of choice at the MCP level. Although fusion of the MCP joint can be performed to obtain finger realignment, preserving MCP joint motion is preferred because it greatly enhances overall grasp. With the arthroplasty techniques available, this can be achieved in a predictable way.

The second-generation flexible silicone rubber implants act as a spacer between resected bone ends of the MP joint and have provided the most predictable results.[3, 45, 46]

## Results of Metacarpophalangeal Joint Arthroplasty

With the flexible implant arthroplasty, the surgeon can, in most cases, correct MCP joint subluxation, dislocations, and ulnar deviation of the fingers.[47, 48] With proper surgical technique, the surgeon should expect to realign the digit, relieve pain, and maintain between 30 and 60 degrees of motion, with an average of 45 degrees.[49–52] Performing surgery earlier is considerably easier than postponing surgical intervention to the point at which the patient has severe deformity, significant bony erosions, severe ulnar drift, and flexion contractures. The results are also better. The polymeric silicone (Silastic) prosthesis is excellent for pain relief and improvement of both appearance and positioning of the fingers, but it does not restore full motion or significantly improve grip or pinched strength. Despite this, patient satisfaction is high.[49–51]

## Proximal Interphalangeal Joint

Like their distal counterparts, the PIP joints are hinged joints allowing flexion and extension. The range of motion at this level is normally full extension or slight hyperextension to 110 degrees of flexion. This mobility, although only slightly greater than that at the distal joint, is far more important than bringing the fingertip to the palm. Therefore, loss of motion at the PIP level is more of a hardship for the patient, and attempts to preserve it are more frequently indicated (Fig. 7–4).

In addition to motion, lateral stability is important, especially in activities involving pinch. The surgeon has a choice between fusion or a flexible implant arthroplasty at this level. Index finger PIP stability is generally more important than motion (compared with the more ulnar digits), so arthrodesis is more often indicated for this joint.

The index finger is used in picking up objects or performing delicate tasks in opposition with the thumb. It is particularly important in lateral pinch when the thumb presses against the radial index finger surface. Most of these functions are carried out with the PIP joint in slight to moderate flexion. For this reason, fusion of the index finger PIP joint is less of a handicap than fusion of the more ulnar digits. In the ring and small fingers, acute flexion of the PIP joint is needed to grasp small objects firmly. For this reason, arthroplasty is likely to be chosen in the ulnar digits.

## Digital Deformities

Digital deformities are classified as boutonnière or swan-neck deformities. The boutonnière deformity is flexion of the PIP joint and hyperextension of the distal interphalangeal (DIP) joint. The cause of boutonnière deformities is a synovitis, with subsequent attenuation of the dorsal capsule of the PIP joint and the overlying central tendon. This allows the lateral bands to slide palmarly, with subsequent extension of the DIP joint. Initially, the boutonnière deformity is passively correctable, although full extension can rarely be achieved with the amount of synovitis present. With time, the deformities become fixed because of changes within the joint and shortening of the capsular structures on the palmar aspect.

Surgical correction of the digital deformity should be carried out only after any MCP joint problems have been taken care of. These procedures can be performed in conjunction with one another, for example, MCP joint arthroplasties with PIP joint fusions. Although the passively correctable or minimally deformed fingers can be corrected with a soft tissue procedure, stiffness often occurs. This stiffness is not only at the PIP joint but also at the DIP joint level because of the nature of the extensor mechanism or dorsal apparatus. Surgery consists of a synovectomy and mobilization of lateral bands, which allows them to be reduced to a more dorsal position. Also, a terminal tenotomy may be required if there is a fixed extension deformity at the DIP joint. If the joint is destroyed, a PIP joint arthroplasty along with a soft tissue reconstruction is indicated. With fixed boutonnière deformities of greater than 50 degrees, the patient and surgeon should seriously consider arthrodesis in the appropriate position depending on the digit.

Swan-neck deformities are the result of hyperextension of the PIP joint and subsequent flexion of the DIP joint. Again, the cause is synovitis, although in this case, the structures that are attenuated are more palmar than dorsal. The primary disease is in the PIP joint, with DIP joint changes occurring as the result of the changes proximally. Again, all MCP deformities must be corrected before the swan-neck deformity is approached surgically. Fixed deformities at the MCP joints are often the cause of swan-neck deformities, and if the MCP joint flexion deformities are not corrected, usually with arthroplasties, swan-neck deformities recur in the PIP joint.

Correction of swan-neck deformities depends on the severity of the changes. If the swan-neck deformity is supple, a flexor digitorum superficialis tenodesis, in combination with the correction of the MCP deformity, suffices. If the swan-neck deformity is fixed, and the joint has an adequate cartilage space, the PIP joint can be manipulated into flexion and held with a percutaneous wire at the same time that the MCP arthroplasties are performed. If this is the chosen procedure, relaxing incisions over the PIP joint are required.

If the PIP joint shows destructive changes, the option of an arthroplasty is raised. If there is such severe

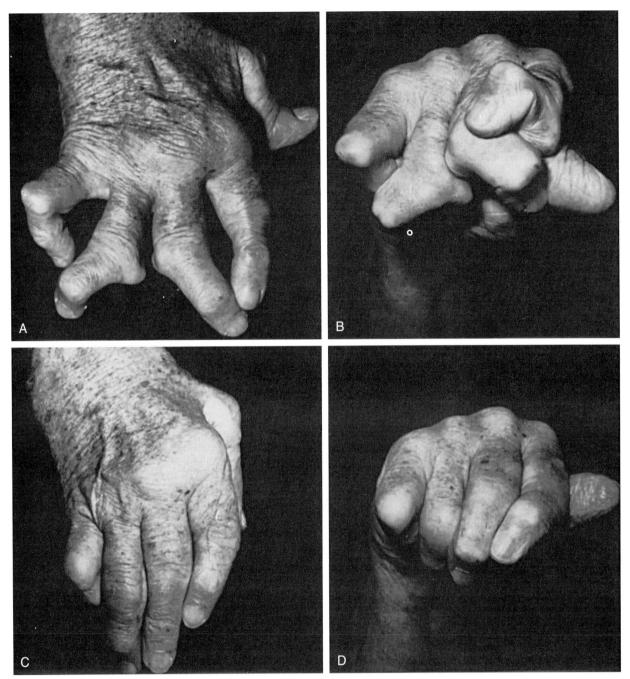

**FIGURE 7–4**
Example of proximal interphalangeal (PIP) joint arthroplasties for severe deformities. *A*, Preoperative view of hand with fingers in extension. Note severe lateral deformities of PIP joints. *B*, Patient's fingers overlap on attempted flexion. Grasping ability is poor. *C*, Postoperative extension after PIP arthroplasties. *D*, Postoperative flexion. (From Kelley WN, Harris ED Jr, Ruddy S, et al [eds]: Textbook of Rheumatology, 5th ed. Philadelphia: WB Saunders, 1997:1659.)

destruction that it is best to accept limited motion of the PIP joints, they can be manipulated and held in flexion and allowed to stiffen in that position. If the physician wants to try to achieve motion at the PIP joint, PIP arthroplasties can be performed. This may or may not be performed at the same time as MCP arthroplasties. The results of either a manipulation or an arthroplasty are limited. At best, a range of 30 to 50 degrees of motion,

ideally from a fixed flexion deformity position of approximately 10 degrees, can be expected.

In general, the results of arthroplasty at the PIP joint level are better with swan-neck deformity than with boutonnière deformity. Although long-term follow-up has not shown a significant increase in range of motion from the preoperative level, pain relief has been good.[53, 54]

## Distal Interphalangeal Joints

Like the PIP joints, the DIP joints of the digits are hinged joints, normally allowing 70 to 80 degrees of flexion. As a result of rheumatoid arthritis, the cartilaginous joint surfaces can be destroyed, which causes pain and limitation of motion. As a result of these changes, either singly or in combination, an unsightly deformity develops that not only is painful but also results in decreased function.

Because of the difficulty involved in restoring active motion and joint stability, and the relative unimportance of mobility of the distal joints, fusion is preferred over arthroplasty of the DIP joint.

The best position for arthrodesis of the DIP joint is 0 to 10 degrees of flexion. In this position, the digit has a relatively normal appearance when the fingers are extended. When the patient makes a fist, the lack of distal joint motion is of little functional significance. Picking up or holding objects between the thumb and the involved digit is not compromised with the distal joint being almost straight. This position enhances "pulp-to-pulp" pinch, which is more useful than the "tip-to-tip" pinch that requires distal joint mobility.

Fusion of the distal joints achieves not only a beneficial effect at the operative site but also function at the more proximal joint level. For example, a distal joint fusion in neutral position balances the extensor and flexor forces. This can be helpful in correcting a mild swan-neck deformity (PIP hyperextension) that is secondary to a distal joint mallet deformity.[55, 56] In addition, fusion in the distal joint simplifies and straightens extensor or flexor forces at the PIP joint level, where active motion is more important than at the distal joint.

## Arthritis Mutilans

Occasionally, patients have such marked destruction of bone that severe deformity and instability exist. In general, arthrodesis with bone grafting is the only salvage procedure available for these patients.

## Summary

Much can be done for the rheumatoid patient with hand involvement. Therapeutic operations on the tendons and nerves can restore lost function, and early prophylactic surgery can slow the progression of deformity. Arthroplasties have also been developed that make it possible to maintain mobility in those joints that must move to maintain significant function. Salvage surgery, such as fusion, can reliably correct deformities and eliminate pain when motion is less predictably restored.

## SYSTEMIC LUPUS ERYTHEMATOSUS

## Clinical Features

Systemic lupus erythematosus (SLE) is a multiple-system connective tissue disease that often has musculoskeletal involvement. Various articular complaints can be some of the most frequent clinical manifestations of the disease. The joints most often involved are the knees, but the small joints of the hands and wrists are also frequently affected.[57, 58] The most typical pattern of involvement is one of migratory arthralgias.

Hand involvement in lupus is generally more benign than that seen in rheumatoid arthritis. Bleifield and Inglis[59] reported some hand involvement in 86% of 50 randomly examined patients with lupus. Most patients reported evanescent arthralgias, although some described definite evidence of swelling and synovitis. The most common cause of symptoms in the hand is Raynaud's phenomenon, occurring in 50% of patients. These deformities can affect any joint in the hand and can cause any rheumatoid deformity.

In contrast to patients with rheumatoid arthritis or osteoarthritis, patients with lupus do not have articular cartilage involvement, unless there is a secondary degenerative type of arthritis from the ligamentous laxity. Because of the ligamentous laxity, however, some of the most severe unstable digital deformities can be seen in these patients. Early reconstructive surgery before severe dislocations and fixed deformities occur is indicated.[60]

## Specific Deformities

### Wrist

Wrist involvement is a frequent radiographic manifestation of the lupus hand but usually is asymptomatic. Most common findings are those of ligamentous laxity. This results in dorsal subluxation of the distal ulna, which can result in pain and limited rotation. Ulnar translocation of the carpus is common and intercarpal dissociation manifested by an increased scapholunate gap and rotation of the scaphoid is also seen. These conditions generally are asymptomatic, and even in the more significant collapse patterns pain is unusual.

### Digital Deformities

The most common digital deformity seen in SLE is secondary to ulnar subluxation of the extensor tendons at the MCP joint and their subsequent overpull at the PIP joints. This picture of MCP flexion deformity with mild ulnar deviation combined with PIP hyperextension and DIP flexion (or swan-neck deformity) is known as *Jaccoud's syndrome*. Initially these deformities are passively correctable, but eventually they become fixed.[60]

The type of surgery performed for lupus deformities depends on whether destructive changes have occurred. With Jaccoud's syndrome, attention must be directed at both the MCP and PIP joints. Soft tissue reconstruction procedures are aimed at providing stability to the PIP and MCP joints. This surgery, although extensive, has relatively good results. Once fixed deformities occur, arthroplasty yields the best results.[60]

### Thumb

The lupus thumb deformity most commonly results from involvement of all three joints: the CMC, MCP, and IP. Soft tissue reconstruction of the CMC or MCP joint provides durable stability provided that the articular surfaces are sound. Otherwise, arthroplasty or fusion is the procedure of choice.[19] IP fusion is frequently needed for marked instability of the IP joint.

## PSORIASIS

### Clinical Features

Approximately 5% of the patients with psoriasis have arthritis, predominantly involving the small bones of the hands and feet. In general, arthropathy develops in a patient with severe skin involvement, although 20% of psoriatic patients come to medical attention with arthritis before the development of skin changes.[61] Unlike rheumatoid arthritis, psoriasis rarely manifests with an exuberant proliferating synovitis or tenosynovitis. Characteristically, there is more diffuse involvement of all soft tissues, which predisposes the patient to scarring.

### Specific Deformities

#### Digital Deformities

Digital stiffness from involvement of the skin is common. Patients classically come to medical attention with a "sausage digit" (finger or toe or both). Articular cartilage and metaphyseal bone changes most often involve the DIP and PIP joints. At the DIP level, the severity of arthritis frequently parallels the degree of nail deformities, such as pitting, ridging, thickening, or detachment. Radiographically, erosive articular destruction in the IP joints (the PIP more than the DIP) predominates. "Pencil-in-cup" deformities are characteristic. Progressive distal phalangeal osteolysis with tuft resorption is highly suggestive of psoriatic arthropathy. Severe resorption may result in an "opera glass hand" with skin collapse over resorbed phalanges. As with other seronegative arthropathies metaphyseal periostitis may develop, with "paintbrush" or "whiskering" of the individual phalanx.[62]

In psoriatic arthritis, spontaneous fusion of the DIP and intercarpal joints often occurs in a functional position, and thus surgical intervention is not needed. The PIP joint is involved most severely, and often flexion contractures greater than 90 degrees develop. On occasion, swan-neck deformities occur. The radiographs frequently show a narrow but not completely destroyed joint space; however, the articular cartilage is involved more significantly than expected, and joint release usually fails. In addition, there may be an adhesive tenosynovitis that prevents good flexor tendon function, predisposing to recurrent contracture and stiffness. Unless there are significant flexion deformities or pain, surgery is usually not advisable. If either is present, arthrodesis in a functional position is advocated.[62] Arthroplasty at the MCP and PIP levels is reserved for patients with severe involvement. At the time of PIP arthroplasty, it is wise to check the excursion of the flexor tendons. MCP arthroplasties are performed for the same indications as in rheumatoid arthritis, that is, pain, deformity, stiffness, and lack of function. However, the rate of infection is slightly higher than in patients with rheumatoid arthritis and lupus, and the eventual range of motion is smaller.[62]

### Wrist

Involvement of the wrist includes carpal erosions, joint space narrowing, and spontaneous intercarpal fusions but generally affects only patients with severe IP involvement. Although surgery is required less frequently at the wrist, the indications and procedures are the same as those in rheumatoid arthritis. Arthrodesis is the procedure of choice.

### Thumb

Arthritic involvement of the IP, MCP, and CMC joints occurs, with the CMC joint affected most severely. CMC destruction with stiffness and decreased opposition may occur. At the CMC level, resection arthroplasty should be performed. At the thumb MCP level, either polymeric silicone arthroplasty or arthrodesis could be performed. We prefer arthroplasty, which may be performed at the same time as the CMC surgery, except when a swan-neck deformity is present. In this situation, MCP arthrodesis has yielded the best results. Problems of the IP joint should be focused on arthrodesis to provide durable relief and function.

As in all arthritides, the results in patient satisfaction are best with thumb and wrist surgery as compared with finger surgery.

## OSTEOARTHRITIS

### Clinical Features

Osteoarthritis of the hand is characterized not by synovial hypertrophy but by gradual loss of articular cartilage. As it relates to the hand and wrist, this condition is most prevalent in postmenopausal women but can appear at a younger age in men, especially those in whom previous joint trauma is thought to be a contributing factor. The onset of this condition is slow, with pain being the chief symptom. Radiographic examination of the involved joint initially shows a loss of joint spaces, followed by the appearance of osteophytes. Sclerosis of adjacent bone is also seen.

Although any joint of the hand or wrist may be involved with the various rheumatic conditions, there are four sites where osteoarthritis is frequently seen: the DIP and PIP joints of the finger (IP joint of the thumb), the CMC joint of the thumb, and the wrist (radiocarpal) joint.

### Specific Deformities

#### Distal Interphalangeal Joint

The DIP joint is the most common location for osteoarthritis, and the typical patient with symptomatic involvement at this level is the postmenopausal woman. Osteophyte formation (enlargement of the joints), or Heberden's nodes, is a typical physical finding, as is pain and mild radial or ulnar deviation. There is a loss of joint motion noted on clinical examination, but this is seldom a concern to the patient. In fact, as the joint loses motion, pain decreases. In these patients with distal joint arthritis, small mucous cysts may develop on the dorsal aspect of the distal phalanx and may gradually enlarge and stretch the overlying skin. Although the cysts originate from the joint, they may appear at the base of the fingernail where pressure against the nail may cause irregular nail growth.

The treatment of arthritis of the DIP joint and IP joint of the thumb includes splinting, analgesics for mild pain, and arthroplasty or arthrodesis with spur removal for unstable or unsightly joints. Bothersome mucous cysts are treated with local excision and removal of any underlying bony spurs that are thought to be contributing factors to their development. Recurrence of the mucous cyst is occasionally seen and can be eliminated by joint fusion. Distal IP joint arthrodesis is a good operation for pain or instability, and the loss of motion is not a problem functionally.

Recently there has been some enthusiasm for DIP arthroplasty.[63, 64] The Swanson polymeric silicone spacer is the implant of choice. Pain relief is excellent, the average active range of motion is 30 degrees, and the patients feel that they have more dexterity than with arthrodesis.

## Proximal Interphalangeal Joint

At the PIP joint level, the gradual loss of joint motion is of major significance, with the patient finding it difficult to grasp small objects. The joints enlarge with spur formation (Bouchard's nodes) and become unsightly. Pain may also be noted with loss of joint articular cartilage. Ulnar deformities of this joint are common, with stretching of the collateral ligaments and bone resorption. This leads to overlapping of the fingers and considerable loss of function. Pain at this level can be controlled by splinting, but restoration of motion can be achieved only by arthroplasty. The use of flexible implants has been worthwhile in this regard. However, achieving more than an average of 30 degrees of motion cannot be expected with this procedure initially. Ulnar deformity tends to recur. Long-term follow-up may show additional loss of 5 to 10 degrees. When patients are being considered for PIP joint arthroplasties because of osteoarthritis, attention should be directed toward the distal joints. If there is distal joint involvement, it is advisable to combine fusion of the distal joint with arthroplasty of the PIP joint. Recently, there has been interest in recreating motion in a fused PIP joint whether the fusion has been spontaneous or surgically induced. Although the procedure is technically more demanding than primary arthroplasty, the results have been comparable.[65]

## Carpometacarpal Joint of the Thumb

The third area of common hand involvement in osteoarthritis is the CMC joint of the thumb. This is the joint that most commonly requires surgery in the osteoarthritic hand. Patients come to medical attention with increasing pain at the base of the thumb and radiographic signs of articular cartilage loss. Rotary motions of the joint are particularly painful. With a gradual lateral subluxation of the joint, the typical patient develops a "shoulder" or a prominence at the base of the thumb. The patient has increasing difficulty applying pressure with the thumb, thus making any activity requiring pinch painful. A simple activity, such as opening a car door or removing a bottle cap, becomes difficult and painful. Secondary deformities include adduction of the metacarpal and MCP hyperextension. These can cause further limitations in the hand, particularly in activities involving grasp.

Rest, nonsteroidal anti-inflammatory drugs (NSAIDs), use of a thumb spica-style thermoplastic splint, and an occasional corticosteroid injection are frequently helpful in relieving pain and certainly should be tried before surgery is contemplated. In patients who do not respond to conservative treatment, arthroplasty affords an excellent solution. Two surgical approaches are commonly used. In one procedure, the trapezium is removed and the space interposed by autogenous soft tissue, such as joint capsule or tendon (resection arthroplasty). In the other procedure, the trapezium is replaced by a prosthesis.

The resection arthroplasty gives predictable relief of pain but some loss of pinch power and some residual proximal migration of the metacarpal. The advantage of this technique is simplicity of surgery and consistency of satisfactory results. Other resection techniques may use a portion of the tendon interposition to reconstruct soft tissues around the CMC joint.[66, 67] Trapezium replacement arthroplasties can also be used to maintain space and thumb alignment. The results of this technique, mainly using the polymeric silicone trapezium prosthesis, were initially encouraging. However, this approach is surgically more demanding, and a longer follow-up has shown increasingly frequent reports of prosthetic erosion or breakage or polymeric silicone synovitis and deterioration of results.[68–70] CMC fusion can be successful in restoring stability and relieving pain in these patients but should be used only in patients who have localized CMC joint involvement and in whom MCP flexion is maintained. CMC fusion is currently advised in traumatic arthritis in the young patient.

## Wrist

Primary osteoarthritis of the wrist is extremely rare. Degenerative changes are usually a sequelae of traumatic injury. Splinting, therapy, and NSAIDs can be helpful. The degenerative patterns and surgical treatment are complex and beyond the scope of this chapter.[71]

# EPICONDYLITIS

Epicondylitis involves soft tissue changes of tendinous origin around the lateral and medial humeral epicondyle. They are commonly associated with overuse and sports-related injuries and are characterized by localized pain around the epicondyles and weakness of the forearm flexors and extensors.

## Lateral Epicondylitis

Lateral epicondylitis (also known as *tennis elbow*) is caused by degeneration at the common extensor origin on the lateral humeral epicondyle. It is characterized by pain and tenderness around the lateral epicondyle. It occurs in more than 50% of tennis players at some point during their playing careers; however, it is known to occur in the non–sports-playing population as well.

Pathologic studies have shown that the extensor carpi radialis brevis (ECRB) tendon is the site where tendon degeneration is most commonly present. Microscopic studies revealed infiltration of normal tendon by a process termed *angiofibroblastic hyperplasia*. A degenerative process is more likely the cause rather than an inflammatory process.[72, 73]

The diagnosis of lateral epicondylitis is noted by maximal tenderness just slightly anterior and distal to the lateral epicondyle at the origin of the ECRB. Increased pain as extension of the wrist is resisted is a provocative test. Degenerative changes in the radiocapitellar joint of the elbow mimics lateral epicondylitis. Radiographs can differentiate between the two. A compressive neuropathy involving the radial nerve around the elbow leads to pain in a similar area. However, pain from the radial nerve compression is usually more distal than that of lateral epicondylitis. Compression of the radial nerve or its branches (posterior interosseus nerve) can be seen in the rheumatoid arthritis patient resulting from synovial hypertrophy at the elbow.

Nonoperative treatment is successful for the majority of patients, although a prolonged course, 12 to 18 months, of treatment may be necessary until resolution of pain and return to activity are possible. Rest from offending activities, NSAIDs, and ice applications are frequently helpful. Once discomfort has abated, range of motion exercises can be started, followed by a progressive strengthening program. Counterforce bracing has also been used.[74]

Local corticosteroid injections should be reserved for more sedentary individuals or patients not responding to the standard nonoperative treatment. As the pathologic condition involves the ECRB tendon, cortisone injections should be directed slightly anterior and distal to the epicondyle, trying to inject into the subaponeurotic fatty recess below the ECRB tendon. Care should be taken to avoid intratendinous injections, as well as subcutaneous injections that may lead to subdermal atrophy and depigmentation.

Patients who fail to respond to a program of rehabilitation are candidates for operative intervention, involving débridement of the degenerative changes in the ECRB and extensor tendons.

## Medial Epicondylitis

Medial epicondylitis is less common than the lateral epicondylitis and is referred to as *golfer's elbow*. The symptoms of pain and weakness are similar to those in lateral epicondylitis but are located at the flexor-pronator origin around the medial humeral epicondyle.

Tenderness around the medial epicondyle is not a specific finding because ulnar nerve inflammation in the cubital tunnel and ulnar collateral (or medial collateral) ligament disorders of the elbow leads to pain there. Tinel's percussion test of the ulnar nerve in the cubital tunnel can be helpful to differentiate medial epicondylitis from ulnar neuropathy. Pain with resisted wrist flexion and forearm pronation are signs of medial epicondylitis. To rule out ulnar collateral ligament disorders, placing the arm in a slightly flexed position with the wrist flexed and forearm pronated relaxes the flexor-pronator muscle mass, thus allowing the examiner to place a valgus stress to the elbow to see whether the pain is referable to the collateral ligament.

Nonoperative treatment is similar to that for lateral epicondylitis, with range of motion and certain exercises emphasizing wrist flexion and forearm pronation. There is no place for corticosteroid injections because of the proximity of the ulnar nerve at the medial epicondyle. If after a several-month course of therapy, resolution of pain and weakness is not resolved, operative intervention is called for. In a manner similar to operative treatment of lateral epicondylitis, the flexor-pronator mass is identified, and degenerative tendinous structures are débrided with reattachment to their bony origins. Rehabilitation once again is a prolonged course and may take 3 to 6 months before patients feel they are at baseline level.[73]

# BURSITIS

Bursae are sacs of synovial tissue that serve to reduce friction between bones and tendons or bones and skin. The most commonly afflicted bursa in the upper extremity is the subcutaneous olecranon bursa. Bursitis can be secondary to trauma, metabolic disorders, systemic diseases such as rheumatoid arthritis, dialysis, and infection. There are also occupational links with carpet layers, construction workers, and gardeners.[75] Subcutaneous bursae do not typically communicate with adjacent joints. Bursal disorders are soft tissue disorders and can be treated as such. Olecranon bursitis can be classified into the aseptic or septic variety.

## Aseptic Olecranon Bursitis

Aseptic olecranon bursitis accounts for the majority of cases and typically follows a course of self-resolution. Manifestation usually involves subcutaneous swelling over the proximal subcutaneous ulna and olecranon process. Occasionally, erythema may be present. The patient is afebrile, and active motion may be slightly limited. Passive range of motion is normal.

Observation, rest, and mild compression can be useful in the initial or mild case. Aspiration of an olecranon bursa may be performed for recurrent or recalcitrant cases. If soft tissue lesions such as rheumatoid nodules or gouty tophi are present, care should be taken to ensure that open lesions do not form. If open soft tissue lesions are present, treating them with simple dressing changes until acute inflammation subsides and performing elective bursectomy are recommended.

If aspiration is to be performed, establishment of sinus tracts through aspiration puncture should be avoided. By guiding the aspiration needle through normal tissue, such as the lateral edge of the triceps in a semiflexed elbow, this can be avoided.

Corticosteroid injections into bursal sacs have been suggested as a way to resolve aseptic bursitis. However, as the majority of the cases are self-limiting with good results, the routine use of corticosteroid injection is not recommended because there is a noted complication rate.[76] The realcitrant or recurrent case can be managed well with surgical excision.[77]

## Septic Olecranon Bursitis

Septic bursitis is usually the result of penetrating trauma, open lesions, or a foreign body. Hematogenous spread, or spread from contiguous soft tissues, is rare. Spreading erythema, fever, and discomfort are common signs. Aspiration of the bursa, via the technique outlined earlier, can be helpful in establishing the diagnosis of septic bursitis, as well as providing identification of the offending organism. *Staphylococcus aureus* and *Streptococcus* species are the most common offending agents. However, polymicrobial infections can be present in the immunocompromised, rheumatoid, or diabetic patient or in the intravenous drug abuser.

If there is no evidence of systemic symptoms, a 2-week course of oral antibiotics can be started. If there is no improvement or evidence of spreading infection, parenteral antibiotics should be used. Clinical symptoms of bursitis may not resolve for 1 to 2 months.[75]

We would not recommend routine incision and drainage of septic bursae in the office, rather preferring to keep skin integrity intact and treat with antibiotics and occasional aspiration, if needed. If there is loss of skin integrity from penetrating trauma or other causes, treating the patient with dressing changes and antibiotics until the acute symptoms subside, followed by bursectomy, would be preferred. Surgical excision is also recommended for the situation that does not show response to antibiotics.

## DE QUERVAIN'S TENOSYNOVITIS

de Quervain's tenosynovitis is an inflammatory disorder involving the synovial lining of the tendons of the first dorsal compartment of the wrist.[78] These are the abductor pollicus longus and extensor pollicus brevis tendons in the area of the radial styloid. Clinical manifestation involves pain around the base of the thumb or the radial styloid area, typically with thumb grasping and pinching activities. There may also be catching of tendons in the area of the radial styloid or a sense of crepitus. Localized swelling in the area of the radial styloid is also common.

Although onset is usually in the fourth to fifth decades, it occurs most frequently in new mothers (new mother disease). It is more prevalent in women. It can be associated with systemic disease such as rheumatoid arthritis, and overuse syndromes. Disorders of the CMC joint of the thumb or scaphoid fractures can also manifest with pain in this region and should be ruled out.

The modified Finkelstein's test is a provocative maneuver to help diagnose de Quervain's tenosynovitis.[79] As the thumb is placed in the palm and the fingers are gently closed around it, the hand is forced into ulnar deviation. Pain elicited in the area of the radial styloid is indicative of de Quervain's tenosynovitis. The patient may also note some discomfort or tenderness along the course of the abductor pollicis longus or extensor pollicis longus tendons along the dorsum of the thumb metacarpal joint.

Nonoperative treatment involves a removable thermoplastic thumb spica splint, activity modification, and NSAIDs. Corticosteroid injection to the first dorsal compartment can also be performed. For the rare recalcitrant case, operative release of the first dorsal compartment is called for.[78]

## REFERENCES

1. Flatt AE: The Care of the Rheumatoid Hand. St. Louis: CV Mosby, 1963.
2. Millender LH, Nalebuff EA: Evaluation and treatment of early rheumatoid hand involvement. Orthop Clin North Am 1975; 6:697.
3. Swanson AB: Flexible Implant Resection Arthroplasty in the Hand and Extremities. St. Louis: CV Mosby, 1973.
4. Millender LH, Nalebuff EA: Preventive surgery—Tenosynovectomy and synovectomy. Orthop Clin North Am 1975; 6:765.
5. Kessler L, Vainio K: Posterior (dorsal) synovectomy for rheumatoid involvement of the hand and wrist: A follow-up study of sixty-six procedures. J Bone Joint Surg Am 1966; 48:1048.
6. Linscheid RL: Surgery for rheumatoid arthritis—Timing and techniques: The upper extremity. J Bone Joint Surg Am 1968; 50:605.
7. Nalebuff EA, Potter TA: Rheumatoid involvement of tendons and tendon sheaths in the hand. Clin Orthop 1968; 59:147.
8. Lipscomb PR: Surgery for rheumatoid arthritis—Timing and techniques: Summary. J Bone Joint Surg Am 1968; 50:614.
9. Brown FE, Brown ML: Long-term results after tenosynovectomy to treat the rheumatoid hand. J Hand Surg Am 1988; 13:704.
10. Williamson SC, Feldon P: Extensor tendon ruptures in rheumatoid arthritis. Hand Clin 1995; 11:449–459.
11. Cracchiolo A III, Marmor L: Resection of the distal ulna in rheumatoid arthritis. Arthritis Rheum 1969; 12:415.
12. Vaughan-Jackson OJ: Attrition ruptures of tendons in the rheumatoid hand. In Proceedings of the Joint Meeting of the Orthopaedic Association of the English-Speaking World. J Bone Joint Surg Am 1958; 40:1431.

13. Vaughan-Jackson OJ: Rupture of extensor tendons by attrition at the inferior radioulnar joint: Reports of two cases. J Bone Joint Surg Br 1948; 30:528.

14. Straub LR, Wilson EH Jr: Spontaneous rupture of extensor tendons in the hand associated with rheumatoid arthritis. J Bone Joint Surg Am 1956; 38:1208.

15. Nalebuff EA: Surgical treatment of tendon rupture in the rheumatoid hand. Surg Clin North Am 1969; 49:811.

16. Nalebuff EA, Patel MR: Flexor digitorum sublimis transfer for multiple extensor tendon ruptures in rheumatoid arthritis. Plast Reconstr Surg 1973; 52:530.

17. Nalebuff EA: Surgical treatment of rheumatoid tenosynovitis in the hand. Surg Clin North Am 1969; 49:799.

18. Mannerfelt L, Norman O: Attrition ruptures of flexors tendons in rheumatoid arthritis caused by bony spurs in the carpal tunnel: A clinical and radiologic study. J Bone Joint Surg Br 1969; 51:270–277.

19. Simmons BP, Smith GR: The hand and wrist. In Harris ED, Kelley WN, Ruddy S, et al (eds): Textbook of Rheumatology, vol 2, 5th ed. Philadelphia: WB Saunders, 1997:1647.

20. Nalebuff EA, Garrod KJ: Present approach to the severely involved rheumatoid wrist. Orthop Clin North Am 1984; 15:369.

21. Dupont M, Vainio K: Arthrodesis of the wrist in rheumatoid arthritis: A study of 140 cases. Ann Chir Gynecol Fenn 1968; 57:513.

22. Mannerfelt L, Malmsten M: Arthrodesis of the wrist in rheumatoid arthritis: A technique without external fixation. Scand J Plast Reconstr Surg 1971; 5:124.

23. Millender LH, Nalebuff EA: Arthrodesis of the rheumatoid wrist: An evaluation of sixty patients and a description of a different surgical technique. J Bone Joint Surg Am 1973; 55:1026.

24. Ishikawa H, Hanyu T, Saito H, et al: Limited arthrodesis for the rheumatoid wrist. J Hand Surg Am 1992; 17:1103.

25. Taleisnik J: Subtotal arthrodeses of the wrist joint. Clin Orthop 1984; 187:81.

26. DellaSanta D, Chamay A: Radiologic evolution of the rheumatoid wrist after radiolunate arthrodesis. J Hand Surg Br 1995; 20:146.

27. Fatti JP, Palmer AK, Mosher JF: The long-term results of Swanson silicone rubber interpositional wrist athroplasty. J Hand Surg Am 1986; 11:166.

28. Goodman MJ, Millender LH, Nalebuff EA, et al: Arthroplasty of the rheumatoid wrist with silicone rubber: An early evaluation. J Hand Surg Am 1980; 5:115.

29. Brase DW, Millender LH: Failure of silicone rubber wrist arthroplasty in rheumatoid arthritis. J Hand Surg Am 1986; 11:175.

30. Haloua JP, Collin, JP, Schernberg F, et al: Athroplasty of the rheumatoid wrist with Swanson implant: Long-term results and implications. Ann Chir Main 1989; 8:124.

31. Jolly SL, Ferlic DC, Clayton ML, et al: Swanson silicone arthroplasty of the wrist in rheumatoid arthritis: A long-term follow-up. J Hand Surg Am 1992; 17:142.

32. Meuli HC: Meuli total wrist arthroplasty. Clin Orthop 1984; 187:112.

33. Volz RG: The development of the total wrist arthroplasty. Clin Orthop 1976; 116:209.

34. Volz RG: The development of the total wrist arthroplasty. Clin Orthop 1984; 187:112.

35. Beckenbaugh RD, Linscheid RL: Total wrist arthroplasty: A preliminary report. J Hand Surg Am 1977; 2:339.

36. Cooney WP, Beckenbaugh RD, Linscheid RL: Total wrist arthroplasty: Problems with implant failures. Clin Orthop 1984; 187:121.

37. Figgie MP, Ranawat CS, Inglis AE, et al: Trispherical total wrist arthroplasty in rheumatoid arthritis. J Hand Surg Am 1990; 15:217.

38. Lirette R, Kinnard P: Biaxial total wrist arthroplasty in rheumatoid arthritis. Can J Surg 1995; 38:51.

39. Cobb TK, Beckenbaugh RD: Biaxial total-wrist arthroplasty. J Hand Surg Am 1996; 21:1011.

40. Darrach W: Partial excision of lower shaft of ulna for deformity following Colles' fracture. Ann Surg 1913; 57:764.

41. Nalebuff EA: Diagnosis, classification, and management of rheumatoid thumb deformities. Bull Hosp Joint Dis 1968; 29:119.

42. Figgie MP, Inglis AE, Sobel, M, et al. Metacarpal-phalangeal joint arthroplasty of the rheumatoid thumb. J Hand Surg Am 1990; 15:210.

43. Kvarnes L, Reikeras O: Rheumatoid arthritis at the base of the thumb treated by trapezium resection or implant arthroplasty. J Hand Surg Br 1985; 10:95.

44. Wood VE, Ichterz DR, Yahiku H: Soft tissue metacarpophalangeal reconstruction for treatment of rheumatoid hand deformity. J Hand Surg Am 1989; 14:163.

45. Simmons BP, de la Caffiniere JY: Physiology of flexion of the fingers. In Tubiana R (ed): The Hand, vol 1. Philadelphia: WB Saunders, 1981:377.

46. Neibauer JJ: Dacron-silicone prosthesis for the metacarpophalangeal and interphalangeal joints. In Cramer LH, Chase RA (eds): Symposium on the Hand, vol 3. St. Louis: CV Mosby, 1971:96.

47. Beckenbaugh RD, Linscheid RL: Arthroplasty in the hand and wrist. In Green DP (ed): Operative Hand Surgery. New York: Churchill Livingstone, 1988:167.

48. Steffee AD, Beckenbaugh RD, Linscheid RL, et al: The development, technique, and early clinical results of total joint replacement for the metacarpophalangeal joint of the fingers. Orthopaedics 1981; 4:175.

49. Bieber EJ, Welland AJ, Volenec-Dowling S: Silicone-rubber implant arthroplasty of the metacarpophalangeal joints for rheumatoid arthritis. J Bone Joint Surg Am 1986; 68:206.

50. Kirschenbaum D, Schneider LH, Adams DC, et al: Arthroplasty of the metacarpal phalangeal joints with use of silicone rubber implants in patients who have rheumatoid arthritis: Long-term results. J Bone Joint Surg Am 1993; 75:3–12.

51. Blair WF, Shurr DG, Buckwalter JA: Metacarpophalangeal joint implant arthroplasty with a Silastic spacer. J Bone Joint Surg Am 1984; 66:365.

52. Wilson YG, Sykes PJ, Niranjan NS: Long term follow-up of Swanson's Silastic arthroplasty of the metacarpal phalangeal joints in rheumatoid arthritis. J Hand Surg Br 1993; 18:81.

53. Swanson AB, Maupin BK, Gajjar NV, et al: Flexible implant arthroplasty in the proximal interphalangeal joint of the hand. J Hand Surg Am 1985; 10:796.

54. Linn HH, Wyrick JD, Stern PJ: Proximal interphalangeal joint silicone replacement arthroplasty: Clinical results using an anterior approach. J Hand Surg Am 1995; 20:123.

55. Nalebuff EA, Millender LH: Surgical treatment of the boutonnière deformity in rheumatoid arthritis. Orthop Clin North Am 1975; 6:753.

56. Nalebuff EA, Millender LH: Surgical treatment of swan neck deformity in rheumatoid arthritis. Orthop Clin North Am 1975; 6:753.

57. Green N, Osmer JC: Small bone changes secondary to systemic lupus erythematosus. Radiology 1968; 90:118.

58. Weisman BN, Rappaport MBB, Sosman JL, et al: Radiographic findings in the hands in patients with systemic lupus erythematosus. Radiology 1978; 126:313.

59. Bleifield CJ, Inglis AE: The hand in systemic lupus erythematosus. J Bone Joint Surg Am 1974; 56:1207.

60. Dray GJ, Millender LH, Nalebuff EA: The surgical treatment of hand deformities in systemic lupus erythematosus. J Hand Surg Am 1981; 6:339.

61. Resnick D, Niwayama G: Diagnosis of bone and joint disorders. Philadelphia: WB Saunders, 1988:1171–1198, 1267–1292.

62. Belsky M, Feldon P, Millender LH, et al: Hand involvement in psoriatic arthritis. J Hand Surg Am 1982; 7:203.

63. Brown L: Distal interphalangeal joint flexible implant arthroplasty. J Hand Surg Am 1989; 14:653.

64. Zimmerman NB, Suhey PV, Clark GL, et al: Silicone implant arthroplasty of the distal interphalangeal joint. J Hand Surg Am 1989; 14:882.

65. Iselin F, Pradet G, Gouet O: Conversion to arthroplasty from proximal interphalangeal joint arthrodesis. Ann Chir Main 1988; 7:115.

66. Pelligrini VD: The basal articulations of the thumb: Pain, instability, and osteoarthritis. In Peimer CA (ed): Surgery of the Hand and Upper Extremity, vol 1. New York: McGraw-Hill, 1995: 1019.

67. Eaton RG, Glickel SZ, Littler JW: Tendon interposition arthroplasty for degenerative arthritis of the trapeziometacarpal joint of the thumb. J Hand Surg Am 1985; 10:645.

68. Smith RJ, Atkinson RE, Jupiter JB: Silicone synovitis of the wrist. J Hand Surg Am 1985; 10:45.

69. Hofammann DY, Ferlic DC, Clayton ML: Arthroplasty of the basal joint of the thumb using a silicone prosthesis: Long-term follow-up. J Bone Joint Surg Am 1987; 69:993.

70. Sollerman C, Herrlin K, Abrahamsson SO, Lindholm A: Silastic replacement of the trapezium for arthrosis: A twelve-year follow-up study. J Hand Surg Br 1988; 13:426.

71. Cooney WP, DeBartolo T, Wood M: Post-traumatic arthritis of the wrist. *In* Cooney WP, Dobyns JH, Linscheid RL (eds): The Wrist: Diagnosis and Operative Treatment, vol 1. St. Louis: CV Mosby, 1998:588.

72. Kraushaar BS, Nirschl RP: Tendinosis of the elbow (tennis elbow). J Bone Joint Surg Am 1999; 81:259.

73. Jobe FW, Ciccotti MG: Lateral and medial epicondylitis of the elbow. J Am Acad Orthop Surg 1994; 2:1.

74. Groppel JL, Nirschl RP: A mechanical and electromyographical analysis of the effects of various joint counterforce braces on the tennis player. Am J Sports Med 1986; 14:195.

75. Boutin FJ Sr, Boutin RD, Boutin FJ Jr: Bursitis. *In* Chapman MW (ed): Operative Orthopaedics, vol 4. Philadelphia: JB Lippincott, 1993:3419.

76. Weinstein PS, Canoso JJ, Wohlgethan JR: Long-term follow-up of corticosteroid injection for traumatic olecranon bursitis. Ann Rheum Dis 1984; 43:44.

77. Stewart NJ, Manzanares JB, Morrey BF: Surgical treatment of aseptic olecranon bursitis. J Shoulder Elbow Surg 1997; 6:49.

78. Weiss APC, Akelman E, Tabatabai M: Treatment of de Quervain's disease. J Hand Surg Am 1994; 19:595.

79. Finkelstein H: Stenosing tendovaginitis at the radial styloid process. J Bone Joint Surg 1930; 12:509.

# 8 | Lumbar Spine Disease

*Jeffrey N. Katz and Nathaniel P. Katz*

Many clinicians find the management of low back pain daunting, perhaps for good reason. The pathophysiology of low back syndromes is poorly understood, the physical examination is seldom rewarding, diagnostic test results are frequently misleading, treatments are poorly studied and often marginally useful at best, and some patients have perverse disincentives to improve. Discouraged by these and other factors, many clinicians never develop a systematic approach to low back pain. Consequently patients with low back pain are often managed haphazardly and suboptimally.

Our goal in this chapter is to present a systematic classification system for low back disorders that will allow the clinician to place each patient within a conceptual framework. We then discuss the management of patients within each category, including medications, rehabilitation, local injections, chronic pain management, and surgery.

## CLASSIFICATION OF LOW BACK DISORDERS

In more than 80% of patients with low back disorders, the precise cause and pathogenesis of the symptoms are not known. Therefore, classification systems are necessarily phenomenologic rather than pathophysiologic. In a landmark study of the classification and management of low back disorders, the Quebec Task Force on Spinal Disorders devised an 11-category classification system distinguished principally by clinical manifestations rather than presumed pathophysiology.[1] We have adopted an analogous but simpler system, which is presented in Table 8–1. The major entities include lumbago, sciatica, neurogenic claudication, chronic low back, inflammatory back pain, and osseous pain syndromes, including fractures, infections, and tumors. Inflammatory back pain and osteoporotic fractures are covered elsewhere in this book and are not discussed in detail in this chapter.

## LUMBAGO

**EPIDEMIOLOGY.** Lumbago simply indicates pain in the back and is by far the most common low back pain syndrome. More than 80% of individuals acquire

lumbago over the course of a lifetime. The prevalence of lumbago at any given point in time is about 15% in adults older than 30 years.[2] These episodes typically start in the teenage years. By age 20, 50% of men and women have had an episode of low back pain.[3] Approximately 80% of episodes resolve within 2 weeks and more than 90% resolve over a period of several months.[2] Less than 1% of patients with lumbago experience progression to a chronic pain syndrome. In the workplace setting, 5% to 10% of persons with episodes of low back pain acquire chronic back pain.[4] Although the natural history of a particular episode of lumbago is excellent, the likelihood of recurrence in the subsequent year is 50%.[5] Thus, lumbago should be viewed as a chronic disorder characterized by recurrent self-limited episodes.

Risk factors for low back pain include obesity, alcohol use, smoking, low income, and limited education.[6, 7] In addition, occupational exposure to heavy lifting, spinal loading, postural stress, and vibration are associated with low back pain[8]. For example, workers performing heavy industrial tasks have twice the prevalence of low back pain as do bank clerks.[9] Decreased satisfaction with work is also associated with greater low back disability,[10] as is monotonous work, a high perceived workload, lack of control over tasks, and a hectic workplace[4, 11]

**PATHOPHYSIOLOGY.** The term *lumbago* is entirely descriptive and implies nothing about pathophysiology. In fact, lumbago likely represents a collection of diverse disorders with distinct pathologic mechanisms. The tissues responsible for mechanical low back pain syndromes include muscles, tendons, ligaments, discs, and facet joints. In some instances, the clinician can make an educated guess about which tissues are responsible for symptoms. For example, low back pain exacerbated by the Valsalva maneuver and sitting or leaning forward may emanate from the intervertebral disc.

**DIAGNOSTIC FEATURES.** Lumbago is generally centered in the lower lumbar region. Radiation into the sacroiliac and coccygeal regions and the buttocks occurs frequently and does not necessarily indicate involvement of nerve roots.[12] Stiffness lasting up to 30 minutes is common, particularly in the setting of degenerative disc disease or facet arthropathy. Patients with lumbago typically have normal straight leg raising tests and have normal lower extremity neurologic

## TABLE 8–1
## A Simple Classification System for Select Low Back Pain Syndromes

| SYNDROME | CLINICAL FEATURES | RADIOGRAPHIC FEATURES | RESOLVED AT 3 MONTHS |
|---|---|---|---|
| Lumbago | Central low back pain<br>Nondermatomal radiation<br>Neurologic examination normal<br>Ubiquitous | Nonspecific | 90% |
| Sciatica | Dermatomal distribution<br>Worse with Valsalva maneuver, flexion<br>Monoradicular neurologic deficit in 50%<br>Straight leg raise in 80–90%<br>Peak incidence in the fourth decade | Herniated disc<br>Foraminal stenosis | 60–80% |
| Neurogenic Claudication | Dermatomal, nondermatomal symptoms<br>Comfortable in flexion<br>Polyradicular neurologic deficits<br>Peak incidence in the sixth and seventh decades | Lumbar stenosis | <10% |
| Chronic Low Back Pain | Duration >6 mo<br>Psychosocial features common<br>Occurs in all ages | Varies | Nil |
| Osseous Pain | Constant<br>No comfortable position<br>Systemic features | Destruction, fracture | Varies |
| Inflammatory Back Pain | Stiffness<br>Improves with exercise, NSAIDs<br>Onset before 30 yr; HLA-B27 association | Sacroiliitis | Nil |

NSAIDs = nonsteroid anti-inflammatory drugs.

examinations, unless a primary neurologic disorder is present such as diabetic neuropathy. Radiography is generally unrevealing in patients with mechanical low back pain. Authoritative low back pain management guidelines emphasize that radiographs should be ordered only to rule out infections, tumors, and other ominous or unusual problems in patients with suggestive clinical findings such as systemic features, abnormal laboratory test results, known primary tumors, or new-onset back pain in older persons.[13]

## SCIATICA

EPIDEMIOLOGY. *Sciatica* refers to pain radiating down the lateral or posterior thigh and calf, often into the foot, in a sciatic nerve distribution. The lifetime prevalence of sciatica is approximately 40%, with a peak prevalence in the fourth and fifth decades. Approximately 1% to 2% of Americans have had surgery for herniated lumbar discs. More than 90% of patients with sciatica resulting from herniated disc syndromes improve by 6 months; however, up to 10% do not and often consider more invasive interventions, including lumbar disc surgery.[2, 9]

PATHOGENESIS. Most episodes of sciatica arise from nerve root impingement from a herniated lumbar intervertebral disc. In older individuals, sciatica can also arise from nerve root irritation by osteophytes in the neural foramina.[14] Disruption of the disc annulus without frank disc bulges or protrusions may also be associated with radiating leg pain.[15] The pain may be referred from the disc in these cases or may result from leakage of material from the nucleus pulposus in the vicinity of the nerve root. More than 90% of herniated discs occur in the L4 5 and L5–S1 interspaces, affecting the L5 and S1 nerve roots. A variety of inflammatory cytokines have been identified at the junction of disc material and the nerve root in patients with disc herniation, supporting an inflammatory mechanism of pain generation.[16] Central disc herniation may rarely cause cauda equina syndrome, characterized by saddle anesthesia and bowel and bladder incontinence. The differential diagnosis of sciatic pain in the absence of structural disc herniation includes extraspinal sciatic nerve compression, such as the piriformis syndrome, and irritation of the sciatic nerve by metabolic or inflammatory processes. Finally, pain that radiates in a sciatic distribution may simply arise from irritation of non-neural spinal structures.[12]

DIAGNOSTIC FEATURES. Sciatica from a herniated disc results in pain and paresthesia that occurs in a dermatomal distribution, usually corresponding to the L5 or S1 nerve root. Neurologic findings are typically monoradicular and dermatomal. The sensitivity and specificity of sensibility deficits are 0.50. The sensitivity of radicular muscle weakness is 0.10 to 0.40, whereas the specificity is 0.50 to 0.90. The straight leg raising test, considered positive when pain radiates to the popliteal fossa or distally, has a sensitivity of 0.80 in patients with documented herniated discs, with a specificity of about 0.40. The crossed straight leg raising test, in which raising the contralateral leg causes ipsilateral radiating pain, is less sensitive (0.2 to 0.3 in surgically confirmed cases, but probably lower in typical outpatient settings) but is highly specific (0.9 to 1.0).[17]

Plain radiographs generally are not helpful in the diagnosis of disc herniation. Half of asymptomatic adults have disc bulges on magnetic resonance imaging (MRI), and one quarter have frank disc protrusions.[18] This poor specificity is a warning that imaging tests should be used to confirm a diagnosis, not to reach for one.

## NEUROGENIC CLAUDICATION

EPIDEMIOLOGY. The syndrome of neurogenic claudication most frequently arises from lumbar spinal stenosis, which usually presents in older patients. More than 20% of asymptomatic adults have lumbar stenosis on MRI.[18] There are no reliable data on the incidence or prevalence of symptomatic lumbar spinal stenosis. Approximately 1 in 1000 individuals older than 65 years undergoes laminectomy for spinal stenosis each year. The natural history of spinal stenosis is much less favorable than that of lumbago and sciatica. After a follow-up period of 3 years in one study of 19 patients treated nonsurgically,[19] 32% rated their overall status improved, 58% rated it unchanged, and 10% said their overall condition was worse.

PATHOGENESIS. Numerous causes of spinal stenosis exist, including congenital, degenerative, postsurgical, metabolic, and inflammatory processes.[20] The most common is degenerative lumbar spinal stenosis with or without an accompanying degenerative spondylolisthesis. Disc degeneration leads to loss of disc height, osteophyte formation, and sclerosis of the vertebral endplates. Loss of height anteriorly loads the facet joints posteriorly, leading to degenerative facet arthropathy. Osteophytes from facet arthropathy can project centrally into the spinal canal. In addition, the ligamentum flavum hypertrophies. The combination of posteriorly protruding disc material, ligamentum flavum and facet joint hypertrophy, and osteophyte formation all lead to a reduction in the cross-sectional area available for the contents of the spinal canal. The stenotic process can occur both centrally and in the neural foramina. These degenerative changes can also lead to degenerative spondylolisthesis, which may also exacerbate nerve root compression.

The 20% prevalence rate of stenosis in asymptomatic adults older than 65 years indicates that these structural abnormalities are not sufficient to produce symptoms of neurogenic claudication. It is believed that symptoms develop when pressure in the epidural space rises sufficiently to impede venous outflow.[21] For this reason, postures that increase epidural pressure, such as standing or lumbar extension, worsen symptoms, whereas lumbar flexion reduces epidural pressure, relieving symptoms.

DIAGNOSTIC FEATURES. Neurogenic claudication consists of pain that radiates into the buttocks and lower extremities and is exacerbated by lumbar extension and improved with lumbar flexion.[22] Patients prefer to sit down and stoop forward and avoid walking and standing. Absence of pain when seated is the most specific finding on taking the history.[22] The pain, numbness, and tingling usually occur in a polyradicular distribution, as multiple nerve roots are often involved. Discomfort radiates below the knees in 50% of cases. Patients also have nonradicular back and lower extremity pain from degenerative disc disease and facet arthropathy. Loss of sensation and position sense in the lower extremities typically causes a wide-based, pseudocerebellar gait.

The physical examination[22] generally reveals limitation in lumbar extension, with radiation of pain into the buttocks and legs on prolonged lumbar extension and relief with flexion. Neurologic findings are often bilateral and polyradicular. Neurologic deficits to pinprick and vibration as well as weakness occur in just half of patients. An abnormal Romberg sign and wide-based gait occur later in the course and have high specificity.[22]

These data suggest that the syndrome has three distinct aspects: pain that typically is worsened with extension and improves with flexion; neurologic deficits to pinprick, vibration, and reflex, and strength findings; and a pseudocerebellar syndrome caused by involvement of proprioceptive fibers.[23] The pain syndrome is typically the presenting feature, whereas neurologic deficits and the pseudocerebellar syndrome become more prominent as the disorder progresses. The stenotic process can be confirmed with imaging modalities—computed tomography, myelography, or MRI. Because more than 20% of asymptomatic older adults have lumbar stenosis on MRI,[18] the imaging results should be interpreted carefully.

## CHRONIC LOW BACK PAIN (CHRONIC PAIN SYNDROME)

Chronic low back pain is a back pain syndrome that has lasted longer than about 6 months. In some patients, chronicity of symptoms is associated with increased prominence of psychosocial features and the dissociation of documented physiologic impairment from reported symptoms.[24] The chronic pain syndrome is multidimensional; its principal features are listed in Table 8–2. They include physical manifestations, such as muscle atrophy and deconditioning; cognitive phenomena, such as exaggerated fear of activity; affective symptoms, including depression and anxiety; the emergence of primary or secondary gain; and social dysfunction, including disruption of work and marital and family relationships as well as sexual dysfunction.

The disability resulting from chronic low back pain is costly: The likelihood of a return to work is about 50% for workers with 6 months of back disability, 20% after 1 year of disability, and essentially nil after 2 years of low back disability.[2, 9]

The explanations for the poor prognosis and prominence of psychosocial features are complex. Deconditioning resulting from bed rest and inactivity leads to rapid loss of muscle strength, flexibility, and general cardiovascular fitness.[25] "Catastrophizing" about the consequences of specific activities and the exaggerated fear of physical activity compound the problem. Loss

## TABLE 8–2
## Features of the Chronic Pain Syndrome

**Physical**

Deconditioning
Muscle atrophy, stiffness, spasm
Poor posture
Inappropriate signs (e.g., nondermatomal deficits)

**Cognitive**

"Catastrophizing"
Exaggerated fear of activity

**Affective**

Depression
Anxiety
Anger, hostility

**Psychodynamic**

Primary or secondary gain
Drug dependence

**Social**

Disrupted marital and family relationships
Sexual dysfunction
Loss of provider role
Unemployment, Worker's Compensation, legal difficulties

of work results in loss of income, self-esteem, and role as provider in the family. This may produce anxiety, frustration, and depression, as well as a very realistic fear of the future. This is particularly true in laborers with limited resources to explore alternative employment opportunities. Some patients find that pain satisfies deeply hidden primary needs such as self-punishment. Other patients derive secondary gain from work absence, compensation, attention from others, or a combination of these things.

From a clinical standpoint, chronic guarding of the painful part further exacerbates muscle stiffness and spasm. Anxiety and emotional stress may further promote pain and spasm. Thus a vicious cycle ensues in which physical and psychological causes of disability potentiate each other. Insomnia and inappropriate use of narcotics and sedative medications may worsen these problems still further.

The clinical evaluation often uncovers emotional distress rather than physical impairment. For example, numbness or pain may be reported over an entire leg rather than in a dermatomal distribution. Similarly, rotation of the pelvis with no lumbar rotation may cause back pain. Sensory or motor deficits may be reported in nondermatomal locations. Straight leg raising or weakness may be inconsistently reported if the examiner attempts to distract the patient during the examination. These inappropriate signs and symptoms are clues to psychosocial distress.[24]

## OSSEOUS PAIN

The most common cause of osseous bone pain is vertebral fractures, particularly osteoporotic compression fractures. Osteoporosis and attendant vertebral fractures have been associated with a greater prevalence of back pain, even in patients who do not have discreet episodes of painful acute fracture.[26] Osteoporosis and fractures are covered in detail in Chapter 40. Tumors and infections are rare causes of back pain but are extremely important to identify. Tumors in the spine are generally metastatic, arising from common solid tumors such as prostate cancer, myeloma, and lung or breast cancer. Infections may occur in the vertebrae, disc spaces, or epidural spaces. They may be caused by pyogenic infections, typically *Staphylococcus aureus*, or to chronic granulomatous processes such as tuberculosis or fungi.

Several key historical features point to the presence of tumors and infections. Patients generally have unrelenting pain in virtually all positions. In most other types of low back pain, patients can find a position that makes them relatively comfortable. Systemic symptoms, including weight loss, generalized fatigue, fever, and sweats, are also associated with tumors and infections. On physical examination, direct palpation over the spine may reveal bony tenderness. Plain radiographs ultimately reveal bony lesions but computed tomography or MRI may be required to detect tumors and infections earlier in the course of these disorders. As symptoms, physical signs, and radiographs are insensitive and nonspecific for ominous spinal lesions, the clinician must maintain a low threshold for obtaining imaging tests among patients with troubling presentations.

## POSTSURGICAL BACK PAIN

The existence of "failed back surgery syndrome" speaks to the frequency of unsuccessful operations on the lumbar spine and the importance of identifying preoperatively those patients who are likely to benefit. Inadequate decompression, postsurgical scarring, recurrent disc protrusion, arachnoiditis, and psychosocial features have all been implicated as causes of surgical failure. The most important reasons for surgical failure may be that the surgery was performed for improper indications, such as discectomy for patients whose symptoms did not in fact arise from a disc protrusion.

## MANAGEMENT OF LOW BACK PAIN

### General Approach

In the first 4 weeks of an episode of low back pain, more than 90% of patients improve. There is little evidence that specific treatments administered during this acute period are better than observation of the natural history alone. In fact, passive treatments such as prescribed bed rest appear to delay recovery.[27] Diagnostic tests are not indicated unless a thorough history and physical examination raise the question of infection or tumor. The clinician should reassure patients about the excellent prognosis of the acute episode but should also alert them to the high likelihood of recurrence.

Risk factors for back pain should be addressed, including smoking, lack of exercise, improper posture and lifting mechanics, and ergonomic aspects of the work environment.

Patients whose symptoms fail to resolve after 1 month are much more likely to experience chronic problems. A more intensive approach is indicated, including physiotherapy to reverse deconditioning and intensive efforts to return the patient to his or her usual work environment. Tasks should be modified if the patient cannot perform usual duties.

Patients who remain disabled and symptomatic beyond 3 months are unlikely to recover or return to work and should be referred to a multidisciplinary functional restoration program. These programs address physical deconditioning and a range of social, psychological, and work environment issues that may complicate the return to usual activities.

This general approach to the treatment of lumbago (Table 8–3) also can be applied to the management of sciatica, but there is less empirical evidence to support this recommendation. Patients with sciatica typically respond more slowly.

This section reviews treatment approaches to the low back pain syndromes discussed in the preceding section. Tables 8–4 and 8–5 summarize the results of randomized controlled trials of a range of therapies for acute (Table 8–4) and chronic (Table 8–5) low back pain. The review of randomized trials from which these tables are derived[28] is highly recommended.

## Lumbago: Acute Low Back Pain

Because acute low back pain improves within weeks to months in more than 90% of patients, therapies must be highly effective to be superior to the natural history. Table 8–4 summarizes controlled trials of therapy for acute low back pain and documents that some traditionally recommended therapies for acute low back pain, such as exercises and bed rest, do not appear

### TABLE 8–3
### General Approach to Management of Low Back Pain

| PHASE | PERCENT RESOLVED AT 6 MONTHS | APPROACH |
|---|---|---|
| Acute (0–4 wk) | >95% | Usual activities<br>Minimal tests and interventions<br>Address risk factors for recurrence |
| Subacute (4–12 wk) | 70% | Above plus intensive physical therapy to strengthen and recondition<br>Work conditioning |
| Chronic (>12 wk) | <50% | Above plus multidisciplinary functional restoration program |

beneficial in the acute setting. The high rate of recurrent episodes indicates that treatment of lumbago should emphasize the prevention of recurrence.

BED REST. The lost productivity and reinforced sense of disability that accompany prescribed bed rest can be more devastating than the backache itself. Deyo and colleagues showed that a recommendation of 2 days of bed rest, rather than 7 days, resulted in 45% fewer days of work missed and no differences in other functional or subjective outcomes.[27] Malmivaara and associates demonstrated that continuing ordinary activities as tolerated led to more rapid recovery from acute low back pain than did 2 days of bed rest or prescribed exercises.[29] In fact, five of six randomized controlled trials of bed rest for treatment of low back pain showed that bed rest was not useful in the management of low back pain (see Table 8–4).[28] The message is that bed rest appears to have few benefits and major costs, including increased work absenteeism and muscle atrophy and deconditioning among others. Clinicians should not prescribe disability in their efforts to prevent it.

MEDICATIONS. The most commonly prescribed medications for patients with acute low back pain include nonsteroidal anti-inflammatory drugs (NSAIDs) and muscle relaxants. The benefit from these medications is generally modest, and side effects are not trivial. Acetaminophen is a good choice in the elderly. When NSAIDs are used in older patients, agents with long half-lives (such as piroxicam) should be avoided.

Patients with prominent muscle spasm frequently appear to benefit most from muscle relaxants such as cyclobenzaprine, methocarbamol, carisoprodol, and others. These medications all have the potential to cause sedation. Carisoprodol may be habit forming. Tricyclic and other antidepressants should not be used in acute low back pain unless there is a more specific indication such as depression, fibromyalgia, or painful neuropathy.[13]

Although clinicians are generally reluctant to use narcotics for back pain, the risk of addiction in properly selected patients without a prior history of substance abuse appears to be low.[30] The issues involved in prescribing narcotics are discussed in the section of this chapter on chronic back pain management.

EXERCISES AND MODALITIES. A variety of exercise programs has been advocated for acute low back pain, including Williams flexion exercises, MacKenzie extension exercises, and aerobic conditionings. Of ten randomized, controlled trials of exercise programs for acute low back pain, three showed benefit from an exercise program, whereas seven reported no benefit (see Table 8–4). The exercise regimens used in these various studies differed markedly, including stretching, abdominal flexion, and back extension along with a variety of modalities. Thus, the role of exercises in the management of acute low back pain is uncertain. At this writing, there is little evidence that exercises are better than simply advising patients to continue their usual activities as tolerated.[29] "Back schools," which offer exercise programs and education regarding posture and back protection, have been examined

**TABLE 8–4**

**Efficacy of Treatment for *Acute* Low Back Pain: Evidence from Randomized Trials**

| TREATMENT | NO. TRIALS SUPPORTING | NO. NOT SUPPORTING | PERCENT SUPPORTING |
|---|---|---|---|
| Analgesics | 1 | 5 | 17% |
| NSAIDs | 7 | 11 | 39% |
| Muscle relaxants | 11 | 3 | 79% |
| Bed rest | 1 | 5 | 17% |
| Exercise | 3 | 7 | 30% |
| Back school | 2 | 2 | 50% |
| Manipulation | 10 | 5 | 67% |
| TENS | 1 | 1 | 50% |
| Traction | 2 | 0 | 100% |

TENS = transcutaneous electrical nerve stimulation.
From Van Tulder M, Koes BW, Bouter LM: Conservative treatment of acute and chronic low back pain: A systematic review of randomized controlled trials of the most common interventions. Spine 1997; 22:2128–2156.

in four randomized controlled trials, two of which showed benefit (see Table 8–4).

The rehabilitative approach to low back pain often includes various modalities such as heat, cold, ultrasonography, and vapocoolant spray. In general, these strategies have not been evaluated critically. There is little evidence or rationale supporting the administration of passive modalities such as ultrasonography or hot or cold packs by professionals. Patients can certainly apply heat or cold treatments themselves.[13] Similarly, traction and lumbar corsets appear to have no proven role in the management of low back pain.[1, 13, 31] Transcutaneous electrical nerve stimulation (TENS) appears to have essentially no proven role in acute mechanical low back pain because of the favorable natural history of the disorder.

MYOFASCIAL TRIGGER POINT INJECTION. Myofascial pain is thought to arise from trigger points. A trigger point is defined as a nodule that upon palpation, reproduces the quality, location, and referral pattern of the patient's pain.[32] There are no reliable diagnostic criteria for this syndrome; thus, its prevalence is unknown.[33] Similarly, there have been no properly controlled trials of this disorder.

Patients may experience prolonged, tender muscle spasm as a result of, rather than a cause of, their underlying back pain problem. This phenomenon may be referred to as secondary myofascial pain. A number of different treatments are used for myofascial pain,[33] including ultrasonography, stretching and strengthening exercises, general aerobic conditioning, stretch, and spray and trigger point injections.

In trigger point injections, a small volume of local anesthetic is injected through a narrow-gauge needle into the trigger points. Administration of local anesthetic is more effective and comfortable than simple dry needling.[33] Therapy should be geared to the complexity of the patient's condition. Simple trigger point injections are appropriate for patients with isolated, localized myofascial pain, whereas a stretching and strengthening program, full reconditioning program, and multidisciplinary rehabilitation can be prescribed as well for patients with greater levels of disability and psychological and other needs.

CHIROPRACTIC MANIPULATIONS. Chiropractic manipulation involves abrupt movement of vertebrae beyond their physiologic but not their anatomic range of motion. Well-designed randomized, controlled trials have

**TABLE 8–5**

**Efficacy of Treatment for *Chronic* Low Back Pain: Evidence from Randomized Controlled Trials**

| TREATMENT | NO. TRIALS SUPPORTING | NO. NOT SUPPORTING | NO CONCLUSION | PERCENT SUPPORTING |
|---|---|---|---|---|
| Antidepressants | 1 | 2 | 1 | 25% |
| NSAIDs | 3 | 1 | 2 | 50% |
| Manipulation | 6 | 2 | 1 | 67% |
| Back school | 5 | 3 | 2 | 50% |
| EMG biofeedback | 1 | 4 | 0 | 20% |
| Exercise | 8 | 8 | 0 | 50% |
| Behavior therapy | 8 | 3 | 0 | 73% |
| TENS | 1 | 2 | 0 | 33% |
| Acupuncture | 4 | 2 | 0 | 67% |

EMG = electromyographic.
From Van Tulder M, Koes BW, Bouter LM: Conservative treatment of acute and chronic low back pain: A systematic review of randomized controlled trials of the most common interventions. Spine 1997; 22:2128–2156.

shown that chiropractic manipulation leads to faster improvement in symptoms than does placebo in patients with acute low back pain without nerve root involvement (see Table 8–4). Chiropractic manipulation also appears beneficial for chronic low back pain (see Table 8–5). A recent comparison of chiropractic manipulation, MacKenzie extension exercises, and a simple educational pamphlet showed no difference in functional outcomes and pain between the chiropractic and exercise groups. Both of these interventions resulted in slightly greater pain relief and functional improvement than the pamphlet alone, and both were more expensive.[34] Patients also appear to be more satisfied with chiropractic care and with an exercise program than with simple educational advice for low back pain.[34] Specifically, patients value the chiropractor's confidence in the accuracy of diagnosis and efficacy of prescribed treatment,[35] even though chiropractic diagnostic findings have poor reproducibility.[36] The style of chiropractic practice, as well as technical aspects of manipulation, appear to underlie the improved outcomes of chiropractic care. These data suggest that patients appreciate a more positive and knowledgeable discussion of low back pain therapy and its likely outcomes.

ALTERNATIVE THERAPIES. One third of Americans use some form of alternative therapy. By far, the most common problem treated with alternative therapies is back pain.[37, 38] The most frequent alternative treatments include massage, relaxation, chiropractic care, and acupuncture. Chiropractic appears to be beneficial in acute lumbago, as noted earlier. Other alternative treatments are less well studied.

EPIDURAL AND FACET INJECTIONS. Epidural steroid injections appear to be most useful for patients with evidence of nerve root irritation.[39] Facet joint injections are occasionally used in patients with lumbago but usually after months to years of symptoms. Steroid injections into the epidural space and facet joints are discussed in the sections of this chapter on the management of sciatica and chronic back pain, respectively.

SURGERY. Some patients with severe radiographic degenerative disc disease and central low back pain, without objective evidence of nerve root impingement or dynamic spondylolisthesis, are offered lumbar fusion. The specific advantages and drawbacks of this controversial approach to acute low back pain are beyond the scope of this chapter.

## Sciatica

As with lumbago, management of sciatica should begin with a clear explanation of the likely natural history. Resolution of symptoms is slower and less complete than in most cases of lumbago. One study[40] showed that 44% of patients were free of pain 1 month after an episode of sciatica, and 55% were pain free at 1 year. By 1 year, 7.5% were out of work, and 45% had some restriction in work. Thus, the natural history is generally favorable and interventions must be quite effective to be superior to simple observation alone.

Conservative management of sciatica parallels that of lumbago. In general, patients should attempt to remain active. Although a short period (1 or 2 days) of bed rest may be useful in patients with severe pain and disability, the potential for muscle atrophy and lost productivity must be weighed against the benefits.

Medications are prescribed for sciatica in much the same manner as for mechanical low back pain. Some physicians prescribe short courses of systemic oral corticosteroids for sciatica. This strategy has not been studied critically. Pain should be treated with analgesics, including acetaminophen or NSAIDs, or both. Short courses of narcotics may be necessary for patients with severe pain who are at low risk of addiction.

The rehabilitative approach to patients with herniated disc syndromes generally includes a program that emphasizes the use of lumbar extension, modeled after the work of McKenzie and others.[41] Extension exercises are purported to accelerate resorption of the protruding disc material. Accordingly, symptoms "centralize," with radiating leg pain shifting to central low back pain.[41] Strengthening programs are indicated for patients with functionally limiting weakness arising from radiculopathy.

Chiropractic manipulation is frequently administered to patients with sciatica caused by herniated disc syndromes. There is less scientific information on the value of manipulation in this setting.

EPIDURAL STEROID INJECTIONS. Injection of a combination of local anesthetic and steroid into the epidural space of the spine is widely performed by anesthesiologists and other practitioners. More than a dozen controlled trials have been performed in patients with radicular pain syndromes.[42, 43] The results are conflicting, partly because of differences in study design. A rigorous randomized, controlled trial of epidural steroid injection in patients with sciatica caused by herniated discs showed that the patients receiving epidural steroids had slightly more improvement in leg pain at 6 weeks.[44] However, there was no difference in pain or function at 3 months between steroid and placebo injections, and there was no difference in the two groups in frequency of subsequent discectomy.[44] We interpret these data to suggest that epidural steroid injections may be beneficial for a few weeks to months in patients with radicular pain. However, it appears that by 3 months after epidural injection, there is no difference between epidural steroid injections and control injections. Two meta-analyses of controlled trials have been published,[45, 43] the most recent of which included trials meeting analytic criteria through 1997. The authors analyzed two end points: 75% relief of pain in the short term and 50% relief in the long term. The meta-analysis demonstrated significant benefits in both end points for epidural injections compared with placebo. A "numbers needed to treat" analysis showed that for every 7 patients treated, 1 will achieve greater than 75% short-term relief, and 1 in 13 will achieve 50% long-term relief. Thus, the benefits of epidural injections are modest, but patients and their clinicians should discuss whether the limited benefit is worth the small risk of the injections.

The safety of epidural injections is well documented.[46, 47] Fewer than 1% of patients have an unintentional dural puncture with the resulting possibility of spinal headache. Patients with steroid-sensitive illnesses, such as diabetes or congestive heart failure, may experience brief exacerbations after an epidural steroid injection. In rare cases, patients may experience prolonged exacerbation of pain after epidural steroid injection.[42] Infection and permanent nerve damage are documented, but very rare, complications.

## Surgery

More than 200,000 lumbar discectomies are performed annually in the United States, and the rate appears to be increasing about 10%/year.[48] Striking variations exist in discectomy rates across small geographic regions and also across large regions of the United States, suggesting considerable uncertainty among physicians about the appropriate indications for surgery.

Cauda equina syndrome, consisting of bowel and bladder dysfunction and saddle anesthesia, is an absolute indication for surgery in patients with disc herniations. Less dramatic urinary abnormalities, such as hesitancy and poor sensation of bladder filling, may be much more common.[49] The natural history of these less disabling forms of sacral root involvement is not well studied. They should by managed on a case-by-case basis in consultation with a spine surgeon and, we would suggest, a clinician with expertise in distinguishing nerve root from other causes of bladder dysfunction. The critical step is to recognize that a wide range of bladder dysfunction syndromes can arise from disc protrusions. Progressive muscle weakness that becomes functionally disabling is also a strong indication for lumbar disc surgery. Cauda equina syndrome and progressive weakness account for less than one fifth of surgeries for disc herniations.

Weber performed an elegant randomized trial of discectomy versus conservative therapy in patients who did not have cauda equina syndrome or progressive neuromuscular deficits.[50] Of patients randomized to receive conservative treatment, 33% were completely satisfied with their status after 1 year, 51% were satisfied after 4 years, and 55% were satisfied after 10 years of conservative therapy. Of patients initially randomized to surgical therapy, 66% were completely satisfied at 1 year, 66% were satisfied at 4 years, and 58% were satisfied after 10 years. Twenty-six percent of patients initially randomized to conservative therapy opted for surgery during the first year and experienced results similar to the surgical group. Thus, although surgical therapy was associated with greater patient satisfaction in the first years, there appears to be little difference in outcome between surgery and conservative care by 4 and 10 years of follow-up. These results indicate that in patients without cauda equina syndrome or rapidly progressive neurologic deficit, the decision to operate should be made on the basis of patient preferences regarding the risks and benefits of the operation.

A review of 81 studies of discectomy showed that, on average, operative mortality was 0.15%, dural tears were reported in 3.7%, and permanent nerve root injuries were seen in 0.8% of patients. Thrombophlebitis was reported in 1.6%, pulmonary emboli were seen in 0.6%, and wound infections were reported in 2% of patients. Reoperation rates increased with a longer duration of follow-up, reaching 10% by 10 years. The review noted success rates of about 70%, on average, for standard discectomy, microdiskectomy, and percutaneous discectomy.[51]

Given the substantial proportion of patients (up to 30%) with poor discectomy outcomes, identification of prognostic factors is crucial. Psychological and social factors associated with poor prognosis include elevated hysteria or hypochondriasis scores on the Minnesota Multiphasic Personality Inventory and the presence of litigation or Worker's Compensation claims.[52, 53] Favorable prognostic features include a positive straight leg raising sign, neurologic deficit, and evidence on imaging studies of a pathologic condition at the corresponding nerve root. Patients with negative prognostic factors such as Worker's Compensation, depression, or lack of neurologic deficits should not necessarily be denied surgery, but their expectations should be adjusted accordingly.

Lumbar discectomy appears to be relatively cost-effective compared with other medical and surgical interventions, with a cost of $30,000 (1993 dollars) per quality adjusted life-year gained.[54]

Several surgical alternatives to conventional discectomy have been introduced, including microdiskectomy, percutaneous discectomy, and chymopapain injections. Microdiskectomy utilizes microsurgical techniques, leaving a smaller wound and leading to earlier mobilization and less postoperative disability. Surgical outcomes appear to be comparable to those of traditional discectomy.[55] Percutaneous discectomy involves suctioning disc material from the body of the herniated disc, thereby decompressing the disc and presumably relieving pressure on the nerve root. This procedure is also associated with a low complication rate and rapid rehabilitation. Open series suggest success that is comparable to traditional discectomy.[56] Chemonucleolysis involves introduction of a proteolytic enzyme, typically chymopapain, into the nucleus of the affected disc. The proteolytic enzyme digests disc material and apparently decompresses the disc in a manner analogous to that of percutaneous discectomy. Randomized, controlled trials have found that standard discectomy is superior to chemonucleolysis.[57, 58] The technique is not employed frequently in the United States because of reports of complications, including anaphylaxis in about 0.3% of patients, and rare but potentially devastating neurologic complications.

## Neurogenic Claudication

Rapid neurologic deterioration is rare among patients with spinal stenosis and neurogenic claudication, and spontaneous, sustained symptomatic improvement is unusual.[19] Disability is driven primarily by symptoms and not neurologic findings.[59] Thus, symptoms, and not subtle neurologic deficits, should trigger treatment.

The typical amelioration of symptoms with lumbar flexion provides a rationale for the use of lumbar corsets. Because older patients are less tolerant of NSAIDs, we use acetaminophen and narcotics frequently for symptomatic degenerative lumbar stenosis. There is no critical literature on the value of an exercise program among patients with spinal stenosis. Patients' inclination to maintain a posture of lumbar flexion suggests that a bicycle exercise program might be useful, but this hypothesis has not been tested.

Lumbar epidural steroid injections are used frequently in patients with spinal stenosis. The literature on epidural steroids in spinal stenosis is sparse, and studies are not of high quality. It appears that only about half of patients report benefit 2 weeks after the injection.[60] Patients with multiple comorbidities who are poor surgical candidates may receive epidural steroid injections every 4 months or so on an ongoing basis as an alternative to decompressive surgery.

Surgical therapy consists of decompressive laminectomy with medial facetectomy and occasionally spinal fusion. The indications for fusion are controversial. It appears that patients with spinal stenosis and concomitant degenerative spondylolisthesis benefit from stablization.[61, 62] In patients with multilevel stenosis and no evidence of spondylolisthesis, fusion does not enhance outcome.[63] Fusion is associated with a higher risk of mortality, medical complications, and subsequent reoperations and higher costs.[64] There is heated debate about the relative merits of performing fusion with autologous bone graft alone versus augmenting fusion with pedicle screw (or other) instrumentation systems. Instrumentation leads to a higher rate of healing the fusion but is associated with greater expense and complications. Two randomized, controlled trials found no benefit for the addition of instrumentation to autologous bone graft fusion and decompression for spondylolisthesis with stenosis.[65, 66]

A literature synthesis of the outcome of decompressive surgery for spinal stenosis reported a success rate of 64%.[67] In a retrospective study by Katz and colleagues, 31% of patients had severe back or buttock pain after an average of 4.5 years of follow-up, and 17% required reoperation for recurrent stenosis or symptomatic instability.[68] At 7 to 10 years after operation, a third of the patients had severe pain, 24% had received reoperation, and 85% said the procedure relieved their pain for at least some time, with relief lasting an average of 3 years.[69] Patients with spinal stenosis often have nonspinal problems, including osteoarthritis of the hips or knees, cardiac or pulmonary disease, and visual problems, among others. Thus, some patients may experience functional decline after surgery for stenosis despite resolution of back symptoms.

Worse function and symptomatic outcomes after surgery for stenosis are predicted by several preoperative factors, including greater comorbidity (particularly cardiovascular problems), worse self-perceived health, and worse functional status.[68, 69]

## Chronic Pain Syndrome

Management of chronic pain syndromes involves the conservative therapies listed previously along with several specific modalities that are discussed in detail in this section, including multidisciplinary pain treatment centers, narcotic use, facet injections, and spinal cord stimulators.

CHRONIC PAIN TREATMENT CENTERS. Table 8–5 provides data on the results of randomized, controlled trials of chronic low back pain. Exercises have a clearer role in chronic back pain, as do behavioral approaches. Acupuncture has been noted to be effective in most acupuncture trials.

Patients with disabling chronic pain are best managed in a multidisciplinary program, which typically involves evaluation by a psychologist or psychiatrist, physical therapist, and physician.[70] The physician reviews the diagnostic work-up, ensuring that no specifically treatable cause for the back pain has been overlooked. The next step typically is to optimize the use of medications. This usually involves streamlining multiple medications and weaning patients from narcotics or benzodiazepines. Insomnia, depression, and anxiety are addressed with medications as well. The psychologist evaluates the person for behavioral factors that may be perpetuating the pain, such as secondary gain in the workplace or in the family. The patient is also assessed for psychological comorbidity, such as anxiety, post-traumatic stress, panic, or depression. The patient is then treated with a variety of cognitive and behavioral techniques, often in combination with medications, for their psychological symptoms. Patients are trained to manage their lives despite their pain with coping strategies, nonpharmacologic therapy for insomnia, and other approaches. The physical therapist assesses the patient's rehabilitative needs and attempts to restore functional status, usually relying on active rather than passive conditioning programs. In a full service program, the patient undergoes triage into a return-to-work program, often in conjunction with employers or payors. Patients may also be screened for more sophisticated pain management techniques such as spinal cord stimulation, implantable opiate pumps, or chronic oral narcotic therapy.

Numerous studies have been conducted on the efficacy of the components of multidisciplinary pain management (exercise, functional restoration, cognitive techniques, behavioral techniques, and so on), and several reviews have been published.[71-74] The overall success rate for interdisciplinary pain clinics varies depending on the population studied and the outcome measure.[75] Return-to-work rates for patients with chronic pain are in the range of 15% to 25%. Select programs report return-to-work rates of 85%.[76] Return to work is not the sole important outcome, since restoration of activity of daily living and reduction in suffering are laudable goals as well.

CHRONIC NARCOTIC THERAPY. It is often assumed that a significant percentage of patients given narcotics for pain become addicted. This is not true in the acute pain setting[77] and the incidence of addiction in the chronic pain setting has been poorly studied. The only randomized, controlled trial with follow-up of 1 year showed that patients with chronic pain treated with opioids were more satisfied and experienced improvements in mood and a slight reduction in pain when compared with controls, with no differences in activity level.[78]

The following are generally regarded as risk factors for narcotic addiction: previous history of substance abuse, ongoing substance abuse, high levels of psychosocial distress, psychological symptoms that may respond to narcotics (e.g., anxiety, panic attacks), use of short-acting narcotics, and prescribing on an as-needed basis rather than a fixed schedule.

A reasonable approach to patient selection for chronic narcotic therapy involves a mental health evaluation before the initiation of therapy. Narcotics should be administered strictly on a trial basis at first, perhaps for several months, with outcomes documented and under strictly supervised conditions. If the patient's clinical status is not improved during the trial, narcotic therapy can justifiably be stopped.

Narcotics can be administered by a number of different routes if the oral route is unavailable or nonviable, including sublingual, rectal, vaginal, cutaneous, intravenous, or transdermal. There is no obvious advantage to the transdermal patch in patients who tolerate oral narcotics.

SPINAL OPIATE ADMINISTRATION. Administration of spinal opiates has been recognized for several decades as a useful technique in the management of selected patients with cancer pain. Patients usually obtain equal or superior analgesia compared with systemic opiate administration, with fewer side effects.[79] The use of this modality has been expanded to the noncancer population.[80] These patients undergo a trial with a temporary spinal catheter, and those patients with a successful response may then undergo implantation of an opiate pump connected to an intrathecal catheter. The pumps must be refilled monthly. Although there is a small incidence of infection, the procedure is generally safe in experienced hands.[81] Although morphine is the only agent approved for infusion via intrathecal pumps, several agents are used in practice, including other opioids, local anesthetics, clonidine, and investigational agents. There are neither large series nor controlled studies of opiate pumps for noncancer conditions; hence, many questions regarding effectiveness and complications remain unanswered. Several survey studies have been published on the use of intrathecal analgesics for chronic pain in nonmalignant conditions.[81–86] These studies generally show pain reduction, whereas data on improvement in activity level are conflicting. No controlled studies have been conducted. At present, intrathecal opioids should be viewed as indicated only in highly selected patients in whom all reasonable alternatives have failed, including multidisciplinary rehabilitative efforts.

TRANSCUTANEOUS ELECTRIC NERVE STIMULATION. TENS has been studied critically in three randomized, controlled studies of patients with chronic low back pain. For two of these studies, TENS was no more effective than sham TENS and offered no advantage over simple exercises alone. However, TENS has not been subject to randomized control trials in patients with spinal stenosis, disc syndromes, or osteoporotic fractures, and its utility in these settings should be considered uncertain.

FACET INJECTIONS. The lumbar facet joints are thought to give rise to clinical low back pain. Pain syndromes that emanate from the facet joints consist of a dull ache radiating into the low back, buttocks, hips, or thigh, and even beyond the knee. Pain is worsened by back extension or rotation, such as rolling over in bed, and can be reproduced on physical examination by prolonged back extension. Radiographic abnormalities of the facet joints are common but only loosely correlated with clinical symptoms, which suggests that this diagnosis should be made with caution and on the basis of congruent radiographic and clinical findings.

In patients with pain that seems to emanate from facet joints, facet joint injections would appear, at least conceptually, to have a role. Carrette and associates[87] studied the efficacy of facet joint injections in a randomized, controlled trial. Patients were selected for participation if they had greater than 50% pain relief after a facet joint injection with a local anesthetic. Even in this select group enriched for presumed facet joint syndrome, facet joint injections with corticosteroids led to improvement at 6 months in only 20% of subjects versus 10% in patients injected with saline placebo. Thus, even in patients with back pain that appears to arrive from true facet arthropathy, injection with corticosteroid was of limited value. It should be noted that less than half of patients in the study had radiographic evidence of degenerative changes at the facet joint. Thus, the role of facet injections in patients with suspected symptomatic degenerative arthropathy of the facet joints remains unproved. Data on complications of facet joint injections are sparse and would be useful in evaluating the relative costs and benefits of the procedure.

Radiofrequency denervation of the facet joints is performed in some centers as an alternative approach to the management of patients with suspected symptomatic facet arthropathy.[47] The facet joints are innervated by the medial branches of the dorsal rami of the spinal nerves. These medial branches are blocked with local anesthetic. If this rather simple procedure is successful in temporarily relieving the patient's pain, it can be followed with radiofrequency denervation in which the medial branches are coagulated using a radiofrequency probe. Radiofrequency ablation appears to be superior to a sham procedure.[88]

SPINAL CORD STIMULATION. Spinal cord stimulation has been used since the early 1970s for treatment of chronic pain. A number of well-designed trials have demonstrated that in 20-year follow-up, spinal cord stimulation is highly effective for neuropathic pain, including radicular pain.[89] The technique is relatively straightforward and quite safe. All patients undergo a temporary trial with an externalized stimulating electrode. If the trial is not successful, the electrode can be easily removed. Patients who do respond become candidates for the implantable stimulator. Carefully selected patients enjoy an average of 50% improvement in their pain activity level, which can be maintained even during long-term follow-up. Patients with pain primarily in the extremities, and minimal axial pain, are most likely to benefit. Spinal cord stimulation is probably the most effective treatment for properly selected patients with failed back surgery syndrome.[90]

# REFERENCES

1. Quebec Task Force on Spinal Disorders report. Spine (suppl) 1987; 12:S9–S53.
2. Frymoyer JW: Back pain and sciatica. N Engl J Med 1988; 318:291–300.
3. LeBoeuf-Yde C, Kyvik KO: At what age does low back pain become a common problem? Spine 1998; 23:228–234.
4. Frank JW, Kerr MS, Brooker AS, et al: Disability resulting from occupational low back pain. Part I. What do we know about primary prevention? A review of scientific evidence on prevention before disability begins. Spine 1996; 21:2908–2917.
5. Von Korff M, Saunders K: The course of back pain in primary care. Spine 1996; 21:2833–2839.
6. Deyo RA, Tsui-Wu YJ: Descriptive epidemiology of low back pain and its related medical care in the United States. Spine 1987; 12:264–268.
7. Deyo RA, Bass JE: Lifestyle and low back pain. The influence of smoking and obesity. Spine 1989; 14:501–506.
8. Kelsey JL, Githens PB, O'Conner T, et al: Acute prolapsed lumbar intervertebral disc. An epidemiologic study with special reference to driving automobiles and cigarette smoking. Spine 1984; 9:608–613.
9. Andersson GBJ: The epidemiology of spinal disorders. In Frymoyer JW (ed): The Adult Spine: Principles and Practice. New York: Raven Press, 1991:107–146.
10. Bigos SJ, Battie MC, Spengler DM, et al: A prospective study of work perceptions and psychosocial factors affecting the report of back injury. Spine 1991; 16:1–6.
11. Bongers PM, de Winter CR, Kompier MAJ, et al: Psychosocial factors at work and musculoskeletal disease. Scand J Work Environ 1993; 19:297–312.
12. Kellgren JH: On the distribution of pain arising from deep somatic structures with charts of segmented pain areas. Clin Sci 1939; 4:35–46.
13. Bigos S, Bowyer O, Braen G, et al: Acute low back problems in adults: Clinical Practice Guideline No. 14. Agency for Health Care Policy and Research, Publication No. 95-0642. Rockville, MD: Agency for Health Care Policy and Research, Department of Health and Human Services, 1994.
14. Epstein NE, Epstein JE: Lumbar decompression for spinal stenosis. In Frymoyer JW (ed). The Adult Spine, 2nd ed. Philadelphia: Lippincott, 1997:2055–2088.
15. Ohnmeiss DD, Vanharanta H, Ekholm J: Degree of disc disruption and lower extremity pain. Spine 1997; 22:1600–1605.
16. Gordon SL, Weinstein JN: A review of basic science issues in low back pain. Phys Med Rehab Clin North Am 1998; 9:323–342.
17. Deyo RA, Rainesville J, Kent DL: What can the history and physical examination tell us about low back pain? JAMA 1992; 268:760–765.
18. Jensen MC, Brant-Zawadzki MN, Obuchowski N, et al: Magnetic resonance imaging of the lumbar spine in people without back pain. N Engl J Med 1994; 331:69–73.
19. Johnsson KE, Uden A, Rosen I: The effect of decompression on the natural course of spinal stenosis. A comparison of surgically treated and untreated patients. Spine 1991; 16:15–19.
20. Moreland LW, Lopez-Mendez A, Alarcon GS: Spinal stenosis: A comprehensive review of the literature. Semin Arthritis Rheum 1989; 19:127–149.
21. Porter RW: Spinal stenosis and neurogenic claudication. Spine 1996; 21:2046–2052.
22. Katz JN, Dalgas M, Bayley J, et al: Degenerative lumbar spinal stenosis: Diagnostic value of the history and physical examination. Arthritis Rheum 1995; 38:1236–1241.
23. Katz JN, Dalgas M, Stucki GH, et al: The diagnosis of lumbar spinal stenosis. Rheum Dis Clin North Am 1994; 20:471–483.
24. Waddell G: A new clinical model for the treatment of low back pain. Spine 1987; 12:632–644.
25. Bortz WM: The disuse syndrome. West J Med 1984; 141:691–694.
26. Nevitt MC, Ettinger B, Black DM, et al: The association of radiographically detected vertebral fractures with back pain and function: A prospective study. Ann Intern Med 1998; 128:793–800.
27. Deyo RA, Diehl AK, Rosenthal M: How many days of bed rest for acute low back pain? A randomized controlled clinical trial. N Engl J Med 1986; 315:1064–1070.
28. Van Tulder M, Koes BW, Bouter LM: Conservative treatment of acute and chronic nonspecific low back pain: A systematic review of randomized controlled trials of the most common interventions. Spine 1997; 22:2128–2156.
29. Malmivaara A, Hakkinen U, Aro T, et al: The treatment of acute low back pain—Bed rest, exercises, or ordinary activity? N Engl J Med 1995; 332:351–355.
30. Portenoy RK: Chronic opioid therapy in nonmalignant pain. J Pain Symptom Manage 1990; 5:546–562.
31. Deyo RA: Non-operative treatment of low back disorders: Differentiating useful from useless therapy. In Frymoyer JW (ed): The Adult Spine: Principles and Practice. New York: Raven Press, 1991:1567–1580.
32. Travell JG, Simons DG: Myofascial Pain and Dysfunction: The Trigger Point Manual. Baltimore: Williams & Wilkins, 1983.
33. Fricton JR: Myofascial pain syndrome: Characteristics and epidemiology. In Fricton JR, Awad E (eds): Advances in Pain Research and Therapy, vol 17. New York: Raven Press, 1990.
34. Cherkin D, Deyo RA, Battie M, et al: A comparison of physical therapy, chiropractic manipulation and provision of an educational booklet for the treatment of patients with low back pain. N Engl J Med 1998; 339:1021–1029.
35. Cherkin DC, MacCornack FA: Patient evaluations of low back pain care from family physicians and chiropractors. West J Med 1989; 150:351–355.
36. Haas M, Nyiendo J, Peterson C, et al: Interrater reliability of roentgenological evaluation of the lumbar spine in lateral bending. J Manipulative Physiol Ther 1990; 13:179–189.
37. Eisenberg DM, Davis RB, Ettner SL, et al: Trends in alternative medicine use in the United States, 1990–97. JAMA 1998; 280:1569–1575.
38. Eisenberg DM, Kessler RC, Foster C, et al: Unconventional medicine in the United States: Prevalence, costs, and patterns of use. N Engl J Med 1993; 328:246–252.
39. Ferrante FM, Wilson SP, Iacobo C, et al: Clinical classification as a predictor of therapeutic outcome after cervical epidural steroid injection. Spine 1993; 18:730–736.
40. Weber H, Holme I, Amlie E: The natural course of acute sciatica with nerve root symptoms in a double blind placebo controlled trial evaluating the effect of piroxicam. Spine 1993; 18:1433.
41. Donelson RG, McKenzie R: Mechanical assessment and treatment of spinal pain. In Frymoyer JW (ed): The Adult Spine: Principles and Practice. New York: Raven Press, 1991.
42. Benzon H: Epidural steroid injections for low back pain and lumbosacral radiculopathy. Pain 1986; 24:277–295.
43. McQuay H, Moore A: Epidural corticosteroids for sciatica. In McQuay H, Moore A (eds): An Evidence-Based Resource for Pain Relief. Oxford, UK: Oxford University Press, 1998:216–218.
44. Carette S, Leclaire R, Marcoux S, et al: Epidural corticosteroid injections for sciatica due to herniated nucleus pulposus. N Engl J Med 1997; 336:1634–1640.
45. Watts RW, Silagy CA: A meta-analysis on the efficacy of epidural corticosteroids in the treatment of sciatica. Anaesth Intensive Care 1995; 23:564–549.
46. Manning DC, Rowlingson JC: Back pain and the role of neural blockade. In Cousins MJ, Bridenbaugh PO (eds): Neural Blockade

in Clinical Anesthesia and Management of Pain, 3rd ed. Philadelphia: Lippincott-Raven, 1998.

47. Bogduk N: Zygapophyseal blocks and epidural steroids. *In* Cousins MJ, Bridenbaugh PO (eds): Neural Blockade in Clinical Anesthesia and Management of Pain, 2nd ed. Philadelphia: JB Lippincott, 1988:935–954.

48. Graves EJ: National hospital discharge survey. Vital Health Stat 1992; 13(100).

49. Perner A, Andersen JT, Juhler M: Lower urinary tract symptoms in lumbar root compression syndromes. Spine 1997; 22:2693–2697.

50. Weber H: Lumbar disc herniation. A controlled prospective study with ten years of observation. Spine 1983; 8:131–140.

51. Hoffman RM, Wheeler KJ, Deyo RA: Surgery for herniated lumbar discs: A literature synthesis. J Gen Intern Med 1993; 8:487–496.

52. Spengler DM: Degenerative stenosis of the lumbar spine. J Bone Joint Surg Am 1987; 69:305–308.

53. Herron LD, Turner J. Patient selection for lumbar laminectomy and discectomy with a reviewed objective rating system. Clin Orthop 1985; 199:145–152.

54. Malter AD, Larson EB, Urban N, et al: Cost effectiveness of lumbar discectomy for the treatment of herniated intervertebral disc. Spine 1996; 21:1048–1055.

55. Williams RW: Microlumbar discectomy: A 12 year statistical review. Spine 1986; 11:851.

56. Schaffer JL, Kambin P: Percutaneous posterolateral lumbar discectomy and decompression with a 6.9 millimeter cannula. Analysis of operative failures and complications. J Bone Joint Surg Am 1991; 73:822–831.

57. Ejeskar A, Nachemson A, Herberts P, et al: Surgery versus chemonucleolysis for herniated lumbar disks: A prospective study with random assignment. Clin Orthop 1983; 174:236–242.

58. Crashaw C, Frazer AM, Merriam WF, et al: A comparison of surgery and chemonucleolysis in the treatment of sciatica. A prospective randomized trial. Spine 1984; 9:195–198.

59. Stucki G, Liang MH, Lipson SJ, et al: Contribution of neuromuscular impairment to physical functional status in patients with lumbar spinal stenosis. J Rheumatol 1994; 21:1338–1343.

60. Rivest C, Katz JN, Ferrante FM, et al: Effects of epidural steroid injection on pain due to lumbar spinal stenosis or herniated disks: A prospective study. Arthritis Care Res 1998; 11:291–297.

61. Herkowitz HN, Kurz LT: Degenerative lumbar spondylolisthesis with spinal stenosis. A prospective study comparing decompression with decompression and intertransverse process arthrodesis. J Bone Joint Surg Am 1991; 73:802–808.

62. Katz JN, Lipson SJ, Lew RA, et al: Lumbar laminectomy alone or with instrumented or noninstrumented arthrodesis in degenerative lumbar spinal stenosis. Spine 1997; 22:1123–1131.

63. Grob D, Jumke T, Dvorak J: Degenerative lumbar stenosis: Decompression with and without arthrodesis. J Bone J Surg Am 1995; 77:1036–1041.

64. Deyo RA, Ciol MA, Cherkin DC, et al: Lumbar spinal fusion: A cohort study of complications, reoperations, and resource use in the Medicare population. Spine 1993; 18:1463–1470.

65. Fischgrund JS, Mackay M, Herkowitz HN, et al: Degenerative lumbar spondylolisthesis with spinal stenosis: A prospective, randomized study comparing decompressive laminectomy and arthrodesis with and without spinal instrumentation. Spine 1997; 22:2807–2812.

66. Thomsen K, Christensen FB, Eiskjaer SP, et al: The effect of pedicle screw instrumentation on functional outcome and fusion rates in posterolateral lumbar spinal fusion: A prospective, randomized clinical study. Spine 1997; 22:2813–2822.

67. Turner JA, Ersek M, Herron L, et al: Surgery for lumbar spinal stenosis: Attempted meta-analysis of the literature. Spine 1992; 17:1–8.

68. Katz JN, Lipson SJ, Larson MG, et al: The outcome of decompressive laminectomy for degenerative lumbar spinal stenosis. J Bone Joint Surg Am 1991; 73:809–816.

69. Katz JN, Lipson SJ, Chang LC, et al: Seven to ten year outcome of decompressive surgery for degenerative lumbar spinal stenosis. Spine 1996; 21:92–98.

70. Ng LKY (ed): New Approaches to Treatment of Chronic Pain: A Review of Multidisciplinary Pain Clinics and Pain Centers (National Institute of Drug Abuse Research Monograph 36). Rockville, MD: National Institute of Drug Abuse, 1981.

71. Turk DC: Efficacy of multidisciplinary pain centers in the treatment of chronic pain. *In* Cohen MJM, Campbell JN (eds): Pain Treatment Centers at a Crossroads: A Practical and Conceptual Reappraisal. Progress in Pain Research and Management, vol 7. Seattle: IASP Press, 1996:257–274.

72. Scheer SJ, Watanabe TK, Radack KL: Randomized controlled trials in industrial low back pain: Part 3. Subacute/chronic pain interventions. Arch Phys Med Rehabil 1997; 78:414–423.

73. Bendix T, Bendix AF, Busch E, et al: Functional restoration in chronic low back pain. Scand J Med Sci Sports 1996; 6:88–97.

74. Hazard RG: Chronic low back pain and disability: The efficacy of functional restoration. Bull Hosp Joint Dis 1996; 55:213–216.

75. Aronoff GM, Evans WO, Enders PL: A review of follow-up studies of multidisciplinary pain units. Pain 1983; 16:1–11.

76. Mayer TG, Gatchel RJ, Mayer H, et al: A prospective two-year study of functional restoration in industrial low back injury. An objective assessment procedure. JAMA 1987; 258:1763–1767.

77. Porter J, Jick H: Addiction rare in patients treated with narcotics. N Engl J Med 1980; 302:123.

78. Jamison RN, Raymond SA, Slawsby EA, et al: Opioid therapy for chronic noncancer back pain: A randomized prospective study. Spine 1998; 23:2591–2600.

79. Coombs DW, Maurer LH, Saunders RL, et al: Outcomes and complications of continuous intraspinal narcotic analgesia for cancer pain control. J Clin Oncol 1984; 2:1414–1420.

80. Magora F, Olshwang D, Eimerl D, et al: Observations on extradural morphine analgesia in various pain conditions. Br J Anaesth 1980; 52:247–252.

81. Waldman SP, Coombs DW: Selection of implantable narcotic delivery systems. Anesth Analg 1989; 68:377–384.

82. Krames ES, Lanning RM: Intrathecal infusional analgesia for nonmalignant pain: Analgesic efficacy of intrathecal opioid with or without bupivacaine. J Pain Symptom Manage 1993; 8:539–548.

83. Hassenbusch SJ, Stanton-Hicks M, Covington EC, et al: Long-term intraspinal infusions of opioids in the treatment of neuropathic pain. J Pain Symptom Manage 1995; 10:527–543.

84. Angel IF, Gould HJ Jr, Carey ME: Intrathecal morphine pump as a treatment option in chronic pain of nonmalignant origin. Surg Neurol 1998; 49:92–98 (discussion 49:98–99).

85. Follett KA, Hitchon PW, Piper J, et al: Response of intractable pain to continuous intrathecal morphine: A retrospective study. Pain 1992; 49:21–25.

86. Tutak U, Doleys DM: Intrathecal infusion systems for treatment of chronic low back and leg pain of noncancer origin. South Med J 1996; 89:295–300.

87. Carrette S, Marcour S, Truchon R, et al: A controlled trial of corticosteroid injections into facet joints for chronic low back pain. N Engl J Med 1991; 325:1002–1007.

88. Lord SM, Bannsley L, Wallis BJ, et al: Percutaneous radiofrequency neurotomy for chronic zygapophyseal joint pain. N Engl J Med 1996; 335:1721–1726.

89. North RB, Kidd DH, Zahurak M, et al: Spinal cord stimulation for chronic, intractable pain: Experience over two decades. Neurosurgery 1993; 32:384–395.

90. De La Porte C, Siegfried J: Lumbosacral spinal fibrosis (spinal arachnoiditis): Its diagnosis and treatment by spinal cord stimulation. Spine 1983; 8:593–603.

# Reflex Sympathetic Dystrophy (Complex Regional Pain Syndrome-I)

*Erik Peterson and Kenneth Saag*

Reflex sympathetic dystrophy (RSD) or complex regional pain syndrome (CRPS) type I defines a group of heterogenous clinical conditions united by features of chronic extremity pain associated with vasomotor and trophic skin changes. CRPS affects persons of all ages and of either sex. Symptoms most commonly follow surgery or extremity trauma, but a wide range of medical conditions has also been associated with CRPS. Although the pathophysiology remains poorly understood, recent work challenges the traditional hypothesis that disturbed sympathetic nervous outflow causes the pain and disability of CRPS. Attempts to define evidence-based standard treatment approaches are hampered by the predominance of small, often uncontrolled or retrospective studies that draw conclusions about patients who satisfy differing case definitions. Principles of management include an early aggressive approach to treatment and sampling of a wide range of sympatholytic, anti-inflammatory, neuropsychiatric, analgesic, and physical therapeutic modalities. Despite therapy, a significant proportion of affected patients acquire irreversible loss of limb function and chronic incapacity.

## HISTORY AND TERMINOLOGY

The earliest report of CRPS described Civil War soldiers with gunshot wound–associated peripheral nerve injuries.[1] These men often experienced burning pain and hyperalgesia, as well as skin temperature, color, and sweating abnormalities in affected limbs. Later, an association of the "causalgia" symptom complex with regional osteoporosis or "bony atrophy" was described.[2] Citing these clinical features of "sympathetic stimulation," and noting the dramatic symptom reductions seen in several of these patients after surgical sympathectomy,[3] Evans introduced the term *reflex sympathetic dystrophy*.[4] Bonica and Buckley later contributed influential reports advocating sympathetic blockade as the primary diagnostic and therapeutic intervention for RSD.[5, 6] RSD-CRPS continues to have numerous synonyms: shoulder-hand syndrome, causalgia, Sudek's atrophy, algoneurodystrophy,

clenched-fist syndrome, reflex neurovascular dystrophy, and "sympathetically maintained pain." Unfortunately, RSD has come to serve as a "wastebasket" label for many types of ill-defined postsurgical or posttraumatic pain.[7]

Widespread disagreement over the case definition and taxonomy of chronic limb pain spurred the development of a classification scheme that replaces the confusing spectrum of diagnostic terms with the phrase *complex regional pain syndrome*.[8] CRPS is defined as "a painful condition following injury that appears regionally, having a distal predominance of abnormal findings exceeding in both magnitude and duration the expected clinical course of the inciting event, often resulting in significant impairment of motor function, and showing variable progression over time."[8] Notably, the term *CRPS* maintains neutrality toward any one putative pathogenic influence. Demonstration of sympathetic involvement is not required for the diagnosis of CRPS; rather, CRPS diagnoses are clinically based. Clinical features of the syndrome previously termed *RSD* are best encompassed by the defining features of CRPS, type I:

1. Pain develops after an initiating or noxious event.
2. Spontaneous pain, allodynia (pain resulting from a non-noxious stimulus), or hyperalgesia occurs; it is not limited to the territory of a single peripheral nerve; and it is disproportionate to the inciting event.
3. There is or has been evidence of edema, skin blood flow abnormality, or abnormal sudomotor (stimulation of sweat gland) activity in the region of the pain since the inciting event.
4. The diagnosis is excluded by the existence of conditions that would otherwise account for the degree of pain and dysfunction.

CRPS, type II, often synonymously referred to as *causalgia*, is distinguished from type I only by the history of documented peripheral nerve injury before symptom onset.[8] Given significant overlap in therapeutic approach to CRPS I and CRPS II, the two conditions are not distinguished in this discussion.

## CLINICAL FEATURES AND NATURAL HISTORY

In an effort to place patients in a probable chronologic framework and to assist with prognostication, Steinbrocker proposed a staging system for RSD-CRPS[9]:

*Acute stage:* Beginning days to weeks after injury, the acute phase is notable for constant, burning pain; allodynia; hyperalgesia; localized edema; and decreased mobility of the limb. Skin is typically red, hot, and dry. Plain radiographs are normal at this stage, but a triple-phase bone scan may show increased radiotracer uptake in the affected limb.

*Dystrophic stage:* Two to 6 months after injury, the onset of the dystrophic stage is heralded by cool, cyanotic, moist skin over the affected part. Nails may become brittle and grooved. Burning pain, allodynia, and hyperpathia persist.

*Atrophic stage:* Irreversible skin and skeletal changes occur 6 to 12 months after the inciting incident. Skin is typically smooth, glossy, and cool; muscle atrophy parallels progressive limitation of motion and claw-like deformities in affected limbs. Patchy osteoporosis is commonly observed radiographically.

Many authorities now question the clinical relevance of temporal staging because many patients do not exhibit organized progression of disease over time.[10] Importantly, the more recently proposed CRPS classification (described earlier) does not emphasize discrete disease stages.

CRPS has been linked to a wide range of inciting stimuli. Historically, 45 to 65% of CRPS cases follow trauma (usually fractures),[4, 10] and another 20% occur after surgical procedures, such as release for carpal tunnel syndrome or Dupuytren's contracture.[11] In 10% of cases, no inciting factor is identified, and the remaining cases are associated with myocardial infarction, cerebrovascular accident with hemiplegia, head injury, inflammatory arthritis, and peripheral nerve entrapment syndromes.[12] Interestingly, the incidence of CRPS in association with specific pathologic states varies widely. For example, after Colles' fracture of the wrist, several studies set the incidence of CRPS at 7 to 35%.[10, 13, 14] In contrast, when all extremity fractures are considered together, CRPS complicates only 1 to 2%.[10] In an era of aggressive cardiac rehabilitation, the incidence of CRPS associated with post–myocardial infarction is extremely low, whereas 12 to 23% of patients with hemiplegia continue to experience CRPS.[15, 16] These data suggest a potential contribution of limb immobilization to the risk of CRPS.

Conflicting information exists concerning natural history and long-term treatment outcomes of CRPS. Epidemiologic studies are hampered because the etiopathogenesis of CRPS is likely heterogenous, and there is no universally accepted set of diagnostic criteria. Investigations of CRPS symptom duration highlight the contradictory nature of the literature: One group reported that more than 85% of CRPS patients had spontaneous resolution of pain and swelling 13 months after diagnosis.[17] In contrast, a separate contemporary study revealed that a majority of CRPS patients still had pain, cold sensitivity, and decreased strength in the affected limb after 5 to 9 years.[11] Supporting the latter notion of CRPS chronicity, Poplawski and colleagues found that nearly all of 62 patients with CRPS had persistent symptoms during 10 years of follow-up.[18]

While the natural history of CRPS remains controversial, there is little dispute that CRPS results in significant psychosocial and socioeconomic consequences. CRPS causes upheaval in employment. In the short term, at least one third of CRPS sufferers cannot work for more than a year after symptom onset.[19] Less than a third of patients eventually return to their premorbid occupation.[12, 18]

A minority of patients with long-standing CRPS experience medical complications. Infection of the affected limb is the most common adverse event and is often preceded by skin ulceration.[20] Dystonia may occur, manifested by finger flexion contractures leading to a "clenched fist" in the upper extremity, or by inversion and equinus positioning of the foot. Less commonly, myoclonus or chronic edema ensue in limbs with little or no residual function after CRPS.[20] The skin temperature of the affected limb at onset is one prognostic factor that appears to predict the development of complications in CRPS. In one study, 62% of patients with a severe complication had "primarily cold skin" at syndrome onset, compared with only 30% of patients without complications.[20]

## PATHOPHYSIOLOGY

The cause of CRPS remains uncertain. CRPS has most commonly been attributed to one or both of two major causal influences: abnormalities in the sympathetic nervous system or poorly controlled regional inflammatory responses to injury.[21] An understanding of these leading theories of CRPS pathogenesis helps guide a rational therapeutic approach.

Many writers have observed that CRPS pain frequently does not conform to the distribution of a peripheral sensory nerve, that its magnitude appears out of proportion to the severity of the initial insult, and that it often persists long after healing of an inciting wound or event.[22] A theory of a "vicious circle of reflexes" was developed to explain these observations.[21] According to the vicious circle model, CRPS pain begins with chronic irritation of a peripheral nerve. The resulting augmentation of afferent impulses enhances activity in internuncial pools of the spinal cord. Continuous increased sympathetic tone springs from synapses between neurons in the anterior horn neurons and in sympathetic ganglia. Chronically elevated sympathetic tone induces both cross-stimulation of nociceptive neurons and increased somatic afferent impulses, leading to pain and completing the "vicious" cycle.[23]

The long-held theory that CRPS is a disorder of pathologically hyperactive sympathethic nervous activity has been based on features of vasomotor instability in CRPS limbs and reports of pain amelioration after sympathectomy.[24] However, clinical and mechanistic studies have questioned the importance of the sympathetic system in CRPS. Several prospective, double-blind, placebo-controlled trials found no difference between sympathetic blockade and placebo in reducing CRPS symptoms.[25–27] Verdugo and Ochoa reported that fewer CRPS patients derived pain relief from phentolamine infusion (alpha blocker) than from placebo.[28]

Several physiologic lines of evidence also argue against simple, unrestrained sympathetic activity as the underlying cause of CRPS. Skin blood flow is increased in limbs with acute CRPS, a finding opposite to that expected in a limb with enhanced sympathetic tone.[29] Similarly, the documented supersensitivity of nociceptive nerve endings and $\alpha$-adrenergic receptors to noradrenaline stimulation in CRPS typically indicates hypoactive rather than overactive sympathetic function.[30] Other work found paradoxically diminished serum concentrations of sympathetically driven neuropeptide Y and norepinephrine in CRPS-affected limbs.[31, 32]

Symptoms of stiffness and pain and classic signs of swelling, warmth, and redness suggest that a pathologic inflammatory response may be present in CRPS. Increased vascular permeability in CRPS suggests activity of inflammatory mediators.[33] Bradykinin, a pro-inflammatory nonapeptide, is found in increased concentrations in CRPS serum.[21] Skin from affected limbs contains markedly increased numbers of Langerhans' or dendritic cells compared with non-CRPS biopsy specimens.[34] Finally, reports of CRPS improvement after treatment with anti-inflammatory medication[35] or free radical scavengers such as mannitol[36] and dimethyl sulfoxide (DMSO)[37] lend weight to the "exaggerated inflammatory response" hypothesis.

Nociceptive sensitization in CRPS is a more recent concept introduced to explain allodynia and hyperpathia associated with CRPS. Neurogenic inflammation stimulated by trauma to peripheral C-fibers may be mediated by histamine. One study found enhanced dysesthetic response to histamine in CRPS limbs, which suggests nociceptive sensitization.[38]

Personality and other psychiatric disorders have been reported in patients with CRPS. In one study, one third of the patients had psychiatric diagnoses.[39] In another group of CRPS patients, 45% needed psychiatric referral, usually for management of mania.[40] Tendencies toward hypochondriasis and depression seen on personality testing have been found in one third of CRPS patients.[12] However, none of these studies can document a causal relationship between psychiatric illness and CRPS because they do not establish the presence of premorbid personality or psychiatric disorders.[41] Therefore, evidence that CRPS has psychopathologic roots is lacking.[42]

# DIAGNOSIS

Although CRPS is primarily a clinical diagnosis, a number of bedside maneuvers and laboratory tests may be helpful for confirmation.

To help guide therapy, some authors emphasize the distinction between CRPS patients experiencing "sympathetically maintained pain" (SMP)—pain that is most clearly attributable to sympathetic efferent function in peripheral tissues—and "sympathetically independent pain".[7, 43] Those with definite SMP may be more likely to respond to therapy directed at interruption of sympathetic flow. Sensitivity to mild cooling stimuli may assist in identification of SMP. In several studies, all patients with SMP exhibited hyperalgesia to the cooling stimulus of acetone placed on the affected limb, whereas only about 50% of patients with sympathetically independent pain displayed hyperalgesia to cold.[44, 45] Extremity swelling seen on physical examination and symptom duration less than 6 months are two additional clinical factors predictive of a response to sympathetic blockade.[46]

Temporary sympatholysis achieved through local anesthetic ganglion blocks[6] or intravenous infusions of $\alpha$-adrenergic antagonists such as phentolamine[47, 48] have also been used as indicators of CRPS patient responsiveness to sympathetic manipulation. However, data suggest that results of such sympatholytic procedures are difficult to interpret because of high rates of placebo response and false-negative results.[7, 28, 49] Diagnostic sympatholysis does little to further refine a clinical diagnosis of CRPS or define a subset of patients likely to benefit from particular management strategies.[28] In one large study, only 62% of clinically diagnosed CRPS patients at a tertiary center responded to sympathetic blockade, whereas 43% of patients who did not meet criteria for CRPS also responded.[46] Thus, the positive predictive value of sympathetic blockade for susceptibility to therapeutic sympathetic manipulation in CRPS is low.

Identification of autonomic functional abnormalities may help predict response to sympathetic blockade in CRPS patients. An elevated resting skin temperature (RST) in the affected limb was found in 75% of patients with chronic limb pain who responded to sympathetic block; less than half of those without increased RST responded to block.[46] In addition, positive findings on two tests of autonomic function, resting sweat output and quantitative sudomotor axon reflex testing (QSART) together predicted a diagnosis of RSD with 98% specificity.[46] However, resting sweat output and QSART have poor sensitivity and thus are useful for confirming, but not excluding, the diagnosis of CRPS.

Common radiographic findings in established CRPS include "patchy" demineralization of bone in painful limbs and abnormal bone scintigraphy. Kozin and colleagues reported osteoporosis or enhanced tracer uptake, or both, in two thirds of limbs affected by CRPS.[50] Some authors report that diffuse, increased tracer uptake in the delayed phase of triple-phase scintigraphic scanning can establish CRPS with high specificity and sensitivity.[51, 52] However, other studies suggest that triple-phase scanning suffers from poor specificity.[46, 53, 54]

In summary, no single test or maneuver can reproducibly identify the group of patients most likely to benefit from CRPS-directed therapy. Recognizing the poor predictive value of any one sign or symptom, Gibbons and Wilson proposed use of an "RSD score," which is calculated using the presence of key clinical and laboratory findings.[55] Although no prospective validating studies have been performed, the RSD score serves as a useful adjunct to the earlier-mentioned CRPS diagnostic criteria (Table 9–1). The scoring system assigns 1 point for the definite presence of each criterion, no points for absence, and ½ point for equivocal findings. Patients are considered to have "probable RSD" (CRPS) if they have a score of greater than 5, and "possible RSD" with a score of 3 to 4.5.

A time- and cost-efficient approach to diagnosis begins with a careful history and physical examination, including assessment of criteria 1 to 5 in Table 9–1. Objective testing should start with assessment of RST and QSART.[46] Plain radiography and scintigraphy should be undertaken if insufficient criteria for "probable" disease are met or if the expertise for assessment of autonomic dysfunction is not immediately available. Response to sympathetic block should be used as a diagnostic criterion only when clinical suspicion of SMP remains high in the absence of other satisfied criteria.

Careful consideration should be given to differential diagnosis. Conditions that may mimic CRPS include chronic arterial insufficiency, Raynaud's phenomenon, entrapment neuropathies, venous thrombosis, infection, and primary systemic rheumatic disorders.[56]

# TREATMENT

## Pharmacologic Approaches

CHEMICAL SYMPATHECTOMY. Historically, direct sympathetic blockade of areas such as the stellate ganglion with local anesthetics has been widely used for CRPS. Significant improvements in pain were reported in many patients,[6, 57–60] but few prospective, controlled trials exist. Postganglionic segmental blockade has

## TABLE 9–1
### Reflex Sympathetic Dystrophy Score Criteria

1. Allodynia
2. Burning pain
3. Edema
4. Color or hair growth changes
5. Sweating changes
6. Temperature changes
7. Radiographic changes (demineralization)
8. Quantitative measurement of vasomotor/sudomotor disturbance
9. Bone scan consistent with RSD
10. Response to sympathetic block

For each criterion, patient is assigned one point for positive findings or one-half point for equivocal findings. Total score of <3 = "RSD absent"; total score of 3–4.5 = "possible RSD"; total score of >5 = "probable RSD."
RSD = reflex sympathetic dystrophy.
Used with permission from Gibbons JJ, Wilson PR: RSD score: Criteria for the diagnosis of reflex sympathetic dystrophy and causalgia. Clin J Pain 1992; 8:260–263.

now largely replaced ganglionic blockade because of (1) concern about uncommon complications such as severe malaise, loss of consciousness, seizures, and postsympathectomy neuralgia; (2) a lack of common expertise in direct sympathetic ganglion injection techniques; and (3) a significant symptom recurrence rate.[61]

Postganglionic sympatholysis, accomplished by intravenous regional sympathetic blockade (Bier's block or IRSB), was first introduced for CRPS in 1983.[18] Adrenergic blocking agents used in this clinical setting have included guanethidine,[62–66] phenoxybenzamine,[67] bretylium,[68, 69] ketanserin,[70] droperidol,[71] and reserpine[65, 72, 73]; see Table 9–2, for a comparison of adrenergic blocking agents.

IRSB requires limb exsanguination followed by prolonged tourniquet time, and this may result in transient extremity pain, particularly in patients with preexistent hyperesthesia.[27] As such, a local anesthetic is usually administered initially. Guanethidine (10 to 30 mg/block) is the most commonly used adrenergic blocking agent. Guanethidine displaces epinephrine from storage sites and prevents its reuptake, inducing a depletion of norepinephrine at the postganglionic nerve endings. More recently, IRSB with bretylium has been performed. Bretylium accumulates in postganglionic adrenergic neurons and inhibits conduction by preventing norepinephrine release. In high concentrations, bretylium also demonstrates local anesthetic and neuromuscular blocking properties. Bretylium infusion produced a 3-week relief period compared with a 3-day relief period accomplished with lidocaine infusion alone.[69] Nonadrenergic agents, such as ketorolac,[74] have also been used for regional blocks.

After tourniquet removal, patients undergoing IRSB must be observed for the development of adverse effects such as orthostatic hypotension, anticholinergic symptoms (dry mouth, nausea, diarrhea, bradycardia, dizziness), and generalized weakness.[25] These potential complications are primarily of concern if patients have underlying cardiovascular disease. Other adverse events may include headaches, rash, thrombophlebitis, and protracted ischemia of an extremity. In general, side effects with IRSB are uncommon. Tricyclic antidepressants, phenothiazines, sympathomimetic agents, and oral adrenergic blockers or agonists may interfere with IRSB and should usually be stopped several weeks before the procedure.

Several reports have questioned the value of postganglionic chemical sympathectomy (IRSB) in CRPS.[75, 76] At least two randomized, double-blind, controlled studies failed to find consistent or dose-responsive benefits.[26, 27] These results concur with a larger uncontrolled trial that found unchanged or worsened pain in 75% of guanethidine-treated CRPS patients at a mean of 3 months of follow-up. A systematic review of randomized, controlled trials of treatment with guanethidine IRSB showed no difference in response between placebo and treatment.[25] Of further concern, at least one group reported significant adverse effects in 34% of CRPS patients receiving IRSB.[75]

These data notwithstanding, it appears that for a subset of CRPS patients, IRSB can produce dramatic

**TABLE 9–2**
## Pharmacologic Agents in the Therapy of Complex Regional Pain Syndrome

| DRUG | DOSAGE | ADVERSE EFFECTS |
|---|---|---|
| **Regional Intravenous Therapy** | | |
| α-Adrenergic antagonists | | |
| Guanethidine | 20–40 mg, administered with lidocaine | Postural hypotension, dizziness, diarrhea, weakness, headache |
| Bretylium | 1.5 mg/kg, administered with lidocaine | Postural hypotension, headache, abdominal cramping |
| Phenoxybenzamine | 5 mg, administered with lidocaine | Postural hypotension, reflex tachycardia, miosis, sedation, inhibition of ejaculation |
| Reserpine | 0.5 mg | Sedation, abdominal cramps, diarrhea, flushing, congestion |
| 5-Hydroxytryptamine antagonists | | |
| Ketanserin | 10–20 mg | Headache, sedation, dry mouth, dizziness |
| Nonsteroidal agents | | |
| Ketorolac | 60 mg, administered with lidocaine | Increased bleeding propensity, abdominal pain |
| **Glucocorticoids** | | |
| Prednisone | 0.25–0.5 mg/kg PO, tapering over 3 mo | Fluid retention, dysphoria, flushing |
| Methlyprednisolone | 80 mg IM depot, every 2 wk up to 12 wk | Long-term: glucose intolerance, fractures, weakness, cataracts, infection |
| **Calcitonin** | 100 units SQ every day | Nausea, vomiting; flushing |
| **Bisphosphonates** | | |
| Alendronate | 7.5 mg/day IV every day for 3 days | Postinjection fever, hypertension, headache, arthralgia, hypocalcemia |
| Pamidronate | 30 mg IV for 3 days | |
| **Anticonvulsants** | | |
| Carbamazepine | 200–800 mg every day in BID/TID dosing | Drowsiness, dizziness, nausea, hepato- and myelotoxicity |
| Gabapentin | 900–3000 mg every day in divided doses | Fatigue, somnolence, nystagmus |
| Phenytoin | 100–300 mg every day | Nystagmus, ataxia, confusion, nausea, gingival hyperplasia, hypertrichosis |
| **Oral Sympathetic Blockade and Vasodilation** | | |
| Phenoxybenzamine | 10 mg every day TID | See preceding section |
| Nifedipine | 10–30 mg TID | Peripheral edema, headache, flushing, hypotension |

and long-lasting benefit with relatively low risk.[62, 63, 66, 72, 77] At a minimum, IRSB may provide temporary pain relief sufficient to allow initiation of a rigorous physical therapy program,[78] although not all authors advocate aggressive therapy after IRSB.[64] Should benefit occur with initial IRSB, repeat injections may then be warranted. The literature does not support firm guidelines regarding an optimal number of infusions or treatment duration.

Some evidence suggests that when chemical sympathectomies are instituted "the earlier the better" improvement potential is maximized. In Steinbrocker and Argyros' study, 92% of patients treated in "acute" phase and 79% of patients in "dystrophic stage" had satisfactory response on late follow-up.[58] No patients treated while in the "atrophic" stage benefited from sympathectomy. Retrospective study of patients treated with a combination of chemical and surgical sympathectomy found that those with satisfactory outcome were treated a mean of 6.8 months after the incit-

ing injury.[24] In contrast, patients with poor outcomes began treatment an average of 24 months after symptom onset.

ANALGESICS. Early in the course of CRPS, short courses of narcotic analgesics may be warranted when pain hinders sleep, activities of daily living, or appropriate limb mobilization. However, narcotics should almost never play a major role in a long-term CRPS pain management plan.[79] Although epidural and intrathecal morphine and ketamine[80] have been employed for refractory pain in several patients, their long-term usefulness has not been studied.

ANTI-INFLAMMATORY AGENTS. A number of CRPS trials have found benefit in the use of glucocorticoids. Steinbrocker and associates recognized potential benefits of steroids as early as 1953, when they were used in combination with stellate ganglion blocks for CRPS.[81] In 1991, methylprednisolone was used in combination Bier's blocks followed by physical manipulation, leading to short-term benefit in uncontrolled trials.[82, 83] Oral prednisone in daily doses of 20 to 40 mg produced better and faster pain relief than did placebo in a number of nonblinded small trials[35, 84, 85] (see Table 9–2). In 1996, an uncontrolled series of acute upper extremity CRPS patients treated with bi-weekly intramuscular methylprednisolone found that nearly 70% achieved marked improvement in night and rest pain as well as in joint motion and grip strength.[86]

DMSO is a novel anti-inflammatory agent that may work by scavenging hydroxyl radicals. A small, randomized trial of DMSO cream found a more rapid and complete improvement in indices of CRPS disease activity than seen with placebo cream.[87]

CALCITONIN. Conflicting data exist about the efficacy of salmon calcitonin and carbocalcitonin in CRPS. Potential beneficial effects of calcitonin may result from its analgesic properties or its bone antiresorptive activity, or both. Calcitonin may decrease pain indicators in acute-phase CRPS, but there is little evidence that it improves joint mobility or disability in the long term.[61, 88–90] One report showed calcitonin to be equal to placebo for short-term pain relief.[91] In sum, the literature suggests that calcitonin may be an effective analgesic in CRPS, but that the drug should be employed early in the disease course and only briefly.

BISPHOSPHONATES. Enthusiasm for bisphosphonates derives from their known antiresorptive effects, their proven analgesic efficacy in patients with Paget's disease and bony metastasis, and the frequent observation of periarticular osteoporosis in CRPS.[92] The usefulness of bisphosphonate in CRPS was initially suggested by several small, short-term, prospective trials of intravenous pamidronate.[93, 94] Although significant pain reduction was realized in a majority of patients, including several refractory cases, adverse events were seen in 50%.[93] In 1997, CRPS patients taking part in a blinded, placebo-controlled trial of intravenous alendronate had significant improvement in spontaneous pain, swelling, and mobility of affected limbs over several months. Marked increases in the bone mineral density of affected limbs were seen 6 weeks after the trial.[95] Strong recommendations favoring the use of these agents in CRPS must await results of larger, longer trials.

ANTICONVULSANTS AND NEUROTROPICS. Phenytoin,[96] carbamazepine,[97] and gabapentin[98]—agents that are commonly employed against neuropathic pain—have putative benefits in CRPS. In a small case series of patients with refractory CRPS, all patients experienced substantial rapid reduction (60% to 100%) in pain with gabapentin monotherapy.[99] Gabapentin is safer than other anticonvulsants because of absent hepatotoxicity and myelotoxicity and few if any interactions with other drugs. Uncommon side effects of gabapentin (<2%) include somnolence, dizziness, ataxia, and fatigue.

EPIDURAL AND PERIPHERAL NERVE BLOCKADE. Blockade of peripheral or epidural sites can produce effects similar to direct paravertebral or IRSB. Epidural clonidine produced mild improvement in visual analog scale scores compared with placebo in patients with CRPS who responded to sympathectomy.[100] Several small reports describe blockade of peripheral nerves such as the brachial plexus leading to marked improvement in CRPS patients.[101, 102]

ORAL SYMPATHETIC BLOCKADE AND VASODILATION. Oral strategies aimed at treating sympathetic hyperactivity include the use of β blockers, calcium channel blocking agents, and α-adrenergic blockers such as phenoxybenzamine.[103] Several trials suggested the efficacy of nifedipine or phenoxybenzamine, especially in "acute" CRPS.[104, 105] Phenoxybenzamine, however, is poorly tolerated because of common orthostatic hypotension, dizziness, nausea, diarrhea, and reversible impotence among male patients.[104] Case reports and uncontrolled trials also favor the use of β blockers in CRPS.[106, 107]

## Physical Modalities

Early physical therapy with limb mobilization in CRPS is nearly universally recommended, although controlled trials documenting the effectiveness of physiotherapy do not exist. A number of writers emphasize that the maxim "control pain to obtain gain," rather than "no pain, no gain," holds best with CRPS sufferers.[79, 108, 109] Therefore, pain exacerbated by physical therapy should be aggressively managed with short courses of narcotics, intravenous regional anesthesia, use of contrast baths (alternating hot and cold), ultrasonography, or repeated sympathetic blocks.[78, 79, 108] Control of extremity edema through support hose or other types of body compression garments also may alleviate pain. Transcutaneous nerve stimulation may provide added benefit in some cases.[108] Intermittent cold applications offer modest benefit during the acute period of active inflammation.[61]

## Surgical Approaches

SURGICAL SYMPATHECTOMY. Historically, surgical sympatholysis via resection of sympathetic ganglia was the treatment of choice for CRPS patients who initially responded to sympathetic anesthetic blockade.[6, 109] Thoracic sympathectomy for upper extremity CRPS, performed either via thoracotomy or more recently using video-assisted thoracoscopy, has been advocated despite an absence of compelling data.[110] Potential complications of sympathectomy include postsympathetectomy neuritis, permanent heart rate regulation problems, Horner's syndrome, cholestasis, and ejaculatory dysfunction.[111] Major limitations include the irreversibility of the surgery and the gradual recurrence of symptoms over periods ranging from months to years.[112, 113]

NEUROAUGMENTATION. For refractory, chronic CRPS pain, several small series suggest the efficacy of techniques collectively known as *neuroaugmentation*. To achieve analgesia, neuroaugmentation relies on the use of spinal cord stimulation (SCS) and other devices that deliver electrical impulses to peripheral nerves.[113, 114] For SCS, electrodes are implanted epidurally with leads tunneled either out of the skin (if an external generator is used) or to an implantable generator placed below the clavicle or in the right iliac fossa. Several small studies have documented marked pain relief and decreasing narcotic requirements in 30 to 50% of refractory CRPS patients, with some responses durable for several years.[114–116] Complications associated with stimulation techniques include lead migration, lead fracture, prolonged pain at the surgical site, and surgical complications of infections and bleeding.[114] Because of the potential for long-term waning effectiveness[117] and the interventional nature of SCS, this modality should be reserved for CRPS that is refractory to other medical and neuromodulatory therapy.[113, 114]

CORRECTIVE SURGERY AND AMPUTATION. In rare cases, release of fixed flexion deformities of the extremities may be required to improve functional status for patients with late-stage, atrophic CRPS.[109] Although intractable pain alone should not serve as an indication, amputation may improve residual function and decrease the rate of recurrent infections in a small, severely affected subgroup of CRPS patients.[118]

## Psychological Interventions

Although most evidence suggests that CRPS is not a primary psychiatric disorder,[42, 119] chronic pain frequently leads to clinical depression or other psychiatric illness. In addition, personality traits may predispose to or exacerbate CRPS.[120, 121] Patients with underlying psychiatric disorders display lower treatment response rates.[72] Judicious use of psychotropic agents (antidepressants, anxiolytic agents) in conjunction with counseling or behavioral modification, or both, may have value in selected patients.

# AUTHORS' APPROACH AND RECOMMENDATIONS

A rational approach to the management of CRPS is confounded by a heterogenous case definition coupled with a lack of large, carefully controlled clinical trials. Although it is difficult to extract strong data-driven recommendations from the literature, a number of broad therapeutic themes emerge.

Early, aggressive management of CRPS is likely to yield better outcomes than is treatment of patients with "atrophic" stage or long-standing disease.[122, 123] Initial treatment should include early mobilization (with analgesia sufficient to facilitate range of motion exercise), moderate doses of glucocorticoids (0.25 to 0.5 mg/kg/day of prednisone), and a trial of IRSB with guanethidine or bretylium. Given growing recognition that mechanisms other than sympathetic hyperactivity may play pathogenic roles in CRPS, response to one application of IRSB should guide plans for protracted blockade. At a minimum, IRSB may provide a period of pain relief lasting several days to weeks, which is sufficient to permit aggressive physical therapy. Preventive measures (bone mass measurement and, at a minimum, administration of calcium and vitamin D supplements) should be taken whenever glucocorti-

coids are employed, given their predictable side effects. Steroids should be tapered and discontinued over a 3-month period.

In the absence of clinical response to initial therapy in 4 to 6 weeks, additional treatment for CRPS is indicated. Antiresorptive agents such as calcitonin or the bisphosphonates may rapidly alleviate symptoms or retard progression, or both. Agents used commonly to manage other chronic neuropathic pain syndromes, such as anticonvulsants, are appropriate as well.

Attention should be directed to the patient's psychological and emotional well-being. Concomitant depression or personality or anxiety disorders, if present, should be directly addressed and appropriately managed. The chronic use of narcotic analgesics should be eschewed.

Refractory, severe CRPS symptoms; progressive loss of function; or complications (i.e., infection) 3 to 6 months after symptom onset should prompt consideration of invasive approaches such as surgical sympathectomy, neuroaugmentation (spinal cord stimulation), epidural infusions, plexus blocks and, in limbs afflicted with severe, recurrent infection, amputation.

*Acknowledgments*

*The authors thank B. Porter, M.D., and H. Peterson, M.D., for critical review of this chapter and E. Ward for clerical assistance.*

# REFERENCES

1. Mitchell S, Morehouse G, Keen W: Gunshot wounds and other injuries of nerves. Philadelphia: JB Lippincott, 1864.
2. Sudeck P: Ueber die akute entzundliche Knochenatrophie. Arch Klin Chir 1900; 62:147–156.
3. Spurling R: Causalgia of the upper extremity. Treatment by dorsal sympathetic ganglionectomy. Arch Neurol Psychiatr 1930; 23:784–788.
4. Evans JA: Reflex sympathetic dystrophy: Report on 57 cases. Ann Intern Med 1947; 26:417–426.
5. Bonica J, Buckley F: Regional analgesia with local anesthetics. *In* Bonica J (ed): The management of pain, 2nd ed. Philadelphia: Lea & Febiger, 1990:883–966.
6. Bonica J: Causalgia and other reflex sympathetic dystrophies. *In* Bonica J, Liebeskind J, Albe-Fessard L (eds): Advances in Pain Research and Therapy, vol 3. New York: Raven Press, 1979.
7. Campbell J, Raja S, Selig D, et al: Diagnosis and management of sympathetically maintained pain. *In* Fields H, Liebeskind J (eds): Progress in Pain Research and Management, vol 1. Seattle: IASP Press, 1994:85–100.
8. Stanton-Hicks M, Janig W, Hassenbusch S, et al: Reflex sympathetic dystrophy: Changing concepts and taxonomy. Pain 1995; 63:127–133.
9. Steinbrocker O: The shoulder-hand syndrome. Associated painful homolateral disability of the shoulder and hand with swelling and atrophy of the hand. Am J Med 1947; 3:402–407.
10. Veldman PH, Reynen HM, Arntz IE, et al: Signs and symptoms of reflex sympathetic dystrophy: Prospective study of 829 patients. Lancet 1993; 342:1012–1016.
11. Geertzen JH, Dijkstra PU, Groothoff JW, et al: Reflex sympathetic dystrophy of the upper extremity—A 5.5-year follow-up: Part I. Impairments and perceived disability. Acta Orthop Scand Suppl 1998; 279:12–18.
12. Subbarao J, Stillwell GK: Reflex sympathetic dystrophy syndrome of the upper extremity: Analysis of total outcome of

management of 125 cases. Arch Phys Med Rehabil 1981; 62:549–554.

13. Atkins RM, Duckworth T, Kanis JA: Features of algodystrophy after Colles' fracture. J Bone Joint Surg Br 1990; 72:105–110.

14. Bickerstaff DR, Kanis JA: Algodystrophy: An under-recognized complication of minor trauma. Br J Rheumatol 1994; 33:240–248.

15. Davis SW, Petrillo CR, Eichberg RD, et al: Shoulder-hand syndrome in a hemiplegic population: A 5-year retrospective study. Arch Phys Med Rehabil 1977; 58:353–356.

16. Van Ouwenaller C, Laplace PM, Chantraine A: Painful shoulder in hemiplegia. Arch Phys Med Rehabil 1986; 67:23–26.

17. Zyluk A: The natural history of post-traumatic reflex sympathetic dystrophy. J Hand Surg Br 1998; 23:20–23.

18. Poplawski ZJ, Wiley AM, Murray JF: Post-traumatic dystrophy of the extremities. J Bone Joint Surg Am 1983; 65:642–655.

19. Geertzen JH, Dijkstra PU, Groothoff JW, et al: Reflex sympathetic dystrophy of the upper extremity—a 5.5-year follow-up: Part II. Social life events, general health and changes in occupation. Acta Orthop Scand Suppl 1998; 279:19–23.

20. van der Laan L, Veldman PH, Goris RJ: Severe complications of reflex sympathetic dystrophy: Infection, ulcers, chronic edema, dystonia, and myoclonus. Arch Phys Med Rehabil 1998; 79:424–429.

21. van der Laan L, Goris RJ: Reflex sympathetic dystrophy. An exaggerated regional inflammatory response? Hand Clin 1997; 13:373–385.

22. Blumberg H, Janig W: Clinical manifestations of reflex sympathetic dystrophy and sympathetically maintained pain. *In* Wall P, Melzack R (eds): Textbook of Pain, 3rd ed, Edinburgh: Churchill Livingstone, 1994:685–697.

23. Livingstone W: Pain mechanisms: A Physiologic Interpretation of Causalgia and Its Related States. New York: MacMillan, 1943.

24. AbuRahma AF, Robinson PA, Powell M, et al: Sympathectomy for reflex sympathetic dystrophy: Factors affecting outcome. Ann Vasc Surg 1994; 8:372–379.

25. Jadad AR, Carroll D, Glynn CJ, et al: Intravenous regional sympathetic blockade for pain relief in reflex sympathetic dystrophy: A systematic review and a randomized, double-blind crossover study. J Pain Symptom Manage 1995; 10:13 20.

26. Blanchard J, Ramamurthy S, Walsh N, et al: Intravenous regional sympatholysis: A double-blind comparison of guanethidine, reserpine, and normal saline. J Pain Symptom Manage 1990; 5:357–361.

27. Ramamurthy S, Hoffman J: Intravenous regional guanethidine in the treatment of reflex sympathetic dystrophy/causalgia: A randomized, double-blind study. Guanethidine Study Group. Anesth Analg 1995; 81:718–723.

28. Verdugo RJ, Ochoa JL: "Sympathetically maintained pain." I. Phentolamine block questions the concept. Neurology 1994; 44:1003–1010.

29. Kurvers HA, Jacobs MJ, Beuk RJ, et al: Reflex sympathetic dystrophy: Evolution of microcirculatory disturbances in time. Pain 1995; 60:333–340.

30. Arnold JM, Teasell RW, MacLeod AP, et al: Increased venous alpha-adrenoceptor responsiveness in patients with reflex sympathetic dystrophy. Ann Intern Med 1993; 118:619–621.

31. Drummond PD, Finch PM, Edvinsson L, et al: Plasma neuropeptide Y in the symptomatic limb of patients with causalgic pain. Clin Auton Res 1994; 4:113–116.

32. Drummond PD, Finch PM, Smythe GA: Reflex sympathetic dystrophy: The significance of differing plasma catecholamine concentrations in affected and unaffected limbs. Brain 1991; 114:2025–2036.

33. Oyen WJ, Arntz IE, Claessens RM, et al: Reflex sympathetic dystrophy of the hand: An excessive inflammatory response? Pain 1993; 55:151–157.

34. Calder JS, Holten I, McAllister RM: Evidence for immune system involvement in reflex sympathetic dystrophy. J Hand Surg Br 1998; 23:147–150.

35. Christensen K, Jensen EM, Noer I: The reflex dystrophy syndrome response to treatment with systemic corticosteroids. Acta Chir Scand 1982; 148:653–655.

36. Goris RJ, Dongen LM, Winters HA: Are toxic oxygen radicals involved in the pathogenesis of reflex sympathetic dystrophy? Free Radic Res Commun 1987; 3:13–18.

37. Geertzen JH, de Bruijn H, de Bruijn-Kofman AT, et al: Reflex sympathetic dystrophy: Early treatment and psychological aspects. Arch Phys Med Rehabil 1994; 75:442–446.

38. Birklein F, Claus D, Riedl B, et al: Effects of cutaneous histamine application in patients with sympathetic reflex dystrophy. Muscle Nerve 1997; 20:1389–1395.

39. Pak TJ, Martin GM, Magness JL, et al: Reflex sympathetic dystrophy. Review of 140 cases. Minn med 1970; 53:507–512.

40. Omer G, Thomas S: Treatment of causalgia. Review of cases at Brooke General Hospital. Tex Med 1971; 67:93–96.

41. Haddox J: Psychological aspects of reflex sympathetic dystrophy. *In* Stanton-Hicks M (ed): Pain and the Sympathetic Nervous System. Boston: Kluwer Academic, 1990.

42. Convington E: Psychological issues in reflex sympathetic dystrophy. *In* Stanton-Hicks M, Janig W (eds): Reflex Sympathetic Dystrophy: A Reappraisal, vol. 6. Seattle: IASP Press, 1996;191–215.

43. Stanton-Hicks M, Prithvi Raj P, Racz G: Use of regional anesthetics for diagnosis of reflex sympathetic dystrophy and sympathetically maintained pain: A critical evaluation. *In* Janig W, Stanton-Hicks M (eds): Reflex Sympathetic Dystrophy: A Reappraisal, vol. 6. Seattle: IASP Press, 1996:217–237.

44. Frost S, Raja S, Campbell J, et al: Does hyperalgesia to cooling stimuli characterize patients with sympathetically maintained pain (reflex sympathetic dystrophy)? *In* Dubner R, Gebhart G, Bond M (eds): Proceedings of the 5th World Congress on Pain. Amsterdam: Elsevier, 1988:151–156.

45. Wahren LK, Torebjork E, Nystrom B: Quantitative sensory testing before and after regional guanethidine block in patients with neuralgia in the hand. Pain 1991; 46:23–30.

46. Chelimsky TC, Low PA, Naessens JM, et al: Value of autonomic testing in reflex sympathetic dystrophy. Mayo Clin Proc 1995; 70:1029–1040.

47. Raja SN, Treede RD, Davis KD, et al: Systemic alpha-adrenergic blockade with phentolamine; A diagnostic test for sympathetically maintained pain. Anesthesiology 1991; 74:691–698.

48. Arner S: Intravenous phentolamine test: Diagnostic and prognostic use in reflex sympathetic dystrophy. Pain 1991; 46:17–22.

49. Charlton J: Current views on the use of nerve blocking in the relief of chronic pain. *In* Swerdlow M (ed): The Therapy of Pain. Lancaster, U.K.: MTP Press, 1986:133–164.

50. Kozin F, Soin JS, Ryan LM, et al: Bone scintigraphy in the reflex sympathetic dystrophy syndrome. Radiology 1981; 138:437–443.

51. Nath RK, Mackinnon SE, Stelnicki E: Reflex sympathetic dystrophy. The controversy continues. Clin Plast Surg 1996; 23:435–446.

52. Mackinnon SE, Holder LE: The use of three-phase radionuclide bone scanning in the diagnosis of reflex sympathetic dystrophy. J Hand Surg Am 1984; 9:556–563.

53. Maurer AH, Holder LE, Espinola DA, et al: Three-phase radionuclide scintigraphy of the hand. Radiology 1983; 146:761–775.

54. Mailis A, Meindok H, Papagapiou M, et al: Alterations of the three-phase bone scan after sympathectomy. Clin J Pain 1994; 10:146–155.

55. Gibbons JJ, Wilson PR: RSD score: Criteria for the diagnosis of reflex sympathetic dystrophy and causalgia. Clin J Pain 1992; 8:260–263.

56. Rosenthal AK, Wortmann RL: Diagnosis, pathogenesis, and management of reflex sympathetic dystrophy syndrome. Compr Ther 1991; 17:46–50.

57. TB R, Alessi A: Chemical production of prolonged sympathetic paralysis. Surgery 1948; 20.

58. Steinbrocker O, Argyros T: The shoulder-hand syndrome: Present status as a diagnostic and therapeutic entity. Med Clin North Am 1958; 42:1533–1553.

59. Linson MA, Leffert R, Todd DP: The treatment of upper extremity reflex sympathetic dystrophy with prolonged continuous stellate ganglion blockade. J Hand Surg Am 1983; 8:153–159.

60. Wang JK, Johnson KA, Ilstrup DM: Sympathetic blocks for reflex sympathetic dystrophy. Pain 1985; 23:13–17.

61. Arlet J, Mazieres B: Medical treatment of reflex sympathetic dystrophy. Hand Clin 1997; 13:477–483.

62. Hannington-Kiff JG: Relief of Sudeck's atrophy by regional intravenous guanethidine. Lancet 1977; 1:1132–1133.
63. Driessen JJ, van der Werken C, Nicolai JP, et al: Clinical effects of regional intravenous guanethidine (Ismelin) in reflex sympathetic dystrophy. Acta Anaesthesiol Scand 1983; 27:505–509.
64. Glynn CJ, Basedow RW, Walsh JA: Pain relief following postganglionic sympathetic blockade with I.V. guanethidine. Br J Anaesth 1981; 53:1297–1302.
65. Rocco AG, Kaul AF, Reisman RM, et al: A comparison of regional intravenous guanethidine and reserpine in reflex sympathetic dystrophy. A controlled, randomized, double-blind crossover study. Clin J Pain 1989; 5:205–209.
66. Holland AJ, Davies KH, Wallace DH: Sympathetic blockade of isolated limbs by intravenous guanethidine. Can Anaesth Soc J 1977; 24:597–602.
67. Malik VK, Inchiosa MA Jr, Mustafa K, et al: Intravenous regional phenoxybenzamine in the treatment of reflex sympathetic dystrophy. Anesthesiology 1998; 88:823–827.
68. Dzwierzynski WW, Sanger JR: Reflex sympathetic dystrophy. Hand Clin 1994; 10:29–44.
69. Hord AH, Rooks MD, Stephens BO, et al: Intravenous regional bretylium and lidocaine for treatment of reflex sympathetic dystrophy: A randomized, double-blind study. Anesth Analg 1992; 74:818–821.
70. Hanna MH, Peat SJ: Ketanserin in reflex sympathetic dystrophy. A double-blind placebo controlled cross-over trial. Pain 1989; 38:145–150.
71. Kettler RE, Abram SE: Intravenous regional droperidol in the management of reflex sympathetic dystrophy; A double-blind, placebo-controlled, crossover study. Anesthesiology 1988; 69:933–936.
72. Eulry F, Lechevalier D, Pats B, et al: Regional intravenous guanethidine blocks in algodystrophy. Clin Rheumatol 1991; 10:337–383.
73. Chuinard RG, Dabezies EJ, Gould JS, et al: Intravenous reserpine for treatment of reflex sympathetic dystrophy. South Med J 1981; 74:1481–1484.
74. Vanos DN, Ramamurthy S, Hoffman J: Intravenous regional block using ketorolac: Preliminary results in the treatment of reflex sympathetic dystrophy. Anesth Analg 1992; 74:139–141.
75. Kaplan R, Claudio M, Kepes E, et al: Intravenous guanethidine in patients with reflex sympathetic dystrophy. Acta Anaesthesiol Scand 1996; 40:1216–1222.
76. Schott GD: Interrupting the sympathetic outflow in causalgia and reflex sympathetic dystrophy. BMJ 1998; 316:792–793.
77. Farcot JM, Mangin P, Laugner B, et al: Regional intravenous guanethidine for sympathetic block in algodystrophic syndromes [Author's translation]. Anesth Analg (Paris) 1981; 38:383–385.
78. Muramatsu K, Kawai S, Akino T, et al: Treatment of chronic regional pain syndrome using manipulation therapy and regional anesthesia. J Trauma 1998; 44:189–192.
79. Cooney WP: Somatic versus sympathetic mediated chronic limb pain. Experience and treatment options. Hand Clin 1997; 13:355–361.
80. Lin TC, Wong CS, Chen FC, et al: Long-term epidural ketamine, morphine and bupivacaine attenuate reflex sympathetic dystrophy neuralgia. Can J Anaesth 1998; 45:175–177.
81. Steinbrocker O, Neustadt D, Lapin L: Shoulder hand syndrome. JAMA 1953; 153:788–791.
82. Duncan KH, Lewis RC Jr, Racz G, et al: Treatment of upper extremity reflex sympathetic dystrophy with joint stiffness using sympatholytic Bier blocks and manipulation. Orthopedics 1988; 11:883–886.
83. Tountas AA, Noguchi A: Treatment of posttraumatic reflex sympathetic dystrophy syndrome (RSDS) with intravenous blocks of a mixture of corticosteroid and lidocaine: A retrospective review of 17 consecutive cases. J Orthop Trauma 1991; 5:412–419.
84. Schutzer SF, Gossling HR: The treatment of reflex sympathetic dystrophy syndrome. J Bone Joint Surg Am 1984; 66:625–629.
85. Kozin F, McCarty DJ, Sims J, et al: The reflex sympathetic dystrophy syndrome: I. Clinical and histologic studies: Evidence for bilaterality, response to corticosteroids and articular involvement. Am J Med 1976; 60:321–331.
86. Grundberg AB: Reflex sympathetic dystrophy: treatment with long-acting intramuscular corticosteroids. J Hand Surg Am 1996; 21:667–670.
87. Zuurmond WW, Langendijk PN, Bezemer PD, et al: Treatment of acute reflex sympathetic dystrophy with DMSO 50% in a fatty cream. Acta Anaesthesiol Scand 1996; 40:364–367.
88. Nuti R, Vattimo A, Martini G, et al: Carbocalcitonin treatment in Sudeck's atrophy. Clin Orthop 1987; 215:217–222.
89. Gobelet C, Meier JL, Schaffner W. et al: Calcitonin and reflex sympathetic dystrophy syndrome. Clin Rheumatol 1986; 5:382–338.
90. Hamamci N, Dursun E, Ural C, et al: Calcitonin treatment in reflex sympathetic dystrophy: A preliminary study. Br J Clin Pract 1996; 50:373–375.
91. Bickerstaff DR, Kanis JA: The use of nasal calcitonin in the treatment of post-traumatic algodystrophy. Br J Rheumatol 1991; 30:291–294.
92. Schott GD: Bisphosphonates for pain relief in reflex sympathetic dystrophy? Lancet 1997; 350:1117.
93. Cortet B, Flipo RM, Coquerelle P, et al: Treatment of severe, recalcitrant reflex sympathetic dystrophy: Assessment of efficacy and safety of the second generation bisphosphonate pamidronate. Clin Rheumatol 1997; 16:51–56.
94. Maillefert JF, Chatard C, Owen S, et al: Treatment of refractory reflex sympathetic dystrophy with pamidronate. Ann Rheum Dis 1995; 54:687.
95. Adami S, Fossaluzza V, Gatti D, et al: Bisphosphonate therapy of reflex sympathetic dystrophy syndrome. Ann Rheum Dis 1997; 56:201–204.
96. Chaturvedi SK: Phenytoin in reflex sympathetic dystrophy. Pain 1989; 36:379–380.
97. Gallien P, Nicolas B, Robineau S, et al: The reflex sympathetic dystrophy syndrome in patients who have had a spinal cord injury. Paraplegia 1995; 33:715–720.
98. Mellick GA, Mellicy LB, Mellick LB: Galbapentin in the management of reflex sympathetic dystrophy. J Pain Symptom Manage 1995; 10:265–266.
99. Mellick GA, Mellick LB: Reflex sympathetic dystrophy treated with gabapentin. Arch Phys Med Rehabil 1997; 78:98–105.
100. Rauck RL, Eisenach JC, Jackson K, et al: Epidural clonidine treatment for refractory reflex sympathetic dystrophy. Anesthesiology 1993; 79:1163–1169.
101. Ribbers GM, Geurts AC, Rijken RA, et al: Axillary branchial plexus blockade for the reflex sympathetic dystrophy syndrome. Int J Rehabil Res 1997; 20:371–380.
102. Klein DS, Klein PW: Low-volume ulnar nerve block within the axillary sheath for the treatment of reflex sympathetic dystrophy. Can J Anaesth 1991; 38:764–766.
103. Ghostine SY, Comair YG, Turner DM, et al: Phenoxybenzamine in the treatment of causalgia. Report of 40 cases. J Neurosurg 1984; 60:1263–1268.
104. Muizelaar JP, Kleyer M, Hertogs IA, et al: Complex regional pain syndrome (reflex sympathetic dystrophy and causalgia): Management with the calcium channel blocker nifedipine and/ or the alpha-sympathetic blocker phenoxybenzamine in 59 patients. Clin Neurol Neurosurg 1997; 99:26–30.
105. Prough DS, McLeskey CH, Poehling GG, et al: Efficacy of oral nifedipine in the treatment of reflex sympathetic dystrophy. Anesthesiology 1985; 62:796–799.
106. Visitsunthorn U, Prete P: Reflex sympathetic dystrophy of the lower extremity: A complication of herpes zoster with dramatic response to propranolol. West J Med 1981; 135:62–66.
107. May V, Aristoff H, Glowinski J, et al: Beta blocking agents in the treatment of algo-neuro-dystrophies. Apropos of 34 cases. Rev Rhum Mal Osteoartic 1977; 44:249–252.
108. Bengtson K: Physical modalities for complex regional pain syndrome. Hand Clin 1997; 13:443–454.
109. Lankford L: Reflex sympathetic dystrophy. In Green DP (ed): Operative Hand Surgery. New York: Churchill Livingstone, 1993:627–660.
110. Krasna MJ, Demmy TL, McKenna RJ, et al: Thoracoscopic sympathectomy: The U.S. experience. Eur J Surg Suppl 1998; 580:19–21.
111. Urschel HC, Jr: Dorsal sympathectomy and management of thoracic outlet syndrome with VATS. Ann Thorac Surg 1993; 56:717–720.

112. Munn JS, Baker WH: Recurrent sympathetic dystrophy: Successful treatment of contralateral sympathectomy. Surgery 1987; 102:102–105.

113. Kumar K, Nath RK, Toth C: Spinal cord stimulation is effective in the management of reflex sympathetic dystrophy. Neurosurgery 1997; 40:503–508 [discussion 40: 503–508].

114. Barolat G, Schwartzman R, Woo R: Epidural spinal cord stimulation in the management of reflex sympathetic dystrophy. Stereotact Funct Neurosurg 1989; 53:29–39.

115. Calvillo O, Racz G, Didie J, et al: Neuroaugmentation in the treatment of complex regional pain syndrome of the upper extremity. Acta Orthop Belg 1998; 64:57–63.

116. Sanchez-Ledesma MJ, Garcia-March G, Diaz-Cascajo P, et al: Spinal cord stimulation in deafferentation pain. Stereotact Funct Neurosurg 1989; 53:40–45.

117. North RB, Kidd DH, Zahurak, M, et al: Spinal cord stimulation for chronic, intractable pain: Experience over two decades. Neurosurgery 1993; 32:384–394 [discussion 32:394–395].

118. Dielissen PW, Claassen AT, Veldman PH, et al: Amputation for reflex sympathetic dystrophy. J Bone Joint Surg Br 1995; 77:270–273.

119. Lynch ME: Psychological aspects of reflex sympathetic dystrophy: A review of the adult and paediatric literature. Pain 1992; 49:337–347.

120. Bruehl S, Carlson CR: Predisposing psychological factors in the development of reflex sympathetic dystrophy. A review of the empirical evidence. Clin J Pain 1992; 8:287–299.

121. Van Houdenhove B, Vasquez G, Onghena P, et al: Etiopathogenesis of reflex sympathetic dystrophy: A review and biopsychosocial hypothesis. Clin J Pain 1992; 8:300–306.

122. Kozin F: Reflex sympathetic dystrophy syndrome: A review. Clin Exp Rheumatol 1992; 10:401–409.

123. Field J. Warwick D, Bannister GC: Features of algodystrophy ten years after Colles' fracture. J Hand Surg Br 1992; 17:318–320.

# 10 | Rheumatologic Consultations in Organ Transplant Recipients

*L. B. Klickstein*

Organ transplantation procedures are more successful than ever. Organ transplant recipients experience a unique set of musculoskeletal problems as a consequence of the underlying disease that led to transplantation, the transplantation surgery, and the perioperative period, as well as immunosuppressive therapy. Musculoskeletal complications are frequently the major issues that limit activities of daily life in long-term transplant recipients.[1] General complications of steroid therapy are well known to rheumatologists and are not discussed here. Organ transplant recipients are generally monitored closely by the physicians responsible for the transplanted organ. These physicians refer patients for rheumatologic consultation under a relatively limited set of circumstances, as outlined in Table 10–1. This chapter focuses on the unique elements of the differential diagnosis and distinct treatments relevant to organ transplant recipients.

## FRACTURE, PAIN, AND BONE MINERAL DENSITY ISSUES

Osteoporosis is a well-documented complication of organ transplantion and is the most common musculoskeletal condition encountered in this population. Contributing factors include prolonged immobility, preexisting illnesses, inadequate calcium and vitamin D intake, sex hormone deficiency, high-dose steroid use before and after transplantation, and chronic steroid use. Patients at highest risk are those who have many or all of these features.

A prospective study of cardiac transplant recipients found a new fracture incidence of 36% among the 47 patients studied despite therapy with calcium and vitamin D.[2] Conversely, an open-label, prospective randomized study of 40 cardiac transplant recipients found improved bone mineral density (BMD) in the lumbar vertebra and a corresponding decreased incidence of fractures in the group treated with calcidiol, in comparison with patients treated with calcitonin or etidronate.[3] This suggests that the form of vitamin D supplementation may be important. Osteoporosis, presumably causally related to fracture, is common in the population of cardiac transplant recipients. A prospec-

tive study of 61 patients noted a 33% decrease in absolute trabecular bone density as assessed by quantitative computed tomography.[4] When assessed by dual energy absorptiometry, using a Z score less than 2 standard deviations below age- and sex-matched normals as the definition of osteoporosis, the prevalence of osteoporosis was found to be 30% in the population of cardiac transplant recipients.[9]

Case-control studies in renal transplant recipients found a fracture prevalence of up to 45% in diabetic recipients and 11% in nondiabetic renal transplant recipients.[5] The issues of bone loss and fracture in renal transplant recipients are extraordinarily complex because most patients have preexisting bone disease from uremia and dialysis and their complications before transplantation and because there are many distinct immunosuppressive regimens in use, each with its own unique complications and toxicities. So-called renal osteodystrophy is actually the sum of the cumulative effects of several concurrent and independent insults to bone, as summarized in Table 10–2.[6]

There are fewer data for lung transplant recipients; however, the problems of osteoporosis and fracture are severe in this population.[7] Many of the patients referred for lung transplantation have had steroid-dependent chronic obstructive pulmonary disease or cystic fibrosis, both of which are associated independently with low BMD and fractures.[8] In one retrospective study of 33 patients who survived at least 1 year after lung transplantation, 42% had suffered at least one fracture.[9]

Liver transplant recipients also have a substantial frequency of osteoporosis and fracture. In a recent prospective study of 58 cirrhotic patients, 43% had osteoporosis at the lumbar spine by dual energy absorptiometry criteria *before transplantation*.[10] In this study, as in most others, the causes were multifactorial as noted earlier, with the additional issue of chronic alcoholism in a subset of patients. An independent, prospective study found a prevalence of osteoporosis of 23% among 56 patients before liver transplantation.[11] After liver transplantation, up to 38% of patients may suffer fractures.[12]

Interestingly, a retrospective study of 29 patients monitored for approximately 5 years after autologous

**TABLE 10–1**
**Rheumatologic Consultations in Organ Transplant Patients**

Fracture, pain, and bone mineral density issues
Inflammatory arthritis
Rule out vasculitis
Miscellaneous conditions, e.g., fever and elevated ESR
Management of preexisting systemic rheumatic disease

bone marrow transplantation found no apparent decrease in BMD[13] despite the fact that these patients had some of the same risk factors as did the organ transplant recipients noted earlier. However, the study did not specifically study patients who received steroids for graft-versus-host disease.

The mechanisms for bone loss in the population of transplant recipients are complex and multifactorial. In 50 male cardiac transplant recipients in a case-control study, renal impairment and steroids were the most important factors.[14] Biochemical[15] and morphometric[16] studies of bone around the time of transplantation support a state of increased bone turnover, with an overall imbalance favoring bone loss. The subject of osteoporosis after organ transplantation has been reviewed.[5, 17]

There are few studies that address the treatment of osteoporosis in the context of organ transplantation, although from one small trial in heart transplant recipients it seems clear that calcium and vitamin D alone are inadequate.[2] Calcitriol in liver transplantation was safe and may have some benefit.[18] A similar finding was described in heart transplant recipients.[3] A small pilot study compared intravenous pamidronate before transplantation followed by cyclic etidronate for 1 year after transplantation plus daily oral calcitriol, calcium, and vitamin D with historical controls who received calcium and vitamin D alone.[19] There was minimal bone loss in the first group and substantially lower bone turnover in comparison with the controls. Of importance, there were 90% fewer fractures in the treatment group than in the controls over the course of the study (3 vs 34 patients with fractures). Similar results were observed in a larger trial of liver transplant recipients.[20] Pamidronate was administered before transplantation and for 9 months afterward in patients with a lumbar BMD lower than 0.84 g/cm². These patients were compared with historical controls; no fractures were observed in the treatment group, whereas 11 of

**TABLE 10–2**
**Elements of Renal Osteodystrophy**

Hyperparathyroidism
Vitamin D deficiency, osteomalacia
Aluminum toxicity
Adynamic bone disease
Hypogonadism
Relative immobility
Medicines for renal failure (loop diuretics, immunosuppressive agents)

29 untreated patients with similar BMD suffered symptomatic vertebral fracture.[20] In a small trial of renal transplant recipients,[21] 46 patients were randomly assigned to receive oral clodronate, nasal calcitonin, or no therapy. All patients received 500 mg of calcium daily. All three groups had increased BMD after 1 year, with the largest increase in the clodronate group (4.6%); however, because of the small number of patients, there was no significant difference among groups. There are only case reports regarding the use of pamidronate in children,[22] so no conclusions or recommendations may be made. In a published prospective trial of injectable calcitonin in heart transplant recipients, no benefit was observed, in comparison with placebo, when the drug was given as 40 MRC units daily in 14-day cycles.[4]

A recent prospective study in 60 heart transplant recipients found that hypomagnesemia was associated with lower parathyroid hormone levels, less calcium excretion, and overall less bone loss.[23] It is well established that magnesium regulates calcium excretion,[24] and magnesium is required for parathyroid hormone release in humans[25] as in animals. Although the potential adverse effects on cardiac rhythm outweigh any potential benefit of therapeutic lowering of patients' total body magnesium, this study was valuable because it indicated indirectly that inhibition of osteoclast activity should be an effective strategy to prevent bone loss in this population. The potential value of calcitonin and bisphosphonates in this setting has been reviewed.[26] A potential concern with calcium supplementation among kidney transplant recipients is stone formation, which might not cause pain because of the denervated state of the organ but would cause graft failure. Clinically, this is not seen when patients receive high doses of calcium carbonate to limit phosphate absorption in the setting of graft dysfunction. Furthermore, there was not a significant difference between kidney transplant recipients and normal individuals with respect to their handling of short-term oral calcium salts under experimental circumstances.[27] In summary, the available data best support the use of intravenous pamidronate to prevent bone loss and fracture in organ transplant recipients.

On the basis of the preceding studies, therapeutic intervention *before transplantation* is recommended to prevent bone loss. An outline of this approach is provided in Table 10–3. The presence and severity of pretransplantation osteoporosis should be assessed by measurement of BMD. Patients should always receive calcium, 1000 to 1500 mg daily, and vitamin D, 400 to 800 IU daily. Hypogonadism is common in chronically ill patients. Luteinizing hormone, follicle-stimulating hormone, estradiol, or total and free testosterone should be measured when appropriate and hormone replacement therapy instituted when indicated. Once a patient is listed for transplantation, treatment with pamidronate, 60 to 90 mg intravenously, should be given every 3 months. Alendronate and risedronate are contraindicated in many patients in the immediate post-transplantation period because these individuals are often intubated and sedated and clearly unable to

## TABLE 10–3
## Suggested Strategy to Prevent Osteoporosis in Patients Around the Time of Transplantation

1. Measure bone density to provide reference for comparison later.
2. Measure serum calcium, phosphorus, magnesium, and albumin levels.
3. Measure serum gonadotropins, estradiol, or free and total testosterone. Treat hypogonadism if present.
4. Consider measurement of urinary N-telopeptides as a baseline to enable assessment of response to therapy. The N-telopeptides of type I collagen decrease with effective antiresorptive therapy.
5. Encourage physical activity to the extent possible.
6. Administer pamidronate, 60–90 mg intravenously every 3 mo while the patient is listed for transplantation.

remain upright for 30 minutes. Furthermore, surgical and critical care physicians and nurses may not be familiar with postural requirements for the safe use of oral bisphosphonates. Calcitonin, either as a nasal spray of 200 IU daily or subcutaneous injections of 100 IU three times a week, is probably not as effective as pamidronate but is an alternative. No significant interactions of alendronate, pamidronate, or calcitonin with immunosuppressive medicines have been reported or noted by the author in clinical practice. All of these agents have the potential to cause hypocalcemia.

Bone loss can occur in the post-transplantation setting from chronic, low-dose steroid use. The standard therapies discussed in Chapter 41 are appropriate. Once a fracture has occurred, the treatment of transplant recipients is no different from that for other persons. Vertebral compression fractures, as noted earlier, are probably the most common fractures in this patient population and may respond well to the analgesic effects of calcitonin in addition to more conventional strategies for pain control.

## INFLAMMATORY ARTHRITIS

The second most common musculoskeletal problem seen in organ transplant recipients is inflammatory arthritis. Gout is by far the most common inflammatory arthritis in this patient group and has been recognized from the earliest days of organ transplantation.[28] Because of the substantial immunosuppression in these patients, infectious arthritis must also be seriously considered. Systemic rheumatic diseases that lead to organ transplantation, such as lupus, are not specifically discussed here.

Randomized, controlled trials of immunosuppression in renal transplant recipients, in which cyclosporine plus prednisone was compared with azathioprine plus prednisone, convincingly demonstrated the necessary (but not sufficient) role for cyclosporine in the development of hyperuricemia and gout. In the earliest published study of 243 patients, hyperuricemia was found in 55% patients treated with cyclosporine, and gout was diagnosed in 12% of

cyclosporine-treated patients. In contrast, hyperuricemia was found in 25% of azathioprine-treated patients and of 32 of azathioprine-treated patients, none acquired gout over the average 3 years of follow-up.[29] In a second group of patients,[30] 80% of 131 cyclosporine-treated patients acquired hyperuricemia in comparison with 55% of azathioprine plus antilymphocyte globulin–treated patients. Six patients in the cyclosporine group acquired gout over the course of the study in comparison with none of the azathioprine-treated patients. In a third study of 297 renal transplant recipients, hyperuricemia was found in 84% of the cyclosporine-treated patients but in only 30% of those who received azathioprine.[31] Over the follow-up period, gout developed in 7% of the cyclosporine-treated group and none of the azathioprine-treated group. A fourth study of 60 patients found gout in 11% of 37 cyclosporine-treated patients and in none of 23 azathioprine-treated patients.[32] There is also a role for diuretics in the development of gout in renal transplant recipients, which was noted in all the studies mentioned and in others because diuretic use was more common among gout patients than in patients without gout.

The cyclosporine effect may not be reversible after 3 months of treatment. In a study that measured the fractional urate clearance in cyclosporine-treated renal transplant recipients, 24% of 55 patients acquired gout at least 2 years after transplantation. There was no change in the fractional urate clearance in the seven patients who were switched to azathioprine.[33] This may indicate an irreversible renal toxicity caused by cyclosporine. In summary, although the criteria for hyperuricemia and even for gout varied among the studies, it is unequivocally clear that cyclosporine plays a major role in the development of hyperuricemia and gout. A role for azathioprine as an inhibitor of uric acid formation, to explain the lack of symptoms, is unlikely.

Hyperuricemia and gout are even more common among heart transplant recipients, all of whom receive cyclosporine or tacrolimus (FK506). A retrospective study in Paris found hyperuricemia in 76% of 365 patients and polyarticular gout in 17.3% of patients monitored for an average of 3 years.[34] As in other studies, the prevalence of gout in men (58 of 292 patients) was higher than that in women (5 of 73 patients). A retrospective study in Pittsburgh of 196 patients reported hyperuricemia in 78% and found an 18% overall prevalence of gout within 1.5 years after transplantation.[35]

Although gout is diagnosed in up to 20% of male heart transplant recipients[35] and 15% of male renal transplant recipients, it is relatively uncommon among patients who receive liver and lung transplants. The difference between these groups of patients that likely explains this finding is underlying renal insufficiency, independent of the nephrotoxic effects of cyclosporine. Heart failure patients typically are managed medically for a prolonged period before transplantation, and during that time, renal insufficiency often develops because of chronic underperfusion and perhaps occasional acute tubular necrosis. Renal transplant recipients receive an organ that has been deprived of all blood flow for hours. In contrast, renal function in patients receiving other organs, and in bone marrow transplant recipients, is usually good before transplantation and, in fact, is often an element in the selection criteria. All liver and lung transplant recipients with gout seen by the author have had some degree of renal insufficiency and are often treated with loop diuretics.

The pace of gout in organ transplant recipients is accelerated, as noted more than 10 years ago.[33] The interval between the initial acute attacks and chronic, polyarticular tophaceous gout is sometimes shortened to less than a year. Management of gout in these patients is particularly challenging because of drug interactions between gout therapies and immunosuppressive medicines. These interactions may be fatal; hence, treatment of gout in organ transplant recipients should be undertaken by physicians knowledgeable in this area.

## DIAGNOSIS AND TREATMENT OF ACUTE GOUT IN THE ORGAN TRANSPLANT RECIPIENT

It is important to first confirm the diagnosis of gout, as in any other patient. The presence of monosodium urate crystals is the sine qua non of the diagnosis, as always. Tophi are more frequent in transplant recipients, and a careful search is warranted. Transillumination of the fingers, toes, and helices of the ear readily allows distinction between lucent tissues and the relatively more opaque tophi. Infection should be considered and joints aspirated to obtain specimens for cultures and stains in appropriate circumstances, despite an established history of gout, for example, a diabetic patient with a foot wound, an unusual joint for gout, or the presence of systemic symptoms beyond those usually seen in gout. Other causes of arthritis or joint pain should be considered in appropriate clinical circumstances. For example, other causes of podagra seen in organ transplant recipients by the author have included septic arthritis, hallux rigidus, and osteonecrosis of a metatarsophalangeal sesamoid.

Management of acute gout in transplant recipients can be performed successfully, with appropriate attention to drug interactions. There are no absolute contraindications to steroid therapy. Relative contraindications include infection, poorly controlled diabetes, uncompensated heart failure, recent myocardial infarction, some major surgery, and severe osteopenia with fractures. A starting dose of prednisone, 40 mg/day or the equivalent, should be tapered to the patient's basal steroid dose over 7 to 10 days. In patients with heart failure for whom the associated fluid retention would be potentially serious, dexamethasone is substituted (8 mg/day initially and tapered by 1 mg daily) to minimize mineralocorticoid effects. Adrenocorticotropic hormone, 40 to 80 units intramuscularly or subcutaneously, is an effective alternative if the basal steroid dose is 10 mg/day or less and may be repeated once or twice as needed.[36] An intramuscular or subcutaneous injection of a depot formulation of methylprednisolone or triamcinolone is also effective.[37] It should be emphasized that the chronic, low-dose steroid therapy used as an immunosuppressant therapy in organ transplantation does not prevent attacks of acute gout or the progression to chronic tophaceous gout.

There is a predictable interaction between nonsteroidal anti-inflammatory drugs (NSAIDs) and cyclosporine or tacrolimus. The glomerular filtration rate in cyclosporine-treated patients is maintained in part by postglomerular vasoconstriction mediated by prostaglandins. Inhibition of this effect with NSAIDs predictably increases serum creatinine levels. Nevertheless, infrequent use of a 1- to 2-day course of NSAID therapy in patients with serum creatinine levels less than or equal to 2 mg/dL is generally safe and effective. Examples include indomethacin, 25 to 50 mg orally twice daily for two to three doses only, or naproxen (Naprosyn), 375 to 500 mg orally twice daily for two to three doses only. This is particularly effective when combined with low-dose colchicine (see further on). Some nephrologists may not find this strategy acceptable under any circumstances for their renal transplant recipients.

Oral colchicine remains an effective therapy for acute gout, although it must be used differently in the transplant recipient to avoid serious toxicity.[37] Intravenous administration of colchicine is potentially hazardous and should be prescribed only by clinicians experienced with this drug, if at all. Although colchicine is effective, there is a significant interaction with cyclosporine or tacrolimus that requires a substantial downward dose adjustment of the colchicine. There are two mechanisms by which cyclosporine potentiates colchicine's effects. First, cyclosporine and tacrolimus are chemosensitizers that block the actions of the multidrug resistance (MDR) glycoprotein.[38] This transporter protein is responsible for most of the hepatic transport and clearance of colchicine.[38] The MDR glycoprotein is also involved in renal clearance of colchicine.[39] Hence, the bioavailability of colchicine is much higher in the presence of cyclosporine. Combinations of chemosensitizers, such as cyclosporine plus verapamil, might render patients extraordinarily susceptible to colchicine toxicity[40]; however this has not been specifically studied in humans. Furthermore, cyclosporine causes dose-dependent renal insufficiency independently of any specific effect on the MDR glycoprotein. Thus, cyclosporine alone causes the combination of renal and specific hepatic insufficiency in which colchicine therapy is recognized as potentially hazardous. Patients may experience profound toxicity manifested as myopathy, neuropathy, granulocytopenia, heart failure, and arrhythmias on colchicine doses as low as 0.6 mg daily. Early findings include an ascending absence of deep tendon reflexes. The serum creatine kinase (CK) level is always elevated over the patient's baseline, although it may be within the normal range.[41] The latter is an important point that bears some elaboration. Chronically ill and debilitated patients may have a baseline serum CK in the 10 to 50 U/L range.

A CK value of 100 to 200 U/L is substantially elevated for these patients but not out of the normal range for most laboratories and, hence, may be misinterpreted. An effective strategy for colchicine therapy in acute gout is to use very low-dose colchicine, 0.15 to 0.3 mg orally once daily for up to a week, in combination with the 1- to 2-day NSAID regimen described earlier. This has been effective, with minimal toxicity, in the author's experience.

Finally, consideration should be given to simple pain control in some cases. Acute gout is generally self-limited and resolves without any treatment within 1 to 3 weeks, so no therapy or narcotics alone may be acceptable to the physician concerned about drug interactions. However, no therapy is generally less acceptable for the patients. Side effects of narcotics are well recognized and are not discussed further.

## MANAGEMENT OF CHRONIC GOUT IN ORGAN TRANSPLANT RECIPIENTS

The goals of therapy are the same as always: to lower serum uric acid, prevent acute attacks, and mobilize the uric acid in tophi. *All commonly used uric acid–lowering therapies have significant drug interactions with immunosuppressive medicines.* These interactions must be considered to implement uric acid–lowering therapy safely. As in other patients, suppressive therapy is usually required to prevent gout flares in the setting of lowering uric acid. This is generally accomplished with colchicine, 0.15 to 0.3 mg daily, because chronic NSAID use is contraindicated, as described earlier.

The only absolute contraindication to allopurinol is hypersensitivity to the drug. Allopurinol is generally used for tophaceous gout, gout with a history of uric acid renal stones, gout in patients with significant renal insufficiency, and in patients with gout who are otherwise unable to take a uricosuric agent. There are two major relevant drug interactions, most importantly with azathioprine. Azathioprine is a prodrug for 6-mercaptopurine, which is metabolized in part by xanthine oxidase. Thus, the inhibition of xanthine oxidase by allopurinol potentiates the effect of azathioprine, typically two- to threefold. This is adequate to cause pancytopenia, in particular profound granulocytopenia, and all the ensuing complications. The granulocytopenia is more likely in the setting of other agents that cause dose-related bone marrow toxicity, in particular colchicine and ganciclovir. Allopurinol may be used safely by lowering the dose of azathioprine by 50% to 75% when the allopurinol is started and monitoring the complete blood count after 1 and 3 weeks. The initial dose of allopurinol should be 100 to 150 mg daily, with periodic increases until the uric acid is less than 6.5 mg/dL. The maximal allopurinol dose is 600 mg daily; however, doses greater than 300 mg daily should be used with caution in the setting of renal insufficiency. The second drug interaction is that allopurinol increases 12-hour trough cyclosporine levels by 10% to 30%, and cyclosporine dose reductions are often required on institution of allopurinol therapy.

Allopurinol should be stopped immediately if a rash appears and the patient evaluated, because the allopurinol hypersensitivity syndrome (exfoliative dermatitis, fever, and hepatitis) has a significant mortality rate. An alternative to adjusting azathioprine doses when starting allopurinol is to replace the azathioprine with mycophenolate mofetil, 1000 mg orally twice daily. Mycophenolic acid is not a purine and not a substrate for xanthine oxidase and thus does not require any dose adjustment. A description of this strategy has been published at the case report level.[42]

The two uricosuric agents available in the United States are probenecid and sulfinpyrazone. Contraindications include allergy to the drugs and renal stones. Note that probenecid is a tertiary sulfonamide. Renal transplantation is considered an absolute contraindication to uricosuric therapy by the author because stone formation is a recognized side effect. When there is a single, transplanted kidney, an obstructing stone may not be painful because of the denervated state of the organ and would cause graft failure. Only a single study, read in abstract only, has suggested the use of a potent uricosuric in this setting.[43] Sulfinpyrazone and probenecid lower 12-hour trough cyclosporine levels, and a 20% to 40% increase in the dose of cyclosporine is usually required. Aspirin antagonizes the uricosuric effect of these drugs and should not be used concurrently. Of the two agents, sulfinpyrazone is more potent and thus more effective in renal insufficiency. It also has mild antiplatelet activity, which may be helpful in some patients unable to tolerate aspirin. Accordingly, sulfinpyrazone is relatively contraindicated in patients receiving chronic warfarin or heparin therapy. A typical dosing schedule is sulfinpyrazone, 100 mg orally twice daily for 1 week and then 200 mg orally twice daily. Probenecid is used at 500 mg orally twice daily. Either drug should be given with calcium citrate, 1 to 2 tablets orally twice daily as a source of alkali to keep the urine in a slightly less acidic range to promote solubility of monosodium urate. Potassium bicarbonate may be substituted for calcium citrate if the patient is taking diuretics and requires potassium supplementation. Magnesium salts and sodium salts (e.g., Alka-Seltzer) are to be avoided in renal insufficiency. The physician should not attempt to produce alkaline urine, as this requires inducing a hypochloremic metabolic alkalosis, which may be dangerous under some circumstances.

A more potent uricosuric agent, benzbromarone, is available in Europe and Japan and may be more effective than allopurinol for the treatment of gout in patients with creatinine clearance as low as 20 mL/1.73 m$^2$.[44] A parenteral formulation of urate oxidase is available in Europe. This is an enzyme that breaks down uric acid to allantoin and carbon dioxide. In a report of three cases of tophaceous gout associated with heart transplantation, urate oxidase, 1000 units, was administered for 7 days each month. Improved hand function and smaller tophi were observed.[45] This treatment, which is not available in the United States, may be effective as an adjunct to standard uric acid–lowering therapy when the burden of tophi is large.[45, 46]

## Musculoskeletal Infections

Obviously infection must not be missed, and the principles of treatment are the same for transplant recipients as for anyone else. Fungal arthritis, particularly in liver and lung transplant recipients, should always be considered and specifically sought with appropriate cultures. Atypical mycobacteria include the rapidly growing species such as *Mycobacterium chelonei, M. abscessus,* and *M. marinum,* as well as the more familiar *M. avium-intercellulare* and others. The major risk factor is steroid use. These relatively infrequent causes of septic arthritis and bursitis are more common in the southern United States. Atypical mycobacterial infections are often indolent but may disseminate and cause serious morbidity or death, particularly in immunosuppressed patients.[47, 48] Joint fluid leukocyte counts may be less than $2000/mm^2$, as in other mycobacterial infections. Therapies for tuberculous and atypical mycobacterial infections are the same in transplant recipients as in others, with appropriate attention to drug interactions and hepatic toxicity. The newer, broad-spectrum macrolides such as clarithromycin may be effective, relatively nontoxic alternatives to the current standard of an aminoglycoside plus cephalosporin for the rapidly growing mycobacteria. Finally, it should be emphasized that functional leukocytes are required for arthritis pain. Granulocytopenia is not uncommon in the immediate post-transplantation period, often in the context of azathioprine and ganciclovir. These patients also receive high-dose glucocorticoids. Thus, in this setting, septic arthritis may occur without the usual dramatic presentation. The key to successful diagnosis and treatment is a high index of suspicion.

## Joint and Limb Pains

There are a few special considerations among organ transplant recipients. Lung and liver transplant recipients have a higher incidence of hypertrophic osteoarthropathy than do other transplant recipients. This may be a sign of chronic rejection,[49, 50] but it is relatively uncommon; in one large series it was described in only 2 of 396 patients.[49] Successful transplantation or retransplantation improves the symptoms.[49, 51–53]

Avascular necrosis or osteonecrosis is a fairly common cause of joint pains in the population of patients receiving organ and bone marrow transplants. This was recognized early in the organ transplantation era.[54] A large case-control study of bone marrow transplant recipients found that osteonecrosis developed in 88 of 1939 patients.[55] Steroids used for graft-versus-host disease were a highly significant risk factor, whereas cyclosporine use was not.[55] Diagnosis and treatment are no different than those for other patients; however, there may be more complications from surgery. In a retrospective study of joint replacement among transplant recipients, the risk of infection was high.[56] Of 27 joint replacements among 16 patients, 5 joints devel-

oped late infection between 1 and 6 years postoperatively. One author has suggested that osteonecrosis in the transplant population may not require surgery as often as is currently recommended.[57]

It is important to recognize the so-called acute bone pain syndrome in recipients of recently transplanted renal allografts and distinguish this from osteonecrosis. The former is a usually self-limited illness and may be associated with non–weight-bearing pain, unlike osteonecrosis.[57] Serial magnetic resonance imaging studies have been suggested as a way to make the distinction radiologically.[58]

A unique arthropathy among patients who are or have been receiving chronic dialysis is $\beta_2$-microglobulin–associated amyloidosis. Symptoms most commonly include carpal tunnel syndrome, and they may improve in the setting of a functioning renal allograft[59] or they may not.[60] Consequently, temporizing measures should be considered and surgery avoided, at least in the short term. Conversely, biopsy is often required for diagnosis of this condition.

## Vasculitis and Pseudovasculitic Syndromes

Transplant recipients in whom vasculitis is suspected should be referred for emergent rheumatologic consultation. The most common cause of vasculitis in this patient population is the underlying illness that led to organ transplantation in the first place. Some examples include systemic lupus in the case of renal transplant recipients, recurrent hepatitis C with associated cryoglobulinemia in liver transplant recipients, and sarcoid in heart transplant recipients. Diagnosis and treatment of vasculitis are considered in Chapter 27 and are not addressed further here. This section focuses on the various pseudovasculitic syndromes that may be more common in the population of organ transplant recipients.

Infection should be considered whenever vasculitis is suspected. Fever, purpuric rash, and arthritis are common symptoms of bacterial endocarditis (SBE). Immunosuppressed patients with symptoms compatible with a systemic vasculitis should always have multiple blood cultures performed to address the possibility of

**TABLE 10–4**

**Adverse Drug Interactions with Immunosuppressants: Gout Drug Effects on Steady-State Cyclosporine Levels**

| DRUG | CHANGE IN CYCLOSPORINE 12-HOUR TROUGH LEVEL | CHANGE (% OF BASELINE) |
|---|---|---|
| Allopurinol | ⇑ | 10%–30% |
| Sulfinpyrazone | ⇓ | 20%–40% |
| Probenecid | ⇓ | 20%–30% |
| Glucocorticoids | ⇑ | 10%–30% |
| Colchicine | No effect | |

**TABLE 10–5**

**Adverse Drug Interactions with Immunosuppressants: Other Important Interactions of Gout Drugs**

| DRUG COMBINATION | | ADVERSE EFFECT | SOLUTION |
|---|---|---|---|
| Allopurinol + azathioprine | ⇒ | Pancytopenia | Lower azathioprine dose by 50%–75% or Δ to mycophenolate |
| NSAIDs + cyclosporine (or FK506) | ⇒ | Renal toxicity | Avoid NSAIDs or use low dose for short period, such as three doses only |
| Colchicine + cyclosporine (or FK506) | ⇒ | Myoneuropathy | Lower colchicine dose to 0.15– 0.3 mg PO daily |

NSAIDs = nonsteroidal anti-inflammatory drugs.

SBE. A favorable response to high-dose steroids or cytotoxic agents, or both, does not rule out SBE.[61, 62] Pulmonary nodules, renal insufficiency, and nasal septum destruction may be manifestations of invasive infection such as mucormycosis.[63–65] Acute cytomegalovirus infection may be associated with a thrombotic microangiopathy and purpuric lesions in human immunodeficiency virus–infected patients, and this is now recognized in organ transplant recipients as well.[66]

Among the population of patients who receive renal transplants and dialysis, livedo and gangrenous cutaneous ulcers may be manifestations of calciphylaxis, a syndrome characterized by extensive vascular calcifications that cause peripheral ischemia. Calciphylaxis has a mortality rate that approaches 50% and may sometimes be treated by parathyroidectomy.[67, 68] Adult-onset primary hyperoxaluria should be considered in patients with renal failure who have symptoms suggestive of calciphylaxis.[69] This may be treated successfully with liver transplantation.

Some herpesvirus infections in immunocompromised transplant recipients may be mistaken for systemic vasculitis. Kaposi's sarcoma is highly correlated with human herpes virus-8 (HHV-8) infection and is established as a complication of solid organ transplantation.[70–72] The purple, firm, and nontender lesions of Kaposi's sarcoma should be recognized as distinct from palpable purpura. (See the following section for a discussion of HHV-6 in the transplant population.)

Schamberg's disease, or progressive pigmented purpura, is a relatively benign capillaritis that may be associated with the onset of pedal edema. It is often bilateral and is seen in children as well as adults.[73] In white persons, the lesions are most commonly café-au-lait–colored macules containing 0.1- to 0.5-mm purpuric spots; however, there are several subtypes. Treatment, if necessary, includes topical steroids and pentoxifylline.[74]

## ELEVATED ERYTHROCYTE SEDIMENTATION RATE

An elevated erythrocyte sedimentation rate (ESR) is a common issue for rheumatologists because a very elevated ESR often prompts referral of patients. The usual algorithm[75] remains appropriate, with additional considerations of unusual problems that are relatively more common among organ transplant recipients. Lymphoma is much more common in immunosuppressed transplant recipients than in the general population. B-cell lymphomas are related to Epstein-Barr virus and cyclosporine administration. Primary effusion lymphomas or body cavity lymphomas are related to HHV8 and present with constitutional symptoms, high ESR, and pleural effusion or ascites.[76] Pancytopenia, rash, and interstitial pneumonitis with a high ESR are the clinical features of acute HHV-6 infection.[77] This increasingly recognized pathogen is susceptible to ganciclovir and foscarnet; thus, routine cytomegalovirus prophylaxis in the immediate post-transplantation period should be effective for HHV-6, too.

Transplant recipients receive many drugs, and adverse drug reactions may present initially with an elevated ESR. A drug-related interstitial nephritis may cause an elevated ESR. The chronic steroid therapy used in these patients may not prevent the problem but may lower urinary eosinophils and make the diagnosis more difficult to recognize. In cardiac patients, amiodarone pulmonary toxicity characteristically causes a very elevated ESR, often greater than 100 mm/hour.[78] These conditions generally respond to withdrawal of the offending agent.

In summary, musculoskeletal problems are prevalent among organ transplant recipients. The most common issues, osteoporosis and gout, often can be prevented. Established osteoporosis and gout can be treated successfully, with care to avoid the pitfalls noted in Tables 10–4 and 10–5. Careful attention to the relevant differential diagnosis and potential drug interactions enables successful treatment of other problems as they arise.

## REFERENCES

1. Braun WE, Richmond BJ, Protiva DA, et al: The incidence and management of osteoporosis, gout, and avascular necrosis in recipients of renal allografts functioning more than 20 years (level 5A) treated with prednisone and azathioprine. Transplant Proc 1999; 31:1366.
2. Shane E, Rivas M, Staron RB, et al: Fracture after cardiac transplantation: A prospective longitudinal study. J Clin Endocrinol Metab 1996; 81:1740.

3. Garcia-Delgado I, Prieto S, Gil-Fraguas L, et al: Calcitonin, etidronate, and calcidiol treatment in bone loss after cardiac transplantation. Calcif Tissue Int 1997; 60:155.

4. Cremer J, Struber M, Wagenbreth I, et al: Progression of steroid-associated osteoporosis after heart transplantation. Ann Thorac Surg 1999; 67:130.

5. Nisbeth U, Lindh E, Ljunghall S, et al: Fracture frequency after kidney transplantation. Transplant Proc 1994; 58:912.

6. Dissanayake IR, Epstein S: The fate of bone after renal transplantation. Curr Opin Nephrol Hypertens 1998; 7:389.

7. Maurer JR, Tewari S: Nonpulmonary medical complications in the intermediate and long-term survivor. Clin Chest Med 1997; 18:367.

8. Ott SM, Aitken ML: Osteoporosis in patients with cystic fibrosis. Clin Chest Med 1998; 19:555.

9. Aringer M, Kiener HP, Koeller MD, et al: High turnover bone disease following lung transplantation. Bone 1998; 23:485.

10. Monegal A, Navasa M, Guanabens N, et al: Osteoporosis and bone mineral metabolism disorders in cirrhotic patients referred for orthotopic liver transplantation. Calcif Tissue Int 1997; 60:148.

11. Hussaini SH, Oldroyd B, Stewart SP, et al: Regional bone mineral density after orthotopic liver transplantation. Eur J Gastroenterol Hepatol 1999; 11:157.

12. Carson KL, Hunt CM: Medical problems occurring after orthotopic liver transplantation. Dig Dis Sci 1997; 42:1666.

13. Keilholz U, Max R, Scheibenbogen C, et al: Endocrine function and bone metabolism 5 years after autologous bone marrow/blood-derived progenitor cell transplantation. Cancer 1997; 79:1617.

14. Guo CY, Johnson A, Locke TJ, et al: Mechanisms of bone loss after cardiac transplantation. Bone 1998; 22:267.

15. Shane E, Rivas M, McMahon DJ, et al: Bone loss and turnover after cardiac transplantation. J Clin Endocrinol Metab 1997; 82:1497.

16. Vedi S, Greer S, Skingle SJ, et al: Mechanism of bone loss after liver transplantation: A histomorphometric analysis. J Bone Miner Res 1999; 14:281.

17. Rodino MA, Shane E: Osteoporosis after organ transplantation. Am J Med 1998; 104:459.

18. Neuhaus R, Kubo A, Lohmann R, et al: Calcitriol in prevention and therapy of osteoporosis after liver transplantation. Transplant Proc 1999; 31:472.

19. Shane E, Rodino MA, McMahon DJ, et al: Prevention of bone loss after heart transplantation with antiresorptive therapy: A pilot study. J Heart Lung Transplant 1998; 17:1089.

20. Reeves HL, Francis RM, Manas DM, et al: Intravenous bisphosphonate prevents symptomatic osteoporotic vertebral collapse in patients after liver transplantation. Liver Transplant Surg 1998; 4:404.

21. Grotz WH, Rump LC, Niessen A, et al: Treatment of osteopenia and osteoporosis after kidney transplantation. Transplantation 1998; 66:1004.

22. Sellers E, Sharma A, Rodd C: The use of pamidronate in three children with renal disease. Pediatr Nephrol 1998; 12:778.

23. Boncimino K, McMahon DJ, Addesso V, et al: Magnesium deficiency and bone loss after cardiac transplantation. J Bone Miner Res 1999; 14:295.

24. Sullivan JM, Dluhy RG, Wacker WE, et al: Interrelationships among thiazide diuretics and calcium, magnesium, sodium and potassium balance in normal and hypertensive man. J Clin Pharmacol 1978; 18:530.

25. Fatemi S, Ryzen E, Flores J, et al: Effect of experimental human magnesium depletion on parathyroid hormone secretion and 1,25-dihydroxyvitamin D metabolism. J Clin Endocrinol Metab 1991; 73:1067.

26. Moe SM: The treatment of steroid-induced bone loss in transplantation. Curr Opin Nephrol Hypertens 1997; 6:544.

27. Dumoulin G, Hory B, Nguyen NU, et al: Lack of increased urinary calcium-oxalate supersaturation in long-term kidney transplant recipients. Kidney Int 1997; 51:804.

28. Nelson CL, Evarts CM, Popowniak K: Musculoskeletal complications of renal transplantation. Surg Clin North Am 1971; 51:1205.

29. West C, Carpenter BJ, Hakala TR: The incidence of gout in renal transplant recipients. Am J Kidney Dis 1987; 10:369.

30. Gores PF, Fryd DS, Sutherland DE, et al: Hyperuricemia after renal transplantation. Am J Surg 1988; 156:397.

31. Lin HY, Rocher LL, McQuillan MA, et al: Cyclosporine-induced hyperuricemia and gout. N Engl J Med 1989; 321:287.

32. Tiller DJ, Hall BM, Horvarth JS, et al: Gout and hyperuricaemia in patients on cyclosporin and diuretics [Letter]. Lancet 1985; 1:453.

33. Noordzij TC, Leunissen KM, Van Hooff JP: Renal handling of urate and the incidence of gouty arthritis during cyclosporine and diuretic use. Transplantation 1991; 52:64.

34. Rozenberg S, Frih L, Lang T, et al: Manifestations rhumatologiques chez les transplantes cardiaques. Etude transversale de 365 patients. (Rheumatologic manifestations in heart transplant recipients. A cross-sectional study of 365 patients.) Rev Rhum Ed Fr 1993; 60:10.

35. Burack DA, Griffith BP, Thompson ME: Hyperuricemia and gout among heart transplant recipients receiving cyclosporine. Am J Med 1992; 92:141.

36. Axelrod D, Preston S: Comparison of parenteral adrenocorticotropic hormone with oral indomethacin in the treatment of acute gout. Arthritis Rheum 1988; 31:803.

37. Alloway JA, Moriarty MJ, Hoogland YT, et al: Comparison of triamcinolone acetonide with indomethacin in the treatment of acute gouty arthritis. J Rheumatol 1993; 20:111.

38. Kuncl RW, Duncan G, Watson D, et al: Colchicine myopathy and neuropathy. N Engl J Med 1987; 316:1562.

39. Speeg KV, Maldonado AL, Liaci J, et al: Effect of cyclosporine on colchicine secretion by a liver canalicular transporter studied in vivo. Hepatology 1992; 15:899.

40. DiDiodato G, Sharom FJ: Interaction of combinations of drugs, chemosensitizers and peptides with the P-glycoprotein multidrug transporter. Biochem Pharmacol 1997; 53:1789.

41. Cook M, Ramos E, Peterson J, et al: Colchicine neuromyopathy in a renal transplant patient with normal muscle enzyme levels. Clin Nephrol 1994; 42:67.

42. Jacobs F, Mamzer-Bruneel MF, Skhiri H, et al: Safety of the mycophenolate mofetil–allopurinol combination in kidney transplant recipients with gout [Letter]. Transplantation 1997; 64:1087.

43. Imanishi M, Ikegami M, Ishii T, et al: Clinical studies on hyperuricema and gout after transplantation [In Japanese with English abstract only]. Hinyokika Kiyo 1990; 36:893.

44. Perez-Ruiz F, Calabozo M, Fernandez-Lopez MJ, et al: Treatment of chronic gout in patients with renal function impairment. An open, randomized, actively controlled study. J Clin Rheumatol 1999; 4:49.

45. Rozenberg S, Roche B, Dorent R, et al: Urate-oxidase for the treatment of tophaceous gout in heart transplant recipients. A report of three cases. Rev Rhum Engl Ed 1995; 62:392.

46. Ippoliti G, Negri M, Campana C, et al: Urate oxidase in hyperuricemic heart transplant recipients treated with azathioprine. Transplantation 1997; 63:1661.

47. Sanger JR, Stampfl DA, Franson TR: Recurrent granulomatous synovitis due to *Mycobacterium kansasii* in a renal transplant recipient. J Hand Surg 1987; 12:436.

48. Zappe CH, Barlow D, Zappe H, et al: 16S rRNa sequence analysis of an isolate of *Mycobacterium haemophilum* from a heart transplant patient. J Med Microbiol 1995; 43:189.

49. Taillandier J, Alemanni M, Samuel D: Complications osteoarticulaires apres transplantation hepatique. (Bone and joint complications after liver transplantation.) Rev Rhum Mal Osteoartic 1991; 58:361.

50. Wolfe SM, Aelion JA, Gupta RC: Hypertrophic osteoarthropathy associated with a rejected liver transplant. J Rheumatol 1987; 14:147.

51. Vickers C, Herbert A, Neuberger J, et al: Improvement in hypertrophic hepatic osteoarthropathy after liver transplantation [Letter]. Lancet 1988; 2:968.

52. Pitt P, Mowat A, Williams R, et al: Hepatic hypertrophic osteoarthropathy and liver transplantation. Ann Rheum Dis 1994; 53:338.

53. Huaux JP, Geubel A, Maldague B, et al: Hypertrophic osteoarthropathy related to end stage cholestatic cirrhosis: Reversal after liver transplantation. Ann Rheum Dis 1987; 46:342.

54. Cruess RL, Blennerhassett J, MacDonald FR, et al: Aseptic necrosis following renal transplantation. J Bone Joint Surg 1968; 50:1577.

55. Fink FC, Leisenring WM, Sullivan KM, et al: Avascular necrosis following bone marrow transplantation: A case-control study. Bone 1998; 22:67.

56. Tannenbaum DA, Matthews LS, Grady-Benson JC: Infection around joint replacements in patients who have a renal or liver transplantation. J Bone Joint Surg 1997; 79:36.

57. Ferrari R: Rheumatologic manifestations of renal disease. Curr Opin Rheumatol 1996; 8:71.

58. Pilmore H, Walker R, McMillan B, et al: Acute bone pain following renal transplantation: Differentiation between benign bone edema and avascular necrosis. Am J Nephrol 1998; 18:57.

59. Tan SY, Irish A, Winearls CG, et al: Long term effect of renal transplantation on dialysis-related amyloid deposits and symptomatology. Kidney Int 1996; 50:282.

60. Julian BA, Quarles LD, Niemann KM: Musculoskeletal complications after renal transplantation: Pathogenesis and treatment. Am J Kidney Dis 1992; 19:99.

61. Lawrence EC, Mills J: Bacterial endocarditis mimicking vasculitis with steroid-induced remission. West J Med 1976; 124:333.

62. Agarwal A, Clements J, Sedmak DD, et al: Subacute bacterial endocarditis masquerading as type III essential mixed microglobulinemia. J Am Soc Nephrol 1997; 8:1971.

63. Martinez EJ, Cancio MR, Sinnott JT, et al: Nonfatal gastric mucormycosis in a renal transplant recipient. South Med J 1997; 90:341.

64. Hammer GS, Bottone EJ, Hirschman SZ: Mucormycosis in a transplant recipient. Am J Clin Pathol 1975; 64:389.

65. Sobol SM, Rakita L: Pneumonitis and pulmonary fibrosis associated with amiodarone treatment: A possible complication of a new antiarrhythmic drug. Circulation 1982; 65:819.

66. Jeejeebhoy FM, Zalzman JS: Thrombotic microangiopathy in association with cytomegalovirus infection in a renal transplant patient: A new treatment strategy. Transplantation 1998; 65:1645.

67. Wenzel-Seifert K, Harwig S, Keller F: Fulminant calcinosis in two patients after kidney transplantation. Am J Nephrol 1991; 11:497.

68. Kafif RA, DeLima C, Silverberg A, et al: Calciphylaxis and systemic calcinosis. Collective review. Arch Intern Med 1990; 150:956.

69. Somach SC, Davis BR, Paras FA, et al: Fatal cutaneous necrosis mimicking calciphylaxis in a patient with type 1 primary hyperoxaluria. Arch Dermatol 1995; 131:821.

70. Alkan S, Karcher DS, Ortiz A, et al: Human herpesvirus-8/Kaposi's sarcoma–associated herpesvirus in organ transplant patients with immunosuppression. Br J Haematol 1997; 96:412.

71. Mendez JC, Procop GW, Espy MJ, et al: Relationship of HHV8 replication and Kaposi's sarcoma after solid organ transplantation. Transplantation 1999; 67:1200.

72. Cathomas G, Tamm M, McGandy CE, et al: Transplantation-associated malignancies: Restriction of human herpes virus 8 to Kaposi's sarcoma. Transplantation 1997; 64:175.

73. Stell JS, Moyer DG: Schamberg's disease. Arch Dermatol 1966; 94:626.

74. Kano Y, Hirayama K, Orihara M, et al: Successful treatment of Schamberg's disease with pentoxifylline. J Am Acad Dermatol 1997; 36:827.

75. Sox HC, Liang MH: The erythrocyte sedimentation rate. Guidelines for rational use. Ann Intern Med 1986; 104:515.

76. Said W, Chien K, Takeuchi S, et al: Kaposi's sarcoma–associated herpesvirus (KSHV or HHV8) in primary effusion lymphoma: Ultrastructural demonstration of herpesvirus in lymphoma cells. Blood 1996; 87:4937.

77. Singh N, Carrigan DR: Human herpesvirus-6 in transplantation: An emerging pathogen. Ann Intern Med 1996; 124:1065.

78. Pollak PT, Sami M: Acute necrotizing pneumonitis and hyperglycemia after amiodarone therapy. Case report and review of amiodarone-associated pulmonary disease. Am J Med 1984; 76:935.

# CHAPTER
# 11 | Fibromyalgia Syndrome

*Robert W. Simms*

Fibromyalgia syndrome is an increasingly recognized chronic musculoskeletal pain disorder of unknown etiology.[1] The American College of Rheumatology (ACR) published the results of a large multicenter study to identify diagnostic criteria for the syndrome, which were shown to have high sensitivity and specificity.[2] A community-based prevalence study conducted in 1993 estimated that approximately 2% of the adult population meets the ACR criteria for the syndrome.[3] This may indicate that fibromyalgia syndrome is twice as common as rheumatoid arthritis. Fibromyalgia syndrome is predominantly a disorder of young and middle-aged women and is the second or third most common diagnosis in rheumatology practices.[1, 4] The clinical presentation of fibromyalgia syndrome is generally that of chronic, diffuse musculoskeletal pain, typically accompanied by fatigue and sleep disturbance, with findings of multiple locations of tenderness, predominantly over muscle insertion sites.[1]

Investigators have studied a variety of pathophysiologic mechanisms, including sleep disturbance, psychological dysfunction, and muscle abnormalities, although no clear understanding of etiology has yet emerged.[1] Much attention has focused on central mechanisms and especially on neurohormonal function. Griep and colleagues[5] have demonstrated that patients with fibromyalgia have enhanced pituitary adrenocorticotropic hormone (ACTH) release in response to ovine corticotropin-releasing hormone (CRH) and to insulin-induced hypoglycemia, although adrenocortical secretion after these neuroendocrine challenge tests did not differ from that in control subjects. The authors suggested that these findings indicated adrenocortical insufficiency in patients with fibromyalgia. Crofford and colleagues[6] also found evidence of low basal hypothalamic-pituitary-adrenal (HPA) function as measured by 24-hour urinary free cortisol levels—findings that are similar to those found in patients with chronic fatigue syndrome.[7] Thus, although patients with both fibromyalgia and chronic fatigue syndrome appear to have significantly lower basal measures of adrenal cortisol output, precise localization of the defect in the HPA axis remains uncertain. Furthermore, it is uncertain whether the observed findings with respect to the HPA axis are primary to fibromyalgia syndrome or are a function of having the disorder.

Although early studies of muscles were thought to demonstrate abnormalities, the weight of evidence suggests that these findings were largely the result of muscle deconditioning[8]. Careful studies of muscle metabolism by means of magnetic resonance spectroscopy have failed to find abnormalities.[9]

Other studies of neurohormonal function include the observation by Bennett and colleagues[10] of low serum levels of the growth hormone analog somatomedin C in fibromyalgia patients in comparison to controls. Bennett and colleagues[10] suggested that reduced growth hormone secretion during disturbed stage IV sleep could explain the muscle pain that characterizes the disorder because growth hormone is involved in muscle homeostasis. Russell and associates[11] found low cerebrospinal fluid levels of biogenic amines in patients with fibromyalgia as compared with controls—a finding that appeared consistent with earlier studies suggesting a deficiency of serotonin metabolism.[1]

Although there are no long-term, population-based prospective studies of natural history, the few available clinic-based studies indicate that the majority of patients have persistent symptoms for many years.[12]

Many studies (both clinic and population-based) have found high rates of major depression in association with fibromyalgia syndrome.[12] Although the nature of this association remains controversial, the frequent coexistence of concomitant migraine headaches, irritable bowel syndrome, chronic fatigue, major depression, and panic disorder suggests that these conditions may share a common physiologic abnormality, what Hudson and Pope termed *affective spectrum disorders*.[13]

Because of the lack of understanding of the basis for fibromyalgia, therapy remains empirical. Available treatments range from conventional medication therapy with tricyclic antidepressants to nonconventional interventions such as biofeedback and electroacupuncture. A substantial number of placebo-controlled trials have demonstrated that many available therapies are effective (Table 11–1). There are, however, few long-term trials, few trials of comparative therapies, and few trials that have assessed the same outcomes and employed the same definitions of response to therapy.[14] In this chapter, we review published controlled and uncontrolled trials of therapy in fibromyalgia syn-

**TABLE 11–1**
**Placebo-Controlled Therapeutic Trials of Medication in Fibromyalgia Syndrome**

| MEDICATION | REFERENCE | TRIAL DURATION (WK) | DOSE (MG/DAY) | BETTER THAN PLACEBO? |
|---|---|---|---|---|
| Amitriptyline | Carrette et al[22] | 9 | 50 | Yes |
| Amitriptyline | Goldenberg et al[23] | 6 | 25 | Yes |
| Amitriptyline | Jaeschke et al[24] | 2 | 10 | Yes |
| Amitriptyline | Carrette et al[28] | 24 | 30 | No |
| Cyclobenzaprine | Bennett et al[26] | 12 | 30 | Yes |
| Cyclobenzaprine | Reynolds et al[27] | 4 | 30 | Yes |
| Cyclobenzaprine | Simms et al[14] | 6 | 30 | Yes |
| Alprazolam | Russell et al[31] | 6 | 0.5–3 | No |
| Temazepam | Hench et al[32] | 12 | 15–30 | Yes |
| Prednisone | Clark et al[33] | 2 | 15 | No |
| Naproxen | Goldenberg et al[23] | 6 | 1000 | No |
| Ibuprofen | Yunus et al[34] | 3 | 2400 | No |
| S-Adenosylmethionine | Tavoni et al[36] | 3 | 200 | Yes |
| Carisoprodol | Vaeroy et al[35] | 8 | 1200 | Yes |
| Fluoxetine | Wolfe et al[29] | 6 | 20 | No |

drome and attempt to identify avenues of future research.

## CONTROLLED TRIALS OF MEDICATION THERAPY

### Psychotropic Agents

Moldofsky and colleagues[15] first identified a sleep electroencephalographic abnormality termed *alpha-delta sleep* in patients with fibromyalgia syndrome. This abnormality consisted of intrusion of the normal awake electroencephalographic pattern (alpha waves) into the deepest non–rapid eye movement (REM) sleep electroencephalographic pattern (delta waves). Moldofsky and Scarisbrick[16] were further able to show that experimentally reproducing alpha-delta sleep in normal subjects resulted in the appearance of musculoskeletal and mood symptoms identical to those of fibromyalgia syndrome. Moldofsky and Scarisbrick[16] hypothesized that fibromyalgia symptoms were the result of this disordered delta sleep and that serotonin, a neurochemical involved in modulation of both sleep and pain, may be deficient in patients with the syndrome. Moldofsky and Lue[17] then performed a clinical trial involving 15 patients with fibromyalgia syndrome who were randomized to receive 5 g of L-tryptophan or 100 mg of chlorpromazine in a 3-week, double-blinded study, with sleep electroencephalograms performed before and after medication. L-tryptophan had no effect on the alpha/delta sleep abnormality or on the patients' symptoms. Chlorpromazine resulted in an increase in delta sleep and an improvement in patient pain rating and tender point scores, although chlorpromazine has since been judged to be too sedating.

### Tricyclic Agents and Other Antidepressants

As inhibitors of serotonin reuptake, tricyclic antidepressants were of interest on the basis of Moldofsky and Scarisbrick's serotonin deficiency hypothesis.[16] At low doses, several tricyclic agents also have hypnotic properties, causing REM suppression and prolongation of stage III and stage IV non-REM sleep.[18] Tertiary amine tricyclics, such as amitriptyline, imipramine, and doxepin, inhibit neuronal uptake of serotonin more than do the secondary amine demethylated metabolites, such as desipramine and nortriptyline.[18] Initial uncontrolled reports suggested that amitriptyline was useful in the management of fibromyalgia syndrome.[19–21]

Carrette and colleagues[22] performed a 9-week double-blind, placebo-controlled trial in 70 patients. Patients were recruited from three centers and met the criteria proposed by Smythe.[20] Patients assigned to the treatment arm received amitriptyline, 10 mg nightly for the first week, 25 mg for the second to fourth weeks, and 50 mg for the final 5 weeks of the trial. Evaluations of efficacy at baseline and at weeks 5 and 9 included duration of morning stiffness, overall pain, sleep quality, and overall disease assessment. Patients who received amitriptyline had significant improvement in their morning stiffness and pain analog scores at 5 and 9 weeks compared with baseline scores, although the placebo group had no changes in these measures. Forty-four percent of the amitriptyline-treated patients had ≥50% improvement in morning stiffness or pain analog, whereas 22% of the placebo patients had ≥50% improvement in these two parameters ($P = NS$). No change was seen in the end-of-trial myalgic scores (defined as the sum of individual tender point scores with a dolorimeter).

Goldenberg and associates[23] randomly assigned 62 patients to receive one of four regimens in a 6-week double-blind trial: (1) 25 mg of amitriptyline at bedtime and 500 mg of naproxen twice daily, (2) amitriptyline alone with naproxen placebo, (3) naproxen alone with amitriptyline placebo, or (4) double placebo. Amitriptyline was used at doses that were believed to be low enough to have no significant effect on depression. At study entry, patients were required to have a score of at least 4 on either the initial pain or global assessment analog scale. Amitriptyline-containing regimens resulted in significant improvements in mean scores of pain, sleep, patient global assessment, and tender point score. There was no association with initial sleep difficulty or preexisting psychopathology in response to amitriptyline. Marginal additional benefit of naproxen was seen. Not determined, however, was the proportion of patients who experienced substantial improvement in one or more outcomes, because of the relatively small numbers of patients in each arm of the study. Dry mouth was the principal adverse side effect attributable to amitriptyline but did not cause discontinuation in any patient. Although the principal therapeutic effect of amitriptyline was thought to be improvement of sleep physiology, there was no association with initial sleep difficulty and response, suggesting a different mechanism of action, possibly via effects on serotonin or endogenous opioids such as endorphins or enkephalins.

Jaeschke and associates[24] conducted 23 N-of-1 randomized, controlled trials of amitriptyline in patients who had shown initial improvement with an open trial of amitriptyline. The N-of-1 design consists of pairs of active-placebo, high or low dose, and first drug-additive combination, with the order of administration determined by random allocation. Assessments are performed in a double-blind fashion, with trial duration determined by both physician and patient. Most of the treatment periods were 2 weeks in duration, with outcome assessment every 2 weeks. The mean difference in multiple symptoms favored amitriptyline over placebo in 18 versus 5 trials. Jaeschke and colleagues[24] noted rapid improvement with amitriptyline, generally occurring within 1 week—a phenomenon also noted by Goldenberg and colleagues.[23] Jaeschke and associates concluded that it is not necessary to give the standard dose of 25 to 50 mg to obtain significant improvement. Smaller doses, such as 10 mg at bedtime, may be effective in some patients, and they avoid the anticholinergic side effects of amitriptyline. Of 23 N-of-1 randomized, controlled trials, 15 resulted in a decision to continue the drug on a long-term basis. The authors of this study concluded that, overall, 25% of patients with fibromyalgia syndrome derived clinically significant benefit from amitriptyline. In eight cases, the N-of-1 randomized, controlled trial was followed by a decision to stop the drug; therefore, these patients were spared long-term or even lifelong therapy, even though the initial open trial suggested improvement with amitriptyline. These data indicate the importance of the N-of-1 randomized, controlled trial format in decisions about long-term continuation of therapy in individual patients.

Of the parallel randomized, controlled trials and the N-of-1 trials published thus far, only a small proportion of patients with fibromyalgia actually appear to achieve clinically significant improvement: on the order of 25% to 30%. Uniformity in defining those patients who undergo significant clinical improvement would provide investigators conducting clinical trials

in fibromyalgia the tools to identify subsets of patients who improve substantially and, eventually, predictors of response to therapy. Along these lines, Simms and colleagues[14] developed a set of preliminary response criteria for use in fibromyalgia clinical trials; they used data from the original trial of Goldenberg and colleagues[23] and determined which combination of outcome measures best distinguished patients treated with amitriptyline from those treated with placebo, using a stepwise logistic regression analysis and receiver-operating characteristic (ROC) curves. An ROC curve is a graphic depiction of the pairing of true-positive and false-positive rates that correspond to each possible cutoff for either diagnostic tests or criteria. The optimal ROC curve comparing different diagnostic tests or response criteria is that which maximizes the area under the curve. The combination of outcome measures with the greatest area under the ROC curve (i.e., that with the highest specificity and sensitivity in distinguishing treated patients from those receiving placebo) consisted of the following: (1) physician global assessment score of 4 (0 = extremely well, 10 = extremely poorly); (2) patient sleep score of 6 (0 = sleeping extremely well, 10 = sleeping extremely poorly); and (3) tender point score of 14 (maximal possible tender point score = 20). Using these criteria, Simms and colleagues[14] analyzed a randomized, double-blind, crossover trial of cyclobenzaprine versus placebo in 24 patients conducted by the same investigators with identical entry criteria and outcome assessment. Sensitivity was defined as the number of patients identified by the criteria as responders divided by the number of patients who received cyclobenzaprine. Specificity was defined as the number of patients not identified by criteria divided by the number who received placebo. The criteria identified 7 of 24 treated patients (sensitivity of 30%), whereas 23 of 24 untreated patients were not identified by the criteria, (specificity of 96%). In the amitriptyline trial, 44% of the amitriptyline-treated patients were identified as responders. To determine the criterion validity of the response criteria, the investigators compared the performance of the criteria in the cyclobenzaprine trial with a composite outcome measure that consisted of a summation of change in visual analog scores of patient global assessment, patient pain assessment, physician global assessment, and tender point score. In this comparison, the criteria identified 11 of 14 patients in the amitriptyline trial and 4 of 6 patients in the cyclobenzaprine trial who had high composite outcome scores, indicating that the criteria had reasonably high criterion validity. Three points can be made from this preliminary attempt to define acceptable response criteria: (1) a small percentage of patients in both analyzed trials met the criteria (44% for amitriptyline-treated patients and 30% for cyclobenzaprine-treated patients); (2) only conventional outcomes were assessed and no psychological or functional outcomes were determined; (3) pain, a cardinal feature of fibromyalgia and a criterion of the ACR diagnostic criteria, did not discriminate as well as other outcome measures.

Cyclobenzaprine is a tricyclic agent that is similar in chemical structure to amitriptyline, which has been marketed as a muscle relaxant on the basis of its ability to reduce brain stem noradrenergic function and motor neuron efferent activity.[25] Several trials have used this agent in fibromyalgia syndrome. Bennett and colleagues[26] conducted a 12-week, double-blind, randomized, controlled trial of 120 patients. Modest efficacy was demonstrated in that the patients' assessment of sleep and pain improved significantly ($P < .02$) in the cyclobenzaprine group compared with the placebo group from weeks 2 to 12. Fatigue improved at weeks 2 to 4 ($P < .02$) but not at weeks 8 to 12. Physician assessment of global pain did not differ between the two treatment groups. Twenty-one of 61 cyclobenzaprine-treated patients and 9 of 57 placebo-treated patients had a moderate or marked overall physician-rated response. In this trial 60% of the placebo-treated patients and 35% of the cyclobenzaprine-treated patients withdrew from the study, with adverse reactions accounting for 8% in the cyclobenzaprine-treated patients and 5% in the placebo-treated patients.

Reynolds and associates[27] evaluated the effect of cyclobenzaprine on sleep physiology in 12 patients who participated in a crossover study of 4 weeks' duration. Patients were treated with 30 mg/day of cyclobenzaprine. With the exception of a decrease in afternoon sleepiness and an increase in total sleep time, no effect of cyclobenzaprine was seen on clinical or sleep parameters. This study, however, was probably too short and of inadequate power for any definite conclusions to be drawn.

Carrette and colleagues[28] conducted the only long-term comparative trial of amitriptyline, cyclobenzaprine, and placebo to date in the treatment of fibromyalgia syndrome. Two hundred eight patients fulfilling the 1990 ACR criteria for the diagnosis of fibromyalgia syndrome were entered into a 6-month double-blind, multicenter trial. Patients assigned to amitriptyline received 10 mg daily at bedtime for the 1st week, 25 mg for the 2nd through the 12th weeks, and 50 mg at bedtime for the last 12 weeks of the trial. Cyclobenzaprine-treated patients received escalating doses beginning at 10 mg at bedtime for the 1st week, 20 mg at bedtime for the 2nd through the 12th week, and 10 mg in the morning with 20 mg at bedtime for the last 12 weeks of the trial. A variety of patient-derived assessments were performed throughout the trial, including visual analog scales evaluating pain, sleep, morning stiffness, and global fibromyalgia symptoms; the McGill Pain Questionnaire; the Sickness Impact Profile; and the Health Assessment Questionnaire (HAQ). Psychological status was also assessed by the anxiety and depression scales of the Arthritis Impact Measurement Scales and the Minnesota Multiphasic Personality Inventory (MMPI). Physician assessments included dolorimeter scores at tender point locations. According to the criteria of Simms and associates[14] for improvement, 21% of amitriptyline-treated patients and 12% of cyclobenzaprine-treated patients experienced significantly more improvement than the placebo-treated patients at 1 month. At 3 months and

at 6 months, however, the proportion of responders was not different among the three groups (19% of the placebo group were classified as responders). Only physician global assessment of treated patients was superior to that of the placebo group at 6 months. Of note, 95% of amitriptyline-treated and 98% of cyclobenzaprine-treated patients experienced side effects, compared with 62% of placebo-treated patients, although only 13% of cyclobenzaprine-treated and 6% of amitriptyline-treated patients withdrew from the study because of side effects. A normal MMPI was the strongest predictor of response to active drug treatment at 1 month.

In summary, as the best studied of the tricyclic agents, both amitriptyline and cyclobenzaprine appear to be effective in the short-term therapy of fibromyalgia syndrome. The overall or mean degree of efficacy is modest, although a subset of patients may have marked improvement on multiple outcome measures. Unfortunately, there are currently no reliable ways to identify responders to these or other tricyclic agents in advance. Although side effects attributable to these agents in both short-term and longer term trials are relatively mild (principally dry mouth and excessive drowsiness) and resolve relatively quickly, maintenance of long-term efficacy compared with placebo remains to be demonstrated.

## Other Antidepressants

Fluoxetine, a selective serotonin reuptake inhibitor and a potent antidepressant agent, has been studied in fibromyalgia syndrome.[29, 30] Wolfe and colleagues studied 42 women with fibromyalgia syndrome who were randomly assigned to receive either fluoxetine at 20 mg daily or a placebo for 6 weeks.[29] At 6 weeks, both Arthritis Impact Measurement Scales depression scores and Beck depression scores as well as sleep quality showed significant improvement in the fluoxetine-treated patients compared with those receiving placebo, although no other studied variables showed improvement.[29] Wolfe and associates concluded that fluoxetine was not an effective agent in the treatment of fibromyalgia syndrome. Unfortunately, 57% of those receiving placebo dropped out of the study before the week 6 assessment (compared with 29% of fluoxetine-treated patients). It is therefore likely that this study had insufficient power to conclude that fluoxetine is an ineffective agent in the therapy of fibromyalgia syndrome.

Goldenberg and colleagues[30] conducted a double-blind, crossover study of four 6-week trials of fluoxetine and amitriptyline in 19 patients. Patients with major depression were excluded. Even though a relatively small number of patients was studied, the crossover design had sufficient power to detect clinically significant differences between the treatments. Both fluoxetine and amitriptyline significantly improved the Fibromyalgia Impact Questionnaire score, pain score, and patient global and sleep scores. Nonsignificant improvements occurred in the Beck Depression Inventory, the physician global score, and scores for fatigue and feeling refreshed on awakening. In combination, fluoxetine and amitriptyline were more effective than either agent alone. This is a promising form of combination therapy, which combines two drugs that have different actions and side effects and which together may be more effective and tolerable than either agent alone.

## Benzodiazepines

Alprazolam is a triazolobenzodiazepine approved for the treatment of anxiety and depression associated with anxiety.[18] Because its antidepressant and antianxiety effects are comparable to those of tricyclic agents, and because alprazolam may be better tolerated, several clinical trials have assessed its efficacy in fibromyalgia syndrome. Russell and colleagues[31] randomly assigned 78 patients into four groups: (1) alprazolam with ibuprofen, (2) alprazolam without ibuprofen, (3) ibuprofen alone, and (4) placebo for 6 weeks followed by 24-week open-label extension for 63 patients. Dolorimeter score, tender point index, patient assessment of pain, physician global assessment, HAQ score, and assessments of depression were determined at weekly intervals during the 6-week trial. All treatment groups improved at week 6 compared with baseline. There was no significant difference in the mean change in outcome variables between the double-placebo group and the other three treatment groups at the end of the 6-week trial, although lower patient rating of diseases severity and lower severity of tenderness on palpation were found in the patients who were receiving the combination of alprazolam and ibuprofen. Power calculations indicated that there was inadequate power in this study to detect improvement of at least 25% in one of the three active treatment arms. Both patient rating of pain and tenderness scores quickly worsened during a brief 2-week cessation of therapy. Among the 52 patients who completed the open-label portion of the study (all patients receiving the combination of ibuprofen and alprazolam), which was 8 weeks in duration, small but statistically significant levels of improvement were seen in several outcomes. With clinically relevant improvement defined as 30% or more at baseline, 7 of 16 patients in the drug-coded trial combination group showed improvement compared with only 4 of 14 in the double-placebo group. With respect to pain assessment, 6 of 15 patients in the combination group compared with only 3 of those in the double-placebo group obtained clinically relevant improvement, suggesting a benefit of the combination over the placebo, at least in a subset of patients. This trial thus illustrates the value of using response criteria to identify a subset of patients who improve, even though mean overall levels of improvement may not differ between treatment and placebo groups.

Hench and associates[32] compared the therapeutic effects of amitriptyline, temazepam, and placebo on clinical and sleep parameters in a double-blind, placebo crossover study of 10 patients for 12 weeks. Temazepam produced significant improvement in physician and patient global assessment, sleep disturbance, and morning stiffness, although paradoxically it appeared to decrease sleep duration and increase sleep latency (the time interval between going to bed and falling asleep). Amitriptyline, in contrast, produced significant improvement only in the number and severity of tender points.

Long-term use of benzodiazepines has been tempered by concern over dependence and possible withdrawal reactions, especially seizures.[18] In the trial of Russell and colleagues[31] there were few side effect–related dropouts attributable to alprazolam, and no information on side effects was reported in the trial of Hench and colleagues,[32] although it is unlikely that either trial was of sufficient duration to assess the issues of dependence and problems caused by withdrawal. Alprazolam should, therefore, be considered an only modestly effective agent that should probably be reserved for only short-term use in the treatment of fibromyalgia syndrome.

## Anti-Inflammatory Agents

Both corticosteroids and nonsteroidal anti-inflammatory drugs (NSAIDs) have been studied in the treatment of fibromyalgia syndrome. Systemic corticosteroids therapy was evaluated by Clark and colleagues[33] in a 2-week double-blind, placebo-controlled crossover trial involving 20 patients. Patients were assigned to treatment with either 15 mg of prednisone/day or placebo. Mean changes in analog scores of pain, sleep, fatigue, and dolorimeter score showed no difference between the prednisone and placebo treatment periods. Several patients who had mild elevation of serum creatine phosphokinase levels also had no significant or consistent improvement in symptom scores during treatment with prednisone.

The apparent lack of improvement in fibromyalgia with the use of systemic corticosteroid therapy is of particular interest in light of studies of chronic fatigue syndrome (a condition with many clinical features that are similar to those of fibromyalgia syndrome) and fibromyalgia syndrome, which have suggested mild perturbations of the HPA axis. Demitrack and colleagues[7] performed a series of assessments of the HPA axis in 30 patients with chronic fatigue syndrome, including measurement of 24-hour urinary free cortisol levels, ACTH and cortisol responses to CRH, and net integrated cortisol response to ACTH. They found reduced pituitary and adrenal responses to CRH and slightly reduced plasma cortisol concentrations, as well as low 24-hour urinary free cortisol levels. Demitrack and colleagues[7] argued that the demonstrated mild glucocorticoid deficiency seen in these patients with chronic fatigue syndrome was most likely the result of a mild central adrenal insufficiency possibly secondary to mild deficiency of CRH. As noted earlier, Griep and associates[5] demonstrated that patients with fibromyalgia have enhanced pituitary ACTH release in response to ovine CRH and to insulin-induced hypoglycemia, and Crofford and colleagues[6] found that basal HPA function as measured by 24-hour urinary free cortisol levels was low when compared with that of normal subjects.

If patients with chronic fatigue syndrome–fibromyalgia syndrome have either mild central or adrenal insufficiency, as is suggested by these studies, one would expect symptomatic improvement with the use of corticosteroids. The results of Clark and colleagues' study[33] are therefore at odds with these findings with respect to he HPA axis and are difficult to reconcile. It may be that Clark and colleagues' study[33] was too short and involved too few patients for definite conclusions to be drawn regarding the efficacy of corticosteroids in these conditions; alternatively, additional studies of the HPA axis in fibromyalgia syndrome may fail to confirm these preliminary findings.

In the earlier trial by Goldenberg and associates[23] of amitriptyline, naproxen, and placebo, naproxen alone (1000 mg/day) was no more effective than placebo, although the combination of amitriptyline and placebo was slightly more effective than amitriptyline alone. Possible synergism of NSAIDs and other "central nervous system (CNS)–active" medication was seen in Russell and colleagues'[31] trial of alprazolam and ibuprofen, in which there was a trend toward greater improvement in patients treated with the combination than in those treated with either agent alone.

Yunus and associates[34] studied the efficacy of ibuprofen in 46 patients with fibromyalgia syndrome in a double-blind, placebo-controlled trial of 3 weeks' duration. Patients receiving a psychotropic drug at a stable dose were allowed to remain on the drug for the duration of the study. At the end of the trial, there were no significant differences in any of the four measured variables (pain, fatigue, sleep difficulty, or total tender points). Both treatment and placebo groups experienced significant improvement compared with baseline in both fatigue and number of tender points, reinforcing the concept that placebo effects of up to 50% improvement in some variables may occur in short-term trials in fibromyalgia syndrome.

In summary, anti-inflammatory agents appear to have little, if any, efficacy alone in the treatment of fibromyalgia syndrome. When combined with other CNS-active agents, NSAIDs may confer slight synergistic analgesic benefit, although it could be argued that the marginal additional benefit of NSAIDs (particularly when used in the long term), given their potential toxicity, is not cost effective. Understandably, corticosteroids have received little attention in fibromyalgia syndrome, given the lack of evidence that there is an inflammatory basis for the disorder and on the basis of the controlled short-term trial by Clark and colleagues.[33] Data suggesting that there is hypofunction of the HPA axis, at least in some patients with fibromyalgia syndrome, may necessitate a re-evaluation of corticosteroids in the disorder, although at this time there remains no indication for the routine use of corticosteroids in clinical practice.

## Other Central Nervous System–Active Medications

Soma, a combination of carisoprodol (1200 mg), acetaminophen, and caffeine, has also been studied in fibromyalgia syndrome and was shown to be more effective than placebo in an 8-week trial of 58 patients.[35] Improved outcome measures in the treatment group included pain, sleep quality, and general feeling of sickness. Also, the pressure pain threshold increased in the treatment group but not in the placebo group, despite the fact that 43% of the patients in the placebo group but none in the active treatment group used tricyclic antidepressants, anxiolytic agents, or sedatives.

S-adenosylmethionine, an antidepressant, was studied in a short-term (3-week) placebo-controlled trial involving 25 patients with fibromyalgia syndrome.[36] Depression as assessed by the Hamilton Depression Rating Scale improved, and decreased trigger point scores were seen after S-adenosylmethionine administration but not after placebo. This agent has not gained acceptance, however, because it requires intramuscular administration and the investigators noted abscesses at injection sites, although the precise number was not detailed.[36]

## Hormone Therapy

With the finding that up to one third of patients with fibromyalgia syndrome have low levels of insulin-like growth factor-1 (IGF-1), Bennett and colleagues conducted a placebo-controlled, randomized trial of growth hormone injections.[37] Fifty women with fibromyalgia and low IGF-1 levels were enrolled in this double-blind study of 9 months' duration. Increases in serum IGF-1 occurred in the treatment group but not the placebo group. A small degree of improvement (approximately 10%) in Fibromyalgia Impact Questionnaire scores occurred in the treatment group at 9 months compared with the placebo group. No change occurred in the other principal outcome measure: the tender point score. Carpal tunnel syndrome occurred in 7 of 25 growth hormone–treated patients. Although this study suggests that a subset of patients with fibromyalgia syndrome may have secondary growth hormone deficiency, treatment of fibromyalgia syndrome with growth harmone is limited by the high risk of carpal tunnel syndrome and the monthly cost of this therapy, which currently is approximately $1500.

## Exercise Therapy

In light of the observation by Moldofsky and Scarisbrick[16] that interference with stage IV sleep in trained athletes did not lead to an overnight increase in musculoskeletal symptoms, McCain and colleagues[38] performed a 20-week trial comparing the efficacy of cardiovascular fitness training (CVR) with simple flexibility and stretching (FLEX) in 42 patients with fibromyalgia syndrome (Table 11–2). The CVR pro-

**TABLE 11–2**
**Nonmedication-controlled Therapeutic Trials in Fibromyalgia Syndrome**

| INTERVENTION | COMPARISON INTERVENTION | REFERENCE | DURATION (WK) | INTERVENTION EFFICACY |
|---|---|---|---|---|
| Cardiovascular fitness training | Flexibility and stretching | McCain et al[38] | 20 | Yes |
| EMG-biofeedback | Sham | Ferraccioli et al[41] | 24 | Yes |
| Electroacupuncture | Sham | Deluze et al[48] | 3 | Yes |
| Hypnotherapy | Physical therapy | Haanen et al[49] | 12 | Yes |

EMG = electromyography.

gram consisted of supervised aerobic fitness training for 20 minutes three times weekly and was designed to result in an increase in heart rate to 75% of the predicted maximum. The FLEX program consisted of a supervised stretching and flexibility program. At the end of the study, patients assigned to the CVR program exhibited increased cardiovascular fitness as determined by an aerobic fitness test, and there were significant improvements in both patient and physician global assessments and tender point pain thresholds. Also, a greater proportion of the CVR program patients experienced moderate or marked improvement compared with the FLEX group, although patients assigned to the CVR group had higher pain scores at study entry and therefore may have had a greater tendency to "regress to the mean" or improve spontaneously. Despite this favorable effect of the CVR program, patients did experience immediate postexertional worsening of symptoms, and few patients continued with long-term aerobic fitness at the conclusion of the trial. This observation tends to mirror the clinical experience with aerobic fitness programs: Relatively few patients are able to comply with a long-term aerobic activity, and many patients are not able to participate at all because of immediate postexertion exacerbation of symptoms. Nevertheless, among patients who are able to participate in long-term aerobic activity, many are able to wean off other medication successfully and are able to avoid the vicious cycle of worsening pain and muscle deconditioning, which unfortunately may occur in patients with more severe symptoms.

Mengshoel and Førre[39] performed a clinical trial of low-intensity endurance training in 25 patients with fibromyalgia syndrome. Eleven patients were randomly assigned to a modified low-impact aerobic dance program twice weekly for 20 weeks. Each session lasted 60 minutes, although the training intensity was kept at a heart rate level not exceeding 150 beats per minute. Fourteen patients randomly assigned to the control group did not change their level of physical activity. At the end of 20 weeks, there was no change in the level of pain (as assessed by the McGill Pain Questionnaire) or fatigue (as assessed by visual analog scales) in the training group from the beginning to the end of the training period nor was there any detectable difference between the training and control groups with respect to either the pain or the fatigue variables. The small sample sizes, the uncertain level of baseline fitness in either the experimental or control group (both groups may have had relatively high levels of physical fitness, and therefore the experimental group would not be expected to improve significantly), and the lack of measurement of other outcomes such as sleep or overall symptom severity make it difficult to conclude that low-level physical activity is ineffective. In clinical practice, many patients experience significant benefit from low-level aerobic fitness, which can be accomplished with simple activities such as a regular walking program.

## Long-Term Experience

As indicated earlier, only two trials have been reported with significant long-term experiences.[28, 37] In the amitriptyline and cyclobenzaprine trial of 6 months' duration, no difference in the proportion of responders between the two active treatments and placebo was noted at the conclusion of the trial.[28] In the growth hormone trial, the modest improvement was tempered by the high rate of carpal tunnel syndrome.[37]

## CONTROLLED TRIALS OF NONCONVENTIONAL THERAPY

### Malic Acid and Magnesium

Malic acid (an organic dicoboxylic acid) and magnesium are involved in the generation of mitochondrial adenosine triphosphate synthesis. A combination proprietary tablet, Super Malic, containing 200 mg malic acid and 50 mg magnesium, was studied in a 4-week, placebo-controlled trial in 24 patients at a dose of three tablets twice daily.[40] The primary outcome measures were those of pain and tenderness. No clear treatment effect of Super Malic was detected, but a longer term, higher dose trial was suggested given improvements that occurred in a 6-month open-label extension of the trial at six tablets twice daily.[40]

### Electromyography-Biofeedback

Electromyography-biofeedback has been shown to be of benefit in psychosomatic disorders such as functional diarrhea and tension headache. With this procedure, patients receive auditory feedback of ongoing muscle tension in scalp muscles determined with the use of surface electrodes placed on the forehead. Typically, the feedback is presented in the form of pulse sounds that are proportional to the level of scalp muscle tension; patients then attempt to control their muscle tension to obtain relief. Under the presumption that fibromyalgia may have a psychosomatic basis, Ferraccioli and colleagues[41] performed a controlled study of biofeedback in 12 patients, following an open study in 15 patients in which they reported a 50% clinical improvement in nine patients at 6 months (see Table 2–2). Biofeedback therapy was conducted in 20-minute sessions twice weekly for a total of 15 sessions. In the controlled trial, patients who received biofeedback demonstrated improvement in all outcome variables, which was apparently sustained for 6 months, although patients who received sham biofeedback (they were disconnected from the recording of muscle tension and therefore had no acoustic signal to determine progressive relaxation) experienced improvement only in tender point counts. Using the MMPI, Ferraccioli and colleagues[41] surprisingly found no correlation between depression or "an overt psychosomatic background" and response to electromyography-biofeedback. As Wolfe[42] pointed out, the blinding status of patients in this study is uncertain and the psychiatric instrument may have been inappropriate. Therefore, the role of biofeedback in fibromyalgia syndrome remains uncertain, and additional studies are required.

## Acupuncture and Electroacupuncture

Despite its apparent popularity, the role of acupuncture, particularly in the therapy of chronic pain, remains controversial. Two meta-analyses reached opposite conclusions regarding the efficacy of acupuncture in the therapy of chronic pain. Patel and colleagues pooled the results of 14 randomized trials and concluded that "while few individual trials had statistically significant results, pooled results of many subgroups attained statistical significance in favour of acupuncture."[43] ter Riet and colleagues[44] performed a criteria-based meta-analysis of 51 controlled studies, which emphasized an assessment of study design and assigned a possible maximum of 100 points based on four main categories: (1) comparability of prognosis, (2) adequate intervention, (3) adequate effect measurement, and (4) data presentation. No study in their analysis earned more than 62% of the maximal score. The results of the better studies (>50% of the maximal score) were contradictory, and a separate subgroup analysis of studies employing sham procedures showed a comparable number of positive and negative results.[44] The authors concluded that "the efficacy of acupuncture in the treatment of chronic pain remains doubtful."[44]

Considerable research has been conducted into the possible mechanism of acupuncture. Most data after 1990 appear to favor a neurohumoral explanation with activation of endogenous pain control mechanisms such as via the opioid or serotoninergic pathways.[45, 46] Acupuncture may work by activation of these endogenous pain-modulating systems through the noxious stimulation of heterotopic body areas at the segmental level or via the systemic release of peptides by the adrenal glands.[47] Electroacupuncture or application of an electric current at the site of application of the acupuncture needle has physiologic effects similar to those of traditional acupuncture.

Deluze and associates[48] reported the only randomized clinical trial of electroacupuncture in the treatment of fibromyalgia (see Table 11–2). In this study, 36 patients were randomly assigned to receive electroacupuncture and 34 were randomly assigned to receive a sham procedure for 3 weeks. Treatment consisted of six sessions of electroacupuncture spread over 3 weeks, with the application of electroacupuncture at four common acupuncture points (dorsal interosseus muscle of the hand and the inferior knee bilaterally) and up to six empirically chosen sites, "depending on the patient's symptoms and pain pattern." The sham procedure consisted of needle insertion approximately 20 mm away from the point that would have been chosen for the real procedure with the application of a weaker electric current. Although seven of eight outcome measures showed improvement in the active treatment group, none was improved in the sham treatment group. Pain threshold, which was considered the principal outcome measure, improved by 70% in the electroacupuncture group and 4% in the control group ($P = .03$). There were several limitations to this study: (1) It is unclear whether electroacupuncture is equivalent to conventional acupuncture (some acupuncturists claim that electroacupuncture provides only short-term analgesic benefit, whereas conventional acupuncture may provide longer-lasting analgesia); (2) patients may not have been optimally blinded in this study, because the sham protocol involved a shallower needle insertion and a weaker electric current; (3) there was no measure of functional or psychological status; and (4) the time that assessments were performed after the treatment was not detailed. This latter point is crucial because the analgesic effect of acupuncture may be short-lived, particularly for protocols involving less than 4 weeks of treatments.

## Hypnotherapy

On the basis of the utility of hypnotherapy in disorders such as asthma, peptic ulcer disease, and irritable bowel syndrome, in which psychological factors may contribute to pathogenesis, Haanen and colleagues performed a controlled trial of hypnotherapy in fibromyalgia (see Table 11–2).[49] Forty patients were randomized to either hypnotherapy or physical therapy for 12 weeks with follow-up at 24 weeks. Patients in the hypnotherapy group experienced significantly greater improvement in pain, fatigue, and global assessment at both 12 and 24 weeks.[49] Hypnotherapy, therefore, may be a useful intervention in some patients with particularly refractory symptoms.

## UNCONTROLLED THERAPIES
(Table 11–3)

Local injection of tender points has been advocated by several authors.[50–52] In general, a local anesthetic with

**TABLE 11–3**
**Uncontrolled Interventions in Fibromyalgia Syndrome**

| INTERVENTION | REFERENCE |
| --- | --- |
| Transcutaneous nerve stimulation | Kaada[54] |
| Local injection | Masi and Yunus,[50] Sheon et al,[51] Yunus[52] |
| Cognitive-behavioral therapy | Nielson et al,[56] Goldenberg et al[59] |
| Multidisciplinary therapy | Bennett et al[60] |

or without local depot corticosteroid administration has been advocated and may provide relief for up to 2 months.

Low-frequency transcutaneous electrical nerve stimulation (TENS) may increase skin and muscle microcirculation and also activate endogenous opioids.[53] TENS was administered to 40 patients with fibromyalgia syndrome and appeared to produce transient benefit in 70% of the patients, although the long-term benefits are unknown.[54] A controlled trial is needed, however, given the lack of benefit of TENS observed in low back pain.[55]

Cognitive-behavioral treatment (CBT) of chronic pain involves a set of interventions that address the sensory, affective, cognitive, and behavioral components of chronic pain and has been effective in a variety of disorders such as low back pain, headache, and temporomandibular joint pain.[56] This approach has also been shown to be useful in the treatment of rheumatoid arthritis, demonstrating improvement not only in psychological outcomes but also in measures of disease activity such as joint tenderness and swelling.[57, 58] Nielson and colleagues[56] studied 30 patients who met ACR criteria for the diagnosis of fibromyalgia. Patients were excluded if they were unable to attend the daily sessions or were unwilling to stop narcotic medication for control of pain. The CBT intervention consisted of a 3-week inpatient program that combined educational techniques (including the use of a videotape in which chronic pain was portrayed as a multidimensional phenomenon that involved cognitive, affective, sensory, and behavioral components), cognitive techniques, aerobic exercises and stretching, pacing and enhancement of pain tolerance, and family education (with at least one family member). Twenty-five patients completed the program, and "target" variables such as pain severity, perceived interference with life, sense of control over pain, and emotional distress all showed statistically significant improvement after the CBT program compared with baseline measures. "Nontarget" variables, such as perceived support by others, response by significant others to pain, marital adjustment, and activity level, did not change with the CBT program. Thus, in this short-term, inpatient trial, CBT appears to be effective, although precisely which components of the program were effective is uncertain. Also, the confounding effects of cardiovascular train-

ing and concomitant use of medication hinder interpretation of the results.

Other groups have used similar combination therapy approaches that employ CBT, physical therapy, and cardiovascular exercise as well as medication in outpatient settings.[59, 60] It appears that these approaches demonstrate improvement in the majority of patients in uncontrolled settings, although the long-term cost-effectiveness of these intensive programs is not known.

Other commonly employed therapies, such as chiropractic manipulation and myofascial therapy (including "spray and stretch" techniques), have been advocated on the basis of anecdotal experience.[50, 60]

## AUTHOR'S APPROACH TO MANAGEMENT

Education is an important component of any therapeutic regimen for patients with fibromyalgia syndrome. Patients and their families should be instructed to view fibromyalgia as a disorder that is not crippling. Although fibromyalgia is generally a chronic condition, effective therapy is available, although there is no specific cure. When possible, patients should be encouraged to take an active, self-help–oriented approach, rather than a passive, physician- or health provider–dependent approach to the treatment of their condition. Emphasis should be placed on the positive or "well" role, as opposed to the negative or "sick" role. Enrollment in patient support groups is to be encouraged.

After the diagnosis is established, it is useful to assess the severity of the condition (Fig. 11–1). Although there is currently no optimal measure of severity, assessment of the functional impact of the condition appears most appropriate (see Fig. 12–1).[64] For patients with mild symptoms that have minimal functional impact, patient education and low-level aerobic exercise may be sufficient. For the majority of patients, the use of antidepressant therapies form the cornerstone of current treatment approaches. For these patients, initiating therapy with low-dose tricyclic agents in addition to low-level aerobic exercise is reasonable. The starting dose of amitriptyline should generally be 10 mg given at bedtime. Occasionally, in patients who are particularly sensitive to side effects, as little as 5 mg/day may be effective. Nortriptyline may be better tolerated than amitriptyline by some patients and should be tried at the same doses as amitriptyline. If there is no response to the initial 10-mg dose, and side effects are tolerable (frequently, side effects such as dry mouth or drowsiness will subside with continued treatment) after 1 week, the dose should be increased in 10-mg increments on a weekly basis thereafter. In general, doses that exceed 50 mg/day, confer little additional benefit if there is no response to lower doses. For patients with more severe symptoms and for those with associated depression without agitation or severe anxiety, a specific serotonin reuptake inhibitor (SSRI) combined with a low-dose tricyclic agent appears to be most effective. For patients with more severe or agitated depression,

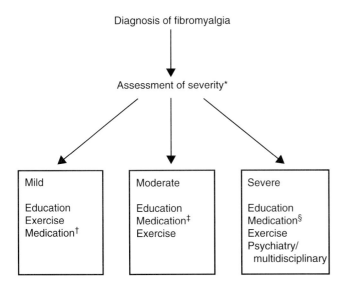

Diagnosis of fibromyalgia

↓

Assessment of severity*

**Mild**

Education
Exercise
Medication[†]

**Moderate**

Education
Medication[‡]
Exercise

**Severe**

Education
Medication[§]
Exercise
Psychiatry/
multidisciplinary

\* Assessment of severity includes evaluation of pain, sleep, and fatigue symptoms as
   well as functional impairment (e.g., impact of symptoms on employment).
[†] Medication for mild symptoms might include only low-dose tricyclic agents.
[‡] Medication for moderately severe symptoms might include a combination of an SSRI
   with a low-dose tricyclic agent.
[§] Medication regimen for severe symptoms would initially include that recommended
   for moderate symptoms but may require revision in coordination with a psychiatrist.

**FIGURE 11–1**
Management of the fibromyalgia syndrome. SSRI = specific
serotonin reuptake inhibitor.

psychiatric input may be required for optimal management. For a minority of symptomatic patients with or without major depression, pain management or multidisciplinary approaches may be required.

Low-level aerobic exercise, such as walking or riding a stationary bicycle, on a regular basis is a useful adjunct to medication therapy and may be advised either concurrently with or shortly after initiation of medication therapy. Frequently, patients who are able to engage in regular aerobic exercise may be able to taper off medication eventually. Muscle strengthening exercises should be employed cautiously.

Judicious use of local anesthetic injections (with or without depot corticosteroid injection) may be helpful in selected patients who have local symptoms that are particularly severe at times.

## DRUG SIDE EFFECTS AND RECOMMENDED MONITORING SCHEDULES

The most common side effects experienced with drug therapy of fibromyalgia syndrome are outlined in Table 11–4. Additional side effects noted with the use of tricyclic agents in low doses include weight gain, nightmares or vivid dreaming, and occasionally paradoxic reactions such as insomnia. The SSRIs as a class may exacerbate anxiety and also produce insomnia. An SSRI discontinuation reaction, consisting of disequilibrium symptoms (e.g., dizziness, vertigo), nausea and

vomiting, flu-like symptoms (e.g., fatigue, lethargy), anxiety, and irritability, has been reported after abrupt discontinuation of these agents.[65] This reaction is generally mild and short-lived but can be distressing. It may be reversed by reintroduction of the medication or one that is pharmacologically similar. It is minimized by a slow taper or by using a drug that has an extended half-life. Tricyclic agents, even at low doses, should be used with extreme caution in patients with a history of urinary retention or narrow-angle glaucoma. As noted earlier, abrupt discontinuation of these agents may produce rebound insomnia. These agents should be used with extreme caution in elderly patients because of the increased potential for confusion, disorientation, and hallucinations. Routine laboratory monitoring is generally not necessary for drug therapies used in the treatment of fibromyalgia (with the possible exception of NSAIDs, for which periodic monitoring of the hematocrit, liver function studies, and renal function is recommended), although it is recommended that initially patients be surveyed at least quarterly to monitor for side effects.

## PERTINENT CLINICAL PHARMACOLOGY AND DRUG INTERACTIONS

Many of the antidepressant agents employed in the therapy of fibromyalgia syndrome may potentiate CNS depression that may occur with alcohol, sedative-hypnotic agents, and other CNS-depressant drugs and should therefore be used with extreme caution, if at all, in these settings. The tricyclic agents are contraindicated in the presence of monoamine-oxidase inhibitors. In conjunction with anticholinergic agents, they may cause acute glaucoma, urinary retention, and paralytic ileus. Concomitant use of the tricyclic drugs with clonidine and guanethidine may reduce the antihypertensive effect of the latter. All these agents have unknown effects on the fetus and are therefore contraindicated during pregnancy. Anecdotally among my patients, pregnancy usually results in spontaneous improvement of symptoms, and withdrawal of medication during pregnancy is generally well tolerated.

## SUMMARY AND CONCLUSIONS

Many different interventions have been reported in the fibromyalgia syndrome (see Tables 11–1 through 11–3). Although many have been effective, trials in general of therapy have been of short duration. Furthermore, important or substantial improvement, when it has been assessed, occurs in only small proportions of patients. Long-term comparative trials of both efficacy and toxicity are necessary, although trials such as these require large numbers of patients and therefore are expensive and difficult to accomplish. Two other approaches offer potential solutions to the problem of adequate long-term comparative trials: (1) N-of-1 trials and (2) meta-analysis. N-of-1 trials have the

**TABLE 11–4**

**Side Effects of Central Nervous System–Active Drugs for Fibromyalgia Syndrome**

| DRUG | SEDATION | INSOMNIA | ANTICHOLINERGIC EFFECTS |
|------|----------|----------|------------------------|
| Amitriptyline | +++ | 0 | +++ |
| Desipramine | + | + | + |
| Doxepin | +++ | 0 | ++ |
| Imipramine | ++ | 0 | ++ |
| Nortriptyline | ++ | 0 | + |
| Protriptyline | + | ++ | ++ |
| Fluoxetine | 0 | ++ | 0 |
| Alprazolam | + | 0 | 0 |
| Cyclobenzaprine | ++ | 0 | ++ |

0 = no side effect; + = a minor side effect; ++ = a moderate side effect; +++ = a major side effect.
Adapted with permission from Potter WZ, Rudorfer MV, Manji H: The pharmacologic treatment of depression. N Engl J Med 1993; 325:633–642.

advantage of random assignment, double-blinding, and multiple potential comparisons in the same patient. Meta-analysis involves combining the results of studies (which individually may have conflicting results and lack adequate statistical power) to reach an overall result with sufficient statistical power to make meaningful conclusions, especially with respect to comparative efficacy. Lack of uniformity in the use of outcome measures hinders the application of meta-analytic methods, and for this reason future clinical trials in the fibromyalgia syndrome should ideally employ the same outcome measures.[61]

Few trials have assessed improvement in functional status. Functional status measures such as the HAQ[62] the Fibromyalgia Impact Questionnaire,[63] or similar instruments should be employed in future studies of therapy in fibromyalgia.

No studies have yet assessed the comparative cost-efficacy of available treatments. Studies that address the cost-efficacy of commonly employed but unproven treatments, such as physical therapy and chiropractic manipulation, are urgently needed.

## REFERENCES

1. Bennett RM: The fibromyalgia syndrome: Myofascial pain and the chronic fatigue syndrome. *In* Kelly WN, Harris ED, Ruddy S, et al (eds): Textbook of Rheumatology, 4th ed. Philadelphia: WB Saunders, 1992:471.
2. Wolfe F, Smythe HA, Yunus MB, et al: The American College of Rheumatology 1990 criteria for the classification of fibromyalgia. Arthritis Rheum 1990; 33:19.
3. Wolfe F: The prevalence and characteristics of fibromyalgia in the general population. Arthritis Rheum 1993; 36:S48.
4. Goldenberg DL: Fibromyalgia syndrome: An emerging but controversial condition. JAMA 1987; 257:2782.
5. Griep EN, Boersma JW, De Kloet ER: Altered reactivity of the hypothalamic-pituitary-adrenal axis in the primary fibromyalgia syndrome. J Rheumatol 1993; 20:469.
6. Crofford L, Pillemer SR, Kalogeras KT, et al: Perturbations of hypothalamic-pituitary-adrenal axis function in patients with fibromyalgia [Abstract]. Arthritis Rheum 1993; 36:S220.
7. Demitrack MA, Dale JK, Straus SE, et al: Evidence for impaired activation of the hypothalamic pituitary-adrenal axis in patients with chronic fatigue syndrome. J Clin Endocrinol Metab 1991; 73:1224.
8. Simms RW: Fibromyalgia is not a muscle disorder. Am J Med Sci 1998; 315:346–350.
9. Simms RW, Roy SH, Hrovat M, et al: Lack of association between fibromyalgia syndrome and abnormalities in muscle energy metabolism. Arthritis Rheum 1994; 37:794.
10. Bennett RM, Clark SR, Campbell SM, et al: Low levels of somatomedin C in patients with the fibromyalgia syndrome: A possible link between sleep and muscle pain. Arthritis Rheum 1992; 35:1113.
11. Russell IJ, Vaeroy H, Javors M, et al: Cerebrospinal fluid biogenic amine metabolites in fibromyalgia/fibrositis syndrome and rheumatoid arthritis. Arthritis Rheum 1992; 35:550.
12. Simms RW: Fibromyalgia syndrome: Current concepts in pathophysiology, clinical features, and management. Arthritis Care Res 1996; 9:315.
13. Hudson JI, Pope HG: The concept of affective spectrum disorder: Relationship to fibromyalgia and other syndromes of chronic fatigue and chronic muscle pain. Ballières Clin Rheumatol 1994; 8:839.
14. Simms RW, Felson DT, Goldenberg DL: Development of preliminary criteria for response to treatment in fibromyalgia syndrome. J Rheumatol 1991; 18:1558.
15. Moldofsky H, Scarisbrick P, England R, et al: Musculoskeletal symptoms and non-REM sleep disturbance in patients with fibrositis syndrome and healthy subjects. Psychosom Med 1975; 37:341.
16. Moldofsky H, Scarisbrick P: Induction of neurasthenic musculoskeletal pain syndrome by selective sleep stage deprivation. Psychosom Med 1976; 38:35.
17. Moldofsky H, Lue LA: The relationship of alpha and delta EEG frequencies and mood in "fibrositis" patients treated with chlorpromazine and L-tryptophan. Electroencephalogr Clin Neurophysiol 1980; 50:71.
18. Potter WZ, Rudorfer MV, Manji H: The pharmacologic treatment of depression. N Engl J Med 1993; 325:633.
19. Yunus M, Masi AT, Calabro JJ, et al: Primary fibromyalgia (fibrositis): Clinical study of 50 patients with matched normal controls. Semin Arthritis Rheum 1981; 11:151.
20. Smythe HA: Fibrositis and other diffuse musculoskeletal syndromes. *In* Kelly WN, Harris ED, Ruddy S, et al (eds): Textbook of Rheumatology. Philadelphia: WB Saunders, 1981:485.
21. Connolly RG: Treatment of fibromyositis with fluphenazine and amitriptyline: A preliminary report. Del Med 1981; 53:189.
22. Carrette S, McCain GA, Bell DA, et al: Evaluation of amitriptyline in primary fibrositis: A double blind, placebo-controlled study. Arthritis Rheum 1986; 29:655.
23. Goldenberg DL, Felson DT, Dinerman H: A randomized controlled trial of amitriptyline and naproxen in the treatment of fibromyalgia syndrome. Arthritis Rheum 1986; 29:1371.
24. Jaeschke R, Adachi J, Guyatt G, et al: Clinical usefulness of amitriptyline in fibromyalgia: The results of 23 N-of-1 randomized controlled trials. J Rheumatol 1991; 18:447.

25. Barnes CD, Fung SJ, Gintautus J: Brainstem noradrenergic system depression by cyclobenzaprine. Neuropharmacology 1980; 19:221.
26. Bennett RM, Gatter RA, Campbell SM, et al: A comparison of cyclobenzaprine and placebo in the management of fibrositis: A double-blind controlled study. Arthritis Rheum 1988; 31:1535.
27. Reynolds WJ, Moldofsky H, Saskin P, et al: The effects of cyclobenzaprine on sleep physiology and symptoms in patients with fibrositis. Arthritis Rheum 1989; 32:B115.
28. Carrette S, Bell MJ, Reynolds WJ, et al: Comparison of amitriptyline, cyclobenzaprine and placebo in fibromyalgia: A randomized double-blind clinical trial. Arthritis Rheum 1994; 37:32.
29. Wolfe F, Cathey MA, Hawley DJ: A double-blind placebo controlled trial of fluoxetine in patients with fibromyalgia. Arthritis Rheum 1993; 36 (suppl): S220.
30. Goldenberg D, Mayskiy M, Mossey C, et al: A randomized, double blind trial of fluoxetine and amitriptyline in the treatment of fibromyalgia. Arthritis Rheum 1996; 39:1852.
31. Russell IJ, Fletcher EM, Michalek JE, et al: Treatment of primary fibrositis/fibromyalgia syndrome with ibuprofen and alprazolam: A double-blind, placebo-controlled study. Arthritis Rheum 1991; 34:552.
32. Hench PK, Cohen R, Mitler MM: Fibromyalgia: Effects of amitriptyline, temazepam and placebo on pain and sleep. Arthritis Rheum 1989; 32(suppl):S47.
33. Clark S, Tindall E, Bennett RM: A double blind crossover trial of prednisone versus placebo in the treatment of fibrositis. J Rheumatol 1985; 12:980.
34. Yunus MB, Masi AT, Aldag JC: Short-term effects of ibuprofen in primary fibromyalgia syndrome: A double blind, placebo controlled trial. J Rheumatol 1989; 16:527.
35. Vaeroy H, Abrahamsen A, Førre O, et al: Treatment of fibromyalgia (fibrositis syndrome): A parallel double blind trial with carisoprodol, paracetamol and caffeine (Somadril comp) versus placebo. Clin Rheumatol 1989; 8:245.
36. Tavoni A, Vitali C, Bombardieri S, et al: Evaluation of s-adenosylmethionine in primary fibromyalgia: A double-blind crossover study. Am J Med 1987; 83(suppl 5A):107.
37. Bennett RM, Clark SC, Walczyk MS: A randomized, double-blind, placebo controlled study of growth homone in the treatment of fibromyalgia. Am J Med 1998; 104:227.
38. McCain GA, Bell DA, Mai FM, et al: A controlled study of the effects of a supervised cardiovascular fitness training program on the manifestations of primary fibromyalgia. Arthritis Rheum 1991; 31:1135.
39. Mengshoel AM, Førre Ø. Physical fitness training in patients with fibromyalgia. J Musculoskeletal Pain 1993; 1:267.
40. Russell IJ, Michalek JE, Flechas JD, et al: Treatment of fibromyalgia syndrome with Super Malic. A randomized, double blind, placebo controlled, crossover pilot study. J Rheumatol 1995; 22:953.
41. Ferraccioli G, Ghirelli L, Scita F, et al: EMG-biofeedback training in fibromyalgia syndrome. J Rheumatol 1987; 14:820.
42. Wolfe F: Fibromyalgia: Whither treatment? J Rheumatol 1988; 15:1047.
43. Patel MS, Gutzwiller F, Pacaud F, et al: A meta-analysis of acupuncture for the treatment of pain: A review of evaluative research. Pain 1986; 24:15.
44. ter Riet G, Kleijnen J, Knipshild P: Acupuncture and chronic pain: A criteria-based meta-analysis. J Clin Epidemiol 1990; 43:1191.
45. Han JS: Central neurotransmitters and acupuncture analgesia. In Pomeranz B, Stux G (eds): Scientific Bases of Acupuncture. Berlin: Springer-Verlag, 1989:7.
46. Fields HL, Basbaum A: Endogenous pain control mechanisms. In Wall PD, Melzack R (eds): Textbook of Pain. Edinburgh: Churchill Livingstone, 1989:206.
47. Ho WKK, When HL: Opioid-like activity in the cerebrospinal fluid of pain patients treated by electroacupuncture. Neuropharmacology 1991; 28:961.
48. Deluze C, Bosia L, Zirbs A, et al: Electroacupuncture in fibromyalgia: Results of a controlled trial. BMJ 1992; 305:1249.
49. Haanen HCM, Hoenderdos HTW, Van Romunde LKJ, et al: Controlled trial of hypnotherapy in the treatment of refractory fibromyalgia. J Rheumatol 1991; 18:72.
50. Masi AT, Yunus MB: Fibromyalgia—Which is the best treatment? A personalized, comprehensive, ambulatory, patient-involved management programme. Ballières Clin Rheumatol 1990; 4:333.
51. Sheon RP, Moskowitz RW, Goldberg VM: Intralesional soft tissue injection technique. In Sheon RP (ed): Soft Tissue Rheumatic Pain: Recognition, Management, Prevention, 2nd ed. Philadelphia: Lea & Febiger, 1987:293.
52. Yunus MB: Diagnosis, etiology and management of fibromyalgia syndrome: An update. Compr Ther 1988; 14:8.
53. McCain GA: Non-medicinal treatments in primary fibromyalgia. Rheum Dis Clin North Am 1989; 15:73.
54. Kaada B: Treatment of fibromyalgia by low-frequency transcutaneous nerve stimulation. Tidsskrift Nor Laegeforen 1989; 109:2992.
55. Deyo RA, Walsh NE, Martin DC, et al: A controlled trial of transcutaneous electrical nerve stimulation (TENS) and exercise for chronic low back pain. N Engl J Med 1990; 322:1627.
56. Nielson WR, Walker C, McCain GA: Cognitive behavioral treatment of fibromyalgia syndrome: Preliminary findings. J Rheumatol 1992; 19:98.
57. Bradley LA, Young LD, Anderson KO, et al: Effects of pschological therapy on pain behavior of rheumatoid arthritis patients: Treatment outcome and six month follow-up. Arthritis Rheum 1987; 30:1105.
58. Parker JC, Frank RG, Beck NC, et al: Pain management in rheumatoid arthritis patients: A cognitive-behavioral approach. Arthritis Rheum 1988; 31:593.
59. Goldenberg DL, Kaplan KH, Nadeau MG: The impact of cognitive-behavioral therapy on fibromyalgia. Arthritis Rheum 1991; 34(suppl):S190.
60. Bennett RM, Campbell S, Burckhardt C, et al: A multidisciplinary approach to fibromyalgia management. J Musculoskel Med 1991; 8:21.
61. Peluso P, Bombardier C, Guillemin F: A meta-analysis of controlled trials in the treatment of fibromyalgia syndrome [Abstract]. Arthritis Rheum 1993; 36:S49.
62. Fries JF, Spitz PW, Kraines RG: Measurement of patient outcome in arthritis. Arthritis Rheum 1980; 23:137.
63. Burckhardt CS, Clark SR, Bennett RM: The fibromyalgia impact questionnaire (FIQ): Development and validation. J Rheumatol 1991; 18:728.
64. Simms RW: Treatment of fibromyalgia. Rheumatol Musculoskeletal Med Primary Care 1998; 1:19.
65. Schatzberg AF: Antidepressant discontinuation syndrome: An update on serotonin reuptake inhibitors. J Clin Psychiatry 1997; 58(suppl 7):3.

# 12 | Developing Medical Documentation for Rheumatology Encounters

*Clifford D. Locks and Robin K. Dore*

The purpose of this chapter is to help the rheumatologist develop a strategy for adequately recording medical encounters with patients. Rheumatologists and other physicians are under increasing pressure to record more and more information pertaining to such encounters.[1] This results largely from changes in reimbursement policies and the requirements of third-party payors, particularly the US government. Demand for information will increase as more information is sought for purposes other than direct patient care or physician reimbursement, such as to obtain data for outcomes research.[2]

The rheumatologist developing medical documentation must ultimately satisfy the information requirements of third parties that have an interest in the patient's health and health care in general. Third parties rely on medical records to make payments (1) to physicians, (2) to *others* for goods or services provided to the patient on the basis of the physician's documentation (e.g., prescription medications, appliances, and physical therapy), and (3) to *patients* on the basis of their medical condition, such as disability payments. In addition, third parties rely prospectively on medical records for financial underwriting purposes, including health and disability insurers, life insurers, and, a relative newcomer, insurers who write policies for long-term care insurance. Finally, third parties may audit the records to evaluate the quality or economy of the physician's performance. An unsatisfactory audit may prevent a physician from providing services to patients who are insured by that third party.[3]

Although the demands for centralized databases may pressure the physician to move the focus of medical documentation away from the patient, the medical records must remain "patient-oriented": addressing the patient's interests first and other interests secondarily.

Recording the treatment rendered to a patient has always been an essential element of medical care. The physician who develops forms (on paper or on a computer screen) must understand the general principles applicable to medical records documentation, whether paper or electronic. The medical record should be complete and legible and displayed in a chronological manner. The reason for the encounter needs to be documented, as should relevant history, physical examination, and prior diagnostic test results. An assessment or clinical impression needs to be made, and a diagnosis must be listed. The plan for future care of the patient needs to be documented. The rationale for ordering diagnostic and other ancillary services should be implied if not documented. Past and present diagnoses should be accessible to the treating and/or consulting physician, and appropriate health risk factors should be identified. The patient's progress and response to therapy, changes in therapy, and revision of diagnoses need to be documented. Finally, the codes reported on the health insurance claim form or billing statement need to be supported by the documentation in the medical record.[4]

The most frequent encounter between the rheumatologist and patient is a follow-up visit: a physician-recommended return visit with an established patient who is seen regularly for a known diagnosis. Formulating an approach for recording this interaction is the focus of this chapter. This approach must satisfy many interests, including those of the patient and of third-party insurers and government entities who indemnify the patient from the cost of medical services incurred. Because of the need to bill and receive payment from third parties, the rheumatologist must comply with reporting conventions established by the American Medical Association (AMA). These conventions, contained in Current Procedural Terminology, Fourth Edition 1999 (CPT) published by the AMA, reflect a long effort to establish a system that will accurately identify the services provided.

CPT is a complex document that contains definitions and algorithms relating to classification of types and levels of medical services. Included in CPT are detailed documentation requirements relating to patient evaluation and management that must be satisfied in order to charge for services at a given level. Although these requirements are broad, some are essentially a codification of recording practices already used by physicians. The additional and more complex documentation requirements result from efforts to devise a mechanism for valuing, and equalizing payment for, diverse medical services. Because of the importance of CPT, using CPT framework to structure the record of the patient encounter is practical. For the same reason, CPT nomenclature is used when appropriate.

Three forms are presented in this chapter as the basis for developing an effective medical record strategy: a *progress note* (Appendix 12–1), a *patient update* (Appendix 12–2), and a *face sheet* (Appendix 12–3). These forms have been developed over many years of clinical practice. The forms may appear unfamiliar to many rheumatologists, but the rationale for selection of information in the forms will not. These forms may be used to develop the rheumatologist's own forms, evaluate or establish requirements for computer programs,[5] or create an outline or template for dictation.[6]

Each rheumatologist must define, record, and report data in a manner that satisfies his or her own documentation objectives. The rheumatologist must first definitively answer the next two questions: (1) What information does the rheumatologist require before the encounter? (2) What information does the rheumatologist want to have recorded at the end of the encounter? The resulting documentation should record and report this information on paper in the desired format? The emphasis on a paper report reflects the fact that most physicians are still using paper forms in their practices. We believe that although most computer programs can record "good" data, some cannot produce good reports, practical patient summaries, or useful progress notes.

Medical records should be designed to help physicians find relevant information rapidly and interpret it without error.[7] Forms are valuable tools for arranging information: Important data (allergies, current medications) appear first; fixing the position of data items is advantageous (i.e., it is easier to find an item by location than by label); standardized headings help physicians orient themselves in lengthy documents; structured text and tables reduce the risk of "losing" important details by laying out data; and the presence of data in a particular area of a form makes it easy to determine whether a clinical finding was made.[8]

Because proper information presentation complements form design, the rheumatologist should (1) identify the main purpose of the encounter; (2) use informative headings that aid interpretation and retrieval; (3) limit the information under a given heading (more subheadings with fewer data under each will be easier used than the reverse); (4) use specific locations for certain kinds of information; (5) mark abnormal values or adverse reactions with a highlighter or margin symbol; (6) use visual separators, such as lines or boxes, to distinguish instructions to other professionals, such as physical therapy or nurse orders, from other information; and (7) use vertical spacing and horizontal indenting to indicate the relationship between different parts of the record.[9]

The foregoing discussion assumes that questions have been asked to elicit the information necessary to complete the forms. Forms also serve as a reminder to ask the patients certain questions. The patient update, for example, ensures that the patient will always be asked a battery of questions regarding past medical, family, and social history. This questionnaire can be as elaborate as the rheumatologist prefers, allowing a trained medical assistant to perform a significant history and ensuring consistency in the quality of that history. The forms may also be useful in training. Structured forms may serve as reminders to perform examinations, assessments, and interventions.[10]

Like any business form, the template used to record medical information (paper or electronic) has basic requirements. A revision date should appear on the form, so that older forms are destroyed. A computer-generated form should contain the file name and the print date. Identifying information should appear uniformly on each form, preferably at the bottom for paper forms, and should include the name of the form, the name of the patient, the date of encounter, and a place

| ALLERGIES: | | | | | | |
|---|---|---|---|---|---|---|
| USING: ☐ WHEEL CHAIR ☐ WALKER ☐ CRUTCH(ES) ☐ CANE ☐ BRACE ☐ SPLINT    WITH: | | | | | | |
| VITAL SIGNS | BP SITTING | BP STANDING | | PULSE | PULSE REGULAR ☐ Y ☐ N | |
| | RR | HEIGHT    IN | | WEIGHT    LBS | TEMP    F | |
| MEDICATIONS (Rx and NON-Rx) | | | | | | |
| DMARDs/STEROIDS/NSAIDs/ANALGESICS | OTHER | | ANTIRESORPTIVE/BIRTH CONTROL/OTHER | | VITAMINS/SUPPLEMENTS | |
| | | | | | CALCIUM | |
| | | | | | MVI | |
| | | | | | | |
| | | | | | | |
| | | | | | | |
| | | | | | | |
| | | | | | | |

**FIGURE 12–1**
Progress Note: Allergies, assistive devices, vital signs, and medications.

for initial or signature by the provider. In large facilities, a unique patient identifying number may be necessary, although many practices can achieve this objective simply by using the patient's name and social security number. The names of the facility and the provider involved in each encounter should also appear on the form.[11]

In 1991, a committee of the Institute of Medicine proclaimed the computerized medical record as the standard for medical and all other records related to patient care.[12] Transition to computerized records seems inevitable, in view of the many benefits conferred by computerized data; however, it will be expensive and difficult.[13] It is not clear that computerization will be beneficial, inasmuch as more data do not guarantee better decisions or decision makers,[14] and the transition may take decades.[15] For most physicians, changing from a system with data maintained in paper records to computerized records will therefore be best achieved in a series of small, discrete, and manageable steps.[16] Indeed, for most rheumatologists, a combination of paper records and computerized data may be the most efficient system for the first few years of the transition.

Certain information is conducive to storage on a computer.[5] Patient-identifying information, demographics, diagnoses, and records of medications and allergies to medications are reproduced in one way or another at every encounter. Some of this information can be thought of as "static" data (i.e., data that does not have to be changed by the physician or office staff frequently). The names and dosages of medications tend to be "dynamic" data (i.e., information that changes frequently). Information can be stored in a database (where records for many patients are kept in one or more files) or simply in a "flat file," which is a word processing or spreadsheet format whereby each file contains the information on one patient. In either case, a data entry clerk can update the information after each encounter. It is considerably more cost effective for a clerk to perform data entry than for a physician to do so. The information is then available for the next encounter.

The progress note is actually used in this manner: The form is preprinted except for a blank area for medications, allergies, and the chief complaint (i.e., Figs. 12–1 and 12–2 are not on the preprinted form). Figures 12–1 and 12–2, containing the patient's medications, allergies, and established diagnoses, are stored on computer and printed on the form before the patient's visit. The form is therefore *independent* of the data. It can be designed quickly and changed easily to add or delete items. A physician with a computer can almost immediately implement this system. For even greater flexibility, a blank space can be left on the form for inserting dictation, allowing the rheumatologist to dictate portions of the encounter. From an efficiency standpoint, it takes significantly less time to "write" the medications and allergies in the progress note by computer than it does by hand; the time can be better spent confirming that the medication and allergy information recorded is correct.

## PROGRESS NOTE

The progress note is organized to monitor the patient through the office and to generally follow the traditional subjective, objective, assessment, and plan (SOAP) format familiar to all physicians.[17] Like most chart notes, allergies, medications, and vital signs precede the SOAP format to reflect workflow. They are followed by the chief complaint; history of present illness; review of systems; past medical, family, and social history; physical examination; assessment; and plan. The progress note is reviewed by section in the following discussion. Note that the objective section of the progress note in Appendix 12–1 does not contain all the detail included in the sections in the text.[18] The rheumatologist can decide whether a complex or simple objective section is preferable.

The progress note may be completed entirely by hand, or portions may be typed or inserted from computerized data. The items appearing at the top of the progress note (see Fig. 12–1) can be completed by a nurse or medical assistant. The nurse or medical assistant records allergies and whether any assistive devices are being used, the presence of which can indicate the functional level of the patient. The name of any person accompanying the patient into the examination room is also recorded after the designation "With:." An "observer" or "recorder" with the patient can help patient recall at a future time the information covered at the time of the encounter.[19] This person may also be a caregiver who can provide additional history or a family member who needs to be counseled with regard to the patient's limitations.

Allergies and medications are listed on the form before the visit, and each allergy and medication is reviewed individually with the patient. A check mark is placed by each allergy and medication to show that it is unchanged, or an appropriate annotation is added to indicate that the medication has been changed or discontinued and to indicate the reason for the change

| CHIEF COMPLAINT | |
| --- | --- |
| | |
| FOLLOW-UP (DIAGNOSIS): | |

**FIGURE 12–2**
Progress Note: Chief complaint.

(e.g., rash, taking too many medications, forgot to fill prescription). Vital signs are taken (weight is measured before the patient is brought to the examination room).

Many rheumatology patients are taking multiple medications as a consequence of their diagnosis, the effects of medications taken to treat the diagnosis, or both. The progress note makes it easier to review medications by providing four columns for medications under the following headings: (1) DMARDs/Steroids/NSAIDs/Analgesics,* (2) Other, (3) Antiresorptive/Birth Control/Other, and (4) Vitamins/Supplements. Of course, not all means of contraception are medications. Because knowledge of contraceptive practices is important, the absence of birth control is recorded (as "BC None") and the use of devices (condoms, diaphragms, intrauterine device) or vasectomy is listed. In recognition of the need for calcium and vitamin D supplementation by a significant portion of rheumatology patients and the elderly population in general, the right column has Calcium and MVI (for multivitamin) preprinted at the top of the column, which can be crossed out if not taken. Chart reminders such as this increase patient counseling.[19]

The advantages of this approach are obvious. The Vitamins/Supplements column of progress notes of patients taking methotrexate or leflunomide can be checked quickly to see whether the patient is receiving folic acid. For the patient taking prednisone, the rheumatologist can see quickly whether the Antiresorptive column lists estrogen or a bisphosphonate, and calcium and multivitamin use is immediately apparent. Computers offer the additional option of organizing the order of presentation of medications within each column as a further aid to the rheumatologist. For example, in the first column, the order would be DMARDs, prednisone, NSAIDs, and finally analgesics. An intended consequence of this uniform approach is that the rheumatologist can easily review every chart before seeing the patient, prompting the rheumatologist to ask certain questions, point out potential drug interactions, or counsel the patient to supplement his or her diet with additional calcium or vitamin D.

## Subjective

Documentation of the history includes the chief complaint; a history of present illness; review of systems; and past medical, family, and social history. The extent to which each type of history is documented is dependent on clinical judgment and the nature of the presenting problem.[20]

### Chief Complaint

The chief complaint is a "concise statement describing the symptom, problem, condition, diagnosis, physician-recommended return, or other problem that is the reason for the encounter."[21]

In a rheumatology practice, the chief complaint for the visit is usually the reason for the physician's recommendation of a return to monitor disease activity, response to therapy, medication toxicity, and the result of other services, such as orthopedic or other consultation, physical therapy, or counseling. If, however, the visit was scheduled for a new or worsening problem, the chief complaint should be described for the visit (e.g., worsening knee pain). The primary rheumatology diagnosis (e.g., rheumatoid arthritis) might also be evaluated at this "extra" visit, if medically necessary, in which case an assessment would be made for each diagnosis.

The next portion of the progress note (Fig. 12–2) incorporates information obtained from the update form (Appendix 12–2) completed by the patient at the time of the visit while in the waiting room. This patient-generated document includes an interim history (review of the past medical history, family history, and social history), the patient's assessment of his or her disease activity, and a review of systems. The nurse or medical assistant reviews the information with the patient to determine its accuracy and to obtain additional information.

### History of Present Illness

The history of present illness is a chronological description of the patient's present illness from the first sign or symptom, or from the previous encounter, to the present.[22] It includes the following elements: location (e.g., worst joint), quality (e.g., average overall quality of life), severity (e.g., pain and swelling), duration (e.g., morning stiffness), timing (e.g., frequency of flares), content, modifying factors (e.g., heat or cold), and associated signs and symptoms (e.g., fatigue) (Fig. 12–3).

### Review of Systems

A review of systems is "an inventory of body systems obtained through a series of questions seeking to identify signs and/or symptoms that the patient may be experiencing or has experienced."[23] For the purpose of the review of systems, the following systems are recognized: constitutional symptoms (e.g., weight loss, fever), eyes (e.g., dry, red, consistent with sicca syndrome), ear, nose, mouth, throat (e.g., oral ulcers found with lupus or methotrexate toxicity; tinnitus caused by NSAIDs), cardiovascular (e.g., chest pain secondary to pleuritis/pericarditis; palpitations caused by corticosteroids; hyperthyroidism), respiratory (e.g., cough, shortness of breath secondary to rheumatoid or methotrexate lung), gastrointestinal (e.g., stomach upset caused by NSAIDs, diarrhea caused by misoprostol), genitourinary (e.g., dysuria seen in Reiter's syndrome, hematuria seen in lupus), musculoskeletal (included in history of present illness for rheumatology patients), integumentary (skin; e.g., rash secondary to sun exposure in lupus patients), neurologic (e.g., headache caused by medications, insomnia secondary to fibromyalgia), psychiatric (e.g., depression secondary to chronic disease, anxiety secondary to denial of dis-

---

* DMARDs: disease-modifying antirheumatic drugs; NSAIDs: nonsteroidal anti-inflammatory drugs.

| HPI | 0 Not present | N New problem | Severity of Existing Problem | | Rate as compared to last visit | 1 Much Better | 2 Better | 3 Same | 4 Worse | 5 Much Worse |
|---|---|---|---|---|---|---|---|---|---|---|
| | Pain Severity: | | Swelling Severity: | AM Stiffness Duration: | Fatigue Associated s/sx: | | Worst Joint Location: | | Pt Assessment Quality: | |
| | | | | | | | | | | |
| | | | | | | | | | | |
| | | | | | | | | | | |

| ROS | ENMT | GI | Skin | Heme/Lymph | Neurologic | Respiratory | Eyes | Cardiovascular | Constitutional |
|---|---|---|---|---|---|---|---|---|---|
| | Tinnitus | GI upset | Rash | Bruising | Difficulty sleeping | Cough | Red | Chest pain | Fever |
| | Oral ulcer | Diarrhea | Ulcers | Swollen glands | Headache | SOB | Dry | Palpitations | Weight loss |
| | | | | | | | | | |
| | | | | | | | | | |
| | | | | | | | | | |

© Robin K. Dore, M.D., Inc. 1993, 1999 Reproduced with permission.

**FIGURE 12–3**
Progress Note: History of present illness and review of symptoms.

ease), endocrine (e.g., Hashimoto's thyroiditis, steroid-induced diabetes), heme/lymph (e.g., easy bruising caused by aspirin, swollen glands secondary to lupus), and allergy/immunology (e.g., recurrent infections, urticaria).

## Past Medical History, Family History, and Social History

The patient's past medical history, family history, and social history (Fig. 12–4) are initially elicited through the series of questions that are included on the patient update form (Appendix 12–2).

PAST MEDICAL HISTORY. A patient's past medical history includes prior illnesses, operations, injuries, hospitalizations, and treatment, including current medications.[24] This part of the patient update form is reviewed with the patient to make sure that medications are being taken as prescribed and to ascertain whether other medications have been prescribed, changed, or discontinued by another physician. Frequently this information discloses that the patient has decided to take or discontinue a medication without a physician's advice. If any proce-

dures or tests have been performed between visits, the medical assistant can request a copy of the results while the physician is examining the patient. Relevant data could include an upper gastrointestinal series demonstrating an ulcer, a peripheral dual energy x-ray absorptiometry (DEXA) or ultrasound study indicating that the patient is at risk for osteoporosis, or an elevated blood glucose level in a patient taking corticosteroids.

The repeated inquiry into the patient's medications, both prescription and nonprescription, as part of the medical history acknowledges that patients are sometimes reluctant to admit that they have discontinued medications or are not taking medications as prescribed. A patient may not want to hurt the physician's feelings or may be embarrassed to admit the inability to afford a medication. The reference to nonprescription medications may elicit admissions of over-the-counter NSAID use that may be contraindicated by prescription therapy.

FAMILY HISTORY. The patient's family history includes medical events in the patient's family, including death and health status, diseases that may be hereditary or could place the patient at risk, and diseases related to

| PFSH | Past Medical History (Since your last visit have you:) | Family/Social History | Allergy/Medication Changes |
|---|---|---|---|
| | ☐Yes ☐No Had any illnesses, injury | ☐Yes ☐No Any change in family history | ☐Yes ☐No Any new allergies or reaction to medication |
| | ☐Yes ☐No Seen any health care providers | ☐Yes ☐No Any change in social history | |
| | ☐Yes ☐No Had any ☐x-ray ☐lab ☐other proc | ☐Yes ☐No ☐N/A Are you postmenopausal | ☐Yes ☐No Any Rx or non-Rx meds not listed above |
| | | ☐Yes ☐No ☐N/A Are your menstrual periods regular | |
| | | | |
| | | | |
| | | | |

© Robin K. Dore, M.D., Inc. 1993, 1999 Reproduced with permission.

**FIGURE 12–4**
Progress Note: Past medical, family, and social history.

the patient's medical problems.[25] The occurrence of lupus in a sibling, a fracture in the mother, and a recent breast cancer in a first-degree relative are all relevant changes in family history that may influence a rheumatologist's care of a patient.

SOCIAL HISTORY. The patient's social history includes significant information about marital status; living arrangements; jobs; occupational exposure; use of drugs, alcohol, and tobacco; level of education; and sexual history.[26] Relevant changes in social history would include discontinuation of smoking or alcohol use, the latter enabling the patient to start methotrexate therapy. A patient's menopausal status should alert the rheumatologist to evaluate the patient for osteoporosis or consider whether some musculoskeletal symptoms may be menopause related.

## Objective

The objective portion of the rheumatology progress note reflects the detailed examination performed by the rheumatologist as part of the evaluation of a patient with chronic musculoskeletal disease and is, of necessity, complicated.

The progress note divides this examination into a vertical list (Fig. 12–5), to record notes on various organ systems/body areas, and grids (Figs. 12–6 and 12–7), to record findings of joint, spine, and nonarticular examinations. Lists of significant findings or exceptions to the norm are provided in Figure 12–5.[27] Selection of items listed for the organ systems/body areas examination reflects a significant subjective judgment regarding the items that are most frequently relevant to the rheumatology examination. Additional pertinent findings are added in writing at the time of the examination.

For a given disease, not all organ systems/body parts may be examined. For a patient with osteoarthritis, the pertinent part of the examination usually includes the abdomen (because obesity is a risk factor for osteoarthritis), the extremities (because varicosities can be seen in the obese osteoarthritis patient), constitutional (whether the patient appears to be in pain), skin (presence of a rash could indicate a drug reaction), psychiatric (whether the patient is depressed by the chronic pain), and musculoskeletal. Additional areas of examination of the patient with osteoarthritis with degenerative disc disease may include neurologic to evaluate the possibility of peripheral neuropathies, myelopathies, entrapment syndromes, and spinal stenosis. For the patient with fibromyalgia, the relevant body areas usually include constitutional, eyes (dry),

---

**OBJECTIVE**

| CONSTITUTIONAL        WNL ND | RESPIRATORY        WNL ND | SKIN        NL ND | PSYCHIATRIC        WNL ND | MUSCULOSKELETAL        WNL ND |
|---|---|---|---|---|
| VITAL SIGNS  See above | ☐ COUGH | ☐ DISCOID | ☐ AGITATED | GAIT ☐ ANTALGIC ☐ KYPHOTIC |
| GENERAL APPEARANCE | ☐ RUB | ☐ DRY | ☐ ANXIOUS | ☐ SLOW ☐ BROAD BASED |
| ☐ OLDER TSA | ☐ ACCESSORY MUSCLE USE | ☐ E NODOSUM | ☐ FLAT AFFECT | ☐ STANCE |
| ☐ YOUNGER TSA | ☐ WHEEZES | ☐ ECCHYMOSIS | | |
| ☐ CHRONICALLY ILL | ☐ RALES | ☐ ERYTHEMA | NEUROLOGIC        WNL ND | DEFORMITY/STABILITY   WNL ND |
| | ☐ RHONCHI | ☐ HIVES | ☐ CRANIAL NERVE PALSY | ☐ SHOULDER  SUBLUXATION |
| HEAD & FACE        WNL ND | ☐ ⇓ BREATH SOUNDS | ☐ JAUNDICE | ☐ DISORIENTED AS TO | ☐ ELBOW        HYPERMOBILE |
| ☐ ALOPECIA | ☐ TACTILE FREMITUS | ☐ MACULAR RASH | ☐ TIME ☐ PLACE ☐ PERSON | ☐ WRIST        RADIAL DEVIATION |
| ☐ CUSHINGOID | ☐ ABNL LUNG PERCUSSION | ☐ MALAR RASH | ☐ TREMOR | ☐ THUMB        SUBLUXATION |
| ☐ TEMPORAL ARTERIES TENDER | | ☐ NAIL PITTING | ☐ SPASTICITY | ☐ FINGERS        ULNAR DEVIATION |
| | CARDIOVASCULAR        WNL ND | ☐ ONYCHOLYSIS | ⇓ COORDINATION | SWAN-NECK    R 2 3 4 5  L 2 3 4 5 |
| EYES        WNL ND | ☐ IRREGULAR RHYTHM | ☐ PALE | ☐ UPPER  ☐ LOWER | BOUTONNIÈRE R 2 3 4 5  L 2 3 4 5 |
| ☐ CONJUNCTIVITIS | ☐ MURMUR | ☐ PETECHIAE | ⇓ DTRS | ☐ HIP        DISLOCATION |
| ☐ DRY EYES | ☐ RUB | ☐ PSORIASIS | ☐ UPPER  ☐ LOWER | KNEE |
| ☐ EPISCLERITIS | ☐ GALLOP | ☐ PURPURA | ⇓ PIN SENSATION | ☐ GENU VALGUS |
| ☐ IRITIS | | ☐ SCARS | ☐ UPPER  ☐ LOWER | ☐ GENU VARUS |
| | GI/ABDOMEN        WNL ND | ☐ SCLERODACTYLY | ⇓ PROPRIOCEPTION | ☐ BAKER'S CYST |
| ENMT        WNL ND | ☐ HEPATOMEGALY | ☐ TELANGIECTASIA | ☐ FINGER/NOSE ☐ HEEL/TOE | ☐ DRAWER SIGN |
| ☐ ⇓ HEARING | ☐ SPLENOMEGALY | ☐ ULCERS | ⇓ VIBRATION | ☐ MCMURRAY'S SIGN |
| ☐ NASAL POLYPS | ☐ MASSES | | ☐ UPPER  ☐ LOWER | ☐ HYPERMOBILE PATELLA |
| ☐ GINGIVITIS | ☐ TENDER | | ☐ MUSCLES  ☐ TENDER | ☐ SUBTALAR SUBLUXATION |
| ☐ ORAL ULCERS | ☐ OBESE | EXTREMITIES        WNL ND | ☐ ATROPHY ☐ FLACCID | ☐ FOOT    BUNION DEFORMITY |
| ☐ DRY MOUTH | ☐ PROTUBERANT | ☐ CLUBBING | ☐ WEAKNESS | HAMMER TOES R 2 3 4 5  L 2 3 4 5 |
| ☐ ABNL TYMPANIC MEMBRANE | ☐ ABNL BOWEL SOUNDS | ☐ CYANOSIS | ☐ UPPER ☐ Proximal ☐ Distal | |
| ☐ SALIVARY GLAND ENLARGED | ☐ HERNIA | ☐ EDEMA | ☐ LOWER ☐ Proximal ☐ Distal | MS EXAM CONTINUED ON NEXT PAGE |
| | | ☐ LEG LENGTH ≠ | | © ROBIN K. DORE, M.D., INC 1993 1999 |
| NECK        WNL ND | LYMPHATIC        WNL ND | ☐ PERIUNGUAL ERYTHEMA | EXTREMITIES        CONT'D | |
| ☐ THYROID ENLARGED | ☐ AXILLA | ☐ PULSES ⇓ UPPER LOWER | ☐ TEMP ⇑ UPPER LOWER | BREAST, RECTAL |
| ☐ THYROID TENDER | ☐ GROIN | ☐ RHEUMATOID NODULES | ☐ TEMP ⇓ UPPER LOWER | AND GENITOURINARY |
| ☐ MASSES | ☐ NECK | FINGER        COCCYX | ☐ TOPHI | NOT EXAMINED |
| | ☐ SUPRACLAVICULAR | ELBOW        KNEE | ☐ VARICOSITIES | WNL  WITHIN NORMAL LIMITS |
| | | OCCIPUT        FOOT | | ND    NOT DONE |

© Robin K. Dore, M.D., Inc. 1993, 1999 Reproduced with permission.

**FIGURE 12–5**
Progress Note: Examination of organ systems/body areas.

Items not marked are normal.   Items crossed through not examined.          CH PN Form Page 2 AA doc February 27, 1999 2/27/99 8:15 AM  Page 2 of 2

| | □WNL □ND | Swelling | | Tender | | | | | | ROM □ROM not examined | | | | | | | Fingers/Toes | | | | | | | | | | | | |
|---|---|---|---|---|---|---|---|---|---|---|---|---|---|---|---|---|---|---|---|---|---|---|---|---|---|---|---|---|---|
| | Joint | R | L | R | L | Warm | Ery | Eff | Pain | Crep | ↓Fl/DF | ↓Ex/PF | ↓InRot | ↓ExRot | ↓ABd | Joint | S | 1 | 2 | 3 | 4 | 5 | T | 1 | 2 | 3 | 4 | 5 |
| JOINT EXAM | TMJ | | | | | | | | | | | | | | | MCP | R | | | | | | R | | | | | |
| | GHJ | | | | | | | | | | | | | | | | L | | | | | | L | | | | | |
| | SCJ | | | | | | | | | | | | | | | PIP | R | | | | | | R | | | | | |
| | ACJ | | | | | | | | | | | | | | | | L | | | | | | L | | | | | |
| | Elbow | | | | | | | | | | | | | | | DIP | R | | | | | | R | | | | | |
| | Wrist | | | | | | | | | | | | | | | | L | | | | | | L | | | | | |
| | CMCs | | | | | | | | | | | | | | | MTP | R | | | | | | R | | | | | |
| | Hip | | | | | | | | | | | | | | | | L | | | | | | L | | | | | |
| | Knee | | | | | | | | | | | | | | | IP | R | | | | | | R | | | | | |
| | Ankle | | | | | | | | | | | | | | | | L | | | | | | L | | | | | |
| | Subtalar | | | | | | | | | | | | | | | Warm | Right | □Hand □Foot | | | | Left | □Hand □Foot | | | | | |

© Robin K. Dore, M.D., Inc. 1993, 1999 Reproduced with permission.

**FIGURE 12–6**
Progress Note: Joint examination.

mouth (dry), extremities (leg length discrepancy), skin (mottled), psychiatric (depressed), neurologic (hypesthesia), and the nonarticular examination (to be discussed). These same body areas are usually examined in patients with rheumatoid arthritis and ankylosing spondylitis, except with emphasis on deformities, the spine, and synovitis in the musculoskeletal examination. Most of the body areas are examined in patients with lupus, scleroderma, Sjögren's syndrome, polymyositis, reactive arthritis, and vasculitis.

The joint examination (see Fig. 12–6) is documented by recording significant findings or exceptions to the norm. This format is used because it offers the opportunity to count tender and swollen joints, providing the rheumatologist with a means of assessing the patient's disease activity. Other diagrammatic options include a homunculus. In Figure 12–6, the total numbers of tender and swollen joints are recorded. Swollen joints may be checked to indicate the presence or absence of soft tissue or bony swelling and the degree of swelling may be scored by a predefined scale, such as 1 to 4. Warmth, erythema, and effusion may be recorded for certain joints. Range of motion is also examined, allowing for recording of pain or crepitation on range of motion and decreased range of motion.

The spine examination and the nonarticular examination are reported (see Fig. 12–7). Tenderness, range of motion, and deformities of the spine may be recorded. The nonarticular examination contains a column to record the results of an 18-item tender point examination. In the assessment (see Fig. 12–9), the total of tender points can be recorded.

## ASSESSMENT

The rheumatologist's clinical impression is frequently based on information obtained from diagnostic tests performed by the rheumatologist or others or from evaluations performed by others, such as consultations or diagnostic reports. Additional information is sometimes obtained from a review of additional records pertaining to the patient or from discussions with caregivers, such as family members or friends of the patient. Written and oral communications with other health care providers, including physicians, physical therapists, and home health nurses, may also be a source of relevant clinical information. Review of this material can be recorded in Figure 12–8. If the recom-

| | □WNL □ND | Tender | | ROM↓ | Pain | Crep | Deformity/Stability | | □WNL □ND | T | S | Tense | | T | S | |
|---|---|---|---|---|---|---|---|---|---|---|---|---|---|---|---|---|
| SPINE EXAM | C Spine | C3  C4 | | R Lat | □ | □ | Buffalo hump | NONARTICULAR EXAM | Occiput | | | Bicipital tendon | | | | KEY |
| | | C5  C6 | | L Lat | □ | □ | Straightening | | Low cervical | | | Subdeltoid bursa | | | | |
| | | C7 | | Flexion | □ | □ | Lordosis | | Trapezius | | | Achilles tendon | | | | S = SWELLING |
| | | | | Extension | □ | □ | | | Supraspinatus | | | Olecranon bursa | | | | |
| | D Spine | T 1 2 3 4 | | Chest | □ | | Kyphosis | | Second rib | | | | | | | |
| | | 5 6 7 8 9 | | expansion | | | Scoliosis | | Lateral epicondyle | | | | | | | T = TENDER |
| | | 10 11 12 | | | | | | | Gluteal | | | | | | | |
| | L/S Spine | L1  L2 | | R Lat | □ | | Lordosis | | Gr trochanter femur | | | | | | | |
| | | L3  L4 | | L Lat | □ | | Scoliosis | | Anserine bursa | | | | | | | |
| | | L5  S1 | | Flexion | □ | | | | | | | | | | | |
| | | | | Extension | □ | | | | | | | | | | | |
| | S/I Joints | □ Right □ Left | | Compression sign | | | | | | | | | | | | |

© Robin K. Dore, M.D., Inc. 1993, 1999 Reproduced with permission.

**FIGURE 12–7**
Progress Note: Spine examination; nonarticular examination.

| REVIEW | INSIDE | ☐DEXA   ☐LAB THIS VISIT: ☐CBC   ☐UA   ☐ESR   LAST VISIT: ☐CBC   ☐UA   ☐ESR | | |
|---|---|---|---|---|
| | OUTSIDE: | ☐LAB   CBC  UA  ESR  HEMOCCULT RA  ANA  CMP  CPK  CRP  Lipid HLA B27  C3  C4  DNA  ACLA  SSA  SSB  CRYOS  OTHER | | |
| | | ☐REPORT ☐MRI ☐CT ☐X-ray ☐DEXA ☐PT ☐Consultation ☐Other | | |
| | REQUEST RECORDS:         ADDITIONAL RECORDS REVIEWED: | | RELEVANT FINDINGS: ☐NO ☐YES: | |
| | OBTAIN ADDITIONAL HISTORY FROM FAMILY/CAREGIVER: | | RELEVANT FINDINGS: ☐NO ☐YES: | |
| | REVIEW RESULTS WITH PHYSICIANS WHO PERFORMED/INTERPRETED TESTS: | | | |
| | DIRECT VISUALIZATIONS OF X-RAY/INDEPENDENT INTERPRETATION OF IMAGE, TRACING, OR SPECIMEN:         OTHER: | | | |

© Robin K. Dore, M.D., Inc. 1993, 1999 Reproduced with permission.

**FIGURE 12–8**
Progress Note: Diagnostic and other review.

mendations of a consultant are not followed, it should be documented why a different course is taken.[18]

After the rheumatologist has completed review of the patient's history and available diagnostic tests and has examined the patient, an assessment or clinical impression of the patient's status must be made. Most encounters involve an established diagnosis, which is the first column in the assessment table shown in Figure 12–9. The heading Presenting Problem/Established Diagnosis is derived from the CPT Assistant, as are the values "worse," "improved," and "stable." The difficulty with the term *stable* is that many diseases may be stable, *active* diseases, and a stable disease involves ongoing disease activity and progression. The term *stable* must therefore be understood to mean stable disease with ongoing disease activity. The reason for improvement or worsening is sometimes evident from the patient's history and may be noted next to the assessment. Intense physical activity (such as moving furniture), extended care of a family member, and failure to take medications are frequently reasons why a patient's condition worsens.

If the patient has developed a new problem, assessment can include whether to perform a work-up for the problem, to refer the patient to another physician for evaluation, or to perform no evaluation but to treat the patient empirically. The need to seek advice from others may be an indication of complex management options. The number of possible diagnoses or the number of management options that must be considered adds to the complexity of medical decision making. Problems that are improving or resolving are less complex than those that are worsening or failing to improve

as expected. The number and type of diagnostic tests ordered may be an indication of the complexity of the patient's problem.

## PLAN

After the diagnoses and the data that support them are listed, the plan for future care of the patient needs to be documented. Room is provided for documenting the reason for ordering further tests and ancillary services. Plan documentation traditionally focused on the management and treatment steps, which were discussed with the patient. It is now necessary to document these *discussions* as well as the diagnostic aspects of the plan.

*Counseling* is the umbrella term that has been selected by CPT to cover this very broad range of physician-patient discussions.[28] Because these discussions logically follow assessment and management, they are located in the plan area of the progress note under a counseling sidebar. Because of the length of the plan portion of the note, it is separated into two figures: Plan Management (Fig. 12–10) and Plan Counseling (Fig. 12–11).

The management portion of the plan can be organized in any sequence satisfactory to the rheumatologist. "Lab" is listed first because laboratory studies may need to be performed at the beginning of the visit in order to make determinations about patient treatment and side effects. "Lab today," "interim lab," and "lab at the next visit" are plan options. Although this form lists various laboratory actions, others can

| | Presenting Problem/Established Diagnosis | Worse | Improved | Stable | New Diagnosis | New Diagnosis | New Presenting Problem Undiagnosed |
|---|---|---|---|---|---|---|---|
| ASSESSMENT | | | | | Self-Limited | No workup planned | Possible Dx |
| | | | | | Minor | | Probable Dx |
| | | | | | SWOLLEN JOINTS | | Rule out Dx |
| | | | | | TENDER JOINTS | | Differential diagnosis |
| | | | | | TENDER JOINTS | | |

© Robin K. Dore, M.D., Inc. 1993, 1999 Reproduced with permission.

**FIGURE 12–9**
Progress Note: Assessment.

| PLAN | LAB | TODAY | ☐ TOXICITY ☐ DZ ACTIVITY ☐ Dx  CBC  UA  ESR  HEMOCCULT RA  ANA  CMP  CPK  CRP  Lipids  Hepatic profile  Creatinine  OTHER |
|------|-----|-------|------------------------------|
| | | INTERIM | ☐ TOXICITY ☐ DZ ACTIVITY ☐ Dx  CBC  UA  ESR  HEMOCCULT RA  ANA  CMP  CPK  CRP  Lipids  Hepatic profile  Creatinine  OTHER |
| | | NEXT VISIT | ☐ TOXICITY ☐ DZ ACTIVITY ☐ Dx  CBC  UA  ESR  HEMOCCULT RA  ANA  CMP  CPK  CRP  Lipids  Hepatic profile  Creatinine  OTHER |

**MEDICATION**

| CURRENT MEDICATIONS | NEW MEDICATIONS |
|---|---|
| ☐ No change   ☐ Change   ☐ Change: Problem requiring change | ☐ No   ☐ New Meds Rxed   ☐ Problem requiring medication |
| | |
| | |
| | |

Samples:                                    Gave patient: ☐ Package insert  ☐ Pamphlet:

**INJECTION**

TRIGGER-POINT INJECTION: After sterile preparation ☐ 2 cc of 1% Xylocaine and 1 cc of Aristospan 20 mg per cc or ☐ 3 cc of 1% Xylocaine were injected into:

ASPIRATION:       Aspiration: ☐ No fluid or ☐    cc of fluid was aspirated prior to the injection
                              Fluid was ☐ clear ☐ yellow ☐ thick ☐ thin ☐ cloudy ☐ bloody.
FOLLOWED BY                   ☐ Patient told to apply heat 2x today, 20 min each time, to inj site.
INJECTION:       Injection:   After sterile preparation ☐ 1/4 cc ☐ 1/2 cc ☐ 1 cc of each of 1% Xylocaine
                              and Aristospan 20 mg per cc were injected into:

**REFERRAL**

☐ MEDICAL   ☐ SURGICAL   ☐ PHYSICAL THERAPY
☐ MENTAL HEALTH COUNSELING

☐ EXERCISE CLASS   ☐ SUPPORT GROUP
☐ OTHER

**ORDER**

☐ X-RAY   ☐ MRI   ☐ CT
☐ DEXA   ☐ APPLIANCES   ☐ OTHER

**RETURN**     DAYS |     WEEKS |     MONTHS | ☐ OTHER:        SIGNED ROBIN K. DORE, M.D.

**PROGRESS NOTE**     PATIENT NAME                              DATE OF VISIT

© Robin K. Dore, M.D., Inc. 1993, 1999 Reproduced with permission.

**FIGURE 12–10**
Progress Note: Plan—management.

| PLAN | COUNSELING | Risk Factor ⇓ Education | ☐ Diet   ☐ Wt Loss <br> ☐ Exercise  ☐ Other |
|------|-----------|----|----|

☐ BROCHURES     ☐ MATERIALS |

**Advice**

Discussed with patient ☐ NEW MED ☐ EXISTING MED ☐ INJECTION ☐ REFERRAL ☐ ORDER ☐ OTHER
☐ Diagnosis/suspected Dx     ☐ Nature/purpose     ☐ Risks/side effects
☐ Monitoring requirements - visits and lab tests
☐ Probability of success     ☐ Reasonable alternatives
☐ Possible consequences if advice/referral/order not followed/no treatment
☐ Review the diagnosis/purpose/risks/prob of success/alternatives etc of surgery/procedure with the surgeon/provider.

**Visit summary:**

REVIEWED WITH PATIENT  ☐ EXAMINATION/FINDINGS
☐ ASSESSMENT/PROGNOSIS     ☐ PLAN

**Patient Questions**

**RETURN**     DAYS |     WEEKS |     MONTHS | ☐ OTHER:        SIGNED ROBIN K. DORE, M.D.

**PROGRESS NOTE**     PATIENT NAME                              DATE OF VISIT

© Robin K. Dore, M.D., Inc. 1993, 1999 Reproduced with permission.

**FIGURE 12–11**
Progress Note: Plan—counseling.

be listed or laboratory tests simply recorded. Of importance are the reasons for the laboratory test. Laboratory tests may be ordered to monitor toxicity of medications, to monitor disease activity, or to make a diagnosis. This distinction is important because the diagnosis code may differ for the same laboratory test, depending on the purpose of the test. Recording the laboratory test for the encounter date is, in effect, the written order for that test. Recording the laboratory test for the next visit allows the laboratory technician to draw appropriate specimens at the next visit without awaiting additional instructions from the rheumatologist. Interim laboratory tests may be required to monitor disease activity or toxicity between visits or may be ordered in advance of the next visit so that laboratory results are available to the rheumatologist before the visit.

Medication changes that are based on the rheumatologist's evaluation of the effectiveness or toxicity of a medication are an important part of most patient encounters. The decision to change a current medication is considered more complex. Plans regarding medications may be documented simply by checking "No change" in current medications and "No" to new medications. If a current medication is changed, the reason for the change should be recorded. The reason for prescribing a new medication should be recorded (e.g., gastrointestinal toxicity with previous NSAID). Ideally, the indication for use should be listed for each new medication. Because patients frequently stop medications that they are then instructed to restart, it is common to note under current medications "Restart NSAID," often accompanied by the notation "Don't self medicate!" Samples are frequently dispensed to patients. A place to record this activity and whether the patient was given product information and relevant pamphlets for the medication is provided in the plan.

Trigger-point injections and joint aspirations are frequently required at patient encounters. Although these may be documented separately, it is sometimes convenient to record them in the progress note. If an injection is documented in this manner, the specific medications used by the rheumatologist should be included on the template. If the injection is given for a problem separate from the reason for the visit, a separate diagnosis should be listed as the reason for the injection (e.g., knee pain in a patient with rheumatoid arthritis).

Areas to record referrals and orders are also provided. These are somewhat arbitrarily separated; referrals are more likely to involve interaction between a caregiver and the patient.

The counseling (or patient discussion) portion of the plan follows. Risk factor reduction is an important component of patient care; such "counseling" deals with "interventions that address patients' personal health practices": that is, prevention strategies or risk factor reduction, particularly in areas likely to contribute to premature death, such as tobacco use, diet, and physical activity patterns; alcohol use; ingestion of antimicrobial agents and toxic agents; use of firearms; sexual behavior; and use of illicit drugs.[29] Educating patients about their chronic disease is also an important element of patient care. Use of patient education materials, particularly Arthritis Foundation pamphlets, is common among rheumatologists.

The advice portion of the plan may pertain to the prescription of new medications and to discussions regarding existing medications, injections, referrals, or orders. The purpose of this area is to document discussions between the rheumatologist and the patient addressing the actions taken by the rheumatologist. Because this discussion has medical-legal implications, it should be reviewed to ensure that it meets the requirements of the laws and customs applicable to the community in which the rheumatologist practices.[30]

In the context of the medications, it is important to discuss the patient's diagnosis or suspected diagnosis, the nature and purpose of the medications, the risks and side effects of the medications, monitoring requirements, probability of success, treatment alternatives, and possible consequences of no treatment. In the case of surgical or other procedures, it may be appropriate to remind the patient to discuss these issues with the surgeon or other provider.

The plan concludes with a visit summary notation, an area for patient questions, and provisions for when a return visit will take place. The purpose of the visit summary is to document that the rheumatologist has reviewed with the patient the results of the examination; laboratory, other diagnostic, and nondiagnostic findings; and the rheumatologist's assessment of the patient and treatment plan. Although this has always been performed in the course of an encounter, the traditional SOAP note did not contain a separate note to this effect. After the rheumatologist's summary of the visit, it is logical for the patient to have questions. Indeed, it is common to complete the summary with the inquiry to the patient, "Do you have any questions?" If the answer is no, the rheumatologist simply checks that response. Otherwise, the patient's questions and the rheumatologist's responses should be recorded.

## PATIENT UPDATE AND FACE SHEET

The patient update has been discussed in the context of the progress note. When use of a patient questionnaire was initiated, there was some concern about whether patients would be willing to complete this form. It was correctly concluded that because others had successfully incorporated sophisticated self-report questionnaires into their clinical practice,[31] there would be little resistance by patients to this short inquiry. Although such questionnaires are currently not used by many rheumatology practices, it is anticipated that low-cost software, combined with scannable forms or touch-screen devices, will lead to wider use.

The face sheet is somewhat analogous to what has been described as a datasheet and may be useful in the care of some or all patients. In this practice it differs from a datasheet because it does not list the patient's allergies and medications. These are instead listed on the progress note. The face sheet contains pertinent diagnoses and laboratory results relating to rheumatic diseases. A list of the patient's medical problems is included under "comorbid conditions," which can serve as evidence of the severity of the patient's overall medical condition. Fractures, surgeries, injuries, and hospitalizations may also be listed, together with pertinent family and social history. Signs and symptoms of rheumatoid arthritis, lupus, seronegative spondyloarthropathies, or fibromyalgia syndrome may be identified. This information can be updated concurrently from the progress note or periodically.

The face sheet is particularly useful for responding to third-party requests for information. Disability is frequently equated with positive results of laboratory serologic tests. Summarization of laboratory information answers many information requests. Medication formulary restrictions and prior approval by insurers of medication prescriptions have greatly increased the need for lists of discontinued medications. Use of certain antiresorptive agents requires evidence of low bone mass.

## CONCLUSION

Fortunately for the rheumatologist, it is not necessary to convert overnight to electronic medical records. To do so would not be possible or prudent. Instead, the rheumatologist must consider the best interests of his or her patients, carefully review his or her documentation needs and available resources, and plan accordingly.

For most practices, implementation of a system of preprinted forms that, at once or over time, may be completed in part from a computerized database or by word processor should increase the efficiency of the practice. This system also provides an introduction into the new so-called science of clinical informatics: the application of information technologies to improve how data, information, and knowledge are managed, in the interest of continuously improving patient care processes and outcomes.[14] Building on this experience, the rheumatologist will be able to evaluate his or her documentation requirements and to determine whether and to what degree additional computerization of the practice's medical records is required.

A look back over the 1990s suggests that rheumatologists have adapted fairly well to their changing environment and should be somewhat circumspect about changes that "must be made" in health care or things that "must be done" in order to survive. The key is to remember Dr. John Sergent's admonition in his presidential address to the American College of Rheumatology, which needs no citation: that it is "the patient" we must satisfy.[32]

## REFERENCES

1. Hand RW: Editorial: E&M Guidelines: Is the medical record a database repository or a communications tool? Chest 1998; 113(6):1432.
2. Liang MH, Shadick N: Feasibility and utility of adding disease-specific outcome measures to administrative databases to improve disease management. Ann Intern Med 1997; 127:739–742.
3. Nathan R: Are we taking care of our patients—or charts? Med Economics 1997; 74(8):201–203.
4. American Medical Association: Revised Documentation Guidelines for Evaluation and Management Services. CPT Assistant 1997; 7(7):3 (Revised October 1997).
5. Fischer JS, Blonde L: Electronic medical records in clinical practice. Clin Diabetes 1999; 17(1):43.
6. Ewy GA: Patient datasheet and generic evaluation tools. Clin Cardiol 1997; 20(3):273.
7. Wyatt JC, Wright P: Design should help use of patients' data. Lancet 1998; 352:1375–1378.
8. Nygren E, Wyatt JC, Wright P: Helping clinicians find data and avoid delays. Lancet 1998; 352:1462–1466.
9. Wright P, Jansen C, Wyatt JC: How to limit clinical errors in interpretation of data. Lancet 1998; 352:1539–1543.
10. Shiffman RN, Brandt CA, Freeman BG: Transition to computer-based records using scannable, structured encounter forms. Arch Pediatr Adolesc Med 1997; 151(12):1247–1253.
11. Rhodes HB: Issue: Developing information capture tools. J AHIMA, Practice Briefs 1997; page 2.
12. The Institute of Medicine: The Computer-Based Patient Record, an Essential Technology for Health Care. Washington, DC: National Academy Press, 1991.
13. Powsner SM, Wyatt JC, Wright P: Opportunities for and challenges of computerisation. Lancet 1998; 352:1617–1622.
14. Kibbe DC, Bard M: Applying clinical informatics to health care improvement: Making progress is more difficult than we thought it would be. J Qual Improv 1997; 23(12):619–622.
15. Kibbe DC, Bard M: A roundtable discussion: Have computerized patient records kept their promise of improving patient care? J Qual Improv 1997; 23(12):695–702.
16. Weintraub WS: A "wheel and spoke" network for medical records: The Emory Heart Center experience. J Invas Cardiol 1998; 10(8):501–505.
17. Weed LL: Records that guide and teach. N Engl J Med 1968; 30(5):593–600.
18. Burton K: Your memory/your patient's memory and your medical records. W Va Med J 1997; 92(6):308–309.
19. Chang JC, Zimmerman LJ, Beck JM: Impact of chart reminders on smoking cessation practices of pulmonary physicians. Am J Respir Crit Care Med 1995; 152(3):984–987.
20. American Medical Association: Current Procedural Terminology, 4th ed (professional edition). Chicago: American Medical Association, 1999:6.
21. American Medical Association: Chief complaint. In Current Procedural Terminology, 4th ed (professional edition). Chicago: American Medical Association, 1999:1.
22. American Medical Association: History of present illness. In Current Procedural Terminology, 4th ed (professional edition). Chicago: American Medical Association, 1999:2.
23. American Medical Association: System review (review of systems). In Current Procedural Terminology, 4th ed (professional edition). Chicago: American Medical Association, 1999:3.
24. American Medical Association: Past history. In Current Procedural Terminology, 4th ed (professional edition). Chicago: American Medical Association, 1999:3.
25. American Medical Association: Family history. In Current Procedural Terminology, 4th ed (professional edition). Chicago: American Medical Association, 1999:2.
26. American Medical Association: Social history. In Current Procedural Terminology, 4th ed (professional edition). Chicago: American Medical Association, 1999:3.
27. Charles EJ: Charting by exception. J Am Dent Assoc 1997; 97(10):S131.
28. American Medical Association: Counseling. In Current Procedural Terminology, 4th ed (professional edition). Chicago: American Medical Association, 1999:2.
29. Introduction. In Clinician's Handbook of Preventive Services, 2nd ed. Washington, DC: US Department of Health and Human Services, 1998:xxiv.
30. Gibofsky A: Liability issues in the treatment of patients with rheumatic diseases. Am J Med 1997; 102(suppl 1A):40S–42S.
31. Pincus T: Documenting quality management in rheumatic disease: Are patient questionnaires the best (and only) method? Arthritis Care Res 1996; 9(5):339–348.
32. Sergent JS: It's the patient, stupid. Arthritis Rheum 1994; 37: 449–453.

# APPENDIX 12–1: PROGRESS NOTE

| ALLERGIES: | | | | | | | |
|---|---|---|---|---|---|---|---|
| USING: | ☐ WHEEL CHAIR | ☐ WALKER | ☐ CRUTCH(ES) | ☐ CANE  ☐ BRACE | ☐ SPLINT | WITH: | |

| VITAL SIGNS | BP SITTING | BP STANDING | PULSE | PULSE REGULAR  ☐ Y  ☐ N |
|---|---|---|---|---|
| | RR | HEIGHT          IN | WEIGHT          LBS | TEMP                    F |

## MEDICATIONS

| DMARDs/Steroids/NSAIDs/Analgesics | Other | Antiresorptive/Birth Control/Other | Vitamins/Supplements |
|---|---|---|---|
| | | | CALCIUM |
| | | | MVI |
| | | | |
| | | | |

### SUBJECTIVE: CHIEF COMPLAINT

### FOLLOW-UP (DIAGNOSIS):

0 Not present   N New problem   Severity of Existing Problem.   Rate as compared to last visit   1 Much Better   2 Better   3 Same   4 Worse   5 Much Worse

**HPI**

| Pain Severity: | Swelling Severity: | AM Stiffness Duration: | Fatigue Associated s/sx: | Worst Joint Location: | Pt Assessment Quality: |
|---|---|---|---|---|---|

**ROS**

| ENMT | GI | Skin | Heme/Lymph | Neurologic | Respiratory | Eyes | Cardiovascular | Constitutional |
|---|---|---|---|---|---|---|---|---|
| Tinnitus | GI upset | Rash | Bruising | Difficulty sleeping | Cough | Red | Chest pain | Fever |
| Oral ulcer | Diarrhea | Ulcers | Swollen glands | Headache | SOB | Dry | Palpitations | Weight loss |

**PFSH**

Past Medical History (Since your visit have you:)
☐ Yes ☐ No   Had any illnesses, injury
☐ Yes ☐ No   Seen any health care providers
☐ Yes ☐ No   Had any ☐ x-ray ☐ lab
                     ☐ other procedures

Family/Social History
☐ Yes ☐ No   Any change in family history
☐ Yes ☐ No   Any change in social history
☐ Yes ☐ No ☐ N/A   Are you postmenopausal
☐ Yes ☐ No ☐ N/A   Are your menstrual
                                 periods regular

Allergy/Medication Changes
☐ Yes ☐ No   Any new allergies or reaction to
                     medication
☐ Yes ☐ No   Any Rx or non-Rx meds not listed
                     above

---

CONSTITUTIONAL          WNL ND

HEAD & FACE          WNL ND

EYES          WNL ND

ENMT          WNL ND

NECK          WNL ND

RESPIRATORY          WNL ND

CARDIOVASCULAR          WNL ND

GI/ABDOMEN          WNL ND

LYMPHATIC          WNL ND

EXTREMITIES          WNL ND

SKIN          WNL ND

PSYCHIATRIC          WNL ND

NEUROLOGIC          WNL ND

BREAST, RECTAL
AND GENITOURINARY
NOT EXAMINED

WNL   WITHIN NORMAL LIMITS
ND    NOT DONE

PAGE 1 OF 2

MUSCULOSKELETAL          WNL ND

GAIT ☐ ANTALGIC ☐ KYPHOTIC
          ☐ SLOW ☐ BROAD BASED
☐ STANCE

DEFORMITY/STABILITY   WNL ND
☐ SHOULDER          SUBLUXATION
☐ ELBOW               HYPERMOBILE
☐ WRIST                RADIAL DEVIATION
☐ THUMB               SUBLUXATION
☐ FINGERS             ULNAR DEVIATION
SWAN-NECK      R 2 3 4 5   L 2 3 4 5
BOUTONNIÈRE   R 2 3 4 5   L 2 3 4 5
☐ HIP                       DISLOCATION
KNEE
          ☐ GENU VALGUS
          ☐ GENU VARUS
          ☐ BAKER'S CYST
          ☐ DRAWER SIGN
          ☐ MCMURRAY'S SIGN
          ☐ HYPERMOBILE PATELLA
☐ SUBTALAR SUBLUXATION
☐ FOOT               BUNION DEFORMITY
HAMMER TOES   R 2 3 4 5   L 2 3 4 5

MS EXAM CONTINUED ON NEXT PAGE

| PROGRESS NOTE          PATIENT: | SEX:          AGE:          DATE: | RKD INITIALS: |
|---|---|---|

Items not marked are normal.  Items crossed through not examined                    CH PN Form Page 2 AA. doc February 27, 1999 2/27/99 8:15:00 AM Page 2 of 2

## JOINT EXAM

| Joint | □WNL □ND Swelling R | L | Tender R | L | Warm | Ery | Eff | ROM Pain | Crep | ↓Fl/DF | ↓Ex/PF | ↓InRot | ↓ExRot | ↓ABd | Joint | S | 1 | 2 | 3 | 4 | 5 | T | 1 | 2 | 3 | 4 | 5 |
|---|---|---|---|---|---|---|---|---|---|---|---|---|---|---|---|---|---|---|---|---|---|---|---|---|---|---|---|
| TMJ | | | | | | | | | | | | | | | MCP R | | | | | | | R | | | | | |
| GHJ | | | | | | | | | | | | | | | L | | | | | | | L | | | | | |
| SCJ | | | | | | | | | | | | | | | PIP R | | | | | | | R | | | | | |
| ACJ | | | | | | | | | | | | | | | L | | | | | | | L | | | | | |
| Elbow | | | | | | | | | | | | | | | DIP R | | | | | | | R | | | | | |
| Wrist | | | | | | | | | | | | | | | L | | | | | | | L | | | | | |
| CMCs | | | | | | | | | | | | | | | MTP R | | | | | | | R | | | | | |
| Hip | | | | | | | | | | | | | | | L | | | | | | | L | | | | | |
| Knee | | | | | | | | | | | | | | | IP R | | | | | | | R | | | | | |
| Ankle | | | | | | | | | | | | | | | L | | | | | | | L | | | | | |
| Subtalar | | | | | | | | | | | | | | | Warm Right □Hand □Foot  Left □Hand □Foot | | | | | | | | | | | | |

ROM □ROM not examined                    Fingers/Toes

## SPINE EXAM

| □WNL □ND Tender | ROM↓ Pain Crep | Deformity/Stability |
|---|---|---|
| C Spine  C3 C4 / C5 C6 / C7 | R Lat □ □ / L Lat □ □ / Flexion □ □ / Extension □ □ | Buffalo hump / Straightening / Lordosis |
| D Spine  T 1 2 3 4 / 5 6 7 8 9 / 10 11 12 | Chest □ expansion | Kyphosis / Scoliosis |
| L/S Spine  L1 L2 / L3 L4 / L5 S1 | R Lat □ / L Lat □ / Flexion □ / Extension □ | Lordosis / Scoliosis / Schober's |
| S/I Joints  □ Right □ Left | Compression sign | |

## NONARTICULAR EXAM

| □WNL □ND | T | S | Tense | | T | S |
|---|---|---|---|---|---|---|
| Occiput | | | Bicipital tendon | | | |
| Low cervical | | | Subdeltoid bursa | | | |
| Trapezius | | | Achilles tendon | | | |
| Supraspinatus | | | Olecranon bursa | | | |
| Second rib | | | | | | |
| Lateral epicondyle | | | | | | |
| Gluteal | | | | | | |
| Gr trochanter femur | | | | | | |
| Anserine bursa | | | | | | |

KEY  T = TENDER  S = SWELLING

## REVIEW

INSIDE          □ Lab     □ X-ray     □ DEXA                        CLINICALLY SIGNIFICANT FINDINGS:

OUTSIDE:     □ Lab     □ Report     □ MRI     □ CT     □ X-ray     □ DEXA     □ PT     □ Consultation     □ Other                        CLINICALLY SIGNIFICANT FINDINGS:

REQUEST RECORDS:                    ADDITIONAL RECORDS REVIEWED:                        RELEVANT FINDINGS: □ No  □ Yes

OBTAIN ADDITIONAL HISTORY FROM FAMILY/CAREGIVER:                        RELEVANT FINDINGS: □ No  □ Yes

REVIEW RESULTS WITH PHYSICIANS WHO PERFORMED/INTERPRETED TEST:

DIRECT VISUALIZATION OF X-RAY/INDEPENDENT INTERPRETATION OF IMAGE, TRACING, OR SPECIMEN:                        OTHER:

## ASSESSMENT

| Presenting Problem/Established Diagnosis | Worse | Improved | Stable | New Diagnosis | New Diagnosis | New Presenting Problem Undiagnosed |
|---|---|---|---|---|---|---|
| | | | | Self-Limited | No workup planned | Possible Dx |
| | | | | Minor | | Probable Dx |
| | | | | SWOLLEN JOINTS | | Rulo out Dx |
| | | | | TENDER JOINTS | | Differential diagnosis |
| | | | | TENDER JOINTS | | |

## PLAN

LAB       TODAY          □ TOXICITY     □ DZ ACTIVITY     □ Dx
         INTERIM         □ TOXICITY     □ DZ ACTIVITY     □ Dx
      NEXT VISIT        □ TOXICITY     □ DZ ACTIVITY     □ Dx

MEDICATION     CURRENT     □ No change     □ Change: Problem requiring change          NEW     □ No     □ New Meds Rxed     □ Problem requiring medication

Samples:                                        Gave patient:  □ Package insert     □ Pamphlet:

INJECTION     TRIGGER-POINT INJECTION:                              IM INJECTION:

ASPIRATION FOLLOWED BY INJECTION:

REFERRAL
ORDER

COUNSELING:
Risk Factor ⇓
Education
Advice     Discussed with patient     □ NEW MED     □ EXISTING MED     □ INJECTION     □ REFERRAL     □ ORDER     □ OTHER
Visit Summary:
Patient Questions

RETURN                    DAYS|          WEEKS|          MONTHS| □ OTHER:  SIGNED ROBIN K. DORE, M.D.

PROGRESS NOTE     PATIENT NAME                              DATE OF VISIT

© Robin K. Dore, M.D., Inc. 1993, 1999

## APPENDIX 12–2: PATIENT UPDATE

### Patient Update

**What's Happened Since I Saw You Last?  Since your last visit, have you:**

☐ Y ☐ N    1. Had any illnesses?

☐ Y ☐ N    2. Seen any health care providers?

☐ Y ☐ N    3. Had any
              ☐ lab ☐ x-ray or ☐ other procedure?

☐ Y ☐ N    4. Had a change in your family medical history?

☐ Y ☐ N    5. Had a change in your social history?

☐ Y ☐ N    6. Had any new allergies or reactions to medications?

☐ Y ☐ N    7. Started, changed, or stopped any medications?

**If yes, please describe below:**

| 1. Illnesses | 2. Health care provider seen | 3. Lab, x-ray, procedure |
|---|---|---|
|  |  |  |
|  |  |  |

| 4. New diseases or illnesses developed by relatives, parents, children, aunts, uncles, brothers, sisters | 5. Change in your social situation: work, relationships, residence, smoking, alcohol consumption | 6. New allergies or reactions to medications |
|---|---|---|
|  |  |  |

| 7. Name of medication which is NEW, CHANGED, or STOPPED: (Since last visit) | N=New C=Changed S=Stopped | For dose change or a new medication, indicate current dosage below | If changed or new, doctor who prescribed? If you made the change, put self | Why new medication taken? or Why medication changed or stopped? 1. No longer needed 2. No longer effective 3. Not effective 4. Side effects 4a GI upset  4b Liver 4c Lungs      4d Lab abnl |
|---|---|---|---|---|
|  |  |  |  |  |
|  |  |  |  |  |

### How Do You Feel Today?  Please help me evaluate you by completing the following:

Put "0" for Problems **not** present today
Put "N" for **New** problems not present last visit
For problems present last visit and today, rate on a 1-to-5 scale as follows:

Estimate the duration of your morning stiffness
Tell me your worst joint
Make an overall assessment of how you feel relative to your last visit

1 = Much better  2 = Better  3 = Same  4 = Worse  5 = Much worse

| Pain | Swelling | Morning stiffness (min) | Fatigue | Worst joint | Overall assessment |
|---|---|---|---|---|---|

| Ringing in ears | GI upset | Skin rash | Bruising | Difficulty sleeping | Cough | Eyes red | Chest pain | Fever |
|---|---|---|---|---|---|---|---|---|
| Oral ulcers | Diarrhea | Skin ulcers | Swollen glands | Headache | Shortness of breath | Eyes dry | Heart palpitations | Weight loss |

Name: ———————————————— Age: ————

# APPENDIX 12–3: FACE SHEET

## Face Sheet

| Test | Result | Date | Test | Result | Date | Prior DMARDs | Date | Comorbid Conditions | Date | Comorbid Conditions | Date |
|---|---|---|---|---|---|---|---|---|---|---|---|
| RA | | | | | | | | | | | |
| ANA | | | | | | | | | | | |
| DNA | | | | | | | | | | | |
| C3 | | | | | | | | | | | |
| C4 | | | | | | | | | | | |
| SM | | | | | | | | | | | |
| RNP | | | | | | | | | | | |
| SSA | | | | | | | | | | | |
| SSB | | | | | | | | | | | |
| ACLA | | | | | | | | | | | |
| HLA B27 | | | | | | | | | | | |
| | | | | | | | | | | | |
| | | | | | | | | | | | |
| | | | | | | | | | | | |

| Fracture/Surgery | Date | Injury/Hospitalization | Date | Prior NSAIDs | Date | Family History | Date | Social History | Date |
|---|---|---|---|---|---|---|---|---|---|
| | | | | | | | | | |

| Other Events | Date | Procedure | Date | Procedure | Date |
|---|---|---|---|---|---|
| GI Ulcer | | Chest x-ray | | DEXA | |
| GI Bleed | | | | | |
| Menopause | | | | | |
| ERT start | | | | | |
| ERT end | | | | | |
| Used corticosteroids | | | | | |

| Rheumatoid arthritis | Date | Lupus | Date | Lupus (cont) | Date | Seroneg. spond. | Date | Fibromyalgia | Date |
|---|---|---|---|---|---|---|---|---|---|
| 1 hr am stiffness | | Malar rash | | Neurologic disease | | +HLA B27 | | _ of 18 tender points | |
| Arthritis 3/+ joints | | Discoid rash | | Seizures | | Diarrhea | | Nonrestorative sleep | |
| Arthritis hand joints | | Photosensitivity | | Psychosis | | Mucocutaneous lesions | | Depression | |
| Symmetric arthritis | | Oral ulcers | | Hematology | | Urogenital | | Fatigue | |
| +RA factor: | | Arthritis 2/+ joints | | Hemolytic anemia | | Eye involvement | | Headache | |
| Nodules: | | Serositis | | Leukopenia | | Enthesopathy | | IBS | |
| | | Pleurisy | | Thrombocytosis | | Spinal disease | | PMS | |
| X-ray changes | | Pericarditis | | Lab  Sm  LE Prep | | Asymmetric arthritis | | Raynaud's | |
| | | Renal disease | | DNA  ACLA | | | | Dry eyes/mouth | |
| | | Proteinuria >.5 g | | ANA | | | | Paresthesias | |
| | | Cellular casts | | | | | | | |

| Primary Care Provider | | Tel | Fax | |
|---|---|---|---|---|
| Gynecologist | | Tel | Fax | |
| Orthopedist | | Tel | Fax | |

Patient Name: _____ DOB: _____ SSN: _____ Home tel: _____ Work tel: _____

# 13 | The Effectiveness of Cognitive-Behavioral and Psychoeducational Interventions in the Management of Arthritis

*Perry M. Nicassio and Melanie A. Greenberg*

On the basis of data from multiple sources, including epidemiologic research conducted in the United States and abroad, as well as findings from clinical studies, the economic, social, and psychological costs of rheumatic disease are enormous.[1] Yelin and Callahan noted that the costs of arthritis, including all rheumatic conditions, were $64.8 billion in 1992.[2] Moreover, estimates of the actual degree of indirect costs in rheumatoid arthritis (RA) may be underestimated because of its higher prevalence in women and the historically lower participation of women in the work force.[3]

The costs of arthritis reflect, in large part, the disabling impact of illness, coupled with refractory treatment response. This is especially true for RA. Reporting on a longitudinal data set of more than 1200 RA patients, Wolfe and Cathey[4] reported that half their sample experienced severe functional loss based on Health Assessment Questionnaire functional disability scores 10 years after the first clinic visit. From studies of a community cohort of more than 300 persons with definite or classic RA, Leigh and Fries[5] found that prior disability accounted for almost 60% of the variance in disability scores 8 years later, reflecting the unremitting impact of the condition. Monitoring a cohort of 112 RA patients who had been treated aggressively with pharmacologic treatment consisting of gold, chloroquine, steroids, penicillamine, and cytotoxic agents over a 20-year period, Scott and colleagues[6] found that function declined markedly between 10 and 20 years, and that 35% of their sample had died.

## PAIN AND COMORBIDITY

Although destruction of cartilage and bone and joint damage are endemic to arthritic conditions and a major contributing factor to functional declines, pain is the most noxious physical symptom and the major reason for the patient's seeking treatment. Pain is a significant factor in the prediction of disability in RA, independent of disease-related factors and drug treatment.[7] Chronic joint pain, combined with episodic, sudden increases in pain severity resulting from disease flare-ups, can lead to significant emotional distress and may contribute to the high levels of psychiatric comorbidity that have been found in arthritis studies.[8] Data on the comorbidity of arthritis with psychiatric disturbances are striking. For example, Wells and associates[9] found a lifetime prevalence rate of psychiatric disorder of 63% in persons with arthritis based on data from the National Institutes of Mental Health catchment area study. This rate was higher than that found in persons with conditions such as cancer, diabetes, and stroke. Furthermore, as many as one third of RA patients have been found to suffer from major depressive disorder or dysthymia, according to interview-based and self-reported criteria.[10] In an effort to determine the direction of the pain-depression relationship, Brown[11] found greater evidence for pain predicting depression than for depression predicting pain in a longitudinal study of more than 300 RA patients followed over a 3-year period.

Depression and psychosocial impairment, however, are not the inevitable consequences of arthritic pain and other illness stressors, but they are dependent on the patient's illness beliefs and pain coping mechanisms. Perceived helplessness,[12] cognitive distortions,[13] and "catastrophizing" (e.g., thinking that pain will never end)[14] in the presence of pain have been found to contribute to mood disturbance and disability independent of pain and, in some instances, to mediate the impact of pain.[15] Helplessness is also associated with passive pain coping efforts that may lead to more depression over time.[16] The obverse of this pattern also has been found to be true in that greater perceived control over pain and the belief in one's coping efficacy may lead to more active coping efforts that may reduce pain, disability, and psychological distress.[17, 18]

Although they result partly from the biologic impact of arthritis, patients' beliefs and coping practices are best conceptualized as learned reactions that are subject to myriad psychological, cultural, and social influences. Characterological traits such as dependency and low levels of resourcefulness, lack of medical knowledge, coping skill deficits, and reactions from significant others that thwart independence and create conflict may all potentially lead to self-defeating cognition and ineffective efforts to manage arthritis.[19] The process of coping with arthritic pain is dynamic and constantly evolving, reflecting incipient changes in biologic activity, the reactions of the family and other persons to the patient's complaints of pain, the patient's beliefs and coping responses, and the impact of environmental demands and challenges.[17–19]

## THE NEED FOR PSYCHOSOCIAL MANAGEMENT

The significant literature, accumulated since 1980, that has highlighted the role of psychological and social variables in the psychosocial impact of arthritis has confirmed the importance of the biopsychosocial model[20] as a conceptual framework for understanding the adjustment process and the design of treatment and management approaches. A major premise of this model is that since numerous variables may affect the process of adjustment to chronic illness, treatment approaches should be broad enough to address these variables in an effort to strengthen the patient's coping skills, reduce disability, and diminish psychological distress. In contrast, the biomedical model has focused on the treatment of underlying disease activity and difficult symptoms (pain) resulting from disease processes such as inflammation and cartilage damage. The limited efficacy of pharmacologic, disease-modifying agents,[21, 22] along with evidence that disease activity in RA may be only modestly associated with pain, psychological, and behavioral parameters of the condition,[23] further underscores the need for alternate treatment conceptualizations. Although somewhat interlocking and interdependent, the biologic, psychological, and behavioral aspects of the adjustment process are unique, highly individualized, and subject to different causal and maintaining factors.[20] Treatment strategies that are sufficiently inclusive to address the various components of the adjustment process have thus been recommended. Psychosocial and biomedical treatment approaches share complementary roles in the management of arthritis patients in that their combination ensures that biologic, psychological, and behavioral dimensions of the adjustment process are addressed and managed.

Cognitive-behavior therapy (CBT) and psychoeducational treatment interventions emphasizing self-management principles have been developed and empirically evaluated since the 1970s in response to emerging theories and findings on the adjustment process. In the following sections of this chapter, we provide a review of the clinical trials evaluating the efficacy of these approaches and make suggestions that will guide further outcomes of research and clinical applications. Our review focuses on the research con-

ducted in RA and osteoarthritis (OA) because these conditions have been the main focus of behavioral and educational treatment interventions.

## THE COGNITIVE-BEHAVIORAL APPROACH

Turk and Salovey[24] noted that there are five central assumptions that provide a rationale for adopting CBT approaches for patients with chronic illness.

1. Patients actively process information about environmental contingencies, their medical conditions, and their treatment.
2. Thoughts (e.g., appraisals, beliefs) can influence affective states and behavior.
3. Individuals both affect and are affected by their environment (reciprocal influence process).
4. Treatment approaches should specifically target maladaptive ways of thinking, feeling, and responding in reaction to illness.
5. Patients are seen as active change agents in their treatment.

To a large extent, the CBT approach recognizes that treatment is a collaborative process between the health care provider and the patient. This process involves explaining the purposes of CBT strategies and their relationship to medical treatment, development of effective coping skills, and application of coping skills on an everyday basis and in problematic situations.

Accordingly, the treatment goals of CBT for persons with chronic medical illness have traditionally been to reduce the stress associated with disease processes, medical treatment, or environmental demands; gain control over difficult symptoms (e.g., pain, fatigue); reduce disability and improve physical functioning and psychological functioning; and limit inappropriate use of medical care.[24] The specific techniques that have been implemented encompass an extensive range of strategies, including biofeedback, relaxation training, cognitive restructuring and cognitive coping, activity pacing, behavioral goal-setting, stress management, and problem-solving. Table 13–1 lists common CBT intervention strategies and their treatment goals.

Although the majority of studies adopting CBT strategies have focused on the management of pain and its impact, other trials have taken a broader approach, emphasizing the management of stress or the development of more general life management skills that have been designed to help patients acquire better control over problems and obstacles created by their medical conditions.

## TRIALS FOCUSING ON THE MANAGEMENT OF PAIN AND ITS CONSEQUENCES

Biofeedback approaches were incorporated in earlier behavioral trials for RA. The rationale for using bio-

**TABLE 13–1**
## Overview of Common CBT Strategies

| STRATEGY | TREATMENT GOAL |
| --- | --- |
| Cognitive restructuring | Reduce dysfunctional thinking |
| | Promote control over coping process |
| | Reduce depression |
| Cognitive coping (e.g., imagery, distraction) | Divert attention from pain |
| | Reduce dysfunctional thinking about symptoms, illness |
| Biofeedback | Control over ANS arousal |
| | Reduce disease activity |
| Relaxation training | Reduce physiological responsivity to stress |
| | Increase positive affect |
| | Decrease negative affect |
| Activity pacing | Increase activity level |
| | Reduce disability |
| | Control over fatigue |
| Pleasant events scheduling | Increase positive affect |
| | Decrease depression |
| Problem-solving | Control over life stressors |
| | Application of coping skills |
| Relapse prevention training | Treatment adherence |
| | Independent self-management |

feedback is that RA patients may learn to acquire control over autonomic nervous system functioning and reduce stress responsivity that may contribute to inflammatory processes and disease activity.

A study by Achterberg and colleagues[25] evaluated the effects of temperature biofeedback training in a sample of 25 RA patients. This research was conducted in two phases. The first phase compared the effects of either increasing or decreasing skin temperature after patients learned general relaxation skills, whereas the second phase compared a combined biofeedback group, based on a subset of patients from the first phase, with a physiotherapy intervention involving the application of heat and cold treatments, exercise, and instruction activities of daily living. Interestingly, both thermal warming and cooling led to improvement in pain, tension, and sleep. The second phase of the study favored biofeedback over physiotherapy on indices of physical functioning and pain. In addition, biofeedback subjects had fewer disability-related work changes at the end of treatment. Major limitations of the study, however, precluded definitive conclusions from being made about the effects of biofeedback treatment. Biofeedback and physiotherapy groups were not formed randomly, and no follow-up of treatment effects was reported.

A better controlled clinical trial was conducted by Bradley and associates[26] in which three treatment conditions were compared in 53 RA patients: (1) a CBT treatment package that included thermal biofeedback, relaxation training, and instruction in behavioral goal setting and use of self-rewards; (2) structured group therapy, incorporating education and discussion of coping methods; and (3) no treatment. The results of this study clearly supported the efficacy of the CBT intervention over the other two conditions on stan-

dardized measures of pain behavior, pain intensity, and disease activity. The group therapy intervention did not prove superior to no treatment. Depression, however, did not respond to CBT treatment. Six-month follow-up data tended to favor the CBT group on outcome criteria, but statistically significant differences were not maintained. A later report,[27] however, demonstrated a substantial reduction in health care utilization and medical costs for CBT patients, as reflected in data collected 7 to 12 months after the end of the intervention. Outpatient office visits decreased 13.1% in the CBT group, whereas outpatient visits increased in the other two conditions.

Applebaum and colleagues[28] compared CBT with a symptom-monitoring condition for 18 RA patients. These investigators also employed thermal biofeedback and combined it with instruction in progressive relaxation, cognitive restructuring in the presence of pain, and problem-solving. After treatment, the CBT group showed greater improvement in weekly pain ratings, McGill Pain Questionnaire scores, and functional measures than did the control group. Neither group improved on measures of anxiety and depression. Eighteen-month follow-up findings did not confirm the continued superiority of CBT. This study, however, was hindered by small sample size and a high rate of attrition (10 subjects) during follow-up.

O'Leary and colleagues[29] compared an omnibus CBT intervention involving relaxation, cognitive coping techniques (e.g., distraction, imagery, relabeling), and tailoring of coping skills to problematic pain situations, with an education control group in which patients were provided with copies of *The Arthritis Helpbook*.[30] CBT led to significant improvement in general pain indices, joint impairment, and self-efficacy. Despite these improvements, no changes in numbers or functions of T-cell subsets or on indices of psychological functioning were found. Importantly, self-efficacy was correlated with less pain and disability after treatment, indicative of the potential mediational role of this variable. Unfortunately, the authors did not report follow-up data on the trial.

Parker and colleagues[31] reported on a comprehensive pain management program in which a 1-week hospital stay was followed by an outpatient group support phase designed to maintain treatment gains. This program was compared with (1) an arthritis education "placebo" group in which didactic information was reviewed and discussed in a supportive group format and (2) a no-treatment control condition. The educational intervention also began with a 1-week hospital stay followed by outpatient maintenance sessions. Findings at the end of 6 and 12 months indicated greater adaptive pain coping and perceived control over pain in the CBT groups, although treatment differences were not found on measures of pain and disability. However, when subjects in the CBT condition were divided into low- and high-adherence groups, those who exhibited high adherence reported less pain and helplessness than did those with low adherence. The authors suggested that the lack of overall efficacy of the CBT intervention may have been a result of the lower educational status, advanced age, and high degree of disease severity in this male veteran sample.

Radojevic and colleagues[32] examined the thesis that family support may augment the clinical effectiveness of CBT treatment for RA. The authors reasoned that family support may assist the patient in applying pain management skills, reducing sick role behaviors, and enhancing adherence responses.[33] This research compared (1) a pain management protocol, emphasizing relaxation and cognitive coping techniques with and without a family support person present, with (2) an arthritis education condition with family support, and (3) no treatment. The behavioral interventions yielded greater treatment gains on joint examination pain at 2-month follow-up and on degree of joint swelling and number of swollen joints after treatment and at follow-up. The CBT with family support condition had significantly lower joint swelling scores after treatment than did the other conditions. However, despite these provocative findings on disease measures, the groups did not differ on indices of self-reported pain. The arthritis education condition did not improve on any clinical criteria.

A study conducted in Holland by Kraaimaat and associates[34] reported null results in a trial comparing a comprehensive CBT pain management protocol with occupational therapy and a no-treatment control group. The authors found no differences on health status measures between groups after treatment and at 6-month follow-up and noted that a progressive deterioration in clinical and laboratory measures of disease had occurred over the course of the trial for the entire sample. Furthermore, with the exception of one pain coping index, the CBT intervention was not successful in facilitating adaptive coping skills. Thus, the failure of CBT could have resulted from the inability of patients to acquire and implement effective pain management or because their disease was not being adequately controlled by standard rheumatologic care.

## COGNITIVE-BEHAVIOR STUDIES WITH OSTEOARTHRITIS PATIENTS

Keefe and colleagues[35] reported on the first clinical trial evaluating the effects of CBT for patients with OA. The study included 99 patients with persistent knee pain and compared the effects of (1) an intensive CBT protocol involving relaxation, cognitive restructuring, coping methods, and activity pacing with behavioral goal setting and (2) arthritis education, in which didactic lectures about OA and medical management took place in a supportive group format, and (3) no treatment. CBT patients experienced significantly larger reductions in pain and psychological disability than did the patients in the education and control groups after treatment. Furthermore, increases in perceived control over pain and rational thinking in CBT patients were associated with improvement in disability over the course of the trial. Although the CBT group had difficulty in maintaining treatment gains at 6-month follow-up, patients who had shown the largest improvement in

pain control and rational thinking had the greatest degree of change for the better in pain, psychological disability, and pain behavior at follow-up.[36]

Calfas and associates contrasted the effects of a CBT regimen for managing pain and disability with a lecture-based education condition in a sample of 40 OA patients.[37] Both groups demonstrated improvement in pain, depression, and quality of well-being after treatment, but the groups did not differ significantly from one another. The data indicated that the CBT group showed a trend for maintaining higher quality of well-being scores through the 2-month follow-up period. Depression remained improved for both groups after 1 year. In comparison to the study by Keefe and colleagues[35] this research was limited by marginal statistical power for examining group differences and the lack of attention to measuring pain coping strategies and pain perception.

In a well-designed and well-executed study, Keefe and associates[38] attempted to determine the incremental benefit of spouse involvement in the CBT intervention for pain management modeled after their previous work.[35, 36] The couple's intervention was based on the premise that OA may have an adverse impact on the marital relationship and that education about how to improve the management of OA and its interpersonal impact would benefit both the patient and the spouse. The couple's intervention involved training in communication skills regarding the practice of pain coping strategies, joint behavioral rehearsal of how to support the implementation of pain coping strategies, mutual goal setting, and maintenance of the couple's skills. As in Radojevic and colleagues'[32] investigation, the two behavioral groups were compared with an arthritis education condition that also included participation of the spouse. After treatment, the spouse-assisted coping skills group was superior to the arthritis education support group on measures of pain, pain behavior, psychological disability, self-efficacy, and marital adjustment. The behavioral intervention without the spouse led to significantly greater gains in self-efficacy and marital adjustment and showed evidence of a trend of greater improvement in pain, psychological disability, and self-efficacy than did the arthritis education support. Although statistical differences were not found between the behavioral groups, spouse-assisted CBT showed consistent superiority on five of the six outcome measures. The study revealed that increases in marital adjustment were associated with improvements in pain behavior and psychological functioning for the sample as a whole. The authors also reported that increases in self-efficacy and perceived control and rational thinking were correlated with decreases in pain and disability.

## STRESS MANAGEMENT INTERVENTIONS

The stressful impact of arthritis on psychosocial adjustment has already been duly noted in an earlier section of this chapter. A review by Huyser and Parker[39] also demonstrated the important role of stress-induced changes in the hypothalamic-pituitary-adrenal axis and sympathetic-adrenal-medullary system that may lead to immune system dysregulation and contribute to inflammatory processes in RA. The authors pointed to evidence indicating abnormally low production of cortisol during periods of disease flare, which is suggestive of the inability of cortisol to down-regulate immune system activity, thus potentially contributing to increased disease activity. Other research[40] has shown that interpersonal conflict is associated with the production of immunostimulatory hormones such as prolactin and estradiol which, in turn, have been correlated with physician ratings of disease activity. Huyser and Parker noted that the research on the role of stress in RA is at an early stage of development and is in need of integrative models in which the causal mechanisms linking environmental events and psychological variables to changes in disease activity are delineated and empirically evaluated. Nonetheless, clinical investigators have applied stress concepts in the design and implementation of intervention protocols that have attempted to modify patients' responses to stressful events through the development of effective coping skills and adaptive appraisal processes.

The first clinical trial evaluating a stress management paradigm was conducted by Shearn and Fireman[41] in a sample of 105 RA patients. The intervention helped patients identify sources of stress, learn relaxation techniques, and identify the use of effective coping methods. The stress management group was compared with a mutual support group intervention that was designed to enhance self-responsibility, exchange information, and build relationships, and compared with a no-treatment control group. The results indicated that the stress management and mutual support groups experienced equivalent improvement in joint tenderness after treatment but did not show a superior therapeutic treatment outcome on measures of self-reported pain, disability, and psychological functioning when compared with the no-treatment group. Although the authors interpreted the outcome of this trial as being unsupportive of the stress management model, it is noteworthy that change was found on joint tenderness, an objective measure of disease activity. However, the lack of information on the specific procedures of the stress management condition and absence of follow-up data were weaknesses of this trial.

In contrast, a more definitive outcome study evaluating the effects of a stress management intervention, an attention control group, and standard care control in a sample of 141 RA patients was reported by Parker and colleagues.[42] The stress management program employed a computer-facilitated multimedia component to teach stress concepts and facilitate skill acquisition. The intervention was broadly structured, encompassing treatment elements such as relaxation training, instruction in coping strategies to deal with common RA-related stressors, assessment of life goals, and optimizing interpersonal relationships. Treatment sessions were administered individually over a 10-week period, followed by a 15-month maintenance phase to sustain

treatment gains. The attention placebo group consisted of a computer-assisted educational program based on Arthritis Foundation materials and had the same number of treatment and maintenance sessions as did the stress management group. The stress management intervention led to significantly greater improvement in helplessness, self-efficacy, coping attempts, self-reported pain, and lower extremity functioning than did the attention placebo and no-treatment groups after treatment. Treatment gains were maintained over 3- and 15-month follow-up on most coping and psychological indices and McGill Pain Questionnaire scores. Treatment differences were not found, however, on joint pain and depression. Unfortunately, neuroendocrine and immune system indices underlying stress responsivity were not reported in the trial. Nevertheless, the study provided strong evidence for the clinical significance of stress management for RA on other health outcomes.

## INTERVENTIONS EMPHASIZING PERCEIVED CONTROL

The studies discussed in this section evaluated behavioral interventions to help RA patients deal with the various lifestyle problems associated with the condition and to enhance a sense of personal mastery and perceived control. In contrast to other CBT protocols, their major focus was not on the management of pain or stress.

DeVellis and associates[43] evaluated the effects of a problem-solving intervention in a sample of 101 RA patients. After a psychosocial interview during which a major compliance problem and a major lifestyle problem were assessed and potential resources were identified for managing them, patients participated in a 1-hour problem-solving intervention led by a health educator. The intervention consisted of teaching patients skills related to identifying and evaluating strategies for problem resolution, developing an action plan, and follow-up. Patients who practiced problem-solving were compared with patients who participated in pre- and post-treatment interviews only. After treatment, a greater percentage of treated patients reported that they had resolved their compliance and lifestyle problems than did control patients. Although no significant differences were found between the two groups in clinical functioning, decreases in pain and physical impairment as measured by the Arthritis Impact Measurement Scale and improvement in symptom ratings for fatigue, stiffness, swelling, and depression were found across the 4-month treatment period. Although the treatment was inconclusive in documenting the effect of problem-solving methodology, the psychosocial interview itself could have stimulated the coping resources of control patients, thereby contributing to their improvement. Despite such ambiguity, it is noteworthy that a moderate amount of clinical improvement occurred as a result of such brief contact with patients.

On the basis of the premise that loss of perceived control and erosion of coping resources contribute to maladaptive coping and negative psychological and physical functioning in RA, Sinclair and colleagues[44] evaluated the effects of the intervention program *Rising Above Arthritis,* which was designed to help women with RA develop better competence in managing the impact of RA and other life obstacles. Nurses administered the intervention to 90 patients who were seen in a small group format in a within-subjects design over an 18-month period. The intervention focused on issues such as establishing reasonable boundaries regarding the demands and expectations of others; developing healthier attributions for stressful life events and difficult symptoms; avoiding a pessimistic, helpless explanatory style; and coping effectively with anger and resentment. The authors reported significant improvement on all measures of coping resources (e.g., health competence, helplessness, self-efficacy), pain coping behaviors, general psychological well-being, and fatigue from before treatment to after treatment. The effects of the intervention on pain were inconclusive because pain began to decline during the preintervention period. The efficacy of this unique approach to arthritis management awaits replication in a between-groups, controlled clinical trial.

## SUMMARY OF COGNITIVE-BEHAVIOR THERAPY APPROACHES

With the exception of the study by Kraaimaat and colleagues,[34] the literature reflects a moderate amount of clinical benefit from CBT interventions. However, the effects of CBT are not consistent across studies, and they show substantial variability on different clinical outcomes. For example, whereas some research shows that CBT may be effective in reducing pain but not underlying disease processes,[29] other research has indicated that CBT may lead to reductions in disease activity without affecting pain.[32] Although such discrepancies may result from methodologic differences involving the assessment of constructs and the design of treatments, the independence of biologic, psychological, and behavioral outcomes in arthritis, and their lack of responsivity to the same therapeutic approaches, may account for such findings. Clearly, the assumption cannot be made from the studies reviewed that improvement in one clinical outcome will be associated with improvement in others after administration of CBT strategies.

Several trends are evident that highlight the clinical significance and value of CBT interventions. First is the finding that CBT interventions generally elicit more healthy and adaptive ways of appraising difficult symptoms and engender more efficacious coping responses.[26, 29, 31, 42] Furthermore, evidence indicates that such change may be a central mechanism that mediates improvement in clinical outcomes.[29, 36] Second, many of the trials[26, 32, 35] have shown the beneficial effects of CBT on objective measures of disease or pain behavior, or both, indicating that the effects of treatment cannot

be accounted for by demand characteristics in which patients report improvement in pain and other symptoms in an attempt to match the expectations of the clinicians administering the protocol. Third, the better designed studies with better controls, adequate sample sizes, and more thoroughly described assessment and treatment protocols[26, 32, 35, 38, 42] have generally produced the strongest clinical findings. Fourth, there is a trend in the literature that intensive CBT approaches are superior to attention control or didactic control interventions, or both, in which education is imparted and group discussion takes place.[32, 38, 42] Thus, there appear to be active treatment elements in CBT that are responsible for clinical change.

Despite these advances, some important questions need to be addressed in future CBT trials. Greater emphasis should be placed on evaluating and ensuring the long-term benefit of CBT interventions. Many trials have not included a follow-up period, whereas others reflect a diminution of treatment gains over time. In addition, it is unclear what specific treatment components in the interventions described are responsible for clinical improvement. CBT interventions have generally encompassed many different treatment elements with the expectation that the overall package will be sufficiently robust to catalyze improvement. Studies with component control groups are needed to tease apart selected elements of omnibus treatment protocols and evaluate their independent effects. This information is especially helpful for strategizing clinical interventions that need to optimize efficacy in light of economic and logistical constraints commonly faced by practitioners. Furthermore, although affective disorders are prevalent in arthritis, CBT has generally had minimal impact on reducing depression, particularly in RA samples. This finding is surprising in that the CBT approach largely evolved from studies on the cognitive biases of depressed patients. It is encouraging to note, however, that the presence of depression does not appear to inhibit the effect of CBT on other health outcomes. Further discussion of the treatment of depression is found in the summary section of this chapter.

## THE SELF-MANAGEMENT TREATMENT APPROACH

The self-management approach to the treatment of arthritis was developed by Lorig and Holman at the Stanford Arthritis Center[45] in the early 1980s and has been tested and refined for almost 20 years. The original impetus for this treatment was more practical than theoretical; the desire to create a low-cost treatment that could be implemented by trained lay individuals and made available to large numbers of patients. The treatment was originally based on broad psychoeducational principles. The rationale was that providing information about the disease and teaching skills in problem-solving, communication, and disease management should enhance the patient's ability to practice self-care. Enhanced self-management should, in turn, reduce pain, disability, and depression and lower health-care utilization. More recently, however, Lorig and Gonzalez[46] adopted self-efficacy theory[47] as the theoretical basis for this treatment, and the treatment protocol was changed to incorporate self-efficacy–enhancing principles.

Self-efficacy theory is a component within the broader framework of social-learning theory,[47] which assumes that thoughts, behavior, other personal characteristics, and the environment all mutually influence one another. In other words, a person's health status can be a function of their thoughts, behaviors, and physical-social environment. Self-efficacy expectations refer to a person's beliefs in his or her ability to execute a desired behavior, achieve a specific cognitive-emotional state, or master a specific skill. These personal estimates of efficacy are made in relation to a specific situation or problem—for example, one's ability to reduce arthritis pain or increase physical activity. In relation to health, it is thought that individuals with higher self-efficacy are more likely to choose, expend effort, and persist in health-promoting behaviors such as exercise or in compliance with treatment regimens. Higher self-efficacy is also thought to reduce anxiety and depression and prevent chronic stress.[48] Applying this theory to self-management programs leads to the rationale that a treatment that enhances a patient's self-efficacy for managing disease should improve health status over time.

Both the original and revised Arthritis Self-Management Programs (ASMP) have a similar structure. The 12-hour course is taught in six weekly 2-hour sessions held in community settings. Each course is taught by a pair of lay leaders, one of whom generally has arthritis and both of whom receive 18 hours of training and standardized teaching manuals. Participants in each course consist of 15 to 20 individuals who include arthritis patients and family members, if desired. Participants with any type of arthritis may enroll. Patients are generally recruited via the mass media and community groups rather than from medical settings. In clinical trials, patient diagnoses have been confirmed by physicians.

The original ASMP focused on the nature and types of arthritis, range of motion and isometric exercises, relaxation techniques, arthritis medications, joint protection, nutrition, evaluating nontraditional treatments, problem-solving strategies, and patient-physician communication. All participants received a copy of *The Arthritis Helpbook*,[30] which contains the course content. Teaching methods were generally interactive rather than didactic and included group discussion, feedback, practice, demonstrations, and self-monitoring of behavior between sessions.

The revised ASMP[46] incorporates specific intervention techniques to enhance patients' self-efficacy to manage disease. These techniques are based on Bandura's[47] delineation of the factors that can enhance self-efficacy judgments. These include actual performance and mastery, modeling (observing similar others perform successfully), verbal persuasion, physiologic feedback indicating that one is calm, and

cognitive appraisal or changing one's beliefs in a positive direction. Table 13–2 presents an overview of self-management strategies and their treatment objectives.

The revised ASMP includes techniques to address each of these factors. To enhance mastery, participants sign written contracts to perform a specific self-management behavior of their choice each week. Participants also learn specific skills (e.g., relaxation and exercise) in session. They receive direct feedback and problem-solving suggestions regarding these activities. Role modeling occurs when participants observe group leaders coping successfully with their arthritis. Participants also help each other solve problems during group discussions. Verbal persuasion occurs when leaders urge participants to increase their goals and when they display confidence in participants' abilities. Physiologic feedback techniques include the use of thermometers to demonstrate the results of relaxation and tape measures to demonstrate increased range of motion. Finally, to change cognitive appraisal, patients are taught that their thoughts and behaviors can influence their physical symptoms, and they learn to think

**TABLE 13–2**
**Overview of Common Self-Management Strategies**

| STRATEGIES | TREATMENT GOAL |
|---|---|
| **Information provision** | |
| Nature and types of arthritis | Enhance knowledge about arthritis |
| Joint protection | Promote self-management behaviors |
| Nutrition | |
| **Treatment information** | |
| Arthritis medications | Facilitate active patient participation in treatment planning |
| Evaluating nontraditional treatments | |
| Patient-physician communication | |
| **Problem-solving** | Enhance coping skills |
| **Performance and feedback** | |
| Behavioral contracts | Promote self-management behaviors |
| Relaxation training | Facilitate mastery |
| Exercise practice (ROM and isometric) | |
| **Modeling** | |
| Group leaders as role models | Enhance self-efficacy |
| Group members share coping strategies | |
| **Verbal persuasion** | |
| Group leaders encourage goal setting | Enhance self-efficacy |
| Group leaders display confidence in participants' abilities | |
| **Cognitive reappraisal** | Promote more positive appraisals of arthritis |

ROM = range of motion

about arthritis and self-management in more positive ways.

The original and revised ASMPs are now offered both nationally and internationally. In 1984, the Arthritis Foundation began offering these programs throughout the United States. More recently, the ASMP has been offered in Australia, New Zealand, Canada, and Europe. Hundreds of thousands of persons with arthritis have taken this course.[45] In the following sections, clinical trials and long-term follow-up studies of the ASMP with mixed arthritis patients are reviewed and empirical support for the relationship between increased self-efficacy and improved health status after the ASMP is completed are discussed. Next, clinical trials of self-management interventions with RA patients are reviewed. Finally, a summary and integration are provided.

## CLINICAL TRIALS OF THE ARTHRITIS SELF-MANAGEMENT PROGRAM WITH MIXED ARTHRITIS PATIENTS

The original ASMP was first tested in a 4-month randomized, controlled clinical trial involving 190 participants with arthritis.[49] The course was given in six weekly sessions, and participants were randomly assigned to receive treatment either immediately or after 4 months (waiting list control). The ASMP led to increased knowledge and self-management behaviors and decreased pain at 4 months relative to controls. There were no significant effects on disability or physician visits.

The ASMP differed from the traditional intervention format by using lay rather than professional course leaders. The question of whether groups taught by professionals would be even more effective was addressed both by Lorig and colleagues[50] and by other researchers.[51] In both studies, mixed arthritis patients were randomly assigned to the lay-taught or professionally taught groups or the waiting list control group. The lay-taught groups in both studies used the standard ASMP content and format. Although the professionally taught groups in both studies focused on the ASMP content areas, only one study[50] used the standard ASMP protocol. In the other study,[51] lectures and demonstrations were the major teaching methods. In both studies, the majority of participants had OA. Overall, few differences were found between the lay-taught and professionally taught groups. Both studies demonstrated beneficial effects of treatment on knowledge and exercise and in one study,[50] the lay-taught group also increased their relaxation practice, relative to controls. In contrast to the earlier study, no beneficial effects were found on pain or other health outcomes.

In a randomized study,[46] three self-efficacy–enhancing versions of the ASMP were compared with a control condition. The three treatments emphasized exercise, cognitive pain management, and a combination of the two, respectively. At 4-month follow-up, no differences were found among the three interventions, yet all three led to significant decreases in pain relative to the control condition.

Lorig and Holman[45] reported between-groups comparisons at 4 months for all randomized participants taking the original ASMP (N = 707). Participants had physician-confirmed diagnoses of arthritis and the majority had OA. Results were similar to those of Lorig and colleagues[49] and indicated significant improvements in exercise and relaxation and decreases in pain for treatment group participants relative to controls. In the intervention group, exercise and relaxation increased by 80% and pain decreased by 12%. There were no treatment effects on disability or depression. Results for knowledge were not reported. This is not a pure replication because participants from the Lorig and associates'[49] clinical trial were included in these analyses. Nonetheless, the large study population and the clinically significant decreases in health behaviors increase confidence in the findings.

## LONG-TERM FOLLOW-UP STUDIES OF THE ARTHRITIS SELF-MANAGEMENT PROGRAM

Several uncontrolled longitudinal studies have evaluated long-term maintenance of treatment gains with the ASMP. Demographic characteristics of 1058 participants in various studies have been reported.[45] These were individuals with physician-confirmed arthritis diagnoses, the majority of whom (about 70%) had OA. Participants were mostly female (about 80%), older (mean age = 64 years), and well educated (mean = 14 years). In a study of 115 treatment group participants,[49] assessments occurred at 4, 8, and 20 months after treatment ended. Treatment gains in knowledge, relaxation, and exercise and decreases in pain from baseline to 4 months were all maintained at 20 months. There was, however, some attenuation between 8 and 20 months. Disability decreased significantly from baseline only at 4 months, but this was not maintained.

Lorig and Holman[52] examined 20-month maintenance of treatment gains in 589 ASMP participants. They also assessed whether post-treatment reinforcement would enhance maintenance of treatment effects. Therefore, at 12 months after baseline, participants were randomized to receive a 12-hour Arthritis Reinforcement Course (ARC), four editions of a bimonthly newsletter, or no reinforcement. Surprisingly, the newsletter group had a greater decrease of depression than did the reinforcement group; however, participant selection factors may have influenced this outcome because participants whose depression had not decreased after treatment were more likely to attend the Arthritis Reinforcement Course. Unlike the previous study,[49] there was no attenuation of treatment gains in this study. Between baseline and 20 months, pain decreased by 20%, depression decreased by 13%, and physician visits decreased by 35%. Disability was not significantly improved. These decreases are large enough to be clinically significant. In the absence of a control group, however, alternative explanations for the findings were not ruled out.

The effects of the ASMP were also evaluated 4 years after baseline. The length of the follow-up period is notable because most studies of psychosocial interventions do not carry out such lengthy follow-ups. In one study, 233 of 280 participants (83%) in the ASMP were evaluated.[53] Results indicated that relative to baseline, pain decreased by 18% and physician visits decreased by 34%, despite a 9% increase in disability. All these changes reached statistical significance. Using comparison group data, the authors estimated 4-year savings due to reductions in physician visits as $343/RA patient and $120/OA patient.

Another 4-year follow-up study[54] used 224 ASMP participants who had completed the reinforcement study (group 1) and 177 participants who were not offered reinforcement (group 2). Results replicated and exceeded the previous study.[53] In groups 1 and 2, pain decreased by 19% and 22%, respectively, and physician visits decreased by 42% and 44%, respectively. Both these decreases were statistically significant. No effect was found on depression, and disability increased slightly. Other analyses compared ASMP participants with comparison groups for whom data were available over the same period. Pain and physician visits in comparison groups remained fairly stable over the 4-year period, despite the fact that more comparison group participants (17%) than ASMP participants (12%) with RA began a course of methotrexate. Cost savings from the ASMP over the 4 years were estimated as $648/RA patient and $189/OA patient.

## THE ARTHRITIS SELF-MANAGEMENT PROGRAM AND SELF-EFFICACY

Does increased self-efficacy mediate the effects of the ASMP on health outcomes? Although there is not currently a definitive answer to this question, existing data support the relationship between increased self-efficacy and improved health in ASMP participants.

At first, the health benefits of the ASMP were assumed to result from increases in health-enhancing behaviors. Changes in behavior after completion of the ASMP were, however, only weakly related to changes in health status.[55] Subsequent qualitative interviews with 50 ASMP participants revealed that patients' perceptions of control may be implicated in health changes.[46] "People who had improved consistently said they felt they had more control over their symptoms, while those who had not improved felt there was little one could do about arthritis."[55] This led the investigators to hypothesize that the ASMP may work by increasing patients' self-efficacy for managing arthritis. They constructed three reliable and valid scales to assess self-efficacy in relation to pain, physical functioning, and other arthritis symptoms, respectively.[56] These scales assessed participants' degree of certainty that they could decrease their pain, perform specific functional tasks or decrease fatigue, depression, and other symptoms.

Subsequent empirical studies indicated that self-efficacy might be involved in treatment gains. In one study using the original ASMP,[56] self-efficacy for both pain and other symptoms increased significantly from baseline to 4-month follow-up in the treatment group but did not change over time in the control group. Between-group differences were not statistically significant, however. More notably, increases in self-efficacy were significantly related to improvements in health outcomes. These results do not, however, establish that self-efficacy causes the health outcomes. It could be that persons with worse health to begin with feel less confident of their ability to control arthritis.

The revised ASMP was specifically designed to enhance self-efficacy and seems to be effective in doing so. In a study of 127 arthritis patients,[45] self-efficacy was enhanced by 15% in the treatment group, which was a significantly greater change than occurred in the control group. Furthermore, the efficacy-enhancing ASMP has been shown to decrease pain at more than twice the rate of the original ASMP (29% vs 12%). No direct statistical comparisons between the two treatments have been conducted, however. Another unresolved issue is how these changes in self-efficacy occur, because they are not related to changes in the practice of exercise or cognitive pain management.[45]

## CLINICAL TRIALS OF THE ARTHRITIS SELF-MANAGEMENT PROGRAM WITH RHEUMATOID ARTHRITIS PATIENTS

In the United States, the ASMP was designed for individuals with any type of arthritis. Investigators in the Netherlands[57] developed a version of the ASMP that is specific to RA patients. This treatment is similar to the ASMP[49] except that it is conducted by health professionals rather than lay leaders. In addition, patients in the RA program develop individualized exercise programs with a physiotherapist rather than practicing physical exercise in the groups. The RA program is delivered in five weekly 2-hour sessions with six to eight patients and, if desired, partners.

A randomized clinical trial of the self-management intervention was conducted with 57 physician-referred RA patients. Treatment participants received the intervention and physiotherapy, whereas control participants received only physiotherapy. After 4 months, the intervention had beneficial effects on knowledge, exercise, functional disability, and physician-assessed joint tenderness, relative to the control condition. At 14-month follow-up, intervention effects on knowledge and exercise were maintained, and self-efficacy for function was also enhanced for treatment participants relative to controls. For joint tenderness, there was a trend in the expected direction. There were no treatment effects on pain or laboratory tests to assess disease progression.

More recently, this same group[58] conducted a well-designed clinical trial of a modified RA self-management program, without supplemental physiotherapy but with reinforcement meetings at 4 and 8 months after the conclusion of treatment. The treatment program included medication compliance, physical exercise, endurance activities, energy conservation and joint protection, information about RA, cognitive restructuring, problem-solving, goal-setting, and feedback. Participants included 55 patients who had RA for less than 3 years and were receiving disease-modifying antirheumatic drug therapy with sulfasalazine. The control group received a brochure on RA. The design was a randomized, assessor-blinded clinical trial with a 1-year follow-up period. Contrary to expectations, education did not lead to enhanced compliance with sulfasalazine; medication compliance was greater than 80%, regardless of condition. The treatment group did demonstrate enhanced compliance with exercise, energy conservation, and joint protection relative to controls, but this did not lead to improved health status at follow-up.

## SUMMARY OF SELF-MANAGEMENT APPROACHES

The effects of self-management interventions have been examined in both randomized, controlled, clinical trials and uncontrolled, long-term follow-ups of treatment group participants. The majority of clinical trials have used community volunteers with arthritis (mainly OA). Two studies used RA patients recruited via physician referral. Both lay and professional leaders have administered the interventions. Follow-up periods ranged from 4 months to 1 year for controlled studies and up to 4 years for uncontrolled studies. Outcome measures included self-reports of arthritis knowledge, health behaviors, pain, depression, self-efficacy, and disability; objective measures of physician visits and RA disease status; and behavioral measures of compliance (e.g., pill counting).

Taken together, these studies indicate that self-management can have beneficial effects on knowledge and health behaviors in both RA and mixed arthritis groups. Surprisingly, changes in knowledge and health behaviors were not associated with changes in health status. Nevertheless, enhanced health behaviors are beneficial because they can increase physical conditioning, prevent further injury, and indicate active disease management by the patient.

Regarding psychosocial adjustment, there is no evidence from controlled studies for decreased depression in either RA or mixed arthritis groups. In one uncontrolled study,[52] depression decreased significantly from baseline to 20 months in the treatment group. Self-management interventions do, however, enhance arthritis patients' self-efficacy, or confidence, to manage pain, function, and other symptoms of arthritis, and this effect seems stronger for the revised ASMP.[46]

Regarding health status, self-management interventions decrease pain relative to control groups. Decreases in pain of 15 to 20% have been maintained for years after treatment. These effects were found in mixed arthritis patients but not in RA patients. More studies of self-management with RA patients are needed to confirm this differential effect because differences could also be due to sampling factors.

In studies with mixed arthritis patients, physician visits declined by 30 to 45% in the 4 years after treatment, whereas visits remained stable in nonrandomized comparison groups. Regression to the mean is a potential confounding factor with this design. Patients may seek self-management treatment when their symptoms are most severe, and therefore symptoms and health care use would be lower later on, even without such treatment. Also, patients with more severe illness may be more likely to seek treatment. Lorig and colleagues[54] reported that OA patients in their sample had physician visit rates similar to the national average on study entry, but visits were higher than average for RA patients. Furthermore, ASMP participants had more severe pain to begin with than did comparison-group patients. Thus, regression to the mean cannot be ruled out.

Other indicators of health status are functional disability and disease status. No self-management studies have found long-term decreases in disability. Without treatment, we would expect arthritis patients to become more disabled over time as a result of worsening disease. Shorter term decreases in disability were sometimes found, but this effect was not consistent. Few studies have used objective measures of disease status; thus, the effects of self-management on this variable are not properly known. There is some suggestion that self-management may reduce joint swelling in RA patients, at least in the short term.

The literature provides empirical support for the efficacy of self-management interventions, primarily in relation to arthritis knowledge, compliance with exercise and disease self-management, self-efficacy, health care utilization, and pain. These benefits occurred over and above any effects of concurrent medical treatment. Furthermore, self-management can be administered by lay leaders and is therefore cost-effective and suitable for broad dissemination. Self-management is also based on a theory that specifies self-efficacy as the mediator of health status changes, and the specific treatment components are geared toward enhancing self-efficacy. This conceptual focus may enhance the clarity and strength of the intervention.

There are still some issues that need to be addressed. The majority of studies have been conducted by Lorig and colleagues. More independent replications should be conducted by other investigators. In long-term follow-up studies, regression to the mean has not been ruled out. Another issue concerns the representative nature of participants. Community volunteers may be individuals who cope more actively with their problems or are more motivated than the average patient. Further, the majority of participants were older white women, of higher than average education, and with OA or RA. As we discuss later, Lorig and colleagues are in the process of modifying their intervention for minorities. In the future, researchers should also examine the suitability of these interventions for individuals with less common forms of arthritis. Self-management also consists of many diverse components and it is not clear which components are most effective. With a few exceptions, the effects of self-management have been evaluated mainly by self-report measures of health status, which could be subject to demand characteristics. Researchers could use performance measures of exercise or pain behavior, objective measures of medication use, or spousal reports of disability. In addition, because self-efficacy does not account for all the variance in health status, researchers should examine other potential psychological mediators. Perhaps treatment works by helping patients devise more positive identities, by giving them emotional support and validation, or by enhancing their problem-solving and stress management skills. Finally, self-management seems to be less effective at decreasing depression, and treatment components could be added to address this variable. For example, patients could be encouraged to engage in more positive and enjoyable activities, take better care of themselves, or use their illness as an opportunity for personal and spiritual growth.

## Treatment Interventions for Diverse Ethnic Groups

Issues of cultural diversity have received little attention in the literature on psychosocial treatments for arthritis. In a review of arthritis intervention studies from 1987 to 1993,[59] we found only two needs assessment studies[60,61] and one intervention study[60] geared toward ethnic minorities. White older women with OA or RA were by far the most frequent participants in psychosocial treatment studies. More recently, a few investigators have examined ethnic minority populations with arthritis, mostly Latinas (Hispanic women). In this section we discuss correlational and needs assessment studies that provide guidelines for research and treatment with ethnic minority arthritis patients as well as a handful of intervention studies.

One group of investigators[62,63] studied psychosocial functioning in a sample of low-income Latinas with arthritis. The first study[62] examined the relationship of illness symptoms to social roles, perceived competence, and psychological well-being. In Hispanic and other ethnic minority groups, individuals are not regarded as autonomous but as members of collective units (e.g., family or community) with associated role obligations.[64] Chronic illnesses should be a risk factor for psychological distress to the extent that they interfere with effective role performance. The data supported this theoretical perspective. Greater arthritis pain was related to more intrusions of illness into valued social roles (e.g., mother or worker). Pain and role intrusions also had a negative effect on well-being, which was mediated by decreases in perceived competence. One limitation is that the data were cross-sectional; thus, reverse causality was not ruled out. The second study[63] assessed coping with arthritis. The most frequent coping response was engagement in activities to maintain a sense of competence or to distract oneself from the symptoms. Many patients prayed to God for help or maintained religious faith. Other cop-

ing strategies were distraction, seeking social support, positive reappraisal, and thinking about family as a source of strength.

These studies suggest important Hispanic cultural values and resources that could be incorporated into treatment interventions. These include "*familialism*, which is valuing family relationships and viewing the family as a source of support, strength, and inspiration; religion and spirituality; and an active coping stance when faced with problems."[65]

Investigators conducting research in minority populations need to address issues of recruitment. Traditional recruitment sources, such as hospital records, physician referrals, and clinics, are less efficacious with minorities.[66] Instead, investigators need to use a broad range of strategies, including community outreach, public awareness campaigns, and methods targeted at individuals. Establishing personal contacts with community leaders and service providers enhances community trust and provides credibility. In one study,[67] community talks about arthritis and word of mouth discussion by participants to friends and relatives were the most effective recruitment efforts. The authors noted that provision of information about arthritis represented a service to the community and enhanced community commitment to the project.

Only a few studies have examined treatment interventions with minority or low income populations. One quasi-experimental study[60] evaluated the effects of a 10-hour education course for older, low-income patients with OA. The majority of participants (66%) were black. Course goals were set based on input from both community leaders and professionals. Classes were conducted by trained community leaders and focused on activities and skill-building. The program resulted in increases in knowledge, exercise, positive attitudes, and use of adaptive equipment. Function improved among those receiving self-help aids.

Investigators at the Stanford Arthritis Center[67-70] designed a Spanish Arthritis Self-Management Program, which is a cultural adaptation of the ASMP for Spanish-speaking individuals. The Spanish Arthritis Self-Management Program is a 12-hour (2 hours/week for 6 weeks) community-based, lay teacher-led program. Various arthritis self-report measures were translated and validated for Hispanics to facilitate assessment. In a randomized trial with a 4-month follow-up period, treatment participants reported reduced pain and increased exercise and self-efficacy relative to controls. Results mirror those found for the original ASMP, suggesting that this program can be adapted for Hispanic participants.

Research on psychosocial interventions for arthritis is in its infancy. Most studies have focused on Hispanic populations. Much less is known about how to adapt these interventions for other minority groups, such as Asian Americans or Native Americans. Future research should focus on the appropriateness of group interventions in cultures (e.g., Asian Americans) in which privacy is valued above self-disclosure and in which there is a tradition of solving problems within the family rather than through professional consultation. Studies with Hispanics have identified important cultural values and have established preliminary efficacy of self-management interventions. There is a need to investigate the applicability of CBT interventions to ethnic minorities.

## SUMMARY OF COGNITIVE-BEHAVIOR THERAPY AND PSYCHOEDUCATIONAL TREATMENT

CBT and psychoeducational treatment approaches have had a significant impact on the clinical management of patients with arthritis and on professional and patient views of the adjustment process. Aside from their impact on health outcomes, perhaps the most important contribution of these approaches is that they have changed the role of the patient in arthritis care and in so doing have broadened the model for service delivery and management. By emphasizing the importance of active patient self-management and the learning and acquisition of specific coping skills, patients are encouraged to assume greater responsibility for their health and the management of their medical condition. Greater interdisciplinary involvement by other health professionals, such as psychologists and nurse educators, is fostered in an effort to promote skill development and effective self-management practices. This process results in patients feeling that they have greater mastery over their lives, are more efficacious in the performance of specific health behaviors, and are consequently less dependent on traditional medical treatment. There is evidence that both approaches reduce medical care utilization and health care costs.[54]

CBT and psychoeducational treatments share many important similarities in their underlying philosophy and management approach. Both strategies emphasize the role of learning in the adjustment process to chronic illness, particularly in reference to the development of effective coping skills that are integrated with everyday functioning. They espouse the principle that patients must be actively engaged in their own treatment and be effective problem-solvers in the management of pain and other obstacles resulting from illness. CBT and psychoeducational treatments incorporate many of the same behavioral strategies in their intervention programs. However, the emphasis on enhanced control and effective coping is seen as the key element in leading to beneficial health outcomes. Although occupying unique roles in health care services delivery, both approaches are also seen as enhancing the effectiveness of standard biomedical treatment and other allied health interventions for arthritis patients.

The differences between these approaches are also worth noting because they illustrate somewhat divergent functions in arthritis care. Psychoeducational interventions have tended to be more community-focused and group-oriented and to possess a more public health orientation. A significant advantage of this approach is its use of treatment manuals that ensure standardization of treatment procedures and replicability across different patient groups. Lay leaders serve as effective role models to patients, and somewhat greater emphasis on patient decision-making and empowerment is found in this treatment paradigm. In contrast, CBT methods have been delivered primarily to clinic patients and have been more specifically directed to the management of core difficulties such as pain and stress. CBT interventions have been more commonly administered by psychologists or psychology trainees who are skilled at recognizing individual differences in adjustment problems in patients with chronic illness. As such, these methods have been more tailored to individual patient needs.

Although outcome research has not compared CBT and psychoeducational interventions within the same trial, an optimal integration of these approaches seems warranted in the future. Although the ASMP and other similar psychoeducational interventions may provide an effective general foundation for self-management, more intensive CBT may be applied to the management of pain, disability, and other adjustment problems that reflect the needs and demands of individual patients. To the extent that patients with arthritis differ markedly from one another in pain, disability, and psychological functioning, there will continue to be a need for effective CBT interventions to be tailored to individual patient profiles.

Despite the optimism created by the emergence of these intervention approaches, neither method has been shown to be effective in reducing depression. A possible reason why depression has remained refractory to treatment is that despite its prevalence, depression has not been regarded as an independent therapeutic target. Although investigators have implicitly assumed that depression may improve in response to reductions in pain and disease activity, unfortunately, this has not been found to be true. A different model for the treatment of depression in arthritis should be considered, one in which attention is given to a greater range of variables. For example, CBT approaches have not specifically addressed the loss experienced by patients who find themselves unable to work, ambulate effectively, or participate in social activities, nor have they addressed the harmful effects of such loss on identity and self-esteem. Greater attention may need to be given to the acceptance of loss and its meaning as patients acquire skills in managing the pain and functional impairment of the medical condition. Increased use of behavioral strategies such as scheduling of pleasant events[71] in which patients are directed to increase the frequency of reinforcing behaviors is warranted. Likewise, there is a greater need in CBT and psychoeducational treatment to address the interpersonal dimensions of arthritis. Depression in some patients, for example, may be related to loss of social support, spousal and family conflict, or social isolation resulting from limitations in work and activity. Finally, patients with histories of recurrent depression should be identified as early as possible in treatment so that effective pharmacologic treatment and psychological care can be implemented immediately and aggressively to prevent problems in medical management and adherence.

CBT and psychoeducational interventions also need to concentrate more definitively on the prevention of disability. Long-term follow-up studies of the effects of CBT on disability have not been conducted, and Lorig's ASMP has not been successful in controlling disability over lengthy time intervals. Earlier intervention with these approaches to promote more effective coping and management practices may forestall the progressive, degenerative impact of arthritis after patients have been newly diagnosed but before they have undergone significant life changes. Furthermore, during the earlier stages of illness, it may be possible to prevent the development of negative illness beliefs and helplessness that over time have been shown to be associated with functional declines and maladaptive coping mechanisms.[12, 14] As is the case with depression, future interventions should focus more specifically on the management and prevention of disability. Increased research and clinical attention needs to be devoted to the role of exercise and shaping increases in activity level and role performances through the establishment of behavioral standards and rewards. Family members and spouses of patients need to be educated on the coping process and integrated more consistently into treatment as early as possible to facilitate optimal adjustment in the patient and to encourage personal mastery. As a means of preventing functional declines, effective behavioral and psychoeducational treatment needs to be made a staple of the ongoing management of the arthritis patient. After an initial intervention period, patients may need several trials of these strategies over the course of illness to reinforce adaptive coping and prevent adjustment problems.

In summary, CBT and psychoeducational approaches have assumed an important role in the management of arthritis. This role will continue to evolve as new scientific findings regarding their clinical effectiveness emerge from controlled clinical trials. In the meantime, these approaches are providing greater opportunities for effective clinical care, creating greater hope and optimism in patients, and shaping the development of interdisciplinary models of service delivery that may have far-reaching implications for the management of other chronic medical conditions.

## APPROACH TO THE PATIENT

It is highly important for rheumatologists to communicate directly with patients about the nature of their medical condition in order to establish appropriate expectations regarding the clinical course and goals of treatment. Because rheumatic conditions are routinely treated but not cured, patients must fully understand that the effective management of a chronic illness is an ongoing process in which they may have to make certain adaptations in order to maximize their functioning and well-being over a long period. Such adaptations may involve changes to career plans, roles, and social relationships resulting from the impact of diffi-cult symptoms and functional declines that may be anticipated. These accommodations may be more difficult to accept for some patients than for others, depending on factors such as age, career aspirations, and personal interests. If patients are particularly resistant to discussing such issues or appear unduly anxious or distressed, a referral for psychological management is recommended.

Along with the establishment of appropriate expectations and goals, the importance of effectively managing pain, stress, and disability cannot be emphasized enough. Rheumatologists should convey to patients the importance of effective self-management practices and alert them to the need for the development of skills in these areas that will complement their medical treatment. On the basis of research evidence, the case has been made in this chapter that effective psychosocial treatment should be made a more common element, if not a staple, of arthritis care. Patients should be informed that other professionals may play useful roles in helping them manage the demands of their condition and that there are limitations to biomedical treatment. In particular, rheumatologists should ask patients about their experiences with pain coping skills training or previous participation in arthritis psychoeducational programs. If patients have no experience in these strategies, have refractory pain, or feel helpless in the presence of their medical condition or not in control of difficult symptoms, participation in psychosocial treatments is critical. Referral to the ASMP, which may be offered through the local chapter of the Arthritis Foundation, may be highly useful to patients who lack basic understanding about how to manage arthritis and are without appropriate support for coping with their medical problems.

In other instances, referral for more intensive CBT interventions and related psychotherapeutic treatment is necessary. The psychologist should be knowledgeable about health psychology and behavioral medicine and, if possible, have special expertise in chronic illness. Psychologists with this background may be found in departments of psychiatry or attached to other medical units within major medical centers. They may also be found in private practice or in specialty clinics. In particular, intensive psychological intervention is required for the effective evaluation and management of depression and severe pain. Brief, self-report measures of depression and pain are available and can be used as potential screening devices and integrated with the acquisition of other medical history information. Patients with problems in these areas may be identified immediately. The rheumatologist should communicate directly with the patient and psychologist about the need for adjunctive treatment to set the stage for an effective collaborative effort. Patients tend to be more receptive to psychological referrals if they are clear about the need for treatment and the role of the psychosocial intervention in their medical management. Psychological intervention is also recommended when patients are debilitated by significant life stress or family conflict or when characterological problems such as dependency or passive-aggression are impediments to medical treatment and compliance. Overuse or inappropriate use of medical services may also signal the need for psychological evaluation and management.

Psychosocial treatment is recommended for all patients, regardless of the stage of their medical condition and type of arthritis, if they lack appropriate knowledge and skill in coping with the condition. Early intervention, however, may be instrumental in instilling in the patient appropriate expectations and management skills that may contribute to a higher quality of life and help mitigate adverse psychological reactions and functional declines. In this manner, the appropriate synergy between psychosocial and biomedical approaches to arthritis treatment may be achieved over time.

*Acknowledgment*

*We thank Ms. Jagruti Bhakta for her assistance in evaluating the literature and preparing the manuscript.*

# REFERENCES

1. Felts W, Yelin E: The economic impact of the rheumatic diseases in the United States. J Rheumatol 1989; 16:867–884.
2. Yelin E, Callahan LF: The economic cost and social and psychological impact of musculoskeletal conditions. Arthritis Rheum 1995; 38:1351–1362.
3. Callahan LF: The burden of rheumatoid arthritis: Facts and figures. J Rheumatol 1998; 25(53, Suppl):8–12.
4. Wolfe F, Cathey MA: The assessment and prediction of functional disability in rheumatoid arthritis. J Rheumatol 1991; 18:1298–1306.
5. Leigh PJ, Fries JF: Predictors of disability in a longitudinal sample of patients with rheumatoid arthritis. Ann Rheum Dis 1992; 51:581–587.
6. Scott DL, Symmons DPM, Coulton BL, et al: Long-term outcome of treating rheumatoid arthritis: Results after 20 years. Lancet 1987; 1:1108–1111.
7. Gibson T, Clark B: Use of simple analgesics in rheumatoid arthritis. Ann Rheum Dis 1985; 44:27–29.
8. Young LD: Psychological factors in rheumatoid arthritis. J Consult Clin Psychol 1992; 60:619–627.
9. Wells KB, Golding JM, Burnham MA: Psychiatric disorders in a sample of the general medical population with and without medical disorders. Am J Psychiatry 1988; 145:976–981.
10. Frank RG, Beck NC, Parker JC, et al: Depression in rheumatoid arthritis. J Rheumatol 1988; 15:920–925.
11. Brown G: A causal analysis of chronic pain and depression. J Abnorm Psychol 1990; 99:121–137.
12. Nicassio PM, Wallston KA, Callahan LF, et al: The measurement of helplessness in rheumatoid arthritis. The development of the Arthritis Helplessness Index. J Rheumatol 1985; 12:462–467.
13. Smith TW, Peck JR, Milano RA, et al: Cognitive distortion in rheumatoid arthritis: Relation to depression and disability. J Consult Clin Psychol 1988; 56:412–416.
14. Keefe FJ, Brown GK, Wallston KA, et al: Coping with rheumatoid arthritis pain: Catastrophizing as a maladaptive strategy. Pain 1989; 37:51–56.
15. Smith TW, Peck JR, Ward JR: Helplessness and depression in rheumatoid arthritis. Health Psychol 1990; 9:337–389.
16. Brown GK, Nicassio PM: Development of a questionnaire for the assessment of active and passive coping strategies in chronic pain patients. Pain 1987; 31:53–64.
17. Manne SL, Zautra AJ: Coping with arthritis. Arthritis Rheum 1992; 35:1273–1280.
18. Buckelew SP, Parker JC: Coping with arthritis pain: A review of the literature. Arthritis Care Res 1989; 2:136–145.
19. Zautra AJ, Manne SL: Coping with rheumatoid arthritis: A review of a decade of research. Ann Behav Med 1992; 14:31–39.
20. Engel GL: The clinical application of the biopsychosocial model. Am J Psychiatry 1980; 137:535–544.
21. Fries JF: Reevaluating the therapeutic approach to rheumatoid arthritis: The "sawtooth" strategy. J Rheumatol 1990; 17(22, Suppl):12–15.
22. Wolfe F: 50 years of antirheumatic therapy: The prognosis of rheumatoid arthritis. J Rheumatol 1990; 17(22, Suppl):24–31.
23. Parker J, Frank R, Beck N, et al: Pain in rheumatoid arthritis: Relationship to demographic, medical, and psychological factors. J Rheumatol 1988; 15:433–437.
24. Turk DC, Salovey P: Cognitive-behavioral treatment of illness behavior. *In* Nicassio PM, Smith TW (eds): The Management of Chronic Illness: A Biopsychosocial Perspective. Washington, DC: American Psychological Association, 1995:245–284.
25. Achterberg J, McGraw P, Lawlis GF: Rheumatoid arthritis: A study of relaxation and temperature biofeedback training as an adjunctive therapy. Biofeedback Self Regul 1981; 6:207–223.
26. Bradley LA, Young LD, Anderson KO, et al: Effects of psychological therapy on pain behavior of rheumatoid arthritis patients. Arthritis Rheum 1987; 30:1105–1114.
27. Young LD, Bradley LA, Turner RA: Decreases in health care resource utilization in patients with rheumatoid arthritis following a cognitive behavioral intervention. Biofeedback Self Regul 1995; 20:259–286.
28. Applebaum KA, Blanchard EB, Hickling EJ, et al: Cognitive behavioral treatment of a veteran population with moderate to severe rheumatoid arthritis. Behav Ther 1988; 19:489–502.
29. O'Leary A, Shoor S, Lorig K, et al: A cognitive-behavioral treatment for rheumatoid arthritis. Health Psychol 1988; 7:527–544.
30. Lorig K, Fries JF: The Arthritis Helpbook. Reading, MA: Addison-Wesley, 1980.
31. Parker JC, Frank RG, Beck NC, et al: Pain management in rheumatoid arthritis patients. A cognitive-behavioral approach. Arthritis Rheum 1988; 31:593–601.
32. Radojevic V, Nicassio PM, Weisman MH: Behavioral intervention with and without family support for rheumatoid arthritis. Behav Ther 1992; 23:13–30.
33. Turk DC, Flor H, Rudy TE: Pain and families: Part I. Etiology, maintenance, and psychosocial impact. Pain 1987; 30:3–27.
34. Kraaimaat FW, Brons MR, Geenen R, et al: The effect of cognitive behavior therapy in patients with rheumatoid arthritis. Behav Res Ther 1995; 33:487–495.
35. Keefe FJ, Caldwell DS, Williams DA, et al: Pain coping skills training in the management of osteoarthritic knee pain: A comparative study. Behav Ther 1990; 21:49–62.
36. Keefe FJ, Caldwell DS, Williams DA, et al: Pain coping skills training in the management of osteoarthritic knee pain: II. Follow-up results. Behav Ther 1990; 21:435–447.
37. Calfas KJ, Kaplan RM, Ingram RE: One-year evaluation of cognitive-behavioral intervention in osteoarthritis. Arthritis Care Res 1992; 5:202–209.
38. Keefe F, Caldwell D, Baucom D, et al: Spouse-assisted coping skills training in the management of osteoarthritic knee pain. Arthritis Care Res 1996; 9:279–291.
39. Huyser B, Parker JC: Stress and rheumatoid arthritis: An integrative review. Arthritis Care Res 1998; 11:135–145.
40. Zautra A, Burleson MH, Matt KS, et al: Interpersonal stress, depression, and disease activity in rheumatoid arthritis and osteoarthritis patients. Health Psychol 1994; 13:139–148.
41. Shearn MA, Fireman BH: Stress management and mutual support groups in rheumatoid arthritis. Am J Med 1985; 78:771–775.
42. Parker JC, Smarr KL, Buckelew SP, et al: Effects of stress management on clinical outcomes in rheumatoid arthritis. Arthritis Rheum 1995; 38:1807–1818.
43. DeVellis BM, Blalock SJ, Hahn PM, et al: Evaluation of a problem-solving intervention for patients with arthritis. Patient Educ Couns 1988; 11:29–42.
44. Sinclair VG, Wallston KA, Dwyer KA, et al: Effects of a cognitive-behavioral intervention for women with rheumatoid arthritis. Res Nurs Health 1998; 21:315–326.
45. Lorig K, Holman H: Arthritis self-management studies: A twelve-year review. Health Educ Q 1993; 20:17–28.
46. Lorig K, Gonzalez V: The integration of theory with practice: A 12-year case study. Health Educ Q 1992; 19:355–368.

47. Bandura A: Social Foundations of Thought and Action: A Social Cognitive Theory. Englewood Cliffs, NJ: Prentice-Hall, 1986.

48. O'Leary A: Self-efficacy and health. Behav Res Ther 1985; 23:437–451.

49. Lorig K, Lubeck D, Kraines RG, et al: Outcomes of self-help education for patients with arthritis. Arthritis Rheum 1985; 28:680–685.

50. Lorig K, Feigenbaum P, Regan C, et al: A comparison of lay-taught and professional-taught arthritis self-management courses. J Rheumatol 1986; 13:763–767.

51. Cohen J, Van Houten Sauter S, DeVellis R, et al: Evaluation of arthritis self-management courses led by laypersons and by professionals. Arthritis Rheum 1986; 29:388–393.

52. Lorig K, Holman H: Long-term outcomes of an arthritis self-management study: Effects of reinforcement efforts. Soc Sci Med 1989; 29:221–224.

53. Holman H, Mazonson P, Lorig K: Health education for self-management has significant early and sustained benefits in chronic arthritis. Trans Assoc Am Phys 1989; 10:206–208.

54. Lorig K, Mazonson P, Holman H: Evidence suggesting that health education for self-management in patients with chronic arthritis has sustained health benefits while reducing health care costs. Arthritis Rheum 1993; 36:439–446.

55. Lorig K, Seleznick M, Lubeck D, et al: The beneficial outcomes of the arthritis self-management course are not adequately explained by behavior change. Arthritis Rheum 1989; 32:91–95.

56. Lorig K, Chastain RL, Ung E, et al: Development and evaluation of a scale to measure perceived self-efficacy in people with arthritis. Arthritis Rheum 1989; 32:37–44.

57. Taal E, Riemsma R, Brus H, et al: Group education for patients with rheumatoid arthritis. Patient Educ Couns 1993; 20:177–187.

58. Brus H, Van de Laar M, Taal E, et al: Effects of patient education on compliance with basic treatment regimens and health in recent onset active rheumatoid arthritis. Ann Rheum Dis 1998; 57:146–151.

59. Hirano P, Laurent D, Lorig K: Arthritis patient education studies, 1987–1991: A review of the literature. Patient Educ Couns 1994; 24:9–54.

60. Bill-Harvey D, Rippey R, Abeles M, et al: Outcome of an osteoarthritis education program for low-literacy patients taught by indigenous instructors. Patient Educ Couns 1989; 13:133–142.

61. Robbins L, Allegrante J, Paget S: Adapting the systemic lupus erythematosus self-help (SLESH) course for Latino SLE patients. Arthritis Care Res 1993; 6:97–103.

62. Abraido-Lanza A: Latinas with arthritis: Effects of illness, role, identity, and competence on psychological well-being. Am J Community Psychol 1997; 25:601–627.

63. Abraido-Lanza A, Guier C, Revenson T: Coping and social support resources among Latinas with arthritis. Arthritis Care Res 1996; 9:501–508.

64. Landrine H: Clinical implications of cultural differences: The referential versus the indexical self. Clin Psychol Rev 1992; 12:401–415.

65. Abraido-Lanza A, Guier C, Colon RM: Psychological thriving among Latinas with chronic illnesses. J Soc Issues 1998; 54:405–424.

66. Murdaugh C: Recruitment issues in research with special populations. Cardiovasc Nurs 1990; 4:51–55.

67. Nacif de Brey V, Gonzalez V: Recruiting for arthritis studies in hard-to-reach populations: A comparison of methods used in an urban Spanish-speaking community. Arthritis Care Res 1997; 10:64–71.

68. Gonzalez V, Lorig K: Spanish arthritis self-management studies: Description and outcomes. Ann Behav Med 1997; 19(Suppl): S074.

69. Gonzalez V, Stewart A, Ritter P, et al: Translation and validation of arthritis outcome measures into Spanish. Arthritis Rheum 1995; 38:1429–1446.

70. Lorig K, Gonzalez V: Spanish arthritis self-management study: Description and outcomes. Arthritis Rheum 1997; 40(9 Suppl):S175.

71. Lewinsohn P: The behavioral study and treatment of depression. In Hersen M, Eisler R, Miller P (eds): Progress in Behavior Modification. New York: Academic Press, 1975:19–65.

CHAPTER

**14**  The Treatment of Rheumatic Diseases During Pregnancy

*Bonnie L. Bermas*

The systemic rheumatic diseases have a predilection for women of child-bearing age. These rheumatic disorders are affected differently by pregnancy. Rheumatoid arthritis (RA) generally improves, whereas systemic lupus erythematosus either ameliorates or worsens.[1] Other diseases, such as progressive systemic sclerosis, dermatomyositis, and relapsing polychondritis, can become active during pregnancy, and patients may require aggressive therapy. Clinicians treating these patients are faced with a difficult dilemma: how to balance the need to control disease in the mother against the potential risk of therapy to both the mother and the fetus.

Pregnancy induces immunologic changes that can potentiate a drug's toxicity and have an impact on disease activity. These alterations include increased complement levels, decreased circulating CD4 cells, and attenuated natural killer cell activity.[2] It has been hypothesized that T helper 1–type cytokines such as interleukin-$\gamma$ and tumor necrosis factor-$\alpha$ (TNF-$\alpha$) are down-regulated in pregnancy.[3] The success of biologic agents that block TNF-$\alpha$ in the treatment of RA may provide one clue as to why RA improves during pregnancy.[4]

The approach to the patient with a rheumatic disease who wishes to become pregnant is complex. Ideally, the pregnancy should be planned when the disease is in remission or well controlled, but this is not always possible given that roughly one half of pregnancies in the general population are unplanned.[5] Assessing a medication's true toxicity is difficult at best. We are dependent on drug testing, which often entails supra-pharmacologic dosing and may not adequately assess real risk.[6] Furthermore, pharmaceutical companies are reticent to test medications for teratogenicity because of their potential liability. The only antirheumatic medications definitively shown to be teratogenic are some

nonsteroidal anti-inflammatory drugs (NSAIDs), leflunomide, methotrexate, and cyclophosphamide,[5] but guidelines developed by the American College of Rheumatology suggest that many other medications currently used to treat rheumatic conditions are not compatible with pregnancy (Table 14–1).[7] Therefore, clinicians are left to sift through conflicting and inconclusive data to assess a medication's true risk during pregnancy.[8–10]

This chapter discusses the impact of pregnancy on RA and progressive systemic sclerosis (systemic lupus erythematosus in pregnancy is discussed in Chapter 23). The safety of antirheumatic therapies in pregnancy and breast-feeding is also reviewed. Medications discussed include aspirin and the NSAIDs, the glucocorticoids, the antimalarials, gold salts, penicillamine, the immunosuppressive agent cyclosporine, the purine analogs azathioprine and 6-mercaptopurine, the alkylating agents chlorambucil and cyclophosphamide, the folate antagonist methotrexate, intravenous immune globulin (IVIG), and the newer agents etanercept and leflunomide.

## PREGNANCY AND RHEUMATOID ARTHRITIS

Most patients with RA improve during pregnancy. This was first observed by Hench, who described amelioration of RA symptoms in 22 pregnant women.[11] In another review of 308 RA patients who became pregnant, 73% had a disease remission.[12] It is now accepted that 70% to 80% of patients with RA undergo remission during pregnancy.[13] In general, symptoms start improving in the first trimester and this improvement continues through delivery, although there is a risk of postpartum flare in most patients.[12, 13] The

**TABLE 14–1**
**Antirheumatic Drug Therapy in Pregnancy and Lactation, and Effects on Fertility**

| DRUG | FOOD AND DRUG ADMINISTRATION USE-IN-PREGNANCY RATING* | CROSSES PLACENTA | MAJOR MATERNAL TOXICITIES | FETAL TOXICITIES | LACTATION | FERTILITY |
|---|---|---|---|---|---|---|
| Aspirin | C; D in third trimester | Yes | Anemia, peripartum hemorrhage, prolonged labor | Premature closure of ductus, pulmonary hypertension, ICH | Use cautiously; excreted at low concentration; doses >1 tablet (325 mg) result in high concentrations in infant plasma | No data |
| NSAIDs | B; D in third trimester | Yes | As for aspirin | As for aspirin | Compatible according to AAP | No data |
| Corticosteroids: |  |  |  |  |  |  |
| Prednisone | B | Dexamethasone and beta-methasone | Exacerbation of diabetes and hypertension, PROM | IUGR | 5%–20% of maternal dose excreted in breast milk; compatible, but wait 4 hr if dose >20 mg | No data |
| Dexamethasone | C |  |  |  |  |  |
| Hydroxychloroquine | C | Yes: fetal concentration 50% of maternal | Few | Few | Contraindicated (slow elimination rate, potential for accumulation) | No data |
| Gold | C | Yes | No data | One report of cleft palate and severe CNS abnormalities | Excreted into breast milk (20% of maternal dose); rash, hepatitis, and hematologic abnormalities reported, but AAP considers it compatible | No data |
| D-Penicillamine | D | Yes | No data | Cutis laxa connective tissue abnormalities | No data | No data |
| Sulfasalazine | B; D if near term | Yes | No data | No increase in congenital malformations, kernicterus if administered near term | Excreted into breast milk (40%–60% maternal dose); bloody diarrhea in 1 infant; AAP recommends caution | Females: no effect; males: significant oligospermia (2 months to return to normal) |

164

| Drug | FDA rating | | | | | |
|---|---|---|---|---|---|---|
| Azathioprine | D | Yes | No data | IUGR (rate up to 40%) and prematurity, transient immunosuppression in neonate, possible effect on germlines of offspring | No data; hypothetical risk of immunosuppression outweighs benefit | Not studied; can interfere with effectiveness of IUD |
| Chlorambucil | D | Teratogenic effects potentiated by caffeine | No data | Renal angiogenesis | Contraindicated | No data |
| Methotrexate | X | No data | Spontaneous abortion | Fetal abnormalities (including cleft palate and hydrocephalus) | Contraindicated; small amounts excreted with potential to accumulate in fetal tissues | Females: infrequent long-term effect; males: reversible oligospermia |
| Cyclophosphamide | D | Yes: 25% of maternal level | No data | Severe abnormalities; case report: male twin developed thyroid papillary cancer at 11 yr and neuroblastoma at 14 yr | Contraindicated; has caused bone marrow depression | Females: age >25 yr, concurrent radiation, and prolonged exposure increase risk of infertility; males: dose-dependent oligospermia and azoospermia regardless of age or exposure |
| Cyclosporine | C | Yes | No data | IUGR and prematurity; 1 case report: hypoplasia of right leg; not an animal teratogen and unlikely to be a human one | Contraindicated due to potential for immunosuppression | No data |

* Food and Drug Administration use-in-pregnancy ratings are as follows: A = Controlled studies show no risk. Adequate, well-controlled studies in pregnant women have failed to demonstrate risk to the fetus. B = No evidence of risk in humans. Either animal findings show risk but human findings do not or, if no adequate human studies have been performed, animal findings are negative. C = Risk cannot be ruled out. Human studies are lacking and results of animal studies are either positive for fetal risk or lacking as well. However, potential benefits may justify the potential risk. D = Positive evidence of risk. Investigational or postmarketing data show risk to the fetus. Nevertheless, potential benefits may outweigh the potential risk. X = Contraindicated in pregnancy. Studies in animals or humans, or investigational or postmarketing reports, have shown fetal risk that clearly outweigh any possible benefit to the patient.

ICH = intracranial hemorrhage; AAP = American Academy of Pediatrics; PROM = premature rupture of membranes; IUGR = intrauterine growth retardation; CNS = central nervous system; IUD = intrauterine device.

From American College of Rheumatology Ad Hoc Committee on Clinical Guidelines: Guidelines for monitoring drug therapy in rheumatoid arthritis. Arthritis Rheum 1996; 39:723–731.

amount of improvement in RA symptoms appears to be related to the degree of HLA disparity between the mother and the fetus.[14] There is no increased fetal wastage or morbidity in women with RA.[15] Some of the antirheumatic medications can be continued in patients who do experience disease flare during pregnancy (see further on). In general, I counsel patients to discontinue their medications during pregnancy because they have a good chance of the disease going into remission.

## PROGRESSIVE SYSTEMIC SCLEROSIS DURING PREGNANCY

Progressive systemic sclerosis (scleroderma) is an uncommon systemic illness whose peak incidence is in the fourth to fifth decades of life. As of 1971, there were only 12 reported cases of pregnancy in scleroderma patients.[16] As the age for child bearing extends, more patients with progressive systemic sclerosis will desire pregnancy and more data on the activity of this disease will be available.

A study by Steen and Medsger retrospectively reviewed reproductive histories in 214 women with progressive systemic sclerosis, 167 patients with RA, and 105 neighborhood controls. They found no overall difference in miscarriage rate, prematurity, or small for gestational age babies between these groups. However, patients who became pregnant after the onset of disease had slightly higher miscarriage rates, prematurity, and infants who were small for gestational age.[17]

Few studies are available evaluating the activity of scleroderma during pregnancy. Although one case report discussed two pregnancies in scleroderma patients that were complicated by hypertension and congestive heart failure,[18] another study showed that the frequency of complications in scleroderma patients was not higher than that seen in RA patients.[19] However, occasionally scleroderma is complicated by renal crisis during pregnancy, and complications are high in these patients.[20]

## OTHER RHEUMATIC DISEASES

There are limited data on other rheumatic diseases during pregnancy. Only case reports or limited case series are available. What is clear is that all of the rheumatic diseases can flare during pregnancy, and medications may be necessary.

## MEDICATIONS

## Aspirin and Nonsteroidal Anti-inflammatory Drugs

ASPIRIN. Aspirin and NSAIDs are a critical aspect of therapy in rheumatic conditions. In animal studies, high doses of aspirin have been found to be terato-

genic.[21] In humans, there have been case reports of fetal malformations with aspirin use[22] (Table 14–2), but in a series of 5128 pregnancies in which high-dose aspirin exposure occurred, there was no increased incidence in teratogenesis.[23]

Daily baby aspirin is used for the treatment of the pregnancy complications seen in the antiphospholipid antibody syndrome.[24] No fetal malformations have occurred, and currently such treatment is recommended to patients through term despite the theoretical risk of intracranial hemorrhage during delivery.[25]

Aspirin is excreted in low concentrations in breast milk. There is one case report of infant toxicity after salicylate exposure from breast milk, but the American Academy of Pediatrics concludes that aspirin is compatible with breast-feeding.[26]

NONSTEROIDAL ANTI-INFLAMMATORY DRUGS. In animal studies, high doses of indomethacin have been shown to be teratogenic.[27] Some of the other nonsteroidal agents such as ibuprofen do not cause fetal malformations.[28] In humans, NSAIDs do cross the placenta. Although NSAIDs are not associated with increased fetal malformation, exposure during the third trimester increases the risk of patent ductus arteriosus.[28]

In conclusion, the limited data suggest that low doses of aspirin and NSAIDs can be used during the first two trimesters. Use of these agents during the third trimester should be avoided because they may interfere with closure of the ductus arteriosus and the progression of labor. Baby aspirin may be used for the treatment of the antiphospholipid antibody syndrome throughout pregnancy. The teratogenicity of the newer cyclooxygenase-2 inhibitors is unknown. These medications can prevent implantation, so they probably should be avoided in patients with fertility issues.[29]

Ingestion of high doses of aspirin should be avoided by nursing mothers because platelet function in the infant may be impaired. Lower doses of aspirin and NSAIDs are compatible with breast-feeding.[26]

## Glucocorticoids

Glucocorticoids are used in treating rheumatic diseases and asthma and in transplant recipients. There is now substantial clinical experience with the use of these medications during pregnancy. There are many preparations of glucocorticoids available. The most commonly used shorter acting agents are prednisone, prednisolone, and methylprednisolone. Radioactively labeled prednisone and prednisolone are found in cord blood at a level that is 8- to 10-fold lower than that seen in the mother's blood.[30] Dexamethasone and betamethasone are less effectively metabolized by the placenta and therefore reach the fetus at higher concentrations, presumably because they are fluorinated. Thus, these latter agents are used to treat fetal disorders such as lung immaturity, whereas the shorter acting agents are used in treating maternal disease.[31]

In animal studies, cleft palates have been seen in offspring exposed to prednisone in utero.[32] In humans, there have been case reports of cleft palates, mental retardation, and fatal adrenal hypoplasia after intra-

# TABLE 14-2
## Summary of Toxicities of Antirheumatic Therapies in Animals and Humans

| DRUG | ANIMALS Embryotoxic | ANIMALS Fetal | HUMANS Maternal | HUMANS Fetal | BREAST-FEEDING |
|---|---|---|---|---|---|
| Aspirin and NSAIDs | No | In high doses—teratogenic | No | Premature closure of the ductus arteriosus | Aspirin: Use cautiously; excreted at low concentrations NSAIDs: Compatible |
| Glucocorticoids | No | Cleft palate Aggressive behavior | PROM Hypertension Glucose intolerance Osteoporosis Osteonecrosis | SGA Adrenal hypoplasia Promotes lung maturity Cleft palate* Still birth* | Crosses into breast milk at low concentration, well tolerated |
| Antimalarial agents | No | Chorioretinotoxicity | No | Case reports of pigment deposition in the retina, cochleovestibular paresis, dorsal column disease, and mental retardation | Crosses into breast milk, contraindicated |
| Gold | No | Teratogenic in rats | No | One report of cleft palate and central nervous system abnormality | Compatible |
| Penicillamine | No information available | Teratogenic in rats | No | Cutis laxa, connective tissue abnormalities | No data |
| Sulfasalazine | No information available | Teratogenic in rats | No | Cleft palate VSD Coarctation of the aorta Macrocephaly Oligospermia | Crosses into breast milk at low concentrations |
| Cyclosporine | Yes | Renal tubular cell damage Skeletal abnormalities Cleft palate Decreased thymic development and hematopoiesis | Renal insufficiency | Spontaneous abortions | Contraindicated |
| Azathioprine | Yes | | No information available | Diminished fertility in offspring* | Contraindicated† |
| 6-Mercaptopurine | Yes | Cleft palate | No information available | SGA Prematurity Intrauterine growth retardation Cleft palate | No information available |
| Methotrexate | Yes | Skeletal abnormalities Cleft palate | No information available | Embryotoxic Skeletal abnormalities Facial abnormalities | Contraindicated† |
| Cyclophosphamide | Yes | SGA Skeletal abnormalities Cleft palate Exophthalmos Decreased fertility | Decreased fertility in males and females | SGA Limb abnormalities Coronary artery agenesis Tumors in offspring* | Contraindicated |
| Chlorambucil | Yes | SGA Skeletal abnormalities Renal agenesis | No information available | SGA Skeletal abnormalities Renal agenesis | Contraindicated* |
| Intravenous immune globulin | No information available | No information available | No information available | SGA Autoantibodies | No information available |
| Leflunomide | No information available | Teratogenic | No information available | Currently FDA class X | Contraindicated |
| Etanercept | No information available | No information available | No information available | Currently FDA class B | Contraindicated |

* Theoretical risk or case reports only.
† Conflicting information.
NSAIDs = nonsteroidal anti-inflammatory drugs; PROM = premature rupture of membranes; SGA = small for gestational age; VSD = ventricular septal defect; FDA = Food and Drug Administration.

uterine exposure to steroids.[33–35] Controlled studies in asthmatic patients receiving low-dose corticosteroid therapy (mean dose of 10 mg/day) during pregnancy failed to show an increased incidence of congenital malformations when compared with that in the general population.[36, 37] Offspring of women with the antiphospholipid antibody syndrome who were treated with steroids during pregnancy did not have increased fetal anomalies, although there was a higher rate of small for gestational age infants. Maternal complications after glucocorticoid exposure include an increased risk of preeclampsia, gestational hypertension, and diabetes.[24] In contrast, in a recent meta-analysis of more than 20,000 pregnancies in which the fetus was exposed to corticosteroids in utero, there was an increased relative risk of 4 of cleft palate formation in the newborns (A. Pastuszak, personal communication).

In conclusion, glucocorticoids appear to be compatible with pregnancy. There is an increased incidence of cleft palate, although the overall rate is still low. In patients receiving glucocorticoid therapy who then have a prolonged or complicated labor or require cesarean section, 100 mg of hydrocortisone sodium succinate, administered intravenously every 8 hours, should be given at delivery. Neonates should be monitored for adrenal insufficiency.

Only 10% of the prednisone and prednisolone ingested is secreted into breast milk; therefore, these medications are considered to be compatible with nursing. In patients who receive greater than 20 mg a day of these medications, the recommendation is to wait 4 hours after dosing to resume breast-feeding.[26]

## Antimalarial Agents

Perhaps no medication better demonstrates prescription difficulties during pregnancy than the 4-aminoquinoline antimalarial agents hydroxychloroquine (Plaquenil) and chloroquine. There are limited controlled studies that adequately address the safety of these drugs during pregnancy, and many of the available data have been extrapolated from the malarial endemic areas of the world where these medications are used for chemoprophylaxis of parasitic infection.

The antimalarial agents have been shown to cross the placenta in animals and cause chorioretinotoxicity.[38] Similarly chloroquine and its metabolites were found to cross the placenta in humans. Concentrations found in the neonatal circulation are approximately 50% that found in the maternal circulation.[39] There is a large body of literature showing that chloroquine phosphate and hydroxychloroquine can be taken safely during pregnancy as malarial prophylaxis.[40] However, doses for malarial prophylaxis are generally in the range of up to 300 mg weekly, whereas doses for rheumatic therapy are more likely to be 200 to 500 mg/day.

Despite the encouraging data from the literature on malaria, there have been case reports of fetal toxicities after in utero exposure to these medications during antirheumatic therapy. In one study of congenital deafness, 4% of cases were thought to be due to prenatal chloroquine exposure (dose unknown).[41] The most alarming data come from the case of a single patient who took chloroquine phosphate, 250 mg twice daily, for discoid lupus for part or all of four pregnancies. These pregnancies resulted in one miscarriage and three children with congenital defects. Abnormalities seen in the children included pigment deposition in the retina, cochleovestibular paresis, dorsal column disease, and mental retardation. In the three pregnancies in which the patient was not taking this medication, no malformations were seen.[42]

There are now several series in which patients with rheumatic diseases continued taking antimalarial agents during pregnancy without adverse outcome. Parke and Rothfield at the University of Connecticut described 16 lupus patients who had continued taking hydroxychloroquine during pregnancy. No ocular or oral defects or other congenital abnormalities were seen in the offspring.[43] Khamashta and colleagues likewise monitored 33 women who had taken hydroxychloroquine during pregnancy and reported no teratogenicity.[44]

In animal models, there is evidence that hydroxychloroquine may reverse the thrombotic properties of anticardiolipin antibodies. Thus in patients with rheumatic diseases and coexisting antiphospholipid antibody syndrome, there may be a stronger rationale for maintaining antimalarial therapy during pregnancy.[45]

There is no clear consensus on the use of antimalarial agents during pregnancy. Although these medications are rated a risk level C by the Food and Drug Administration for use during pregnancy, the half-life of the drugs is so long that discontinuing these medications soon before conception does not necessarily eliminate exposure. I recommend that patients with systemic lupus erythematosus whose disease is well controlled with antimalarial agents remain on medication during pregnancy. Careful prenatal counseling about the theoretical risks to the fetus (retinal and aural in particular) should be carried out so that the patient can participate in the decision regarding treatment. Patients with RA are likely to go into remission during pregnancy and should discontinue these medications when they become pregnant.

Hydroxychloroquine crosses the placenta in small amounts. Although the American Academy of Pediatrics considers this medication compatible with breast-feeding, the slow accumulation of this medication and the higher doses used in the treatment of rheumatic conditions supported the American College of Rheumatology's decision to state that this medication was incompatible with breast-feeding.[7, 26] I believe that antimalarial agents should be avoided in nursing mothers.

## Gold

Gold has been used for the therapy of RA, and less frequently for psoriatic arthritis, for many years. Animal studies have shown that rats exposed to suramin and aurothiomalate sodium in utero have a risk of congenital malformations. The proposed mechanism of toxicity is the interference with the yolk sac nutritional pathway.[46]

In humans, there has been one case report of multiple congenital malformations in the offspring of a mother who received intramuscular gold therapy for the first 20 weeks of gestation.[47] A subsequent case series of 128 children exposed to gold in utero failed to show any increased risk of congenital malformations.[48]

Given the selection of alternative therapies, and the paucity of information regarding the safety of gold during pregnancy, I would recommend avoiding gold during pregnancy. In reality, however, the half-life of gold is so long that discontinuation of this therapy does not significantly reduce body stores during pregnancy.

Gold is concentrated in milk and can reach detectable levels in the infant's serum.[49] Nonetheless, this medication is considered compatible with breast-feeding by the American Academy of Pediatrics.[26]

## Penicillamine

Penicillamine is teratogenic in animals.[50] There are limited data on the use of penicillamine during pregnancy in humans. Although there have been case series of safety during pregnancy, there have also been reported cases of connective tissue defects such as cutis laxa.[51, 52] As a result, penicillamine is rated class D for use during pregnancy. Given the wide variety of alternative therapies, this medication should be avoided during pregnancy.

There are no data on whether penicillamine is secreted in breast milk. Given the lack of data, the American Academy of Pediatrics advises against the use of penicillamine for breast-feeding.

## Sulfasalazine

Sulfasalazine is used for the treatment of RA, psoriatic arthritis, and inflammatory bowel disease. Sulfasalazine and its metabolite sulfapyridine cross the placenta.[53] Sulfapyridine displaces small amounts of bilirubin from albumin, which could potentially lead to kernicterus, although this is not thought to be clinically relevant.[54]

In rats, sulfasalazine is teratogenic.[55] There have been case reports of cleft lip and palate, hydrocephalus, macrocephaly, ventricular septal defect, and coarctation of the aorta after sulfasalazine exposure in utero.[56, 57] However, larger case series have failed to demonstrate an increased risk of congenital anomalies in offspring of mothers treated with this medication. In one study of 137 patients with ulcerative colitis and 107 patients with Crohn's disease, there were 135 and 105 births, respectively.[58] There was no increased rate of fetal anomalies or jaundice in the offspring. Other series have substantiated the safety of this medication during pregnancy.[59] Thus, although case reports of fetal anomalies in offspring exposed to sulfasalazine in utero exist, larger series show no increased incidence of adverse pregnancy outcomes. Because this medication can interfere with folic acid absorption, supplemental folic acid beyond the standard amount used in pregnancy is recommended.[60]

Sulfasalazine also induces oligospermia and decreased sperm motility. Normal sperm function appears to return about 3 months after discontinuation of this medication.[61] Therefore we recommend the cessation of this medication in males 3 months before attempting conception. For women with active arthritis who require treatment during pregnancy, sulfasalazine therapy may be a viable option with relatively low risk.

Although the amount of sulfasalazine found in the breast milk and serum of nursing babies is minimal,[62, 63] the American Academy of Pediatrics warns against its use in nursing mothers because of a case report of bloody diarrhea in a breast-fed infant receiving sulfasalazine therapy.[52]

## Cyclosporine

Cyclosporine is a cyclic 11–amino acid peptide used as an essential component of immunosuppressive therapy for solid organ transplant recipients. In mice, radioactive-labeled cyclosporine does not cross the placenta.[64] In contrast, in two pregnant women receiving cyclosporine, high levels of cyclosporine were found in the cord blood and the placenta.[65]

In animals given high doses of cyclosporine (25 mg/kg/day) from conception to 20 days after mating, there were increased fetal mortality and kidney abnormalities.[66] In another study of rat embryos, cyclosporine had no effect on organogenesis.[67]

Transplant registries provide information on a large number of women who have taken cyclosporine while pregnant. In one series of 154 pregnancies in 115 female renal transplant recipients, there were two sets of twins and 155 live births in women taking cyclosporine.[68] These pregnancies were compared with 146 pregnancies during which the mothers received azathioprine and steroids, azathioprine alone, or steroids alone. In the cyclosporine group, the patients had a higher incidence of diabetes and hypertension. Offspring were more likely to be premature and have a lower birth weight. There were neonatal complications in 22%, including respiratory distress syndrome, one case of kidney malformation, one ventricular septal defect, and one patent ductus arteriosus. In Norway, the experience has been similar. There was no increase in fetal malformations in pregnant patients taking cyclosporine, although there was an increase in the spontaneous abortion rate and preterm deliveries.[69] Liver transplant recipients treated with cyclosporine during pregnancy were more likely to have preeclampsia, hypertension, and infants who were small for gestational age than were pregnant liver transplant recipients given tacrolimus, another immunosuppressive agent.[70] Finally, in the National Transplantation Pregnancy Registry in the United States, 500 pregnancies have been reported thus far.[71] The live birth rate is slightly lower in the kidney patients receiving cyclosporine than in patients receiving other immunosuppressive regimens. These results must be interpreted with caution, as those patients who are sicker or at greater risk of losing their grafts are more likely to be treated with cyclosporine. There is a hypothetical risk that exposure to cyclosporine in utero when the thymus is developing could predispose to subsequent autoimmune disease. This concern is substantiated in at least one animal model in which mice exposed to cyclosporine in utero had thymuses that were partially depleted of some sets of T cells. Two animals also had evidence of mononuclear cell infiltrates in the gastric mucosa.[72] In humans, two babies born to mothers who had received cyclosporine had some differences in T-cell subpopulations in comparison with control infants, but the profile was not suggestive of chronic immunosuppression.[73] In another case report, an infant born to a mother receiving cyclosporine after liver transplantation had low levels of all lymphocyte subsets for the first 2 years of life.[74]

In conclusion, cyclosporine is considered to be safe during pregnancy. Teratogenicity is low, but intrauterine growth retardation and infants small for gestational age are seen. Although there is a hypothetical risk for long-term immunologic suppression, to date there are no data available to address this issue adequately. Cyclosporine is thus a viable alternative when immunosuppression is required during pregnancy.

Cyclosporine crosses into breast milk. The American Academy of Pediatrics does not consider this medication compatible with breast-feeding, as there is a risk of immunosuppression in the infant.[26]

## Azathioprine

The purine analog azathioprine and its major metabolite 6-mercaptopurine have been used for the treatment of cancer and rheumatic diseases and in transplant recipients. Azathioprine is metabolized to 6-mercaptopurine, and the metabolites of 6-mercaptopurine are thiouric acid and inorganic sulfate.

In rats treated with high doses of azathioprine during pregnancy (20 mg/kg/day), reduced fetal and placental size was observed.[75] Lower doses (2 to 4 mg/kg/day) did not have an impact on trophoblastic development.[76]

When radioactively labeled azathioprine is administered during pregnancy, the majority of the compound appears in the fetal blood in the form of the inactive metabolite thiouric acid. The authors concluded that azathioprine was not effectively metabolized to 6-mercaptopurine by the fetus.[77] In humans, there have been case reports of adverse outcomes in babies exposed to azathioprine in utero. One preterm baby boy had severe pancytopenia and combined immunodeficiency after his mother received azathioprine and prednisone throughout pregnancy.[78] A mother who took azathioprine before and during pregnancy gave birth to a male infant with a chromosomal abnormality manifested by microcephaly, unusual facial features, and micropenis.[79]

Despite the preceding case reports, larger studies involving transplant recipients receiving azathioprine

who have become pregnant have yielded more favorable results. One problem in interpreting the literature is that most transplant recipients receive combinations of cyclosporine, azathioprine, and prednisone, which makes attribution of teratogenesis to any one drug difficult.

Armenti and colleagues followed 146 renal allograft recipients during pregnancy; 90% received azathioprine and prednisone, 2% received azathioprine alone, and 8% received glucocorticoids alone. There was a 52% incidence of prematurity and low birth weight seen in 40% of patients. Isolated cases of craniosynostosis, hypoplasia of the frontal lobe, and ventriculomegaly were reported, but because there was no consistent pattern to these malformations, they were not directly attributed to azathioprine.[68] The Norway Transplant Registry reported similar findings.[69] In 43 pregnancies in which azathioprine was used alone or in combination with prednisolone and cyclosporine for transplant organ maintenance, offspring had low birth weights and high rates of prematurity but did not have fetal malformations.

Azathioprine has also been well tolerated as a treatment for pregnant patients with rheumatic and inflammatory bowel diseases. Ramsey-Goldman and associates monitored six patients with systemic lupus erythematosus treated with azathioprine through nine pregnancies.[80] No congenital malformations were found but there was one miscarriage at 12 weeks, one preterm neonatal death at 28 weeks, and two other preterm deliveries. Of the five full-term deliveries, two infants were small for gestational age. The offspring of patients treated with azathioprine had an overall increased rate of survival when compared with patients not treated with this medication. No congenital malformations were seen in 14 patients with inflammatory bowel disease treated with azathioprine during 16 pregnancies.[81]

In addition to the case of pancytopenia noted earlier, other incidences of immunosuppression in offspring exposed to azathioprine in utero have been reported. In a series of seven patients who received azathioprine during pregnancy, one mother and her baby had IgA deficiency.[82] Others have also described transient lymphopenia and lower IgG and IgM levels but absent IgA after 1 year.[83] The significance of these findings in the long term is unclear.

Despite the above data, the *Physician's Desk Reference* still classifies azathioprine as a class D drug during pregnancy. Although the transplant and rheumatology literature would suggest that there is no increased risk of fetal malformations, higher rates of prematurity and infants small for gestational age are seen. There have been isolated reports of fetal immunosuppression, but the long-term impact on the immune system after in utero exposure to azathioprine is unknown. This medication may be used cautiously during pregnancy when immunosuppression is necessary.

## 6-Mercaptopurine

6-Mercaptopurine, the active metabolite of azathioprine, is used to treat rheumatic diseases and inflammatory bowel disease. Animal studies clearly show that this medication is teratogenic, with a high incidence of fetal resorption and cleft palate formation.[84, 85]

Data in humans are more confounding. Unfortunately, we do not have the availability of large case series with this agent as we do with the transplant registries and azathioprine. In a literature review of 79 pregnancies in which there had been some exposure to 6-mercaptopurine, there was one case of fetal malformations including cleft palate, microphthalmia, hypoplasia of the thyroid and ovaries, corneal opacity, and cytomegaly.[52] A case series of 15 infants exposed to this medication throughout gestation showed no fetal malformations (D. Present, personal communication). Whether 6-mercaptopurine is more toxic than azathioprine during pregnancy is unclear. Given the inconclusive nature of the available data, and alternatives such as azathioprine, 6-mercaptopurine should be avoided during pregnancy.

Both azathioprine and 6-mercaptopurine pass into breast milk. Because of the theoretical risk of immunosuppression, these medications should be avoided during breast-feeding.

## Methotrexate

Methotrexate, a folic acid antagonist, works by binding to dihydrofolate reductase and was initially developed as a chemotherapeutic agent. Since the early 1980s, this medication has been used for the treatment of RA and other rheumatic disorders.[86] A potent abortigenic agent, it is now the treatment of choice for the therapy of trophoblastic gestational tumors, ectopic pregnancies, and other conditions necessitating early termination of pregnancy.[87]

Animals exposed to methotrexate in utero show limb bud malformation, craniofacial abnormalities, and an increased fetal resorption rate.[88, 89] One possible mechanism of the skeletal anomalies is that methotrexate has been shown to reduce osteoblastic matrix production by osteoblasts.[90]

In humans, several of the reports of teratogenicity have been in offspring who survived abortogenic attempts by the mother who ingested methotrexate.[91, 92] These offspring suffered from the fetal methotrexate syndrome, which includes craniofacial and digital anomalies and growth retardation. Feldkamp and Carey reported a woman who took one dose of 7.5 mg of methotrexate at less than 6 weeks of gestation and had a healthy baby. They reviewed the literature and concluded that the critical period for exposure is 6 to 8 weeks after conception at a dose of 10 mg/week to produce the aminopterin syndrome.[93] In Kozlowski and colleagues' series of eight patients (10 pregnancies) who were taking methotrexate for rheumatic diseases and who became pregnant, there were three spontaneous abortions, two elective abortions, and five full-term healthy babies.[94] Donnenfeld and associates found a high rate of spina bifida in children exposed to methotrexate in utero. They also reported a high spontaneous abortion rate of 44% in patients taking this medication before conception and concluded that this medication

should be discontinued 12 weeks before conception.[95] In men treated with methotrexate there are no data on the teratogenicity of this medication if taken at conception. However, oligospermia does occur, and it can take up to 3 months after the discontinuation of therapy for sperm counts to return to normal.[96] Therefore, I recommend that male patients stop taking methotrexate 3 months before attempting conception. The package insert recommends discontinuing this medication in women for one complete menstrual cycle, although others advocate discontinuing this medication for at least two complete cycles because of the risk of pulmonary problems in the neonate.[97] Extremely reliable contraceptive methods should be used in patients taking this medication. Should pregnancy inadvertently occur, patients should be counseled that the risk of teratogenicity is high.

Although methotrexate is excreted in small amounts in breast milk, it is considered incompatible with breast-feeding by the American Academy of Pediatrics.[26]

## Cyclophosphamide

Cyclophosphamide, a chemotherapeutic agent, is used in severe vasculitic conditions such as Wegener's granulomatosis, lupus nephritis, and life-threatening cases of rheumatic diseases.

i Treatment of male rats for 4 weeks before fertilization resulted in abnormal implantation secondary to inner cell mass–denied embryonic cells.[98] In another study of pregnant female mice, high doses but not lower doses of cyclophosphamide induced multiple teratogenic abnormalities including limb abnormalities and cleft palate.[99]

Cyclophosphamide does cross the placenta in humans, achieving amniotic fluid levels of about 25% of maternal plasma levels.[100] There have been case reports of both limb abnormalities and coronary artery problems in the offspring of mothers treated with cyclophosphamide during pregnancy[101] as well as a report of a child who acquired thyroid papillary cancer at age 11 and a neuroblastoma at age 14 after in utero exposure to cyclophosphamide.[102]

There have been a few case series of women who were treated with cyclophosphamide during the second and third trimesters of pregnancy. In one case, a 23-year-old woman with Wegener's granulomatosis was treated from week 17 of pregnancy and gave birth to a healthy baby boy at 33 weeks.[103] Similarly, a woman with lymphoma treated during the third trimester of pregnancy gave birth to a normal infant.[104]

Given the alternative medications and the high potential of teratogenicity, cyclophosphamide should be avoided during pregnancy except in life-threatening circumstances.

Cyclophosphamide is transferred into breast milk and should be avoided by nursing mothers.

## Chlorambucil

Chlorambucil is an alkylating agent that is occasionally used to treat a variety of autoimmune diseases. In

rodents, chlorambucil has been shown to be teratogenic, causing skeletal malformations and renal disease.[105, 106]

Data in humans are limited. There has been one case
of renal agenesis in an infant exposed to this medication in utero,[107] but normal infants have also been born
to mothers taking this drug.[108] Given the many available alternative therapies and the limited data regarding this medication's safety, chlorambucil should be
avoided during pregnancy. There are no data available
on this medication during breast-feeding, but given its
potential for high toxicity, it should not be used by
nursing mothers.

### Intravenous Immune Globulin

IVIG is used to treat severe dermatomyositis-
polymyositis, juvenile RA, and the antiphospholipid
antibody syndrome. This medication was well tolerated in mice with induced antiphospholipid antibody syndrome.[108]

In humans, IVIG is transferred to the placenta.[109] This
medication has been used to treat pregnant women
with complications of the antiphospholipid antibody
syndrome.[110] It has been used successfully for the
treatment of idiopathic thrombocytopenic purpura
and Rh immunization and for the prevention of intrauterine infection after premature rupture of the membranes.[111–113] Although there appears to be no fetal toxicity with this therapy, there have been case reports of
hepatitis C seroconversion in individuals who have
received IVIG.[114] There has also been a case of hemolytic disease in the newborn after in utero exposure to
this treatment.[115]

In conclusion, IVIG appears to be compatible with
pregnancy. There is no information on breast-feeding
with this therapy.

### Newer Medications

Etanercept is a human monoclonal antibody that is
directed against the TNF-$\alpha$ receptor.[4] Although this
drug could hypothetically be helpful in the maintenance of pregnancy, there are currently no available
data on its safety during pregnancy. Therefore, this
medication should be avoided during pregnancy and
during breast-feeding.

Leflunomide is a newer drug used to treat RA.[116]
This medication is extremely teratogenic (risk category
X). Leflunomide has a long half-life, underscoring the
importance of contraceptive counseling in patients taking this medication. A drug elimination program using
cholestyramine is recommended in women of child-
bearing potential at the time that leflunomide is discontinued. It is recommended by the manufacturer that
cholestyramine, 8 g three times/day, be administered
for 11 days. After drug therapy, blood tests to ensure
that levels of the active metabolite are less than
0.02 mg/L should be obtained in two tests 14 days
apart. Once this is achieved, the woman can attempt
conception without undue risk to the fetus. Without
the drug elimination program, it may take up to 2

years to reach the acceptable plasma metabolite level
of less than 0.02 mg/L.

## CONCLUSIONS

Treating the pregnant patient with a rheumatic disease
remains a challenge. Clinicians must constantly weigh
the risks and benefits of potential therapy. This chapter
has reviewed the safety in pregnancy of the most common medications used in the treatment of rheumatic
diseases. All these drugs have the potential for toxicity,
but because patients can have active disease during
pregnancy, I recommend the following approach to
treatment. For mild disease, low doses of corticosteroids can be used. For more severe disease that requires
immunosuppression, higher doses of prednisone, azathioprine, and cyclosporine can be used. Patients with
conditions that are well controlled with antimalarial
agents can probably continue taking their medications.
In severe disease, IVIG, pulse steroid therapy, azathioprine, and cyclosporine can be used. In all cases, a
frank discussion with the patient, preferably before
conception, about the potential hazard of all therapies
to both the mother and the fetus should occur.

## REFERENCES

1. Cerere PA, Persellin RH: The interaction of pregnancy and the
   rheumatic diseases. Clin Rheumatol 1981; 7:747–768.
2. Branch DW: Physiologic adaptations of pregnancy. Am J Reprod Immunol 1992; 28:120–122.
3. Raghupathy R: Th1-type immunity is incompatible with successful pregnancy. Immunol Today 1997; 18:478–482.
4. Moreland LW, Baumgartner SW, Schiff MH, et al: Treatment of
   rheumatoid arthritis with a recombinant human tumor necrosis
   factor receptor (p75)-Fc fusion protein. N Engl J Med 1997;
   337:141–147.
5. Koren G, Patuszak A, Ito S: Drugs in pregnancy. N Engl J Med
   1998; 338:1128–1137.
6. Tuchmann-Duplessis H: Teratogenic drug screening: Present
   procedures and requirements. Teratology 1972; 5:271–285.
7. American College of Rheumatology Ad Hoc Committee on
   Clinical Guidelines: Guidelines for monitoring drug therapy in
   rheumatoid arthritis. Arthritis Rheum 1996; 39:723–731.
8. Roubenoff R, Hoyt J, Petri M, et al: Effects of antiinflammatory
   and immunosuppressive drugs on pregnancy and fertility.
   Semin Arthritis Rheum 1988; 18:88–110.
9. Bermas BL, Hill JA: Effects of immunosuppressive drugs during
   pregnancy. Arthritis Rheum 1995; 38:1722–1732.
10. Ramsey-Goldman R, Schilling E: Immunosuppressive drug use
    during pregnancy. Rheum Dis Clin North Am 1997; 23:149–167.
11. Hench PS: The ameliorating effect of pregnancy on chronic
    atrophic (infectious rheumatoid) arthritis, fibrosis and intermit-
    tent hydrarthrosis. Proc Mayo Clin 1938; 13:161.
12. Perselin RH: The effect of pregnancy on rheumatoid arthritis.
    Bull Rheum Dis 1977; 27:922.
13. Nelson JL, Ostensen M: Pregnancy and rheumatoid arthritis.
    Rheum Dis Clin North Am 1997; 23:195.
14. Nelson JL, Hughes KA, Smith AG, et al: Maternal-fetal disparity
    in HLA class II alloantigens and the pregnancy-induced amelio-
    ration of rheumatoid arthritis. N Engl J Med 1993; 329:466.
15. Ostensen M, Husby G: A prospective clinical study of the effect
    of pregnancy on rheumatoid arthritis and ankylosing spondyli-
    tis. Arthritis Rheum 1983; 26:1155.
16. Knupp MZ, O'Leary JA: Pregnancy and scleroderma: Systemic
    sclerosis. J Fla Med Assoc 1972; 58:28.

17. Steen VD, Medsger TA: Fertility and pregnancy outcome in women with systemic sclerosis. Arthritis Rheum 1999; 42:763–768.
18. Ballou SP, Morley JJ, Kushner I: Pregnancy and systemic sclerosis. Arthritis Rheum 1984; 27:295.
19. Steen VD, Conte C, Day N, et al: Pregnancy in women with systemic sclerosis. Arthritis Rheum 1989; 32:151–157.
20. Steen V: Pregnancy in systemic sclerosis. Rheum Dis Clin North Am 1997; 23:133–148.
21. Warkary J, Takacs E: Experimental production of congenital malformations in rats by salicylate poisoning. Am J Pathol 1959; 35:315–319.
22. Mandelcorn MS, Merin S, Cardarelli J: Goldenhar's syndrome and phocomelia: Case report and etiologic considerations. Am J Ophthalmol 1971; 72:618–621.
23. Slone D, Heinonen OP, Kaufman DW, et al: Aspirin and congenital malformations. Lancet 1976; 1:1373–1375.
24. Cowchuck FS, Reece EA, Balaban D, et al: Repeated fetal losses associated with antiphospholipid antibodies: A collaborative randomized trial comparing prednisone with low-dose heparin treatment. Am J Obstet Gynecol 1992; 166:1318–1323.
25. Rumack CM, Guggenheim MA, Kumack BH, et al: Neonatal intracranial hemorrhage and maternal use of aspirin. Obstet Gynecol 1981; 58:52S–56S.
26. American Academy of Pediatrics Committee on Drugs: Transfer of drugs and other chemicals into human milk. Pediatrics 1989; 84:924–936.
27. Klein KL, Scott WJ, Clark KE, et al: Placental transfer, cytotoxicity, and teratology in the rat. Am J Obstet Gynecol 1981; 141:448–452.
28. Schoenfeld A, Bar Y, Merlob P, et al: NSAIDs: Maternal and fetal considerations. Am J Reprod Immunol 1992; 28:141–147.
29. Lim H, Paria BC, Das SK, et al: Multiple female reproductive failures in cyclooxygenase 2–deficient mice. Cell 1997; 91:197–208.
30. Beitins IZ, Bayard F, Ances IG, et al: The transplacental passage of prednisone and prednisolone in pregnancy near term. J Pediatr 1972; 81:936–945.
31. Blanford AT, Murphy BE: In vitro metabolism of prednisolone, dexamethasone, betamethasone, and cortisol by the human placenta. Am J Obstet Gynecol 1977; 127:264–267.
32. Pinsky L, DiGeorge AM: Cleft palate in the mouse: A teratogenic index of glucocorticoid potency. Science 1965; 147:402–403.
33. Harris JWS, Ross IP: Cortisone therapy in early pregnancy: Relation to cleft palate. Lancet 1956; 1:1045–1047.
34. Chhabria S: Aicardi's syndrome: Are corticosteroids teratogens? Arch Neurol 1981; 38:70.
35. Oppenheimer EH: Lesions in the adrenals of an infant following maternal corticosteroid therapy. Bull Johns Hopkins Hosp 1964; 114:146–151.
36. Schatz M, Patterson R, Zeitz S, et al: Corticosteroid therapy for the pregnant asthmatic patient. JAMA 1975; 233:804–807.
37. Schatz M, Zeiger RS, Harden K, et al: The safety of asthma and allergy medications during pregnancy. J Allergy Clin Immunol 1997; 100:301–306.
38. Ullberg S, Lindquist NG, Sjostrand SE: Accumulation of chorioretinotoxic drugs in the foetal eye. Nature 1970; 2227:1257–1258.
39. Essien EE, Afamefuna GC: Chloroquine and its metabolites in human cord blood, neonatal blood, and urine after maternal medication. Clin Chem 1982; 28:1148–1152.
40. Steketee R, Wirima J, Slutsker L, et al: Malaria treatment and prevention in pregnancy: Indications for use and adverse events associated with use of chloroquine or mefloquine. Am J Trop Med Hyg 1996; 55:50–56.
41. Ganga N, Rajogopal B, Rajendran S, et al: Deafness in children—An analysis. Indian Pediatr 1991; 28:273–276.
42. Hart C, Naunton R: The ototoxicity of chloroquine phosphate. Arch Otolaryngol 1964; 80:407–412.
43. Parke A, Rothfield N: Antimalarial drugs in pregnancy: The North American experience. Lupus 1996; 5(suppl 1):S67–S69.
44. Khamashta MM, Buchanan M, Hughes G: The use of hydroxychloroquine in lupus pregnancy: The British experience. Lupus 1996; 5(suppl 1):S65–S66.
45. Edwards MH, Pierangeli S, Liu ZW, et al: Hydroxychloroquine reverses thrombogenic properties of antiphospholipid antibodies in mice. Circulation 1997; 96:4380–4394.
46. Freeman SJ, Lloyd JB: Evidence that suramin and aurothiomalate are teratogenic in rat by disturbing yolk sac–mediated embryonic protein nutrition. Chem Biol Interact 1986; 58:149–160.
47. Fuchs U, Lippert T: Gold therapy and pregnancy. Dtsch Med Wochenschr 1986; 111:31–34.
48. Miyamoto T, Miyaji S, Horiuchi Y, et al: Gold therapy in bronchial asthma with special emphasis upon blood levels of gold and its teratogenicity [In Japanese]. Nippon Naika Gakkai Zasshi 1974; 63:1190–1197.
49. Bennett P, Humphries S, Osborne J, et al: Use of sodium aurothiomalate during lactation. Br J Clin Pharmacol 1990; 29:777–779.
50. Keen C, Mark-Savage P, Lonnerdal B, et al: Teratogenic effects of D-penicillamine in rats: Relation to copper deficiency. Drug Nutr Interact 1983; 2:17–34.
51. Scheinberg I, Sternlieb I: Pregnancy in penicillamine-treated patients with Wilson's disease. N Engl J Med 1975; 65:273–285.
52. Briggs GG, Freeman RK, Yaffe SJ: Drugs in Pregnancy and Lactation. Baltimore: Williams & Wilkins, 1998.
53. Jarnerot G, Into-Malmberg MB, Esbjorner E: Placental transfer of sulfasalazine and sulfapyridine and some of its metabolites. Scand J Gastroenterol 1981; 16:693–697.
54. Jarnerot G, Andersen S, Esbjorner E, et al: Albumin reserve for binding of bilirubin in maternal and cord serum under treatment with sulphasalazine. Scand J Gastroenterol 1981; 16:1049–1055.
55. Korelitz BI: Pregnancy, fertility, and inflammatory bowel disease. Am J Gastroenterol 1985; 80:365–370.
56. Hoo JJ, Hadro TA, Von Behren P: Possible teratogenicity of sulfasalazine [Letter]. N Engl J Med 1988; 318:1128.
57. Craxi A, Pagliarello F: Possible embryotoxicity of sulfasalazine. Arch Intern Med 1980; 140:1674.
58. Mogadam M, Dobbins WOI, Korelitz BI, et al: Pregnancy in inflammatory bowel disease: Effect of sulfasalazine and corticosteroids on fetal outcome. Gastroenterology 1981; 80:72–76.
59. Levy N, Roisman I, Teodor I: Ulcerative colitis in pregnancy in Israel. Dis Colon Rectum 1981; 24:351–354.
60. Byron MA: Prescribing in pregnancy: Treatment of rheumatic diseases. BMJ 1987; 294:236–238.
61. Chatzinoff M, Guarino JM, Corson SK, et al: Sulfasalazine induced abnormal sperm penetration assay reversed on changing to 5-aminosalicylic acid enemas. Dig Dis Sci 1988; 33:108–110.
62. Esbjorner E, Jarnerot G, Wranne L: Sulphasalazine and sulphapyridine serum levels in children to mothers treated with sulphasalazine during pregnancy and lactation. Acta Paediatr Scand 1987; 76:137–142.
63. Jarnerot G, Into-Malmberg MB: Sulphasalazine treatment during breast feeding. Scand J Gastroenterol 1979; 14:869–871.
64. Backman L, Brandt I, Appelkvist E-L, et al: Tissue and subcellular localization of 3H-cyclosporin A in mice. Pharm Toxicol 1988; 62:110–117.
65. Venkataramanan R, Koneru B, Wang C-CP, et al: Cyclosporine and its metabolites in mother and baby. Transplantation 1988; 46:468–469.
66. Mason RJ, Thomson AW, Whiting PH, et al: Cyclosporine-induced fetotoxicity in the rat. Transplantation 1985; 39:9–12.
67. Schmid BP: Monitoring of organ formation in rat embryos after in vitro exposure to azathioprine, mercaptopurine, methotrexate or cyclosporin A. Toxicology 1984; 31:9–21.
68. Armenti VT, Ahlswede KM, Ahlswede BA, et al: National transplantation pregnancy registry—Outcomes of 154 pregnancies in cyclosporine-treated female kidney transplant recipients. Transplantation 1994; 57:502–506.
69. Haugen G, Fauchald P, Sodal G, et al: Pregnancy outcome in renal allograft recipients in Norway. Acta Obstet Gynecol Scand 1994; 73:541–546.
70. Casele HL, Laifer SA: Pregnancy after liver transplantation. Semin Perinatol 1998; 22:149–155.
71. Radomski JS, Ahlswede BA, Jarrell BE, et al: Outcomes of 500 pregnancies in 335 female kidney, liver, and heart transplant recipients. Transplant Proc 1995; 27:1089–1090.
72. Classen JB, Shevach EM: Evidence that cyclosporine treatment during pregnancy predisposes offspring to develop autoantibodies. Transplantation 1991; 51:1052–1057.

73. Rose ML, Dominguez M, Leaver N, et al: Analysis of T cell subpopulations and cyclosporine levels in the blood of two neonates born to immunosuppressed heart-lung transplant recipients. Transplantation 1989; 48:223–226.

74. Baarsma R, Kamps WA: Immunological responses in an infant after cyclosporin A exposure during pregnancy. Eur J Pediatr 1993; 152:476–477.

75. Connon AF: Effects of azathioprine on reproduction in rats. J Reprod Fertil 1964; 18:165–166.

76. Gross A, Fein A, Serr DM, et al: The effect of Imuran on implantation and early embryonic development in rats. Obstet Gynecol 1977; 50:713–718.

77. Saarikoski S, Seppala M: Immunosuppression during pregnancy: Transmission of azathioprine and its metabolites from the mother to the fetus. Am J Obstet Gynecol 1973; 115:1100–1106.

78. DeWitte DB, Buick MK, Cyran SE, et al: Neonatal pancytopenia and severe combined immunodeficiency associated with antenatal administration of azathioprine and prednisone. J Pediatr 1984; 105:625–628.

79. Ostrer H, Stamberg J, Perinchief P: Two chromosome aberrations in the child of a woman with systemic lupus erythematosus treated with azathioprine and prednisone. Am J Med Genet 1984; 17:627–632.

80. Ramsey-Goldman R, Mientus JM, Kutzer JE, et al: Pregnancy outcome in women with systemic lupus erythematosus treated with immunosuppressive drugs. J Rheumatol 1993; 20:1152–1156.

81. Alstead EM, Ritchie JK, Lennard-Jones JE, et al: Safety of azathioprine in pregnancy in inflammatory bowel disease. Gastroenterology 1990; 99:443–446.

82. Cederqvist LL, Markatz IR, Litwin SD: Fetal immunoglobulin synthesis following maternal immunosuppression. Am J Obstet Gynecol 1977; 129:687–690.

83. Cote CJ, Meuwissen HJ, Pickering RJ: Effects on the neonate of prednisone and azathioprine administered to the mother during pregnancy. J Pediatr 1974; 85:324–328.

84. Burdett DN, Waterfield JD, Shah RM: Vertical development of the secondary palate in hamster embryos following exposure to 6-mercaptopurine. Teratology 1988; 37:591–597.

85. Reimers TH, Sluss PM: 6-Mercaptopurine treatment of pregnant mice: Effects on second and third generations. Science 1978; 201:65–67.

86. Weinblatt ME, Coblyn JS, Fox DA, et al: Efficacy of low-dose methotrexate in rheumatoid arthritis. N Engl J Med 1985; 312:818–822.

87. Hoppe DE, Bekkar BE, Nager CW: Single-dose systemic methotrexate for the treatment of persistent ectopic pregnancy after conservative surgery. Obstet Gynecol 1994; 83:51–54.

88. Wilson JG, Scott WJ, Ritter EJ, et al: Comparative distribution and embryotoxicity of methotrexate in pregnant rats and rhesus monkeys. Teratology 1979; 19:71–80.

89. Lecuru F, Querleu D, Buchet-Bouverne B, et al: The effect of tubal injection of methotrexate on fertility in the rabbit. Fertil Steril 1992; 57:422–424.

90. May KP, Mercill D, McDermott MT, et al: The effect of methotrexate on mouse bone cells in culture. Arthritis Rheum 1996; 39:489–494.

91. Bawle E, Conard J, Weiss L: Adult and two children with fetal methotrexate syndrome. Teratology 1998; 57:51–55.

92. Thiersch JB: Early experiences with antimetabolites as abortifacient agents in man. Acta Endocrinol 1956; 28:37–45.

93. Feldkamp M, Carey JC: Clinical teratology counseling and consultation case report: Low dose methotrexate exposure in the early weeks of pregnancy. Teratology 1993; 47:533–539.

94. Kozlowski RD, Steinbrunner JV, MacKenzie AH, et al: Outcome of first-trimester exposure to low-dose methotrexate in eight patients with rheumatic disease. Am J Med 1990; 88:589–592.

95. Donnenfeld AE, Pastuszak A, Noah JS, et al: Methotrexate exposure prior to and during pregnancy. Teratology 1994; 49:79–81.

96. Sussman A, Leonard JM: Psoriasis, methotrexate, and oligospermia. Arch Dermatol 1980; 116:215–217.

97. Ramsey-Goldman R, Schilling E: Immunosuppressive drug use during pregnancy. Rheum Dis Clin North Am 1997; 23:149–167.

98. Kelly SM, Robaire B, Hales BF: Paternal cyclophosphamide treatment causes postimplantation loss via inner cell mass-specific cell death. Teratology 1992; 45:313–318.

99. Francis BM, Rogers JM, Sulik KK, et al: Cyclophosphamide teratogenesis: Evidence for compensatory responses to induced cellular toxicity. Teratology 1990; 42:473–482.

100. D'Incalci M, De Palo G, Semprini AE: Transplacental passage of cyclophosphamide. Cancer Treat Rep 1982; 8:1681–1682.

101. Toledo TM, Harper RC, Moser RH: Fetal effects during cyclophosphamide and irradiation therapy. Ann Intern Med 1971; 74:87–91.

102. Zemlickis D, Lishner M, Erlich R, et al: Teratogenicity and carcinogenicity in a twin exposed in utero to cyclophosphamide. Teratog Carcinog Mutagen 1993; 13:139–143.

103. Fields CL, Ossorio MA, Roy TM, et al: Wegener's granulomatosis complicated by pregnancy: A case report. J Reprod Med 1991; 36:463–466.

104. Hardin JA: Cyclophosphamide treatment of lymphoma during third trimester of pregnancy. Obstet Gynecol 1972; 39:850–851.

105. Brummett ES, Johnson EM: Morphological alterations in the developing fetal rat limb due to maternal injection of chlorambucil. Teratology 1979; 20:279–287.

106. Kavlock RT, Rehnberg BI, Rogers EH: Chlorambucil induced congenital renal hypoplasia: Effects on basal renal function in the developing rat. Toxicology 1986; 40:247–258.

107. Steege JF, Caldwell DS: Renal agenesis after first trimester exposure to chlorambucil. South Med J 1980; 73:1414–1415.

108. Jacobs C, Donaldson SS, Rosenberg SA, et al: Management of the pregnant patient with Hodgkin's disease. Ann Intern Med 1981; 95:669–675.

109. Hockel M, Queiber-Luft A, Beck T, et al: The effect of antenatal intravenous immunoglobulin on ascending intrauterine infection after preterm premature rupture of the membranes: A pilot study. J Perinat Med 1992; 20:101–110.

110. Parke A: The role of IVIG in the management of patients with antiphospholipid antibodies and recurrent pregnancy losses. *In* Ballow M (ed): IVIG Therapy Today. Totowa, NJ: Humana Press, 1992:105–118.

111. Fabris P, Quaini R, Coser P, et al: Successful treatment of a steroid-resistant form of idiopathic thrombocytopenic purpura in pregnancy with high doses of intravenous immunoglobulins. Acta Hematol 1987; 77:107–110.

112. De La Camara C, Arrieta R, Gonzalez A, et al: High-dose intravenous immunoglobulin as the sole prenatal treatment for severe Rh immunization. N Engl J Med 1988; 318:519–520.

113. Hockel M, Queiber-Luft A, Beck T, et al: The effect of antenatal intravenous immunoglobulin on ascending intrauterine infection after preterm premature rupture of the membranes: A pilot study. J Perinat Med 1992; 20:101–110.

114. Outbreak of hepatitis C associated with intravenous immunoglobulin administration, United States: October 1993–June 1994. MMWR Morb Mortal Wkly Rep 1994; 43:505–509.

115. Potter M, Stockley R, Storry J, et al: ABO alloimmunization after intravenous immunoglobulin infusion. Lancet 1988; 1:932–933.

116. Smolen JS, Kalden JR, Scott DL, et al: Efficacy and safety of leflunomide compared with placebo and sulphasalazine in active rheumatoid arthritis: A double-blind randomized, multicenter trial. European Leflunomide Study Group. Lancet 1999; 353:259–266.

# 15 | Treatment of Cutaneous Disease Associated with Rheumatic Disease*

*Jeffrey P. Callen*

Cutaneous disease is frequent in many rheumatic disorders.[1] Some of these disorders, such as lupus erythematosus (LE), dermatomyositis, scleroderma, vasculitis, neutrophilic dermatoses, panniculitis, and psoriasis, are defined by their cutaneous manifestations. As investigation increases our understanding of these disorders, available therapy becomes more logical and less empirical. Unfortunately, few controlled clinical trials have been published, and thus much of the treatment selection is based on anecdotal observations or small case studies.

## CUTANEOUS LUPUS ERYTHEMATOSUS

There are multiple cutaneous manifestations of LE. These have been divided arbitrarily into those with histopathologic features that are LE-specific, represented by an interface dermatitis (discoid LE [DLE], subacute cutaneous LE [SCLE], and malar and photosensitive erythemas) and those with non–LE-specific histopathologic features. In this section we concentrate on the LE-specific lesions, including the clinical subsets—chronic cutaneous LE (CCLE) and SCLE.

Without therapy, CCLE results in scarring, permanent alopecia, or atrophy of the skin (Fig. 15–1). Rare patients have a hypertrophic variation (Fig. 15–2).[2] Over a prolonged period, some patients acquire malignancy in the chronic scars of DLE lesions.[3] It appears that these changes can be prevented with therapy. Although lesions that are already scarred cannot be reversed, it does appear that extension of the disease can be prevented.

Patients with SCLE have more transient disease (Figs. 15–3 and 15–4) that is distinguished from DLE by its lack of atrophy or scarring.[4] However, in some SCLE patients who do not receive therapy, it is possible for them to develop lesions that are characterized by atrophy and scarring.

One concern expressed by most patients is whether their cutaneous disease is reflective of systemic disease. In most cases of CCLE the patients have few, if any, systemic manifestations.[5] In contrast, patients with SCLE often have some systemic disease, but it is usually limited to serologic, mild hematologic, or joint involvement.[6,7] It is possible that patients with either variant may display characteristics of severe systemic disease including central nervous system or renal involvement, but these instances are uncommon. LE is a dynamic disorder and thus some patients in whom the skin condition is the only manifestation will eventually experience systemic involvement. This phenomenon is rare in DLE, but is more common in SCLE patients. However, the risk of severe involvement developing is limited. Thus, most patients can be reassured at the time of their diagnosis.

### Standard Therapy

Cosmetic disfigurement is often of major importance. Dyspigmentation may be covered with make-up such as Covermark or Dermablend. Inactive lesions that lead to scarring may be excised; however, the possibility of reactivation of the lesions exists. Patients with scarring alopecia may wish to use hairpieces or wigs.

Because photosensitivity is a well-documented phenomenon in patients with LE, sunscreen is recommended for daily use. The wavelength of light that exacerbates LE is within the ultraviolet B (UVB) or ultraviolet A (UVA) spectrum, or both.[8] Therefore, it is best to select an agent with a broad spectrum for UVA coverage and a high sun protective factor for UVB protection. There are many such agents available as over-the-counter products.

In controlled trials, topical corticosteroids are clearly beneficial[9], however, in practice they do not provide control in most patients, perhaps because of their messiness and cost. When choosing a corticosteroid, the clinician should consider the area being treated, for example, selection of a lotion for hair-bearing areas or low potency for facial lesions versus high potency for hypertrophic lesions or palmar lesions.

Intralesional corticosteroids are often effective in patients with refractory individual lesions.[10] Lesions injected intradermally with diluted triamcinolone acetonide (3 mg/mL) often respond within several days and may remain quiescent for several weeks (Fig. 15–5). Care must be taken to avoid atrophy by limiting the amount of corticosteroid injected.

---

* All figures in this chapter also appear in color following page 188.

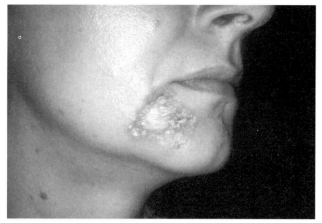

**FIGURE 15–1**
Chronic cutaneous lupus erythematosus. This lesion of discoid lupus erythematosus was present for a long time before treatment was initiated. The result was atrophy and scarring.

Antimalarial therapy is the first line of systemic therapy. Demonstration of efficacy dates back to the 1950s and 1960s, and these agents are approved for use by the Food and Drug Administration. Hydroxychloroquine in doses of 200 to 400 mg/day (<6.5 mg/kg/day) is effective in decreasing the appearance of new lesions, controlling the photoexacerbation and improving existing lesions in about 80% to 90% of patients. The response is not immediate, thus evaluation at 6 to 8 weeks is most appropriate. Risks inherent to hydroxychloroquine include blood dyscrasias, cutaneous dyspigmentation (Fig. 15–6), gastrointestinal effects, and ophthalmic toxicity. The prevalence of ocular toxicity is low, and studies have questioned the value of routine eye examinations.[11] However, because of the litigious nature of American society and the existence of guidelines suggested in the package insert, it is still prudent to involve an ophthalmologist in the patient's care.

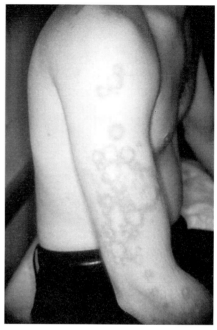

**FIGURE 15–3**
An annular variant of subacute cutaneous lupus erythematosus.

Patients who do not respond to hydroxycloroquine fully may be switched to chloroquine phosphate, 250–500 mg/day. Chloroquine is clearly associated with a higher prevalence of ocular toxicity. It has also been stated that chloroquine is more efficacious than hydroxychloroquine; however, the evidence for this statement is anecdotal.

One study compared the effects of smoking on the efficacy of antimalarial agents in lupus and found that

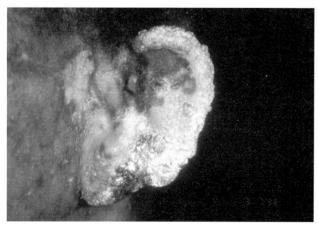

**FIGURE 15–2**
This patient with long-standing lesions of discoid lupus erythematosus failed to follow medical advice and his lesions became verrucous over an 18-year period. Subsequent to this picture he has developed multiple squamous cell carcinomas.

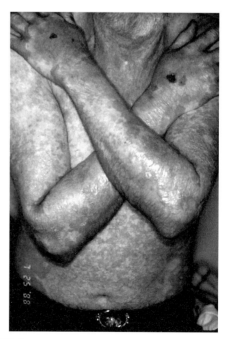

**FIGURE 15–4**
Papulosquamous variant of subacute cutaneous lupus erythematosus.

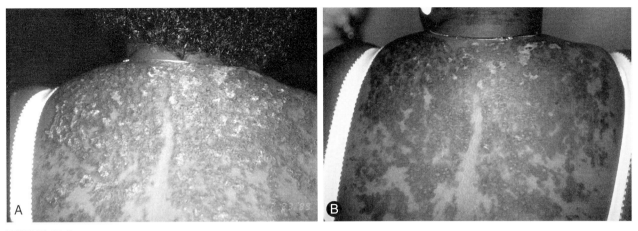

**FIGURE 15–5**
Chronic cutaneous lupus erythematosus before (A) and 1 month after (B) intralesional triamcinolone treatment.

smoking appears to interfere with the efficacy of therapy.[12] However, the explanations for this observation may be (1) that smoking results in more severe cutaneous disease,[13] (2) that it is caused by blockade of antimalarial action, or (3) that it is caused by increased metabolism of antimalarial agents.

In patients who fail to respond fully to either hydroxychloroquine or chloroquine, the addition of quinacrine, 100 to 200 mg per day, may enhance the effect.[14] Quinacrine is no longer manufactured by a pharmaceutical company in the United States, and thus it must be obtained from a compounding pharmacy.

## Alternative Therapies

Many other approaches have been developed for treating difficult cases of cutaneous LE. In general, low-dose systemic corticosteroids have been ineffective in

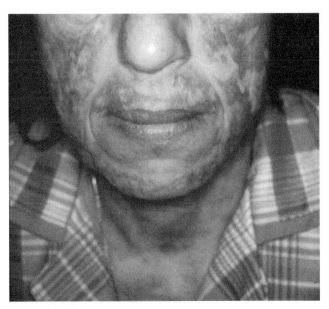

**FIGURE 15–6**
Pigmentation resulting from hydroxychloroquine therapy of subacute cutaneous lupus erythematosus.

treating my patients with DLE. Corticosteroids do seem to be effective in some patients with SCLE and particularly in those who have an acute photosensitivity eruption.

### Cytotoxic Agents

Several cytotoxic agents (azathioprine in particular) have been reported to be beneficial in patients with cutaneous disease. My experience with azathioprine in six patients with refractory disease and the experience of several other groups demonstrated improvement in most patients within 4 to 8 weeks (Fig. 15–7).[15, 16] Nonscarring lesions of SCLE also responded well. Several of my patients noted no change in photosensitivity while taking azathioprine; thus sunscreen and sun avoidance remain an integral part of therapy. Azathioprine may be used long term (>2 years).

Small open trials and individual cases of successful treatment with methotrexate (10 to 20 mg/week),[17] cyclophosphamide, cytarabine,[18] or cyclosporine have been reported. I have not observed the same type of results with the use of methotrexate, cyclophosphamide, or chlorambucil in a limited number of my patients. I have recently observed a beneficial effect with mycophenolate mofetil, similar to the results with azathioprine.

Lagrange and coworkers reported their experience with high-dose intravenous immunoglobulin in nine patients with refractory cutaneous LE.[19] They gave 1 g/kg/day for 2 consecutive days each month. Three of their patients improved, but relapses occurred within 1 to 10 months. Toxic effects were minimal. Perhaps future use of this therapy will allow control to be maintained with less expensive and less toxic agents after an induction with intravenous immunoglobulin.

### Antilepromatous Agents

Dapsone given in oral doses of 25 to 200 mg/day has been useful in patients with vasculitic lesions complicating LE, nonscarring cutaneous LE, bullous LE, and

**FIGURE 15-7**
Before (*A*) and after (*B*)
azathioprine therapy of
papulosquamous subacute
cutaneous lupus erythematosus.

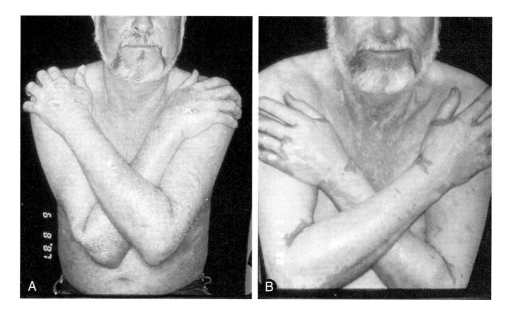

oral ulcerations.[20, 21] Dapsone has also led to improvement in some patients with DLE or SCLE[22]; however, the level of benefit has been judged as "excellent" in only about 25% of patients. In general, my impression of dapsone as a therapy for cutaneous LE is not favorable. In addition, toxic reactions associated with dapsone may result in exacerbation of systemic manifestions of LE.

Clofazimine is another antilepromatous agent that has been used successfully for treating cutaneous LE. In open trial of oral clofazimine (100 mg/day) for periods of 3 to 6 months, about two thirds of patients have benefited.[23] Minimal toxic effects occur with clofazimine, the most notable of which is a pinkish to reddish discoloration of the skin. My limited experience with this agent has not been encouraging.

Thalidomide has been difficult to obtain in the United States; however, it has been remarketed for graft-versus-host disease and human immunodeficiency virus–related aphthosis and may be used in selected patients with LE. European, South American, and US investigators demonstrated excellent results in patients whose LE was refractory to antimalarial drugs.[24–26a] Induction with 100 to 300 mg daily resulted in improvement in 90% of patients able to tolerate the drug. Toxic effects include drug eruptions, drowsiness, and headache. Neuropathy, which is idiosyncratic, can occur and may be irreversible. Thalidomide is a potent teratogen, so it must not be used in women of childbearing age. A program for guaranteeing safety, known as the System for Thalidomide Education and Prescribing Safety (STEPS) program, is mandatory. Although it may bring improvement in cutaneous lesions, thalidomide does not appear to have much effect on the systemic features of LE.

## Auranofin

Oral gold has been used for cutaneous LE.[27] Complete remission occurs in a minority of patients (about 20%), whereas a partial response has been noted in about two thirds of those treated. My experience has been encouraging in a limited number of patients (Fig. 15–8). Auranofin is used as it would be in patients with rheumatoid arthritis. Responsiveness is believed to be best in nonscarring forms of cutaneous LE. A referred patient on auranofin had lichenoid skin lesions that complicated her "refractory" LE. Cessation of the drug led to control of her disease, indicating that the auranofin was the cause of the lichenoid skin lesions.

## Phenytoin

Rodriguez-Castellanos and coworkers reported their results with phenytoin.[28] They studied 93 patients with CCLE and observed excellent control of disease in 90% of the patients. They administered oral phenytoin (300 mg/day) for up to 6 months. Relapse occurred in at least one third of the patients for whom follow-up data were available, but prolonged remissions of 6 to 12 months were noted in 33 patients. Toxic effects were minimal in prevalence and severity. Thus far, I have not prescribed phenytoin, perhaps because about one third to one half the cases of toxic epidermal necrolysis I see are caused by phenytoin administration.

## Cytokine Therapy

Use of cytokine therapy for cutaneous LE has been reported. Interferon-$\alpha$ has been used successfully; however, all patients on this regimen experience toxic effects, and long-term remission is rarely achieved.[29] In contrast, Prinz and colleagues have used chimeric CD4 monoclonal antibody infusions in five patients with severe and refractory cutaneous LE.[30] Long-lasting improvement was noted, with a reconstitution of responsiveness to "conventional" treatments. This is promising therapy for patients in whom responsiveness to less toxic therapy is lost.

**FIGURE 15–8**
Before (*A*) and after (*B*) auranofin therapy for subacute cutaneous lupus erythematosus.

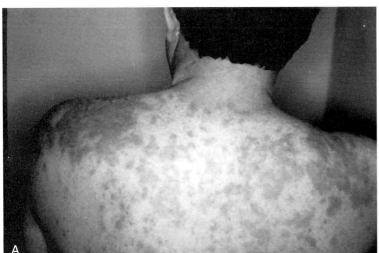
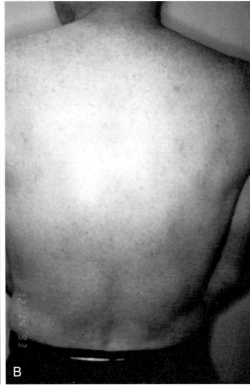

## *Retinoids*

Various retinoids used topically or orally have been found to be effective in treating patients with cutaneous LE. In individual patients, I have noted benefits from tretinoin cream or gel applied topically to resistant individual lesions. Newton and colleagues reported that oral isotretinoin not only cleared cutaneous lesions clinically but also altered results of histopathologic and immunopathologic examinations of the skin.[31] Their data were short term, and it is not known whether long-term isotretinoin therapy would continue to be effective and safe.

In a patient with disease of the palms and soles that was recalcitrant to therapy with corticosteroids, dapsone, combinations of antimalarial agents, colchicine, and azathioprine, we noted a dramatic and rapid response to 40 mg/day of oral isotretinoin (Fig. 15–9). After this short-term use, control of this patient's disease with "standard" therapy was again possible. Similar results have been noted when oral etretinate was used.

In summary, patients with cutaneous lesions of lupus erythematosus should be treated with sunscreens, topical and intralesional corticosteroids, and antimalarial agents as standard therapy. The choice of alternative therapy is personal, and discussions of the risks and benefits should be carefully documented. Successful therapy for cutaneous LE is possible in almost all well-motivated, cooperative patients.

## CUTANEOUS DERMATOMYOSITIS

Therapy for cutaneous disease in patients with dermatomyositis is often difficult because even though the myositis may respond to treatment with corticosteroids or immunosuppressive drugs, or both, the cutaneous lesions often persist. Although cutaneous disease may be of minor importance in patients with serious fulminant myositis, in many patients cutaneous disease becomes the most important aspect of their disorder.

Most patients with cutaneous lesions are photosensitive[32]; thus, the daily use of a broad-spectrum sunscreen with a high sun protective factor is recommended. Hydroxychloroquine given as a steroid-sparing agent in dosages of 200 mg to 400 mg/day is effective in approximately 80% of patients treated (Fig. 15–10).[33, 34] Patients who do not respond well to hydroxychloroquine can be switched to chloroquine phosphate, 250 to 500 mg/day, or quinacrine, 100 mg twice daily, can be added to the regimen. Patients receiving continuous antimalarial therapy should be evaluated in a manner similar to that in LE patients (see earlier). It appears that patients with dermatomyositis (DM) have a greater frequency of drug eruptions from antimalarials, thus patients should be warned about this possibility.

Recently methotrexate in doses of 15 to 35 mg/week have been reported to be useful for DM[35, 36] (Fig. 15–11).

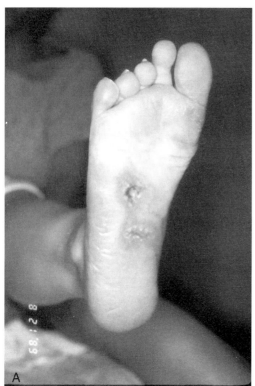

FIGURE 15-9
Before (*A*) and 4 weeks after (*B*) oral isotretinoin therapy for plantar lesions of lupus erythematosus.

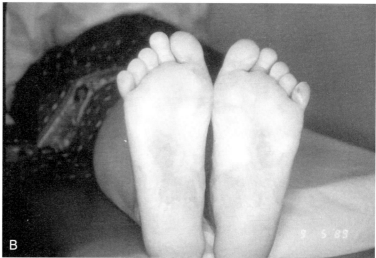

These studies, however, are in uncontrolled, open-label observations. The need for routine liver biopsy in the DM patient treated with methotrexate is controversial, but patients who are obese or diabetic or who have abnormal liver function test results should probably have periodic liver biopsies. Other immunosuppressive agents have not been systematically studied as treatment of cutaneous lesions of DM, but some anecdotes suggest that mycophenolate mofetil might be beneficial (H. Nousari, personal communication). Lastly, intravenous immune globulin administered monthly can result in clearing in patients with cutaneous lesions.[37]

Calcinosis is a complication of disease in children and adolescents. This process may be prevented by aggressive early treatment. Preliminary analysis of the use of intravenous methylprednisolone suggested that this therapy might lessen the frequency and severity of this process. Other authorities have suggested that immunosuppressive agents may similarly reduce the chance of calcinosis. Once established, calcinosis is difficult to treat. Reports of long-term administration of diltiazem are promising.[38]

## LOCALIZED SCLERODERMA

Localized scleroderma refers to primary involvement of the skin with minimal, if any, systemic features.[39] Only rarely have patients with localized scleroderma

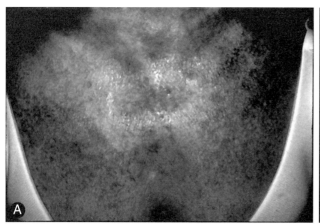

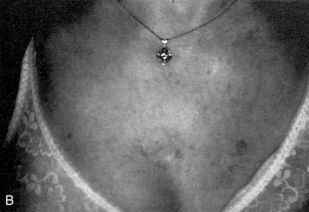

FIGURE 15-10
Before (*A*) and after (*B*) hydroxychloroquine therapy for dermatomyositis.

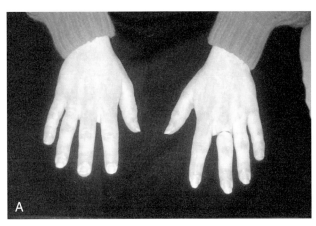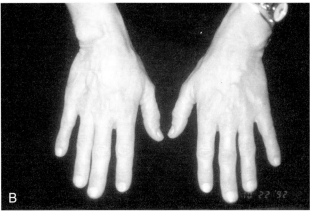

**FIGURE 15–11**
Before (A) and after (B) methotrexate therapy for cutaneous lesions of dermatomyositis.

acquired systemic sclerosis.[40] Three major types of localized scleroderma exist: morphea, generalized morphea, and linear scleroderma (Fig. 15–12). Morphea is represented by indurated dermal or subcutaneous plaques. The disease is most common in young women. Morphea sometimes overlaps or coexists with another cutaneous condition known as lichen sclerosus et atrophicus (Fig. 15–13). In contrast, a small number of patients acquire numerous larger lesions that coalesce. These individuals are said to have generalized morphea. Patients with morphea usually have a benign course, characterized by softening of lesions with time.

Scleroderma is a disease of unknown cause, and its pathogenesis is poorly understood. Therapy is directed at symptoms and at alteration of collagen metabolism. Advances are often serendipitous, but with a better understanding of the disease perhaps more specific therapies can be developed.

Localized scleroderma is usually not associated with life-threatening complications and therefore local forms of therapy that have limited toxicity are usually suggested. Some patients, however, particularly those with linear lesions, can be left with deformity or may lose function.

Oral 1,25-dihydroxyvitamin $D_3$ (calcitriol) has been reported to be an effective therapy in both adults and children.[41, 42] Calcitriol is metabolized in the skin, but the skin may also be a target organ for its effects. Calcitriol may affect the function of lymphocytes or fibroblast proliferation or may regulate collagen gene expression. In a recent open-label study, Elst and colleagues treated seven children with linear scleroderma with calcitriol.[43] They began therapy with 0.25 μg/day and raised the dose to a maximum of 1.25 μg/day in 0.25-μg increments each week. Dietary calcium intake was restricted to 600 mg/day, and calcium levels in the blood and urine were measured repeatedly. They also performed repeated renal ultrasonographic scans to exclude stone formation. Effects were measured clinically in this study and six of seven patients seemingly responded within 3 months. Therapy was continued

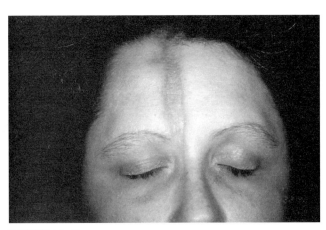

**FIGURE 15–12**
En coup de sabre: a form of linear scleroderma.

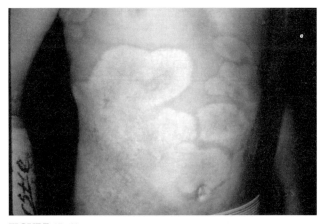

**FIGURE 15–13**
Widespread morphea. This patient has the surface characteristics of lichen sclerosus et atrophicus. Four years after diagnosis, this child acquired an interstitial pneumonitis that was consistent with scleroderma pulmonary disease. This progression to systemic manifestations is exceedingly rare.

safely for up to 10.5 months. Similar results have been reported in adults with localized scleroderma.

Noting these studies, Cunningham and colleagues reported that topical application of calcipotriene under occlusion is effective in some patients with morphea or linear scleroderma.[43] This group treated 12 patients (both children and adults) in an open-label trial for up to 3 months. Statistical improvement was observed based on a clinical scoring system in which dyspigmentation, induration, erythema, and telangiectasias were noted. No systemic adverse effects were noted, but some patients may experience local irritation. In one patient with two affected sites, only the treated site improved.

Oral methotrexate use has been reported in an open-label prospective study of widespread morphea.[44] Methotrexate has been reported to be useful in a controlled trial for progressive systemic sclerosis. These authors used oral methotrexate, 15 mg/week, and measured clinical response by a modified skin score, a visual analog scale for tightness and itching, and a durometer score for induration. In addition, they measured serum levels of aminoterminal propeptide of type III procollagen. They found significant improvement in the modified skin score and visual analog scale for tightness and a positive trend for itching and the durometer score. There was no change in type III procollagen levels. Adverse events did not occur. They suggested that this therapy may be beneficial.

Both high-dose and low-dose UVA-1 have been reported to be of benefit for localized scleroderma in 17 and 20 patients.[45, 46] In one study, high doses (130 J/cm$^2$) were compared with low doses (20 J/cm$^2$).[45] The high-dose therapy resulted in reduced thickness and increased elasticity in all 10 patients and complete clearance in 4 patients. The response continued even 3 months after the therapy was stopped in 9 of 10 patients. It was demonstrated subsequently that UVA-1 induces interstitial collagenase production, which may explain the clinical results noted.[47] Unfortunately, UVA-1 phototherapy is not widely available worldwide, and the cost of these bulbs precludes the development of this therapy in the United States. Currently, psoralen plus UVA phototherapy is available; however, it has not been reported to have similar effects.

Localized scleroderma may have overlapping features with lichen sclerosus et atrophicus. The latter often responds to superpotent topical corticosteroids such as clobetasol or halobetasol ointment. Individual cases of morphea may also respond. Physical therapy is useful in patients with morphea that occurs over a joint, and it was useful in at least one patient with a lesion on the foot; physical therapy alone led to improvement.

In Europe, localized scleroderma may be associated with *Borrelia* infection, and some patients have responded to penicillin. Studies in the United States have routinely failed to demonstrate *Borrelia* in morphea or linear scleroderma. A short course of penicillin is often used but has rarely been reported to be effective. Other therapies suggested include antimalarial agents, vita-min E, phenytoin, colchicine, cyclosporine, interferon-α, penicillamine, and plasmapheresis.

## CUTANEOUS VASCULITIS

The term *cutaneous vasculitis* may refer to a number of syndromes.[48] *Leukocytoclastic vasculitis* is a term that specifies a histopathologic pattern. This pattern is observed in many of the vasculitic syndromes that affect the small vessels of the skin. Although circulating immune complexes are involved in the pathogenesis of many of the vasculitic syndromes, the exact pathogenetic mechanisms have not been fully elucidated. However, even when the skin is seemingly the only system organ involved, vasculitis should be thought of as a systemic process.

Syndromes that can involve the small cutaneous vessels include hypersensitivity vasculitis, Henoch-Schönlein purpura, vasculitis associated with paraproteinemias, vasculitis as part of a collagen-vascular disorder, and hypocomplementemic (or urticarial) vasculitis.[49] In addition, many patients with Wegener's granulomatosis, microscopic polyarteritis, and other vasculitides involving small to medium-sized vessels have cutaneous small vessel disease. Therefore, before any pharmacologic therapy is instituted, a thorough evaluation should be performed.

### Evaluation

Evaluating the patient with cutaneous vasculitis is useful in determining possible causative factors or associated processes, assessing for the presence of systemic disease, and formulating a prognosis. Historical information can reveal the presence of a preexisting disorder or disease, medications taken before the onset of vasculitis, the presence of infection, and symptoms suggestive of systemic involvement. On physical examination, both the type of cutaneous lesion and the extent of disease are of prognostic importance. Purpura, livedo reticularis, subcutaneous nodules, and ulcerations may be manifestations of noninflammatory vascular compromise such as in hypercoagulable states, scurvy, left atrial myxoma, atheromatous emboli, or calciphylaxis; these conditions should be ruled out. Immunofluorescence microscopy is helpful when the possibility of Henoch-Schönlein purpura is considered, particularly in adults. Tissue confirmation of vasculitis is almost always necessary, and biopsy should be performed on an early lesion (<48 hours old) if possible. A complete laboratory evaluation is also helpful and should include a complete blood count, urinalysis, cryoglobulin determination, serum protein electrophoresis, hepatitis B surface antigen test, hepatitis C antibody test, antinuclear antibody test and possibly an anti-Ro (SS-A) test, tests of renal function, and a chest film. The presence of cytoplasmic antineutrophil cytoplasmic antibody (ANCA) has been closely associated with Wegener's granulomatosis and may be predictive of the activity of the disease. Perinuclear ANCA may be present in other vasculitic syndromes such as polyarteritis nodosa and microscopic polyarteritis but may also be present in nonvasculitic conditions such as Sweet's syndrome, pyoderma gangrenosum, and ulcerative colitis.

## Treatment

GENERAL MEASURES. If an associated condition or causative factor is present, its removal or treatment can result in a cure of the process. Identification and treatment of an infection, discontinuation of offending medications or other ingestants, and therapy directed against the production of an abnormal protein are most important. An open-label trial in Italy studied the effect of an elimination diet on five patients.[50] With reintroduction of foods and food dyes, the offending agent was identified, and sustained control of the disease was possible. Dietary restriction has been of limited value in my practice. Because lesions are more frequent or more severe in the skin overlying dependent areas and on cooler acral regions of the body, frequent turning, the use of compression stockings, elevation, and a warm environment are helpful.

DISEASE-SPECIFIC CONSIDERATIONS. Hypersensitivity vasculitis and Henoch-Schönlein purpura are often self-limited, and only symptomatic therapy may be required.[51] Polyarteritis nodosa, Wegener's granulomatosis, and systemic necrotizing vasculitis are potentially life-threatening conditions and without treatment, patients may die of renal or central nervous system involvement.[52] Thus, aggressive therapy is often necessary. Urticarial vasculitis may be a chronic condition with a benign course or, in the presence of hypocomplementemia, may be complicated by chronic obstructive pulmonary disease.[53] The chronic nature of the process necessitates continual suppressive therapy. Manifestations of vasculitis complicating rheumatoid arthritis, systemic lupus erythematosus (SLE), or Sjögren's syndrome range from benign palpable purpura to severe life-threatening disease, and therapy should be based on the severity of the process. In patients with paraproteinemias, therapy required for suppression of the abnormal protein may be more aggressive than that for the cutaneous vasculitis. It has been recognized that many patients with cryoglobulinemia-associated vasculitis also have hepatitis C virus infection.[54] Currently available antiviral agents are occasionally effective.[55, 56]

NONIMMUNOLOGIC DRUG THERAPY. Administration of antihistamines has often been suggested as a first line of therapy based on the observation that injected histamine allows deposition of immune complexes in the vessel walls with the eventual development of leukocytoclastic vasculitis. In patients with palpable purpura, antihistamines have rarely, if ever, been effective in my practice. However, in patients with urticarial vasculitis, I generally begin therapy with a nonsoporific agent such as loratadine (Claritin) each morning and $H_1$ inhibitor in the evening. An agent such as doxepin (Sinequan) may have both $H_1$- and $H_2$-inhibiting effects and is preferable in some cases.

Various nonsteroidal anti-inflammatory drugs (NSAIDs) have been used in the treatment of vasculitic syndromes. In particular, patients with urticarial vasculitis may respond to ibuprofen or indomethacin.[57] The therapeutic benefit of NSAIDs comes from their effect on prostaglandins and leukotrienes and possibly on platelet aggregation. In my experience, NSAIDs have not been particularly effective in any vasculitic syndrome.

Pentoxifylline (Trental) has been reported to be useful in some patients.[58] In particular, patients with evidence of an occlusive vasculopathy such as livedo vasculitis may respond.

Antimalarial agents such as hydroxychloroquine (Plaquenil) and chloroquine (Aralen), have been used for some patients with vasculitis. Although they are effective for the cutaneous lesions of SLE, they have not been effective for vasculitis, even in my patients with SLE.

Diaminodiphenylsulfone (i.e., dapsone) has received some attention. It is effective in dermatitis herpetiformis (a disease characterized by neutrophilic papillitis) and has various effects on leukocytes. It is the agent of choice for treatment of the rare cutaneous vasculitic syndrome of erythema elevatum diutinum.[59] In selected patients it has been effective in controlling the manifestations of palpable purpura in doses of 100 to 200 mg/day.[60] One report suggested that there may be a synergistic effect between pentoxifylline and dapsone.[61]

Colchicine has been reported to be effective in open-label trials for cutaneous vasculitis as manifested by palpable purpura or urticarial lesions (Fig. 15–14).[62] Colchicine is an alkaloid derived from a crocus-like plant, *Colchicum autumnale*. Its effects in vasculitis may be related to a blockade of disease expression. Colchicine inhibits leukocyte chemotaxis, blocks the release of lysosomal enzymes, inhibits DNA synthesis and cell proliferation, and may inhibit the effects of prostaglandins. Of the more than 50 patients I have treated and observed, colchicine has been effective in about 35, nonevaluable in about 5, and ineffective in the remaining 10 patients. The only double-blind placebo-controlled trial failed to demonstrate a positive benefit[63]; however, the colchicine-treated group included all the dapsone failures and thus there may have been some inadvertent selection bias. I use a dose of 0.6 mg given orally twice daily. If this dose is tolerated, effects are usually observed within 7 to 14 days. In patients with associated arthralgias or arthritis, colchicine may also be of benefit. Immune complexes are unaffected by the drug, and this leads to my belief that the mechanism of action is a suppression of disease expression. Long-term effective use (up to 10 years) has been possible in some of my patients without serious side effects. These patients should be regularly monitored with complete blood counts.

CORTICOSTEROIDS. Systemic corticosteroids are useful in most patients with vasculitis, but because of multiple potential toxic effects, their use should be limited to patients with severe disease or when their use is expected to be short term. The absolute indica-

**FIGURE 15–14**
Before (*A*) and 4 weeks (*B*) after oral colchicine therapy for small vessel cutaneous vasculitis.

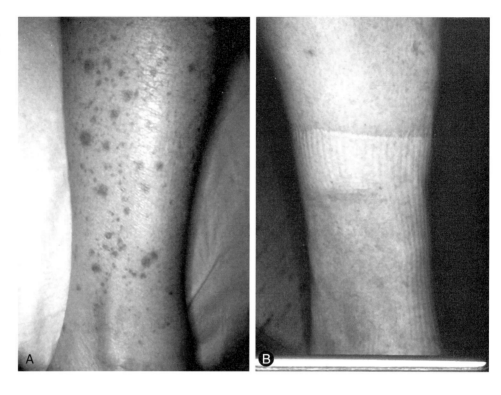

tions for systemic corticosteroids include a rapidly progressive course, neurologic involvement, renal involvement with loss of function, carditis or coronary vasculitis, and severe pulmonary disease with cavitation or infiltration. Among the relative indications are chronic cutaneous disease that is unresponsive to other agents, peripheral neuropathy, chronic lung disease, weight loss, and fever.

Corticosteroids should be given in moderate to high daily dosages. I use prednisone; when there are strong indications for its use, a starting dose of 60 to 80 mg/day is given in divided doses. Divided doses are clinically more effective than a single morning dose, even in equivalent milligram-for-milligram doses. However, in addition to the greater clinical efficacy, the divided dosage schedule has more chance of toxicity. Prednisone is continued until the signs and symptoms of vasculitis have been controlled. At this point, a switch to a single morning dose should be attempted, and the drug can then be slowly tapered. Tapering should take place over a period of about twice the length of the active treatment phase. If reactivation of the disease occurs, the original dosage should be reinstituted, followed by a slow taper.

Intravenous administration of methylprednisolone in high doses (1 g/day for 5 days) has been used in patients with acute fulminating vasculitis. This therapy is not without risk: sudden electrolyte shift, cardiac arrhythmia, and cardiac arrest have been reported. The patients should be carefully monitored throughout the therapy. This approach constitutes a stopgap measure for the management of severe disease and other means of disease suppression are necessary for long-term control of the vasculitic process.

Corticosteroid therapy, as mentioned, is frequently accompanied by side effects. Careful monitoring for diabetes mellitus, hypertension, peptic ulcer disease, osteoporosis, cataract formation, and glaucoma is important. Also, reactivation of *Mycobacterium tuberculosis* infection is possible, and attempts to identify the patient at risk should be made at the onset of therapy. It has been pointed out that reliable purified protein derivative skin testing can be performed during the first days to weeks of therapy with systemic corticosteroids, and thus the patient in need of rapid treatment need not wait for the result of the skin test before initiation of therapy.

IMMUNOSUPPRESSIVE AGENTS. Patients who fail to respond to systemic corticosteroids, who experience steroid-related side effects, or in whom the disease is severe may be given an immunosuppressive agent. The agents most often used in vasculitis are alkylating agents such as cyclophosphamide (Cytoxan) and chlorambucil (Leukeran), antimetabolites such as azathioprine (Imuran), the folate antagonist methotrexate (Rheumatrex), and cyclosporine (Sandimmune, Neoral). Earlier studies suggested that cyclophosphamide was the agent of choice in conditions such as severe necrotizing vasculitis and Wegener's granulomatosis,[64] but later reports suggested that methotrexate may be equally effective in maintaining a control for Wegener's granulomatosis.[65] Cyclophosphamide has been used in a daily oral dose of 1 to 2 mg/kg. It is administered in the morning, and the patient is given adequate hydration throughout the day to prevent hemorrhagic cystitis. This agent should not be given during pregnancy. Its beneficial effects are often delayed, beginning within 4 to 6 weeks. Cyclophosphamide has been administered in intermittent intravenous pulses. This method avoids some of the potential long-term toxicity, but hemorrhagic cystitis remains a possibility. Chlorambucil is an agent with a presumably similar mechanism of action without associated bladder toxicity, but it has been much less well studied. Both cyclophosphamide and chlorambucil have been linked to an increased risk of neoplasia—in particular, lymphoreticular malignancies (both agents), skin cancer (chlorambucil), and bladder cancer (cyclophosphamide).

Azathioprine has been reported to be useful in patients with severe refractory cutaneous vasculitis (Fig. 15–15)[66] and in patients with rheumatoid vasculitis.[67] It has also been used in severe necrotizing vasculitis, polyarteritis nodosa, and Wegener's granulomatosis but is probably less effective than cyclophosphamide in these conditions. It is administered in a single oral dose of 1 to 2 mg/kg. The primary toxic effects that occur are drug-induced fever, pancreatitis, hepatitis, and bone marrow toxicity. The onset of its action is also delayed, occurring within 4 to 6 weeks. Long-term toxic effects such as potential neoplasia have been studied in patients with rheumatoid arthritis, and the risk of subsequent malignancy was no greater in the patients receiving azathioprine than in those with similar disease levels who were not given azathioprine.

Low-dose weekly methotrexate (7.5 to 15 mg) has been used to treat patients with Wegener's granulomatosis, rheumatoid vasculitis, and cutaneous polyarteritis nodosa.[68] Methotrexate can be administered orally, intramuscularly, or intravenously. Renal function should be carefully assessed before initiating methotrexate therapy because an inability to excrete the drug increases the potential for severe toxicity. Initial monitoring of patients receiving methotrexate should in-

clude frequent complete blood counts and liver function tests. Patients receiving long-term therapy will need periodic liver biopsies to monitor for potential fibrosis or cirrhosis, or both.

Cyclosporine is a relatively new agent developed to prevent transplant rejection. The mechanism of its action is unknown. It is administered in doses of 3 to 5 mg/kg/day, with effects and side effects closely linked to one another. Nephrotoxicity is a limiting factor, and careful monitoring of renal function and blood pressure is necessary. Blood levels (trough) can be obtained, but it is not clear how meaningful they are in terms of toxicity or effect. Clinical experience with cyclosporine therapy for vasculitis is anecdotal.

PLASMAPHERESIS. Plasma exchange can be an adjunct to therapy for severe diseases characterized by circulating immunoreactants, such as vasculitis. A number of exchanges are required, and the procedure must be performed in a hospital setting. This therapy can protect patients through a severe flare of disease, although systemic therapy with corticosteroids or immunosuppressives, or both, is required for long-term control of the disease process.

## PSORIASIS

Psoriasis is a chronic inflammatory condition of the skin characterized by localized to widespread scaly plaques (papulosquamous lesions). There is a genetic predisposition for psoriasis, but the exact cause and pathomechanisms are still not fully understood. It does appear that psoriasis is a disorder in which there is epidermal proliferation that is T-cell driven.[69] Psoriasis is common, affecting 1% to 2% of the general popula-

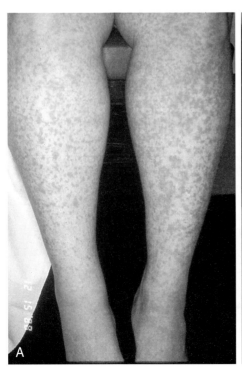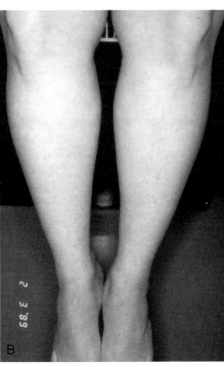

**FIGURE 15–15**
Before (A) and 6 weeks after (B) azathioprine therapy of small vessel cutaneous vasculitis. This patient had chronic disease limited to the skin, but it caused such psychological distress that she was not socially functional. With therapy she resumed her usual daily routines.

tion. There is no known cure, but prolonged remission is possible in some patients.

The diagnosis of psoriasis is best made by an experienced clinician and is based on clinical findings. Skin biopsy findings are characteristic in patients with clinically typical lesions of psoriasis, although microscopic features are less specific when clinically atypical lesions are sampled. Other papulosquamous disorders that may simulate psoriasis include seborrheic dermatitis, superficial dermatophyte infection, and Reiter's disease. In some patients, it may be virtually impossible to distinguish psoriasis from seborrheic dermatitis; thus, the term *sebopsoriasis*. In addition, patients with psoriasis and arthritis may manifest findings similar to those seen in Reiter's disease, and some authorities have suggested that there is a disease continuum among psoriasis, psoriatic arthritis, and Reiter's disease.

Psoriasis is characterized by scaly papules and plaques. In an untreated patient, the scale is silvery and thick. When the scale is removed, there is often pinpoint bleeding—the so-called Auspitz sign. Psoriasis may be manifested in various forms. Plaque-type psoriasis (psoriasis vulgaris) is the most common type and affects the elbows, knees, scalp, lower back, and nails. A variant characterized by small but widespread "drop-like" plaques is known as guttate psoriasis. This form is common in adolescents and is often triggered by an upper respiratory tract infection, particularly a streptococcal pharyngitis. Finally, erythrodermic and pustular variants can be life-threatening.

The choice of therapy for the patient with psoriasis involves an assessment of the extent of disease and the character of the disease. Limited involvement (<10% of the body surface) should be treated with topical agents. Corticosteroid preparations are mainstays of treatment, and their selection is based on the desired potency and formulation needed to control the disease. For example, plaques on the knees and elbows require a potent preparation in an ointment or cream base. Facial lesions should be treated with low-potency creams. Scalp disease is best treated with a mid- to high-potency solution or gel. Other topical preparations are available, including calcipotriene (Dovonex), which is a vitamin D analog that is available as an ointment, cream, and scalp solution; tazarotene (Tazorac), which is a retinoid; anthralins; and various tar preparations. Patients who do not respond to topical corticosteroids should be referred for dermatologic care because many of the alternative preparations are potentially irritating even when used properly.

Psoriasis that affects greater than 20% of the body surface should be approached with systemic therapies. UVB phototherapy is often useful. This therapy may be delivered in an outpatient setting or hospital but is not available in a "tanning" salon. As tanning salon UV light is primarily UVA, it causes tanning, and without a photosensitizer it has limited or no benefit for psoriasis. Oral psoralen in combination with UVA light is beneficial for psoriasis, but appropriate monitoring is necessary. Psoralen should not be given to a patient planning on visiting a tanning salon because of severe burns and even deaths that have occurred. Patients who fail to respond to phototherapy may be considered for systemic pharmacotherapy. There is a large experience with oral low-dose weekly methotrexate.[70] Methotrexate is used in dosages of 10 to 25 mg/week. Concomitant administration of other folic acid inhibitors such as trimethoprim is contraindicated. Most dermatologists still have their patients undergo liver biopsy at cummulative doses of 1 to 1.5 g.[71] Mycophenolate mofetil has been used as an alternative to methotrexate. It is administered in oral doses of 1 to 1.5 g twice daily. There are open-label studies that have documented the usefulness of this agent.[72] The recognition that cyclosporine was of benefit to patients with psoriasis led investigators to new therapies that affect the T cell and led to new insights into the pathogenesis of psoriasis. Cyclosporine (in the new formulation Neoral) is now approved by the US Food and Drug Administration for the treatment of psoriasis.[73] It is administered in doses of 3 to 5 mg/kg/day and is effective in about 80% of patients. Patients treated with cyclosporine must be monitored carefully for blood pressure elevation and renal dysfunction. The oral retinoids acitretin (Soriatane) and isotreninoin (Accutane) can be used safely. They are particularly useful in erythrodermic or pustular forms of psoriasis, and benefits have been demonstrated in plaque-type disease as well. The retinoids are also useful as adjunctive therapy in patients receiving phototherapy.

## PYODERMA GANGRENOSUM

Pyoderma gangrenosum is an uncommon, ulcerative cutaneous condition with distinctive clinical characteristics.[74, 75] Frequently there is an associated systemic disease. The diagnosis is made by exclusion of other processes that may cause cutaneous ulcers. Patients with pyoderma gangrenosum are often pathergic, with lesions sometimes developing after minor trauma.

The ulcerations of classic pyoderma gangrenosum frequently are clinically characteristic. The border is well defined with a deep erythematous to violaceous color. The lesion extends peripherally, and often the border overhangs the ulceration (undermined) as the inflammatory process spreads within the dermis, only secondarily causing necrosis of the epidermis. The lesions may be single, or may occur in crops, often beginning as a discrete pustule with a surrounding inflammatory erythema. The lesions may occur on any surface but are most common on the legs. Pain is a prominent feature and is sometimes so severe that narcotics are required for symptomatic relief. As the lesion heals, scar formation occurs and the resulting scar is often described as cribriform.

Initial reports of pyoderma gangrenosum emphasized the association with ulcerative colitis.[76] Eventually, it became recognized that regional enteritis and Crohn's disease (granulomatous colitis) are found with pyoderma gangrenosum as often as with ulcerative colitis.[75] In the most recent accounts, inflammatory bowel disease has constituted about 15% to 20% of the associated phenomena. In addition, early reports stressed the relationship of pyoderma gangrenosum to the activity of the bowel disease and even suggested that some patients' pyoderma gangrenosum lesions may benefit from surgical resection of the inflamed bowel (ulcerative colitis only). Callen and colleagues reported pyoderma gangrenosum in associated with inactive terminal ileitis,[77] and Talansky and associates also reported lack of effect of bowel resection in some patients with pyoderma gangrenosum and ulcerative colitis.[78]

Arthritis is a frequent finding with pyoderma gangrenosum. In some of the later reports, arthritis was the most frequent associated condition.[79] Five of the nine patients with arthritis reported by Prystowsky and colleagues[79] had inflammatory bowel disease–associated arthritis. In general, the arthritis associated with pyoderma gangrenosum is a symmetrical polyarthritis that may be seronegative or seropositive. Spondylitis and psoriatic arthritis have been reported in conjunction with pyoderma gangrenosum in individual cases.[80, 81]

The differential diagnosis of ulcerative cutaneous lesions includes the following conditions: infectious diseases, halogenodermas, vasculitis, insect bites, venous or arterial insufficiency (including antiphospholipid antibody–associated occlusive disease), and factitial ulcerations. Specimens for culture should be taken from both exudate and tissues.

To test for the presence of an associated disorder, another series of examinations should be performed. A thorough historical evaluation and examination of the gastrointestinal tract should be undertaken in consultation with a gastroenterologist. Radiographic procedures may include an upper gastrointestinal series and a barium enema. Flexible sigmoidoscopy or colonoscopy, or both, may also be performed, with appropriate biopsy specimens being taken. A complete blood count, careful evaluation of the peripheral smear, and possibly a bone marrow aspirate or biopsy helps rule out the presence of an associated hematologic malignant process. Serum protein electrophoresis, serum immunodiffusion studies, and possibly serum and urine immunoelectrophoresis help eliminate a diagnosis of associated monoclonal gammopathy or myeloma. Multiple reports of pyoderma gangrenosum–like leg ulcers in patients with antiphospholipid antibodies have appeared and tests such as the VDRL (Venereal Disease Research Laboratory), anticardiolipin antibody, and partial thromboplastin time are now standard in the evaluation of a patient with pyoderma gangrenosum.[82]

There is no specific, uniformly effective treatment for pyoderma gangrenosum. Although systemic treatment may affect the underlying disease process in some patients with chronic ulceration, it sometimes becomes necessary to consider colectomy.[83] Some patients' skin lesions respond to bowel resection, but there are patients in whom total colectomy, including removal of the rectosigmoid colon, does not lead to a remission.[78] In one report, a patient acquired pyoderma gangrenosum 10 years after total colectomy.[84] In mild cases, local

measures, such as dressings, elevation, rest, topical agents, or intralesional injections may be sufficient to control the disease process. Compresses, wet-to-dry dressings, or the newer biooclusive semipermeable dressings may be useful. Cleansing or therapy with antibacterial agents such as hydrogen peroxide or benzoyl peroxide has been reported to be beneficial in an occasional patient. Hyperbarbic oxygen therapy has also been reported to be effective in a small number of cases. Superpotent topical corticosteroids and intralesional injections of corticosteroids may be beneficial in some patients. Care must be taken to avoid introducing infection and to limit the potential systemic effects of corticosteroids that arise from injecting large doses intralesionally. In general, the periphery of the lesion is injected, but the agent may also be introduced into the ulcer base. Other topical approaches include the use of sodium cromoglycate, nitrogen mustard, and 5-aminosalicylic acid.[85, 86]

In patients who do not respond to topical or local therapies or patients whose severe, rapid course warrants the use of a systemic agent, sulfonamides, sulfones, or corticosteroids have been the most commonly used agents. Perry reported that oral sulfasalazine is effective in patients both with and without inflammatory bowel disease.[76] Dapsone has often been used as a monotherapy, or as an adjunctive steroid-sparing agent. Usually the drug is administered in lower dosages (100 to 150 mg/day), and the usual precautions and pretherapy evaluation are necessary. The mechanism of action of the sulfonamides and sulfones in this process is not understood, but effects on the polymorphonuclear leukocyte may be a factor. Another antileprosy agent, clofazimine, has also been reported to be successful in some patients with pyoderma gangrenosum. Thalidomide was reported to be useful in one report.[88] Finally, several other antibiotics have been used successfully in individual cases, including minocycline and rifampin.

Systemic corticosteroids have been used extensively in patients with pyoderma gangrenosum and its variants and are generally believed to be very effective. Usually, large dosages (40–120 mg/day) are necessary to induce remission of disease. These dosages, used over the long term, frequently result in steroid-related side effects. In a study by Holt and colleagues, 6 of their 12 patients who were treated with corticosteroids experienced serious steroid complications, and 4 of these 6 individuals died as a result of the therapy.[88] To avoid the complications of long-term steroid use, Johnson and Lazarus, and subsequently others, used pulse therapy with 1 g of methylprednisolone given intravenously each day for a period of 5 days.[89] Maintenance of the remission was accomplished with oral corticosteroids every other day. Prystowsky and associates repeated the experience of Lazarus with a further eight patients.[79] They found that remissions occurred in five of the patients and that they were usually able to discontinue oral corticosteroid therapy and often lower the dose of other medications. Pulse therapy is not without side effects, which include sudden death. In the hands of Prystowsky and associates, and in my experience with three patients, this therapy has primarily resulted in transient hyperglycemia; however, it should only be used with great caution and proper monitoring.

Immunosuppressive agents have been suggested for use in patients who fail to respond to other therapies, particularly systemic corticosteroids, or in who steroid-related side effects develop. Individual reports using oral azathioprine, cyclophosphamide,[90] chlorambucil,[91] cyclosporine (Fig. 15–16)[92] tacrolimus (FK 506),[93] mycophenolate,[94] or methotrexate[95] have suggested that, at least in some patients, these agents may be successful. Intravenous pulses of cyclophosphamide[96] or immune globulin[97] have also been successful in individual patients. The mode of action of the immunosuppressive agent is not understood.

## SWEET'S SYNDROME (ACUTE FEBRILE NEUTROPHILIC DERMATOSIS)

In 1964, R.D. Sweet described a group of patients with one or more attacks of painful, erythematous plaques accompanied by fever, arthralgias, and leukocytosis.[98] The histopathologic correlate was a massive neutrophilic infiltration of the dermis in the absence of vessel wall destruction or demonstrable infection. Sweet termed the process *acute febrile neutrophilic dermatosis,* but it has become known as Sweet's syndrome. Since Sweet's original description, more than 500 cases have been reported.[99]

Sweet's syndrome has been reported with a variety of diseases. von den Driesch suggested that Sweet's syndrome can be subdivided into four groups: (1) classic or idiopathic, (2) parainflammatory, (3) para-

neoplastic, and (4) associated with pregnancy.[99] Although idiopathic cases are most frequent, paraneoplastic Sweet's syndrome is the most frequently identified association and myelogenous leukemia or preleukemia account for most of the paraneoplastic conditions.[100] Sweet's syndrome is not clinically or histopathologically different among the four groups; however, in the presence of leukemia, the patients more frequently tend to be anemic or thrombocytopenic and may have hemorrhagic lesions. Other associated processes in paraneoplastic Sweet's syndrome include benign monoclonal gammopathy, lymphoma, myelodysplastic disorders, and various solid tumors (breast, stomach, genitourinary, and colon most commonly).[101] Parainflammatory Sweet's syndrome has also been reported in conjunction with lupus erythematosus, rheumatoid arthritis, Sjögren's syndrome, inflammatory bowel disease (Crohn's disease and ulcerative colitis), Behçet's disease, thyroiditis, various infections (including human immunodeficiency virus, hepatitis, mycobacterial infection, cytomegalovirus, salmonellosis), and drug hypersensitivity. It is not known how frequently paraneoplastic Sweet's syndrome occurs, but most authorities quote a figure ranging from 10% to 20%, with about 40% to 50% of these patients having a hemtologic malignancy.

Sweet's syndrome is usually an acute, steroid-responsive, self-limited disease. In general, a 2-week tapering course of oral prednisone (40 to 60 mg/day) is effective (Fig. 15–17). One or more exacerbations requiring brief reinstitution of corticosteroids are common. From Sweet's initial report and the many later ones, it appears that the process can follow a chronic course, and the use of steroid-sparing agents should be considered. In reports of individual or small groups

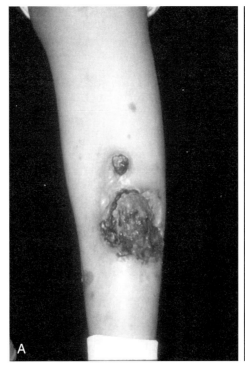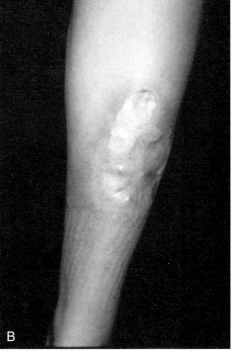

**FIGURE 15–16**
Before (*A*) and after (*B*) oral cyclosporine therapy (5 mg/kg/day) for pyoderma gangrenosum. At this time, the patient had no systemic disease. She later acquired a lupus nephritis.

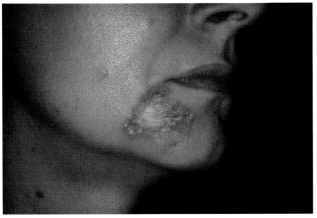

**FIGURE 15–1**
Chronic cutaneous lupus erythematosus. This lesion of discoid lupus erythematosus was present for a long time before treatment was initiated. The result was atrophy and scarring.

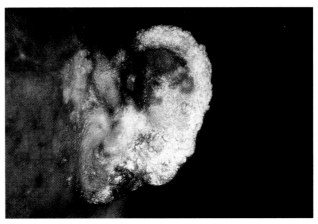

**FIGURE 15–2**
This patient with long-standing lesions of discoid lupus erythematosus failed to follow medical advice, and his lesions became verrucous over an 18-year period. Subsequent to this picture, he has developed multiple squamous cell carcinomas.

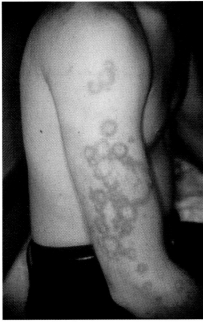

**FIGURE 15–3**
An annular variant of subacute cutaneous lupus erythematosus.

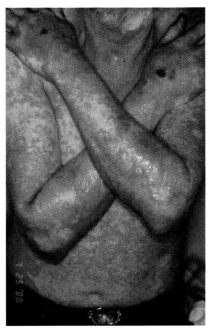

**FIGURE 15–4**
Papulosquamous variant of subacute cutaneous lupus erythematosus.

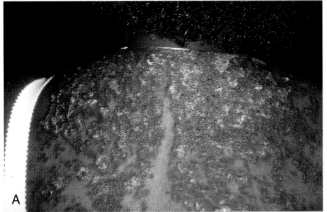

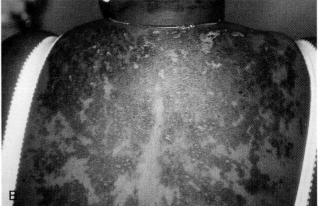

**FIGURE 15–5**
Chronic cutaneous lupus erythematosus before (*A*) and 1 month after (*B*) intralesional triamcinolone treatment.

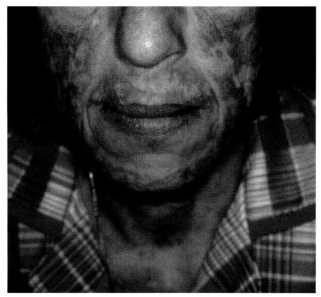

**FIGURE 15–6**
Pigmentation resulting from hydroxychloroquine therapy of
subacute cutaneous lupus erythematosus.

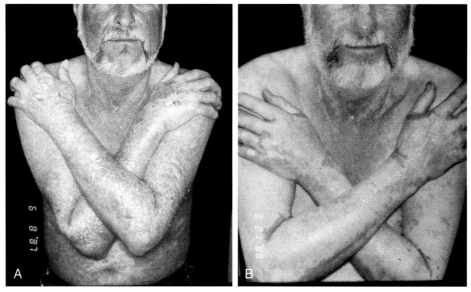

**FIGURE 15–7**
Before (*A*) and after (*B*) azathioprine therapy of papulosquamous subacute cutaneous lupus
erythematosus.

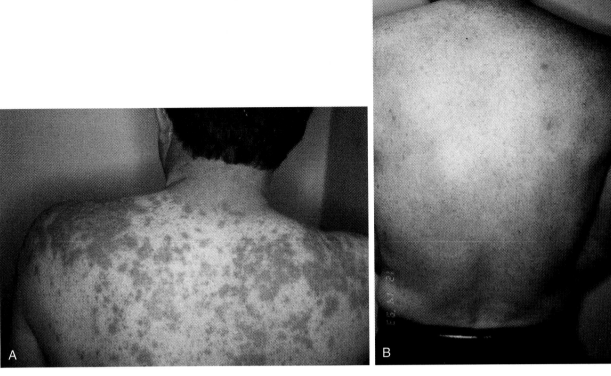

**FIGURE 15–8**
Before (*A*) and after (*B*) auranofin therapy for subacute cutaneous lupus erythematosus.

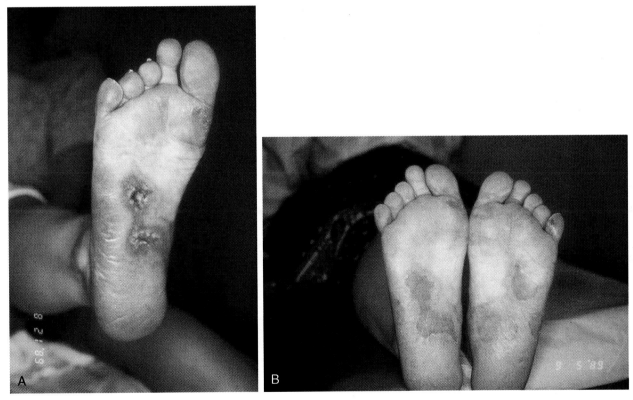

**FIGURE 15–9**
Before (*A*) and 4 weeks after (*B*) oral isotretinoin therapy for plantar lesions of lupus erythematosus.

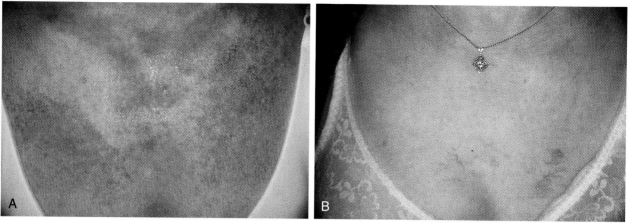

**FIGURE 15–10**
Before (A) and after (B) hydroxychloroquine therapy for dermatomyositis.

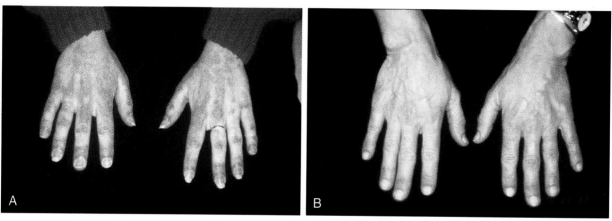

**FIGURE 15–11**
Before (A) and after (B) methotrexate therapy for cutaneous lesions of dermatomyositis.

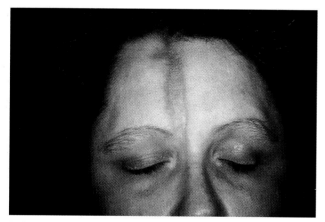

**FIGURE 15–12**
En coup de sabre: a form of linear scleroderma.

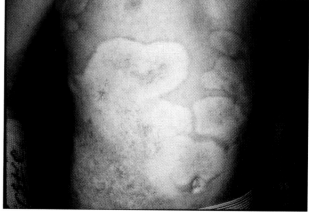

**FIGURE 15–13**
Widespread morphea. This patient has the surface characteristics of lichen sclerosus et atrophicus. Four years after diagnosis, this child acquired an interstitial pneumonitis that was consistent with scleroderma pulmonary disease. This progression to systemic manifestations is exceedingly rare.

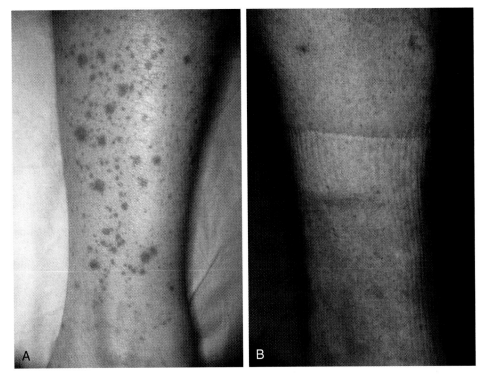

**FIGURE 15–14**
Before (*A*) and 4 weeks after (*B*) oral colchicine therapy for small vessel cutaneous vasculitis.

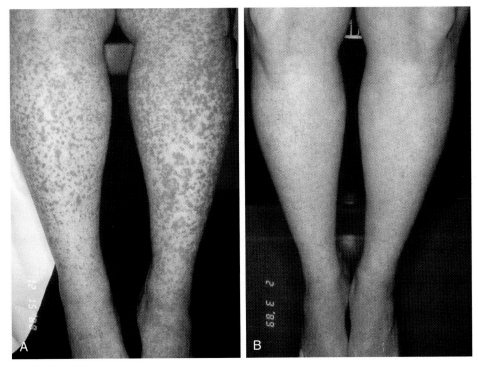

**FIGURE 15–15**
Before (*A*) and 6 weeks after (*B*) azathioprine therapy for small vessel cutaneous vasculitis. This patient had chronic disease limited to the skin, but it caused such psychological distress that she was not socially functional. With therapy she resumed her usual daily routines.

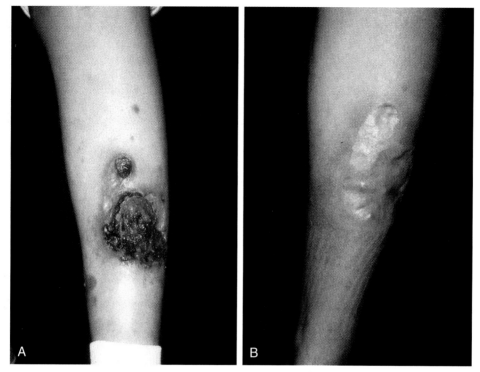

**FIGURE 15–16**
Before (*A*) and after (*B*) oral cyclosporine therapy (5 mg/kg/day) for pyoderma gangrenosum. At this time, the patient had no systemic disease. She later acquired a lupus nephritis.

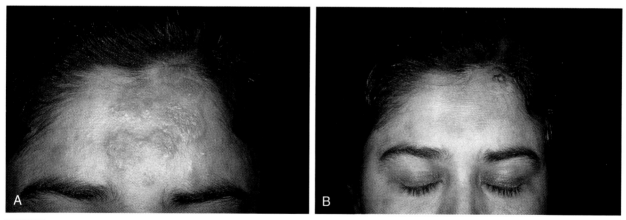

**FIGURE 15–17**
Before (*A*) and 1 week after (*B*) oral prednisone therapy for Sweet's syndrome.

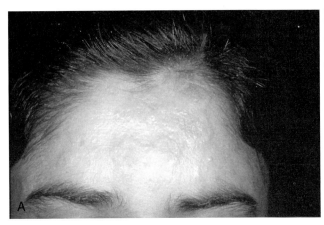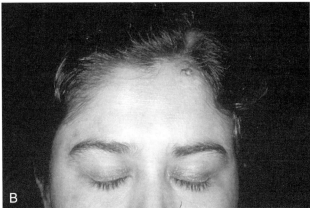

**FIGURE 15-17**
Before (*A*) and 1 week after (*B*) oral prednisone therapy of Sweet's syndrome.

of patients, dapsone, potassium iodide, indomethacin, doxycycline, clofazimine, colchicine, metronidazole, isotretinoin, methotrexate, chlorambucil, cyclosporine, and pulse dosing of methylprednisolone have been used successfully.[99, 101–105]

## PANNICULITIS

Panniculitis refers to inflammation within the subcutaneous fat. It is probably a dynamic process that progresses from inflammation with neutrophils to inflammation with lymphocytes, and then to inflammation with histiocytes, ending with fibrosis. The panniculitis can become granulomatous when in the histiocytic phase. The exact nature of the infiltrate perhaps depends on when the biopsy specimen is taken in relation to the age of the lesion being sampled. The panniculitides have been divided into four categories on the basis of histopathologic criteria: (1) septal panniculitis, (2) lobular panniculitis, (3) mixed with septal and lobular components, and (4) panniculitis with vasculitis. Frequently the panniculitides are associated with systemic disease. Often the distinction of one syndrome from another is possible only after a period of observation.

The treatment of erythema nodosum and other panniculitides first involves assessment of a causative disease and its treatment. In the absence of a treatable disorder, therapy is symptomatic.[106] Acute erythema nodosum is often self-limited; thus, nontoxic therapies are advised. Bed rest and leg elevation are helpful in controlling symptoms. In patients who need to continue to be ambulatory, support stockings or tights may be helpful.[107] Aspirin or other nonsteroidal anti-inflammatory agents may be helpful. My experience with aspirin has not produced results before it produces toxicity, and therefore my choice is to use oral indomethacin at a dosage of 25 to 75 mg/day.[108]

In patients with chronic erythema nodosum or frequent recurrences, oral potassium iodide at a dosage of 325 to 975 mg/day has been useful in open clinical trials.[109] My experience with 15 patients with erythema

nodosum treated with oral potassium iodide has yielded control of the disease in 10 patients (unpublished observation). Furthermore, in some of the responding patients, when the drug is stopped or the dosage is lowered, the disease has relapsed only to respond again with reinstitution of therapy. Other drugs that may be considered include oral corticosteroids, colchicine,[110] or an immunosuppressive agent. Systemic corticosteroid therapy, which is almost always effective, is often complicated by iatrogenic Cushing's syndrome. Colchicine has not been effective in any of the patients that I have treated. Azathioprine and cyclosporine have been used successfully in some patients. One adjunctive therapy that can be helpful is intralesionally injected triamcinolone acetonide (3 to 5 mg/mL).

There is no specific therapy for Weber-Christian disease. Reports have centered on the use of anti-inflammatory drugs, oral corticosteroids, antimalarial agents, and immunosuppressive drugs including cyclophosphamide and cyclosporine.[111] In addition, colchicine, dapsone, and potassium iodide may be effective in individual cases.

## REFERENCES

1. Callen JP: Collagen vascular diseases. Med Clin North Am 1998; 82:1217–1237.
2. Spann CR, Callen JP, Klein JB, et al: Clinical, serologic and immunogenetic studies in patients with chronic cutaneous (discoid) lupus erythematosus who have verrucous and/or hypertrophic skin lesions. J Rheumatol 1988; 15:256–261.
3. Millard LG, Barker DJ: Development of squamous cell carcinoma in chronic discoid lupus erythematosus. Clin Exp Dermatol 1978; 3:161.
4. Sontheimer RD, Thomas JR, Gilliam JN: Subacute cutaneous lupus erythematosus: A cutaneous marker for a distinct lupus erythematosus. Arch Dermatol 1979; 115:1409–1415.
5. Callen JP: Systemic lupus erythematosus in patients with chronic cutaneous (discoid) lupus erythematosus. J Am Acad Dermatol 1985; 12:278–288.
6. Cohen MR, Crosby D: Systemic disease in subacute cutaneous lupus erythematosus: A controlled comparison with systemic lupus erythematosus. J Rheumatol 1994; 21:1665–1669.
7. Chelbus E, Wolska H, Blaszcyk M, et al: Subacute cutaneous lupus erythematosus versus systemic lupus erythematosus: Di-

agnostic criteria and therapeutic implications. J Am Acad Dermatol 1998; 38:405–412.

8. Lehmann P, Hölzle E, Kind P, et al: Experimental reproduction of skin lesions in lupus erythematosus by UVA and UVB radiation. J Am Acad Dermatol 1990; 22:181–187.

9. Roenigk HH Jr, Martin JS, Eichorn P, et al: Discoid lupus erythematosus. Diagnostic features and evaluation of topical corticosteroid therapy. Cutis 1980; 25:281–285.

10. Callen JP: Intralesional triamcinolone is effective for discoid lupus erythematosus of the palms and soles. J Rheumatol 1985; 12:630–633.

11. Levy GD, Munz SJ, Paschal J, et al: Incidence of hydroxychloroquine retinopathy in 1,207 patients in a large multicenter outpatient practice. Arthritis Rheum 1997; 40:1482–1486.

12. Rahmann P, Gladman DD, Urowitz MB: Smoking interferes with efficacy of antimalarial therapy in cutaneous lupus. J Rheumatol 1998; 25:1716–1719.

13. Gallego H, Crutchfield CE III, Lewis EJ, et al: Report of an association between discoid lupus erythematosus and smoking. Cutis 1999; 63:231–234.

14. Feldmann R, Salomon D, Saurat J-H: The association of the two antimalarials—chloroquine and quinacrine—for treatment of treatment-resistant chronic and subacute lupus erythematosus. Dermatology 1994; 189:425–427.

15. Callen JP, Spencer LV, Burruss JB, et al: Azathioprine: An effective, corticosteroid sparing therapy for patients with recalcitrant cutaneous lupus erythematosus or with recalcitrant cutaneous leukocytoclastic vasculitis. Arch Dermatol 1991; 127:515–522.

16. Tsokos GC, Caughman SW, Klippel JH: Successful treatment of generalized discoid skin lesions with azathioprine. Arch Dermatol 1985; 121:1323–1325.

17. Boehm IB, Boehm GA, Bauer R: Management of cutaneous lupus erythematosus with low-dose methotrexate: Indication for modulation of inflammatory mechanisms. Rheumatol Int 1998; 18:59–62.

18. Yung RL, Richardson BC: Cytarabine therapy for refractory cutaneous lupus erythematosus. Arthritis Rheum 1995; 38:1341–1343.

19. Lagrange S, Frances C, Roy S, et al: High dose intravenous immune globulin in the treatment of refractory severe discoid lupus erythematosus. J Am Acad Dermatol, in press.

20. Holtman J, Neustadt D, Callen JP: Dapsone is an effective therapy for the skin lesions of subacute cutaneous lupus erythematosus and urticarial vasculitis in a patient with C2 deficiency. J Rheumatol 1990; 17:1222–1225.

21. Hall RP, Lawley TJ, Smith HR, et al: Bullous eruption of systemic lupus erythematosus: Dramatic response to dapsone therapy. Ann Intern Med 1982; 97:165–170.

22. Neri R, Mosen M, Bernacchi E: A case of systemic lupus erythematosus with acute, subacute, and chronic cutaneous lesions successfully treated with dapsone. Lupus 1999; 8:240–243.

23. Krivanek JFC, Paver WKA: Further study of the use of clofazimine in discoid lupus erythematosus. Australas J Dermatol 1980; 21:169–171.

24. Grosshans E, Illy G: Thalidomide therapy for inflammatory dermatoses. Int J Dermatol 1984; 23:598–602.

25. Atra E, Sato EI: Treatment of the cutaneous lesions of systemic lupus erythematosus with thalidomide. Clin Exp Rheumatol 1993; 11:487–493.

26. Warren KJ, Nopper AJ, Crosby DL: Thalidomide for recalcitrant discoid lesions in a patient with systemic lupus erythematosus. J Am Acad Dermatol 1998; 39:293–295.

26a. Duong DJ, Spigel GT, Moxley RT III, Gasparita A: American experience with low-dose thalidomide therapy for severe cutaneous lupus erythematosus. Arch Dermatol 1999; 135:1079–1087.

27. Steinjker B: Auranofin in the treatment of discoid lupus erythematosus. J Dermatol Treat 1991; 2:27–29.

28. Rodriguez-Castellanos MA, Barba Rubio J, Barba Gomez JF, et al: Phenytoin in the treatment of discoid lupus erythematosus. Arch Dermatol 1995; 131:620–621.

29. Tebbe B, Lauy M, Gollnick H: Therapy of cutaneous lupus erythematosus with recombinant interferon alpha-2a: A case report. Eur J Dermatol 1992; 2:253–255.

30. Prinz JC, Meurer M, Reiter C, et al: Treatment of severe cutaneous lupus with a chimeric CD4 monoclonal antibody, cM-T412. J Am Acad Dermatol 1996; 34:244–252.

31. Newton RC, Jorizzo JL, Solomon AR, et al: Mechanism-oriented assessment of isotretinoin in chronic or subacute lupus erythematosus. Arch Dermatol 1986; 122:180–186.

32. Cheong WK, Hughes GRV, Norris PG, et al: Cutaneous photosensitivity in dermatomyositis. Br J Dermatol 1994; 131:205–208.

33. Woo TY, Callen JP, Voorhees JV, et al: Cutaneous lesions of dermatomyositis are improved by hydroxychloroquine. J Am Acad Dermatol 1984; 10:592–600.

34. Olson NY, Lindsley CB: Adjunctive use of hydroxychloroquine in childhood dermatomyositis. J Rheumatol 1989; 16:1545–1547.

35. Kasteler JS, Callen JP: Low-dose methotrexate administered weekly is an effective corticosteroid-sparing agent for the treatment of cutaneous manifestations of dermatomyositis. J Am Acad Dermatol 1997; 36:67–71.

36. Zieglschmid-Adams ME, Pandya, Cohen SB, et al: Treatment of dermatomyositis with methotrexate. J Am Acad Dermatol 1995; 32:754–757.

37. Dalakas MC, Illa I, Dambrosia JM, et al: A controlled trial of high-dose intravenous immune globin infusions as a treatment for dermatomyositis. N Engl J Med 1993; 329:1993–2000.

38. Oliveri MB, Palermo R, Mantalen C, et al: Regression of calcinosis during diltiazem treatment in juvenile dermatomyositis. J Rheumatol 1996; 23:2152–2155.

39. Uziel Y, Krafchik BR, Silverman ED, et al: Localized scleroderma in childhood: A report of 30 cases. Semin Arthritis Rheum 1994; 23:328–340.

40. Dehen L, Roujeau JC, Cosnes A, et al: Internal involvement in localized scleroderma. Medicine 1994; 73:241–245.

41. Humbert P, Delaporte E, Dupond JL, et al: Treatment of localized scleroderma with oral 1,25-dihydroxyvitamin $D_3$. Eur J Dermatol 1994; 4:21–23.

42. Elst EF, van Suijlekom-Smit LWA, Oranje AP: Treatment of linear scleroderma with oral 1,25-dihydroxyvitamin $D_3$ (calcitriol) in seven children. Pediatr Dermatol 1999; 16:53–58.

43. Cunningham BB, Landells IDR, Langman D, et al: Topical calcipotriene for morphea/linear scleroderma. J Am Acad Dermatol 1998; 39:211–215.

44. Seyger MB, van den Hoogen FHJ, de Boo T, et al: Low-dose methotrexate in the treatment of widespread morphea. J Am Acad Dermatol 1998; 39:220–225.

45. Stege H, Berneburg M, Humke S, et al: High dose UVA-1 radiation therapy for localized scleroderma. J Am Acad Dermatol 1997; 35:938–944.

46. Kerscher M, Volkenandt M, Gruss C, et al: Low-dose UVA-1 phototherapy for treatment of localized scleroderma. J Am Acad Dermatol 1998; 38:21–26.

47. Gruss C, Reed JA, Altmeyer P, et al: Induction of interstitial collagenase (MMP-1) by UVA-1 phototherapy in morphea fibroblasts. Lancet 1997; 350:1295–1296.

48. Callen JP: Cutaneous vasculitis: Relationship to systemic disease and therapy. Curr Prob Dermatol 1993; 2:45–80.

49. Jorizzo JL: Classification of vasculitis. J Invest Dermatol 1993; 100:106S–110S.

50. Lunardi C, Bambara LM, Biasi D, et al: Elimination diet in the treatment of selected patients with hypersensitivity vasculitis. Clin Exp Rheumatol 1992; 10:131–135.

51. Blanco R, Martínez-Taboada VM, Rodrígues-Valverde V, et al: Cutaneous vasculitis in children and adults. Associated diseases and etiologic factors in 303 patients. Medicine 1998; 77:403–418.

52. Fauci AS, Katz P, Haynes BF, et al: Cyclophosphamide therapy of severe systemic necrotizing vasculitis. N Engl J Med 1979; 301:235–238.

53. Wisnieski JJ, Baer AN, Christensen J, et al: Hypocomplementemic urticarial vasculitis syndrome. Medicine 1995; 74:24–41.

54. Karlsberg PL, Lee WM, Casey DL, et al: Cutaneous vasculitis and rheumatoid factor positivity as presenting signs of hepatitis C virus–induced mixed cryoglobulinemia. Arch Dermatol 1995; 131:1119–1123.

55. Misani R, Bellavita P, Fenili D, et al: Interferon alfa-2a therapy in cryoglobulinemia associated with hepatitis C virus. N Engl J Med 1994; 330:751–756.

56. Durand JM, Cacoub P, Lunel-Fabiani F, et al: Ribavirin in hepatitis C related cryoglobulinemia. J Rheumatol 1998; 25:1115–1117.

57. Millns JL, Randle HW, Solley GO, et al: The therapeutic response of urticarial vasculitis to indomethacin. J Am Acad Dermatol 1980; 31:349–355.

58. Wahba-Yahav AV: Chronic cutaneous leukocytoclastic vasculitis associated with polycythemia vera: Effective control with pentoxifylline. J Am Acad Dermatol 1992; 26:1006–1007.

59. Katz SI, Gallin JI, Hertz KC, et al: Erythema elevatum diutinum: Skin and systemic manifestations, immunologic studies, and successful treatment with dapsone. Medicine 1977; 56:443–455.

60. Muramatsu C, Tanabe E: Urticarial vasculitis: Response to dapsone and colchicine. J Am Acad Dermatol 1985; 13:1055.

61. Nürnberg W, Grabbe J, Czarnetzki BM: Synergistic effects of pentoxifylline and dapsone in leucoclastic vasculitis. Lancet 1994; 343:491.

62. Callen JP: Colchicine is effective in controlling chronic cutaneous leukocytoclastic vasculitis. Arch Dermatol 1991; 127:515–522.

63. Sais G, Vidaller A, Jucglá A, et al: Colchicine in the treatment of cutaneous leukocytoclastic vasculitis: Results of a prospective, randomized controlled trial. Arch Dermatol 1995; 131:1399–1402.

64. Hoffman GS, Kerr GS, Leavitt RY, et al: Wegener's granulomatosis: An analysis of 158 patients. Ann Intern Med 1992; 116:488–498.

65. Hoffman GS, Leavitt RY, Kerr GS, et al: The treatment of Wegener's granulomatosis with glucocorticoids and methotrexate. Arthritis Rheum 1992; 35:1322–1329.

66. Callen JP, Spencer LV, Burruss JB, et al: Azathioprine: An effective, corticosteroid sparing therapy for patients with recalcitrant cutaneous lupus erythematosus or with recalcitrant cutaneous leukocytoclastic vasculitis. Arch Dermatol 1991; 127:515–522.

67. Heurkens AHM, Westedt ML, Breedveld FC: Prednisone plus azathioprine treatment in patients with rheumatoid arthritis complicated by vasculitis. Arch Intern Med 1991; 151:2249–2254.

68. Jorizzo JL, White WL, Wise CM, et al: Low-dose weekly methotrexate for unusual vascular reactions: Cutaneous polyarteritis nodosa and Behçet's disease. J Am Acad Dermatol 1991; 24:973–978.

69. Stern RS: Psoriasis. Lancet 1997; 350:349–353.

70. Jeffes EWB III, Weinstein GD: Methotrexate and other chemotherapeutic agents used to treat psoriasis. Dermatol Clin 1995; 13:875–890.

71. Roenigk H, Auerbach R, Weinstein G, et al: Methotrexate in psoriasis: Revised guidelines. J Am Acad Dermatol 1988; 19:145–156.

72. Haufs MG, Beissert S, Grabbe S, et al: Psoriasis vulgaris treated successfully with mycophenolate mofetil. Br J Dermatol 1998; 138:179–181.

73. Lebwohl M, Ellis C, Gottlieb A, et al: Cyclosporine consensus conference: With emphasis on the treatment of psoriasis. J Am Acad Dermatol 1998; 39:464–475.

74. Callen JP: Pyoderma gangrenosum. Lancet 1998; 351:581–585.

75. Powell FC, Su WPD, Perry HO: Pyoderma gangrenosum: Classification and management. J Am Acad Dermatol 1996; 34:395–409.

76. Perry HO: Pyoderma gangrenosum. South Med J 1959; 62:899–908.

77. Callen JP, Case JD, Sager D: Chlorambucil: An effective corticosteroid sparing therapy for pyoderma gangrenosum. J Am Acad Dermatol 1989; 21:515–519.

78. Talansky AL, Meyer S, Greenstein AJ: Does intestinal resection heal the pyoderma gangrenosum of inflammatory bowel disease? J Clin Gastroenterol 1983; 108:580–581.

79. Prystowsky JH, Kahn SN, Lazarus GS: Present status of pyoderma gangrenosum. Review of 21 cases. Arch Dermatol 1989; 125:57–64.

80. Oliveri I, Costa AM, Cantini F, et al: Pyoderma gangrenosum in association with undifferentiated seronegative spondyloarthropathy. Arthritis Rheum 1996; 39:1062–1065.

81. Smith DL, White CR Jr: Pyoderma gangrenosum in association with psoriatic arthritis. Arthritis Rheum 1994; 37:1258–1260.

82. Babe KS Jr, Gross AS, Leyva WH, et al: Pyoderma gangrenosum associated with antiphospholipid antibodies. Int J Dermatol 1992; 31:588–590.

83. Mir-Madjlessi SH, Taylor JS, Farmer RG: Clinical course and evolution of erythema nodosum and pyoderma gangrenosum in chronic ulcerative colitis: A study of 42 patients. Am J Gastroenterol 1985; 80:615–620.

84. Cox NH, Peebles-Brown DA, MacKie RM: Pyoderma gangrenosum occurring 10 years after proctocolectomy for ulcerative colitis. Br J Hosp Med 1986; 36:363.

85. DeCock KM, Thorne MG: The treatment of pyoderma gangrenosum with sodium cromoglycolate. Br J Dermatol 1980; 102:231–233.

86. Tsele E, Yu RCH, Chu AC: Pyoderma gangrenosum response to topical nitrogen mustard. Clin Exp Dermatol 1992; 17:437–440.

87. Harris MN, Farmer ER: Thalidomide treatment in pyoderma gangrenosum. J Am Acad Dermatol, in press.

88. Holt PJA, Davies MG, Saunders KC, et al: Pyoderma gangrenosum. Medicine 1980; 59:114–133.

89. Johnson RB, Lazarus GS: Pulse therapy: Therapeutic efficacy in the treatment of pyoderma gangrenosum. Arch Dermatol 1982; 118:76–84.

90. Newell LM, Malkinson FD: Pyoderma gangrenosum: Response to cyclophosphamide therapy. Arch Dermatol 1983; 119:495–497.

91. Burruss JB, Farmer ER, Callen JP: Chlorambucil is an effective corticosteroid-sparing agent for recalcitrant pyoderma gangrenosum. J Am Acad Dermatol 1996; 35:720–724.

92. Matis WL, Ellis CN, Griffiths CEM, et al: Treatment of pyoderma gangrenosum with cyclosporin. Arch Dermatol 1992; 182:1060–1064.

93. Weichert G, Sauder DN: Efficacy of tacrolimus (FK506) in idiopathic treatment-resistant pyoderma gangrenosum. J Am Acad Dermatol 1998; 39:648–650.

94. Nousari HC, Lynch W, Anhalt G, et al: The effectiveness of mycophenolate mofetil in refractory pyoderma gangrenosum. Arch Dermatol 1998; 134:1509–1511.

95. Teitel AD: Treatment of pyoderma gangrenosum with methotrexate. Cutis 1996; 57:326–328.

96. Reynoso-von Drateln C, Perla-Navarro AV, Gamez-Nava JI, et al: Intravenous cyclophosphamide pulses in pyoderma gangrenosum: An open trial. J Rheumatol 1997; 24:689–693.

97. Gupta AK, Shear NH, Sauder DN: Efficacy of human intravenous immune globulin in pyoderma gangrenosum. J Am Acad Dermatol 1995; 32:140–142.

98. Sweet RD: An acute febrile neutrophilic dermatosis. Br J Dermatol 1964; 74:349–356.

99. von den Driesch P: Sweet's syndrome (acute febrile neutrophilic dermatosis). J Am Acad Dermatol 1994; 31:535–556.

100. Cohen PR, Kurzrock R: Sweet's syndrome and cancer. Clin Dermatol 1993; 11:149–157.

101. Aram H: Acute febrile neutrophilic dermatosis (Sweet's syndrome): Response to dapsone. Arch Dermatol 1984; 120:245–247.

102. Horio T, Imamura S, Danno F, et al: Treatment of acute febrile neutrophilic dermatosis (Sweet's syndrome) with potassium iodide. Dermatologica 1980; 160:341–347.

103. Hoffman GS: Treatment of Sweet's syndrome (acute febrile neutrophilic dermatosis) with indomethacin. J Rheumatol 1977; 4:201–206.

104. Case JD, Smith SZ, Callen JP: The use of pulse methylprednisolone and chlorambucil in the treatment of Sweet's syndrome. Cutis 1989; 44:125–129.

105. Banet DE, McClave SA, Callen JP: Metronidazole is an effective treatment for Sweet's syndrome in a patient with associated inflammatory bowel disease. J Rheumatol 1994; 21:1766–1768.

106. Callen JP: Panniculitis. In Madison PJ, Isenberg DA, Woo P, et al (eds): Oxford Textbook of Rheumatic Diseases, 2nd ed. Oxford University Press, Oxford, England, 1998:1450–1457.

107. Lehman DW: Control of chronic erythema nodosum with naproxen. Cutis 1980: 26:66–67.

108. Bar WB, Robinson JA: Chronic erythema nodosum treated with indomethacin. Ann Intern Med 1981; 95:661.

109. Marshall JK, Irvine EJ: Successful therapy of refractory erythema nodosum associated with Crohn's disease using potassium iodide. Can J Gastroenterol 1997; 11:501–502.

110. Lupton GP, Slagel JA, Diskelmeier MR: Treatment of nodular vasculitis with colchicine. J Assoc Mil Dermatol 1988; 14:24–26.

111. Usuki K, Kitamura K, Urabe A, et al: Successful treatment of Weber-Christian disease by cyclosporin A. Am J Med 1988; 85:276–278.

# 16 | Inflammatory Eye Disease: Uveitis and Scleritis

## *James T. Rosenbaum*

*Uveitis* is a descriptive term for intraocular inflammation. Symptoms vary but may include pain, redness, photophobia, floaters, or visual loss. Like arthritis, uveitis has many etiologies (Table 16–1). Iritis, iridocyclitis, pars planitis, and chorioretinitis are types of uveitis named for the portion of the uveal tract most affected by the inflammation (Fig. 16–1). The causes of uveitis include infections and systemic immune-mediated diseases. Many forms of uveitis are clinically confined to the eye; most of these are presumed to have an immune-mediated cause as well. About 25% of patients with uveitis have a disease that does not fit well within a diagnostic category.[1] These patients frequently receive a diagnosis of an idiopathic disease, and an immunologic mechanism is, again, presumed to be causally related to the inflammation. So-called masquerade syndromes are noninflammatory conditions, such as lymphoma, and are often treated incorrectly because of their ability to mimic inflammatory disease.

The therapy for uveitis should obviously be tailored to some extent to the specific diagnosis. Etiology is critical; an infectious disease should clearly be treated differently from an autoimmune disease. Among the autoimmune causes, the choice of therapy is influenced by the location of the inflammation (anterior uveitis, which is synonymous with iritis, may respond to topical therapy far better than does posterior uveitis); by the prognosis (human leukocyte antigen [HLA] B27–associated iritis, for example, tends to resolve completely over weeks, whereas sarcoid associated uveitis tends to persist for months or years); by the severity; and by individual doctor and patient preferences. Only a few studies have addressed the possibility that specific subtypes of uveitis such as Behçet's disease might respond to specific approaches with immunotherapy. In general, the treatment of immune-mediated uveitis is empirical. There is a paucity of data from randomized, controlled clinical trials on which to base therapeutic decision making.[2, 3]

## GENERAL TREATMENT GUIDELINES

The therapy for uveitis may involve a combination of topical medications, periocular corticosteroid injections, oral corticosteroids, and oral immunosuppres-

sives. The rheumatologist or internist normally becomes involved in therapeutic decision making only if the ophthalmic physician has determined that the clinical response to topical and periocular medications has been inadequate. In this process, the ophthalmologist has needed to consider the possibility of an active infectious process such as herpes simplex or toxoplasmosis, both of which are relatively common causes of uveitis. In some instances, an infectious etiology is present but not apparent; it may take special alertness to the diagnosis in order to confirm the infection by appropriate culture or serologic technique. The therapy for infectious causes of uveitis is outside the scope of this chapter.

Uveitis is also not, in general, a surgically treated disease, although vitrectomy or cryotherapy (freezing a portion of the peripheral retina) has a limited role in some instances. Complications of uveitis such as cataract, vitreous hemorrhage, or retinal detachment may necessitate surgical intervention.

Uveitis is not a common disease. Epidemiologic studies have been limited. One of the better studies found an incidence of 17 new cases per 100,000 individuals living in Olmsted County, Minnesota, per year.[4] Many of these patients had anterior uveitis, which can generally be managed with topical corticosteroids alone. The rarity of uveitis, especially the rarity of specific subsets of uveitis, means that randomized clinical trials are difficult to conduct. In addition, some form of immunosuppression has become generally accepted as part of the therapy for severe, active, noninfectious causes of uveitis. Therefore, it would be ethically questionable to attempt to prove the efficacy of immunosuppression on the basis of current acceptance of this approach. However, the therapy for uveitis is certainly imperfect and clearly involves a risk/benefit ratio. Patients who are considering the use of a medication such as prednisone or methotrexate need to assess the degree of visual loss as well as the potential risks of the medication. For many practitioners, the threshold for recommending systemic immunosuppression is similar to the threshold for the use of an immunosuppressive agent in rheumatoid arthritis: the presence of disease that has an impact on activities of daily living. With uveitis, this often means bilateral disease with

## TABLE 16–1
## Diagnostic Categorization of Uveitis

**Infectious Causes (Agent or Disease)**

Viral
  Cytomegalovirus
  Herpes simplex
  Herpes zoster
  Human immunodeficiency virus-1
Bacterial or spirochetal
  Atypical Mycobacteria
  Bartonella
  Brucellosis
  Leprosy
  Leptospirosis
  Lyme disease
  Propionibacterium
  Syphilis
  Tuberculosis
  Whipple's disease
Parasitic (protozoan or helminthic)
  Acanthamoeba
  Cysticercosis
  Onchocerciasis
  Pneumocystis carinii
  Toxocariasis
  Toxoplasmosis
Fungal
  Aspergillosis
  Blastomycosis
  Candidiasis
  Coccidioidomycosis
  Cryptococcosis
  Histoplasmosis
  Sporotrichosis

**Suspected Immume-Mediated Diseases**

Ankylosing spondylitis
Behçet's disease
Crohn's disease
Drug or hypersensitivity reaction
Interstitial nephritis

Juvenile rheumatoid arthritis
Kawasaki disease
Multiple sclerosis
Psoriatic arthritis
Reactive arthritis
Relapsing polychondritis
Rheumatic fever
Sarcoidosis
Sjögren's syndrome
Systemic lupus erythematosus
Ulcerative colitis
Vasculitis
Vitiligo
Vogt-Koyanagi-Harada syndrome

**Syndromes Confined Primarily to the Eye**

Acute multifocal placoid pigmentary epitheliopathy
Acute zonal outer retinal necrosis
Birdshot choroidopathy
Fuchs' heterochromic cyclitis
Glaucomatocyclitic crisis
Lens-induced uveitis
Multifocal evanescent white dot syndrome
Pars planitis
Punctate inner choroidopathy
Serpiginous choroiditis
Sympathetic ophthalmia
Trauma

**Masquerade Syndromes**

Juvenile xanthogranuloma
Leukemia
Lymphoma
Ocular ischemia
Ocular melanoma
Retinal tear
Retinitis pigmentosa
Retinoblastoma

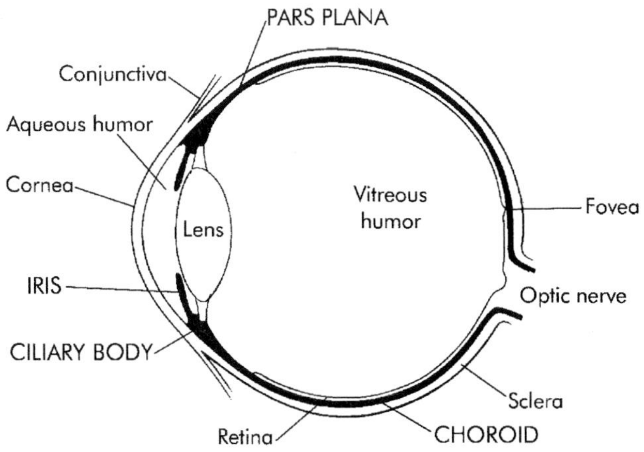

**FIGURE 16–1**
Schematic diagram of the eye. Capital letters indicate that the structure is part of the uveal tract.

visual acuity in the better eye of approximately 20/40, close to the threshold for safely operating a motor vehicle. Visual loss in uveitis can be caused by scarring or fibrosis in the macula, as well as by glaucomatous nerve damage and cataract. The treating physician must make a decision as to whether there are reversible inflammatory causes of the visual loss.

In general, the therapy for uveitis is designed to control rather than to cure. In this sense, the goal of therapy is similar to that in treating rheumatoid arthritis. It is important for the patient to recognize that therapy does not usually restore vision to completely normal levels and that the duration of therapy can be lengthy. The final choice of therapy is very much a matter of personal preference for both the patient and physician. Individual situations such as a history of hepatitis in a particular patient might sway the physician away from prescribing methotrexate, whereas a patient's history of diabetes might dissuade the practitioner from aggressive use of prednisone. Some patients wish to avoid the long-term risk of an alkylating agent, whereas others are willing to accept this risk if it means a shorter duration of therapy. Some of these issues are discussed further as follows.

## Topical Medications

Most of the decisions about topical therapy are generally made by the treating ophthalmologist. Topical corticosteroids are a mainstay of therapy in most instances. The absorption of topical steroids is such that it usually can treat anterior uveitis effectively, but it generally does not significantly affect inflammation that is posterior to the lens. Suspensions of corticosteroids such as prednisolone acetate generally have better penetration across the cornea than do more soluble corticosteroids such as phosphates and alcohols.[5] Corticosteroid therapy raises intraocular pressure in about 5% of patients, and intraocular pressure must be monitored carefully while patients receive this form of therapy. A family history of glaucoma increases the likelihood that steroid-induced glaucoma will develop.[6] Topical corticosteroids also promote cataract or lens opacification. However, inflammation itself is also cataractogenic, and the steroid risk to the lens is balanced by the reduced risk of cataract if inflammation is reduced. Consequently, the topical steroid dose should be titrated to fit the degree of inflammation. This can be accomplished only by judging inflammatory activity by means of a slit-lamp examination. This procedure entails the use of a biomicroscope that permits an accurate enumeration of cells in the normally acellular aqueous humor. Topical corticosteroids can also interfere with wound healing or the response to an infection such as a bacterial corneal ulcer or a viral corneal infection.

A drop to induce pupil dilation is commonly added to the therapy for anterior uveitis. A dilating drop of an agent such as scopolamine or cyclopentolate helps prevent the formation of posterior synechiae, which are adhesions between the iris and the lens capsule that lock the iris into a fixed position and interfere with the flow of aqueous humor. Sudden-onset anterior uveitis is usually associated with pain that results from spasm of the ciliary musculature. Both this spasm and, consequently, the pain are relieved by a dilating drop.

If the intraocular pressure has risen dangerously, ophthalmologists routinely add therapy to lower intraocular pressure. The majority of this treatment is topical as well and is beyond the scope of this chapter.

Several nonsteroidal anti-inflammatory drugs, including ketorolac, flurbiprofen, and diclofenac, are available for topical administration. Many practitioners add a topical nonsteroidal to other regimens with the belief that the need for topical corticosteroids is consequently reduced. However, the efficacy of topical nonsteroidal anti-inflammatory drugs in the treatment of anterior uveitis has had only limited support in animal models and human trials.[7]

## Periocular Injections

Periocular corticosteroid injections are indicated for posterior inflammation that has not responded to topical therapy. Unlike topical therapy, the periocular injections can be placed at a location in such a way that they considerably affect inflammation behind the lens. Periocular injections can reduce a common complication of uveitis known as macular edema. Periocular corticosteroid injections are somewhat analogous to intra-articular corticosteroid injections. In general, this approach to therapy is safe and well tolerated. In some patients, the injection causes a sustained rise in intraocular pressure, and in rare instances, the depot of corticosteroids must be surgically removed. The injection is usually placed superiorly and posteriorly beneath the conjunctiva or given through the lower lid on the floor of the orbit. These injections cause some fat atrophy on rare occasions. They clearly are contraindicated in cases of uveitis with infectious causes. Some preparations such as dexamethasone have relatively short-lived action, whereas other preparations such as triamcinolone have a very long duration of effect. The discomfort of periocular injection is such that many patients prefer an oral immunosuppressive if the disease is bilateral and if the injections are required frequently. In general, the injections are not as efficacious as orally administered prednisone. Occasionally, a periocular corticosteroid injection is given for anterior uveitis that is especially severe or refractory to topical therapy.

## Oral Corticosteroids

Oral corticosteroids have become the mainstay of therapy for many patients with uveitis that is severe enough to affect activities of daily living. Prednisone is usually begun *as* a single daily dose of 40 to 60 mg/day. Some practitioners prefer a higher dose or a divided-dosage schedule. In an occasional patient, a relatively brief course of oral corticosteroids is remarkably effective, and inflammation may resolve completely, just as a shoulder bursitis can sometimes completely resolve from the limited use of oral or local corticosteroids. In the majority of patients, however, corticosteroid use must be continued for a long duration. The dosage is tapered as tolerated and as mandated by the activity of the inflammation. If possible, an alternate-day schedule is followed. The toxicity of oral corticosteroids is discussed extensively elsewhere in this book.

With regard to ocular disease, steroid-induced glaucoma and cataract can be especially problematic in the treatment of uveitis. Both cataract and glaucoma are recognized complications of uveitis, as well as potential complications of steroid therapy. Accordingly, it is sometimes difficult to ascertain whether the treatment or the underlying disease process has been the prime factor in either of these complications. Oral corticosteroids are generally the fastest acting oral immunosuppressive medication for the treatment of uveitis. For short courses, they are generally well tolerated. If the therapy is sustained for months, however, oral corticosteroids are the oral immunosuppressive agents most likely to be associated with toxicity. As a consequence, additional immunosuppressive medication is frequently given in conjunction with oral corticosteroid therapy. If long-term corticosteroid use is planned, my practice is to assess bone density and to institute prophylactic measures to protect bone mass.

## Antimetabolites

The choice of immunosuppressive is based on the severity of inflammation as well as on patient and physician preference. Few studies have compared the relative efficacy of various immunosuppressive agents for uveitis care. Methotrexate has been used by several investigators in uncontrolled studies.[8–12] I often start with methotrexate as the first choice for an immunosuppressive medication beyond corticosteroid because methotrexate is usually tolerated extremely well. Depending on liver function test findings and the patient's tolerance, the dosage range is usually between 15 and 25 mg per week orally or by injection. In the ideal situation, methotrexate maintains or improves visual acuity and allows corticosteroid dosage to be eliminated or at least minimized. Azathioprine (1.5 mg/kg/day) is a second antimetabolite with probably somewhat comparable potency but it is slightly less well tolerated than methotrexate.[13–15] Mycophenolate (1 g twice a day) has also been used in some preliminary studies with success in the treatment of uveitis.[16] Published reports have not as yet described leflunomide in the treatment of this disease.

## Cyclosporine and FK-506

Cyclosporine is the best studied immunosuppressive agent for the treatment of uveitis.[17–20] Uveitis was perhaps the first autoimmune disease for which cyclosporine was tested. Initial studies for uveitis generally used doses in the range of 7.5 to 12.5 mg/kg/day. Currently, most ophthalmologists use a dose of 2.5 to 5 mg/day divided every 12 hours to treat uveitis. It is usually well tolerated but can certainly cause nephrotoxicity, hypertension, myalgias, gingival hyperplasia, neuropathy, and hair growth.[21] Cyclosporine is generally more expensive than methotrexate or azathioprine. Many authorities also believe that it is somewhat more effective than either methotrexate or azathioprine. In patients who have severe inflammation and whose disease is refractory either to an antimetabolite alone or to cyclosporine alone, my practice is to combine cyclosporine with an antimetabolite. One report found this combination to be dramatically effective for many patients with uveitis,[22] just as the addition of cyclosporine to methotrexate produces additional therapeutic benefit over methotrexate alone in the care of rheumatoid arthritis.[23]

FK-506 (tacrolimus) (up to 0.2 mg/kg/day) has been used to a limited extent in the treatment of uveitis. It appears to be beneficial in animal models as well as in human trials.[24]

## Alkylators

Alkylating drugs such as cyclophosphamide and chlorambucil are also efficacious in the care of patients with uveitis.[13] Because of the chronicity of uveitis and the increased risk that malignancy will develop as a result of the use of these agents, most authorities reserve the use of an alkylating agent for patients in whom antimetabolites, cyclosporine, or the combination has failed. The dosage of an alkylator is adjusted on the basis of careful monitoring of hematologic parameters. I try to keep the neutrophil count above 1500/$\mu$L. The initial dose of cyclophosphamide is 1 to 1.5 mg/kg/day and chlorambucil is begun at 0.1 mg/kg/day. My published experience with intravenous cyclophosphamide for the treatment of uveitis showed only a 30% response rate.[25]

## SCLERITIS: UNIQUE CONSIDERATIONS

Scleritis is a distinct clinical entity that should not be confused with uveitis. Scleritis usually represents a vasculitis of the blood vessels in the sclera, the white outer tunic of the eye (see Fig. 16–1). Scleritis is usually associated with pain and redness, which sometimes affects a wedge-shaped portion of the outer eye. An unusual form of scleritis is scleromalacia perforans. This condition is usually painless, but it may result in loss of vision, secondary to perforation of the globe. The histologic characteristics of scleromalacia perforans are similar to those of a rheumatoid nodule, and this form of scleritis most commonly occurs in the setting of seropositive, nodular rheumatoid arthritis. Some patients with scleritis also have a form of uveitis, just as some patients with arthritis also have a form of tendinitis. Scleritis responds to many of the same approaches used to treat uveitis, but four additional guidelines should be recognized: (1) In general, periocular corticosteroid injections should be avoided in treating anterior scleritis because the steroid promotes scleral thinning and increases the likelihood of globe rupture. (2) Scleritis is frequently associated with a systemic disease, especially rheumatoid vasculitis,[26–29] and it may respond to treatment of the underlying disease. (3) Scleritis may be associated with a systemic necrotizing vasculitis; like vasculitis but unlike uveitis, scleritis is more likely to require an alkylating drug for adequate control. (4) Ironically, despite the tendency to be associated with vasculitis, a subset of patients with scleritis have a dramatic response to oral nonsteroidal anti-inflammatory drugs such as indomethacin.[30]

## FUTURE APPROACHES

Additional innovative forms of therapy are being studied for uveitis. Oral tolerance has been tested as a means to reduce other forms of immunosuppression.[31] Its benefit in the therapy of uveitis was not convincingly proved, but the size of the study is such that a type 2 statistical error was certainly possible. Intravenous immunoglobulin (0.5 g/kg/day, 3 days/month) has been used for patients whose disease is refractory to other modes of immunosuppression.[32] Although some patients have responded, intravenous immunoglobulin (0.5 g/kg/day, 3 days/month) is expensive and carries an unknown risk from potential infectious agents such as prions. Interferon-α (initial dose of 3 to 6 million units/day subcutaneously) may be especially useful in the treatment of the uveitis associated with Behçet's disease.[33, 34] One group has had preliminary success in the use of a monoclonal antibody directed at the interleukin-2 receptor (1 mg/kg intravenously, initially every 2 weeks) as a means of reducing immunosuppression for patients with long-standing uveitis.[35] Most other biologic therapies such as tumor necrosis factor inhibitors have not yet been studied sufficiently in the treatment of uveitis. The inhibition of tumor necrosis factor has been noted to worsen animal models of uveitis, but these models involved acute inflammation paradigms rather than a cell-mediated immune response.[36, 37] An innovative approach to therapy for uveitis is the use of surgically placed implants that could be a continuous source of medication. Such a trial with a cyclosporine implant is currently ongoing.[35] Corticosteroid implants are also being actively assessed.

## DISEASE-SPECIFIC CONSIDERATIONS

The therapy for immune-mediated uveitis is, for the most part, nonspecific; that is, idiopathic uveitis does not merit therapy that would differ substantially from the treatment for sarcoid-associated uveitis or for a common chronic form of uveitis known as pars planitis. The autoimmune disease, Vogt-Koyanagi-Harada syndrome, is characterized by a severe bilateral uveitis with retinal elevation caused by subretinal fluid. Patients may also experience hearing loss, balance difficulties, a sterile meningitis, and depigmentation. The long-term use of oral corticosteroids is especially indicated in the treatment of this entity. A rare form of uveitis known as serpiginous choroiditis has been successfully treated with the combination of prednisone, cyclosporine, and azathioprine.[38] The efficacy of either azathioprine (2.5 mg/kg/day) or cyclosporine (10 mg/kg/day) has been convincingly proved in the treatment of uveitis associated with Behçet's disease on the basis of two separate, well-designed, controlled trials.[39, 40] Both of these randomized, controlled trials used dosages that are approximately twofold greater than my preferred initial dosage of either azathioprine or cyclosporine. Interferon-α may also be effective for this specific diagnosis, as discussed earlier. Sulfasalazine (my preferred dosage is 1 g PO BID) is beneficial in helping to reduce the frequency and severity of recurrent episodes of anterior uveitis associated with ankylosing spondylitis or reactive arthritis.[41]

The treatment of uveitis during childhood poses unique challenges. Oral corticosteroid therapy has the added risk of growth retardation. Children are often unable to cooperate with periocular injections without anesthesia. Furthermore, persistent iridocyclitis is common in association with juvenile rheumatoid arthritis. Because children appear to tolerate methotrex-

ate well when it is used for arthritis,[42] it is also a reasonable choice as a steroid-sparing agent for treating chronic iridocyclitis.[43] Cyclosporine has also specifically been used successfully to treat uveitis in children.[17]

## SUMMARY

The therapy for immune-mediated forms of uveitis differs only slightly from the therapy for other autoimmune diseases. Many of the same principles hold. The therapy involves a risk/benefit ratio and individual choices by both the patient and the physician. The therapy is often efficacious, although the therapy rarely meets the requirement demanded by those who base treatment choices on the gold standard of evidence-based medicine, the randomized controlled trial.

## REFERENCES

1. Rosenbaum JT: Uveitis. An internist's view. Arch Intern Med 1989; 149:1173.
2. Nussenblatt RB, Palestine AG, Chan C-C, et al: Randomized, double-masked study of cyclosporine compared to prednisolone in the treatment of endogenous uveitis. Am J Ophthalmol 1991; 112:138.
3. Nussenblatt RB, de Smet MD, Rubin B, et al: A masked, randomized, dose-response study between cyclosporine A and G in the treatment of sight-threatening uveitis of noninfectious origin. Am J Ophthalmol 1993; 115:583.
4. Darrell RW, Wagener HP, Kurland LT: Epidemiology of uveitis, incidence and prevalence in a small urban community. Arch Ophthalmol 1962; 68:502.
5. Kupferman A, Leibowitz HM: Anti-inflammatory effectiveness of topically administered corticosteroids in the cornea without epithelium. Invest Ophthalmol Vis Sci 1962; 252:255.
6. Becker BH, Hahn KA: Topical corticosteroids and heredity in primary open-angle glaucoma. Am J Ophthalmol 1964; 57:543.
7. Ogawa T, Obara K, Shimizu H, et al: Effects of a combination use of steroidal and nonsteroidal anti-inflammatory drugs on E. coli endotoxin–induced uveitis in pigmented rabbits. Jpn J Ophthalmol 1995; 39:353.
8. Wong VG, Hersh EM: Methotrexate in the therapy of cyclitis. Trans Am Acad Ophthalmol Otolaryngol 1965; 69:279.
9. Lazar M, Weiner MJ, Leopold IH: Treatment of uveitis with methotrexate. Am J Ophthalmol 1969; 67:383.
10. Shah SS, Lowder CY, Schmitt MA, et al: Low-dose methotrexate therapy for ocular inflammatory disease. Ophthalmology 1992; 99:1419.
11. Tamesis R, Rodriquez A, Christen W, et al: Systemic drug toxicity trends in immunosuppressive therapy of immune and inflammatory ocular disease. Ophthalmology 1996; 103:768.
12. Dev S, McCallum R, Jaffe GJ: Methotrexate treatment for sarcoid-associated panuveitis. Ophthalmology 1999; 106:111.
13. Andrasch RH, Pirofsky B, Burns RP: Immunosuppressive therapy for severe chronic uveitis. Arch Ophthalmol 1978; 96:247.
14. Newell FW, Krill AE: Treatment of uveitis with azathioprine (Imuran). Trans Ophthalmol Soc U K 1967; 87:499.
15. Mathews JD, Crawford BA, Bignell JL, et al: Azathioprine in active chronic iridocyclitis. Br J Ophthalmol 1969; 53:327.
16. Larkin GL, Lightman S: Mycophenolate mofetil. A useful immunosuppressive in inflammatory eye disease. Ophthalmology 1999; 106:370.
17. Palestine AG, Nussenblatt RB, Chan C-C: Cyclosporine therapy of uveitis in children. In Saari KM (ed): Uveitis Updates. New York: Excerpta Medica, 1984:499.
18. Wakefield D, McCluskey P, Reece G: Cyclosporin therapy in Vogt Koyanagi Harada disease. Austral N Z J Ophthalmol 1990; 18:137.

19. Nussenblatt RB, Palestine AG, Chan C-C: Cyclosporin A therapy in the treatment of intraocular inflammatory disease resistant to systemic corticosteroids and cytotoxic drugs. Am J Ophthalmol 1983; 96:275.
20. Graham EM, Sanders MD, James DG, et al: Cyclosporin A in the treatment of posterior uveitis. Trans Ophthalmol Soc U K 1985; 104:146.
21. Deray G, Benhmida M, Hoang PL, et al: Renal function and blood pressure in patients receiving long-term, low-dose cyclosporine therapy for idiopathic autoimmune uveitis. Ann Intern Med 1992; 117:578.
22. Pascalis L, Pia G, Aresu G, et al: Combined cyclosporin A–steroid–MTX treatment in endogenous non-infectious uveitis. J Autoimmun 1993; 6:467.
23. Tugwell P, Pincus T, Yocum D, et al: Combination therapy with cyclosporine and methotrexate in severe rheumatoid arthritis. The Methotrexate-Cyclosporine Combination Study Group. N Engl J Med 1995; 333:137.
24. Mochizuki M, Masuda K, Sakane T, et al: A clinical trial of FK506 in refractory uveitis. Am J Ophthalmol 1993; 115:763.
25. Rosenbaum JT: Treatment of severe refractory uveitis with intravenous cyclophosphamide. J Rheumatol 1994; 21:123.
26. McGavin DDM, Williamson J, Forrester JV, et al: Episcleritis and scleritis. A study of their clinical manifestations and association with rheumatoid arthritis. Br J Ophthalmol 1976; 60:192.
27. Foster SC, Forstot SL, Wilson LA: Mortality rate in rheumatoid arthritis patients developing necrotizing scleritis or peripheral ulcerative keratitis. Ophthalmology 1984; 91:1253.
28. Jayson MIV, Jones DEP: Scleritis and rheumatoid arthritis. Ann Rheum Dis 1971; 30:343.
29. Sainz de la Maza M, Foster CS, Jabbur NS: Scleritis asociated with rheumatoid arthritis and other systemic immune-mediated diseases. Ophthalmology 1994; 101:1281.
30. Rosenbaum JT, Robertson JE Jr: Recognition of posterior scleritis and its treatment with indomethacin. Retina 1993; 13:17.
31. Nussenblatt RB, Gery I, Weiner HL, et al: Treatment of uveitis by oral administration of retinal antigens: Results of a phase I/II randomized masked trial. Am J Ophthalmol 1997; 123:684.
32. Rosenbaum JT, George R, Gordon C: The treatment of refractory uveitis with intravenous immunoglobulin. Am J Ophthalmol 1999; 127:545.
33. Kotter I, Eckstein AK, Stubiger N, et al: Treatment of ocular symptoms of Behçet's disease with interferon alpha 2A: A pilot study. Br J Ophthalmol 1998; 82:488.
34. O'Duffy JDC, Calamia K, Cohen S, et al: Interferon-alpha treatment of Behçet's disease. J Rheumatol 1998; 25:1938.
35. Nussenblatt RB: Current research in immunomodulation of uveitis. Invest Ophthalmol Vis Sci 1998; 39:S215.
36. Kasner L, Chan C-C, Whitcup SM, et al: The paradoxical effect of tumor necrosis factor alpha (TNF$\alpha$) in endotoxin-induced uveitis. Invest Ophthalmol Vis Sci 1993; 34:2911.
37. De Vos AF, Van Haren MA, Verhagen C, et al: Systemic anti-tumor necrosis factor antibody treatment exacerbates endotoxin-induced uveitis in the rat. Exp Eye Res 1995; 61:667.
38. Hooper PL, Kaplan HJ: Triple agent immunosuppression in serpiginous choroiditis. Ophthalmology 1991; 98:944.
39. Yazici H, Pazarli H, Barnes CG, et al: A controlled trial of azathioprine in Behçet's syndrome. N Engl J Med 1990; 322:281.
40. Masuda K, Nakajima A, Urayama A, et al: Double-masked trial of cyclosporine versus colchicine and long-term open study of cyclosporine in Behçet's disease. Lancet 1989; 1:1093.
41. Dougados M, Berenbaum F, Maetzel A, et al: Prevention of acute anterior uveitis associated with spondyloarthropathy induced by salazosulfapyridine. Rev Rhum 1993; 60:81.
42. Giannini EH, Brewer EJ, Kuzmina N, et al: Methotrexate in resistant juvenile rheumatoid arthritis. N Engl J Med 1992; 326:1043.
43. Weiss AH, Wallace CA, Sherry DD: Methotrexate for resistant chronic uveitis in children with juvenile rheumatoid arthritis. J Pediatr 1998; 133:266.

# 17 | Hematologic Disease*

*Gordon Starkebaum*

Hematologic abnormalities associated with rheumatic diseases are seen primarily in rheumatoid arthritis (RA) and systemic lupus erythematosus. This chapter discusses the major manifestations and current therapy in these disorders according to the blood cell affected.

## ANEMIA IN RHEUMATOID ARTHRITIS

### Natural History

Anemia is common in RA: Both anemia of chronic disease (ACD) and iron deficiency anemia occur, and they may coexist. In two reports, of a total 341 RA patients, more than 50% had anemia; of that 50%, approximately three quarters had ACD, and one quarter had iron deficiency.[1, 2] ACD patients tended to have more severe RA, with significantly more erosive joint damage and increased concentrations of serum rheumatoid factor in comparison with patients who did not have anemia.[2]

### Mechanism of Anemia of Chronic Disease

Inflammatory cytokines, especially tumor necrosis factor-$\alpha$, interleukin (IL)–1, interferon-$\gamma$, and IL-6 appear to mediate ACD.[3] Supporting this notion, blocking tumor necrosis factor-$\alpha$ with the mouse-human monoclonal antibody cA2 (infliximab) in RA patients with ACD led to a dose-dependent increase in hemoglobin levels in comparison to placebo, and these changes were accompanied by a reduction in serum levels of both erythropoietin (EPO) and IL-6.[4] Conversely, EPO counteracts the inhibitory effect on erythropoiesis mediated by inflammatory cytokines.[3] RA patients with anemia caused by iron deficiency show a rise in their serum EPO levels as the hemoglobin concentration falls, whereas RA patients with ACD do not have an increase in EPO levels.[5] These and other data suggest that the EPO response to ACD in RA is relatively blunted.[6]

## Evaluation of Anemia in Rheumatoid Arthritis

Although bone marrow aspiration has been considered necessary to distinguish iron deficiency from ACD in RA, there are noninvasive means to distinguish the two types of anemia. Usually, ferritin levels are helpful in evaluating iron deficiency; however, in RA, inflammation drives up the ferritin level as part of the acute-phase reactant response, confounding the ability to predict iron deficiency. Nevertheless, in anemic RA patients, ferritin levels of less than 50 ng/mL were predictive of iron deficiency in more than 90% of patients, whereas ferritin levels greater than 100 ng/mL were equally well predictive of ACD.[7] Similarly, according to an algorithm using the serum ferritin, mean corpuscular volume, and iron saturation levels, Mulherin and colleagues[8] correctly classified 94% of RA patients with iron deficiency and 85% of patients with ACD (Fig. 17–1).

## Treating Anemia in Rheumatoid Arthritis

### Anemia of Chronic Disease

Resolution of the ACD is related to success in treating RA. Many RA patients with active disease remain anemic; these patients generally have more severe RA than do those without anemia.[2] Conversely, the majority of iron-deficient RA patients recover with iron supplements,[2] although changes in mucosal ferritin levels may decrease iron absorption in active inflammatory disease.[9] Such patients may require parenteral iron.

### Controlled Trials with Erythropoietin

Several controlled trials have demonstrated the efficacy of EPO in treating the anemia of RA.[10, 11] The necessity of treating iron deficiency along with the use of EPO has been emphasized. Peeters and colleagues performed a double-blind, placebo-controlled trial, using EPO, initially at a dose of 240 units/kg subcutaneously 3 times/week for 52 weeks. Thirty-four patients received EPO, and 36 received placebo. In patients achieving a normal hemoglobin level, the dose of EPO or placebo was adjusted by reducing the frequency of administration. Patients receiving EPO showed a

* This work was supported by the Medical Research Service of the Department of Veterans Affairs.

**FIGURE 17–1**
Algorithm for the identification of iron deficiency in patients with rheumatoid arthritis. (From Mulherin D, Skelly M, Saunders A, et al: The diagnosis of iron deficiency in patients with rheumatoid arthritis and anemia: An algorithm using simple laboratory measures. J Rheumatol 1996; 23:237.)

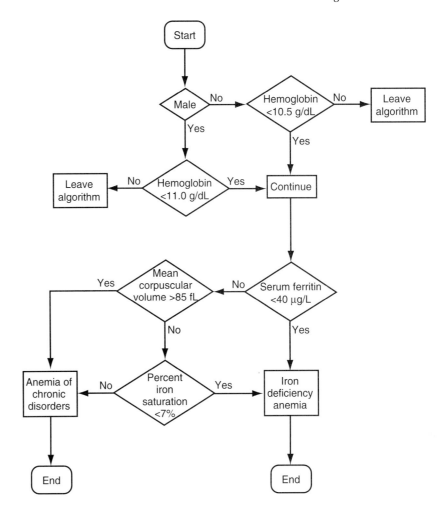

significant increase in hemoglobin levels. In addition, significant improvement in favor of the EPO group was also observed in secondary disease activity measures, including the Ritchie index, number of swollen joints, pain score, erythrocyte sedimentation rate, and patients' global assessment of disease activity.[11]

These results indicate that treatment of ACD with EPO in RA is effective in restoring normal hemoglobin levels and also exerts a beneficial effect on disease activity. Nevertheless, the place for recombinant EPO in the therapy of ACD in RA has not been clearly established; in RA patients with ACD, the best initial therapy remains control of the underlying disease, most commonly with second-line drugs or corticosteroids, or both.

EPO may be useful in preparing RA patients for elective surgery, particularly hip arthroplasty, in which correction of the anemia may decrease the need for transfusion or may allow for donation of blood for purposes of autologous transfusion perioperatively.[12, 13] Furthermore, because serum EPO levels are blunted in ACD, some RA patients with moderate to severe ACD are possible candidates for EPO treatment.

## Author's Approach to Management of Anemia in Rheumatoid Arthritis

1. Evaluate for blood loss and iron stores, checking ferritin, mean corpuscular volume, and percent iron saturation. Bone marrow examination is not essential for distinguishing iron deficiency from ACD (see Fig. 17–1).

2. Treat iron deficiency if present; prescribe oral iron as ferrous sulfate, 325 mg three times daily, or ferrous gluconate, 300 mg three times daily; absorption in iron-deficient patients is generally adequate.[14, 15] Occasionally, patients have decreased iron absorption,[16] and parenteral iron as iron dextran given intramuscularly or with slow intravenous infusion may be necessary.[17, 18] An initial test dose of 25 mg should be given to confirm that the patient is not sensitive to the preparation. The total dose of iron should be calculated on the basis of the level of hemoglobin; however, some patients may experience a flare of RA.[19]

3. Treat active RA; ACD may improve.

Future directions may include the following:

4. Consider using EPO because serum level may be relatively decreased.

5. In EPO doses, some authors have prescribed 50 to 250 units/kg/day subcutaneously, giving injections three to five times/week, whereas others found that 300 to 800 units/kg/week given subcutaneously once or twice a week was effective.[20, 12] Correcting iron deficiency, using either parenteral[21] or oral iron,[22] appears necessary to optimize the benefits of EPO. In one open study, 500 to 1000 units/day given subcutaneously 4 days/week was successful. In the 52-week placebo-controlled trial of Peeter and associates, not only did the anemia subside but RA disease activity was also ameliorated significantly.[11]

## PURE RED CELL APLASIA IN RHEUMATOID ARTHRITIS

More than 20 cases of pure red cell aplasia (PRCA) have been reported in RA. Most cases occur in patients with long-standing RA, but in rare instances patients may have PRCA at the onset of RA. The mechanism of the red cell aplasia appears to result from cell-mediated suppression. Some cases responded to immunosuppressive therapy such as cyclosporine, with initial doses up to 12 mg/kg/day or azathioprine in doses of 200 mg/day.[23, 24] The results of in vitro culture studies of marrow erythroid progenitors appear to be a reliable indicator of response to immunosuppressive therapy in the general population of PRCA patients.[25]

## CHRONIC NEUTROPENIA IN RHEUMATOID ARTHRITIS (FELTY'S SYNDROME)

### Natural History

Felty originally described patients with chronic arthritis who had chronic leukopenia with neutropenia and splenomegaly.[26] There have since been several refinements of Felty's original description. Campion and colleagues found that neutropenic RA patients with and without splenomegaly were indistinguishable; thus, splenomegaly should not be considered an essential feature of this disorder.[27] Patients with clonal expansions of T-cell large granular lymphocytes (LGLs) with chronic neutropenia frequently have RA.[28] Like patients with Felty's syndrome, nearly 90% of RA patients with the LGL syndrome are HLA-DR4-positive.[29] Because the clinical features and response to treatment (see further on) of both disorders appear similar, these findings support the concept that Felty's syndrome and LGL leukemia plus RA are parts of a single disease process rather than two separate disorders.[30]

### Clinical Features

Patients in whom Felty's syndrome develops often have severe, long-standing RA, with nodules, ulcers, splenomegaly, and hyperpigmentation of lower extremities; synovitis may not be active, which is perhaps a reflection of the neutropenia. Other extra-articular features are frequent and include vasculitis, neuropathy, pulmonary fibrosis, hepatomegaly, and Sjögren's syndrome.[27] In rare cases, neutropenia may begin with arthritis. Some patients with Felty's syndrome have nodular regenerative hyperplasia, a form of chronic liver disease, which may progress to portal hypertension, result in variceal bleeding, or complicate treatment with methotrexate (see later text).

Patients with Felty's syndrome tend to have high levels of rheumatoid factor, antinuclear antibodies (often because of antihistone antibodies), and immune complexes (shown by elevated C1q binding) and hypergammaglobulinemia. The leukocyte count is generally less than 4000/$\mu$L, with less than 1500 neutrophils/$\mu$L. Mild anemia, thrombocytopenia, and modest lymphopenia with decreased CD4 counts are also seen. The bone marrow is typically normocellular to hypercellular.[27]

The pathogenesis of neutropenia in Felty's syndrome is multifactorial and reflects both humoral and cellular immune mechanisms.[31–33] Circulating neutrophils from most patients with Felty's syndrome have elevated levels of cell-bound immunoglobulin G (IgG), mainly as a result of immune complexes. Such cell-bound immune complexes may cause functional disturbances of neutrophils in Felty's syndrome.

Neutropenia tends to be chronic and rarely remits spontaneously. Patients with Felty's syndrome are at risk for recurrent pyogenic infections, which reflects both the neutropenia and functional abnormalities of the circulating neutrophils. The risk of infection is particularly increased in patients with neutrophil counts less than 200/$\mu$L.[34] In such patients, the rate of mortality resulting from pneumonia, septic arthritis, or overwhelming sepsis is substantially increased over that of patients with uncomplicated RA.[27] A 12-fold increased risk for the development of non-Hodgkin lymphoma was reported in patients with Felty's syndrome.[35]

### Treatment

The optimal treatment of neutropenia in Felty's syndrome has not been established. Multiple treatment modalities have been reported to improve the neutropenia of some but not all patients with Felty's syndrome. Neutropenia appears to reflect an active rheumatoid process; hence, effective treatments for RA are often useful in treating Felty's syndrome, including gold,[36] D-penicillamine,[37] cyclophosphamide,[38, 39] methotrexate (see next section), cyclosporine,[40–42] corticosteroids,[43] and lithium carbonate.[44] Splenectomy has been reported to be useful in Felty's syndrome, with long-term success rates ranging from 20% to 66%.[43, 45, 46] An increased risk of postsplenectomy sepsis, however, has been suggested to occur in patients who have had recurrent infections before splenectomy.[43] Variations on surgical splenectomy for Felty's syndrome and other conditions have included splenic artery embolization,[47] laparoscopic splenectomy, and splenic irradiation.[48] Conversely, none of the following modalities used to treat Felty's syndrome has worked well: intravenous immune globulin (IVIG), total nodal irradiation, and plasmapheresis.

### Methotrexate in Felty's Syndrome

Several reports indicate a good response to treatment in Felty's syndrome.[49–51] The rise in neutrophils may occur promptly, although some patients respond slowly. Wassenberg and colleagues suggested that methotrexate is the current treatment of first choice in Felty's syndrome.[51] Hepatic dysfunction during methotrexate therapy may result from underlying nodular regenerative hyperplasia.[52]

### Granulocyte Colony-Stimulating Factor or Granulocyte-Macrophage Colony-Stimulating Factor

Patients with Felty's syndrome may respond to granulocyte colony-stimulating factor (G-CSF) or granulocyte-macrophage colony-stimulating factor (GM-CSF) with a rise in neutrophil counts and often a decrease in infections, often without further complications.[53–56] In general, after short-term administration of G-CSF or GM-CSF, the neutrophil count promptly falls to pretreatment levels when the drug is discontinued. However, long-term colony-stimulating factor administration in Felty's syndrome is often effective in increasing patients' neutrophil counts to greater than $1000/\mu L$ and in decreasing infections.[57–59] The frequency of administering G-CSF in these patients was often tapered to two and three times a week.

Complications of both G-CSF and GM-CSF treatment in Felty's syndrome have included flares of arthritis,[55, 60] anemia and thrombocytopenia, and vasculitis.[61, 62] In some patients with Felty's syndrome, treatment with G-CSF in combination with methotrexate,[63] cyclophosphamide,[64] or prednisone[65] was needed to correct the neutropenia.

## Treatment of LGL Leukemia and Rheumatoid Arthritis

Although there has been less experience in treating patients with large granular lymphocytic leukemia and RA, it appears that treatments similar to those used for Felty's syndrome are often effective in these patients. Thus, neutropenia in patients with LGL leukemia, both with and without RA, was reported to respond to methotrexate in a study of 10 patients.[66] Complete clinical remissions in patients receiving methotrexate were observed in five patients; an additional patient had a partial response. Complete and partial responses were maintained with therapy, with a follow-up period ranging from 1.3 to 9.6 years. Some patients with T-cell LGL leukemia and chronic neutropenia have also responded to colony-stimulating factors.[67, 68]

## Author's Approach to Management of Felty's Syndrome

1. Attempt to exclude drug toxicity, usually by discontinuing a possible suspected agent. The absence of splenomegaly should not diminish the diagnosis of Felty's syndrome (see earlier discussion).

2. Perform a bone marrow examination; the marrow should be cellular or hypercellular. Serologic tests are helpful and usually demonstrate high-titer rheumatoid factor, often positive antinuclear antibodies, and elevated immune complexes (C1q binding). If the test is available, it is helpful to demonstrate elevated levels of neutrophil-reactive IgG.

3. Treat patients who have infections regardless of the neutrophil count. Prescribe dosages of G-CSF of 3 $\mu g/kg/day$, which is somewhat less than the usual dosage of 5 $\mu g/kg/day$, to decrease the risk of flare of arthritis or vasculitis; for the same reason, prescribe low to medium doses of prednisone (20 to 30 mg/day) while G-CSF is started.

4. If the patient responds to G-CSF, add methotrexate, starting at 5 to 7.5 mg/week. Confirm that the patient's renal function is normal. Increase the dose by 2.5 mg/week every 3 to 4 weeks to a maximal dose of 15 to 20 mg/week, along with folic acid, 1 mg/day. Thus, it may take several months for the patient to reach the maximal dose of methotrexate. The goal is to induce a stable remission and eliminate the need for chronic G-CSF administration.

5. In asymptomatic patients without infections, the decision about when to treat may be more difficult. If the neutrophil count is persistently less than $200/\mu L$, however, treatment should begin, in view of the high risk of serious infections. Prescribe methotrexate, 5 mg/week and slowly increase the dose as described earlier. In patients with renal insufficiency or hepatic disease, in whom methotrexate is contraindicated, prescribe G-CSF on a long-term basis or perform splenectomy.

6. In all patients, splenectomy should be considered if there is no response to therapy or if complications such as disease flare or vasculitis occur.

## ANEMIA IN SYSTEMIC LUPUS ERYTHEMATOSUS

Hemolytic anemia in systemic lupus erythematosus (SLE) may result from autoimmune or microangiopathic processes. Patients with autoimmune hemolytic anemia (AIHA) alone, immune thrombocytopenia (ITP) alone, or AIHA and ITP together (Evans' syndrome) may later acquire SLE. In SLE, a positive direct antiglobulin (direct Coombs') test and AIHA are associated with antibodies to phospholipids (APLAs), especially IgM APLAs.[69, 70] Patients with ITP generally have IgG APLAs[69]; patients who acquire Evan's syndrome often have both isotypes of APLAs.[71] The diagnosis of AIHA is made by demonstrating a positive direct Coombs' test result in the presence of anemia, an elevated reticulocyte count, spherocytes, and depressed haptoglobin and elevated bilirubin levels. About one third of patients with AIHA, however, may not have an elevated reticulocyte count.[72]

## Author's Approach to Treatment of Autoimmune Hemolytic Anemia in Systemic Lupus Erythematosus

Patients with brisk hemolysis constitute a medical emergency. Finding compatible blood for transfusion may be difficult in such patients because of the presence of a positive indirect Coombs' test result. In this case, "best match" incompatible blood should be given.[73]

1. Give high doses of corticosteroids, in doses of 60 to 80 mg of prednisone/day in divided doses (Fig. 17–2).
2. Occasional patients may respond to IVIG in doses of 0.4 to 1 g/kg/day given over 1 to 2 days, although no controlled trials have compared steroids with IVIG.
3. Although most patients respond to high-dose steroid treatment with an increase in hematocrit, some patients require unacceptably high doses of prednisone to maintain the hematocrit. Such patients are candidates for splenectomy.[73]

## Microangiopathic Hemolytic Anemia in Systemic Lupus Erythematosus

Hemolytic anemia in SLE may be a manifestation of a microangiopathic, thrombotic process. SLE patients in whom a thrombotic microangiopathy develops may also manifest thrombocytopenia, central nervous system dysfunction, fever, and renal insufficiency, that is,

the features of thrombotic thrombocytopenic purpura (TTP). The differential diagnosis in these cases also includes the "catastrophic" antiphospholipid syndrome, disseminated intravascular coagulation, or the hemolytic uremic syndrome. More than 45 cases of TTP associated with SLE have been reported.[74-76] As reviewed by Musio and colleagues, the majority of these cases of TTP occurred in patients with established lupus,[76] but TTP may also precede or begin simultaneously with lupus.

Distinguishing TTP from active SLE can be difficult because thrombocytopenia, anemia, and renal and neurologic dysfunction can be manifestations of both disorders. In the case of TTP, however, the anemia is Coombs' test–negative, and microangiopathic changes are present in the red blood cells, that is, schistocytes. Thrombocytopenia is caused by platelet consumption and not by immune-mediated mechanisms. Renal biopsy in TTP generally shows a thrombotic microangiopathy with arteriolar fibrin thrombi in addition to various glomerular lesions characteristic of lupus nephritis. Disseminated intravascular coagulation, also a differential diagnosis of TTP, shows evidence of a consumptive coagulopathy and generally occurs in the setting of infection or carcinoma (Table 17–1).

The primary antiphospholipid antibody syndrome is also a differential diagnosis of acute thrombocytopenia. Furthermore, more than half of TTP cases associated with SLE have antiphospholipid antibodies, which suggests a potential role for these antibodies. Asherson and colleagues reviewed 50 cases of catastrophic antiphospholipid antibody syndrome; half of these patients had SLE.[77] The majority of patients had acute multiorgan failure with an occlusive microangiopathy affecting kidneys, lungs, brain, heart, and liver.

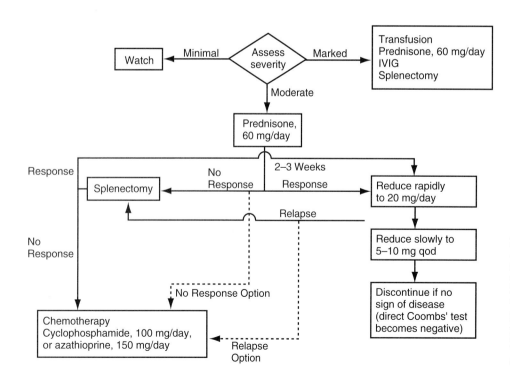

**FIGURE 17–2**
Algorithm for the treatment of autoimmune hemolytic anemia due to IgG antibody. (From Rosse W, Bullel W, Ortel T: Challenges in managing autoimmune disease. *In* McArthur JR, Schecter GP, Platt OS [eds]: Hematology—1997. Washington DC: American Society of Hematology, 1997:93.)

**TABLE 17–1**

**Differential Diagnosis and Clinical Manifestations of Systemic Thrombotic Processes Associated with Systemic Lupus Erythematosus**

| | THROMBOTIC THROMBOCYTOPENIC PURPURA | DISSEMINATED INTRAVASCULAR COAGULATION | CATASTROPHIC ANTIPHOSPHOLIPID SYNDROME* | SYSTEMIC LUPUS ERYTHEMATOSUS |
|---|---|---|---|---|
| Fever | + | + | — | + |
| Central nervous system symptoms | + | + | 56% | + |
| Hemolytic anemia | + | + | 26% | + (Coombs'-positive) |
| Thrombocytopenia | + | + | 68% | + (immune) |
| Schistocytes | + | + | 14% | — |
| Renal abnormalities | + | + | 78% | + |
| Consumptive coagulopathy | — | + | 28% | — |
| Hypocomplementemia | — | — | — | + |
| Hemorrhagic manifestations | + | + | — | + |

* Data in this column from Asherson RA, Cervera R, Piette JC, et al. Catastrophic antiphospholipid syndrome. Clinical and laboratory features of 50 patients. Medicine (Baltimore) 1998; 77:195.

Only a minority had large vessel occlusions. Thrombocytopenia was reported in 34 patients (68%), hemolytic anemia in 13 (26%), disseminated intravascular coagulation in 14 (28%), and schistocytes in 7 (14%) (see Table 17–1).

Patients with idiopathic TTP have been found to have plasma inhibitors, usually IgG antibodies, to the protease that cleaves von Willebrand factor (vWF).[78–80] Inhibition of the vWF protease appears to result in unusually large multimers of vWF in plasma of patients with TTP and probably plays a critical role in the platelet aggregation that leads to microthrombi characteristic of TTP.[79] These findings also appear to account for the observation that TTP can be reversed by infusion of fresh-frozen plasma without concurrent plasmapheresis, presumably by restoring vWF protease.[81]

## Approach to Thrombotic Thrombocytopenic Purpura in Systemic Lupus Erythematosus

TTP is a rapidly developing multisystem disorder that can be fatal. Current therapy for TTP consists of plasma exchange: that is, plasmapheresis with infusion of platelet-depleted fresh-frozen plasma.[82] The rationale for using both modes of therapy has been strengthened by the reports of antibodies to the vWF protease in TTP patients described earlier. Presumably, plasmapheresis removes both the vWF protease inhibitors and the large multimers of vWF that contribute to platelet aggregation and thrombosis, whereas infusion of fresh plasma provides intact vWF protease. In view of the effective therapy noted previously, early recognition of TTP is important. In a lupus patient, a falling platelet count and hematocrit drop with microangiopathic red cell changes and negative Coombs' test results should trigger the initiation of therapy in most cases.[82] It is essential to begin plasma exchange promptly because TTP can progress rapidly. If it is not feasible to initiate

plasma exchange early, fresh-frozen plasma should be given by infusion.

On the basis of the review by Kwaan and Soff,[83] the following steps are recommended:

1. Obtain adequate vascular access with a wide-bore two-lumen catheter. Plasma exchange should be performed by means of a blood cell separator or single-pass discontinuous centrifugation.

2. Initial plasma exchange is performed once daily, replacing 40 mL/kg body mass; the standard replacement fluid is fresh-frozen plasma, although cryosupernatant has been reported to perform as well as fresh-frozen plasma.

3. Plasma infusion alone did not provide as much benefit as plasma exchange in most studies.

4. Platelet transfusions may worsen the manifestations of TTP and should be avoided.

5. Although steroids have not consistently improved outcome in TTP, some studies show benefit, and no studies show an adverse effect. Therefore, it is appropriate to give steroids in doses such as 60 to 80 mg/day of prednisone.

6. Use of antiplatelet therapy and vincristine has been advocated by some investigators, but no conclusive evidence supports their use in all cases of TTP.

7. Plasma exchange should be continued on at least a daily basis for several days after the platelet count, serum lactate dehydrogenase levels, and neurologic status become normal. The frequency of plasma exchange should then be tapered over a period of 1 to 2 weeks because TTP may relapse within 1 to 4 weeks after discontinuation of plasma exchange.

## THROMBOCYTOPENIA AND SYSTEMIC LUPUS ERYTHEMATOSUS

Thrombocytopenia occurs commonly in SLE. Patients may have acute, severe thrombocytopenia or may acquire chronic thrombocytopenia during the course of lupus. Up to 25% of SLE patients acquire thrombocytopenia, although only 5% to 10% experience clinically severe thrombocytopenia. Of patients with idiopathic ITP, about 10% acquire SLE after intervals of up to 10 years. More than half of all lupus patients were found to have elevated platelet-associated IgG levels.[84] Although not all the patients with elevated platelet-bound IgG levels had thrombocytopenia, all the patients with thrombocytopenia had elevated platelet-bound IgG.[84] Macchi and colleagues found that thrombocytopenic SLE patients had antibodies to platelet membrane glycoproteins such as GP IIb/IIIa more often than did nonthrombocytopenic SLE patients.[85] Similar antibodies are found in patients with idiopathic ITP.[86] Other studies have documented depressed platelet survival in SLE. Taken together, these findings are evidence that a humoral immune-mediated process causes thrombocytopenia in SLE.

Thrombocytopenia may also be associated with the antiphospholipid antibody syndrome, with or without SLE. As noted earlier, ITP associated with AIHA is Evans' syndrome.

Treatment of thrombocytopenia with SLE has generally been similar to that of treating idiopathic ITP. Practice guidelines for treating ITP have been published by the American Society of Hematology[87] based mainly on expert opinion rather than conclusive evidence because virtually no controlled trial of any treatment of adult ITP has been carried out. In patients with serious thrombocytopenia (<20,000 to 30,000/$\mu$L or less than 50,000/$\mu$L if there is evidence of bleeding), initial therapy should include hospitalization and prednisone in doses of 1 to 2 mg/kg/day. In patients with severe, life-threatening bleeding, treatment should also include platelet transfusions and IVIG, usually in combination with intravenous methylprednisolone, 1 g/day for 3 days. The subsequent therapy for the majority of ITP patients who do not respond to this initial therapy is a splenectomy according to most authorities. The American Society of Hematology Guidelines panel recommends a splenectomy if a patient's platelet count remains less than 10,000/$\mu$L after 4 to 6 weeks of therapy. Some panelists recommend splenectomy after as little as 2 weeks of unsuccessful therapy.

Some reports indicate that IVIG has limited value in comparison with corticosteroids in treating thrombocytopenia caused by SLE.[88, 89] Conversely, Maier and colleagues reported seven patients with thrombocytopenia and SLE who were treated with IVIG.[90] Five of seven patients had a greater than 50% increase in platelet counts. Four of these patients had a sustained benefit of at least 6 months' duration. How IVIG compares with corticosteroids has not been determined in prospective trials in SLE. However, Jacobs and colleagues, in a randomized trial comparing oral prednisone (1 mg/kg/day) with IVIG (400 mg/kg/day) or with both therapies together in patients with ITP, concluded that IVIG offers no advantage over conventional corticosteroid administration as the primary form of therapy in previously untreated adults with symptomatic ITP. In addition, more intense immunosuppression,

resulting from the use of both agents combined, was no better than single-agent corticosteroid therapy and appeared to be an unnecessary and unwarranted expense.[89]

Although there have been no reports of treating ITP in SLE with anti-D immunoglobulin, there is growing experience with its use in ITP.[91, 92] Anti-D immunoglobulin appears to be effective in raising the platelet count of adults with acute ITP in more than 70% of cases, a level of effectiveness similar to IVIG.[93] The cost of anti-D immunoglobulin is substantially lower than that of IVIG,[94] and anti-D immunoglobulin appears to be well tolerated, although hepatitis C was transmitted by some earlier preparations. A solvent-detergent–treated preparation is now available that is free of hepatitis C.[93] Patients must have an intact spleen and be Rh-positive for anti-D immunoglobulin to be effective.

In lupus patients with severe thrombocytopenia that is not responding to steroids, there are two main options: splenectomy or other immunosuppressive drugs. Splenectomy has been successful for treating thrombocytopenia in SLE in some reports,[95] but other reports indicate that thrombocytopenic SLE patients may not respond to splenectomy or have increased complications from postsplenectomy infections or vasculitis.[96–98] A report of 17 patients with thrombocytopenia by Hakim and colleagues, however, confirms that splenectomy may be useful for treating thrombocytopenia in some patients with SLE.[99] Of 17 patients with severe thrombocytopenia, splenectomy was performed on 13: 9 patients with SLE, 3 patients with primary antiphospholipid antibody syndrome, and 1 patient with lupus-like disease. After splenectomy, six of nine patients with SLE and all three patients with the primary antiphospholipid antibody syndrome gained complete remission of thrombocytopenia. There were no complications from splenectomy. The remaining four patients—three with SLE and one with the primary antiphospholipid antibody syndrome—remained in a stable partial or full remission with oral medication and did not require splenectomy.

In addition to conventional splenectomy, splenic irradiation has been reported to be useful in patients with ITP or secondary immune-associated thrombocytopenia (including SLE) who have contraindications to splenectomy.[48, 100] In neither report were there significant side effects observed from the splenic irradiation. Therefore, splenic irradiation should be considered in thrombocytopenic lupus patients who have contraindications to splenectomy.

Good results occur with danazol therapy for lupus patients with refractory thrombocytopenia.[101–105] Cervera and colleagues treated 16 consecutive thrombocytopenic SLE patients with danazol.[104] Three patients had coexisting autoimmune hemolysis (Evans' syndrome) and five patients had undergone splenectomy. Danazol was started at doses of 200 mg/day and increased gradually to a maximum of 1200 mg/day. All 16 patients had a rise in platelet counts to greater than 100,000/$\mu$L by a mean of 2 months after starting therapy, with remissions persisting during continued danazol therapy for a mean of 18 months. Combining these results with the reports cited earlier, 34 of 36 SLE patients with refractory thrombocytopenia responded to danazol. Two patients acquired rashes while taking danazol. These findings suggest that danazol is effective for the thrombocytopenia of SLE regardless of splenectomy status.

Cyclosporine has also been reported to improve refractory thrombocytopenia in several SLE patients,[106, 107] as well as in patients with ITP.[108, 109]

## Author's Approach to Thrombocytopenia in Systemic Lupus Erythematosus

1. Confirm that the thrombocytopenia is immune-mediated and not part of TTP (see Table 17–1). Examine for schistocytes on smear and check lactate dehydrogenase levels.

2. Begin with corticosteroids, 2 mg/kg/day; they may need to be administered intravenously initially.

3. If there is no response within 3 to 4 days or thrombocytopenia is life-threatening (platelet count $<10,000/\mu L$ or with bleeding) begin IVIG at 400 mg/kg/day; occasionally doses of 1 g/kg/day may be needed. Also use intravenous methylprednisolone 1 g/day for three doses and platelet transfusions as needed to keep the platelet count greater than $20,000/\mu L$.

4. If thrombocytopenia is life-threatening or does not respond to steroids or IVIG, perform splenectomy. Consider splenic irradiation if patient is not a good candidate for surgery.

5. With response to therapy, taper prednisone over 2 to 4 months. If unable to taper, add danazol at 200 mg/day, increasing dose by 200 mg/day every 3 to 4 weeks to a maximum of 1200 mg/day. If patient does not respond to danazol, begin cyclosporine at 1 to 2 mg/kg/day.

## REFERENCES

1. Remacha AF, Rodriguez-de la Serna A, Garcia-Die F, et al: Erythroid abnormalities in rheumatoid arthritis: The role of erythropoietin. J Rheumatol 1992; 19:1687.
2. Peeters HR, Jongen-Lavrencic M, Raja AN, et al: Course and characteristics of anaemia in patients with rheumatoid arthritis of recent onset. Ann Rheum Dis 1996; 55:162.
3. Means RT Jr, Krantz SB: Inhibition of human erythroid colony-forming units by gamma interferon can be corrected by recombinant human erythropoietin. Blood 1991; 78:2564.
4. Davis D, Charles PJ, Potter A, et al: Anaemia of chronic disease in rheumatoid arthritis: In vivo effects of tumour necrosis factor alpha blockade. Br J Rheumatol 1997; 36:950.
5. Takashina N, Kondo H, Kashiwazaki S: Suppressed serum erythropoietin response to anemia and the efficacy of recombinant erythropoietin in the anemia of rheumatoid arthritis. J Rheumatol 1990; 17:885.
6. Means RT Jr, Krantz SB: Progress in understanding the pathogenesis of the anemia of chronic disease. Blood 1992; 80:1639.
7. Porter DR, Sturrock RD, Capell HA: The use of serum ferritin estimation in the investigation of anaemia in patients with rheumatoid arthritis. Clin Exp Rheumatol 1994; 12:179.
8. Mulherin D, Skelly M, Saunders A, et al: The diagnosis of iron deficiency in patients with rheumatoid arthritis and anemia: An algorithm using simple laboratory measures. J Rheumatol 1996; 23:237.
9. O'Toole PA, Sykes H, Phelan M, et al: Duodenal mucosal ferritin in rheumatoid arthritis: Implications for anaemia of chronic disease. Q J Med 1996; 89:509.
10. Pincus T, Olsen NJ, Russell IJ, et al: Multicenter study of recombinant human erythropoietin in correction of anemia in rheumatoid arthritis. Am J Med 1990; 89:161.
11. Peeters HR, Jongen-Lavrencic M, Vreugdenhil G, et al: Effect of recombinant human erythropoietin on anaemia and disease activity in patients with rheumatoid arthritis and anaemia of chronic disease: A randomised placebo controlled double blind 52 week clinical trial. Ann Rheum Dis 1996; 55:739.
12. Saikawa I, Hotokebuchi T, Arita C, et al: Autologous blood transfusion with recombinant erythropoietin treatment: 22 arthroplasties for rheumatoid arthritis. Acta Orthop Scand 1994; 65:15.
13. Mercuriali F: Epoetin alfa for autologous blood donation in patients with rheumatoid arthritis and concomitant anemia. Semin Hematol 1997; 33:18.
14. Benn HP, Drews J, Randzio G, et al: Does active rheumatoid arthritis affect intestinal iron absorption? Ann Rheum Dis 1988; 47:144.
15. Vreugdenhil G, Wognum AW, van Eijk HG, et al: Anaemia in rheumatoid arthritis: The role of iron, vitamin $B_{12}$, and folic acid deficiency, and erythropoietin responsiveness. Ann Rheum Dis 1990; 49:93.
16. Weber J, Werre JM, Julius HW, et al: Decreased iron absorption in patients with active rheumatoid arthritis, with and without iron deficiency. Ann Rheum Dis 1988; 47:404.
17. Bentley DP, Williams P: Parenteral iron therapy in the anaemia of rheumatoid arthritis. Rheumatol Rehabil 1982; 21:88.
18. Merry P, Kidd B, Blake DR: How safe is it to give parenteral iron to a patient with rheumatoid arthritis (RA) and iron deficiency anaemia? Br J Rheumatol 1989; 28:22.
19. Blake DR, Lunec J, Ahern M, et al: Effect of intravenous iron dextran on rheumatoid synovitis. Ann Rheum Dis 1985; 44:183.
20. Pettersson T, Rosenlof K, Friman C, et al: Successful treatment of the anemia of rheumatoid arthritis with subcutaneously administered recombinant human erythropoietin. Slower response in patients with more severe inflammation. Scand J Rheumatol 1993; 22:188.
21. Mercuriali F, Gualtieri G, Sinigaglia L, et al: Use of recombinant human erythropoietin to assist autologous blood donation by anemic rheumatoid arthritis patients undergoing major orthopedic surgery. Transfusion 1994; 34:501.
22. Nordstrom D, Lindroth Y, Marsal L, et al: Availability of iron and degree of inflammation modifies the response to recombinant human erythropoietin when treating anemia of chronic disease in patients with rheumatoid arthritis. Rheumatol Int 1997; 17:67.
23. Dessypris EN, Baer MR, Sergent JS, et al: Rheumatoid arthritis and pure red cell aplasia. Ann Intern Med 1984; 100:202.
24. Fujii T, Yajima T, Kameda H, et al: Successful treatment with cyclosporin A of pure red cell aplasia associated with rheumatoid arthritis. J Rheumatol 1996; 23:1803.
25. Charles RJ, Sabo KM, Kidd PG, et al: The pathophysiology of pure red cell aplasia: Implications for therapy. Blood 1996; 87:4831.
26. Felty AR: Chronic arthritis in the adult associated with splenomegaly and leukopenia. Bull Johns Hopkins Hosp 1924; 35:16.
27. Campion G, Maddison PJ, Goulding N, et al: The Felty syndrome: A case-matched study of clinical manifestations and outcome, serologic features, and immunogenetic associations. Medicine (Baltimore) 1990; 69:69.
28. Loughran TPJ, Starkebaum G: Large granular lymphocyte leukemia. Report of 38 cases and review of the literature. Medicine (Baltimore) 1987; 66:397.
29. Starkebaum G, Loughran TP Jr, Gaur LK, et al: Immunogenetic similarities between patients with Felty's syndrome and those with clonal expansions of large granular lymphocytes in rheumatoid arthritis. Arthritis Rheum 1997; 40:624.
30. Bowman SJ, Sivakumaran M, Snowden N, et al: The large granular lymphocyte syndrome with rheumatoid arthritis. Immuno-

genetic evidence for a broader definition of Felty's syndrome. Arthritis Rheum 1994; 37:1326.

31. Starkebaum G, Singer JW, Arend WP: Humoral and cellular immune mechanisms of neutropenia in patients with Felty's syndrome. Clin Exp Immunol 1980; 39:307.

32. Abdou NI: Heterogeneity of bone marrow–directed immune mechanisms in the pathogenesis of neutropenia of Felty's syndrome. Arthritis Rheum 1983; 26:947.

33. Breedveld FC, Lafeber GJ, de Vries E, et al: Immune complexes and the pathogenesis of neutropenia in Felty's syndrome. Ann Rheum Dis 1986; 45:696.

34. Breedveld FC, Fibbe WE, Hermans J, et al: Factors influencing the incidence of infections in Felty's syndrome. Arch Intern Med 1987; 147:915.

35. Gridley G, Klippel JH, Hoover RN, et al: Incidence of cancer among men with the Felty syndrome. Ann Intern Med 1994; 120:35.

36. Dillon AM, Luthra HS, Conn DL, et al: Parenteral gold therapy in the Felty syndrome. Experience with 20 patients. Medicine (Baltimore) 1986; 65:107.

37. Lakhanpal S, Luthra HS. D-penicillamine in Felty's syndrome. J Rheumatol 1985; 12:703.

38. Neish PR, Fuchs HA: Resolution of Felty's syndrome with cyclophosphamide [Letter]. J Rheumatol 1989; 16:709.

39. Pixley JS, Yoneda KY, Manalo PB: Sequential administration of cyclophosphamide and granulocyte-colony stimulating factor relieves impaired myeloid maturation in Felty's syndrome. Am J Hematol 1993; 43:304.

40. Coiffier B: Cyclosporine in Felty's syndrome [Letter]. N Engl J Med 1986; 314:184.

41. Canvin JM, Dalal BI, Baragar F, et al: Cyclosporine for the treatment of granulocytopenia in Felty's syndrome. Am J Hematol 1991; 36:219.

42. Sood R, Stewart CC, Aplan PD, et al: Neutropenia associated with T-cell large granular lymphocyte leukemia: Long-term response to cyclosporine therapy despite persistence of abnormal cells. Blood 1998; 91:3372.

43. Barnes CG, Turnbull AL, Vernon-Roberts B: Felty's syndrome. A clinical and pathological survey of 21 patients and their response to treatment. Ann Rheum Dis 1971; 30:359.

44. Mant MJ, Akabutu JJ, Herbert FA: Lithium carbonate therapy in severe Felty's syndrome. Benefits, toxicity, and granulocyte function. Arch Intern Med 1986; 146:277.

45. Moore RA, Brunner CM, Sandusky WR, et al: Felty's syndrome: Long-term follow-up after splenectomy. Ann Intern Med 1971; 75:381.

46. Laszlo J, Jones R, Silberman HR, et al: Splenectomy for Felty's syndrome. Clinicopathological study of 27 patients. Arch Intern Med 1978; 138:597.

47. Nakamura H, Ohishi A, Asano K, et al: Partial splenic embolization for Felty's syndrome: A 10-year followup. J Rheumatol 1994; 21:1964.

48. Calverley DC, Jones GW, Kelton JG: Splenic radiation for corticosteroid-resistant immune thrombocytopenia. Ann Intern Med 1992; 116:977.

49. Fiechtner JJ, Miller DR, Starkebaum G: Reversal of neutropenia with methotrexate treatment in patients with Felty's syndrome. Correlation of response with neutrophil-reactive IgG. Arthritis Rheum 1989; 32:194.

50. Isasi C, Lopez-Martin JA, Angeles TM, et al: Felty's syndrome: Response to low dose oral methotrexate. J Rheumatol 1989; 16:983.

51. Wassenberg S, Herborn G, Rau R: Methotrexate treatment in Felty's syndrome. Br J Rheumatol 1998; 37:908.

52. Bills LJ, Seibert D, Brick JE: Liver disease, erroneously attributed to methotrexate, in a patient with rheumatoid arthritis. J Rheumatol 1992; 19:1963.

53. Lubbe AS, Schwella N, Riess H, et al: Improvement of pneumonia and arthritis in Felty's syndrome by treatment with granulocyte-macrophage colony-stimulating factor (GM-CSF). Blut 1990; 61:379.

54. Bhalla K, Ross R, Jeter E, et al: G-CSF improves granulocytopenia in Felty's syndrome without flare-up of arthritis [Letter]. Am J Hematol 1993; 42:230.

55. Stanworth SJ, Bhavnani M, Chattopadhya C, et al: Treatment of Felty's syndrome with the haemopoietic growth factor granulocyte colony-stimulating factor (G-CSF). Q J Med 1998; 91:49.

56. Starkebaum G: Use of colony-stimulating factors in the treatment of neutropenia associated with collagen vascular disease. Curr Opin Hematol 1997; 4:196.

57. Wandt H, Seifert M, Falge C, et al: Long-term correction of neutropenia in Felty's syndrome with granulocyte colony-stimulating factor. Ann Hematol 1993; 66:265.

58. Graham KE, Coodley GO: A prolonged use of granulocyte colony stimulating factor in Felty's syndrome. J Rheumatol 1995; 22:174.

59. Moore DF Jr, Vadhan Raj S: Sustained response in Felty's syndrome to prolonged administration of recombinant human granulocyte-macrophage colony-stimulating factor (rhGM-CSF). Am J Med 1995; 98:591.

60. Hazenberg BP, Van LMA, Van RMH, et al: Correction of granulocytopenia in Felty's syndrome by granulocyte-macrophage colony-stimulating factor. Simultaneous induction of interleukin-6 release and flare-up of the arthritis. Blood 1989; 74:2769.

61. Farhey YD, Herman JH: Vasculitis complicating granulocyte colony stimulating factor treatment of leukopenia and infection in Felty's syndrome. J Rheumatol 1995; 22:1179.

62. Vidarsson B, Geirsson AJ, Onundarson PT: Reactivation of rheumatoid arthritis and development of leukocytoclastic vasculitis in a patient receiving granulocyte colony-stimulating factor for Felty's syndrome. Am J Med 1995; 98:589.

63. Hoshina Y, Moriuchi J, Nakamura Y, et al: CD4+ T cell-mediated leukopenia of Felty's syndrome successfully treated with granulocyte-colony-stimulating factor and methotrexate. Arthritis Rheum 1994; 37:298.

64. Pixley JS, Yoneda KY, Manalo PB: Sequential administration of cyclophosphamide and granulocyte-colony stimulating factor relieves impaired myeloid maturation in Felty's syndrome. Am J Hematol 1993; 43:304.

65. Toshioka K: Combined therapy of G-CSF and prednisolone for neutropenia in a patient with Felty's syndrome [Letter]. Am J Hematol 1995; 48:130.

66. Loughran TPJ, Kidd PG, Starkebaum G: Treatment of large granular lymphocyte leukemia with oral low-dose methotrexate. Blood 1994; 84:2164.

67. Weide R, Heymanns J, Koppler H, et al: Successful treatment of neutropenia in T-LGL leukemia (T gamma-lymphocytosis) with granulocyte colony-stimulating factor. Ann Hematol 1994; 69:117.

68. Stanworth SJ, Green L, Pumphrey RS, et al: An unusual association of Felty syndrome and TCR gamma delta lymphocytosis. J Clin Pathol 1996; 49:351.

69. Deleze M, Alarcon-Segovia D, Oria CV, et al: Hemocytopenia in systemic lupus erythematosus. Relationship to antiphospholipid antibodies. J Rheumatol 1989; 16:926. [Published erratum appears in J Rheumatol 1989; 16:1523]

70. Fong KY, Loizou S, Boey ML, et al: Anticardiolipin antibodies, haemolytic anaemia and thrombocytopenia in systemic lupus erythematosus. Br J Rheumatol 1992; 31:453.

71. Deleze M, Oria CV, Alarcon-Segovia D: Occurrence of both hemolytic anemia and thrombocytopenic purpura (Evans' syndrome) in systemic lupus erythematosus. Relationship to antiphospholipid antibodies. J Rheumatol 1988; 15:611.

72. Liesveld JL, Rowe JM, Lichtman MA: Variability of the erythropoietic response in autoimmune hemolytic anemia: Analysis of 109 cases. Blood 1987; 69:820.

73. Rosse W, Bullel W, Ortel T: Challenges in managing autoimmune disease. In McArthur JR, Schechter GP, Platt OS (eds): Hematology—1997. Washington DC: American Society of Hematology, 1997:93.

74. Caramaschi P, Riccetti MM, Pasini AF, et al: Systemic lupus erythematosus and thrombotic thrombocytopenic purpura. Report of three cases and review of the literature. Lupus 1998; 7:37.

75. Jorfen M, Callejas JL, Formiga F, et al: Fulminant thrombotic thrombocytopenic purpura in systemic lupus erythematosus. Scand J Rheumatol 1998; 27:76.

76. Musio F, Bohen EM, Yuan CM, et al: Review of thrombotic thrombocytopenic purpura in the setting of systemic lupus erythematosus. Semin Arthritis Rheum 1998; 28:1.

77. Asherson RA, Cervera R, Piette JC, et al: Catastrophic antiphospholipid syndrome. Clinical and laboratory features of 50 patients. Medicine (Baltimore) 1998; 77:195.
78. Furlan M, Robles R, Galbusera M, et al: von Willebrand factor—cleaving protease in thrombotic thrombocytopenic purpura and the hemolytic-uremic syndrome. N Engl J Med 1998; 339:1578.
79. Moake JL: Moschcowitz, multimers, and metalloprotease. N Engl J Med 1998; 339:1629.
80. Tsai HM, Lian EC: Antibodies to von Willebrand factor–cleaving protease in acute thrombotic thrombocytopenic purpura. N Engl J Med 1998; 339:1585.
81. Byrnes JJ, Khurana M: Treatment of thrombotic thrombocytopenic purpura with plasma. N Engl J Med 1977; 297:1386.
82. George JN, Gilcher RO, Smith JW, et al: Thrombotic thrombocytopenic purpura–hemolytic uremic syndrome: Diagnosis and management. J Clin Apheresis 1998; 13:120.
83. Kwaan HC, Soff GA: Management of thrombotic thrombocytopenic purpura and hemolytic uremic syndrome. Semin Hematol 1997; 34:159.
84. Pujol M, Ribera A, Vilardell M, et al: High prevalence of platelet autoantibodies in patients with systemic lupus erythematosus. Br J Haematol 1995; 89:137.
85. Macchi L, Rispal P, Clofent-Sanchez G, et al: Anti-platelet antibodies in patients with systemic lupus erythematosus and the primary antiphospholipid antibody syndrome: Their relationship with the observed thrombocytopenia. Br J Haematol 1997; 98:336.
86. Lipp E, von Felten A, Sax H, et al: Antibodies against platelet glycoproteins and antiphospholipid antibodies in autoimmune thrombocytopenia. Eur J Haematol 1998; 60:283.
87. George JN, Woolf SH, Raskob GE, et al: Idiopathic thrombocytopenic purpura: A practice guideline developed by explicit methods for the American Society of Hematology. Blood 1996; 88:3.
88. ter Borg EJ, Kallenberg CG: Treatment of severe thrombocytopenia in systemic lupus erythematosus with intravenous gammaglobulin. Ann Rheum Dis 1992; 51:1149.
89. Jacobs P, Wood L, Novitzky N: Intravenous gammaglobulin has no advantages over oral corticosteroids as primary therapy for adults with immune thrombocytopenia: A prospective randomized clinical trial. Am J Med 1994; 97:55.
90. Maier WP, Gordon DS, Howard RF, et al: Intravenous immunoglobulin therapy in systemic lupus erythematosus–associated thrombocytopenia. Arthritis Rheum 1990; 33:1233.
91. Bussel JB: Recent advances in the treatment of idiopathic thrombocytopenic purpura: The anti-D clinical experience. Semin Hematol 1998; 35:1.
92. Tarantino MD, Goldsmith G: Treatment of acute immune thrombocytopenic purpura. Semin Hematol 1998; 35:28.
93. Smith N: Intravenous anti-D immunoglobulin in the management of immune thrombocytopenic purpura. Curr Opin Hematol 1996; 3:498.
94. Simpson KN, Coughlin CM, Eron J, et al: Idiopathic thrombocytopenia purpura: Treatment patterns and an analysis of cost associated with intravenous immunoglobulin and anti-D therapy. Semin Hematol 1998; 35:58.
95. Coon WW: Splenectomy for cytopenias associated with systemic lupus erythematosus. Am J Surg 1988; 155:391.
96. Rivero SJ, Alger M, Alarcon-Segovia D: Splenectomy for hemocytopenia in systemic lupus erythematosus. A controlled appraisal. Arch Intern Med 1979; 139:773.
97. Hall S, McCormick JL Jr, Greipp PR, et al: Splenectomy does not cure the thrombocytopenia of systemic lupus erythematosus. Ann Intern Med 1985; 102:325.
98. Kueh YK: Adult idiopathic thrombocytopenic purpura (ITP)—A prospective tracking of its natural history. Singapore Med J 1995; 36:367.
99. Hakim AJ, Machin SJ, Isenberg DA: Autoimmune thrombocytopenia in primary antiphospholipid syndrome and systemic lupus erythematosus: The response to splenectomy. Semin Arthritis Rheum 1998; 28:20.
100. Caulier MT, Darloy F, Rose C, et al: Splenic irradiation for chronic autoimmune thrombocytopenic purpura in patients with contra-indications to splenectomy. Br J Haematol 1995; 91:208.
101. Marino C, Cook P: Danazol for lupus thrombocytopenia. Arch Intern Med 1985; 145:2251.
102. West SG, Johnson SC: Danazol for the treatment of refractory autoimmune thrombocytopenia in systemic lupus erythematosus. Ann Intern Med 1988; 108:703.
103. Wong KL: Danazol in treatment of lupus thrombocytopenia. Asian Pac J Allergy Immunol 1991; 9:125.
104. Cervera H, Jara LJ, Pizarro S, et al: Danazol for systemic lupus erythematosus with refractory autoimmune thrombocytopenia or Evans' syndrome. J Rheumatol 1995; 22:1867.
105. Blanco R, Martinez-Taboada VM, Rodriguez-Valverde V, et al: Successful therapy with danazol in refractory autoimmune thrombocytopenia associated with rheumatic diseases. Br J Rheumatol 1997; 36:1095.
106. Manger K, Kalden JR, Manger B: Cyclosporin A in the treatment of systemic lupus erythematosus: Results of an open clinical study. Br J Rheumatol 1996; 35:669.
107. Sugiyama M, Ogasawara H, Kaneko H, et al: Effect of extremely low dose cyclosporine treatment on the thrombocytopenia in systemic lupus erythematosus. Lupus 1998; 7:53.
108. Schultz KR, Strahlendorf C, Warrier I, et al: Cyclosporin A therapy of immune-mediated thrombocytopenia in children [Letter]. Blood 1995; 85:1406.
109. Blanchette V, Freedman J, Garvey B: Management of chronic immune thrombocytopenic purpura in children and adults. Semin Hematol 1998; 35:36.

# 18 | Novel Therapies for Rheumatoid Arthritis

*F. C. Breedveld*

## CYTOKINE-TARGETED THERAPIES

Rheumatoid arthritis (RA) is one of a group of conditions frequently referred to as autoimmune disease in which immunologic activity is involved. Joint pain and joint immobility, which are characteristic of RA, arise from a chronic fluctuating inflammation in the synovial tissue of the joints. The joint lesions are dominated by activated macrophages and fibroblast-like cells, found at the site of bone and cartilage destruction, and are dominated by activated T cells, plasma cells, and B cells in the inflamed synovium and granulocytes in the synovial fluid. Although the mechanism by which this immune-mediated inflammation is triggered and the nature of the target antigen remain to be elucidated, mediators that perpetuate inflammation and destruction of cartilage and bone have been identified. On the basis of this increasing knowledge, new therapeutic principles have been developed with biologic agents that act on more specific targets than do the established antirheumatic drugs. Table 18–1 provides an overview of already investigated approaches to RA. In this chapter, not all approaches for intervention listed in Table 18–1 can be discussed extensively. The focus is mainly on (1) interventions that block the effect of proinflammatory cytokines and (2) interventions targeted at cell surface molecules.

## CYTOKINE-TARGETED THERAPIES

The mediators that received most attention in the 1990s, cytokines, are designed to perform intercellular communication.[1] Cytokines can be categorized as those that enhance inflammation, such as tumor necrosis factor (TNF) or interleukin (IL)–1, and those that decrease inflammation, such as interleukin (IL)–10 or IL-4. Several natural endogenous inhibitors of TNF and IL-1 have been identified, including IL-1 receptor antagonist (IL-1ra), soluble IL-1 receptors, and soluble TNF receptors. These natural inhibitors are present in healthy persons, and even increased levels are found in serum specimens and at sites of inflammation in RA patients. Several lines of evidence suggest that in RA, an imbalance has occurred at the site of inflammation whereby proinflammatory cytokines outnumber antiinflammatory cytokines or natural inhibitors.[2] This has

resulted in the investigation of therapies with products of the biotechnology industry that aim at the restoration of this imbalance.

## Blockage of Tumor Necrosis Factor

The progression of the clinical development of TNF blockage in RA has been impressive. It was only in March 1992 that the first RA patient was treated with a TNF-blocking agent. In 1994 the results of the first placebo-controlled trial became available, and in 1998 sufficient information had been gathered to convince several registration authorities that the efficacy/toxicity ratio was good enough that access to the market was justified. The available information at present suggests that TNF blockage is the first effective targeted therapy with a biologic response modifier in RA; it has the potential to become a milestone in rheumatology, with regard to both the scientific approach toward the disease and the extent of clinical efficacy.

TNF is a pleiotropic cytokine that is of particular interest in RA because it is abundantly produced in the rheumatoid synovium and because preclinical studies have shown that binding of TNF to the surface receptors of cells leads to a pattern of gene activation. This process causes (1) macrophages to produce proinflammatory mediators that amplify the inflammation reaction; (2) endothelial cells to express adhesion molecules that allow access of more inflammatory cells into the site of inflammation; and (3) fibroblasts to produce proteases that can destroy cartilage, bone, and ligaments.[2]

An important role of TNF in arthritis has been further supported by the observations that in mice transgenic for TNF, destructive arthritis developed spontaneously.[3] The administration of TNF monoclonal antibodies (mAb) that bind and inactivate TNF prevented this form of arthritis. Other animal work has further strengthened the view that TNF plays a key role in the pathogenesis of RA. TNF administered intra-articularly induces synovitis. Similarly, in collagen-induced arthritis, TNF administered during the development of arthritis leads to a more severe form of joint inflammation, whereas mice receiving TNF mAb in the same time period show significant amelioration of the

## TABLE 18–1
## Therapies Targeted at Immunologic Mechanisms and Investigated in Rheumatoid Arthritis

**Cytokine Targeted Therapies**
- TNF blockage
- IL-1 blockage
- IL-6 blockage
- Administration of anti-inflammatory cytokines (IL-10, IL-4)

**Cell Surface–Targeted Therapies**
- Anti-adhesion molecules (ICAM-1)
- Anti-CD4
- Anti-CD5, anti-CD7, anti-CD25, anti-CD52
- Anti-CD28
- IL-2 fusion protein

**Administration of Autoantigens (Collagen Type II)**

**T Cell Receptor Vaccination**

**High-Dose Intravenous Immunoglobulins**

**Plasmapheresis, Apheresis, Immunoadsorption Column**

**Autologous Bone Marrow Transplantation**

ICAM-1 = intercellular adhesion molecule-1; IL = interleukin; TNF = tumor necrosis factor.

disease process.[4] TNF may also contribute to systemic features of RA by stimulating acute-phase protein synthesis and inhibiting erythropoiesis.[5]

In the first half of the 1990s, clinical trials using chimeric human/mouse or humanized TNF mAb in RA patients provided the first direct evidence that inhibitors of TNF might be useful therapeutic agents. An open-label trial of the TNF mAb infliximab (Remicade)[6] showed that intravenous administration induced significant improvements in swollen joint counts and serum C–reactive protein levels in all RA patients who received infliximab. In a subsequent double-blind multicenter European trial, patients were randomly assigned to receive single infusions of placebo, low-dose infliximab (1 mg/kg), or high-dose infliximab (10 mg/kg). Of the patients treated with high-dose infliximab, 79% showed a response (20% according to the Paulus response criteria) at 4 weeks after treatment, and of the patients treated with the low dose, 44% responded; both these results were in clear contrast with the 8% of placebo responders.[7] The response was substantial inasmuch as more than 50% of the patients receiving high-dose infliximab achieved a strong response (50% Paulus). Duration of response was related to the persistence of serum levels of infliximab and the original antibody dose; in those who received a single infusion of 10 mg/kg, the median response duration was 8 weeks. The antibody was well tolerated; minor infections and rashes were the most common side effects.

In addition to these short-term studies, a repeated therapy study, which involved eight patients included in the open-label trial, also indicated that infliximab may be useful for controlling disease flares during the long-term management of RA,[8] despite the fact that some patients develop antibodies against infliximab.

The development of a humanized TNF mAb (CDP571) has been part of a strategy directed toward minimizing the development of such antibody responses. A double-blind study performed with CDP571 in 36 patients with RA demonstrated clinical benefit over 8 weeks at the 10-mg/kg dose level.[9] These trials provided the first convincing evidence that blockade of a specific cytokine could be an effective treatment in human autoimmune inflammatory disease.

To determine whether TNF therapy with mAb is efficacious over the long term and may reduce disease activity in patients who do not respond to methotrexate therapy, two placebo-controlled trials have been performed with infliximab. In the first study, the patients with active RA despite methotrexate treatment received five infusions of infliximab during 14 weeks with or without continuation of a fixed low dose (7.5 mg/week) methotrexate therapy; results indicated that TNF mAb in combination with methotrexate markedly suppressed inflammatory disease activity in RA, and the best results occurred with 3 and 10 mg/kg of TNF-mAb.[10] The combination therapy enhanced the degree and duration of efficacy and also appeared to promote immunologic tolerance to infliximab therapy with a reduction in antibodies to the human chimeric monoclonal antibody (HACA). The second study evaluated the effect of placebo injections and 3 or 10 mg/kg of infliximab infused every 4 or 8 weeks in patients with active RA who continued methotrexate therapy. Results indicated that infliximab at all dosages and schedules achieved at 30 weeks a clinical response according to the American College of Rheumatology (ACR) 20% response criteria in 50% to 58% of the patients, which was clearly a higher percentage than the 20% of placebo responders.[10a]

At 54 weeks, impressive clinical effects were still observed in the patients who had received infliximab plus methotrexate, in comparison with those who received methotrexate plus placebo.[10b] In fact, the ACR 20% response was achieved by 42% to 59% of patients in all treatment groups with infliximab, in contrast to 17% of patients who received methotrexate plus placebo. There was a trend toward higher responses in the group receiving 10-mg/kg doses, but it was not statistically significant.

Clinical response was observed early, frequently within 1 week. There was a 60% to 70% improvement in number of swollen and tender joints, fatigue, and acute-phase reactants, including C-reactive protein and sedimentation rate. Approximately 25% to 30% of patients did not respond to therapy (as defined by ACR response), but markers or factors that could identify nonresponders before dosing had not yet been defined.

In addition to the clinical effects, infliximab plus methotrexate had a positive impact on progression as shown by radiography. Significant differences in the Sharp erosion and narrowing score were observed with infliximab plus methotrexate in comparison with methotrexate plus placebo. The data indicate that erosions did not progress in most of the patients receiving infliximab.

Side effects observed in the clinical studies with infliximab have included infusion reactions (similar to those with intravenous immunoglobulin) and were uncommon. Serious infections were rarely observed, but they are a concern with all TNF inhibitors. These agents should not be used in patients with active infection or in patients at increased risk for infection. Such patients include those with a history of untreated tuberculosis, chronic bone or joint infections, and those with recurrent cellulitis or draining nodules. Antibodies against infliximab have been observed with treatment with infliximab alone, but their numbers are reduced with concomitant use of methotrexate. To date, there are no data on an increased risk of lymphoproliferative disorders with this antibody or other TNF inhibitors.

In 1999 the US Food and Drug Administration approved infliximab plus methotrexate for the therapy for active RA. The approved dose of infliximab is 3 mg/kg dosed at 0, 2, 6, and every 8 weeks thereafter. In the United States, the cost of 1 year of therapy at a dose of 3 mg/kg for a 70-kg patient is approximately $9000/year. In clinical studies, doses as high as 10 mg/kg were used. It is not known whether patients who do not respond to 3 mg/kg will have a response at higher doses. It is also not known whether patients who do not respond to one TNF inhibitor, such as an mAb, will respond to another, such as another mAb or a soluble TNF receptor.

Administration of soluble TNF receptors is another therapeutic strategy aimed at TNF blockage. The biologic activities of TNF are mediated through membrane-bound receptors that are expressed by numerous cell types. Biotechnology allows the production of soluble monomeric receptors; in an attempt to increase their half-life and affinity, soluble TNF receptors have been fused to the crystallizable fragment (Fc) portion of an immunoglobulin G1 (IgG1), forming a fully human soluble TNF receptor-Fc fusion protein. The fusion protein investigated most extensively is etanercept (Enbrel). In a dose escalation study in patients with refractory RA, the subcutaneous administration of etanercept twice weekly was well tolerated and strongly decreased the number of painful and swollen joints, as well as the C-reactive protein levels.[11] TNF receptor fusion proteins that have a half-life of 2 to 3 days after administration are therefore given more frequently than the chimeric mAb infliximab, which has a half-life of approximately 10 days. These encouraging initial clinical results were confirmed in a multicenter, randomized, double-blind, placebo-controlled study in which patients received etanercept subcutaneously twice a week during 3 months.[12] Patients who received the highest dose (16 mg/m² = approximately 25 mg) had the greatest decrease in the number of swollen and tender joints. A clinical response according to the ACR 20% response criteria was observed in 75% of patients receiving the highest dose of etanercept but in only 14% of those receiving placebo. Similarly, 57% of the group receiving 16 mg/m² of etanercept had at least 50% improvement, according to ACR criteria, in contrast to only 7% of those receiving placebo. Mean erythrocyte sedimentation rate and C-reactive protein

levels decreased markedly. Etanercept was also well tolerated in this study, and only one patient withdrew (because of a mild injection site reaction).

In another multicenter trial, patients were treated for 6 months with placebo, 10 mg of etanercept, or 25 mg of etanercept subcutaneously twice weekly.[13] At the end of treatment, 51% and 59% of the 10- and 25-mg–treated groups fulfilled the ACR 20% response criteria; these percentages were significantly higher than the 11% of the placebo-treated patients. Of the group receiving 25 mg, 40% achieved a 50% ACR response; this is in sharp contrast to the 5% of the placebo-treated patients.

To study whether addition of etanercept to methotrexate would provide additional benefit to patients who had persistent active RA despite receiving methotrexate (15 to 25 mg/week,) patients received either 25 mg of etanercept or placebo subcutaneously twice a week while continuing to receive methotrexate.[14] At 24 weeks, 71% of the patients receiving etanercept plus methotrexate and 27% of those receiving placebo plus methotrexate met the ACR 20% response criteria. A long-term study has demonstrated that the efficacy and safety of etanercept therapy continued for more than 24 months.[15] Longer term studies have reported continued response with etanercept plus methotrexate over 24 months of dosing.[15a] There was no increase in adverse events with chronic dosing in this cohort.[15a] Sixty-two percent of patients were able to reduce methotrexate dosing, and 10% of patients were able to discontinue methotrexate without a flare of arthritis. TNF blockade with etanercept was also found to be efficacious in patients with polyarticular juvenile chronic arthritis,[15b] and etanercept has since been approved by the US Food and Drug Administration for use in juvenile rheumatoid arthritis at a dose of 0.4 mg/kg subcutaneously twice a week. In a 1-year trial comparing etanercept with methotrexate in 632 patients with early RA (disease duration of less than 3 years), etanercept had a more rapid response and showed greater efficacy than did methotrexate over time, according to an area-under-the-curve analysis. There was less radiographic progression (total Sharp score) at 1 year with etanercept than with methotrexate.[15c] Etanercept was well tolerated in all studies. The only adverse events clearly associated with etanercept were mild injection-site reactions and a small increase in minor upper respiratory tract infections. The induction of antibodies against etanercept was observed in fewer than 16% of patients tested. This low frequency may be related to the agent's fully human derivation. Etanercept was approved by the US Food and Drug Administration in 1998 as therapy for active RA by itself or in combination with methotrexate at a dose of 25 mg injected subcutaneously twice a week. It has also been approved for use in juvenile RA. The cost of 1 year's treatment is approximately $12,000.

These data demonstrate that TNF inhibition is a viable approach to controlling disease activity in RA. TNF blockage induces a rapid improvement in multiple clinical assessments of disease activity and is associated with improvements in biologic parameters. Rheumatologists who participated in the early trials were particularly impressed by the significant decrease in fatigue reported by the patients.

At present, infliximab and etanercept have been investigated most extensively and particularly in RA. Other mAb and soluble receptors are being developed and seem to be therapeutically effective against RA. These successful observations indicate that the unanswered questions about this therapy are becoming more important. For example, the precise mechanism of action remains to be defined. The possibilities include (1) binding and inactivation of TNF in the fluid phase, (2) binding to transmembrane TNF, (3) down-regulation of the expression of proinflammatory cytokines (suggested by the rapid reduction of C-reactive protein production and IL-6), (4) blockage of cell trafficking (suggested by the significant suppression of circulating levels of adhesion molecules and the reduced expression of adhesion molecules in synovial tissue after treatment), and (5) blockage of metalloproteinase production.[2, 16, 17]

It is not yet certain whether there are significant differences among the most important biologic agents being developed. The mAb has the possibility of cytotoxicity to cells that express membrane-bound TNF. Whether this effect as well as the high affinity of the TNF receptor:Fc fusion proteins and the possibility of these proteins to bind TNF in addition to lymphotoxin are relevant to the efficacy remains to be seen.

Another important issue is whether blockade of TNF is merely anti-inflammatory or whether it is able to prevent destruction of the joints. An inhibitory effect on joint destruction is suggested by reduced excretion of surrogate markers of cartilage and bone turnover after treatment.[18] The results of the infliximab clinical trial[10b] and the early rheumatoid study of etanercept[15c] demonstrate a beneficial effect with TNF blockade on radiographic progression.

Furthermore, considerably more information on long-term toxicity is necessary. Experimental data on the biology of TNF suggests that TNF mediates inflammation and modulates cellular immune responses, and therefore it is theoretically possible for anti-TNF therapy to affect immune response involved with host defense against infections and malignancies. The side effect spectrum was found to be benign in short-term studies. Sporadic cases of malignancy or severe infections have been documented in patients treated with TNF blockade, and rare cases of lupus-like disease have occurred. Intriguing is the observation that of the patients treated so far, up to 10% have developed anti-double stranded DNA antibodies. Whether such cases are related to the natural history of RA or to the new treatment can be answered only by well-designed, large, and long-term studies of treated patients. The physicians involved should carefully document adverse effects and should communicate these most ideally to a central database.

The indications and contraindications of TNF blockage will certainly develop in the coming years. At present, candidates for TNF blocking therapy are patients who have active disease despite a full and adequate trial of one or more disease-modifying antirheumatic drugs (DMARDs) unless precluded by toxicity concerns that preclude DMARD use. On an individual patient basis, the aggressiveness of the RA and its effects on quality of life should be considered in order to judge the indication for TNF blockage. TNF-blocking agents can be added to preexisting methotrexate therapy. With the results of studies on the effect of TNF blockage on structural joint damage, application in earlier phases of the disease may be considered in selected populations. It is important to note that TNF blocking compounds should not be continued if severe infections, including joint infections, occur and should be resumed only if such infections have completely healed. In addition, decisions about initiation of these agents should be made in the context of the costs of these drugs ($8000 to $12,000/year in the United States). Pharmacoeconomic data about these exciting new agents are essential, as are data on long-term safety and efficacy, for decision making.

## Interleukin-1 Blockage

In analogy to TNF, IL-1 can be seen as a pivotal proinflammatory cytokine. IL-1 enhances cell migration into the inflamed synovium by up-regulation of adhesion molecules, stimulates the production of prostaglandins and metalloproteinases, inhibits collagen and proteoglycan synthesis, and stimulates osteoclastic bone resorption.[19] IL-1 injection has also been shown to exacerbate the chronic phase of experimental arthritis, and IL-1 inhibition ameliorates the arthritis. Two therapeutic approaches to IL-1 blockage have been used on a trial basis in the treatment of RA. The first approach has been the intra-articular and subcutaneous administration of recombinant human IL-1 receptor. This treatment has achieved limited therapeutic efficacy. More recently, IL-1 blockage was pursued by the subcutaneous administration of recombinant IL-1ra. In a preliminary trial, RA patients received daily injections of IL-1ra for a total of 28 days. After 7 days of treatment, there were reductions in the mean number of painful and swollen joints and acute-phase reactants; 12 of 15 patients showed more than a 50% reduction in serum C-reactive protein levels.[20]

In a subsequent double-blind, placebo-controlled, multicenter trial, RA patients were randomized to receive 20, 70, or 200 mg of IL-1ra with dose intervals varying from daily to once a week for 3 weeks,[21] followed by weekly maintenance for 4 weeks. At the end of the 3 weeks of treatment, daily dosing appeared more effective; patients showed a 50% or more improvement in clinical outcome such as the number of painful and swollen joints and general assessments of disease activity by patient or doctor. This improvement was maintained when patients continued with IL-1ra treatment once daily for 4 weeks. The most frequent side effects were reactions at the site of injection. In a follow-up study, patients with early active RA received daily injections of 30, 75, or 150 mg of IL-1ra or placebo for 24 weeks. In the patients who received 150 mg, a significant improvement of clinical parameters ranging from 20% to 35% was reported[22]; of those patients, 43% met the ACR 20% criteria for response at 24 weeks, and that percentage was significantly higher than the 27% of placebo-treated patients. Studies on synovial biopsies demonstrated a strong decrease in lymphocyte infiltration during treatment.[23] In addition, preliminary data on the evaluation of joint radiographs of treated patients suggest that a significant slowing of the progression of the disease with regard to cartilage and bone destruction occurred in the IL-1ra–treated groups.[24] On the basis of these observations, the investigators concluded that IL-1ra treatment modifies the events that result in articular damage with less striking effects on the clinical parameters of disease activity. If observations such as these can be confirmed, optimal treatment of RA is likely to require combinations of therapeutic compounds that inhibit more than one of the pivotal mediators on the pathogenic network.

A 1999 study compared the combination of IL-1ra plus methotrexate with the combination of methotrexate plus placebo.[24a] In this study, 419 patients on long-term methotrexate were injected with placebo or with IL-1ra at doses that ranged from 0.04 to 2.0 mg/kg. At 24 weeks, an ACR 20% response was observed in 42% of patients who received the combination of IL-1ra plus methotrexate, in contrast to 23% of those treated with methotrexate plus placebo. The most frequent adverse events were injection site reactions.

## Other Cytokine-Targeted Therapies

Several cytokine-targeted therapies are being investigated, but conclusions on efficacy cannot yet be drawn. IL-6, like TNF and IL-1, is produced in high concentrations in the synovial tissue, and increased levels correlate with disease activity. Preclinical work suggests that several characteristic features of RA—including autoantibody production, T cell activation, acute-phase protein production, and osteoclast activation—can be explained by the effect of IL-6. In open-label studies, RA patients have been treated with murine IL-6 mAb or a humanized anti-human IL-6 receptor mAb. These preliminary data suggest that on average the patients showed improvement in clinical variables during such treatment.[25]

The imbalance between proinflammatory and anti-inflammatory cytokines in RA can also be corrected by anti-inflammatory cytokines. Three different anti-inflammatory cytokines have been identified as inhibiting production of proinflammatory cytokines: IL-4, IL-10, and IL-13. These cytokines exhibit numerous effects, including the down-regulation of synthesis of IL-1 and TNF-$\alpha$. Both IL-4 and IL-10 inhibit expression of proinflammatory (IL-1, IL-6, IL-8, TNF-$\alpha$) genes by rheumatoid synovial cells.[26] IL-4 is more potent than IL-10, but the combination has the most profound effects. IL-4 and IL-10 were incubated with pieces of synovium, and both IL-4 and IL-10 reduced IL-1 production.[27] However, IL-4, in contrast to IL-10, increased production of IL-1ra about threefold, which suggests that IL-4 has a greater propensity for shifting the IL-1/IL-1ra production ratio toward an anti-inflammatory

profile. Both IL-4 and IL-10, when added to cultures of synovial fluid mononuclear cells, inhibit the ability of these supernatants to induce cartilage damage.[28] IL-10 seems to be of special importance for joint protection because IL-10 also directly stimulates cartilage proteoglycan synthesis.[28]

In experimental animal models of arthritis, IL-10 has more potent anti-inflammatory effects than does IL-4. IL-10 suppresses development of collagen-induced arthritis and ameliorates sustained arthritis in rats and in several different murine models of arthritis.[29, 30]

On the basis of the experience in animals, IL-10 seems to be an attractive anti-inflammatory cytokine in the treatment of RA. The phase I study of recombinant human IL-10 in active RA was a placebo-controlled, multicenter, randomized, double-blind multidose study.[31] After a 4-week washout period of DMARDs, RA patients received either IL-10 at doses of 0.5, 1, 5, 10, or 20 $\mu$g/kg or placebo by daily subcutaneous injections for 4 weeks. IL-10 was well tolerated and no anti–IL-10 antibodies were detected. A small drop in platelet counts was detected but returned to normal immediately after cessation of therapy. The biologic effect was confirmed by a decrease in plasma concentration of soluble TNF-$\alpha$ receptor and increase in IL-1ra concentration. The clinical observations did not suggest the presence of strong antirheumatic effect.

These observations were expanded in a 4-week multicenter placebo controlled study of IL-10 (1, 4, or 8 $\mu$g/kg/day or 8 or 20 $\mu$g/kg twice a week) or placebo with methotrexate in subjects with active RA.[31a] A trend toward improvement in RA disease activity was observed with IL-10 at doses of 8 $\mu$g/kg/day and doses of 8 and 20 $\mu$g/kg twice a week (50% to 63% of patients receiving active treatment had an ACR 20% response, in contrast to only 10% of those receiving placebo treatment). In these studies, IL-10 was well tolerated and induced no anti–IL-10 antibodies. The role of IL-10 and IL-4 therapy in RA is uncertain.

## CELL-TARGETED THERAPIES

### CD4 mAb

CD4$^+$ T cells have been at the center of thinking about disease pathogenesis in RA. Various pieces of evidence have been cited, some of which have stood the test of time.[32] These include the predominance of CD4$^+$ T cells in the inflamed synovium, their activation state and proximity to antigen presenting cells, and the association between RA and specific major histocompatibility complex (MHC) alleles. At least six different forms of CD4 mAb have been investigated in the treatment of RA. Early studies employed murine antibodies, whereas in more recent studies, chimerized, primatized, and humanized antibodies were employed.

Although early, uncontrolled studies with CD4 mAb almost showed promising results, more recent data from two large, well-controlled clinical trials with the chimeric mAb, cM-T412, failed to show evidence of efficacy in two different RA populations, despite induction of CD4 depletion.[33, 34] A controlled trial of the murine CD4 mAb, B-F5, used at the same dose that had previously been effective in an open-label trial, also produced results no different from those of placebo.[35]

Despite disappointing clinical results from these studies, they have provided some valuable insights into the biologic effects of CD4 mAb. Reduction in synovial cellularity (including T cells and monocyte/macrophages) and synovial adhesion molecule expression has been demonstrated after 5 days of therapy with CD4 mAb, providing support for the notion that CD4+ T cells regulate the influx of other cell types into the joint.[36] Binding of mAb to the CD4 molecules expressed on T cells (CD4 coating) in synovial fluid has been shown to be facilitated by a longer duration of dosing with CD4 mAb, and the percentage of synovial (but not peripheral blood) T cells coated correlated with clinical improvement in an open-label study.[37] It was shown in a subsequent study that injection of CD4 mAb led to dose-related CD4 coating in peripheral blood, which suggested that dose levels or dosing frequency used in CD4 studies may have been inadequate.[34] Studies in preclinical models of autoimmunity showed that depletion of CD4+ T cells was not required for efficacy with CD4 mAb,[38] and the clinical studies confirmed that simple depletion of CD4+ T cells does not guarantee a positive clinical response.

Results of studies with a primatized CD4 mAb (keliximab) also suggested that CD4 coating and not CD4 depletion is a predictor of efficacy.[39] In open-label, uncontrolled, single- and repeat-dose phase I studies in patients with moderate to severe RA, keliximab was well tolerated and induced only transient CD4 depletion.[40, 41] In two studies, the results of which were presented in abstract form, RA patients received multiple dosages of nondepleting CD4 mAb. During 4 weeks patients received placebo twice a week or 40, 80, or 140 mg of keliximab. Seventy-seven percent of the 140-mg cohort, 47% of the 80-mg cohort, 42% in the 40-mg cohort, and 20% in the placebo cohort met the predefined response criteria.[42] In another study that used the CD4 mAb 4162W94, RA patients received on 5 consecutive days 10, 30, 100, or 300 mg/day of the mAb. In contrast to the patients receiving lower dosages, the large majority of patients who received 100 or 300 mg/day fulfilled the response criteria, beginning as early as day 7 and lasting in some patients for more than 3 months.[43] In both studies several patients who received the highest dose of CD4 mAb developed a rash, which was diagnosed as leukocytoclastic vasculitis. It seems reasonable to speculate that effective and sustained interference with CD4/MHC interactions, either by reducing CD4 density or by coating residual CD4 with mAb, is the mechanism of action of CD4 mAb in RA. However, another possible mechanism includes functional modification of CD4+ T cells, resulting in suppression of TH1 cytokine production and induction of TH2 cytokines.[38]

Mounting evidence suggests that the epitope recognized by a CD4 mAb has profound biologic effects. Differences in the antigen-binding fragment (Fab) portions of different forms of mAb tested in RA may explain why earlier studies failed to show efficacy in controlled trials. In addition, CD4 mAb may need to be administered at a sufficient dosage and frequency to sustain CD4 down-modulation and/or coating, in order to be effective. Overall, the findings at present are inconclusive for the hypothesis that appropriate construction and use of CD4 mAb results in clinical improvement in this disease.

## Other Cell Surface Molecules

The cell surface antigens of T cells have also been targeted with mAb directed against CD5, CD7, CD25, and CD52, as well as with IL-2 fusion protein. These studies either showed limited efficacy or revealed serious side effects, including a pronounced cytokine release syndrome and long-lasting lymphopenia, and these methods have not been further developed as treatment for RA.

Other strategies for cell-targeted therapies include interference with cell activation and with migration. Monocyte/macrophage–like cells and dendritic cells are prominently represented in the rheumatoid synovium. These antigen-presenting cells (APCs) express an activated phenotype and express both class II MHC as well as costimulatory molecules such as CD80 (B7-1) and CD86 (B7-2).[44, 45]

Resting T cells require at least two signals for induction of cytokine gene expression and cell proliferation. The first signal is antigen specific and delivered by engagement of the T cell receptor/CD3 complex with peptide presented by an MHC molecule on an APC. The second, or costimulatory signal, is delivered by engagement of a costimulatory ligand on the APC with a coreceptor on the T cell. A key costimulatory signal is provided by the interaction of CD28 on T cells with CD80 (B7-1) or CD86 (B7-2) expressed on APCs.[46, 47] The condition known as anergy (unresponsiveness) can be induced when the T cell receives signal one in the absence of signal two.[48, 49]

CTLA41g can block the interaction of CD28 with CD80/CD86, thus preventing T cells from receiving the requisite costimulatory signal two.[46] Results of animal studies suggest that CTLA4Ig may not completely block T cell activation.[50] In these experiments, profound anti-inflammatory and immunosuppressive activity has been demonstrated. The therapeutic efficacy in patients with RA is being evaluated at present.

## Intercellular Adhesion Molecule-1

The finding that adhesion molecules play a pivotal role in RA has inspired trials with mAb against the intercellular adhesion molecule-1 (ICAM-1).[51] The expression of adhesion molecules on endothelial cells and complementary ligands on the surface of leucocytes allow cell migration into the site of inflammation. In an open-label study, RA patients were treated with different dosages of a murine mAb against ICAM-1.[52] A limited improvement of arthritis was reported in 50% of the patients who were treated with the highest dosage. Because re-treatment resulted in side effects, however, no further studies were organized. Nevertheless, in addition to experimental animal approaches, the observation that the impressive therapeutic effect of TNF blockage is highly associated with a decrease in the expression of adhesion molecules can be interpreted to show that pharmacologic approaches to reduce the expressional function of ICAM-1 might indeed be of therapeutic value.

## Gene Therapy

Instead of administration of proteins, administration of the gene encoding these proteins has several theoretical advantages, such as continuous production of the protein, localized production with high local concentration, and fewer systemic side effects. Moreover, continuous long-term treatment may establish disease modification. Several methods of delivering the genes encoding anti-inflammatory cytokines or decoy proteins for proinflammatory cytokines are available. The methods of gene delivery are rapidly improving. It is not yet clear which gene delivery system is most appropriate for RA.

In bacterial cell wall–induced arthritis in rats, the arthritic joints were shown to contain a population of cells that could be infected with retroviral vectors in vivo.[53] Effectiveness of this method was demonstrated in rabbits with synovial tissue ex vivo transduced by the retrovirus containing the IL-1ra gene, which was subsequently injected intra-articularly into rabbits that then developed arthritis.[54] In these animals, high IL-1ra levels were found in the arthritic joints. In these joints, a clear inhibition of cartilage matrix catabolism was observed; this inhibition was presumably caused by the IL-1ra produced by the synoviocytes.

The first clinical protocol to assess safety, feasibility, and efficacy of gene therapy in RA has been approved,[55] and completed.[56] The trial included patients who required total joint replacement of metacarpophalangeal joints. Synovial fibroblasts that were transduced in vitro with retrovirus containing the IL-1ra gene were injected into the metacarpophalangeal joints in a double-blind manner. One week later, all joints were removed and replaced by prostheses. The retrieved joints were analyzed for evidence of successful gene transfer and gene expression. In the first three patients reported, the data suggest that transfer of the IL-1ra gene to the metacarpophalangeal joints was accomplished and that gene expression was achieved.[57]

## Other Approaches

The increasing knowledge about pathogenetic mechanisms in RA and the increasing technical possibilities of immune intervention proven to be effective in experimental animal work have resulted in the initiation of a variety of early studies in RA. The induction of tolerance for autoantigens by means of oral administration of joint-specific antigens[58] or T cell vaccination,[59] which has been successfully used in a number of animal models for autoimmune disease, has been investigated in RA. The available data do not suggest a clear therapeutic potential in RA, although a subgroup of patients might respond to this type of treatment. Further investigations, including controlled double-blind trials, are necessary to substantiate the reported treatment effects. Other potential strategies such as stem cell transplantation, blood transfusion, administration of human leukocyte antigen peptides, intravenous immunoglobulin administration, or adsorption are in the same stage of early development.

## SUMMARY AND CONCLUSION

The concept of a targeted therapy that could affect one or more specific pathologic processes in RA has enormous implications for the future. Heretofore, all the available therapies have been truly nonspecific, often borrowed from other disciplines (e.g., oncology, infectious diseases) and containing side effect profiles that limit their usefulness. With the new biologic agents on the horizon, several questions need to be addressed before their true role can be clarified:

1. Although immediately effective, will these new drugs continue to exert the same effect over time?
2. Do these agents have the capacity to modify (i.e., prevent structural damage) the course of the disease?
3. In spite of a good safety record before regulatory registration, will the promise of no effect on susceptibility to infection and/or malignancy-causing potential be realized over the long term?
4. Why do some patients respond and others not respond to these agents? Is there a biologic explanation for this diversity?
5. How can the large up-front cost of these agents be justified in terms of impact on the disease process and certainly in comparison with money spent on treatments for other chronic illnesses?
6. Which patients should be selected for these agents: those most in need (with the highest risk) of disease modification, or those with the most devastating symptoms?
7. If questions 1 to 6 are answered, should these agents be given to selected patients as initial therapy, or should they be given to patients who do not respond to single agents or to their combination?

Although these questions are challenging and in many ways not yet answered by the available data, they do represent the conundrum in facing the utility of these new agents. Currently the new drugs (etanercept, infliximab) are approved by the US Food and Drug Administration for patients in whom either a single agent has failed or the disease is insufficiently controlled by standard therapy such as methotrexate. Whether this will change in the near future is unknown.

RA is a severe disease necessitating new therapies because many patients fail to respond to established treatment. The most promising therapies at present include products of biotechnology, particularly the parenterally administered TNF binding proteins and anti–TNF-$\alpha$ antibodies. These therapies, which have become available for the therapeutic armamentarium of the rheumatologist, may certainly be seen as breakthroughs in the treatment of RA and in understanding its pathogenesis. It is expected that these biologic agents will not remain the only tools for achieving a decreased disease activity or decreased destruction. Alternative strategies are being studied intensively. Also, TNF blockade needs much more study. The optimization of TNF blockade through increasing experience and extended careful surveillance of patients should ensure anticytokine agents a pivotal place in the therapy for RA.

# REFERENCES

1. Dayer JM, Arend WP: Cytokines and growth factors. *In* Kelley WN, Harris ED, Ruddy S, et al (eds): Textbook of Rheumatology, 5th ed. Philadelphia: WB Saunders, 1998:267.
2. Feldmann M, Elliott MJ, Woody JN, et al: Anti-tumor necrosis factor-alpha therapy of rheumatoid arthritis. Adv Immunol 1997; 64:310.
3. Keffer J, Probert L, Cazlaris H, et al: Transgenic mice expressing human tumor necrosis factor: A predictive model of arthritis. EMBO 1991; 10:4025.
4. Williams RO, Feldmann M, Maini RN: Anti-tumor necrosis factor ameliorates joint disease in murine collagen induced arthritis. Proc Natl Acad Sci U S A 1992; 89:9784.
5. Vreugdenhill G, Lowenberg B, Van Eijk HG, et al: TNF alpha is associated with disease activity and the degree of anemia in patients with rheumatoid arthritis. Eur J Clin Invest 1992; 22:488.
6. Elliott MJ, Maini RN, Feldmann M, et al: Treatment of rheumatoid arthritis with chimeric monoclonal antibodies to tumor necrosis factor alpha. Arthritis Rheum 1993; 36:1681.
7. Elliott MJ, Maini RN, Feldmann M, et al: Randomised double-blind comparison of chimeric monoclonal antibody to tumour necrosis factor alpha (cA2) versus placebo in rheumatoid arthritis. Lancet 1994; 344:1105.
8. Elliott MJ, Maini RN, Feldmann M, et al: Repeated therapy with monoclonal antibody to tumour necrosis factor alpha (cA2) in patients with rheumatoid arthritis. Lancet 1994; 344:1125.
9. Rankin ECC, Choy EHS, Kassimos D, et al: The therapeutic effect of an engineered anti-TNF antibody (CDP571) in rheumatoid arthritis. Br J Rheumatol 1995; 34:334.
10. Maini RN, Breedveld FC, Kalden JR, et al: Therapeutic efficacy of multiple intravenous infusions of anti–tumor necrosis factor α monoclonal antibody combined with low-dose weekly methotrexate in rheumatoid arthritis. Arthritis Rheum 1998; 41:1552.
10a. Maini R, St Clair EW, Breedveld F, et al: Infliximab (chimeric anti–tumour necrosis factor α monoclonal antibody) versus placebo in rheumatoid arthritis patients receiving concomitant methotrexate: a randomized phase III trial. Lancet 1999; 354:1932.
10b. Lipsky P, St Clair W, Furst D, et al: 54 Week clinical and radiographic results for the Attrack trial: A phase III study of infliximab (Remicade) in patients with active RA despite methotrexate. Arthritis Rheum 1999; 42(suppl 9):S401.
11. Moreland LW, Margolies G, Heck LW Jr, et al: Recombinant soluble tumor necrosis factor receptor (p80) fusion protein: Toxicity and dose finding trial in refractory rheumatoid arthritis. J Rheumatol 1996; 23:1849.
12. Moreland LW, Baumgartner SW, Schiff MH, et al: Treatment of rheumatoid arthritis with a recombinant human tumor necrosis factor receptor (p75)–Fc fusion protein. N Engl J Med 1997; 337:141.
13. Moreland LW, Schiff MH, Baumgartner SW, et al: Etanercept therapy in rheumatoid arthritis. Ann Intern Med 1999; 130:478.
14. Weinblatt ME, Kremer JM, Bankhurst AD, et al: A trial of etanercept, a recombinant tumor necrosis factor receptor:Fc fusion protein, in patients with rheumatoid arthritis receiving methotrexate. N Engl J Med 1999; 340:253.
15. Moreland LM, Cohen SB, Baumgartner M, et al: Long-term use of etanercept in patients with DMARD-refractory rheumatoid arthritis. Arthritis Rheum 1999; 42(suppl 9):S401.
15a. Weinblatt ME, Kremer JM, Lange M, et al: Long-term safety and efficacy of combination therapy with methotrexate (MTX) and etanercept (Enbrel). Arthritis Rheum 1999; 42(suppl 9):S401.
15b. Lovell DJ, Giannini EH, Reiff A, et al: Etanercept in children with polyarticular juvenile rheumatoid arthritis. N Engl J Med 1999; 342:763.
15c. Finck B, Martin R, Fleischmann R, et al: A phase III trial of etanercept vs. methotrexate in early rheumatoid arthritis. Arthritis Rheum 1999; 42(suppl 9):S117.
16. Paleolog E: Target effector role of vascular endothelium in the inflammatory response: Insights from the clinical trial of anti-TNF alpha antibody in rheumatoid arthritis. Mol Pathol 1997; 50:225.
17. Tak PP, Taylor PC, Breedveld FC, et al: Reduction in cellularity and expression of adhesion molecules in rheumatoid synovial tissue after anti–TNF-α monoclonal antibody treatment. Arthritis Rheum 1996; 39:1077.
18. Choy EHS, Kassimos D, Kingsley GH, et al: The effect of an engineered human anti–tumour necrosis factor alpha (TNFα) antibody (A6) on interleukin-6 (IL-6) and bone markers in rheumatoid arthritis (RA) patients. Arthritis Rheum 1995; 38:S185.
19. Arend WP, Malyak M, Guthridge CJ, et al: Interleukin-1 receptor antagonist: Role in biology. Annu Rev Immunol 1998; 16:27.
20. Campion GV, Lesback ME, Lookabaugh J, et al: Dose-range and dose-frequency study of recombinant human interleukin-1 receptor antagonist in patients with rheumatoid arthritis. Arthritis Rheum 1996; 39:1092.
21. Drevlow BE, Lovis R, Haag MA, et al: Recombinant human interleukin-1 receptor type I in the treatment of patients with active rheumatoid arthritis. Arthritis Rheum 1996; 39:257.
22. Bresnihan B, Lookabaugh J, Witt K, et al: Treatment with recombinant human interleukin-1 receptor antagonist (rhIL-1ra) in rheumatoid arthritis (RA): Results of a randomized double-blind, placebo-controlled multicenter trial. Arthritis Rheum 1996; 39(suppl 9):S73.
23. Cunnane G, Madigan A, FitzGerald O, et al: Treatment with recombinant human interleukin-1 receptor antagonist (rhIL-1RA) may reduce synovial infiltration in rheumatoid arthritis (RA). Arthritis Rheum 1996; 39:S245.
24. Watt I, Cobby M, Amgen rhIL-1ra Clinical Research Product Team: Recombinant human IL-1 receptor antagonist (rhIL-1ra) reduces the rate of joint erosion in rheumatoid arthritis (RA). Arthritis Rheum 1996; 39(suppl 9):S123.
24a. Cohen S, Hurd E, Cush JJ, et al: Treatment of interleukin-1 receptor antagonist in combination with methotrexate (MTX) in rheumatoid arthritis (RA) patients. Arthritis Rheum 1999; 42(suppl 9):S273.
25. Yoshizaki K, Nishimoto N, Mihara M, et al: Therapy of rheumatoid arthritis by blocking IL-6 signal transduction with a humanized anti–IL-6 receptor antibody. Springer Semin Immunopathol 1998; 20:247.
26. Sugiyama E, Kuroda A, Taki H, et al: Interleukin 10 cooperates with interleukin 4 to suppress inflammatory cytokine production by freshly prepared adherent rheumatoid synovial cells. J Rheumatol 1995; 22:2020.
27. Chomarat P, Vannier E, Dechanet J, et al: Balance of IL-1 receptor antagonist/IL-1 beta in rheumatoid synovium and its regulation by IL-4 and IL-l0. J Immunol 1995; 154:1432.
28. Van Roon JAG, Van Roy JLAM, Gmelig-Meyling FHJ, et al: Prevention and reversal of cartilage degradation in rheumatoid arthritis by interleukin-10 and interleukin-4. Arthritis Rheum 1996; 39:829.
29. Walmsley M, Katsikis PD, Abney E, et al: Interleukin-10 inhibition of the progression of established collagen-induced arthritis. Arthritis Rheum 1996; 39:495.
30. Joosten LAB, Lubberts E, Durez P, et al: Role of interleukin-4 and interleukin-10 in murine collagen–induced arthritis. Protective effect of interleukin-4 and interleukin-10 treatment on cartilage destruction. Arthritis Rheum 1997; 40:249.
31. Maini R, Paulus H, Breedveld FC, et al: rHUIL-10 in subjects with active rheumatoid arthritis (RA): A phase I and cytokine response study. Arthritis Rheum 1997; 40(suppl 2):S224.

31a. Weinblatt ME, St Clair EW, Breedveld FC, et al: rHUIL-10 (Teno-vil) plus methotrexate (MTX) in active rheumatoid arthritis: A phase I/II study. Arthritis Rheum 1995; 42(suppl 9):S170.

32. Fox DA: The role of T cells in the immunopathogenesis of rheu-matoid arthritis. New perspectives. Arthritis Rheum 1997; 40:598.

33. Van der Lubbe PA, Dijkmans BAC, Markusse HM, et al: A randomized, double-blind, placebo-controlled study of CD4 monoclonal antibody therapy in early rheumatoid arthritis. Ar-thritis Rheum 1995; 38:1097.

34. Moreland LW, Pratt PW, Mayes MD, et al: Double-blind, placebo-controlled multicentre trial using chimeric monoclonal anti-CD4 antibody, cM-T412 in rheumatoid arthritis patients re-ceiving concomitant methotrexate. Arthritis Rheum 1995; 38:1581.

35. Wendling D, Racadot E, Wijdenes J, et al: A randomized, double-blind, placebo-controlled multicenter trial of murine anti-CD4 monoclonal antibody therapy in rheumatoid arthritis. J Rheuma-tol 1998; 25:1457.

36. Tak PP, van der Lubbe PA, Cauli A, et al: Reduction of synovial inflammation after anti-CD4 monoclonal antibody treatment in early rheumatoid arthritis. Arthritis Rheum 1995; 38:1457.

37. Choy, EHS, Pitzalis C, Cauli A, et al: Percentage of anti-CD4 monoclonal antibody–coated lymphocytes in the rheumatoid joint is associated with clinical improvement. Implications for the development of immunotherapeutic dosing regiments. Arthritis Rheum 1996; 39:52.

38. Chu C-Q, Londei M: Induction of Th2 cytokines and control of collagen-induced arthritis by non-depleting anti-CD4 antibodies. J Immunol 1996; 157:2685.

39. Truneh A, MacDonald B, Elliot M, et al: Treatment of rheumatoid arthritis with a primatized® anti-CD4 monoclonal antibody, SB-210396 (IDEC-CE9.1)—Responsiveness correlates with duration of monoclonal antibody coating, CD4 receptor modulation and decrease in number of activated lymphocyte subpopulations. Arthritis Rheum 1997; 40(suppl 9):S191.

40. Yocum DE, Solinger AM, Tesser J, et al: Clinical and immuno-logic effects of a primatized anti-CD4 monoclonal antibody in active rheumatoid arthritis: Results of a phase I, single dose, dose escalating trial. J Rheumatol 1998; 25:1257.

41. Kaine J, Solinger A, Yocum D, et al: Results of a multi-dose protocol 7002 using an immunomodulating, non-depleting primatized anti-CD4 monoclonal antibody in rheumatoid arthri-tis (RA). Arthritis Rheum 1995; 38(suppl 9):S185.

42. Levy R, Weisman M, Wiesenhutter C, et al: Results of a placebo-controlled multicenter trial using a primatized non-depleting, anti-CD4 monoclonal antibody in the treatment of rheumatoid arthritis. Arthritis Rheum 1996; 39(suppl 9):S122.

43. Panayi GS, Choy EHS, Connolly DJA, et al: T cell hypothesis in rheumatoid arthritis (RA) tested by humanized non-depleting anti-CD4 monoclonal antibody (mAb) treatment I: Suppression of disease activity and acute phase response. Arthritis Rheum 1996; 39(suppl 9):S244.

44. Balsa A, Dixey J, Samson DM, et al: Differential expression of the costimulatory molecules B7.1 (CD80) and B7.2 (CD86) in rheumatoid synovial tissue. Br J Rheumatol 1996; 35:33.

45. Sfikakis PP, Zografou A, Viglis V, et al: CD28 expression on T cell subsets in vivo and CD28-mediated T cell response in vitro in patients with rheumatoid arthritis. Arthritis Rheum 1995; 38:649.

46. Linsley PS, Greene JL, Brady W, et al: Human B7-1 (CD80) and B7-2 (CD86) bind with similar avidities but distinct kinetics to CD28 and CTLA-4 receptors. Immunity 1994; 1:793.

47. Young JW, Koulova L, Soergel SA, et al: The B7/BB1 antigen provides one of several costimulatory signals for the activation of CD4+ T lymphocytes by human blood dendritic cells in vitro. J Clin Invest 1992; 90:229.

48. Harding FA, McArthur JG, Gross JA, et al: CD28-mediated sig-naling costimulates murine T cells and prevents induction of anergy in T cell clones. Nature (London) 1992; 356:607.

49. Boussiotis VA, Barber DL, Nakarai T, et al: Prevention of T cell anergy by signaling through the c chain of the IL-2 receptor. Science 1994; 266:1039.

50. Griggs ND, Agersborg SS, Noelle RJ, et al: The relative contribu-tion of the CD28 and gp39 costimulatory pathways in the clonal expansion and pathogenic acquisition of self-reactive T cells. J Exp Med 1996; 183:801.

51. Oppenheimer-Marks N, Lipsky PE: Adhesion molecules as tar-gets for the treatment of autoimmune diseases. Clin Immunol Immunopathol 1996; 79:203.

52. Kavanaugh AF, Cush JJ, St Clair EW, et al: Anti–TNF-alpha monoclonal antibody (mAb) treatment of rheumatoid arthritis (RA) patients with active disease on methotrexate (MTX); results of double-blind, placebo controlled multicenter trial. Arthritis Rheum 1996; 39(suppl 9):S123.

53. Makarov SS, Olsen JC, Johnston WN, et al: Retrovirus-mediated in vivo gene transfer to synovium in bacterial cell wall-induced arthritis in rats. Gene Therapy 1995; 2:424.

54. Otani K, Nita I, Macaulay W, et al: Suppression of antigen-induced arthritis in rabbits by ex vivo gene therapy. J Immunol 1996; 156:3558.

55. Evans CH, Mankin HJ, Ferguson AB, et al: Clinical trial to assess the safety, feasibility, and efficacy of transferring a potentially anti-arthritic cytokine gene to human joints with rheumatoid arthritis. Hum Gene Ther 1996; 7:1261.

56. McCarthy M: Gene therapy for rheumatoid arthritis starts clinical trials. Lancet 1996; 348:323.

57. Ghivizzani SC, Kang R, Muzzonigro T, et al: Gene therapy for arthritis—Treatment of the first three patients. Arthritis Rheum 1997; 40(suppl 9):S223.

58. Kalden JR, Sieper J: Oral collagen in the treatment of rheumatoid arthritis. Arthritis Rheum 1998; 41:191.

59. Moreland LW, Morgan EE, Adamson TC III, et al: T cell receptor peptide vaccination in rheumatoid arthritis. A placebo-controlled trial using a combination of $V_B3$, $V_B14$, and $V_B17$ pep-tides. Arthritis Rheum 1998; 41:1919.

# 19 | Rheumatoid Arthritis

*Mark J. Borigini and Harold E. Paulus*

## NATURAL HISTORY

Rheumatoid arthritis (RA) is a chronic, systemic inflammatory disorder of unknown cause that affects approximately 1% of the world's population.[1] Women are affected two to three times more often than men, but this female preponderance is less impressive when one considers only those patients who are serologically positive for rheumatoid factor and are found to have radiographic evidence of erosive changes of joints.[2] RA can occur at any age; it appears, however, to increase in incidence with advancing age.

There are occasions in which several family members are found to have RA, a greater than expected incidence occurs in monozygotic twins.[3] Studies of the class II gene products (human leukocyte antigen [HLA]-DR,-DQ,-DP) of the major histocompatibility complex have shown that susceptibility to RA is influenced by the immune response genes.[4] HLA-DR4 is the primary susceptibility haplotype in most ethnic groups (black Americans being an exception).[5] Although the relative risk of developing RA is several times greater in DR4 individuals, only a minority are affected. In fact, a significant number of patients with RA have a haplotype other than DR4. Monoclonal antibodies have defined an epitope present on several different classes of HLA-D that confers a higher relative risk for the development of RA. Because class II molecules are involved in antigen presentation, it is possible that further analysis will lead to identification of an infectious or chemical antigen that may be responsible for the development of RA.

Although RA is characterized largely by the manner in which it involves joints, in most patients symptoms begin as gradually increasing malaise and fatigue, likely to be accompanied by diffuse musculoskeletal pain. Joint involvement is appreciated as pain, tenderness, swelling, and redness. Symmetry is characteristic, most commonly involving the joints of the hands, wrists, elbows, and shoulders, but also involving the knees, ankles, and feet: virtually any diarthrodial joint can be affected.[6]

Inactivity such as sleep or prolonged sitting is often followed by stiffness. In fact, the duration of morning stiffness is one measure of the activity of RA. The stiffness—and pain—may increase as the disease progresses, often limiting the patient's ability to perform basic activities of daily living. Other systemic manifestations may include weight loss, depression, and low-grade fever.[2]

In about 20% of patients the onset of RA is acute. Frequently, disease activity is at first intermittent; with the passage of time it becomes more sustained. Some patients may have no more than a few months of discomfort; others become severely disabled. Spontaneous remission is not likely, however, if disease has been continuous for 2 or more years.

Continued articular inflammation results in progressive joint destruction, deformity, and subsequent incapacitation, each to varying degrees. Extra-articular features such as rheumatoid nodules, vasculitis, neuropathy, scleritis, pericarditis, lymphadenopathy, and splenomegaly are other manifestations that are most often associated with more aggressive, rheumatoid factor–positive disease.[7] An individual patient may manifest any or all of these clinical features at any given time.

An analysis of patients with RA monitored prospectively for 6 years showed that 18% had at least one remission; the remission periods comprised 35% of the follow-up period for those in remission, and the mean length of remission was 10 months.[8] Developing rheumatoid arthritis after 60 years of age or being male was found to increase the probability of remission. On the other hand, early development of erosions decreased the probability of remission.

The median life expectancy in established RA is less than in control populations. A 25-year prospective study showed that median life expectancy was shortened by 7 years in men and 3 years in women.[9] Another study showed that 48% of patients were without disability at the onset of the survey period; after 12 years this figure had declined to 17%.[10] At the study's initiation 3% were completely disabled; this increased to 16% at the end of 12 years. Disability developed most rapidly during the first 2 years of disease, progressing less rapidly in subsequent years. Factors that influenced outcome included older age, functional class, radiographic grade, and female sex. Patients with an insidious onset of disease appear to do less well than those with an acute onset.[11]

Potentially morbid complications that may occur in later stages of the disease include atlantoaxial subluxation, cricoarytenoid synovitis, and sepsis of involved joints. Those extra-articular complications that potentially may result in mortality include Felty's syndrome (possible life-threatening infection), Sjögren's syndrome, cardiopulmonary complications, systemic vasculitis, gastrointestinal complications of treatment, amyloidosis, and infection.[12] Chronic inanition and debilitation may increase the risk of death from all causes. Increased mortality associated with RA is equivalent to that of Hodgkin's disease, diabetes mellitus, or stroke (age-adjusted).[13] The education level of patients is reported to be inversely proportional to mortality.[14]

Seropositivity for rheumatoid factor has been associated with a poorer prognosis in RA.[15] These patients have a greater number of involved joints and develop more erosions and greater ligamentous instability.[16] Rheumatoid nodules occur almost solely in patients seropositive for rheumatoid factor, and patients with such nodules have a poorer outcome and more frequent erosions.[16]

# REST

Most would agree that the main objectives in the management of RA should include relief of pain, reduction of inflammation, preservation of muscle strength and joint function, prevention of joint damage, and maintenance of as normal a lifestyle as possible, while minimizing side effects from treatment. All patients should be taught the most basic treatment of joint inflammation: adequate rest.

Whole-body rest can decrease the general systemic inflammatory response; in addition, local rest of an inflamed joint protects the joint to permit repair. Exercise of an inflamed joint is proinflammatory; splinting of a joint is anti-inflammatory (although one must use caution with this practice; initially, splints can increase the sensation of joint stiffness and its duration).[17] When a patient with RA experiences a stroke, the rheumatoid joints on the paralyzed side lose their inflammation. The prescription of rest should be accompanied by the caution that the level of physical activity should not be immediately increased as joint inflammation decreases.

Patients often discover that the fatigue that occurs in the midafternoon can be significantly reduced by a nap. This aids patients in coping with the remainder of the day. A regularly disciplined afternoon nap can be an effective part of any treatment program. Acute exacerbations of disease may require longer periods of rest in bed to suppress the inflammatory process. Nevertheless, full range of motion of joints should be maintained by a graded exercise program.

McCarty suggested that upper extremity joints be rested by splinting for 3 weeks after intra-articular corticosteroid injection. However, the splint should be removed and one full range of motion performed daily in each joint in the fingers and wrists. For joints of the lower extremity, he advises patients to avoid weight-bearing for 8 weeks after the injection. A controlled study showed that 88% of upper extremity joints remained free of inflammation for almost 2 years after local injection of triamcinolone administered in this manner.[18]

# DRUG THERAPY

## Nonsteroidal Anti-inflammatory Drugs

The choice of drug therapy for RA today is more often than not determined by the degree of disease activity, the apparent disease severity, and the adverse effects of the drugs. For example, explosive polyarticular disease with severe systemic symptoms, early extra-articular signs (e.g., serositis, episcleritis), and nodules suggests aggressive disease. Although in most patients the pattern of disease severity is established during the first year, activity can wax and wane over time. Predicting a disease course or eventual outcome may be possible for groups or large numbers of subjects in an epidemiologic study; in an individual patient, it is not so easy. Therefore, careful initial and periodic follow-up assessments are necessary in administering an appropriate drug program.

The traditional approach to the treatment of RA is to begin with symptomatic treatment of inflammation using salicylates or other nonsteroidal anti-inflammatory drugs (NSAIDs) in addition to rest and corticosteroid injections (as needed). As the severity of the disease progresses, the clinician progresses up the "therapeutic pyramid" to drugs that are more effective but possibly more toxic. Much time may be spent at the "base" of the pyramid, prescribing several NSAIDs in sequence in the hope that the patient may undergo a spontaneous remission of disease activity. The assumption of the pyramid approach is that all patients will receive the "basic" therapy and fewer patients will receive more aggressive therapy at a later date. This approach has been challenged, and disease-modifying antirheumatic drugs (DMARDs) such as methotrexate frequently are started as soon as the diagnosis is made (see Treatment Strategies).

By impairing the activity of various natural mediators of inflammation such as bradykinins, prostaglandins, and oxygen radicals, NSAIDs partially impair the final expression of inflammation. Because they act on terminal events in the inflammatory cascade, the benefits of these drugs are quickly evident. However, these drugs do not fully prevent tissue injury, so it is not surprising that joint damage and other evidence of organ damage may progress during therapy. Sustained drug-induced remission usually is not expected with these short-acting antirheumatic agents, which act distally in the inflammatory cascade.

NSAIDs reduce but do not completely eliminate the signs and symptoms of established inflammation. The presence of drug in the blood is associated with a rapid onset of benefit, but exacerbation of signs and symptoms occurs quickly after metabolism or excretion of the drug. NSAIDs have no major effect on the underlying RA disease process. In addition to their anti-inflammatory effects, NSAIDs decrease pain, suppress fever, and decrease platelet adhesiveness, leading to a multitude of short-term and long-term prescribed and nonprescribed uses. In the United States, available NSAIDs include aspirin, salicylsalicylate, magnesium choline salicylate, other salicylates, ibuprofen, phenylbutazone, indomethacin, sulindac, naproxen, tolmetin, fenoprofen, meclofenamate sodium, diflunisal, piroxicam, ketoprofen, diclofenac, flurbiprofen, etodolac, ketorolac, nabumetone, oxaprozin, rofecoxib, and celecoxib (Table 19–1). Many others are under development or available elsewhere.[19]

Most NSAIDs are organic acids and are highly bound to plasma proteins. (Nabumetone, however, is a nonacidic prodrug that is metabolized to an active organic acid.) These properties may enhance drug concentrations in inflamed tissues, which are more permeable to plasma proteins and tend to have a lower pH. Although their chemical structures differ somewhat, the clinical usefulness of available NSAIDs does not relate to their chemical class. It is more useful to remember their plasma half-life, which is related to the frequency of administration and in some instances to the occurrence of adverse reactions, especially in the elderly. NSAIDs have a broad range of pharmacologic activities; they are able to inhibit cyclooxygenase, the enzyme that transforms arachidonic acid via endoperoxides to prostaglandins, prostacyclin, and thromboxanes. Currently available drugs have little direct effect on lipoxygenase, which transforms arachidonic acid to leukotrienes. (Diclofenac has an indirect inhibitory effect on lipoxygenase by stimulating uptake of arachidonic acid into triglycerides.) NSAIDs also have been shown to suppress bradykinin release, alter lymphocyte responses, and limit granulocyte and monocyte migration and phagocytosis under certain laboratory conditions.[19]

## Selective Cyclooxygenase-2 Inhibitors

There are two isoenzymes of cyclooxygenase: COX-1 and COX-2. COX-1 is constitutively present in many tissues; it enables the physiologic production of homeostatic and cytoprotective prostanoids in the gastric mucosa, endothelium, platelets, and kidney. Inhibition of COX-1 is responsible for many of the adverse effects of NSAIDs. COX-2 is expressed by stimulated cells; stimuli such as mitogens, endotoxin, and certain cytokines induce COX-2 in leukocytes, rheumatoid synoviocytes, and vascular smooth muscle cells to produce proinflammatory prostaglandins. COX-2 is also present constitutively in the brain and kidney.[19] Except for rofecoxib and celecoxib, all of the NSAIDs listed in Table 19–1 inhibit both COX-1 and COX-2 at therapeutic doses. Celecoxib and rofecoxib are the first of a new

## TABLE 19–1
## Nonsteroidal Antiinflammatory Drugs used in Rheumatoid Arthritis

| DRUG | DOSE RANGE (MG/D) | HALF-LIFE (H) | COMMENTS |
|---|---|---|---|
| **Salicylates** | | | |
| Aspirin (acetylsalicylic acid) | 1000–6000 | 4–15 | |
| **Nonacetylated Salicylates** | | | |
| Magnesium choline salicylate | 1500–4000 | 4–15 | Decreased effect on platelets, gastric musosa, and (to a |
| Salsalate | 1500–5000 | 4–15 | certain extent) prostaglandin-mediated renal function |
| Sodium salicylate | 3000–5000 | 4–15 | |
| **Short Serum Half-Life NSAIDs** | | | |
| Diclofenac sodium | 75–150 | 2 | Higher incidence of liver function test abnormalities |
| Fenoprofen calcium | 1200–3200 | 2 | Rarely associated with acute T cell–mediated interstitial nephritis with renal failure |
| Flurbiprofen | 100–300 | 3–4 | |
| Ibuprofen | 1200–3200 | 2 | |
| Ketoprofen | 100–400 | 2 | |
| Meclofenamate sodium | 200–400 | 2–3 | Associated with a higher incidence of severe diarrhea |
| Tolmetin sodium | 800–1600 | 1 | Because there is less hepatobiliary recirculation, may cause less gastrointestinal toxicity in the elderly |
| **Long Serum Half-Life NSAIDs** | | | |
| Celecoxib | 200–400 | 11 | Selective COX-2 inhibitor (see text) |
| Diflunisal | 500–1500 | 7–15 | Although a derivative of the salicylates, it does not break down in the body to actually form a salicylate |
| Indomethacin | 50–200 | 3–11 | |
| Nabumetone | 1000–2000 | 24 | Nonacidic prodrug with active acidic metabolite |
| Naproxen | 750–1500 | 13 | |
| Oxaprozin | 600–1200 | 21–25 | |
| Phenylbutazone | 200–800 | 40–80 | |
| Piroxicam | 20 | 30–86 | |
| Sulindac | 300–400 | 16 | Associated with a lower incidence of prostaglandin-mediated renal insufficiency |

COX-2 = cyclooxygenase-2; NSAIDs, nonsteroidal anti-inflammtory drugs.

generation of selective COX-2 inhibitors that inhibit COX-2 at concentrations several hundred-fold to thousand-fold lower than those required to inhibit COX-1. At therapeutic doses, the homeostatic prostaglandins that help to prevent gastric mucosal inflammation and enhance platelet coagulation are not suppressed. Therefore, the selective COX-2 inhibitors should not induce gastritis, peptic ulcer disease, or gastrointestinal bleeding and do not produce platelet anticoagulation. In RA clinical trials, the efficacy of celecoxib, 200 mg twice daily, was superior to that of placebo and equivalent to naproxen, 500 mg twice daily, or diclofenac, 75 mg twice daily, but the incidence of endoscopically observed gastroduodenal ulcers was lower and almost equivalent to that of placebo. However, in acute pain studies, single doses were less effective than naproxen sodium, 550 mg, or ibuprofen, 400 mg.[20]

Other highly selective COX-2 inhibitors are under intensive development. In view of Fries' estimate[21] that NSAID-induced gastropathy is responsible for 76,000 hospitalizations and 7600 deaths each year in the United States, from a public health viewpoint selective COX-2 inhibitors should replace the older mixed COX-1/COX-2–inhibiting NSAIDs. However, it is not yet clear that their efficacy in clinical practice will be equal to or better than current NSAIDs for individual patients. Clinical experience will determine the relative roles of the older NSAIDs and the selective COX-2 inhibitors.

## Nonselective Cyclooxygenase-1 and -2 Inhibitors

Although the standard NSAIDs are generally well tolerated, they are associated with a wide spectrum of potential clinical toxicities. Aspirin is the most difficult to use effectively, has more frequent side effects, and is more dangerous if overdoses are taken. Side effects tend to be dose related.[22] Because NSAIDs suppress prostaglandin synthesis, gastric acid production is increased; also, the production of gastric mucus and bicarbonate is decreased, as is the rate of cellular proliferation of the gastric mucosa, impairing the normal protective mechanisms of the stomach and causing gastric irritation and the exacerbation of peptic ulcers. If gastrointestinal bleeding occurs, it is worsened, because NSAIDs decrease platelet adhesiveness and increase acid production in the stomach. Firmly compressed aspirin tablets may dissolve slowly in the stomach, causing irritation and superficial ulceration of the gastric mucosa directly under the undissolved tablet. Ion trapping of weak organic acids such as NSAIDs in mucosal cells leads to back-diffusion of hydrogen ions and may result in mucosal damage.

NSAIDs may produce two types of anticoagulant effects. First, COX-1 inhibition decreases platelet adhesiveness by inhibiting a prostaglandin-initiated sequence that is necessary for platelet activation. Because platelets lack mitochondria and are unable to synthesize additional cyclooxygenase, acetylation of this enzyme by aspirin irreversibly decreases platelet aggregation in response to various stimuli. This effect persists for about 10 to 12 days until the acetylated platelets are replaced by new platelets that have not been exposed to aspirin. In contrast, cyclooxygenase inhibition by other NSAIDs is reversible, their platelet effects persisting only as long as the drug is present. The second type of anticoagulant effect occurs when protein-bound NSAIDs displace warfarin from plasma protein–binding sites, thus increasing warfarin's anticoagulant effect, a mechanism significant only for phenylbutazone and for salicylates in toxic concentrations.

Reversible hepatocellular toxicity, characterized by elevations of one or more liver enzymes, has been observed in up to 15% of patients treated with NSAIDs.[23, 24] Transaminase elevations usually revert to normal after discontinuation of the drug and sometimes become normal even when the drug is continued. Rarely, hepatic dysfunction is severe and necessitates discontinuation of the drug. Fatal fulminant hepatitis occurs rarely; transaminase levels should be checked on a regular basis during treatment, especially after a change of NSAID or increase in dose.

NSAIDs may decrease creatinine clearance and increase serum creatinine in some patients predisposed by hypovolemia, impaired renal function, or decreased renal blood flow, probably by suppressing the vasodilatory regulatory function of renal prostaglandins. NSAIDs should be used with caution in patients with conditions that impair renal perfusion or function, in those with decreased circulating blood volume, and in the elderly. Acute interstitial nephritis and the nephrotic syndrome rarely occur with NSAIDs; most patients recover when the drug is discontinued, but occasionally dialysis or high-dose corticosteroid therapy is needed to support patients before recovery of renal function.[24]

Other adverse effects include a variety of skin reactions and rashes.[22] Hypersensitivity responses include an aspirin-associated syndrome of rhinitis, nasal polyposis, and asthma. Anaphylaxis has been associated with NSAID use, as have agranulocytosis and aplastic anemia. The latter two are more frequent with phenylbutazone but may also occur rarely with other NSAIDs. Celecoxib is chemically related to the sulfa drugs; it should not be used by persons who are allergic to sulfa.

Salicylates cause blood level–related tinnitus and hearing loss; overdoses can cause a variety of central nervous system manifestations including coma. Headaches occur with indomethacin, and confusion may appear in elderly patients treated with indomethacin, naproxen, or ibuprofen. Although reported more commonly in patients with lupus, aseptic meningitis has occurred in normal subjects treated with ibuprofen, sulindac, or other NSAIDs.

Generally speaking, NSAIDs are completely absorbed shortly after oral administration, unless enteric-coated or sustained-release forms are used. Aspirin, nabumetone, and sulindac have active metabolites with longer half-lives than the parent drugs. Indomethacin, meclofenamate sodium, and sulindac display enterohepatic recirculation. Some metabolites of salicylate and diflunisal exhibit Michaelis-Menten kinetics;

the plasma half-life of the drug increases as the plasma concentration increases. It follows that doses need to be given less frequently when plasma concentrations are high; toxic concentrations take much longer to clear than would be anticipated. The prodrug, nabumetone, is a poor inhibitor of prostaglandin synthesis but is rapidly transformed by the liver to an acidic metabolite with potent inhibitory effects. Virtually all available NSAIDs are eventually converted by the liver to inactive metabolites that are excreted predominantly in urine and bile; however, sulindac may also be converted to an inactive metabolite by the kidney.[19]

It is important to individualize treatment with aspirin and NSAIDs. Substantial individual variability is present with respect to the pharmacology and pharmacokinetics of these drugs, which also vary in effectiveness. Patients with RA usually need prolonged treatment with maximum tolerated doses. Whereas aspirin has a long history of efficacy in the treatment of RA, the agent's side effects, with gastrointestinal distress most prominent, make it intolerable for many patients in the doses required for efficacy. Enteric-coated aspirin preparations somewhat relieve these gastric symptoms. The nonacetylated salicylates have fewer of the side effects that are typically associated with NSAID-induced suppression of prostaglandin production. With all forms of salicylates, it is important to use sufficient amounts to achieve a clinical response. Doses can be adjusted by monitoring serum salicylate levels (a therapeutic level being 20 to 30 mg/dL) during the first 2 to 4 weeks of therapy.[25] Occasional monitoring after 1 to 2 months is also appropriate, because increased metabolism that is caused by the salicylate itself can decrease salicylate levels by 15% to 20%.[26] The nonacetylated salicylates have a prolonged serum half-life at anti-inflammatory concentrations, and studies have shown that they are as effective anti-inflammatory medications as aspirin in patients with RA.[27] Nonacetylated salicylates (except sodium salicylate) are more expensive than aspirin, but they have the advantage of being 25 to 50 times less potent than aspirin as prostaglandin synthetase inhibitors and therefore may be useful in patients with bleeding tendencies or possibly in patients with compromised renal function.[27] They may also have an advantage in patients with a history of NSAID-induced asthma or nasal polyposis, because a correlation exists between potency as a cyclooxygenase inhibitor and induction of asthma (but the first dose should be given under close supervision).[27] Despite the availability of salicylate levels for monitoring purposes, the clinician must remain vigilant for side effects such as hearing loss (mostly in the elderly) and the other laboratory and clinical abnormalities mentioned earlier.

Obviously, the selection of a particular agent depends on a patient's medical history (e.g., history of gastrointestinal bleeding or intolerance) and on the personal preference and previous experience of the prescribing physician and the patient. If the patient has insufficient benefit or intolerable toxicity to a specific NSAID, another NSAID is often substituted, initially at a moderate dose to establish tolerance. (The average RA patient tries more than three NSAIDs before finding the one that is most satisfactory.[28]) The dose is then carefully increased to the maximal dose recommended or tolerated, and continued for at least 2 weeks.[29] The biologic effects of NSAIDs do not depend directly on serum levels but rather on tissue concentrations and the effect that these concentrations have on the inflammatory process. Because these latter effects may require days to appear, a delay can be expected between kinetic equilibrium and maximum clinical response. There is little evidence to suggest that combinations of salicylates and NSAIDs, or one NSAID with another, are more beneficial than full-dose single drug therapy, whereas toxicity is probably additive.[30]

Caution is advised in prescribing NSAIDs to the elderly; to patients with peptic ulcer disease, impairment of renal or hepatic function, dehydration, congestive heart failure, or hypertension; and to those being treated with anticoagulants, oral hypoglycemics, or other drugs that may interact with the NSAID. Because these conditions are frequent in hospitalized patients, great care should be taken when NSAIDs are given to such patients. It should be recalled that any side effect related to serum concentration will be prolonged with those drugs that have a prolonged serum half-life.[22]

Patients should be monitored particularly closely during introduction of an NSAID, when doses are increased, or when the patient's condition changes. Although prostaglandin-mediated or hypersensitivity-mediated renal failure is rare and abnormal liver function tests are uncommon with NSAIDs, it is recommended to check baseline serum creatinine, hemoglobin levels, and liver function tests before starting a new NSAID. It is reasonable to repeat these tests every 2 to 4 weeks for the first 3 to 4 months. Renal function and liver function abnormalities are relatively rare in an uncomplicated case after an NSAID has been used for several months.

Even optimal use of NSAIDs does not completely suppress all evidence of inflammation, particularly in chronic RA. If a spontaneous remission does not develop within a reasonable time, a second-line antirheumatic drug should be added to the continuing maximal NSAID therapy.

## Disease-Modifying Antirheumatic Drugs

The term *DMARDs* refers to a group of medications with diverse mechanisms of action. Other names for these drugs are slow-acting antirheumatic drugs, remission-inducing drugs, and second-line antirheumatic agents. They have traditionally been used when the disease is not responding to NSAIDs and other conservative treatment modalities. DMARDs include gold compounds, chloroquine or hydroxychloroquine, sulfasalazine, D-penicillamine, azathioprine, and methotrexate (Table 19–2), as well as cyclosporine leflunomide, and tumor necrosis factor (TNF) inhibitors such as etanercept and infliximab. They have been demonstrated to produce additional clinical benefit when added to continuing stable background NSAID use and low-dose corticosteroid therapy. DMARDs dif-

**TABLE 19–2**
**Disease-Modifying Antirheumatic Drugs Commonly in Use in the United States**

| DRUG | DOSE | EFFICACY | TOXICITY Treatment-Limiting | TOXICITY Life-Threatening | MONITORING (AUTHORS' RECOMMENDATIONS) |
|---|---|---|---|---|---|
| Methotrexate | 7.5–25 mg PO or IM once weekly | +++ | ++ | Hepatic fibrosis, acute interstitial pneumonia, bone marrow suppression | Baseline chest radiograph and hepatitis B, C serologies; CBC every 2–4 wk for 4 mo, then every 4 wk; Liver function tests every 4–8 wk; Creatinine levels every 4–8 wk |
| Sulfasalazine | 500–3000 mg/d PO | +++ | +++ | Bone marrow suppression | Baseline G6PD; CBC every 2 wk for 8 wk, then monthly for 6 mo, then every 2–3 mo; Liver function tests every 2–3 mo |
| Gold sodium thiomalate | Start with 10, 25, and then 50 mg/wk IM | +++ | +++++ | Aplastic anemia, thrombocytopenia, pneumonitis | CBC and urinalysis before each injection; Liver function tests and creatinine levels every 3 mo |
| D-Penicillamine | 250 mg/d PO for 4–6 wk, then 500–750 mg/d | +++ | +++++ | Aplastic anemia, thrombocytopenia, obliterative bronchiolitis, polymyositis | CBC and urine protein levels every 1–2 wk for 6 mo, then monthly; Liver function tests and creatinine levels every 1–3 mo |
| Hydroxychloroquine sulfate | 400 mg/d PO | ++ | + | Rare | Ophthalmologic examination (baseline, then every 6 mo) |
| Azathioprine | 2–2.5 mg/kg/d (100–150 mg/d, PO) | ++ | +++ | Probable twofold increase in the relative risk of inducing non-Hodgkin's lymphoma | CBC every 1–2 wk for 2 mo, then every other week for 2–4 mo, then every 2–4 wk, liver function tests and creatinine levels every 3 mo |
| Auranofin | 3 mg PO BID | + | ++ | Rare | CBC and urine protein levels every 2–4 wk; Liver function tests every 1–2 mo |
| Cyclosporine | 2.5–4 mg/kg/d PO | ++ | ++ | Renal dysfunction Hypertension | Creatinine every 2 wk for 3 mo, then monthly; Decrease dose if creatinine increases ≥ 30% above baseline |
| Leflunomide | Loading dose: 100 mg/d × 3 d; Maintenance: 20 mg/d | +++ | ++ | New drug; uncertain | Same as methotrexate |
| Etanercept | 25 mg SC twice a week | ++++ | + | New drug; withdraw for major infections | Clinical assessment every 1 to 3 mo |
| Infliximab | 3 mg/kg IV at weeks 0, 2, 6, and then q 8 weeks | ++++ | + | New drug; withdraw for major infections | Clinical assessment every 1–2 months; Always use with concomitant methotrexate |

CBC = complete blood count; G6PD = glucose-6-phosphate dehydrogenase.

Data for efficacy and toxicity estimates from Felson DT, Anderson JJ, Meenan RF. The comparative efficacy and toxicity of second-line drugs in rheumatoid arthritis. Arthritis Rheum 1990; 33:1449 *and* Felson DT, Angerson JJ, Meenan RF. Use of short-term efficacy/toxicity tradeoffs to select second-line agents in rheumatoid arthritis. Arthritis Rheum 1992; 35:1117.

fer from NSAIDs in their usually delayed onset of action and lack of analgesia. They appear to act more proximally on the inflammatory process, perhaps on the immunologic initiators of tissue injury but without actually removing the basic cause of disease. They often affect laboratory tests that measure acute-phase reactants such as C-reactive protein and erythrocyte sedimentation rate and sometimes affect immunoglobulins and rheumatoid factor. Perhaps because their proximal effects take considerable time to influence the intermediate and distal sites of inflammation, it takes weeks or months of DMARD treatment before clinical benefit is recognized, although TNF inhibition may produce recognizable benefit within 24 to 48 hours in some patients. However, they most often only moderate the disease process; some level of chronic inflammation usually persists. Even if a drug-induced remission does occur, it is likely that the disease will recur—with a delay of weeks to months—after the drug is discontinued. Although the phenomenon is not well understood, the disease may be exacerbated even when the drug is being maintained at the same dose. DMARDs may slow the rate of progression of joint erosions or destruction and disability.[31]

### Gold Compounds

Sulfhydryl-containing organic gold compounds were first used to treat arthritis in the 1920s, and Forestier's enthusiastic report[32] stimulated their use. Their value in RA was established in a double-blind trial that was published by the Empire Rheumatism Council in 1960.[33] Intramuscular gold has been found to be beneficial in about 60% to 80% of patients, with the response beginning in 3 to 6 months.[34] Aurothiomalate and aurothioglucose, water-soluble preparations given by intramuscular injection, are 50% gold by weight. Their administration requires regular office visits to monitor for toxicity and efficacy. The standard injection schedule involves respective test doses of 10 and 25 mg in the first 2 weeks, and then a routine dosage of 25 to 50 mg weekly, assuming tolerance has been established. The orally absorbed gold preparation, auranofin, is lipid soluble, 30% gold by weight, and usually given in a dosage of 6 mg/day.[35]

In the case of both aurothiomalate and auranofin, animal studies indicate that gold and the thiomalate or phosphine portions of the respective molecules dissociate within hours after administration and have different tissue distributions and excretion patterns, suggesting that gold is the pharmacologically effective portion of the molecule.[35] Although the exact mechanism of action has not been definitively established, studies have shown that gold compounds diminish acute and chronic inflammatory responses, acting at many points in the sequence of inflammatory events. They may reduce vascular permeability, reduce cell number at sites of inflammation, suppress phagocytosis, prevent protein denaturation, and suppress both lysosomal and nonlysosomal enzymes. Human lymphocyte responses to mitogens and antigens are inhibited by gold in culture conditions. Monocyte participa-

tion in cell-mediated in vitro responses is impaired by gold.[36] In patients, however, there is no evidence of generalized suppression of either inflammatory responses or cellular and humoral immune responses. Still, gold treatment produces major improvement and occasional remission in some patients with RA and may reduce the progression of joint erosions.

About 35% of patients discontinue gold injections because of side effects.[35] The most common side effects are rash and stomatitis, which occur in 15% to 30% of patients.[35] More serious toxic manifestations include an immune complex–mediated membranous glomerular nephritis in 3% to 7% of patients, leukopenia in 2% to 5%, thrombocytopenia in about 3%, and, rarely, aplastic anemia.[35] A minor degree of proteinuria may require only interruption of the treatment, which can be resumed once the urinalysis is again normal. Nitritoid reaction (flushing sometimes accompanied by transient hypotension) immediately after injection occurs only with aurothiomalate and can be relieved by changing to aurothioglucose.[35] Among drug-induced causes of death in the United Kingdom, gold compounds were a major contributor.[35]

In controlled prospective studies, there were fewer withdrawals for toxicity from auranofin than from aurothiomalate. Dose-related loose stools or diarrhea is a frequent complaint with auranofin and can usually be controlled by decreasing the dose.[35] Although stomatitis and rashes are about equally frequent with oral and injectable gold, proteinuria and hematologic toxicity are less common. However, physicians generally believe that auranofin is less effective than intramuscular preparations.

Routine monitoring of the complete blood count (CBC) and urinalysis is required with parenteral gold. At our institution it is mandatory that these studies be obtained before each injection of gold; however, it is recognized that other rheumatologists use different monitoring schedules. When major clinical benefit occurs, the frequency of injections can be reduced to alternate weeks and then, if benefit persists, to every third or fourth week. There is no maximum time limit to intramuscular gold treatment; it is continued as long as it is tolerated and beneficial. Liver function tests should be checked every 1 to 3 months. A CBC and urinalysis should be performed every 2 to 4 weeks for the patient taking auranofin, and liver function tests should be monitored every 1 to 3 months.[37]

### Methotrexate

The earliest use of an antifolate for the treatment of nonmalignant disease was reported by Gubner who, in 1951, successfully treated patients with RA and psoriatic arthritis with aminopterin.[38] The introduction of steroids in the early 1950s diverted attention away from the use of antifolates in RA. At that time, however, aminopterin's less toxic replacement—methotrexate—was used for the treatment of psoriasis. In a subset of patients with psoriasis, improvement in both skin and joints was observed, but it was not until the 1980s that methotrexate become an acceptable option in the treatment of RA, and during the 1990s it became the DMARD of choice for most RA patients.[39]

A number of clinical trials have provided evidence that methotrexate is effective in RA. It has a significant anti-inflammatory effect within 3 to 4 weeks after starting therapy; it is taken once a week in doses of 7.5 to 25 mg, depending on efficacy and toxic reactions.[40] Weinblatt and associates showed that after 84 months of treatment methotrexate remained effective.[41] Methotrexate may be erratically absorbed from the gastrointestinal tract in some patients, perhaps contributing to a diminished efficacy over time. Switching to a parenteral administration may improve benefit. Experienced clinicians sometimes reduce the dosing interval to 10 or 14 days in stable patients.

In RA patients treated with low doses of methotrexate once a week, inhibition of dihydrofolate reductase is incomplete and perhaps is not essential for efficacy.[42] Because polyglutamates of methotrexate are direct inhibitors of thymidylate synthase and folate-dependent enzymes of purine biosynthesis, efficacy of methotrexate may involve blockade of these pathways. It has been hypothesized that one such blockade alters purine biosynthesis, producing immunosuppression by secondary inhibition of crucial enzymes and perhaps also by decreasing leukotriene production and interleukin-1 expression.[43, 44]

Methotrexate is cleared through the kidneys, so the dosage must be decreased in patients with mild renal insufficiency to offset the higher risk of adverse effects. The drug should not be used for patients with more significant renal insufficiency ($C_{creat}$ less than 60% predicted) or those undergoing dialysis. Reported adverse effects include stomatitis, nausea, vomiting, diarrhea, usually reversible bone marrow suppression, teratogenesis, pulmonary symptoms, and, rarely, liver fibrosis and cirrhosis.[40] Rare pulmonary hypersensitivity reactions (cough, progressive dyspnea, and markedly decreased oxygenation) do occur at the 1% to 2% level and usually improve with prompt discontinuation of the drug[39] and treatment with corticosteroids. Methotrexate may be associated with occasional systemic fungal infections and other unusual infections.

The frequent side effects led one group to conclude that toxicity, rather than lack of efficacy, is the major factor limiting the clinical usefulness of methotrexate. However, 1 mg per day of folate reduced the toxicity experienced with a median weekly dose of 7.5 mg, without altering methotrexate's efficacy, and folate supplementation is now standard, markedly decreasing the frequency of annoying side effects.[42] Risk factors for methotrexate-induced hepatic fibrosis include long duration of treatment with methotrexate, age, and ethanol abuse. Coadministration of an NSAID with higher-dose methotrexate has been rarely associated with leukopenia and thrombocytopenia, perhaps because of an NSAID-induced decrease in glomerular filtration and inhibition of renal tubular secretion of methotrexate, both of which cause a reduction in methotrexate clearance.[40] Methotrexate toxicity may be further diminished by giving folinic acid (leucovorin),

5 mg, 8 to 12 hours after the weekly dose of methotrexate.[40]

## Sulfasalazine

Many physicians use the weaker antifolate, sulfasalazine, for patients with mild RA; it is one of the few drugs originally developed to treat RA.[45] It has been postulated that its mechanism of action may be similar to that of methotrexate. Although several studies have indicated that sulfasalazine is effective for RA, one study was unable to separate sulfasalazine from placebo because of an unusually high placebo response.[45] In controlled clinical trials its efficacy is comparable to methotrexate and leflunomide and somewhat stronger than hydroxychloroquine.

Sulfasalazine is a chemical combination of a salicylate and a sulfa moiety and is therefore contraindicated in patients with sulfa or salicylate allergies. Side effects include headache, gastrointestinal upset, rash, hemolytic disease, leukopenia, reversible depression of sperm count, and rare instances of lupus-like illness.[45] A number of studies have indicated that the rate of discontinuation of sulfasalazine is comparable to (or better than) that of other DMARDs. One study showed a continuation rate at 5 years of 22%.[46] (By way of contrast, the continuation rate of gold injections at 5 years was 8%.) The usual starting dose of sulfasalazine is 500 or 1000 mg/day, slowly raised to 2 or 3 g/day over a 4- to 6-week period—an approach that may decrease the incidence of adverse reactions.[45]

Sulfasalazine is an extremely popular drug in Europe for the treatment of RA. In addition, it is used for HLA-B27–related arthropathies and psoriatic arthritis. It is frequently used in combination with other DMARDs, including methotrexate and hydroxylchloroquine. Monitoring of the CBC is recommended on a regular basis, with more frequent monitoring early in the course of treatment because of the rare occurrence of leukopenia and even agranulocytosis. Efficacy with sulfasalazine is generally noted within 12 weeks with a dose of 2 to 3 g/day. Higher doses are not associated with greater efficacy.

## Antimalarials

Antimalarial agents have been used to treat some rheumatic diseases since the 1800s.[47] In 1951, Page first suggested the use of antimalarial agents in patients with other connective tissue diseases, describing remission of "associated rheumatoid arthritis" in his series of patients.[47] Efficacy in RA was shown in several double-blind, placebo-controlled trials that were done in the 1950s and 1960s with chloroquine hydrochloride.[48] Many controlled and uncontrolled trials of hydroxychloroquine have been conducted, with varying results. Some have suggested that hydroxychloroquine is as effective as gold, D-penicillamine, or azathioprine.[48] The meta-analyses by Felson and colleagues[49] suggested that antimalarial drugs have a better risk/benefit ratio than azathioprine or auranofin.

Hydroxychloroquine is probably the least toxic DMARD. It is a member of the quinolone group of drugs, and the dosage is usually 400 mg/day orally.[47] It is well absorbed and extensively distributed into the tissues, with high concentrations in liver, lung, kidney, heart, and pigmented tissue. Excretion is slow and may continue for as long as 5 years after the drug is discontinued. Because the antimalarial compounds are weak bases that lack protons at the neutral pH of serum, they can diffuse into acidic vacuoles where they become protonated. The more polar protonated molecules are unable to diffuse out of the vacuoles, and the pH within the vacuole becomes elevated by 1 to 2 pH units. The elevation of intracytoplasmic pH in turn alters the molecular assembly of $\alpha$-$\beta$-peptide complexes. This may interfere with antigenic processing and lead to a reduced stimulation of autoimmune CD4$^+$ T cells, resulting in a down-regulation of autoimmune responses.[50] Chloroquine has been shown to decrease antigen processing and presentation by both macrophages and lymphoid dendritic cells.[51]

Hydroxychloroquine's onset of action is delayed; response is seen in 40% to 60% of patients by 3 to 6 months, but it may take 9 to 12 months for maximum response to occur.[52] Nevertheless, this drug has relatively few serious side effects.[47] The high concentrations found in the pigment layers of the retina may lead to retinal damage with destruction of rods and cones; however, significant retinopathy is very rare with current dosing regimens.[53] The dose should be kept below 6 mg/kg/day. Early changes can be detected by an electroretinogram or by changes in color vision or visual fields; abnormal results in a sensitive ophthalmologic examination occur in 0.5% to 10% of patients without symptoms. If clinical symptoms of visual impairment occur, the damage may be irreversible; therefore, a patient should undergo an ophthalmologic examination for retinopathy before starting hydroxychloroquine therapy and every 6 months thereafter.[53] The drug should be stopped at the first sign of retinal toxicity. Other side effects include dermatitis, nausea and epigastric pain, insomnia, myopathy, headache, hemolytic anemia, and rare leukopenia. All side effects, however, are extremely infrequent. By life-table analysis, less toxicity was shown with hydroxychloroquine than with intramuscular gold or D-penicillamine.[54] Most clinicians would agree that the place of hydroxychloroquine in the sequence of DMARD use is in early, mild disease, and they often continue it as a background therapy when another DMARD is started.[55]

## D-Penicillamine

D-Penicillamine is a well-established DMARD but is seldom initiated today because of its frequent toxicity. In well-controlled studies comparing gold, D-penicillamine, and azathioprine, no statistically significant differences in clinical response were found.[56] However, in most well-controlled 6- to 12-month trials, between 30% to 50% of patients taking D-penicillamine stopped the drug because of side effects such as leukopenia, rash, thrombocytopenia, and proteinuria.[35] It can also cause rare "autoimmune" side effects, such as conditions resembling systemic lupus erythematosus, polymyositis, myasthenia gravis, and Goodpasture's syndrome. Many physicians believe that it is more toxic than either gold or azathioprine, and this fact limits its usefulness. In addition, it must be taken on an empty stomach without other medications or food to avoid wide swings in intestinal absorption.

The mechanism of action of D-penicillamine on RA is unknown. Some studies demonstrate a suppressant effect of the drug on cellular immune responsiveness; in other situations, immune enhancement was found. It has been reported to selectively inhibit human T helper cell function.[57]

D-Penicillamine is usually started with a single daily dose of 250 mg, but therapy may be started at 125 mg/day to determine early tolerance. Because the clinical response is slow, increments in dosage are usually made in not less than 8-week intervals, up to a daily dose of 750 to 1000 mg/day, since this is the time period required to assess the effectiveness of the newer dosage level.[58] With lower doses, the incidence of adverse reactions is reduced; but using 125 mg/day may be too low a dose.[59] It has been suggested that intermittent therapy can sustain a successful response, at the same time reducing the total dose of drug taken by 75%[60]: Although it has a half-life of less than 24 hours, it does bind strongly to both cellular and serum proteins. The half-life of a D-penicillamine–albumin complex is between 14 and 21 days, which could have a bearing on the effectiveness of intermittent therapy.[61]

It may take more than 12 weeks before there is evidence of a response to the drug. The duration of treatment in a patient who has shown a good response is variable. Some suggest a gradual reduction in decrements of 125 mg/day at intervals of approximately 8 weeks. Some patients can be completely withdrawn and remain in a condition of relative remission for years. However, one study showed a relapse rate of 80% in the first year with gradual withdrawal of the drug; in comparison, 17 of 19 patients remained in remission when no dosage change was made.[62] CBC, platelet count, and urinalysis should be monitored every 2 weeks for 6 months; the interval may be gradually extended thereafter.

## Azathioprine

Azathioprine is an immunosuppressive drug; used in concert with steroids, it has been standard therapy for inhibition of organ transplant rejection. Its use is suggested in RA patients who have not responded to conventional therapy. Dosage usually is begun at 1.0 mg/kg/day and gradually increased to no more than 2.5 mg/kg/day. The leukocyte count should be monitored and should not be allowed to fall below 3000 cells/mm$^3$. Dosage should be increased as tolerated, if necessary, to control the arthritis. Improvement may begin by 12 weeks, but studies have suggested that improvement often does not plateau until 6 months or longer.[63]

The undesirable adverse effect of greatest concern when azathioprine is used chronically is the rare occurrence of lymphoreticular cancer.[69] Other adverse effects include hepatotoxicity, leukopenia (more often than thrombocytopenia or anemia), superimposed opportunistic infections, nausea, and a macrocytic anemia.[65] The clinician may decide to forgo the use of azathioprine in a patient with a strong family history of non-Hodgkin's lymphoma or a personal history of malignant disease. Full discussion of the potential risks is mandatory before prescribing azathioprine or other DMARDs.

## Cyclosporine

Cyclosporine is a standard immunosuppressive drug for the prevention of organ rejection in heart, liver, and kidney transplantation patients. It produces specific reversible inhibition of T lymphocytes and inhibits lymphokine production and release. In doses of 2.5 to 4.0 mg/kg daily in RA patients whose disease has not adequately responded to methotrexate, it is more effective than placebo. Efficacy is usually observed within 8 to 12 weeks of dosing. It is frequently used in combination with methotrexate. Clinical responses after 6 months of treatment with the combination were markedly better than those in patients who continued methotrexate (plus placebo),[67] suggesting a beneficial interaction between cyclosporine and methotrexate.[68] Serum creatinine must be monitored frequently in patients treated with cyclosporine, because it causes dose-related impairment of renal function and hypertension. This can occur with any dose but particularly with doses greater than 5 mg/kg/day. A 30% or greater increase above pretreatment creatinine levels mandates a decrease in dosage, which usually is associated with a decrease in creatinine. Persistent dosing despite rising creatinine values may cause an irreversible decrease of renal function. Other side effects associated with cyclosporine include gastrointestinal intolerance, headaches, paresthesias, tremors, flushing, facial hair growth, and gum hyperplasia. Most of these adverse events are less frequent with the lower doses used to treat RA. The microemulsion preparation of cyclosporine (Neoral) has greater bioavailability than that achieved with the earlier product. Drug interactions may occur with cyclosporine therapy owing to the metabolism of cyclosporine by the P450 isoenzyme system. Drugs that inhibit the P450 isoenzyme, such as erythomycin, lead to elevations in cyclosporine levels, and drugs that activate the P450 system, such as anticonvulsive therapy, may lead to lower levels of the drug. Grapefruit juice also inhibits P450 isoenzymes and leads to higher levels of cyclosporine.

## Leflunomide

Leflunomide is a prodrug; its active metabolite inhibits dihydroorotate dehydrogenase, thereby inhibiting pyrimidine biosynthesis.[69] After oral administration, it is slowly absorbed and converted to the active metabolite during the first pass through the liver. It is slowly excreted in urine and stool with a long half-life of about 16 days, taking about 7 to 8 weeks to reach steady-state levels in the blood. To decrease the time to reach steady state, a loading dose of 100 mg/day for 3 days is recommended, followed by maintenance doses of 10 to 20 mg/day. Cholestyramine can be given to enhance fecal elimination, decreasing the half-life to about 24 hours. Leflunomide is highly protein bound and may increase concentrations of diclofenac, ibuprofen, and tolbutamide, but not of warfarin or methotrexate. Rifampin increases leflunomide concentrations about 40%.

In clinical trials, leflunomide efficacy was similar to that of methotrexate and sulfasalazine. The onset of benefit is relatively rapid, with significant benefit after 2 to 3 months of treatment.[70–72] The rate of progression of radiographic damage to hand/wrist and forefoot joints during a 12-month study was significantly less than that with placebo and comparable to that with methotrexate.[73] Clinical side effects seen with leflunomide include diarrhea, hair thinning, and skin rash. A reduction in the daily dose from 20 to 10 mg/day may reduce these adverse events.

Leflunomide use is not recommended in patients with significant hepatic impairment or positive hepatitis B or C serologies. Abnormal liver function tests (alanine and aspartate aminotransferase) occurred in about 30% of patients taking leflunomide, compared with 11% of those receiving placebo. Most abnormalities reversed with continued treatment, or with lowering of the dose to 10 mg/day, but liver function tests should be monitored monthly initially, and the drug should be discontinued in patients with levels three or more times normal. Cholestyramine may be given to enhance drug excretion. Leflunomide is teratogenic and is contraindicated during pregnancy. Because it may take up to 2 years after discontinuation to completely excrete leflunomide, pregnancy should be avoided until plasma levels are less than 0.03 mg/L. This may be achieved more quickly by giving cholestyramine 8 g three times a day for 11 days.

## Antibiotics

In the late 1960s, several reports described improvement in patients with RA after treatment with tetracycline.[74] Minocycline has been studied in patients with RA. Although some improvement was noted for the patients receiving minocycline in a study undertaken by the National Institutes of Health, placebo response was also high.[75] In a Dutch study, patients with a long history of disease derived significant benefit from treatment with minocycline compared with placebo.[76]

# TNF Inhibitors

## Etanercept

The FDA has approved both etanercept and infliximab for the treatment of RA. TNF is a proinflammatory cytokine involved in the pathogenesis of RA. The TNF antagonist etanercept is a recombinant fusion protein consisting of the soluble TNF receptor (p75) linked to the Fc portion of human immunoglobulin G1 (IgG1), designated TNFR : Fc. Compared with placebo, it has been found to be safe, well tolerated, and associated with improvement in the inflammatory symptoms of RA.[77] Etanercept can be used in combination with methotrexate for patients who do not respond to methotrexate alone.[78] Continued responses have been seen for up to 18 months when patients receive etanercept without interruption; the most frequently reported adverse events in clinical trials were mild to moderate injection site reactions.[79] Etanercept is available as a subcutaneous injection administered twice weekly in a 25-mg dose. Etanercept was originally approved by the FDA with the indication for moderate to severe RA in patients who have had an inadequate response to one or more DMARDs. However, in an FDA ruling based on data from a controlled clinical trial, etanercept was allowed to claim disease modification (ability to retard the rate of radiographic progression) and efficacy in patients with early RA (less than 3 years of disease duration).[79a]

Clinical improvement may occur after the first injection, and maximum responses occur in 3 to 6 months. About 70% of patients achieve 20% or greater improvement; 40% are 50% better; and 15% are near remission with 70% or greater improvement.[78] Inhibition of TNF may impair natural defenses against certain infections; etanercept therapy should be interrupted during treatment of serious infections such as sepsis, septic arthritis, pyelonephriitis, and tuberculosis, and probably also during hospitalizations for major surgical procedures.

### Infliximab

Infliximab is a chimeric IgG1 monoclonal antibody that binds to cell-bound and circulating TNF alpha but not to TNF beta and abrogates the biologic effects of TNF. It has been approved by the FDA to be used in combination with methotrexate for patients who have continued active RA despite an adequate trial of methotrexate.[79b] Antibodies to infliximab are less likely to develop if methotrexate is continued. Infliximab is given intravenously in a dose of 3 mg/kg at weeks 0, 2, and 6. Patients can then be maintained thereafter with infusions every 8 weeks. In one study, 20% responses occurred in 50% of patients, and 50% responses occurred in 27% of patients. Cautions regarding infections are the same as with etanercept. Postinfusion reactions have occurred, but with uninterrupted dosing schedules and the use of concomitant methotrexate these are described as mild. Three patients have developed lupus-like symptoms (migratory arthritis, pleuro-peritonitis, malar rash, anti-dsDNA antibodies) while on the drug.[79c] Important disease modification, as illustrated by stopping radiologic progression in a cohort of methotrexate-treated patients with long-standing disease, has recently been demonstrated in a large multinational clinical trial with this agent.[79d]

## Corticosteroids

Therapeutic administration of corticosteroids produces rapid, potent, and reliable suppression of inflammation, the extent and duration of which depends on the dose, dosing schedule, and length of treatment. Their unsurpassed short-term efficacy and versatility have made corticosteroids a key element in the treatment of many rheumatic diseases.

There have always been rheumatologists who have advocated a disease-modifying role for corticosteroids in RA.[80] A randomized, double-blind, placebo-controlled trial demonstrated decreased progression of radiographic damage in patients treated with prednisolone 7.5 mg/day.[81] Although there is a dearth of published studies on the moderate-term effectiveness of low-dose corticosteroids for RA, a meta-analysis concluded that over a period of about 7 months corticosteroids appeared to be as effective or more effective than alternative therapies in improving several common RA disease activity measures and, in fact, appeared to be about as effective as the traditional DMARDs in terms of the outcomes measured.[82]

Corticosteroids enter target cells and couple with a specific cytoplasmic receptor before transfer to the nucleus, where the corticosteroid-receptor complex binds to chromatin and modulates protein synthesis.[83] Corticosteroids decrease collagen synthesis and impair wound healing; augment gluconeogenesis and glycogen deposition while inhibiting the action of insulin; impair lipogenesis and stimulate lipolysis in adipose tissue; and increase liver synthesis of protein while enhancing its peripheral catabolism. They have a profound effect on bone metabolism through interference with intestinal absorption of calcium, inhibition of osteoblast collagen synthesis, elevation of parathyroid hormone levels resulting in amplification of osteoclast bone resorption, and enhancement of renal calcium excretion.[84]

Corticosteroids have a short-term effect on inflammation, probably mediated by interference with the inflammatory and immune cascade at the following levels[84]:

- Impairment of antigen opsonization
- Interference with inflammatory cell adhesion and migration through vascular endothelium
- Interruption of cell-cell communication by altering the release or antagonizing the action of cytokines
- Impairment of leukotriene and prostaglandin synthesis
- Inhibition of neutrophil superoxide production

Corticosteroids decrease immunoglobulin generation, inhibit immune clearance of sensitized erythrocytes, and impair the transit of immune complexes across basement membranes.[85]

Cortisol is the prototype for the available synthetic corticosteroids. Minor structural modifications of this parent hormone have led to the creation of a panel of drugs with a wide spectrum of plasma half-lives, anti-inflammatory potency, and mineralocorticoid effect (Table 19–3). Corticosteroids have biologic half-lives

## TABLE 19–3
## Glucocorticoid Preparations

| DRUG | RELATIVE ANTI-INFLAMMATORY POTENCY | SODIUM-RETAINING POTENCY | EQUIVALENT DOSE (mg) | BIOLOGIC HALF-LIFE (h) |
|---|---|---|---|---|
| **Short-acting** | | | | |
| Hydrocortisone | 1 | 2+ | 20 | 8–12 |
| Cortisone | 0.8 | 2+ | 25 | 8–12 |
| Prednisone | 4 | 1+ | 5 | 12–36 |
| Prednisolone | 5 | 1+ | 4 | 12–36 |
| Methylprednisolone | 5 | 0 | 4 | 12–36 |
| Triamcinolone | 5 | 0 | 4 | 12–36 |
| **Long-acting** | | | | |
| Betamethasone | 20–30 | 0 | 0.6 | 36–54 |
| Dexamethasone | 20–30 | 0 | 0.75 | 36–54 |

that are 2 to 36 times longer than their plasma half-lives, but the onset of biologic effect lags behind peak plasma levels. Corticosteroids are widely and rapidly distributed in tissues.

In general, increasing doses and dosing frequencies of corticosteroids correspond to enhanced inflammatory suppression, more rapid onset of therapeutic benefits, and increased side effects. Doses given several times a day are more potent than once-a-day dosing. When disease control is required in a timely but nonurgent manner, once-daily oral dosing, given in the morning to minimize adrenal suppression, is adequate. Prednisone is most frequently used for RA, the usual dose being 5 to 10 mg daily, a dose often used for long periods. Tapering should be gradual to avoid disease flares: serial reductions of 0.5 to 1.0 mg/day every few weeks to months should be tried when daily doses are less than 10 to 15 mg/day. Dose reduction should not be more frequent than the time required to detect a steroid dose-related exacerbation of disease activity, which in RA can be as short as a few days. In the case of doses lower than 10 mg/day, the reduction interval must be long enough to allow incremental recovery of adrenal function; the interval increases with the duration of corticosteroid therapy. Alternate-day administration of short-acting preparations such as prednisone usually avoids the cushingoid and adrenal suppressive adverse effects seen with more frequent doses but is of limited usefulness in RA because symptoms usually exacerbate during the day without steroids.

In the situation where rapid amelioration of damaging inflammation is desired, treatment can be initiated with a short course or even a single dose of high-dose corticosteroid. Pulsed doses of methylprednisolone, 1 g intravenously daily for 1 to 3 days, has proven efficacy in the treatment of RA.[86] Profound effects on lymphocyte function may occur, leading to a prolonged effect on disease activity. Doses of 100 and 300 mg given intravenously also have been shown to be as effective, or almost as effective, as 1-g doses.[87] Intravenous therapy appears to relieve symptoms for about 3 to 6 weeks, but there is no evidence that it changes the underlying course of the disease.[87]

Prolonged administration of corticosteroids leads to genralized adrenal suppression and the development of unwanted side effects. The severity of these side effects depends on the maximum dose, dosage schedule, duration of treatment or cumulative dose, and the type of corticosteroid used. Accelerated osteoporosis with pathologic fractures occurs. Supplemental calcium and vitamin D may slow this process.[86]

Exogenous administration of corticosteroids can stop native adrenal corticosteroid production through effects on the pituitary-adrenal axis; in the face of stressors, Addisonian crisis and shock may develop. The chances of developing adrenal suppression increase in the following conditions:

• Doses exceed the average daily equivalent output of the adrenal glands of 5.0 to 7.5 mg prednisone
• Therapy continues for longer than a few weeks or months
• Doses are given late in the day or in split doses
• Long-acting corticosteroid preparations are used

Adrenal suppression can sometimes develop with short courses and low doses of corticosteroid. If doubt exists, an adrenocorticotropic hormone (ACTH) stimulation test, or metyrapone test, may be done to determine whether pituitary and adrenal functions are preserved, before discontinuation of corticosteroid treatment. In patients receiving 10 mg or less of prednisone, with a single injection of synthetic ACTH and measurement of cortisol levels, current steroid therapy was the only significant factor determining hypothalamic-pituitary-adrenocortical axis intergrity. Subjects receiving 5 mg or more had varied responses to ACTH, whereas patients receiving less than 5 mg of prednisone daily displayed a normal stimulation response.[88] The investigators speculated that spontaneous recovery of the hypothalamic-pituitary-adrenocortical axis is to be expected for rheumatic disease patients taking 5 mg or less of prednisone daily. However, normalization of the adrenal response to stress may be markedly delayed, and intravenous administration of hydrocortisone during general anesthesia is prudent for at least 1 year after the last dose of corticosteroids.

The inhibitory effect of corticosteroids on inflammatory and immune responses results in increased risk of bacterial and opportunistic infections such as tuberculosis, *Pneumocystis carinii,* and fungi. Effects on glucose and protein metabolism may cause hyperglycemia, centripetal fat deposition leading to rounded facies and a cervical fat pad, and hyperlipidemia. They can cause hypokalemia, fluid retention, edema, and hypertension. Cutaneous problems include capillary fragility with petechiae and easy bruising, acne, hirsutism, impaired wound healing, hyperhidrosis, and striae. Glaucoma and cataract formation are further complications, as are myopathy, possible ulcerogenicity, pancreatitis, premature atherosclerosis, avascular necrosis of bone, psychiatric disturbances, and bowel or diverticular perforations. High-dose steroids can mask the symptoms of other inflammatory processes, making diagnosis difficult. Pulses of 1 g may induce cardiac arrhythmia in hypokalemic patients and may result in the hematogenous dissemination of previously localized infections. Concomitant illnesses or previous adverse reactions may guide the physician when prescribing corticosteroids. For example, a patient with known hypertension may better tolerate a corticosteroid that has a lower mineralocorticoid effect.

An alternative to (long-term) oral therapy is the occasional use of intra-articular injections.[86] It has been noted that injection of the equivalent of 10 to 20 mg of prednisone (although prednisone itself is not an intra-articular preparation) sometimes gives relief in the injected joint for up to 10 weeks.[86] Because the drug diffuses systemically, systemic effects may occur, including a generalized (albeit short-term) improvement in the patient's arthritis. However, there are no specific side effects. Hollander documented crystal-induced synovitis in about 1% of patients; 0.01% may have intra-articular infections, and a small number of patients may have ligamentous rupture.[86] Apparently, crystal-induced synovitis occurs less often with triamcinolone hexacetonide and other modern intra-articular preparations.[86] The danger here occurs in chronic therapy with repeated, regular monthly intramuscular or intra-articular injections (albeit into different joints). This form of treatment often brings the patient back into the office because of the "wearing off" of systemic effects of glucocorticoids in the weeks after the injection. The use of repeated injections in this manner should be avoided for chronic, long-term therapy because other alternatives are available (see later discussion).

## Combination Therapy with Disease-Modifying Antirheumatic Drugs

The use of combinations of DMARDs when a single DMARD fails to adequately control RA is now generally accepted by rheumatologists. A 1997 survey of 200 US rheumatologists found that combination DMARD therapy was used by 99% of rheumatologists to treat an estimated 24% of their patients with RA.[89] Methotrexate with hydroxychloroquine is the most frequently used combination. A 1990 review found that various DMARD combinations were effective in early anecdotal reports and uncontrolled trials but that balanced, randomized, prospective clinical trials showed no advantage to combinations when compared with their component single DMARDs.[90] More recently, a prospective, randomized study of methotrexate, sulfasalazine, or the combination as the first DMARD therapy in 115 patients with early RA showed no significant differences among the three treatment groups after 1 year, although there was a trend toward greater improvement with the combination.[91] Several prospective, controlled, double-blind but unbalanced studies have supported combination DMARD therapy as more effective (and not more toxic) than standard single agents alone such as methotrexate or sulfasalazine. As discussed earlier, the addition of cyclosporine to methotrexate is clearly more beneficial than the addition of placebo in patients with active RA.[67] Triple-DMARD therapy with methotrexate, sulfasalazine, and hydroxychloroquine was more effective than methotrexate alone or sulfasalazine/hydroxychloroquine in patients who had experienced a poor response to single-DMARD therapy with one or more of the three DMARDs, gold penicillamine.[92] The COBRA trial in 155 patients with only 4 months of RA demonstrated that a step-down combination of high-dose prednisolone (60 mg/day tapering to 7.5 mg after 6 weeks and zero after 35 weeks), methotrexate (7.5 mg/week for 46 weeks), and sulfasalazine, 2 g/day, was more effective than sulfasalazine alone until the prednisolone was stopped. After the prednisolone was stopped, the clinical differences between the treatment arms were no longer significant, but radiographic joint damage was less in the group receiving combined therapy.[93] Addition of the TNF inhibitor etanercept for patients with inadequate responses to methotrexate therapy produces substantial additional benefit, and the combination has been approved by the FDA.[78] The chimeric (mouse/human) monoclonal anti-TNF antibody in infliximab is used in combination with methotrexate. Methotrexate prevents the formation of (anti-mouse) antibodies that decrease the benefit of long-term infliximab monotherapy.[94]

## TREATMENT STRATEGIES FOR RHEUMATOID ARTHRITIS

The traditional pyramid approach to RA therapy has been challenged; earlier use of DMARDs has been suggested. The concept of "waiting" months or years for a natural remission while the patient takes NSAIDs alone is today thought to be counterproductive; disability and functional loss often occur early in RA, and the delay before aggressive management is thought by most rheumatologists to be inappropriate. Moreover, 50% of maximal radiologic damage is observed within the first 2 to 6 years of disease, bolstering the view that RA is particularly aggressive within the first few years.[95] Rheumatologists today institute one or more DMARDs as soon as the diagnosis of RA is secure. Of course, the ideal drug should provide maximal efficacy with minimal toxicity (in both the short and long term). Felson and associates[54] found in a meta-analysis of published clinical trials of single agent therapy published before 1990 that antimalarial drugs and methotrexate had the best balance of efficacy and toxicity in the treatment of RA.[54] Azathioprine scored in the intermediate range in terms of both efficacy and toxicity. Injectable gold was the most toxic drug, and auranofin was among the weakest. Long-term observational studies using drug termination as the measure of overall drug appeal indicate that methotrexate and antimalarial drugs are the ones that patients are the most likely to continue taking for several years. The strong DMARDs were found to be injectable gold, D-penicillamine, methotrexate, and sulfasalazine. We would add leflunomide, etanercept, and infliximab to that list.

Patients with aggressive synovitis develop radiographically evident joint damage in the first 2 years of disease; almost 50% become disabled within 5 years after onset of disease,[96] and 90% by 30 years.[97] Life expectancy may be shortened by 10 to 15 years, particularly in patients with severe disease or extra-articular complications.[14] To prevent such morbidity, early control of inflammation and the disease itself is critical.[98] Several studies revealed that therapy with DMARDs early in the course of RA slowed disease progression more effectively than DMARD use in late RA.[99, 100] In addition, the efficacy of DMARDs is indicated by the increased frequency of exacerbations when these drugs were discontinued in patients with remissions.[101]

Short-term clinical responsiveness to drugs (demonstrated in clinical trials) is not necessarily equivalent to long-term control. The paradox of short-term success and long-term failure is based on several trial-related factors, including strict exclusion criteria, emphasis on marginal benefits that are statistically significant, and failure to adjust for patient drop-out in drug studies.[102, 103] With the exception of methotrexate, most DMARDs have to be stopped within a few months to a few years because of poor efficacy or intolerable side effects.[104, 105] Indeed, 5 years after the initiation of treatment with gold compounds or antimalarials, only 10% to 25% of patients are still taking these drugs; in contrast, this number is 60% in those patients taking methotrexate.[106] Clinical trials demonstrating efficacy usually run for 1 year or less, whereas more protracted observational studies show increasing morbidity after most drugs have been discontinued by patients or have lost their effect.[97] Remission in aggressive RA is un-

usual, and sustained control of inflammation is rare.[107] Many gains in patient function over the past 15 years can be attributed to joint replacement.[108]

It is doubtful that one treatment strategy or a single treatment modality will be the best therapy for all patients with RA. The current consensus is that all therapeutic regimens should emphasize early control of disease, with the hope of a resultant sustained improved function. Most patients favor a more aggressive approach: One study reported that patients would accept a 21% risk of death in exchange for a cure and a 17% risk of death for relief of pain.[109] However, the willingness to accept risk decreases with decreased disease duration and with functional improvement as measured by self-assessment questionnaires.

When we see a patient shortly after the onset of RA symptoms, we determine whether the rheumatoid factor is positive and whether any erosive changes are present on hand/wrist and forefoot radiographs. Basic education about the disease, the importance and use of rest, joint protection and maintenance of motion, and the use of NSAIDs are initiated in all patients. If any erosions are present, the disease is classified as "aggressive" and methotrexate is started at once. If there are no erosions and rheumatoid factor is positive, sulfasalazine or hydroxychloroquine is started. If the disease is nonerosive and rheumatoid factor is negative, the basic regimen is continued for 6 months; if there is no remission after 6 months, sulfasalazine or hydroxychloroquine is started. Joint radiographs are repeated every 6 to 12 months for the first 2 years; when the first erosions are noted, methotrexate is added to the treatment regimen. Even when the disease remains nonerosive, if there is an inadequate response to the first DMARD after 4 to 12 months, the next DMARD is added. Patients who do not develop erosions during the first 2 years are less likely to do so, and the frequency of joint radiographs can then be decreased to every 2 to 3 years.

For patients with established RA with inadequate response to methotrexate, there are a number of options. The methotrexate dose may be increased to 25 or 30 mg/week, if tolerated. One may add sulfasalazine and hydroxychloroquine,[92] cyclosporine,[67] gold, or sulfasalazine. Leflunomide may be substituted for methotrexate.[70–73] Sometimes monthly methylprednisolone pulses are necessary.[86, 87]

The apparent remarkable effectiveness of TNF inhibition in many patients may change the strategies just described; etanercept, infliximab, or another TNF inhibitor may become the first DMARD to add in patients with inadequate response to methotrexate.[77, 78] Since TNF inhibition has been shown to inhibit erosion development or progression in early RA, it may become the first choice for management of aggressive early RA instead of methotrexate. Other biologic agents, such as interleukin-1 inhibitors, are under development and some show promise in RA. These are discussed in detail in Chapter 18.

At least in the immediate future, management of RA will be focused on control as opposed to cure.[110] The therapeutic repertoire will be larger, allowing one to combine or replace older therapies with newer experimental agents.

## AUTHORS' APPROACHES TO MANAGEMENT OF RHEUMATOID ARTHRITIS PATIENTS

Our personal approach to the management of RA is illustrated in the following hypothetical cases. It is risky to describe a "cookbook" approach, because RA management blends the art of medicine and patient preferences with a thorough understanding of the scientific basis of the pharmaceutical and physical interventions available for its treatment. Optimal management requires that both the physician and the patient understand the character of the disease in that particular patient, its interactions with the patient's life situation, the vagaries of the disease course, and its response to treatment. It is essential that the physician and the patient are honest with and trust each other. If this feeling of confidence and trust has not developed after the first few visits, the patient should find a more compatible physician; no single physician can be "right" for all patients.

We will assume that each of the hypothetical patients is coming to us for the first time, although some have had much previous therapy. As discussed earlier in this chapter, whole-body rest is one of the most important and least understood components of RA treatment. For all RA patients, we spend most of the first several visits determining how their life situation affects their ability to obtain adequate rest and to deal with the disease. This includes prescribing specific additional hours of bed rest to demonstrate its value to the patient. Splinting of appropriate inflamed joints, joint protection, and range of motion exercises are initiated at the same time. NSAID doses are optimized; the NSAID is changed and adjunctive therapy to improve gastric tolerance is added if indicated or a selective COX-2 inhibitor is substituted. DMARDs are discussed but are not added or changed until we are satisfied that the patient has mastered the basic program.

### Hypothetical Case 1

New-onset RA; patient seropositive, functional and working. This patient is cautioned to avoid overcommitment that may lead to physical exhaustion and exacerbation of the RA. Additional rest is scheduled, but the patient can continue to work. With relatively mild synovitis and no joint erosions, if spontaneous remission does not occur after 1 or 2 months of basic therapy, we would add a relatively low-risk DMARD such as hydroxychloroquine or sulfasalazine or the combination of the two. In this seropositive patient without joint erosions, x-ray films of hands and feet are obtained every 6 months until the first definite erosion is found. The appearance of the first erosion in a well-functioning patient or an otherwise unacceptable level of pain, stiffness, or diminished function is an indication for a more aggressive approach. At this point, we

usually will add oral methotrexate to the first DMARD in an attempt to produce a drug-induced remission. Etanercept may be an option in some patients for whom methotrexate is either not safe or not tolerated.

### Hypothetical Case 2

New-onset RA; patient nonfunctional, devastated by the illness; many systemic features such as marked fatigue and weight loss. The explosive onset of severe, disabling, polyarticular synovitis does not necessarily imply a poor prognosis, particularly if the rheumatoid factor is negative and no joint erosions are present. Ideally, this patient should receive 10 days to 2 weeks of inpatient treatment with intensive bed rest (up to 16 or 18 hours/day), education, passive and active physical and occupational therapy, and pharmaceutical therapy. However, hospitalization now is rarely practical or affordable. Full-dose NSAID therapy will probably control the fever and help to cool the joints. Corticosteroid injections of several joints, a 1- to 3-day course of intravenous minipulse corticosteroid therapy, or both, could be used to suppress the synovitis and expedite physical therapy. If the patient is seropositive or if erosions or nodules are present, methotrexate is started immediately, with rapid increase to a maximum tolerated dose of 15 to 25 mg/week—parenterally if necessary. Plaquenil could be added to the methotrexate regimen. Folic acid, 1 mg, is given daily, and leucovorin (folinic acid), 5 mg, may be added 8 to 12 hours after the methotrexate dose if needed to improve tolerance. If the patient is seronegative and the disease is nonerosive, hydroxychloroquine is started, with methotrexate held in reserve to use if a lot of improvement is not seen after 3 or 4 months. Joint injections (or intravenous corticosteroid pulses) are given as needed (but cautiously) for the first 3 or 4 months, but we try to avoid daily oral prednisone. Most patients are markedly improved in 3 or 4 months, and some are in remission by the end of the first year. If the disease remains active and disability continues after 3 or 4 months, methotrexate is added to achieve rapid control of the RA. If the disease is still uncontrolled after an additional 3 or 4 months, we would add etanercept or infliximab or initiate therapy with leflunomide.

### Hypothetical Case 3

Active RA after failure of one or two second-line drugs. This is a very common situation among patients with RA who are referred to us, and our response depends on the details of the prior "failed" treatment program. Many patients abandon a DMARD if they have not had dramatic improvement in 3 or 4 months or if they experience relatively minor side effects. Generally, we do not consider a DMARD to have failed until adequate doses have been used for 1 year or a major adverse effect has occurred, so we sometimes continue the "failed" treatment with adjustments in dosage, concomitant therapies, and insistence on the basic program of increased rest and physical therapy. Many patients have a gratifying response to this program. If the RA is particularly active, with rapidly progressing erosions, we would try to control it with higher-dose weekly parenteral methotrexate (20 to 35 mg/week) and, on rare occasions, monthly 1-g pulses of intravenous methylprednisolone. Azathioprine or injectable gold or sulfasalazine may be added to the regimen at this time, or leflunomide may be substituted for methotrexate. With the current availability of etanercept and infliximab, we would add TNF inhibition to this regimen if not satisfied with the observed response.

## Hypothetical Case 4

Long-standing RA, all drugs failed, many steroid side effects, sometimes dependent on increasing doses of narcotics. The general approach is similar to that with case 3, except that we have the additional debilitation of prolonged poorly controlled RA and long-term steroid use. The patient must be considered to have active disease with progressing erosions, even if the steroids are suppressing the usual signs of joint inflammation. (Serial joint radiographs will document the progression of joint damage in these patients.) We start with the basic program of increased bed rest balanced with exercise. In this patient, exercise of some sort is particularly important; we find that pool therapy three times a week is most helpful if it can be arranged. The degree of osteoporosis is documented, and appropriate therapy is initiated (see Chapter 40). For such patients, the benefits of daily prednisone are vanishingly small and the adverse effects are obvious, even to the patient, but attempts to decrease the dose cause immediate flare-ups of discomfort and synovitis. However, if the patient can tolerate it, the withdrawal-induced flare-up will subside after a variable time that depends on the magnitude of the dosage decrement. We explain this to the patient and then try to find a dosage decrement that causes a flare-up for only 3 to 7 days. This decrease in dosage can then be repeated every 2 to 4 weeks without causing any deterioration in the basic control of the RA. If the flare-up has not subsided after 2 to 4 weeks, the next decrease in dose is delayed, but we ask the patient not to increase the prednisone dosage. When the flare-up eventually subsides, the dosage decrease schedule is resumed. The size of the decrements depends partly on the patient's tolerance, the starting dosage, and the duration of prior steroid therapy. Usually we can decrease prednisone by 1 mg at a time if the daily dose is more than 12 mg or by 0.5 if it is between 5 and 12 mg. With daily doses of less than 5 mg, one must allow time for adrenal recovery after each dose reduction, and we often use more gradual dose-reduction programs, sometimes reducing by 0.5 mg on one additional day each week, taking 7 weeks to decrease the daily dose by 0.5 mg. Patients who have taken daily steroids for more than 10 years may have permanently suppressed adrenal glands, in which case they will need 3.5 to 4.5 mg of prednisone daily for life. The steroid-reduction program will not be successful if the disease activity cannot be controlled with other agents.

We review the reasons for failure of the previously tried DMARDs and usually find one or two agents that can be tried again and continued for a longer time at a higher or lower dosage or with adjunctive therapy, such as leucovorin with high-dose methotrexate. If not already tried, new agents such as etanercept, infliximab, or leflunomide may be effective in a substantial proportion of "end-stage" RA patients. Sometimes a patient responds to low-dose cyclosporine or can be entered in a protocol to evaluate a new investigational therapy. Apheresis-based treatments with the staphylococcal protein A immunoabsorption column have been successfully used in some patients who had failed all other treatments.[111] Treating a case 4 patient takes several years and requires a major commitment by both the physician and the patient. The results are usually incomplete, because the patient continues to have substantial disability from the cumulative RA damage, but the patient usually is grateful to have gotten off the slippery slope of ever-increasing steroid side effects and is a much better candidate for reconstructive surgical procedures.

## Hypothetical Case 5

Older male patient with acute seronegative polyarthritis. Rheumatologists in Europe have found sulfasalazine to be a powerful tool in the treatment of the elderly patient with active RA. Some in the United States consider this to be a variant of polymyalgia rheumatica (PMR) and use prednisone to treat it, avoiding NSAIDs because of their increased gastrointestinal toxicity in the elderly. If the major complaints are of shoulder and/or hip girdle pain, associated with a very high erythrocyte sedimentation rate and only mild small-joint synovitis, we would treat the condition like PMR with corticosteroids (see Chapter 29). If small-joint synovitis is prominent and symmetric, we would treat it like RA, using sulfasalazine first and adding small doses of methotrexate if the response is poor. A selective COX-2 inhibitor or small doses of prednisone (5 mg for women, 7.5 mg for men) may be used in a patient who is at high risk for complications of NSAID use or who is intolerant of NSAIDs. If predominantly larger joints are involved, particularly if involvement is asymmetric, we would search diligently for chronic calcium crystal deposition disease and treat with NSAIDs and/or prophylactic colchicine, 0.6 mg once or twice a day.

## SUMMARY

In all cases, we see patients more frequently than the long intervals recommended by managed care algorithms. Frequent hands-on personal interactions between the patient and the physician are essential to maintain the patient's confidence and commitment to the difficult treatment regimens and to permit timely adjustments to deal with changing circumstances. In the long run, these frequent brief outpatient visits are much more cost-effective than the disability and hospitalizations associated with inadequate care.

# REFERENCES

1. Hochberg MC: Adult and juvenile rheumatoid arthritis: Current epidemiologic concepts. Epidemiol Rev 1981; 3:27.
2. Harris ED: The clinical features of rheumatoid arthritis. In Kelly WN, Harris ED Jr, Ruddy S, et al (eds): Textbook of Rheumatology, 4th ed. Philadelphia: WB Saunders, 1993: 874.
3. Harvald B, Hauge M: Genetics and the Epidemiology of Chronic Diseases, Washington DC: US Government Printing Office, 1965:61.
4. Nunez G, Moore SE, Ball GV, et al: Study of HLA antigens in ten multiple-case rheumatoid arthritis families. J Rheumatol 1984; 11:129.
5. Christiansen FT, Kelly H, Dawkins RL: Rheumatoid arthritis. In Albert ED, Baur MP, Mayr WR (eds): Histocompatibility Testing. Berlin: Springer-Verlag, 1984:378.
6. Fleming A, Benn RT, Corbett M, et al: Early rheumatoid disease: II. Patterns of joint involvement. Ann Rheum Dis 1976; 35:361.
7. Hurd ER: Extra-articular manifestations of rheumatoid arthritis. Semin Rheum Dis 1979; 8:151.
8. Wolfe F, Hawley DJ: Remission in rheumatoid arthritis. J Rheumatol 1985; 12:245.
9. Van der Grouche JP, Hazevoct HM, Cats A: Survival and cause of death in rheumatoid arthritis: A 25-year prospective follow-up. J Rheumatol 1984; 11:158.
10. Sherrer YS, Block DA, Mitchell DM, et al: The development of disability in rheumatoid arthritis. Arthritis Rheum 1986; 29:494.
11. Luukkainen R, Isomaki H, Kajander A: Prognostic value of the type of onset of rheumatoid arthritis. Ann Rheum Dis 1983; 42:274.
12. Sharp JT, Calkins E, Cohen AS, et al: Observations on the clinical, chemical, and serologic manifestations of rheumatoid arthritis, based on the course of 154 cases. Medicine (Baltimore) 1964; 43:41.
13. Mitchell DM, Spitz PW, Young DY, et al: Survival, prognosis, and causes of death in rheumatoid arthritis. Arthritis Rheum 1986; 29:706.
14. Pincus T, Callahan LF: Taking mortality in rheumatoid arthritis seriously: Predictive markers, socioeconomic status and comorbidity. J Rheumatol 1986; 13:541.
15. Kellgren JH, O'Brien WM: On the natural history of rheumatoid arthritis in relation to the sheep cell agglutination test. Arthritis Rheum 1962; 5:115.
16. Jacoby RK, Jayson MIV, Cosh TA: Onset, early stages and prognosis of rheumatoid arthritis: A clinical study of 100 patients with 11-year follow-up. Br Med J 1973; 2:96.
17. Gault SJ, Spyker JM: Beneficial effect of immobilization of joints in rheumatoid arthritis and related arthritides: A splint study using sequential analysis. Arthritis Rheum 1969; 12:34.
18. McCarty DJ: Treatment of rheumatoid joint inflammation with triamcinolone hexacetomide. Arthritis Rheum 1972; 15:157.
19. Clements PJ, Paulus HE: Nonsteroidal anti-rheumatic drugs. In Kelley WN, Harris ED Jr, Ruddy S, et al (eds). Textbook of Rheumatology, 5th ed. Philadelphia: WB Saunders, 1997:707.
20. Celecoxib for arthritis. Med Lett Drugs Ther 1999; 41:11.
21. Fries JF: NSAID gastropathy: The second most deadly rheumatic disease? Epidemiology and risk appraisal. J Rheumatol 1991; 18(suppl 28):6.
22. Schlegel SI, Paulus HE: NSAIDs: Use in rheumatic disease, side effects and interactions. Bull Rheum Dis 1986; 36:1.
23. Katz LM, Love PY: NSAIDs and the liver. In Famaey JP, Paulus HE (eds): Clinical Applications of NSAIDs, Subpopulation Therapy and New Formulations. New York: Marcel Dekker, 1992:247.
24. Blackshear JL, Napier JS, Davidman M, et al: Renal complications of NSAIDs. Arch Intern Med 1985; 143:1130.
25. Furst DE, Blocka K, Cassell S, et al: A strategy for reaching therapeutic salicylate levels in patients with rheumatoid arthritis using standardized dosing regimens. J Rheumatol 1987; 14:342.
26. Day RO, Furst DE, Dromgoole SH, et al: Changes in salicylate serum concentration and metabolism during chronic dosing in normal volunteers. Biopharm Drug Dispos 1988; 9:273.
27. Paulus HE: Aspirin versus nonacetylated salicylates [Editorial]. J Rheumatol 1989; 16:264.
28. Cooperating Clinics of the New York Chapter of the Arthritis Foundation. A retrospective look at prescribing practice of NSAIDs in rheumatoid arthritis [Abstract]. In Proceedings of Eighth Pan-American Congress of Rheumatology, San Francisco, June 7, 1982.
29. Broader RN, Heel RL, Speight TM, et al: Tolmetin: A review of its pharmacological properties and therapeutic efficacy in rheumatic diseases. Drugs 1978; 15:429.
30. Furst DE, Blocka K, Cassell S, et al: A controlled study of concurrent therapy with a nonacetylated salicylate and naproxen in rheumatoid arthritis. Arthritis Rheum 1987; 30:146.
31. Iannuzzi L, Dawson N, Zein N, et al: Does drug therapy slow radiographic deterioration in rheumatoid arthritis? N Engl J Med 1983; 309:1023.
32. Forestier J: Rheumatoid arthritis and its treatment with gold salts. J Lab Clin Med 1935; 20:827.
33. Research Subcommittee of the Empire Rheumatism Council: Gold therapy in rheumatoid arthritis. Ann Rheum Dis 1960; 19:95–119.
34. Blocka K, Paulus HE: The clinical pharmacology of the gold compounds. In Paulus HE, Furst DE, Dromgoole SH (eds): Drugs for Rheumatic Disease New York: Churchill Livingstone, 1987:4.
35. Gordon DA: Gold compounds and penicillamine in the rheumatic diseases. In Kelley WN, Harris ED Jr, Ruddy S, et al (eds): Textbook of Rheumatology, 5th ed. Philadelphia: WB Saunders, 1997:759.
36. Lipsky PE, Ugai K, Ziff M: Alterations in human monocyte structure and function induced by incubation with gold sodium thiomalate. J Rheumatol 1979; 6(suppl 5):130.
37. Paulus HE: Government Affaris, FDA Arthritis Advisory Committee Meeting: Auranofin. Arthritis Rheum 1985; 28:450.
38. Gubner R, August S, Ginsburg V: Therapeutic Suppression of tissue reactivity: II. Effect of aminopterin in rheumatoid arthritis and psoriasis. Am J Med Sci 1951; 221:176.
39. Weinblatt ME, Coblyn JS, Fox DA, et al: Efficacy of low-dose methotrexate in rheumatoid arthritis. N Engl J Med 1985; 312:818.
40. Weinblatt ME: Methotrexate. In Kelley WN, Harris ED Jr, Ruddy S, et al (eds): Textbook of Rheumatology, 5th ed. Philadelphia: WB Saunders, 1997:771.
41. Weinblatt ME, Weissman BN, Holdsworth DE: Long-term prospective study of methotrexate in the treatment of rheumatoid arthritis. Arthritis Rheum 1992; 35:129.
42. Morgan SL, Baggott JE, Vaughn WH, et al: The effect of folic acid supplementation on the toxicity of low-dose methotrexate treatment of rheumatoid arthritis. Arthritis Rheum 1990; 30:9.
43. Sperling RI, Benincaso AI, Anderson RJ: Acute and chronic suppression of leukotriene B4 synthesis ex vivo in neutrophils from patients with rheumatoid arthritis beginning treatment with methotrexate. Arthritis Rheum 1992; 35:376.
44. Connolly KM, Stecher VJ, Davis E: Alteration of interleukin-1 production and the acute phase response following medication of adjuvant arthritic rats with cyclosporin-A or methotrexate. Int J Immunopharmacol 1988; 10:717.
45. Day RO: Sulfasalazine. In Kelley WN, Harris ED Jr, Ruddy S, et al (eds): Textbook of Rheumatology, 5th ed. Philadelphia: WB Saunders, 1997:741.
46. Skosey JL: Comparison of responses to and adverse effects of graded doses of sulfasalazine in the treatment of rheumatoid arthritis. J Rheumatol 1988; 16(suppl):5.
47. Wickens S, Paulus HE: Antimalarial drugs. In Paulus HE, Furst DE, Dromgoole SH (eds). Drugs for Rheumatic Disease. New York. Churchill Livingstone, 1987:113.
48. Rynes RI: Antimalarial drugs. In Kelley WN, Harris ED Jr, Ruddy S, et al (eds): Textbook of Rheumatology, 5th ed. Philadelphia: WB Saunders, 1997:747.

49. Felson DT, Anderson JJ, Meenan RF: Use of short-term efficacy/toxicity trade-offs to select second-line drugs in rheumatoid arthritis. Arthritis Rheum 1992; 35:1117.

50. Fox RI, Kang H: Mechanism of action of antimalarial drugs: Inhibition of antigen processing and presentation. Lupus 1993; 2(suppl 1):S-9.

51. Guidos C, Wong M, Lee KC: A comparison of the stimulatory activities of lymphoid dendritic cells and macrophages in T proliferative responses to various antigens. J Immunol 1984; 133:1179.

52. Runge LA: Risk/benefit analysis of hydroxychloroquine sulfate treatment in rheumatoid arthritis. Am J Med 1983; 75(1A):52.

53. Bernstein HN: Ophthalmologic considerations and testing in patients receiving long-term antimalarial therapy. Am J Med 1983; 75(1A):25.

54. Felson DT, Anderson JJ, Meenan RF: The comparative efficacy and toxicity of second-line drugs in rheumatoid arthritis. Arthritis Rheum 1990; 33:1449.

55. Davis MJ, Dawes PT, Fowler PD, et al: Should disease-modifying agents be used in mild rheumatoid arthritis? Br J Rheumatol 1991; 30:451.

56. Day RO, Paulus HE: D-Penicillamine. In Paulus HE, Furst DE, Dromgoole SH (eds): Drugs for Rheumatic Disease. New York: Churchill Livingstone, 1987:85.

57. Lipsky PE: Immunosuppression by D-penicillamine in vitro: Inhibition of human T lymphocyte proliferation by copper- or ceruloplasmin-dependent generation hydrogen peroxide and protection by monocytes. J Clin Invest 1984; 73:53.

58. Scott DL, Williams JD, Greenwood A, et al: Assessing the outcome of penicillamine therapy. Br J Rheumatol 1986; 25(suppl 21):114.

59. Williams HJ, Ward JR, Reading JC, et al: Low dose D-penicillamine therapy in rheumatoid arthritis: A controlled double-blind clinical trial. Arthritis Rheum 1983; 26:581.

60. Doyle DV, Perrett D, Foster OJF, et al: The long-term use of D-penicillamine for treating rheumatiod arthritis: Is continuous therapy necessary? Br J Rheumatol 1993; 32:614.

61. Joyce DA, Day RO, Murphy BR: The pharmacokinetics of albumin conjugates of D-penicillamine in humans. Drug Metab Dispos 1991; 19:309.

62. Ahern MJ, Hall ND, Case K, et al: D-Penicillamine withdrawal in rheumatoid arthritis. Ann Rheum Dis 1984; 43:213.

63. Fauci AS, Young KR Jr: Immunoregulatory agents. In Kelley WN, Harris ED Jr, Ruddy S, et al (eds): Textbook of Rheumatology, 5th ed. Philadelphia: WB Saunders, 1997:805.

64. Kinlen LJ: Incidence of cancer in rheumatoid arthritis and other disorders after immunosuppressive treatment. Am J Med 1985; 78(1A):44.

65. Singh G, Fries JF, Spitz P, et al: Toxic effects of azathioprine in rheumatoid arthritis: A national post-marketing perspective. Arthritis Rheum 1989; 32:837.

66. Tugwell P, Bombardier C, Gent M, et al: Low-dose cyclosporin versus placebo in patients with rheumatoid arthritis. Lancet 1990; 335:1051.

67. Tugwell P, Pincus T, Yocum D, et al: Combination therapy with cyclosporin and methotrexate in severe rheumatoid arthritis. N Engl J Med 1995; 333:137.

68. Fox R, Morgan S, Smith H, et al: Treatment of RA patients with methotrexate plus cyclosporin A leads to elevation of plasma methotrexate levels and decrease of hydroxy-methotrexate levels. Arthritis Rheum 1998; 41(suppl 9):S-138.

69. Fox R, Mahboubi A, Green D, et al: Leflunomide inhibits de novo uridine synthesis and is dependent on p53 for arrest in G1 phase of cell cycle. Arthritis Rheum 1998; 41(suppl 9):S-137.

70. Miladenovic V, Domljan Z, Rozman B, et al: Safety and effectiveness of leflunomide in the treatment of patients with active rheumatoid arthritis. Arthritis Rheum 1995; 38:1595.

71. Weaver A, Caldwell J, Olsen H, et al: Treatment of active rheumatoid arthritis with leflunomide compared to methotrexate. Arthritis Rheum 1998; 41(suppl 9):S131.

72. Smolen JS, Kalden JK, Rozman B, et al: A double-blind randomized, phase III trial of leflunomide vs placebo vs sulfasalazine in rheumatoid arthritis. Arthritis Rheum 1998; 41(suppl 9):S131.

73. Schiff M, Kaine J, Sharp J, et al: X-ray analysis of 12 months treatment of active rheumatoid arthritis with leflunomide compared to placebo or methotrexate. Arthritis Rheum 1998; 41(suppl 9):S155.

74. Kloppenburg M, Breedveld FC, Miltenburg AM, et al: Antibiotics as disease modifiers in arthritis. Clin Exp Rheumatol 1993: 11(suppl 8):S113.

75. Tilley BC, Alarcón GS, Heyse SP, et al: Minocycline in rheumatoid arthritis: A 48-week, double-blind, placebo-controlled trial. MIRA Trial Group. Ann Intern Med 1995; 122:81.

76. Kloppenburg M, Breedveld FC, Terwiel JP, et al: Minocycline in active rheumatoid arthritis: A double-blind, placebo-controlled trial. Arthritis Rheum 1994; 37:629.

77. Moreland LW, Baumgartner SW, Schiff MH, et al: Treatment of rheumatoid arthritis with a recombinant human tumor necrosis factor receptor (p75)-Fc fusion protein. N Engl J Med 1997; 337:141.

78. Weinblatt ME, Kremer JM, Bankhurst AD, et al: A trial of etanercept, a recombinant tumor necrosis factor receptor:Fc fusion protein, in patients with rheumatoid arthritis receiving methotrexate. N Engl J Med 1999; 340:253.

79. Moreland LW, Baumgartner SW, Tindall EA, et al: Longterm safety and efficacy of TNF receptor (P75) Fc protein (TNFR:Fc;Enbrel) in DMARD refractory RA. Arthritis Rheum 1998; 41(suppl 9):S364.

79a. Finck B, Martin R, Fleischmann R, et al: A phase III trial of etanercept vs methotrexate in early rheumatoid arthritis. Arthritis Rheum 1999; 42 (supplement 9):S117.

79b. Cush J, Spiera R: Infliximab (Remicade) approved for use in rheumatoid arthritis. ACR Hotline Feb 29, 2000. American College of Rheumatology, Atlanta, pages 1–2.

79c. Maini R, St Clair EW, Breedveld F, et al: Infliximab (chimeric anti-tumour necrosis factor alpha monoclonal antibody) versus placebo in rheumatoid arthritis patients receiving concomitant methotrexate: a randomised phase III trial. ATTRACT Study Group. Lancet 1999; 354(9194):1932.

79d. Lipsky P, van der Heijde D, St. Clair WE, et al: Sustained clinical benefit and arrest of radiographic joint damage by continued therapy with a chimeric anti-TNF alpha monoclonal antibody, infliximab, in combination with methotrexate. Manuscript submitted for publication.

80. Weiss MM: Corticosteroids in rheumatoid arthritis. Semin Arthritis Rheum 1989; 19:9.

81. Kirwan JR, Arthritis and Rheumatism Council Low Dose Glucocorticoid Study Group: The effect of glucocorticoids on joint destruction in rheumatoid arthritis. N Engl J Med 1995; 333:142.

82. Saag K, Criswell L, Sems K, et al: Low-dose corticosteroids in rheumatoid arthritis. Arthritis Rheum 1996; 39:1818.

83. Chen L, O'Malley BW: Steroid hormone action: Recent advances. Ann Intern Med 1978; 89:694.

84. Weiss MM: Corticosteroids in rheumatoid arthritis. Semin Arthritis Rheum 1989; 19:9.

85. Parrillo JE, Faucci AS: Mechanisms of glucocorticoid action on immune processes. Annu Rev Pharmacol Toxicol 1979; 19:179.

86. Garber EK, Targoff C, Paulus HE: Corticosteroids in the rheumatic diseases: Chronic low doses, chronic high doses, "pulses," intra-articular. In Paulus HE, Furst DE, Dromgoole SH (eds): Drugs for Rheumatic Disease. New York: Churchill Livingstone, 1987:443.

87. Radia M, Furst DE: Comparison of three pulse methylprednisolone regimens in the treatment of rheumatoid arthritis. J Rheumatol 1988; 15:24.

88. La Rochelle GE, La Rochelle AG, Ratner RE, et al: Recovery of the hypothalamic-pituitary-adrenal (HPA) axis in patients with rheumatic disease receiving low dose prednisone. Am J Med 1993; 95:258.

89. O'Dell J: Combination DMARD therapy for rheumatoid arthritis: Apparent universal acceptance. Arthritis Rheum 1997; 40:S50.

90. Paulus HE: Current controversies in rheumatology: The use of combinations of disease-modifying anti-rheumatic agents in rheumatoid arthritis. Arthritis Rheum 1990; 33:113.

91. Haagsma CJ, van Riel PLCM, de Jong AJL, et al: Combination of sulfasalazine and methotrexate versus the single components in early rheumatoid arthritis: A randomized, controlled, double-blind 52 weeks clinical trial. Br J Rheumatol 1997; 36:1082.

92. O'Dell JR, Haire CE, Erikson N, et al: Treatment of rheumatoid arthritis with methotrexate alone, sulfasalazine and hydroxychloroquine or a combination all three medications. N Engl J Med 1996; 334:1287.

93. Boers M, Verhoeven AC, Markusse HM, et al: Randomized comparison of combined step-down prednisolone, methotrexate and sulfasalazine with sulfasalazine alone in early rheumatoid arthritis. Lancet 1997; 350:309.

94. Lipsky P, St. Clair W, Kavanaugh A, et al: Long-term control of signs and symptoms of rheumatoid arthritis with chimeric monoclonal anti-TNF alpha antibody (infliximab) in patients with active disease on methotrexate. Arthritis Rheum 1998; 41(suppl):S364.

95. Fuchs HA, Kaye JJ, Callahan LF, et al: Evidence of significant radiographic damage in rheumatoid arthritis within the first 2 years of disease. J Rheumatol 1989; 16:585.

96. Caruso I, Santandrea S, Sarzi Puttini P, et al: Clinical, laboratory and radiographic features of early rheumatoid arthritis. J Rheumatol 1990; 17:1268.

97. Scott DL, Symmons DPM, Coulton BL, et al: Long-term outcome of treating rheumatoid arthritis: Results after 20 years. Lancet 1987; 1:1108.

98. Wilske KR, Healey LA: Remodelling the pyramid: A concept whose time has come. J Rheumatol 1990; 17:127.

99. Van der Heide A, Jacobs JWG, Bijlsma JWJ: The effectiveness of early treatment with "second-line" antirheumatic drugs: A randomized, controlled trial. Ann Intern Med 1996; 124:699.

100. Egsmose C, Lund B, Borg C, et al: Patients with rheumatoid arthritis benefit from early second line therapy: 5 year follow-up of a prospective double blind placebo controlled study. J Rheumatol 1995; 22:2208.

101. ten Wolde S, Breedveld FC, Hermans J, et al: Randomised placebo-controlled study of stopping second-line drugs in rheumatoid arthritis. Lancet 1996; 347:347.

102. Gabriel SE, Luthra HS: Rheumatoid arthritis. Can the long-term outcome be altered? Mayo Clin Proc 1988; 63:58.

103. Pincus T: Rheumatoid arthritis: Disappointing long-term outcomes despite successful short-term clinical trials. J Clin Epidemiol 1988; 41:1037.

104. Wolfe F: Adverse drug reactions of DMARDs and DCARTs in rheumatoid arthritis. Clin Exp Rheumatol 1997; 15(suppl 15):S75.

105. Hawley DJ, Wolfe F: Are the results of controlled clinical trials and observational studies of second line therapy valid and generalizable as measures of rheumatoid arthritis outcome: Analysis of 122 studies. J Rheumatol 1991; 19:1008.

106. Rau R, Schleusser NB, Herborn G, et al: Longterm treatment of destructive rheumatoid arthritis with methotrexate. J Rheumatol 1997; 24:1881.

107. Thompson PW, Kirwan JR, Barnes CG: Practical results of treatment with disease-modifying anti-rheumatoid drugs. Br J Rheumatol 1985; 24:167.

108. Wolfe F, Hawley DF: Remission in rheumatoid arthritis. J Rheumatol 1985; 12:245.

109. O'Brien BJ, Elswood J, Calin A: Willingness to accept risk in the treatment of rheumatic disease. J Epidemiol 1990; 44:249.

110. Edmonds J: Better guidelines to rheumatoid arthritis therapy. Aust N Z J Med 1993; 23:143.

111. Felson D, Furst D, La Valley M, et al: Results of a randomized double blind trial of the Prosorba® column for treatment of severe rheumatoid arthritis. Arthritis Rheum 1998; 41(suppl): S364.

# 20 | Extra-articular Manifestations of Rheumatoid Arthritis

*Eric L. Matteson and Doyt L. Conn*

Extra-articular features of rheumatoid arthritis (RA) may occur at any time in the course of the disease and may even overshadow the joint disease. An understanding of the systemic nature of RA is essential to its successful treatment. The systemic or extra-articular manifestations may sometimes be the major manifestations necessitating treatment, and at other times they may be in the background, apparent only because of constitutional symptoms such as weight loss, low-grade fever, malaise, and generalized weakness. When systemic features dominate, they may be life-threatening and may constitute true emergencies. These complications must be recognized and treated appropriately, because systemic features of RA are major predictors of overall morbidity and mortality.[1, 2]

## GENERAL PRINCIPLES

The treatment of extra-articular manifestations of RA is guided by the specific organ system involved and by the severity of involvement. In general, therapeutic strategies designed to control the joint involvement are often effective in treating systemic disease. They include the use of nonsteroidal anti-inflammatory drugs (NSAIDs); disease-modifying antirheumatic drugs (DMARDs) such as gold, penicillamine, hydroxychloroquine, methotrexate, sulfasalazine, azathioprine, cyclosporine, leflunomide, tumor necrosis factor antagonists, including etanercept and infliximab; glucocorticosteroids; and in rare cases, other cytotoxic agents such as cyclophosphamide and chlorambucil. In our view, the use of glucocorticosteroids remains the mainstay for management of the systemic inflammatory features of RA. The initial dose of glucocorticosteroid is commensurate with the organ involved and the degree of involvement; it is given orally as a daily divided dose and is tapered according to the response of the organ system involved. At the same time, baseline therapy with NSAIDs and DMARDs is usually continued. In our experience, the rapid tapering or termination of glucocorticosteroid dosage after 1 or 2 weeks results in relapse of the disease manifestation being treated and an unnecessary cycle of "burst and taper" therapy. Many of the manifestations of extra-articular disease necessitate 2 or more months of glucocorticoid therapy and frequently maintenance therapy with low doses of glucocorticoids.

The role of high-dose "pulse" glucocorticosteroid therapy (1 g or more of intravenous methylprednisolone [Solu-Medrol]) is not established and is rarely, if ever, required for treating any disease manifestation, in our experience. In some cases, it is necessary to add cytotoxic agents as adjunctive therapy to facilitate steroid reduction. Surgical management of specific target organ involvement is sometimes necessary (e.g., cervical spine fusion for C1–2 instability, pericardiectomy for restrictive pericarditis). The role of newer agents such as leflunomide and anticytokine therapies such as tumor necrosis factor (TNF) antagonists and others is as yet unclear, although the increased production of proinflammatory cytokines such as TNF-$\alpha$ in involved tissues such as the synovium and lung tissue makes TNF antagonism an attractive additional therapeutic measure.

In this chapter, the treatment of the more characteristic extra-articular manifestations of RA is addressed. Because there are no controlled trials of treatments for extra-articular disease, these recommendations are based on case reports, case series, and the experience of the authors. Skin manifestations characteristic of RA, such as nodulosis and vasculitis with its complications, are addressed, whereas more nonspecific manifestations, such as pyoderma gangrenosum, neutrophilic dermatitis, purpura, and livedo, are not. The management of extra-articular musculoskeletal sequelae such as tendon ruptures is not further discussed; certainly, prevention of these complications by medical interventions and occasionally surgical tenosynovectomy is the best form of treatment.

## PULMONARY DISEASE

Although pulmonary involvement is often not clinically significant in RA, it is a leading cause of death in this disease, perhaps second to infection.[3] In addition to the clinical symptoms and examination with conventional radiography and pulmonary function tests, high-resolution computed tomography is emerging as a useful tool in the diagnosis and management of these manifestations of disease, especially bronchiectasis obstruction, fibrosis, and pulmonary nodulosis.[4] Pulmonary biopsy should be performed if the clinical situation is ambiguous, especially when there are new findings or the cause of the pulmonary nodule or nodules remains unclear.

Pulmonary fibrosis may occur in up to 28% of patients,[5] and it occurs even early in the disease course (14% of patients with disease of less than 2 years' duration).[6] Interstitial pulmonary fibrosis is strongly related to smoking,[7] an even stronger independent predictor of lung disease than RA disease activity or severity.[8] In patients with long-standing disease, the picture of interstitial fibrosis may in rare cases be a result of amyloidosis,[9] with its attendant therapeutic implications. Because smoking can accelerate the development of pulmonary fibrosis, an important therapeutic intervention in these patients is cessation of smoking.

The treatment of pulmonary fibrosis has traditionally focused on the use of glucocorticosteroids.[10, 11] It is unclear whether or how glucocorticoids affect the fibrotic disease process. Short-term high doses of glucocorticosteroids (usually prednisone, 20 to 40 mg/day for 1 to 2 months, then tapering slowly over a 6-month period) have a beneficial effect in improving exercise tolerance.[12, 13] In general, the use of protracted high-dose glucocorticosteroids in patients with interstitial fibrosis does not appear to be justified as long-term therapy if there is no beneficial response in the initial 2 to 4 months. Penicillamine has been used in some patients with interstitial lung disease, cardiovascular diseases, and RA with variable and uncertain success.[14]

Cytotoxic agents are sometimes used in patients with RA to control aggressive pulmonary fibrosis. Numerous case series and case reports of patients treated suggest potential improvement with methotrexate, penicillamine, azathioprine, cyclophosphamide, and cyclosporine.[14–19] As with glucocorticosteroids, there are no controlled studies demonstrating the benefit of this approach.

Symptomatic pleural involvement occurs in 20% of patients with RA, although autopsy studies have shown pleural inflammation or scarring in up to 50%. Male patients with active seropositive nodular disease are often affected. Pleurisy and pleural effusions may improve spontaneously or necessitate treatment, particularly when the pleuritic pain or shortness of breath becomes intolerable. It is important to rule out other causes of pleurisy and pleural effusion, most notably infection. Pleurisy without large pleural effusions frequently responds to the use of NSAIDs for 2 to 4 weeks or to modest doses of prednisone (less than 15 mg/day) for 1 to 2 months, with doses tapered thereafter. Large effusions, particularly those that cause respiratory compromise, may be treated with higher doses of glucocorticosteroids. Prednisone, 40 to 60 mg/day in divided doses, may be given over a 2- to 4-week period, with the dose tapered as the symptoms resolve and the chest roentgenogram clears. Intrapleural glucocorticosteroids are usually without long-term efficacy.[20]

Patients who experience marked shortness of breath may require thoracentesis or continuous suction drainage to evacuate the pleural effusion. Pleurectomy is necessary if persistent effusions lead to pleural fibrosis limiting lung expansion. Intrapleural tetracycline may prevent recurrence.[21] Care must be taken in the evacuation of these effusions because of the risk of lung puncture and infection.[22]

Parenchymal pulmonary nodules are usually asymptomatic and occur in patients with seropositive RA who have widespread synovitis and who usually have nodules elsewhere. These nodules tend to be peripheral in location and are from less than 1 to 8 cm in diameter.[23] Pulmonary nodules can persist unchanged for years, or they may resolve spontaneously. Pulmonary nodules present a dilemma that is more diagnostic than therapeutic, because it is necessary to consider neoplasia, tuberculosis, and fungal infections in the differential diagnosis. In general, rheumatoid pulmonary nodulosis does not necessitate specific therapeutic intervention if asymptomatic; the treatment of the underlying rheumatoid disease frequently results in improvement of the nodules. Cavitation may occur and can be associated with hemoptysis or infection, necessitating surgical therapy. The occurrence of a bronchopulmonary fistula may be life-threatening and necessitate surgical repair. Pneumothorax may occur; this can resolve spontaneously or may necessitate surgical intervention.[23]

Caplan's syndrome, defined as pneumoconiosis in a patient with RA, is characterized by multiple nodules greater than 1 cm in diameter scattered throughout the peripheral lung field.[24] This condition is seen in association with extensive exposure to silica. Some patients with Caplan's syndrome have exacerbations of their RA in association with the development of pneumoconiosis.[24] In addition to treatment of the underlying disease, avoidance of the offending exposure would seem to be the best treatment course.

Obliterative bronchiolitis has been reported in patients with RA.[25] It is not known whether this pulmonary manifestation is a consequence of the rheumatoid inflammatory process, another concomitant process, or medications. Bronchiolitis obliterans can be obstructive or associated with organizing pneumonia.[26, 27] It frequently leads to rapidly progressive respiratory insufficiency.[28, 29]

Bronchiolitis obliterans-organizing pneumonia (BOOP) may respond rapidly to high-dose glucocorticosteroid treatment (60 to 80 mg/day for 2 to 4 weeks), with the dose reduced by about 10% every 1 to 2 weeks according to patient response.[30] The duration of therapy required is not known but may exceed 3 to 6 months, and protracted low-dose glucocorticosteroid therapy may be necessary. Initial antibiotic therapy in BOOP is often attempted because of the frequently unclear clinical situation.[31] Anecdotal experience with cytotoxic agents is also reported. Cyclophosphamide has been successfully used orally and intravenously in patients with bronchiolitis obliterans and interstitial fibrosis refractory to glucocorticoid therapy. The duration of cytotoxic therapy required has not been established, but conventional use is usually over the course of several months and up to 1 year.[32, 33]

The long-term outcome in patients in whom bronchiolitis obliterans develops is unclear; it has been suggested that the disease does not respond to glucocorticosteroids and has an invariably poor, if not fatal, outcome within a few months after diagnosis.[25] Although the outcome of the proliferative form of bronchiolitis obliterans with obstructive pneumonia is often favorable, especially if causative drugs such as penicillamine or gold can be identified and removed, the patient should be given vigorous respiratory support and treated with glucocorticosteroids in high doses. Prognosis of the constrictive form of bronchiolitis is quite poor.[34]

Bronchiectasis has been reported in one third of patients with RA by high-resolution computed tomography,[4] although only somewhat more than 300 cases have been reported in the literature.[35] More than 50% of these patients have other extra-articular manifestations.[35] When appropriate, treatment is with antibiotics, chest physiotherapy, hydration, discontinuation of smoking, bronchodilators, oxygen, and resection.

Pulmonary arteritis is an uncommon complication of RA. Although it may be the sole manifestation of lung disease, it is usually associated with other manifestations of rheumatoid lung disease, such as interstitial fibrosis and nodulosis.[36] The literature reveals virtually no experience with treatment of this disease complication. As an arteritis that may be associated with acrocyanosis and digital infarction, pulmonary arteritis may respond to glucocorticosteroid treatment as well as vasodilatory agents, including calcium channel blockers.

RA involving the larynx may lead to upper airway obstruction and dyspnea. As many as 26% of patients with RA have cricoarytenoid involvement.[37] Moderate obstruction may cause no symptoms, but if laryngeal edema is present the obstruction may interfere with normal tidal breathing.[38] Upper airway obstruction can be of acute onset and constitute an emergency. This is especially true of patients who develop an ordinary upper respiratory tract infection and experience sudden respiratory decompensation.[39] Patients with symptoms of hoarseness, shortness of breath, and laryngeal discomfort or dysphagia should undergo direct laryngoscopy. This may show decreased mobility of the true vocal cords and erythema of the arytenoid mucosa.[37] Initial management should be prompt and should include prednisone, 20 mg three times daily for 1 week and tapered thereafter according to symptoms. Injection of the cricoarytenoid joints with triamcinolone acetonide may greatly accelerate the resolution of inflammation.[40, 41] It must be emphasized that for patients who have a compromised airway a trial of systemic glucocorticosteroids and close observation in the hospital is warranted. In some cases tracheostomy is necessary. Patients in whom cricoarytenoid ankylosis develops may have stable upper airway disease that may not even be symptomatic because of relatively sedentary lifestyles.[38] After the diagnosis of cricoarytenoid ankylosis is established, the degree of laryngeal obstruction should be determined by spirometry and flow-volume loops, and bilateral paralysis of the recurrent laryngeal nerves should be excluded. Surgical interventions to relieve airway obstruction may include lateral fixation.[38, 42, 43] Arytenoidectomy is regarded as definitive therapy and is usually performed unilaterally.[44]

## CARDIAC DISEASE

Cardiac involvement in patients with RA reflects the systemic nature of the underlying disease. Patients may have pericarditis as a form of serositis, nodulosis of the myocardium or valves and conduction pathways, or vasculitis of the coronary arteries. Pericarditis is the most common of these manifestations, occurring in up to 50% of patients.[45]

Pericarditis may be associated with chest pain and dyspnea, usually in the context of active RA, although it can occur in patients with otherwise quiescent disease.[46] In contrast to the high incidence found by electrocardiographic, echocardiographic, or postmortem studies, clinically symptomatic pericarditis is relatively unusual, occurring in approximately 3% of patients.[47, 48] In one large series, three fourths of the patients had acute pericarditis and the remainder had recurrent acute pericarditis and chronic pericarditis with effusion or chronic constrictive carditis.[49] Uncomplicated clinical pericarditis responds to medical management, including the use of NSAIDs, glucocorticosteroids, or both.[48] In general, we favor the use of glucocorticosteroids in moderate doses (10 to 15 mg/day tapering as symptoms tolerate) for the treatment of chest discomfort associated with pericarditis in patients with small, nonconstricting effusions. Patients with tamponade and constrictive pericarditis require pericardiectomy.[49] Emergency pericardiocentesis can be lifesaving. This should be accompanied by high doses of prednisone (20 mg three times daily) and may be followed by intracardiac injections of glucocorticosteroids.[50] These should be regarded as emergency procedures. Patients who have tamponade or impending tamponade require surgical intervention because of the high mortality rate (approaching 100%) of this condition.[50–52]

Although pericardial resection appears to be the treatment of choice, one study failed to find any beneficial effect of pericardiectomy on the survival of patients with RA.[49] The 2-year mortality rate after pericardiectomy was high if cardiac compression had occurred and general debilitation had ensued. Surgical pericardiectomy should be as extensive as possible.[51, 53] A pericardial window is usually inadequate to prevent reaccumulation and should be reserved for ill patients who are unable to tolerate a thoracotomy.[50, 54] Glucocorticosteroid treatment of cardiac tamponade neither prevents its development nor effects its regression. Symptom-free patients without evidence of tamponade in whom small pericardial effusions are found on incidental echocardiographic examinations may not require treatment. Glucocorticosteroid therapy usually reverses the symptoms and signs of rheumatoid pericarditis in 2 to 4 weeks.[55] Reaccumulation of pericardial fluid before significant tapering of the glucocorticoid is accomplished should be considered a strong indication for a pericardiectomy.[55] It has been estimated that approximately one third of patients with pericarditis eventually require pericardiectomy.[56]

Myocardial disease may be focal or diffuse and may lead to frank muscle necrosis.[56] Nonspecific myocarditis is thought to be asymptomatic and rarely affects cardiac size or function. Hence it is rarely recognized, and its natural history and treatment are uncertain. Postmortem examination has revealed nonspecific myocarditis in as many as 19% of autopsy cases.[56]

Myocardial and endocardial disease associated with RA is usually a result of vasculitis with or without nodule formation. Small-vessel vasculitis is seen in up to 20% of cases.[57] Rheumatoid vasculitis in the form of coronary arteritis is also reported. How often this leads to myocardial infarction is not known. One study of 90 patients with rheumatoid vasculitis revealed evidence of myocardial infarction in 5 patients, 1 of whom demonstrated angiitis at autopsy.[58] Vasculitis of the small vessels of the myocardium leading to congestive hart failure has been seen on percutaneous catheter-directed endomyocardial biopsy. A high degree of clinical suspicion is necessary to recognize vasculitis and to institute therapy promptly. Patients may respond well to glucocorticosteroid therapy.[59]

Rheumatoid granuloma in or near the atrioventricular node or bundle of His may result in arrhythmias, including complete heart block and syncope. Some patients with minor degrees of heart block later develop complete heart block, which is usually discovered only after syncope or on physical examination and electrocardiogram of an otherwise symptom-free patient.[60] Patients with complete heart block usually have established erosive nodular disease and test positive for rheumatoid factor. Typically, patients are already undergoing antirheumatic drug therapy with NSAIDs and even glucocorticosteroids when heart block appears. The role of medications, including glucocorticosteroids, in the treatment of arrhythmias in patients with RA is uncertain; cardiac pacemakers are the treatment of choice for complete heart block. Chloroquine has been associated with prolongation of the PR interval[61] and may be a cause of heart block. Rarely would this complication appear to be a clinically significant problem in patients with RA.[62, 63]

Valvular disease is well recognized in patients with RA. The aortic valve shows nodules, cusp thickening, and perforation leading to incompetence in 20% of cases at autopsy.[64, 65] Endocardial disease in the setting of pleurisy and cutaneous vasculitis responds to high doses of glucocorticosteroids (40 to 60 mg/day initially). In the absence of these systemic features, the role of glucocorticosteroids in the treatment of endocardial lesions is uncertain. The heart disease should be managed in conjunction with a cardiologist and cardiac surgeon.

Inflammatory aortic root disease may be asymptomatic at the time of diagnosis, with a typical murmur of aortic regurgitation.[66] Clinically evident aortic incompetence probably affects fewer than 1% of patients who have RA.[67] When active aortitis and dilatation occur, oral prednisone at 60 mg/day and azathioprine or cyclophosphamide are useful at the onset.[66] The treatment response can be monitored according to clinical status, echocardiographic findings, and the erythrocyte sedimentation rate. Some authors have found factor VIII–related antigen levels to be useful in monitoring these patients.[66] Surgery is more successful when aortic root inflammation is suppressed.[67, 68]

## OCULAR DISEASE

Keratoconjunctivitis sicca affects 10% to 35% of patients with RA.[69] Symptoms include pain, visual disturbance, foreign body sensation, and mucoid discharge. Treatment of keratoconjunctivitis sicca remains symptomatic. It is important to emphasize that the treatment of keratoconjunctivitis sicca also has the purpose of preventing scarring because of dryness as well as infection, and even patients with asymptomatic dry eyes should be treated with artificial tears, including methylcellose-containing products. Several preparations are available, including Liquifilm, Liquifilm Forte, Tears Plus, and Tears Naturale. In some cases the preservatives contained in these artificial tears cause topical irritation.[70] Ointments such as Lacri-Lube can be used at bedtime.

Humidifiers, wraparound glasses, and goggles may be useful.[71] In patients who have refractory dryness of the eyes, obliteration of the puncta and canaliculi may be considered. On rare occasions, a partial tarsorrhaphy may become necessary. Unless inflammation is present, topical steroids should be avoided because of the potential for corneal perforation. See Chapter 21 for a detailed discussion of Sjögren's syndrome.

Episcleritis often correlates with the activity of the RA disease. Episcleritis may be nodular or diffuse and may cause eye redness and pain but only rarely causes changes in visual acuity.[69] Improved control of the RA itself may or may not improve the episcleritis. In general, episcleritis is self-limited and usually does not necessitate treatment. When it is recurring or uncomfortable, topical glucocorticosteroids may be employed under the supervision of an ophthalmologist.

As with other extra-articular manifestations, the most severe forms of ocular disease in RA, necrotizing scleritis (NS) and severe peripheral ulcerative keratitis (PUK), occur in patients with longer-standing and widespread systemic disease including systemic vasculitis. Severe PUK and NS may result in intense ocular pain, erythema, and eventually even perforation. In cooperation with an ophthalmologist, prednisone in doses from 40 to 100 mg/day is initiated.[72] In addition to high doses of oral glucocorticosteroids, cytotoxic therapy is always necessary to treat active PUK and NS.[73] In a series of 16 patients (25 eyes), cyclophosphamide was effective in 50% and methotrexate in 38% of patients. Oral and topical cyclosporine may also be effective in the treatment of NS.[73, 74] Topical cyclophosphamide and azathioprine may also be given with good effect, particularly in patients with PUK.[75] Other cytotoxic agents, including nitrogen mustard and duazomycin, have also been used.[76] The key to successful treatment of NS and severe PUK is early recognition of these conditions. The duration of medical therapy with combination glucocorticosteroids and cytotoxic agents for PUK and NS is often about 6 months, depending on the clinical situation.[73, 75] In advanced cases, surgical procedures such as conjunctival resection, cyanoacrylate adhesive, tectonic coronal grafts, conjunctival flaps, scleral grafting, and keratoplasty may be necessary.[73, 76] Even if the globe can be preserved, the visual outcome is often poor despite these measures, with loss of visual acuity in 40% of patients with NS.[77] Other manifestations such as iridocyclitis or choroiditis, which may develop in up to one third of patients,[76] often also necessitate similar intensive therapy but are usually less severe than PUK and NS[73] (see Chapter 16).

It has been thought that cornea and scleral disease in RA may be accelerated by cataract extraction.[78, 79] However, it appears that these problems are no more frequent in patients with RA who undergo cataract surgery than in the general population.[80] However, keratoconjunctivitis sicca should be carefully managed perioperatively because of the increased risk of corneal surface disease, including superficial punctate keratopathy.[80]

Tenosynovitis of the superior oblique tendon sheath may lead to mechanical obstruction when the patient attempts to raise the eye in adduction (Brown's syndrome). Patients have diplopia and pain on attempted upward and inward gaze.[81, 82] This manifestation may improve with oral glucocorticosteroids, although local injection of the tendon sheath or even nodule removal may be necessary.

It has been suggested that the eye is a sensitive indicator of occult systemic vasculitis in patients with RA in whom PUK or NS develops. A nonrandomized trial compared steroid plus NSAID therapy with cytotoxic immunosuppression for 34 patients with RA and PUK or NS; 9 of 17 patients given steroid without cytotoxic therapy died from a vasculitis-related event during the 10-year follow-up period. In 13 of these 17 patients, the ocular inflammatory lesions progressed, and in 5 patients extraocular but nonlethal vasculitis lesions developed. In the group treated with cytotoxic drugs, only 1 of 17 patients died, and this death occurred after cytotoxic therapy was withdrawn. None of the patients given cytotoxic regimens developed extraocular vasculitis or had progression of the ocular destructive lesions while taking cytotoxics.[83]

## NEUROLOGIC DISEASE

Nerve compression is a common cause of neurologic impairment in RA. Peripheral entrapment neuropathies are not related to the duration, degree of activity, or severity of extra-articular manifestations of RA, although they do tend to correlate with the degree and severity of local synovitis. The median, ulnar, posterior tibial, and posterior interosseous branch of the radial nerves are the most commonly involved nerves.[84–86] Although no formal studies have evaluated this question, it is our experience that when active synovitis is present, relief can be afforded by local steroid injection as well as by resting of the adjacent joint and splinting. The use of NSAIDs is also necessary. If unsuccessful, and especially in instances in which there is compression without active synovitis, surgical nerve release will be effective.

It has been estimated that 35% to 40% of patients with RA have peripheral neuropathy that is manifested as paresthesias, dysesthesias, and burning.[87] In addition to treatment of the underlying inflammatory process, the use of thiamine (50 mg/day), diphenylhydantoin (100 mg three times a day), carbamazepine (100 to 800 mg/day), amitriptyline (50 to 150 mg/day),[87] gabapentin (starting at 300 mg at bedtime, increasing the dose every few days to 300 to 600 mg three times a day), or mexiletine (150 mg one to three times a day) may be beneficial in controlling the pain and dysesthesia.

Mononeuritis multiplex and related conditions are discussed in the section on vasculitis.

Atlantoaxial subluxation caused by erosion of the odontoid process and/or the transverse ligament of C1 may allow the odontoid process to slip posteriorly and lead to cervical myelopathy.[88] Basilar invagination may occur, leading to upward impingement of the odontoid process on the foramen magnum and resulting in cord compression.[89] Signs and symptoms of cord compression include hyper-reflexia, motor weakness of the extremities, a positive Babinski sign, Lhermitte's sign, and posterior neck pain. If the posterior cerebral circulation is affected, visual disturbances, vertigo, paresthesias, and paresis may occur. Most patients with cervical subluxation have extensive erosive joint disease and nodulosis with positive rheumatoid factor.[90]

Neck instability and pain can usually be managed conservatively with a collar to immobilize the neck, with the patient instructed to use the collar particularly while riding in motor vehicles and to take care to avoid whiplash injuries and falls. These collars are often burdensome and are frequently rejected by the patient.[91] Patients with progressing spinal cord signs should be considered for surgical cervical immobilization and traction.[92, 93] Surgery should be undertaken before severe myelopathy develops, because it is difficult to reverse and carries a high risk of premature death.[94] The prognosis for pain relief with surgery is generally very good.[95] Surgical stabilization is recommended for patients with subaxial subluxation and a posterior canal diameter of less than 14 mm.[95] C1–2 arthrodesis is also recommended for isolated atlantoaxial subluxation when the posterior atlantodental interval (the distance between the posterior surface of the dens and the anterior margin of the posterior ring of the atlas) is less than 14 mm, because decreases of the posterior atlanto-odontoid space correlate with paralysis more significantly than do decreases of the classical anterior atlanto-odontoid space.[95] Occiput-cervical fusion is recommended for basilar invagination, especially when atlantoaxial instability is present.[96] These recommendations must be seen in the clinical context of the specific patient's medical condition, including comorbidities, personal priorities, and surgical risks.

Several operative techniques have been employed to relieve posterior cervical pain and stabilize neurologic defects. Surgical decompression of the cervical medullary junction is considered for patients with irreducible encroachment.[97] A transoral-transpalatine approach may be used to resect irreducible invaginated odontoid granulation tissue.[98] Stabilization is most frequently attempted by means of posterior occipital cervical fusion with bone grafting, acrylics, and wire. Preoperative halo traction may help reduce cervical subluxation (M. E. Cabanela, Mayo Clinic, Rochester, Minnesota, personal communication, 2000). Occipital cervical fusion is recommended after any of these procedures.[89] These complications must be managed in conjunction with a surgery team skilled in the treatment of RA and related surgical techniques. Such procedures usually lead to excellent fusion rates approaching 100%, although tissue healing may be slowed in patients with RA, and pseudoarthrosis may occur.[99]

## AMYLOIDOSIS

In rare instances, amyloidosis complicates RA in patients with long-standing disease.[100] Secondary amyloidosis in RA occurs in 5% to 15% of patients.[100, 101] The average survival time after the diagnosis of secondary amyloidosis–associated RA is estimated to be about 4 to 5 years.[101, 102] Amyloidosis has been the attributed cause of death in about 8% of patients with RA at autopsy.[103] Renal amyloidosis in particular has been associated with diminished survival.[102, 104] The perinuclear antineutrophilic cytoplasmic antibody (pANCA) is present in up to 21% of patients with RA and renal disease of various causes, including amyloidosis and mesangial, focal segmental, and membranous glomerulonephritis, resulting in hematuria and proteinuria. pANCA may be an independent predictor of nephropathy in amyloidosis even in the absence of systemic vasculitis.[105] In patients with nephrotic syndrome, a renal biopsy is needed to distinguish amyloidosis from the mesangial glomerulonephritis of RA.

There are no controlled studies that address the treatment of amyloidosis in RA. Chlorambucil, cyclophosphamide, and azathioprine are among the drugs whose use has been advocated.[106] The role of these agents is uncertain. A study of 34 patients with RA and renal amyloidosis reported poor survival even in patients receiving alkylating agents; 20 patients died at a mean of 26 months after diagnosis of renal amyloidosis.[96] Of the 14 survivors, 7 were given alkylating agents. Only 3 patients had normal renal function at a mean of 59 months after diagnosis, all of whom had received an alkylating agent; 5 patients were undergoing dialysis.[96]

## FELTY'S SYNDROME

Felty's syndrome is defined as the presence of leukopenia and splenomegaly in RA. It occurs in 1% to 3% of patients with RA. It develops in that subset of patients with long-standing (more than 10 years), seropositive, nodular, and destructive joint disease. These patients usually display extra-articular features of disease, including rheumatoid nodules, skin lesions or nailfold infarcts and leg ulcers, peripheral neuropathy, and sicca syndrome.[107] In addition to Felty's syndrome, they usually have high-titer rheumatoid factor, antinuclear antibodies, cryoglobulins, and a diminished serum complement.[108] There is frequently a family history of RA, and most of the patients have the genetic type human leukocyte antigen (HLA)-DR4 and an increased frequency of the DQW3 variant, 3b.[109] These patients, like those with rheumatoid vasculitis, are homozygous for the HLA-DRB1 allele 0401.[110] Patients with RA and neutropenia without splenomegaly have the same clinical features as the defined Felty's syndrome, including the development of the extra-articular features and an increased susceptibility to infection.[111]

The neutropenia of Felty's syndrome predisposes the patient to infections, and 60% to 95% develop a superficial or deep infection (i.e., pneumonia or joint infection).[112] It is uncertain whether there is a correlation between the neutrophil count and the incidence of infection.[113]

Large granular lymphocyte syndrome (LGL syndrome) is a condition that may accompany RA and Felty's syndrome.[114] Affected patients have lymphocytosis and sometimes neutropenia. They have a subset of lymphocytes that are large with abundant pale blue cytoplasm. Patients with LGL syndrome commonly have splenomegaly and recurrent infections and may or may not have RA. Usually the total leukocyte count is normal, with lymphocytosis. The patients also commonly have rheumatoid factor and antinuclear antibodies.[111] Typing of the lymphocytes in these patients shows that there is a predominance of CD3[+], CD16[+], and CD57[+] types (see also Chapter 17).[115] The lymphocytes have a T-cell receptor gene rearrangement. It is not known whether this occurs because of a reactive change in response to an unknown antigen or a neoplastic change. Most patients have a nonprogressive course.

A study of clonal expansion of CD8[+] and CD57[+] T cells (LGL cells) in patients with RA and neutropenia showed two populations: those with LGL expansion and those without expansion.[116] Another study examined the HLA-DR alleles in patients with the LGL syndrome and Felty's syndrome. There was a high prevalence of HLA-DR4 in patients with Felty's syndrome and in patients with LGL syndrome in RA. The prevalence of DR4 was much less in those who had LGL syndrome without RA.[117] Consequently, Felty's syndrome with or without LGL probably is part of the same disease process (see Chapter 17).

There are patients who have Felty's syndrome with neutropenia for many years without infections. Likewise, there are case reports of patients with neutropenia due to Felty's syndrome who improve spontaneously.[118] There are probably several mechanisms responsible for the clinical finding of Felty's syndrome; spontaneous regression may occur depending on the specific pathogenetic process involved. There are no prospective, controlled treatment studies of Felty's syndrome. In one case control study, the outcome was poor; compared with rheumatoid control subjects without Felty's syndrome, there was an increasing mortality with time.[109] In another study comparing the outcome in patients with Felty's syndrome and matched controls with RA, there was no difference in the incidence of infection or in the death rate.[119] The death rate was increased in both groups.

There is no ideal therapy for Felty's syndrome. The reason for the lack of an effective approach to management is an incomplete understanding of the cause of Felty's syndrome, which may vary from patient to patient. A major mechanism is the presence of immune complex disease. Polymorphonuclear leukocytes (PMNs) phagocytize immune complexes, and these engorged PMNs are removed by the reticuloendothelial system. In addition, there may be decreased cytokine production, humoral inhibition of marrow responsiveness to colony-stimulating activity, and T-cell–mediated immune suppression of granulopoiesis.[111]

Glucocorticoids in higher doses may stimulate neutrophilia, but low doses may not maintain this improvement. Parenteral testosterone may stimulate granulopoiesis but is too toxic, particularly for long-term use in women.[120] Lithium carbonate stimulates granulopoiesis; it is a short-term measure but has no lasting benefit, and any benefit disappears after treatment is discontinued.[121] Intravenous immune globulin is not effective.[122]

Retrospective studies suggest that the best treatment for Felty's syndrome is the use of DMARDs. When this approach was examined in the early 1980s, most patients with Felty's syndrome either had not been given a disease-modifying agent or had been inadequately treated, sometimes because of adverse reactions to this type of drug.[123] This observation raises the possibility that early treatment of RA with DMARDs may prevent the development of Felty's syndrome.

Parenteral gold is the agent most widely used in retrospective studies of treatment of Felty's syndrome. In one study, 80% of patients with Felty's syndrome had improvement of neutropenia and a diminution of infections.[123] Penicillamine has not been as effective, partly because of frequent side effects in these patients.

Methotrexate is probably as effective as parenteral gold for the treatment of Felty's syndrome.[124] Cyclophosphamide has been shown to be effective, but side effects restrict its use to selected cases in which other DMARDs have not been effective.

Granulocyte colony-stimulating factor (CSF) and granulocyte-macrophage CSF have been used to correct neutropenia in Felty's syndrome.[111] The neutrophil count can be stimulated acutely but declines with time. This approach may be used when it is necessary to increase the leukocyte count quickly and for a limited time. In one case study, however, the neutrophil count was maintained for longer than 1 year with weekly injections of granulocyte CSF.[125] With the increase in the neutrophil count, the arthritis may worsen. It has been shown that, despite an increase in the peripheral neutrophil count, the bone marrow shows persistent maturation arrest.

Splenectomy results in an acute resolution of neutropenia, and in 80% of patients, improvement is long lasting. Still, about half of patients continue to have infections, and a small percentage sustain fatal infection.[126]

A reasonable management approach in Felty's syndrome is outlined as follows:

1. RA must be appropriately managed with timely initiation of DMARD therapy and, when needed, low doses of prednisone; this approach may prevent the development of Felty's syndrome.

2. If Felty's syndrome develops despite the use of a DMARD, then another DMARD should be tried.

3. If the patient has Felty's syndrome but no associated infection, then the current management approach should be continued with a DMARD; the neutropenia does not necessitate treatment if there is no apparent increased susceptibility to infections.

4. Patients with properly treated Felty's syndrome and persistent neutropenia who develop infections should be considered for granulocytic CSF therapy.

5. If a patient with Felty's syndrome and recurrent infections has not responded to granulocytic (CSF) therapy or if it is not available, splenectomy should be considered.

## RHEUMATOID VASCULITIS

Rheumatoid vasculitis occurs when small blood vessels, small- and medium-sized arteries outside the joints, become inflamed and result in clinical features of disease. The organs that usually are involved in rheumatoid vasculitis are the skin and peripheral nerves and, less commonly, the viscera, heart, and central nervous system. A small-vessel vasculitis is an early event in the development of rheumatoid nodules.[127] Rheumatoid vasculitis may occur in early RA, but it more commonly occurs later in the course of the disease.[128] The clinical features resulting from rheumatoid vasculitis include nailfold infarcts, livedo reticularis, leg ulcers, digital gangrene, and a peripheral neuropathy. The peripheral nerve involvement may be a sensory neuropathy or a sensory-motor neuropathy.[129] Less commonly, the vasculitis may extend to involve the mesentery, coronary, and cerebral arteries. These manifestations of rheumatoid vasculitis may occur singly or in combination.

Rheumatoid vasculitis occurs in a setting of long-standing RA. Most patients have had their disease for 10 years or longer. Men are affected as commonly as women. Patients in whom rheumatoid vasculitis develops have had more severe joint disease, with destructive changes, rheumatoid nodules, high titers of rheumatoid factor, and a history of smoking.[130–132] Patients with Felty's syndrome are more likely to develop vasculitic complications. There is a genetic predisposition to the development of extra-articular features of RA, particularly rheumatoid vasculitis.[133, 134] Although homozygosity for the HLA-DRB1*0401 allele was common in patients with rheumatoid vasculitis in Minnesota,[133] only skin vasculitis was associated with the DRB1*04 in Europe, and no clear association of the shared epitope with major organ lesions was found.[134]

The initial vascular injury in rheumatoid vasculitis is probably immunologically induced. Indirect evidence of immunologic involvement includes high-titer rheumatoid factor, circulating immune complexes, and a diminished serum complement.[135] Antiendothelial antibodies may be present.[136] The finding of immunoglobulins, complement, and fibrin in acute arterial lesions provides direct evidence of immune-induced injury in rheumatoid vasculitis. In the chronic lesions of arterial intimal proliferation and occlusion, only fibrin was found.[137] This suggests that the immune deposits initiated the injury and then were removed, leaving the fibrin, which must be resistant to normal clearing mechanisms.

Rheumatoid vasculitis comprises a spectrum of clinical features. Some clinical manifestations are benign and probably do not influence outcome. Clinical experience suggests that localized skin lesions and a distal sensory neuropathy are not indicators of a poor outcome.[129, 138] Multiple organ involvement and visceral involvement are major predictors of increased morbidity and decreased survival. Actuarial survival is decreased in patients with clinical rheumatoid vasculitis, similar to survival in classic RA (Table 20–1).

A retrospective study by Vollertsen and colleagues[139] showed that increased age at diagnosis was the best predictor of decreased survival. This study also demonstrated a decrease in actuarial survival in those patients who had not been taking NSAIDs at the time of diagnosis of vasculitis and who had previously taken cytotoxic drugs or glucocorticoids. In contrast, another study of 32 patients with rheumatoid vasculitic neuropathy with frequent skin vasculitis found that the presence of skin involvement, neuropathy affecting more than two extremities, and diminished C4 complement were associated with reduced survival. Age had no effect.[140]

Randomized, controlled treatment trials for rheumatoid vasculitis are not available. The management of RA is based on retrospective studies, the clinical experience of the clinician, and the collective experience of the clinician's institution. Since 1950, glucocorticoids have been used to manage rheumatoid vasculitis. It was observed in the 1950s that rheumatoid vasculitis appeared to be more common in patients who had received glucocorticoids.[141] This observation probably represents a selection bias, because patients with more severe RA and rheumatoid vasculitis were more likely to be prescribed glucocorticoids. Nevertheless, wide fluctuations in glucocorticoid doses, particularly a rapid tapering or switching to an alternate-day dose, may allow the suppressed vasculitis to explode and progress very rapidly. It is also possible that glucocorticoids may control inflammation but allow an occlusive vasculopathy to develop and progress.[142]

Patients who develop rheumatoid vasculitis frequently have never taken disease-modifying agents or have been unable to tolerate them.[139] This raises the possibility that patients with RA treated early in their disease with appropriate DMARDs may not develop rheumatoid vasculitis. Consequently, patients who have manifestations of rheumatoid vasculitis should be given an appropriate DMARD. Additional treatment depends on the particular disease manifestations, extent of disease, tempo of disease, clinical or laboratory evidence of inflammation, and coexisting disease states. Coexisting diseases or factors that influence the final vascular outcome include smoking, hypertension, and diabetes mellitus.

The clinician should attempt to determine whether the vascular lesion is inflammatory. Biopsy of involved tissue is a good way to determine the degree of inflammation if accessible tissue is available. Involved accessible tissue may include the skin or the sural nerve.[143] An estimate of the inflammatory nature of the vascular process can sometimes be made from clinical and laboratory examinations. Certain skin lesions, such as palpable purpura, an expanding ulcer, or progressive mononeuritis multiplex, indicate an active, progressive, inflammatory process. Systemic evidence of inflammation is reflected in the following laboratory abnormalities: an increased erythrocyte sedimentation rate, anemia, thrombocytosis, cryoglobulinemia, diminished serum complement, and elevation of cytokines (e.g., TNF, interleukin-6).[144, 145]

A patient with digital-tip infarcts but no other features of disease and no laboratory evidence of inflammation probably should not be treated with high doses of steroids or cytotoxic drugs. The pathology of this lesion is probably an intimal proliferation process.[146] Treatment should be directed toward reducing vasospasm, inhibiting platelet aggregation, and promoting revascularization. This patient should be given an appropriate DMARD, a vasodilating agent, antiplatelet drugs, and possibly low doses of prednisone.

## TABLE 20–1
## Relative Survival* of 52 Patients with Rheumatoid Arthritis or Rheumatoid Vasculitis

|  | YEARS AFTER DIAGNOSIS | | | | |
| --- | --- | --- | --- | --- | --- |
| TYPE | 1 | 2 | 3 | 4 | 5 |
| **Rheumatoid Arthritis** | | | | | |
| Definite | 101 | 100 | 102 | 103 | 100 |
| Classic | 96 | 95 | 85 | 85 | 85 |
| **Rheumatoid Vasculitis** | | | | | |
| All patients | 82 | 77 | 76 | 72 | 67 |
| Corrected for referral bias† | 95 | 90 | 92 | 93 | 87 |

* Expressed as percentage of expected survival in comparison with age- and sex-matched upper Middle Western control subjects from the general population.

† When corrected for referral distance, the survival time of vasculitis is similar to that of classic rheumatoid arthritis without vasculitis.

From Vollertsen RS, Conn DL, Ballard DJ, et al. Rheumatoid vasculitis: survival and associated risk factors. Medicine (Baltimore) 1986; 65:365–375. Copyright 1986 Williams & Wilkins Company.

For patients who have had a stable mononeuritis multiplex for several months with no other systemic vasculitic manifestations, treatment with DMARDs, NSAIDs, and low doses of prednisone may be sufficient.

It is important to recognize that factors in addition to the vasculitis may influence a final vascular outcome. In patients with leg ulcers there may be an initial underlying vasculitis but its extent and chronicity may be influenced by other factors, including venous insufficiency, ankle arthritis, dependent edema, trauma, and chronic glucocorticoid use.[147] In patients with digital infarcts, other factors that affect the blood vessels, including diabetes mellitus, hypertension, and smoking, may be as important as the vasculitic component.

Over the past two decades, the treatment of rheumatoid vasculitis has focused on the use of D-penicillamine, glucocorticoids, cytotoxic drugs, and plasmapheresis. Retrospective studies have not determined the influence of the extent of disease, the tempo of the disease, or inflammatory features of the disease on outcome. In addition the concept of relapse, long-term toxicity and maintenance of disease control with these agents need to be addressed.[148]

D-Penicillamine has been used in a number of studies for the management of rheumatoid vasculitis.[149] A significant benefit of D-penicillamine on actuarial survival remains to be demonstrated.[150] D-Penicillamine is no more effective than any of the other DMARDs for this condition. The authors do not use penicillamine for rheumatoid vasculitis.

There are small, uncontrolled series demonstrating the effectiveness of cyclophosphamide in the management of rheumatoid vasculitis.[150, 151] Chlorambucil may be equally effective. Although methotrexate has been reported to be beneficial in rheumatoid cutaneous vasculitis,[152] it has also been associated with the development of cutaneous vasculitis and rheumatoid nodules in RA.[153] A study designed to determine the frequency of methotrexate-induced vasculitis in RA failed to show an association compared with other treatments.[154] Azathioprine is the only DMARD that has been tested in a randomized trial for rheumatoid vasculitis.[155] This study failed to demonstrate any benefit but was of brief duration and low power. Another study demonstrated improvement in persons with rheumatoid vasculitis treated with high-dose prednisone and azathioprine.[156] The combination of methotrexate and azathioprine may induce a febrile reaction with cutaneous vasculitis.[157]

Pulsed, high-dose intravenous glucocorticoids, usually 1 g methylprednisolone per day for 1 to 5 days, are used empirically in the treatment of severe rheumatoid vasculitis. There is no established rationale for this therapy and no documentation showing that this dose is more efficacious than a dose in the range of 100 mg prednisone per day. Plasmapheresis used alone is not helpful. When it is used with prednisone and an alkylating agent, there may be improvement, but it is impossible to show any benefit attributable to the plasmapheresis.[158] Plasmapheresis cannot be recommended because of the lack of effectiveness and the expense.

Intravenous immune globulin has been used to treat rheumatoid vasculitis and shows promise.[159] Doses given have been between 0.5 and 1 g/kg/day for 2 days. More experience with this therapy is needed.

A reasonable treatment strategy for the patient with rheumatoid vasculitis is outlined in Table 20–2. These patients should be given a DMARD, including methotrexate or possibly azathioprine. The role of newer drugs such as TNF antagonists and leflunomide is uncertain, but they may be beneficial. There is no established role for the use of immunosorbent column (Prosorba) therapy in the treatment of vasculitis or any other extra-articular disease manifestations of RA. Doses of NSAIDs sufficient to provide anti-inflammatory and particularly antiplatelet effects are necessary. Doses of prednisone commensurate with the activity and extent of the vasculitis are necessary to control the vascular inflammation.

Other nonvasculitic influences on the vascular system should be managed as effectively as possible. Blood pressure should be normalized, diabetes mellitus should be controlled, and smoking should be stopped.

## TABLE 20–2
## Treatment of Rheumatoid Vasculitis

| | |
|---|---|
| General measures | Stop smoking; control hypertension and diabetes mellitus |
| Manage rheumatoid arthritis and constitutional features (in all cases) | NSAIDs, low-dose prednisone, disease-modifying drugs |
| Localized vasculitis manifestations | |
| Nailfold infarcts | Manage the rheumatoid arthritis |
| Distal sensory neuropathy | Manage the rheumatoid arthritis |
| Leg ulcers | Local care for leg ulcers, possibly skin graft |
| Digital-tip gangrene without other manifestations and with no clinical evidence of inflammation | Antiplatelet drugs, vasodilating agents |
| Systemic vasculitis | |
| Progressive manifestations with clinical evidence of inflammation, mononeuritis multiplex, digital-tip infarcts, and central nervous system and/or visceral involvement | High-divided-dose prednisone, azathioprine, chlorambucil, or cyclophosphamide, antiplatelet drugs prednisone 60–80 mg/d divided in three doses and azathioprine 100–150 mg/d or chlorambucil 4–6 mg/d or cyclophosphamide 125–150 mg q AM orally or 500–1250 mg IV q month, or methotrexate 7.5–20 mg once a week |
| Resistant progressive inflammatory multisystem disease | Addition of IV immune globulin 0.5–1 g/kg/d for 2d. Consider use of TNF antagonists. |

AM = morning; IV = intravenously; NSAIDs = nonsteroidal anti-inflammatory drugs; TNF = tumor necrosis factor.

Leg ulcers without any other vasculitic manifestations should be managed with local care. In some cases a skin graft may be necessary. Isolated digital vasculopathy should be treated with DMARDs, NSAIDs, vasodilators, and an appropriate antiplatelet regimen. Rheumatoid vasculitis manifested by distal sensory neuropathy, nailfold infarcts, or both necessitates optimal management for RA, including methotrexate. It is not necessary to use treatments such as high doses of prednisone or cytotoxic agents to treat the nailfold infarcts or sensory neuropathy.

The treatment for patients with more extensive, progressive disease and evidence of inflammation should be more aggressive. This would include those patients with progressive mononeuritis multiplex, coronary angiitis, cerebral vasculitis, or visceral ischemia. They should be given high doses of prednisone (60 to 80 mg/day in three divided doses), as well as an immunosuppressive agent. If they have been taking methotrexate or another DMARD without any benefit, then azathioprine, cyclophosphamide, or chlorambucil can be considered. If they have not been taking methotrexate, it can be considered, but there is no experience to suggest its efficacy in severe vasculitis.

Cyclophosphamide or chlorambucil may have a beneficial effect within weeks; azathioprine requires several months to take effect but can usually be administered for a longer period. Although there is more published experience with cyclophosphamide than with chlorambucil in the treatment of rheumatoid vasculitis, the efficacy and side effects of these two drugs are probably comparable, but cyclophosphamide is also toxic to the bladder.

The toxic effects of cyclophosphamide may be lessened by intravenous administration 1 day per month. There is little convincing evidence to suggest that intravenous pulsed cyclophosphamide is any more efficacious than oral cyclophosphamide in the management of rheumatoid vasculitis, although it is less toxic to the bladder.[151] Other strategies for minimizing toxic effects, especially to the bone marrow, have not been studied. Other strategies of drug administration may be as safe, less expensive, and easier to manage than the intravenous pulsed cyclophosphamide regimen. For example, oral pulse administration of this cytotoxic agent given daily for 2 to 3 weeks and then "resting" of the bone marrow for the remaining days of the month may be as efficacious and safe.

The usual oral doses of these cytotoxic agents in adult patients are as follows: cyclophosphamide, 125 to 150 mg/day given in a single morning dose with liberal fluids (3 to 4 L/day); chlorambucil, 4 to 6 mg/day given either in a single daily dose or in a split dose. The complete blood count should be monitored for the cellular elements and, when cyclophosphamide is used, the urinalysis for microscopic hematuria weekly for the first 1 to 2 months and then monthly. If azathioprine is selected, it can be given orally in a single or divided dose of 100 to 150 mg/day total, with the hematology group and aspartate aminotransaminase monitored monthly. Usually the intravenous pulsed cyclophosphamide is given in doses of 500 to 1250 mg in a vehicle of 5% dextrose and water over 30 to 60 minutes. Initially, it is given 1 day each month for 4 to 6 months and then less frequently, depending on response and toxicity. For an in-depth discussion of the mechanism of action of cytotoxic drugs and immunoregulatory agents, see Kelley and associates, *Textbook of Rheumatology*, Section VI.[160]

As the manifestations of vasculitis are controlled, the prednisone dose can be tapered. As prednisone is tapered, the cytotoxic drug dose may also need to be lowered. This is because the cytotoxic drug may become more suppressive of the bone marrow as the prednisone dose is reduced.

Once the disease is controlled, prednisone can be tapered, so long as disease control is maintained during the taper. In our experience, flares of the vasculitis are less likely with daily doses of prednisone than with an alternate-day regimen.

When the dose of prednisone used to control the disease is 60 mg/day or greater, tapering can be accomplished by decreasing the daily prednisone dose by 10 mg each week to a dose of 40 mg/day. Thereafter, the taper is slowed and the daily prednisone dose is decreased by 5 mg/day each 1 to 2 weeks to a total of 25 mg/day. Thereafter, the daily dose should be tapered by decrements of 2.5 mg each week to a total of 15 mg/day. At this point, the taper is slowed and the daily prednisone dose reduced by 1 mg/day every 2 to 3 weeks in an attempt to achieve the lowest possible prednisone dose. Some patients require a low dose of prednisone indefinitely. The pace of the prednisone taper depends on the clinical and laboratory status of the patient.

If the disease flares during the prednisone taper, the use of prednisone should be increased to the level that allows control of the disease. If the patient is taking a single daily dose of prednisone and experiences worsening of the inflammatory features later in the day, the prednisone should be given in divided doses, usually twice or three times a day.

Assuming that the prednisone has been tapered to less than 10 mg/day while the cytotoxic agent is continued with control of the disease, the regimen should be maintained for approximately 1 year. Thereafter, if the disease remains under control, the cytotoxic agent can be gradually tapered further and stopped altogether. If the cytotoxic agent can be tapered off and the disease remains under control, then a slow prednisone taper is undertaken by decreasing the daily prednisone dose by 1 mg/day each month in an attempt to reach the lowest dose of prednisone that will continue to control the disease.

Any patient receiving chronic glucocorticoid treatment should be advised to take calcium 1 to 2 g/day and a multivitamin with 800 units of vitamin D. Further treatment to prevent osteopenia depends on the patient's sex, age, and bone mineral density.[161]

## REFERENCES

1. Rasker JJ, Cosh JA: Cause and age of death in a prospective study of 100 patients with rheumatoid arthritis. Ann Rheum Dis 1981; 40:115.

 2. Voskuyl AE, Zwinderman AH, Westedt ML, et al: The mortality of rheumatoid vasculitis compared with rheumatoid arthritis. Arthritis Rheum 1996; 39:266.
 3. Anaya JM, Diethelm L, Ortiz LA, et al: Pulmonary involvement in rheumatoid arthritis. Semin Arthritis Rheum 1995; 24:242.
 4. Cortet B, Perez T, Roux N, et al: Pulmonary function tests and high resolution computed tomography of the lungs in patients with rheumatoid arthritis. Ann Rheum Dis 1997; 56:596.
 5. Walker WC, Wright V: Diffuse interstitial pulmonary fibrosis and rheumatoid arthritis. Ann Rheum Dis 1969; 28:252.
 6. Gabbay E, Tarala R, Will R, et al: Interstitial lung disease in recent onset rheumatoid arthritis. Am J Respir Crit Care Med 1977; 156:528.
 7. Geddes DM, Webley M, Emerson PA: Airways obstruction in rheumatoid arthritis. Ann Rheum Dis 1979; 38:222.
 8. Saag KG, Kolluri S, Koehnke RK, et al: Rheumatoid arthritis lung disease. Arthritis Rheum 1996; 10:1711.
 9. Sumiya M, Ohya N, Shinoura H, et al: Diffuse interstitial pulmonary amyloidosis in rheumatoid arthritis. J Rheumatol 1996; 23:933.
10. Walker WC, Wright V: Pulmonary lesions and rheumatoid arthritis. Medicine (Baltimore) 1968; 47:501.
11. Roschmann RA, Rothenberg RJ: Pulmonary fibrosis in rheumatoid arthritis: A review of clinical features and therapy. Semin Arthritis Rheum 1987; 16:174.
12. Turner-Warwick M, Evans RC: Pulmonary manifestations of rheumatoid disease. Clin Rheum Dis 1977; 3:549.
13. Wallaert B, Hatron PY, Grosbois JM, et al: Subclinical pulmonary involvement in collagen vascular diseases assessed by bronchoalveolar lavage. Am Rev Respir Dis 1986; 133:574.
14. Goodman M, Knight RK, Turner-Warwick M: Pilot study of penicillamine therapy in steroid failure patients with interstitial lung disease. *In* Maini RN, Berry H (eds): Modulation of Autoimmunity and Disease: Clinical Pharmacology and Therapeutics Series. New York: Praeger, 1981:41.
15. Scott DGI, Bacon PA: Response to methotrexate in fibrosing alveolitis associated with connective tissue disease. Thorax 1980; 35:725.
16. Lorber A: Penicillamine therapy for rheumatoid lung disease: Effects on protein sulphydryl groups. Nature 1966; 210:1235.
17. Cohen JM, Miller A, Spiera H: Interstitial pneumonitis complicating rheumatoid arthritis. Chest 1977; 72:521.
18. Brown CH, Turner-Warwick M: The treatment of cryptogenic fibrosing alveolitis with immunosuppressant drugs. Q J Med 1971; 158:289.
19. Alegre J, Teran J, Alverez B, et al: Successful use of cyclosporine for the treatment of aggressive pulmonary fibrosis in a patient with rheumatoid arthritis. Arthritis Rheum 1990; 33:1594.
20. Russell MI, Gladman DD, Mintz S: Rheumatoid pleural effusion: Lack of response to intrapleural corticosteroid. J Rheumatol 1986; 13:412.
21. Kelly CA: Rheumatoid arthritis: Classical lung disease. Balliere's Clin Rheumatol 1993; 7:1.
22. Dieppe PA: Empyema in rheumatoid arthritis. Ann Rheum Dis 1975; 34:181.
23. Portner MM, Gracie WA: Rheumatoid lung disease with cavitary nodules, pneumothorax, and eosinophilia. N Engl J Med 1966; 275:697.
24. Caplan A: Certain unusual radiological appearances in the chest of coal-miners suffering from rheumatoid arthritis. Thorax 1953; 8:29.
25. Penny WJ, Knight RK, Rees AM, et al: Obliterative bronchiolitis in rheumatoid arthritis. Ann Rheum Dis 1982; 41:469.
26. Epler RG, Colby TV, McCloud TC, et al: Bronchiolitis obliterans organizing pneumonia. N Engl J Med 1985; 312:152.
27. Gosink BB, Friedman PJ, Liebow AA: Bronchiolitis obliterans: Roentgenologic-pathologic correlation. Am J Roentgenol Radium Ther Nucl Med 1973; 117:816.
28. Geddes DM, Corrin B, Brewerton DA, et al: Progressive airway obliteration in adults and its association with rheumatoid disease. Q J Med 1977; 46:427.
29. Jansen HM, Elema JD, Hylkema BS, et al: Progressive obliterative bronchiolitis in a patient with rheumatoid arthritis. Eur J Respir Dis 1982; 63:43.
30. van Thiel RJ, van der Burg S, Groote AD, et al: Bronchiolitis obliterans organizing pneumonia and rheumatoid arthritis. Eur Respir J 1991; 4:905.
31. Epler G: Bronchiolitis obliterans organizing pneumonia: Definition and clinical features. Chest 1992; 102:2S.
32. Fort JG, Scovern H, Abruzzo JL: Intravenous cyclophosphamide and methylprednisolone for the treatment of bronchiolitis obliterans and interstitial fibrosis associated with cryotherapy. J Rheumatol 1988; 15:850.
33. Van De Laar MAFJ, Westerman CJJ, Wagenaar SS, et al: Beneficial effect of intravenous cyclophosphamide and oral prednisone in D-penicillamine-associated bronchiolitis obliterans. Arthritis Rheum 1985; 28:93.
34. Epler G: Bronchiolitis obliterans organizing pneumonia. Semin Respir Infect 1995; 10:65.
35. Despaux J, Polio J-C, Toussirot E, et al: Rheumatoid arthritis and bronchiectasis: A retrospective study of fourteen cases. Rev Rhum Engl Ed 1966; 63:801.
36. Gardner DL, Duthie JR, MacLeod J, et al: Pulmonary hypertension in RA: Report of a case with intimal sclerosis of pulmonary and digital arteries. Scott Med J 1957; 2:183.
37. Löfgren R, Montgomery W: Incidence of laryngeal involvement in rheumatoid arthritis. N Engl J Med 1962; 267:193.
38. Geterud A, Ejnell H, Mansson I, et al: Severe airway obstruction caused by laryngeal rheumatoid arthritis. J Rheumatol 1986; 13:948.
39. Phellps J: Laryngeal obstruction due to cricoarytenoid arthritis. Anesthesiology 1966; 27:518.
40. Dockery KM, Sismanis A, Abedi E: Rheumatoid arthritis of the larynx: The importance of early diagnosis and corticosteroid therapy. South Med J 1991; 84:95.
41. Habib MA: Intra-articular steroid injection in acute rheumatoid arthritis of the larynx. J Laryngol Otol 1977; 91:909.
42. Montgomery W: Cricoarytenoid arthritis. Laryngoscope 1963; 73:801.
43. Kleinsasser O: Microlaryngoscopy and Endolaryngeal Microsurgery. Philadelphia: WB Saunders, 1968:120.
44. Simpson GT II, Javaheri A, JanFaza P: Acute cricoarytenoid arthritis: Local periarticular steroid injection. Ann Otol Rhinol Laryngol 1980; 89:558.
45. Bonfiglio T, Atwater EC: Heart disease in patients with seropositive rheumatoid arthritis. Arch Intern Med 1969; 124:714.
46. Sigal LH, Friedman HD: Rheumatoid pancarditis in a patient with well-controlled rheumatoid arthritis. J Rheumatol 1989; 16:368.
47. Gordon DA, Stein JL, Broder I: The extra-articular features of rheumatoid arthritis: A systematic analysis of 127 cases. Am J Med 1973; 54:445.
48. Wilkinson M: Rheumatoid pericarditis: A report of four cases. Br Med J 1962; 2:1723.
49. Hara KS, Ballard DJ, Ilstrup DM, et al: Rheumatoid pericarditis: Clinical features and survival. Medicine (Baltimore) 1990; 69:81.
50. Escalante A, Kaufman RL, Quismorio FP Jr, et al: Cardiac compression in rheumatoid pericarditis. Semin Arthritis Rheum 1990; 20:148.
51. Thadani U, Iveson JMI, Wright V: Cardiac tamponade, constrictive pericarditis and pericardial resection in rheumatoid arthritis. Medicine (Baltimore) 1975; 54:261.
52. Thould AK: Constrictive pericarditis in rheumatoid arthritis. Ann Rheum Dis 1986; 45:89.
53. Blake S, Bonar S, O'Neill H, et al: Etiology of chronic constrictive pericarditis. Br Heart J 1983; 50:273.
54. Cameron J, Oesterle SN, Baldwin JC, et al: The etiologic spectrum of constrictive pericarditis. Am Heart J 1987; 113:354.
55. Franco AE, Levine HD, Hall AP: Rheumatoid pericarditis: Report of 17 cases diagnosed clinically. Ann Intern Med 1972; 77:837.
56. Lebowitz WB: The heart in rheumatoid arthritis (rheumatoid disease): A clinical and pathological study of 62 cases. Ann Intern Med 1963; 58:102.
57. Lebowitz WB: The heart in rheumatoid disease. Geriatrics 1966; 21:194.
58. Bacon PA, Scott DGI: La vascularite rhumatoide. *In* Sany J (ed). Polyarthrite Rhumatoide. Paris: Medecine-Sciences, Flammarion, 1987.

59. Slack JD, Waller B: Acute congestive heart failure due to the arteritis of rheumatoid arthritis: Early diagnosis of endomyocardial biopsy. A case report. Angiology 1986; 37:477.

60. Ahern M, Lever JV, Cosh J: Complete heart block in rheumatoid arthritis. Ann Rheum Dis 1983; 42:389.

61. Hess ME: Effect of antimalarial drugs on cardiac muscle. Fed Proc 1954; 13:365.

62. Jurik AG, Moller P: Atrioventricular conduction time in rheumatoid arthritis. Rheumatol Int 1985; 5:205.

63. Whisnant JP, Espinosa RE, Kierland RR, et al: Chloroquine neuromyopathy. Mayo Clin Proc 1963; 38:501.

64. Iveson JMI, Pomerance A: Cardiac involvement in rheumatic disease. Clin Rheum Dis 1977; 3:467.

65. Liew M, Wilson D, Horton D, et al: Successful valve replacement for aortic incompetence in rheumatoid arthritis with vasculitis. Ann Rheum Dis 1979; 38:483.

66. Townend JN, Emery P, Davies MK, et al: Acute aortitis and aortic incompetence due to systemic rheumatological disorders. Int J Cardiol 1991; 33:253.

67. Cosh JA, Lever JV: The aortic valve. In Ansell BM, Simkin PA (eds): The Heart and Rheumatic Disease. Cornwall, UK: Butterworths International Medical Reviews—Rheumatology 2, 1984:83.

68. Isomur T, Hisatomi K, Yanagi I, et al: The surgical treatment of aortic incompetence secondary to aortitis. Ann Thorac Surg 1988; 45:181.

69. Duke-Elder S, Soley RE: Summary of systemic ophthalmology. In Duke-Elder S (ed). System of Ophthalmology. St. Louis: CV Mosby, 1976:139.

70. Wilson F: Adverse external ocular effects of topical ophthalmic medications. Surv Ophthalmol 1979; 24:57.

71. Fox RI, Howell FV, Bone RC, et al: Primary Sjögren's syndrome: Clinical and immunopathologic features. Semin Arthritis Rheum 1984; 14:77.

72. Watson PG, Hayreh SS: Scleritis and episcleritis. Br J Ophthalmol 1976; 60:163.

73. Messmer EM, Foster CS: Destructive corneal and scleral disease associated with rheumatoid arthritis: Medical and surgical management. Cornea 1995; 14:408.

74. Hoffman F, Wiederholt M: Local treatment of necrotizing scleritis with cyclosporin A. Cornea 1985/1986; 4:3.

75. Jifi-Bahlool H, Saadeh C, O'Connor J: Peripheral ulcerative keratitis in the setting of rheumatoid arthritis: Treatment with immunosuppressive therapy. Semin Arthritis Rheum 1995; 25:67.

76. Ferry AP: The eye and rheumatic disease. In Kelley WN, Harris ED, Ruddy S, et al (eds): Textbook of Rheumatology, 4th ed. Philadelphia: WB Saunders, 1993:507.

77. Watson PG, Hayreh SS: Scleritis and episcleritis. Br J Ophthalmol 1976; 60:163.

78. Insler MS, Boutros G, Boulware O: Corneal ulceration following cataract surgery in patients with rheumatoid arthritis. J Am Intraocul Implant Soc 1985; 11:594.

79. Maffett MJ, Johns KJ, Parrish CM, et al: Sterile corneal ulceration after cataract extraction in patients with collagen vascular disease. Cornea 1990; 9:279.

80. Jones RR, Maguire LJ: Corneal complications after cataract surgery in patients with rheumatoid arthritis. Cornea 1992; 11:148.

81. Killian PJ, McClain B, Lawless OJ: Brown's syndrome: An unusual manifestation of rheumatoid arthritis. Arthritis Rheum 1977; 20:1080.

82. Cooper C, Kirwan JR, McGill NW, et al: Brown's syndrome: An unusual ocular complication of rheumatoid arthritis. Ann Rheum Dis 1990; 49:188.

83. Foster CS, Forstot SL, Wilson LA: Mortality rate in rheumatoid arthritis patients developing necrotizing scleritis or peripheral ulcerative keratitis: Effects of systemic immunosuppression. Ophthalmology 1984; 91:1253.

84. Chang LW, Gowans JDC, Granger CV, et al: Entrapment neuropathy of the posterior interosseous nerve: A complication of rheumatoid arthritis. Arthritis Rheum 1972; 15:350.

85. Baylan SP, Paik SW, Barnert AL, et al: Prevalence of the tarsal tunnel syndrome in rheumatoid arthritis. Rheumatol Rehabil 1981; 20:148.

86. Chamberlain MA, Bruckner FE: Rheumatoid neuropathy: Clinical and electrophysiological features. Ann Rheum Dis 1970; 29:609.

87. Nakano KK: Neurologic complications of rheumatoid arthritis. Orthop Clin North Am 1975; 6:861.

88. Lipson SJ: Rheumatoid arthritis of the cervical spine. Clin Orthop 1984; 182:143.

89. Menezes AH, VanGilder JC, Clark CR, et al: Odontoid upward migration in rheumatoid arthritis: An analysis of 45 patients with "cranial settling." J Neurosurg 1985; 63:500.

90. Conlon PW, Isdale IC, Rose BS: Rheumatoid arthritis of the cervical spine: An analysis of 33 cases. Ann Rheum Dis 1966; 25:120.

91. Smith PH, Benn RT, Sharp J: Natural history of rheumatoid cervical luxations. Ann Rheum Dis 1972; 31:431.

92. Santavirta S, Kankaanpää U, Sandelin J, et al: Evaluation of patients with rheumatoid cervical spine. Scand J Rheumatol 1987; 16:9.

93. Crellin RQ, MacCabe JJ, Hamilton EBD: Severe subluxation of the cervical spine in rheumatoid arthritis. J Bone Joint Surg Br 1970; 52:244.

94. Olerud C, Larsson B-E, Rodriquez M: Subaxial cervical spine subluxation in rheumatoid arthritis: A retrospective analysis of 16 operated patients after 1–5 years. Acta Orthop Scand 1997; 68:109.

95. Boden SD, Dodge LD, Bohlman HH, et al: Rheumatoid arthritis of the cervical spine. J Bone Joint Surg Am 1993; 75:1282.

96. Couverchel L, Maugars Y, Prost A: Outcomes of thirty-four rheumatoid arthritis patients with renal amyloidosis, including twelve given alkylating agents. Rev Rhum Engl Ed 1995; 62:79.

97. Menezes AH, VanGilder JC, Graf CJ, et al: Craniocervical abnormalities: A comprehensive surgical approach. J Neurosurg 1980; 53:444.

98. Apuzzo MLJ, Weiss MH, Heiden JS: Transoral exposure of the atlantoaxial region. Neurosurgery 1978; 3:201.

99. Weiland DJ, McAfee PC: Posterior cervical fusion with triple-wire strut graft technique: One hundred consecutive patients. J Spinal Disord 1991; 4:15.

100. Husby G: Amyloidosis in rheumatoid arthritis. Ann Clin Res 1975; 7:154.

101. Lender M, Wolf E: Incidence of amyloidosis in rheumatoid arthritis. Scand J Rheumatol 1972; 1:109.

102. Wegelius O, Wafin F, Falck H, et al: Follow-up study of amyloidosis secondary to rheumatic disease. In Glenner GG, Costa PP, Falcao de Freitas A (eds): Amyloid and Amyloidosis. Amsterdam: Excerpta Medica, 1980:337.

103. Koota K, Isomäki HA, Mutru O: Death rate and causes of death in patients with rheumatoid arthritis. Scand J Rheumatol 1975; 4:205.

104. Husby G: Amyloidosis and rheumatoid arthritis. Clin Exp Rheumatol 1985; 3:173.

105. Mustila A, Korpela M, Mustonen J, et al: Perinuclear antineutrophil cytoplasmic antibody in rheumatoid arthritis. Arthritis Rheum 1997; 40:710.

106. Ahlmen M, Ahlmen J, Svalander C, et al: Cytotoxic drug treatment of reactive amyloidosis in rheumatoid arthritis with special reference to renal insufficiency. Clin Rheumatol 1987; 6:27.

107. Thorne C, Urowitz MB: Long-term outcome in Felty's syndrome. Ann Rheum Dis 1982; 41:486.

108. Weisman M, Zvaifler NJ: Cryoimmunoglobulinemia in Felty's syndrome. Arthritis Rheum 1976; 19:103.

109. Campion G, Maddison PJ, Goulding N, et al: The Felty syndrome: A case-matched study of clinical manifestations and outcome, serologic features and immunogenetic associations. Medicine (Baltimore) 1990; 69:69.

110. Weyand CM, Xie C, Goronzy JJ: Homozygosity for the HLA-DRB1 allele selects for extraarticular manifestations in rheumatoid arthritis. J Clin Invest 1992; 89:2033.

111. Rosenstein ED, Kramer N: Felty's and pseudo-Felty's syndromes. Semin Arthritis Rheum 1991; 21:129.

112. Dillon AM, Luthra HS, Conn DL, et al: Parenteral gold therapy in the Felty syndromes: Experience with 20 patients. Medicine (Baltimore) 1986; 65:107.

113. Breedveld FC, Fibbe WE, Hermans J, et al: Factors influencing the incidence of infections in Felty's syndrome. Arch Intern Med 1987; 147:915.

114. Barton JC, Prasthofer EF, Egan ML, et al: Rheumatoid arthritis associated with expanded populations of granular lymphocytes. Ann Intern Med 1986; 104:314.

115. Loughran TP Jr: Clonal diseases of large granular lymphocytes. Blood 1993; 82:1.

116. Bowman SJ, Geddes GC, Corrigall V, et al: Large granular lymphocyte expansions in Felty's syndrome have an unusual phenotype of activated CD45RA+ cells. Br J Rheumatol 1996; 35:1252.

117. Starkebaum G, Loughran TP Jr, Gaur LK, et al: Immunogenetic similarities between patients with Felty's syndrome and those with clonal expansions of large granular lymphocytes in rheumatoid arthritis. Arthritis Rheum 1997; 40:624.

118. Luthra HS, Hunder GG: Spontaneous remission of Felty's syndrome. Arthritis Rheum 1975; 18:515.

119. Sibley JT, Haga M, Visram DA, et al: The clinical course of Felty's syndrome compared to matched controls. J Rheumatol 1991; 18:1163.

120. Wimer BM, Sloan MW: Remission of Felty's syndrome with long-term testosterone therapy. JAMA 1973; 223:671.

121. Mant MJ, Akabutu JJ, Herbert FA: Lithium carbonate therapy in severe Felty's syndrome: Benefits, toxicity, and granulocyte function. Arch Intern Med 1984; 14:277.

122. Breedveld FC, Brand A, Van Aken WG: High dose intravenous gamma globulin for Felty's syndrome. J Rheumatol 1985; 12:700.

123. Luthra HS, Conn DL, Ferguson RH: Felty's syndrome: Response to parenteral gold. J Rheumatol 1981; 8:902.

124. Fiechtner JJ, Miller DR, Starkebaume G: Reversal of neutropenia with methotrexate treatment in patients with Felty's syndrome. Arthritis Rheum 1989; 32:194.

125. Wandt H, Seifert M, Falge C, et al: Long-term correction of neutropenia in Felty's syndrome with granulocyte colony-stimulating factor. Ann Hematol 1993; 66:265.

126. Rashba EJ, Rowe MH, Pakeman CH: Treatment of the neutropenia of Felty's syndrome. Blood Rev 1996; 10:177.

127. Sokoloff L, Bunim JJ: Vascular lesions in rheumatoid arthritis. J Chronic Disord 1957; 5:668.

128. Lakhanpal S, Conn DL, Lie JT: Clinical and prognostic significance of vasculitis as an early manifestation of connective tissue disease syndromes. Ann Intern Med 1984; 101:743.

129. Conn DL: Rheumatoid neuropathy. *In* Utsinger PD, Zvalifer NJ (eds): Rheumatoid Arthritis. Philadelphia: JB Lippincott, 1985.

130. Voskuyl AE, Zwinderman AH, Westedt ML, et al: Factors associated with the development of vasculitis in rheumatoid arthritis: Results of a case-control study. Ann Rheum Dis 1996; 55:190.

131. Voskuyl AE, Zwinderman AH, Westedt ML, et al: Smoking and the risk of vasculitis in rheumatoid arthritis. Arthritis Rheum 1997; 40:S170.

132. Scott DGI, Bacon PA, Tribe CR: Systemic rheumatoid vasculitis: A clinical and laboratory study of 50 cases. Medicine (Baltimore) 1981; 60:288.

133. Weyand CM, Hicok KC, Conn DL, et al: The influence of HLA-DRB1 genes on disease severity in rheumatoid arthritis. Ann Intern Med 1992; 117:801.

134. Voskuyl AE, Hazes JMW, Schreuder GMT, et al: HLA-DRB1, DQA1, and DQB1 genotypes and risk of vasculitis in patients with rheumatoid arthritis. J Rheumatol 1997; 24:852.

135. Luthra HS, McDuffie FC, Hunder GG, et al: Immune complexes in sera and synovial fluid of patients with rheumatoid arthritis: Radioimmunoassay with monoclonal rheumatoid factor. J Clin Invest 1975; 56:458.

136. Heurkens AHN, Hiemstra PS, Lafeber GJM, et al: Anti-endothelial cells antibodies in patients with rheumatoid arthritis complicated by vasculitis. Clin Exp Immunol 1989; 78:7.

137. Conn DL, McDuffie FC, Dyck PJ: Immunopathologic study of sural nerves in rheumatoid arthritis. Arthritis Rheum 1972; 15:135.

138. Watts RA, Carruthers DM, Scott DGI: Isolated nail fold vasculitis in rheumatoid arthritis. Ann Rheum Dis 1995; 54:927.

139. Vollertsen RS, Conn DL, Ballard DJ, et al: Rheumatoid vasculitis: Survival and associated risk factors. Medicine (Baltimore) 1986; 65:365.

140. Puechal X, Said G, Hilliquin P, et al: Peripheral neuropathy with necrotizing vasculitis in rheumatoid arthritis: A clinico-pathologic and prognostic study of thirty-two patients. Arthritis Rheum 1995; 11:1618.

141. Kemper JW, Baggenstoss AH, Slocumb CH: The relationship of therapy with cortisone to the incidence of vascular lesions in rheumatoid arthritis. Ann Intern Med 1957; 46:831.

142. Conn DL, Tompkins RB, Nichols WL: Glucocorticosteroids in the management of vasculitis: A double-edged sword? J Rheumatol 1988; 15:1181.

143. Dyck PJ, Conn DL, Okazaki H: Necrotizing angiopathic neuropathy: Three-dimensional morphology of fiber degeneration related to sites of occluded vessels. Mayo Clin Proc 1972; 47:461.

144. Deguchi Y, Shibata N, Kishimoto S: Enhanced expression of the tumor necrosis factor/cachectin gene in peripheral blood mononuclear cells from patients with systemic vasculitis. Clin Exp Immunol 1990; 81:311.

145. Dasgupta B, Panayi GS: Interleukin-6 in serum of patients with polymyalgia rheumatica and giant cell arteritis. Br J Rheumatol 1990; 29:456.

146. Bywaters EGL: Peripheral vascular obstruction in rheumatoid arthritis and its relationship to other vascular lesions. Ann Rheum Dis 1957; 16:84.

147. McRorie ER, Ruckley CV, Nuki G: The relevance of large vessel vascular disease and restricted ankle movement to the etiology of leg ulceration in RA. Br J Rheumatol 1998; 37:1295–1298.

148. Gordon M, Luqmani RA, Adu D, et al: Relapses in patients with a systemic vasculitis. Q J Med 1993; 86:779.

149. Jaffe IA: The treatment of rheumatoid arthritis and necrotizing vasculitis with penicillamine. Arthritis Rheum 1970; 13:436.

150. Abel T, Andrews BS, Cunningham PH, et al: Rheumatoid vasculitis: Effect of cyclophosphamide on the clinical course and levels of circulating immune complexes. Ann Intern Med 1980; 93:407.

151. Scott DGI, Bacon PA: Intravenous cyclophosphamide plus methylprednisolone in treatment of systemic rheumatoid vasculitis. Am J Med 1984; 76:377.

152. Upchurch KS, Heller K, Bress NM: Low-dose methotrexate therapy for cutaneous vasculitis and rheumatoid arthritis. J Am Acad Dermatol 1987; 17:355.

153. Segal R, Caspi D, Tishler M, et al: Accelerated nodulosis and vasculitis during methotrexate therapy for rheumatoid arthritis. Arthritis Rheum 1988; 31:1182.

154. Kaye O, Beckers CC, Paquet P, et al: The frequency of cutaneous vasculitis is not increased in patients with rheumatoid arthritis treated with methotrexate. J Rheumatol 1996; 23(2):253–257.

155. Nicholls A, Snaith ML, Maini RN, et al: Controlled trial of azathioprine in rheumatoid vasculitis. Ann Rheum Dis 1973; 32:589.

156. Heurkens AH, Westedt ML, Breedveld FC: Prednisone plus azathioprine treatment in patients with rheumatoid arthritis complicated by vasculitis. Arch Intern Med 1991; 151:2249.

157. Blanco R, Martinez-Taboada VM, Gonzalez-Gay MA, et al: Acute febrile toxic reaction in patients with refractory rheumatoid arthritis who are receiving combined therapy with methotrexate and azathioprine. Arthritis Rheum 1996; 39:1016–1020.

158. Scott DGI, Bacon PA, Bothamley JE, et al: Plasma exchange in rheumatoid vasculitis. J Rheumatol 1981; 8:433.

159. Lockwood, CM: New treatment strategies for systemic vasculitis: Role of intravenous immune globulin therapy. Clin Exp Immunol 1996; 104(suppl 1):77–82.

160. Kelly WN, Harris ED, Ruddy S, et al (eds): Textbook of Rheumatology, 5th ed. Philadelphia: WB Saunders, 1997.

161. American College of Rheumatology Task Force on Osteoporosis Guidelines: Recommendations for the prevention and treatment of glucocorticoid induced osteoporosis. Arthritis Rheum 1996; 36:1791–1801.

# CHAPTER
## 21 | Approaches to the Treatment of Sjögren's Syndrome

*Robert I. Fox, Paul Michelson, and Jryki Tornwall*

Sjögren's syndrome (SS) is characterized by dry eyes (xerophthalmia) and dry mouth (xerostomia); the dryness is caused by lymphocytic infiltrates of the lacrimal and salivary glands. SS is divided into a primary form (first-degree SS) and secondary form (second-degree SS). In second-degree SS, the so-called sicca symptoms are associated with other well-defined autoimmune diseases such as rheumatoid arthritis, systemic lupus erythematosus (SLE), progressive systemic sclerosis, polymyositis, and biliary cirrhosis. Dryness can result from many other causes, including drugs with anticholinergic side effects (including certain herbal supplements), infections such as hepatitis C or retroviruses, autonomic neuropathy, depression, and fibromyalgia. Because patients with SS see a wide variety of health care professionals, it is important that rheumatologists be familiar with the treatments used by ophthalmologists, dermatologists, otolaryngologists, and oral medicine specialists.

Patients may be referred to the rheumatologist by several routes. The traditional route is referral by the primary physician, ophthalmologist, or dentist on the basis of the sicca symptoms. In many instances the patient may have antinuclear antibodies (ANA) and vague symptoms of fatigue or myalgia. The evaluation of these patients (Table 21–1) represents a challenge because fibromyalgia is so common in the population and positive ANA titers are frequently found in the normal population. For example, up to 23% of normal persons have a positive ANA titer of 1:40.[1] Antibody tests performed for anti–Sjögren's syndrome antigens A and B (anti–SS-A and anti–SS-B) by enzyme-linked immunosorbent assay depend heavily on the quality of the antigen used in the assay and have great variability. Even at a higher ANA titer of 1:640, the actual risk for developing SLE (or SS) is less than 1%.[2] The key point for rheumatologists is that not all patients with complaints of dryness suffer from a systemic autoimmune disease. All patients with objective ocular and oral dryness need instruction in conservative treatment. The difficult diagnostic problem is the decision of whether symptoms are caused by a systemic autoimmune process and thus necessitate a more aggressive therapeutic intervention.

Patients with sicca complaints also see rheumatologists through self-referral. There is increasing patient awareness of dry eye syndromes, partly because of increased patient educational programs on radio and television as well as information on the Internet. An editorial in an ophthalmology newsletter called "dry eyes" the fastest growing problem in the writer's practice, now reaching an epidemic proportion.[3] In particular, this article pointed out that people increasingly work for long hours at a computer in a low-humidity environment. The blink rate (the mechanism for spreading tears) is significantly diminished while a person is working at a computer terminal.[4]

The treatment for SS can be separated into conservative therapy (i.e., local replacement therapy for dry eyes, dry mouth, and other dry surfaces), treatment of systemic autoimmune features such as vasculitis, and management of nonspecific symptoms such as fatigue or sleep disorders. In addition, these patients have particular needs at the time of surgery to prevent complications related to dry eyes, mouth, and upper airways. This chapter concentrates on the conservative management of dryness complaints in the Sjögren's patients, because this information is not easily accessible in the rheumatology literature.

## CONTROVERSY REGARDING DIAGNOSTIC CRITERIA

Although the ophthalmic component (i.e., keratoconjunctivitis sicca [KCS]) is well defined, the criteria for classifying the oral component remain controversial, and thus no uniform classification system for SS exists.[5] For example, two very different criteria for SS are listed in a 1998 edition of the *Primer on the Rheumatic Diseases:* one in the text and one in the appendix.[6] On the one hand, the San Diego or San Francisco criteria (to be described) for SS require objective evidence of KCS, xerostomia, and the presence of autoantibodies or histologic evidence such as that from minor salivary gland biopsy.[5] For diagnosis of definite SS, a characteristic minor salivary gland biopsy is suggested for research protocols, but it is not required for routine clinical diagnosis or management. On the other hand, the original pro-

**TABLE 21–1**
**Evaluation of Patient with Dry Eyes and Mouth**

Identify cofactors such as
　Low-humidity environment (airplanes, highly air-conditioned areas)
　Exposure to cigarette smoke, dust, and other irritants
　Medications with anticholinergic side effects
Perform tests of tear volume secretion
　Schirmer I (with or without topical anesthetic)
　Schirmer II (with nasolacrimal reflex stimulation)
　Osmolality of tears (requires particular equipment and artifacts)
Perform tests of ocular surface and tear film integrity
　Rose bengal staining
　Lissamine green
　Fluorescein staining of conjunctiva
　Tear breakup time (von Bijerfeld score)
Perform tests of saliva volume of secretion
　Measure of total saliva expectoration
　Measure of parotid secretion (requires particular collection cups)
　Scintigraphy (excretion rate of technetium)
　Sialography (to be avoided because of risk of complications)
If eye symptoms are out of proportion to the objective findings:
　Rule out blepharitis (inflammation of eyelids)
　Rule out uveitis or retinitis (requires slit-lamp examination)
　Rule out blepharospasm (uncontrolled blink reflex)
　Rule out anxiety or depression

posed SS criteria by the European Community Study group (EEC)[7] can be fulfilled in the absence of biopsy results or autoantibodies. A further difference between the San Diego and EEC criteria is the exclusion of hepatitis C infection or retroviral infection from the San Diego criteria (but not from the EEC criteria). The incidence of SS in the adult population is about 0.5% according to the San Diego criteria, whereas the incidence according to the EEC criteria is 3% to 5%; thus there is almost a 10-fold difference in the number of patients fulfilling criteria.[5] This lack of uniform classification criteria has led to confusion in clinical practice and in the research literature.[8] For example, the incidence of a particular disease association (i.e., liver involvement, neurologic symptoms, or lymphoma) and the response to a particular therapy are directly affected by the inclusion and exclusion criteria for the study group.

One suggestion for modification of the EEC criteria[9]—to require the presence of antibody against SS-A (Ro) antigen or a positive result of a minor salivary gland biopsy (focus score of 1 or greater)—will lead to much closer agreement of criteria for diagnosis. At the present time, however, rheumatologists must review published studies on treatment, with careful attention paid to differences in inclusion and exclusion diagnostic criteria.

## OVERVIEW FOR PATHOGENESIS OF SYMPTOMS IN SJÖGREN'S SYNDROME

It is important to recognize that SS patients complain about their dry, painful eyes and mouth, whereas rheu-matologists talk about the patients' lacrimal and salivary glands, their autoantibodies, and acute-phase reactants. The patient is describing ocular symptoms caused by increased friction as the eyelid (particularly the upper lid) passes over the orbital globe. When the tear film is inadequate and the movement between the eyelid and globe feels rough, the lid adheres to the surface layers of the globe and can actually pull epithelial cells away from the surface layer of the conjunctiva and cornea. It is these epithelial defects that are viewed clinically as KCS and corneal abrasions. As a result of the insult to the epithelial surface, an inflammatory response (release of cytokines and influx of inflammatory cells) occurs. The wounding process continues and the normal healing process is impaired because an adequate tear film is necessary to provide nutritive and anti-inflammatory substances. Thus in SS patients, exposure to certain environmental stresses can lead to KCS lesions that are very slow to heal.

Similarly, the tongue and buccal mucosal surfaces require lubrication for the tongue to move around the mouth and for the actions of speaking and swallowing. However, there are important differences between the oral symptoms and the ocular symptoms. The eye is a "clean" environment (i.e., not colonized), whereas the mouth has high levels of resident aerobic and anaerobic organisms. A dry mouth is not necessarily painful. Common problems in the mouth involve changes in the microbial flora, especially with the emergence of chronic candidiasis (to be discussed) or periodontal disease caused by particular organisms. Furthermore, there are important differences in the types of neural innervation, mucins, cytokines, and enzymes in the secretions of the mouth and the eye.

Normal lacrimal flow and salivary flow are regulated through feedback mechanisms (Fig. 21–1A). The mucosal surfaces of the eye and mouth are heavily innervated by unmyelinated fibers that carry afferent signals to the lacrimatory or salivatory nuclei located in the medulla. These medullary nuclei, which are part of the autonomic nervous system, are influenced by higher cortical inputs, including taste, smell, anxiety, medications, and emotions. The efferent neurons innervate both glandular cells and local blood vessels. The blood vessels provide not only water for tears and saliva but also growth factors, including hormones (e.g., insulin) and matrix proteins (e.g., fibronectin and vitronectin) of the lacrimal and salivary glands. In response to neural stimulation through muscarinic $M_3$ receptors and vasoactive intestinal peptide receptors, glandular acinar and ductal cells secrete water, proteins, and mucopolysaccharides (mucins). This complex mixture forms a hydrated gel that lubricates the ocular surface (i.e., tears) and the oral mucosa (i.e., saliva). In the simplest model of SS (see Fig. 21–1B), the lacrimal or salivary gland is incapable of adequate response to neural signals, as a consequence of local immune infiltrates and their derived cytokines. The actual processes in SS or autonomic neuropathy are more complicated than indicated in these schematic diagrams, which are designed primarily to emphasize

**Normal tear response**

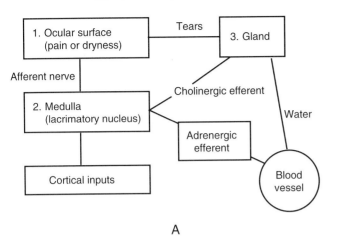

**What happens in Sjögren's syndrome**

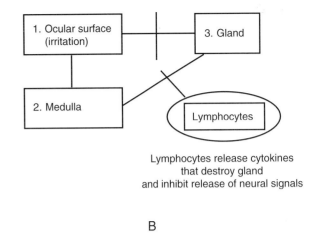

Lymphocytes release cytokines
that destroy gland
and inhibit release of neural signals

**FIGURE 21–1**

*A,* Schematic diagram of a "circuit" that controls normal tear flow or salivation. The stimulation of the ocular or oral mucosal surface leads to afferent nerve signals that reach the lacrimatory or salvatory nuclei in the medulla. Efferent neural signals stimulate both blood vessels and glandular epithelial cells. The medullary signal may be affected by cortical inputs that reflect stimuli such as taste, smell, anxiety, or depression. *B,* Schematic depiction of Sjögren's syndrome, in which the glandular dysfunction prevents the neural signal from initiating glandular secretion.

that salivation and lacrimation are part of a regulatory circuit involving the central nervous system.[10]

# THE PATIENT WITH DRY EYES

## Evaluation of Symptoms

SS patients usually describe a burning or "foreign body" sensation in their eyes. The symptoms are often worse at the end of the day and are relieved by the use of over-the-counter artificial tears (which most patients have tried before seeing a rheumatologist). Symptoms of itching are poorly correlated with objective findings of keratoconjunctivitis.[7] Patients may be relatively free of symptoms until their condition is triggered by the use of medications with anticholinergic side effects (such as over-the-counter cold remedies or prescription medications) or environmental stress to the tear film (such as airline travel or exposure to dry winds). Identification and alteration of the offending medication are often all that are required.

A wide variety of medications have anticholinergic side effects. The most common offenders in rheumatology patients are antidepressants, muscle spasm agents, cold remedies, and urologic and blood pressure agents (Table 21–2). Many cardiac medications and antiseizure medications also have significant anticholinergic side effects.

Contact lenses, especially the soft and gas-permeable types, can contribute to corneal abrasions because adequate tear film may not be available to wash out foreign substances trapped under the lenses. Thus, if contact lenses are worn, they should be taken out at night, and the patient needs to be cautioned about risk of corneal abrasions. One study has suggested that SS patients

should be offered photorefractive surgery (i.e., excimer laser keratectomy) if they do not tolerate contact lenses[11]; however, caution about the use of invasive procedures involving the cornea needs to be exercised until data from long-term follow-up of SS patients with photorefractive surgery (essentially a cosmetic procedure) are available.

**TABLE 21–2**
# Drugs Associated with Increased Dryness

**Blood Pressure Medications**
$\alpha$ Blockers (clonidine [Klonopin])
$\beta$ Blockers (propranolol [Inderal])
Combined $\alpha\beta$ blockers (labetalol [Normodyne])

**Antidepressants**
Amitriptyline (Elavil)
Nortriptyline (Pamelor)

**Muscle Spasm Medications**
Cyclobenzaprine (Flexeril)
Methocarbamol (Robaxin)

**Urologic Drugs**
Bethanechol (Urecholine)
Oxybutynin (Ditropan)

**Cardiac Drugs**
Disopyramide (Norpace)

**Drugs for Parkinson's Disease**
Carbidopa, levodopa (Sinemet)

**Decongestants (Over-the-Counter, Containing Pseudoephedrine)**
Chlorpheniramine (Chlor-Trimeton)
Pseudoephedrine (Sudafed)
Other over-the-counter preparations

## Evaluation of Signs

In evaluating the patient with a complaint of dry eyes, it is important to determine whether the objective signs of dry eyes are commensurate with the patient's symptoms. Methods for measuring the integrity of the corneal surface and tear film, including rose bengal staining, fluorescein staining, lissamine green staining, and the tear breakup time, are described later (Table 21–3). For example, the absence of a significantly abnormal result of an examination with rose bengal staining (a test that is easily performed by the rheumatologist) should suggest a search for additional causes to explain the patient's ocular complaints. These may include eye strain (poor refraction), blepharitis (irritation and low-grade infection of the meibomian glands in the lids), blepharospasm (uncontrolled blinking caused by an increased local neural reflex circuit), and symptoms caused by anxiety or depression.[12]

Unstimulated tear flow is referred to as *basal flow.* This tear secretion derives from the minor tear glands located predominantly in the lower lid. They are probably stimulated by a local reflex arc involving neural receptors in the lid and probably do not involve neural loops that regulate the major salivary glands. This decrease in basal secretion correlates fairly well with symptoms of dryness but not closely with KCS. Decrease in basal tear flow is very common in the general population, especially the elderly, and does not signify an autoimmune condition. A decrease in basal tear flow may also be the initial symptom in SS patients. These symptoms of eye discomfort occur even though the patient can generate tears when he or she cries (i.e., supratentorial stimulation) or is exposed to certain stimuli such as onions (nasal-lacrimal reflexes).

Tear volume is usually measured by the Schirmer test; however, this test is routinely performed in several distinct ways, and the results are often quite different. It is important for the rheumatologist to note the methods of quantitation of tear flow when evaluating patients clinically (or reports by their ophthalmologist) or reviewing the published literature. Many ophthalmologists (and clinical studies) measure the Schirmer I test with topical anesthetic (Ophthaine) and the result reflects the basal secretory rate of the minor lacrimal glands in the eyelids (i.e., not the major lacrimal glands). This test is sensitive but not specific and tear flow rate may be diminished for many reasons.

Most commonly, rheumatologists perform the Schirmer I test in the absence of anesthetic. This value reflects both the minor glands and the stimulation of the major glands. However, the extent of stimulation of the major lacrimal glands is variable.

As an addition to the Schirmer I test (either with or without anesthesia), the Schirmer II test provides a rapid way to measure the "maximal" output of minor plus major lacrimal glands. The Schirmer II test is performed by gently inserting the cotton end of a cotton-tipped swab into the nose, where it stimulates the naso-lacrimal gland reflex.[13] The volume of tearing is measured by Schirmer paper strips without anesthesia. The stimulated tearing reflex involves a neural loop in which afferent fibers from the ocular surface travel to the midbrain (lacrimatory nucleus), where they stimulate efferent adrenergic and cholinergic nerves that travel back to the lacrimal gland (cholinergic) and its blood vessels (adrenergic).[14] A diminished Schirmer II test result has good specificity for SS but lacks sensitivity to early stages of SS. The presence of increased tearing on the Schirmer II test has been a good predictor of response to oral pilocarpine as a way to stimulate secretions, in our experience.

A wide range of tear volume flow (i.e., values on the Schirmer I test with anesthesia) occurs in SS patients as well as in normal people and is poorly correlated with signs and symptoms of KCS. Similarly, the volume of saliva produced as basal secretion or after stimulation correlates poorly with symptoms of dry mouth and objective signs of severe periodontal problems.[15] This suggests that the qualitative content of tears and saliva (i.e., specific glycoproteins and mucins) plays an important role in the maintenance of ocular and oral mucosal integrity and that decreases in tear volume are not the sole cause of problems. An important implication of these findings is that future products of artificial tears, artificial saliva, and toothpastes may contain bioengineered products that provide these important functions lacking in the currently available products.

In addition to the volume of tears, the quality of the tear film is assessed by simple procedures such as rose bengal staining. This material is readily available from pharmacies that carry ocular supplies, and a single drop is administered into the lower eyelid. After the rose bengal is rinsed out with a preservative-free tear, the residual staining of the conjunctiva and cornea can be determined with an ophthalmoscope. Although this evaluation by the rheumatologist does not replace the more accurate evaluation of KCS by slit-lamp examination performed by ophthalmologists, the test does provide a rapid method for assessing the significance of the patient's complaints. The rose bengal should not be left in the patient's eye (before rinsing out with an artificial tear) for a prolonged period, because this may lead to local irritation. In comparison, lissamine green

## TABLE 21–3
## Guidelines for Evaluation and Treatment of Dry Eyes

**Do the Artificial Tears Last Long Enough? If Not:**

Use a more viscous tear
Try a tear with different osmolality
Use a tear with a different vehicle
Ophthalmologist can perform punctal occlusion to make instilled tears last longer
    Punctal plugs
    Permanent occlusion (cautery or laser)

**Do the Tears Burn After Instillation? If So:**

Choose a tear with different preservative
Use a nonpreserved tear

**Anticipate Low-Humidity Environments and Increase Use of Tears in Advance**

is reported to cause less irritation, but a slit-lamp examination is required for adequate quantitation. The results obtained with both rose bengal and lissamine green methods are very dependent both on the methods for performing the test and on the training and skill of the observer. In research studies (or in the rheumatologist's evaluation of published studies), it is important to recognize limitations of the different methods and the variation between different observers.

## Topical Therapy

The mainstay of treatment for the patient with dry eyes is the regular use of artificial tears.[16] When evaluating a particular artificial tear preparation (Table 21–4), the patient must carefully determine (1) whether the tear is beneficial but the benefit does not last long enough or (2) whether the tear burns immediately upon instillation. Artificial tears can be considered to have at least two distinct components: the moisturizing component and the preservative. If the tear is helpful but its effects do not last long enough, a more viscous tear (such as a product with a higher concentration of hydroxymethylcellulose) or a different vehicle to concentrate the moisturizing element (such as a polymer-like dextran) is indicated.

If the tear burns soon after instillation, an irritant reaction to a preservative in the tear must be considered.[17] These reactions were much more frequent in the past when benzalkonium chloride and thimerosal were commonly used in artificial tears. However, it should be remembered that these preservatives are still widely used in other ophthalmologic preparations (particularly topical antibiotics) and may contribute to ocular irritation. Irritation of the eyelids in some patients with blepharitis may be related to the preservatives present in some ocular lubricants (used at night),

as well as the use of excessive amounts of lubricant at night that plug the meibomian glands.

It is important for the patient to identify environmental factors and medications that contribute to dry eye symptoms (see Table 21–1). For example, symptoms of dry eyes are exacerbated by low-humidity environments such as airplanes, highly air-conditioned offices or department stores, and outdoor areas with strong dry winds. The increased use of tears *before* the onset of symptoms is symptomatically helpful and prevents corneal abrasions. The use of cool-mist humidifiers at night (or even in the office) and wrap-around sunglasses outdoors helps retard tear evaporation. Among patients who wear glasses, moisture shields can be added to the frames by the optometrist. In patients who like or need to be outdoors, ski goggles can provide a local "moisture chamber."

If the particular artificial tear seems helpful but benefit does not last long enough, punctal occlusion may be performed on a temporary or permanent basis.[18] The puncta are the small openings at the medial aspects of the lids. The puncta can be blocked with silicone plugs or by electrocautery.[18] Previously, a trial of temporary punctal occlusion with collagen plugs (i.e., occlusion that lasts several days) was advocated. However, clinical experience has indicated that adequate occlusion with collagen plugs is achieved in only a minority of patients, and this procedure is no longer advocated as an adequate trial. In some patients, a prior punctal occlusion may reopen; this can be determined easily by instilling fluorescein in the patient's eye. If the punctum has reopened, the fluorescein drains into the nasopharynx, and the patient experiences the characteristic taste of fluorescein. This simple test reveals the need (or non-necessity) for repeat punctal occlusion.

Topical cyclosporine has been used to ameliorate the keratoconjunctivitis in dogs with dry eyes. High levels of cyclosporine are achieved in the tear film, but there is little absorption into the systemic circulation. The beneficial effects of cyclosporine arise from its ability to serve as an anti-inflammatory agent. Additional benefits may result from stimulation of prolactin receptors on the cell surface of corneal cell and lacrimal gland acinar cells.[19] However, the diluent used to dissolve cyclosporine in the dog models was too irritating to use in SS patients in initial trials; more recently, a new vehicle has allowed cyclosporine to undergo phase III trials in KCS patients. These trials indicated that topical cyclosporine was significantly better than placebo or commercially available tears (M. Stern, personal communication); application to the US Food and Drug Administration is currently pending.

Adjuncts to therapy have included acetylcysteine 10% drops to break up mucus strands, but these drops have the smell of rotten eggs and are thus objectionable to most patients.[20] Vitamin A and related preparations have a theoretical role in the treatment of dry eye, because vitamin A–deficient patients have increased keratinization of the corneal surface[21]; however, more recent studies have not supported the initial enthusiasm for this form of treatment.[16]

## TABLE 21–4
## Artificial Tears

| Preserved Tears | Preservatives |
|---|---|
| Hydroxyethylcellulose (Adsorbotear) | Thimerosal |
| White petrolatum (Duratears) | Methylparaben |
| Polyvinyl alcohol (HypoTears, | Benzalkonium chloride |
| HypoTears PF, | None |
| Liquifilm Forte, | Thimerosal |
| Tears Plus) | Chlorobutanol |
| Methylcellulose (Murocel) | Methylparaben |
| Hydroxypropyl methylcellulose | |
| (Tears Naturale II) | Polyquad |

**Preserved Ocular Ointments**

| | |
|---|---|
| White petrolatum (Lacri-Lube) | Chlorobutanol |

**Nonpreserved Tears**

Polyethylene glycol 400 (AquaSite)
  (Dextran 70 1%)
Hydroxypropyl methylcellulose (Bion Tears)
  (Dextran 70 3%)
Carboxymethylcellulose 0.5% (Refresh Plus)
Polyvinyl alcohol (Hypotears PF)

## Oral Therapy

Pilocarpine, an agonist for the muscarinic $M_3$ receptor, has been used as an oral preparation to stimulate secretion by the salivary and lacrimal glands. Initial studies in 1986 indicated the benefit of pilocarpine in SS patients.[22] The effects on salivation were more marked than were the effects on lacrimal stimulation. Also of note, the relationship between subjective symptoms and objective measurements of saliva flow showed a weak correlation. These results were interpreted to indicate that pilocarpine stimulated "water" flow, but symptoms correlated with mucin secretion, which was not adequately quantitated in the studies. A series of additional studies on oral pilocarpine[23–25] have led to approval to market for symptoms of dry mouth. The available dosage is 5 mg up to four times daily. The most common side effect is increased sweating or gastrointestinal intolerance, which is generally controlled by decreasing the dose.

A clinical study using a different oral muscarinic agonist, cevimeline, was presented in abstract form.[26] In comparison to pilocarpine, cevimeline has (1) a longer half-life (4 hours) than pilocarpine (1.5 hours) and (2) a higher specificity, by about 10-fold, for muscarinic $M_3$ receptor (salivary and lacrimal gland) than for muscarinic $M_2$ receptor (cardiac tissues). This ratio of binding to $M_3$ receptor (i.e., efficacy in treatment of dry eyes and mouth) and $M_2$ receptor (i.e., toxicity to the heart) may prove important. In the clinical studies, an objective improvement in tear film, as measured by exfoliative cytologic study, was reported with cevimeline, which the same investigators had not seen in their prior studies with pilocarpine in the same study population of patients.[26]

Bromhexine, a cough syrup, has been reported to stimulate tear production.[10] Subsequent clinical trials have not been convincing, although some patients report considerable benefit.[4] In an animal model of dry eyes, bromhexine did not significantly increase salivary secretion.[27]

## EVALUATION AND TREATMENT OF DRY MOUTH

The principal oral symptom of SS is mouth dryness, with a broad range of severity. Not all patients complain of dryness specifically; many describe difficulty in swallowing food, problems in wearing dentures, changes in their sense of taste, increased incidence of dental caries, chronic burning symptoms, intolerance of acidic or spicy foods, and the inability to eat dry food or speak continuously for more than a few minutes. Nutrition may be compromised, and patterns of sleep may be disturbed.

On examination of the mouth, the SS patient lacks the normal salivary pooling under the tongue and may have rapidly progressive caries. The mouth frequently exhibits petechial (small, red, nonpalpable) lesions on the hard palate and/or a lichen planus–like appearance (fine, white, lacy strands) on the buccal mucosa.

Also, these lesions may be detected in the recesses of the buccal mucosa only on careful examination. These petechial and lichen planus–like lesions result from chronic oral candidiasis infection in the SS patient; it is uncommon for an SS patient's mouth to exhibit the plaquelike appearance (thrush) found in severely immunocompromised patients. Another manifestation of oral candidiasis in the SS patient is angular cheilitis, a condition that must be treated at the same time as the buccal mucosal candidiasis.

Patients with residual salivary gland function may benefit from either local or systemic methods to stimulate flow (Table 21–5). Gustatory stimulation with sugarless mints is often effective, as is chewing sugarless gum. One caution is that even sugarless gum may contain carbohydrates that have cariogenic potential in the presence of reduced salivary function.[12] Some patients find that chewing on paraffin wax or a fruit pit provides adequate masticatory stimulation without increasing cariogenic potential.

Systemic sialagogues have been used to increase salivation. Three agents have been studied in controlled trials. Bromhexine, a mucolytic agent, was not found to increase salivary flow rate, but patients described subjective benefit.[28] Anetholtrithion (Sialor) showed significant effects on saliva output in one study of SS patients with mild secretory hypofunction[29]; how-

---

**TABLE 21–5**
### Guidelines for Dry Mouth

**A Dry Mouth Is Not Necessarily Painful**
Look for oral yeast (especially under dentures) and angular
  cheilitis (both common after antibiotics or steroids)
Look for nasal congestion that contributes to mouth breathing

**Use of Fluorides, Toothpastes, and Salivary Stimulants**
Fluorides
  Topical applications by toothbrush
  Direct application by dental trays
Toothpastes without detergent
  Biotene toothpaste
  Arm and Hammer
Prevention of periodontal disease
  Regular oral hygiene by trained specialist
  Anti-infective mouthwash
    Peridex
    Retardex

**Saliva Stimulation**
Potassium iodide (SSKI) (10% saturated potassium iodide, 5
  drops QID)
Guaifenesin (Organidin)
Sugarless chewing gum
Soft toothbrush to stimulate buccal mucosa and tongue
Pilocarpine
Cevimeline
Bromhexine

**Mouth Rinses and Gels**
Oral balance gel
Biotene mouth rinse
MouthKote
Salivart
Saliment
Xero-Lube

ever, a later study failed to find a significant response in patients with severe hypofunction.[30] A series of controlled studies have indicated that pilocarpine exerts stimulatory properties in patients with SS and after radiation therapy.[22,31] The drug acts primarily as a muscarinic-cholinergic agonist with mild $\beta$-adrenergic activity. In these studies, pilocarpine, 5 mg three times a day, increased salivary flow for several hours, in comparison with placebo.[32] As noted previously, cevimeline, 30 mg three times a day, also stimulates muscarinic $M_3$ receptors and improves symptoms of dry mouth.[26] Side effects, including sweating, flushing, and increased urination, were common.[32] Further studies are needed to compare these treatments with other agents containing iodide (SSKI) or guaifenesin (Organidin) that are occasionally helpful in some SS patients.

It is common for a Sjögren's patient to develop a low-grade oral yeast infection.[33] Predisposing factors include recent use of antibiotics and/or corticosteroids. Treatment of this problem is particularly difficult in the patient with dentures, because continued excoriation of the mucosal surface occurs. Many topical antifungal drugs (including clotrimazole [Mycelex] troches) are available, but these oral preparations contain a low amount of antifungal agent and a high concentration of glucose (to improve the taste) and thus contribute to dental decay if used chronically.[33] The reason for inclusion of dextrose (rather than aspartame) as a sweetener was the US Food and Drug Administration's concern about long-term effects of aspartame at the time when the drug was first introduced; attempts by the authors to have Mycelex reformulated without dextrose by the manufacturer have not been successful. Both nystatin and clotrimazole (available as vaginal suppositories that can be sucked) are helpful but must be sucked for about 20 minutes twice daily for at least 6 weeks to prevent recurrence of oral candidiasis.[34] Patients with very dry mouths require periodic sips of water to help dissolve the troches. For angular cheilitis, topical antifungal creams are used two to three times per day for several weeks. This must be done concurrently with intraoral candidal treatment because the angular cheilitis serves to reinfect the buccal mucosa (and vice versa).

To permit drug access to all intraoral mucosal sites, patients must remove any dentures while antifungal tablets are dissolving. The dentures also must be treated to remove traces of Candida, and the method of disinfecting must be discussed with the dentist. However, it is usually sufficient to soak the complete denture overnight in benzalkonium chloride (e.g., a 1/700 dilution of the surgical scrub solution benzalkonium chloride [Zephiran Chloride]). The dentures must be carefully cleaned with a toothbrush, and nystatin powder often must be applied to the fitting surfaces of the upper denture before reinserting the denture. In extreme cases, a short course of oral antifungal therapy (such as ketoconazole or fluconazole) may be necessary to control oral candidiasis.

Progressive periodontal disease should be suspected on the basis of an increased need for dental restorations and the presence of cavities at the gum line. The loss

of teeth and requirement for dentures at any age, but particularly in the younger patient, may have significant emotional and economic consequences. Patients with dentures may change their social patterns of interpersonal interactions. For example, their social life may frequently involve eating meals with friends, and the patient may feel uncomfortable about not being able to eat the same foods. Furthermore, the patient's diet may be shifted to preprocessed foods that are often higher in sugars and thus further accelerate the rate of the periodontal problems.

The use of topical fluorides may help protect dental enamel. In some patients, a neutral fluoride drop may be applied by toothbrush or by an oral hygienist. In other patients, direct contact of the dental surfaces and the fluoride gel can be achieved by using dental plates at night to apply the fluoride. These plates are made specifically for each patient by a periodontist.

The use of the correct technique of toothbrushing to massage the gums and remove debris is important, because this function, normally provided by saliva, is diminished in SS patients. In some patients, a rotating toothbrush (such as Oratek) is useful, together with regular oral hygiene from a technician experienced in care of dry mouth.

Several types of toothpastes specially designed for periodontal problems are available for the patient with dry mouth. In the past, Peridex (a fluorine-based product) was popular but occasionally stained the dental enamel. A chlorine-based toothpaste (Retardent) that lacks this problem is in trials. An additional type of toothpaste based on the principle of generating low levels of antibacterial peroxides (Biotene) has been used. Recently, low-dose minocycline, 50 mg twice a day for 1 month, has been approved by the US Food and Drug Administration for periodontal disease. However, long-term treatment with minocycline may lead to tooth discoloration, a problem that seems less frequent with doxycycline. A local delivery system for antimicrobials to the gingival pockets has been advocated[35] but may be limited partially by the development of drug resistance.[36] Part of the benefit of tetracyclines on dental status may involve their ability to inhibit certain metalloproteinases (an activity distinct from their antimicrobial activity); thus, chemically modified tetracyclines may be able to retard periodontal disease without selecting for drug-resistant organisms.[36]

A variety of saliva substitutes is available. They differ in their flavoring agents and preservatives. Mouth-Kote and Salivart sprays contain mucins, which are glycoproteins that help lubricate the mouth and thus provide relief for a longer time than simply rinsing with water.[37] After administration of these sprays, parotid flow rates are increased for 7 to 8 minutes in SS patients; however, the sense of oral well-being may last for several hours. Electrical (vibrating) stimulation was used to stimulate saliva in some patients with mildly decreased flow rates,[38] although the cost of the apparatus has precluded wide usage.

A single-blind controlled trial was conducted to test the efficacy of low-dose oral human interferon alfa (IFN-alfa) to improve salivary function in SS patients.[39]

Fifty-six outpatients with first-degree SS and four patients with second-degree SS were randomly assigned to receive either IFN-alfa or sucralfate (control). The IFN-alfa (150 IU) or sucralfate (250 mg) was given orally three times a day for 6 months. After 6 months of treatment, 15 (50%) of 30 IFN-alfa–treated patients had saliva production increases at least 100% above baseline, whereas only 1 (3.3%) of 30 sucralfate recipients had a comparable increase ($P \le .001$). Serial labial salivary gland biopsies of nine IFN-alfa responders showed that lymphocytic infiltration was significantly decreased ($P \le .02$) and the proportion of intact salivary gland tissue was significantly increased ($P = .004$) after the IFN-alfa treatment. This agent is currently in double-blind trials.

## NASAL DRYNESS AND SINUSITIS

Many SS patients complain of nasal dryness and have symptoms of sinusitis with postnasal drip. It is common for a simple upper respiratory tract or sinus infection to linger for months in SS patients. This probably develops because of decreased secretion of glands lining the nasopharynx, leading to crusting of mucous secretions that block drainage and predispose to subsequent bacterial infection. Our initial approach is to provide increased moisture to this region by use of normal saline sprays and humidifiers during sleep.

It is frequently beneficial for the patient to learn to "lavage" the sinuses to remove the dry, crusted secretions. In patients with persistent sinus symptoms, it is useful to obtain a nasal smear to determine whether allergic factors (indicated by presence of eosinophils on the smear) are playing a role. Topical nasal sprays (such as Beconase Nasal AQ, Rhinocort, Flonase, or Nasalide) may be helpful in these patients. In the setting of sinusitis, it is always important to notice whether the secretions change from clear to yellow or green; the latter situation may indicate the occurrence of bacterial infection and necessitate treatment with antibiotics. For patients taking antibiotics, we frequently prescribe antifungal oral troches and/or yogurt to help prevent oral candidiasis.

## SKIN AND GYNECOLOGIC DRYNESS

Skin dryness is common in SS patients. This may result partly from decreased function of the eccrine glands in some patients. A variety of hydrating creams and ointments are available (Table 21–6). In general, it is best for the patient to soak the hands in water to allow the skin to absorb as much fluid as possible and then seal in the fluid with creams such as Lac-Hydrin, Eucerin, and Aquaphor. The prevention of cracking of the skin from dryness is important in the prevention of chronic skin infections.

Vaginal dryness often leads to painful intercourse (dyspareunia). It is important to reassure the patient that this does not occur in all female SS patients, even those with severe mouth and eye dryness. A gyneco-

## TABLE 21–6
## Treatment for Skin and Mucous Membrane Manifestations

| Skin Creams* | Anticandidal Agents for the Mouth |
|---|---|
| Eucerin | Lotrimin Cream,* external |
| Moisturel | Micatin cream,* external |
| Ticreme | Naftin cream, external |
| Aquaderm | Spectazole cream, external |
| Complex 15 | Loprox cream, external |
| Neutrogena | Clotrimazole cream, external |
| | Gyne-Lotrimin cream,* external |
| **Skin Lotions*** | Nystatin Oral Troche* |
| Keri lotion | Mycelex troches* |
| Carmol 10 | Gyne-Lotrimin vaginal suppositories* |
| Lubriderm | |
| Nutraderm | **Vaginal Lubricants and Anticandidal Agents*** |
| Lac-Hydrin Five | Surgilube |
| LactiCare | K-Y vaginal jelly |
| | Maxilube |
| **Soaps and Shampoos*** | Gyne-Moisture |
| Purpose | Astroglide |
| Dove | Feminase |
| Alpha Keri Moisturizing Soap | Topical estrogens (postmenopausal) |
| Aveeno Cleansing | Gyne-Lotrimin vaginal suppositories or cream |
| **Topical Steroids** | **Sunscreens** |
| 0.5% Hydrocortisone* with LactiCare-HC (2.5% HC) | Any sunscreen with SPF greater than 15 |
| Medium-strength corticosteroids (Kenalog, Aristocort)—not for use on the face | UVA and UVB blockers |
| | Solbar 50 |
| | Photoplex (UVB plus UVA blockers) |

UVA = ultraviolet A; UVB = ultraviolet B.
* Over-the-counter medication.

logic examination is useful for ruling out other causes of painful intercourse and other causes of vaginal dryness. When it does occur as part of SS, the spouse needs to be reassured that this is a physiologic problem and not related to a failure of sexual arousal. Sterile lubricants such as K-Y Jelly or Surgilube are helpful (see Table 21–6). The SS patient currently has multiple options regarding safe and effective vaginal lubrication. Lubricants such as Maxilube and Astroglide have physical characteristics slightly different from those of K-Y Jelly and Surgilube and yet share the common characteristics of being water-soluble and nonirritating. This also holds true for the newer nonhormonal vaginal moisturizer Replens, which may be used without association with intercourse. For patients who do not like the gel-type lubricant, Lubrin (vaginal inserts) is now available. A newer once-a-week vaginal lubricant called Vagikote (in clinical trials) may be added to this. Finding the right preparation for a specific individual is often a matter of trial and error, inasmuch as satisfaction with each lubricant is a matter of personal preference. Patients need to be frank with their physicians with regard to satisfaction or dissatisfaction with a particular preparation. The internal use of preparations containing petrolatum or oils that seal in moisture, such as Vaseline or cocoa butter, may lead to maceration of the vaginal lining and is to be avoided.

Vaginal dryness in perimenopausal or postmenopausal women is often related to vaginal atrophy because of declining estrogen levels and therefore responds to vaginal estrogen creams. Cortisone creams are not beneficial in this situation. If vaginal yeast infection occurs, prompt treatment with clotrimazole cream or suppositories (Gyne-Lotrimin) is effective and safe. On the external vulvar surface, dryness may be treated with lubricating creams, as on other skin surfaces. Several anecdotal reports note satisfaction with the use of a thin film of vitamin E oil used on the vulva once or twice a day.

An issue of concern to female SS patients has been whether estrogen replacement therapy is harmful to their condition. With regard to estrogen replacement in general, the clinical evidence is now convincing that estrogen treatment helps retard osteoporosis, reduces cardiovascular mortality, and improves quality of life by eliminating hot flashes and hormone-related vaginal dryness. Earlier investigators were concerned, on the basis of animal studies, that estrogen might have a negative influence on SS. At our clinic, we have not seen any deterioration of SS in relation to either estrogen replacement therapy or oral contraceptives. Because of this, we encourage adequate estrogen replacement for properly screened postmenopausal SS patients. In animal studies, progesterones may serve to augment secretory function; their better known role is in preventing uterine cancer in patients receiving estrogen. However, patient compliance with estrogens is rather low, because of side effects as well as fear of breast cancer. In some patients, the side effects are minimized by use of a natural estrogen (e.g., Prometrium); in these patients, estradiol levels should be checked to ensure adequate bioconversion to active forms. Many patients find the progesterone (as in Provera) to cause unacceptable side effects, and natural progesterone agents that may have lesser side effects are available.

## FATIGUE

Fatigue is a common complaint in SS. The problem may have many causes and may be related directly or indirectly to SS. Two types of fatigue should be considered. The first type is late morning or early afternoon fatigue. In this case, the patient arises with adequate energy but simply "runs out of gas" in the early afternoon. This type of fatigue suggests an inflammatory or metabolic process. Patients describe this type of fatigue as being accompanied by flu-like symptoms, and these probably result from the active immune system's liberating specific cytokines such as interleukin-1 and tumor necrosis factor. Fatigue caused by active inflammation is often associated with elevated sedimentation rate, elevated levels of C-reactive protein, and polyclonal increase in immunoglobulins. An increased frequency of hypothyroidism is associated with SS, and thus periodic laboratory evaluation rules out this cause of fatigue.

A second type of fatigue is morning fatigue, whereby the patient awakens and does not feel that he or she has obtained adequate sleep. This type of fatigue is also quite common in SS and may exist in addition to "inflammatory" fatigue. For example, sleep may be inadequate because of joint or muscle pain. Also, SS patients often drink a great deal of liquid during the day because of dry mouth and throat; then the patient may awaken three or four times during the night to urinate. This disrupts the sleep pattern and leads to morning fatigue. When this is the case, it is best to treat the symptoms directly, and better sleep should follow. In treating sleep disorders, tricyclic drugs (such as amitriptyline, nortriptyline, and doxepin) should be avoided if possible because they increase dryness through their anticholinergic side effects. A small series of SS patients studied under a research protocol at the Scripps Sleep Research Center has revealed a relatively high frequency of nocturnal myoclonus. In these patients, clonazepam (Klonopin) in low dosages (0.5 to 1 mg at bedtime) has proved helpful (unpublished observations). In comparison to benzodiazepines, clonazepam seems to be most effective in rapid eye movement sleep disorders when the nocturnal myoclonus may be most prominent (personal communication, M. Erman, Director of Sleep Research Center at Scripps Memorial Medical and Research Foundation). In patients with sleep disorders related to nocturia, the use of saliva substitutes (rather than fluid ingestion) after dinner and at night may prove helpful. In patients with severe nocturia that interrupts sleep patterns, agents such as desmopressin (DDAVP) (now available as an oral agent) may prove helpful; oxybutynin (Ditropan) tends to exacerbate the sicca symptoms.

Sometimes initiating good sleep habits is not enough to ameliorate the sense of daytime fatigue and poor sleep. If this is the case, a specific evaluation for sleep disorders can be performed. Certain people may have a higher risk of physiologic sleep disorders such as sleep apnea. Persons over 55 years old who snore loudly and who have had substantial weight gain (often while taking steroids) may be particularly prone to sleep apnea and require C-pap.

Probably the most difficult challenge in the differential diagnosis of SS is to determine the relative contribution of the disease to complaints of vague memory loss and fatigue. This problem is similar to that in SLE patients. It is hoped that the wider availability and better resolution of noninvasive imaging studies in the future will provide more objective guidelines for diagnosis and treatment.

## DEPRESSION IN SJÖGREN'S SYNDROME

Depression can manifest in many clinical forms, including difficulty concentrating, poor appetite, or a sleep disorder. The precise role of inflammation and hormone imbalances associated with SS as factors contributing to depression remains unclear, but depression is certainly caused in part by chemical alterations in the brain. Stress, poor sleep, and chronic illness can all contribute to depression. When antidepressant medications are used to help regulate sleep patterns and treat fatigue, drugs with relatively fewer anticholinergic side effects (such as trazodone, paroxetine [Paxil], and fluoxetine [Prozac], which interfere with serotonin uptake) are preferred. However, sleep disruptions are common with these drugs, and the more selective uptake inhibitors (e.g., citalopram [Celexa]) may be tried.

## SYSTEMIC MEDICATIONS IN PATIENTS WITH SJÖGREN'S SYNDROME

The overall approach to systemic therapy in the SS patient is similar to that in the SLE patient (Table 21–7). Disease manifestations are categorized as nonvisceral (arthralgias, myalgias, skin conditions, fatigue) and visceral (lung, heart, kidney, brain, peripheral nervous system) conditions. Nonvisceral manifestations are generally treated with salicylates, nonsteroidal agents, and often hydroxychloroquine. Particular attention to SS patients' difficulty in swallowing pills is necessary because the decreased salivary content can cause pills to become stuck in the midesophagus, resulting in erosions of the mucosa. Little improvement with salivary or lacrimal flow rates has been noted with nonsteroidal anti-inflammatory drugs (NSAIDs), although some increase in tearing and salivation may occur after systemic corticosteroids. Indomethacin is the only NSAID readily available as a suppository for the SS patient who has difficulty swallowing tablets. Flurbiprofen has been shown in a pilot study to decrease periodontal inflammation and resultant gum disease.

## TABLE 21–7
## Extraglandular Manifestations in Patients with Sjögren's Syndrome

**Respiratory**
Chronic bronchitis secondary to dryness of upper and lower airway with mucus plugging
Lymphocytic interstitial pneumonitis
Pseudolymphoma with nodular infiltrates
Lymphoma
Pleural effusions
Pulmonary hypertension, especially with associated scleroderma

**Gastrointestinal**
Dysphagia associated with xerostomia
Atrophic gastritis
Liver disease, including biliary cirrhosis and sclerosing cholangitis

**Skin and Mucous Membranes**
*Candida* (oral and vaginal)
Vaginal dryness
Hyperglobulinemic purpura
Raynaud's phenomenon
Vasculitis

**Endocrine, Neurologic, and Muscular**
Thyroiditis
Peripheral neuropathy: involvement of hands and/or feet
Mononeuritis multiplex
Myositis

**Hematologic**
Neutropenia, anemia, thrombocytopenia
Pseudolymphoma
Lymphadenopathy
Lymphoma and myeloma

**Renal**
Tubular interstitial nephritis
Glomerulonephritis, in absence of antibodies to DNA
Mixed cryoglobulinemia
Amyloidosis
Obstructive nephropathy caused by enlarged periaortic lymph nodes
Lymphoma
Renal artery vasculitis

Among the slow-acting drugs, antimalarials (e.g., hydroxychloroquine) have proved useful in decreasing the arthralgias, myalgias, and lymphadenopathy in SS patients,[23] which is similar to their benefit in some SLE patients. We have prescribed hydroxychloroquine (6 to 8 mg/kg/day) to SS patients in whom the erythrocyte sedimentation rate (ESR) is elevated and polyclonal hyperglobulinemia is present, because these laboratory abnormalities suggest that symptoms of arthralgia and myalgia may have an "inflammatory" cause. In a European study,[40] hydroxychloroquine improved ESR but did not increase tear flow volumes. Comparison of drug benefit in SS patients in European and US studies is strongly influenced by the very different inclusion criteria for diagnosis of SS (described earlier). When taken at the proper dosage (6 to 8 mg/kg/day), hydroxychloroquine has a very good safety record, although there remains a remote possibility (probably less than 0.1%)[41] of significant build-up in the eye. For this reason, periodic eye checks (generally every 6 to 12 months) are recommended so that the medicine can be discontinued if there is any significant build-up. In patients with cognitive features associated with SS, the use of atabrine has been advocated.[42] However, the patients should be screened for glucose-6-phosphate dehydrogenase deficiency before this drug is taken, and a "yellowing" of the skin is common. This skin change can be partially ameliorated with oral vitamin A. These agents are not readily available from most pharmacies but can be obtained from compounding pharmacies.

For visceral involvement, including vasculitic skin lesions, pneumonitis, neuropathy, and nephritis, corticosteroids are used in a manner similar to that in SLE patients. As in other autoimmune disorders, a key question is how to taper the corticosteroids, because these agents in addition accelerate periodontal problems. Drugs such as hydroxychloroquine, azathioprine, and methotrexate are used to help taper the corticosteroids. In one study, methotrexate appeared most useful.[43] It is likely that several of the newer agents approved for rheumatoid arthritis (leflunomide and the tumor necrosis factor antagonist etanercept) will prove useful in selected SS patients. In some SS patients, cyclosporine may be used,[44] but the tendency for the development of interstitial nephritis in many SS patients limits the usefulness of this drug.

For life-threatening illness, cyclophosphamide is occasionally required. However, the increased frequency of lymphoma in SS patients[45] mandates caution in the use of cyclophosphamide, and its use as a pulse therapy, rather than daily administration, has been suggested.

Painful swelling of the parotid glands may develop in SS patients. The swelling may be unilateral or bilateral, acute or chronic. In the setting of acute, unilateral swelling of the parotid or submandibular gland, an infectious process should be presumed to be the cause. Often, the patient has previously been dehydrated (e.g., after surgical or dental procedures, when the patient is unable or too uncomfortable to eat). The relative dehydrated state may lead to mucus inspissation in the ducts, leading to relatively sudden increase in ductal pressure and painful swelling of the gland. It is important on physical examination to determine that pus can be expressed (and cultured) from the opening of the ducts (i.e., Stensen's duct, which is adjacent to the upper molars, or Warthin's duct, which is under the tongue). If no drainage is noted, infection similar to a closed-space abscess needs to be considered. In some cases, a low dose of corticosteroids (e.g., prednisone, 10 to 15 mg/day) helps decrease swelling of the gland and the duct. In order to facilitate diagnostic coding for conditions associated with SS, a list of ICD-9 codes is provided in Table 21–8.

The patient needs to be advised about the serious nature of major salivary gland infections. Moist heat and adequate hydration are emphasized. In patients too sick to take oral medications and rehydration, intravenous medications and hydration may be required. The agents usually associated with this process are oral

**TABLE 21–8**
**ICD-9 Code Assignments for Sjögren's Syndrome, Manifestations, Symptoms, and Related Disorders**

| | |
|---|---|
| 710.2 | Sicca syndrome (primary Sjögren's syndrome) |
| 714.0 | Rheumatoid arthritis |
| 710.0 | Systemic lupus erythematosus |
| 710.1 | Systemic sclerosis (scleroderma) |
| 710.3 | Dermatomyositis |
| 710.4 | Polymyositis |
| 357.1 | Polyneuropathy in collagen vascular disease |
| 517.8 | Lung involvement in diseases classified elsewhere |
| 112.0 | Candidiasis of mouth (thrush) |
| 112.84 | Candidial esophagitis |
| 202.8 | Lymphoma, malignant (non-Hodgkin) |
| 273.0 | Polyclonal hypergammaglobulinemia |
| 285.9 | Anemia, unspecified |
| 373.0x | Blepharitis, unspecified |
| 443.0 | Raynaud's syndrome |
| 447.6 | Arteritis, unspecified |
| 521.0 | Dental caries |
| 523.4 | Chronic periodontitis |
| 530.81 | Esophageal reflux |
| 571.49 | Other chronic (active) hepatitis |
| 571.5 | Cirrhosis of liver without alcohol (cryogenic) |
| 571.6 | Biliary cirrhosis |
| 595.1 | Chronic interstitial cystitis |
| 135.3 | Dyspareunia |
| 729.1 | Myalgia and myositis, unspecified (fibromyalgia) |
| 375.15 | Tear film insufficiency (dry eye syndrome) |
| 370.33 | Keratoconjunctivitis sicca, *not specified as Sjögren's* [excludes (diagnosed) Sjögren's syndrome] |
| 527.1 | Hypertrophy of salivary glands |
| 527.7 | Disturbance of salivary secretion (xerostomia) |
| 719.4x | Pain in joint (requires fifth digit for site) |
| 780.7 | Malaise and fatigue |
| 785.6 | Enlargement of lymph nodes |
| 797.2 | Dysphagia |
| 790.1 | Elevated sedimentation rate |

organisms, and thus treatment may include penicillin or other broad-spectrum antibiotics. Persistent swelling of the parotid or submandibular gland (over several weeks) should be further evaluated by computed tomographic scan or magnetic resonance imaging of the soft tissues of the neck. The use of retrograde sialography must be avoided during any acute infection. Although this technique is periodically reported in the literature in Europe, the lack of experience in performing and interpreting these studies (in comparison to computed tomographic or magnetic resonance scans) leads to lower yields and higher risk of complications, including chemical sialadenitis resulting from ruptured ducts and the instilled contrast material.

## SPECIAL THERAPEUTIC CONSIDERATIONS IN THE PATIENT WITH SJÖGREN'S SYNDROME

### Anesthesia and Surgery

SS patients have particular problems during the preoperative, perioperative, and postoperative periods. The normal preoperative instruction is "no fluids by mouth" after dinner or midnight on the day before surgery. In the absence of normal saliva flow, these patients have great discomfort that can be reduced by the use of artificial salivas. Because the main concern behind this instruction is aspiration of stomach contents during anesthesia, these patients can safely use oral mouth sprays such as MouthKote (described earlier) without increased risk. These are also useful in postoperative patients, including those who are not able to take food by mouth.

Operating rooms and postoperative recovery areas have extremely low humidity, particularly as nonhumidified oxygen blows over a face mask. Therefore, SS patients have increased risk of developing corneal abrasions during surgery and in the postoperative setting. The decreased blink reflex of the patient during anesthesia also contributes to this problem. The administration of ocular lubricants before surgery and in the postoperative recovery period reduces the chances of this complication. Patients are advised to take Refresh P.M. ointment with them to the hospital; this allows the ointment to be available to the anesthesiologist. It is increasingly common for patients to be told not to bring their medications with them to the hospital (because all medications must be identified by nurses for medical and legal reasons), but specialty medications such as ocular or oral lubricants are not readily available in most hospitals. Patients should bring their medications in labeled containers and become advocates for their illness recognition and treatment.

Upper airway dryness of the SS patient may lead to mucus plug inspissation during the postoperative period, followed by obstructive pneumonias. The use of humidified oxygen and avoidance of medications that excessively dry the upper airways (i.e., used by the anesthesiologist to control secretions) help prevent this problem. Also, adequate hydration and respiratory therapy to keep airways clear are important. This problem has become more common because current practice is for one anesthesiologist to take the history and a different one to perform the procedure. Therefore, we advocate that patients take the "special instructions" page with them at the time of surgery (Table 21–9).

An additional problem for the anesthesiologist is the poor state of teeth in many SS patients. Thus, a higher risk of damage to teeth during intubation must be considered. This can lead to loss of the teeth and their subsequent aspiration. SS patients already incur great expense in dental care, and so needing to prepare dentures as a result of damage to and loss of their remaining teeth will be further burdensome.

In patients with rheumatoid arthritis and second-degree SS, the anesthesiologist must be informed about arthritic involvement of the neck (especially at the C1–2 level). Attempts to hyperextend the neck in order to intubate the patient may result in transection of the cervical spinal cord and paraplegia. When cervical involvement in rheumatoid arthritis is suspected, extreme caution during nasotracheal intubation needs to be taken, and intubation while the patient is wearing a soft cervical collar may avoid this problem.

## TABLE 21–9
## Instructions to the Patient with Sjögren's Syndrome at the Time of Surgery

**Preoperative Period**

Stop aspirin 1 week before surgery
Stop NSAIDs 3 days before surgery
Do not stop steroids
Notify anesthesiologist about specific problems with teeth, dentures, eyes, neck, sinuses, and lungs because such problems may affect the way intubation is performed

**Day of Surgery**

Take all medications with you to hospital in their bottles
Be sure to ask anesthesiologist to use an ocular ointment (such as Refresh P.M.) during surgery and in postoperative recovery room
If receiving steroids, make sure these are taken on day of surgery either orally or IV; in some cases, a higher dose is required
It is all right to use artificial salivas (such as MouthKote) to keep mouth moist on the day of surgery when NPO (nothing per mouth)
Ask anesthesiologist to use humidified oxygen in operating room and postoperative area

**Postoperative Days**

Watch for yeast infections if receiving antibiotics
Use artificial tears and salivas
Use artificial salivas

IV = intravenously; NSAIDs = nonsteroidal anti-inflammatory drugs.

In many surgical procedures, antibiotics are routinely given. In the patient with sicca symptoms, the risk for associated oral candidiasis is greatly increased. The use of topical oral antifungal drugs such as nystatin helps prevent this complication. Precautions regarding steroid coverage are important because patients remain relatively adrenal-insufficient after an extended period on glucocorticoids, depending on the dosage.

Finally, assessment of the fluid status of the SS patient in the postoperative period may be relatively difficult. Normal clinical clues such as the moisture in the ocular and oral membranes may be quite misleading. Furthermore, some SS patients have a tendency to develop interstitial nephritis, which prevents adequate urine concentration and fluid balance. This problem may be exacerbated by antibiotics such as aminoglycosides.

*Acknowledgments*

*The authors greatly appreciate the help of Drs. Lee Kaplan (Dermatology), Ray Steward and Malin Gehrn (Oral Medicine), Ray Vandenburg (Gynecology), John Schleimer and Dee Silver (Neurology), and Milt Erman (Sleep Disorder), all of the Scripps Memorial Medical and Research Foundation.*

# REFERENCES

1. Tan EM, Feltkamp TE, Smolen JS, et al: Range of antinuclear antibodies in "healthy" individuals. Arthritis Rheum 1997; 40:1601.

2. Emlen W, O'Neill L: Clinical significance of antinuclear antibodies: Comparison of detection with immunofluorescence and enzyme-linked immunosorbent assays. Arthritis Rheum 1997; 40:1612.

3. Bekker M: Dry eyes: An emerging epidemic. Ophthalmology Management 1999; 10:4.

4. Yamada F: Frontal midline theta rhythm and eyeblinking activity during a VDT task and a video game: Useful tools for psychophysiology in ergonomics. Ergonomics 1998; 41:678.

5. Fox RI: Sjögren's syndrome. Controversies and progress. Clin Lab Med 1997; 17:431.

6. Fox RI: Sjögren's syndrome. *In* Klippel J (ed): Primer on the Rheumatic Diseases, vol 11. Atlanta: Arthritis Foundation, 1998:283.

7. Vitali C, Moutsopoulos HM, Bombardieri S: The European Community Study Group on diagnostic criteria for Sjögren's syndrome. Sensitivity and specificity of tests for ocular and oral involvement in Sjögren's syndrome. Ann Rheum Dis 1994; 53:637.

8. Fox RI, Maruyami T, Tornwald J: Sjögren's syndrome: Current issues in diagnosis and pathogenesis. Curr Opin Rheumatol 1999; 11:364.

9. Vitali C, Bombardieri S: The European classification criteria for Sjögren's syndrome (SS): Proposal for modification of the rules for classification suggested by the analysis of the receiver operating characteristic (ROCS) curve of the criteria performance. J Rheumatol 1997; 24(suppl):S18.

10. Stern ME, Beuerman RW, Fox RI, et al: A unified theory of the role of the ocular surface in dry eye. Adv Exp Med Biol 1998; 438:643.

11. Toda I, Yagi Y, Hata S, et al: Excimer laser photorefractive keratectomy for patients with contact lens intolerance caused by dry eye. Br J Ophthalmol 1996; 80:604.

12. Pflugfelder SC: Differential diagnosis of dry eye conditions. Adv Dent Res 1996; 10:9.

13. Tsubota K: Tear dynamics and dry eye. Prog Retin Eye Res 1998; 17:565.

14. Stern ME, Beuerman RW, Fox RI, et al: The pathology of dry eye: The interaction between the ocular surface and lacrimal glands. Cornea 1998; 17:584.

15. Atkinson J, Pillemer S, Travis WD, et al: Major salivary gland function in primary Sjögren's syndrome and its relationship to clinical features. J Rheumatol 1990; 17:318.

16. Friedlaender M: Ocular manifestations of Sjögren's syndrome. Rheum Dis Clin North Am 1992; 18:591.

17. Wilson F: Adverse external ocular effects of topical ophthalmic medications. Surv Ophthalmol 1979; 24:57.

18. Friedlaender MH, Fox RI: Punctal occlusion for the treatment of dry eye. Adv Exp Med Biol 1998; 438:1017.

19. Kaswan R: Characteristics of a canine model of KCS: Effective treatment with topical cyclosporine. Adv Exp Med Biol 1994; 350:583.

20. Lemp M: General measures in management of the dry eye. Int Ophthalmol Clin 1988; 27:36.

21. Tseng S: Topical tretinoin treatment for dry-eye disorders. Int Ophthalmol Clin 1987; 27:47.

22. Fox PC, van der Ven PF, Baum BJ, et al: Pilocarpine for the treatment of xerostomia associated with salivary gland dysfunction. Oral Surg Oral Med Oral Pathol 1986; 61:243.

23. Rhodus NL, Schuh MJ: Effects of pilocarpine on salivary flow in patients with Sjögren's syndrome [see comments]. Oral Surg Oral Med Oral Pathol 1991; 72:545.

24. Rhodus NL: Oral pilocarpine HCl stimulates labial (minor) salivary gland flow in patients with Sjögren's syndrome. Oral Dis 1997; 3:93.

25. Papas AS, Fernandez MM, Castano RA, et al: Oral pilocarpine for symptomatic relief of dry mouth and dry eyes in patients with Sjögren's syndrome. Adv Exp Med Biol 1998; 438:973.

26. Fox RI, Pentrone J, Condemi R, et al: Randomized, placebo controlled trial of SNI-2011, a novel $M_3$ muscarinic receptor agonist, for the treatment of Sjögren's syndrome. Arthritis Rheum 1998; 41(suppl):S288.

27. Nanni JM, Nguyen KH, Alford CE, et al: Assessment of bromhexine as a treatment regimen in Sjögren's syndrome–like disease in the NOD (non-obese diabetic) mouse. Clin Exp Rheumatol 1997; 15:515.

28. Fox P: Systemic therapy of salivary gland hypofunction. J Am Dent Assoc 1987; 115:581.

29. Epstein J, Decoteau WE, Wilkinson A: Effect of sialor in treatment of xerostomia in Sjögren's syndrome. Oral Surg 1983; 56:495.

30. Schiodt M, Oxholme P, Jacobsen A: Treatment of xerostomia in patients with primary Sjögren's syndrome with sulfarlem. Scand J Rheumatol 1986; 61:250.

31. Fox P, Atkinson JC, Macynski AA: Pilocarpine treatment of salivary gland hypofunction and dry mouth. Arch Intern Med 1991; 151:1149.

32. Vivino FB, Al-Hashimi I, Khan Z, et al: Pilocarpine tablets for the treatment of dry mouth and dry eye symptoms in patients with Sjögren syndrome: A randomized, placebo-controlled, fixed-dose, multicenter trial. P92-01 Study Group [In Process Citation]. Arch Intern Med 1999; 159:174.

33. Daniels TE, Fox PC: Salivary and oral components of Sjögren's syndrome. Rheum Dis Clin North Am 1992; 18:571.

34. Hernandez YL, Daniels TE: Oral candidiasis in Sjögren's syndrome: Prevalence, clinical correlation and treatment. Oral Surg Oral Med Oral Pathol 1989; 68:324.

35. Killoy WJ: Chemical treatment of periodontitis: Local delivery of antimicrobials. Int Dent J 1998; 48:305.

36. Larsen T, Fiehn NE: Development of resistance to metronidazole and minocycline in vitro. J Clin Periodontol 1997; 24:254.

37. Rhodus N, Schuh M: Effectiveness of three artifical salivas as assessed by mucoprotective relativity. J Dent Res 1991; 70:40708.

38. Steller M, Chou L, Daniels T: Electrical stimulation of salivary flow in patients with Sjögren's syndrome. J Dent Res 1988; 67:1334.

39. Shiozawa S, Tanaka Y, Shiozawa K: Single-blinded controlled trial of low-dose oral IFN-alpha for the treatment of xerostomia in patients with Sjögren's syndrome. J Interferon Cytokine Res 1998; 18:255.

40. Kruize A, Hene R, Kallanberg C, et al: Hydroxychloroquine treatment for primary Sjögren's syndrome: A two year double blind crossover trial. Ann Rheum Dis 1993; 52:360.

41. Bernstein HN: Ocular safety of hydroxychloroquine. Ann Ophthalmol 1991; 23:292.

42. Wallace D: Antimalarial agents and lupus. Rheum Dis Clin North Am 1994; 20:243.

43. Skopouli FN, Jagiello P, Tsifetaki N, et al: Methotrexate in primary Sjögren's syndrome. Clin Exp Rheumatol 1996; 14:555.

44. Dalavanga YA, Detrick B, Hooks JJ, et al: Effect of cyclosporin A (CyA) on the immunopathological lesion of the minor salivary glands from patients with Sjögren's syndrome. Ann Rheum Dis 1990; 46:89.

45. Fox RI, Adamson TC III, Fong S, et al: Lymphocyte phenotype and function of pseudolymphomas associated with Sjögren's syndrome. J Clin Invest 1983; 72:52.

# 22 | The Seronegative Spondyloarthropathies (Ankylosing Spondylitis, Reactive Arthritis, Psoriatic Arthritis)

*Christopher G. Jackson and Daniel O. Clegg*

The seronegative (rheumatoid factor negative) spondyloarthropathies are a group of rheumatic diseases that share clinical, radiologic, and genetic similarities. Included in this group of diseases are ankylosing spondylitis, reactive arthritis (formerly called Reiter's syndrome), psoriatic arthritis, and arthritis associated with inflammatory bowel disease. These diseases are characterized by the absence of serum autoantibodies, including rheumatoid factor. It is important to distinguish them from rheumatoid arthritis because, as will be seen, treatment of the two disorders is often different. The following are some common features that the seronegative spondyloarthropathies share:

- An association with the class I human leukocyte antigen (HLA)–B27.
- A strong predilection for symptomatic disease in young adult males.
- Radiographic evidence of sacroiliitis and spondylitis.
- Oligoarticular peripheral joint involvement.
- Enthesopathy (inflammation at the sites of tendinous insertions).
- Extra-articular manifestations, including oral ulcers, specific dermatologic lesions, uveitis, aortitis, and pulmonary fibrosis.

This chapter addresses the treatment of ankylosing spondylitis, reactive arthritis, and psoriatic arthritis. In general, there is a dearth of carefully controlled clinical trials with sufficient statistical power to address this issue. Where such information exists, we provide an objective summary of the material. In addition, we present published, uncontrolled data in a balanced manner with the caveat that, as a rule, uncontrolled reports in the literature most often document positive outcomes.

## ANKYLOSING SPONDYLITIS

### Definition and Natural History

Ankylosing spondylitis is characterized by sacroiliitis and spondylitis, most commonly involving the lumbar spine and occasionally progressing cephalad to involve the thoracic and cervical spines. A number of criteria sets have been proposed to aid in the diagnosis of ankylosing spondylitis. Most include assessment of the patient for inflammatory low back pain and stiffness, limitation of lumbar spine motion, limitation of chest expansion, and the presence of radiographic sacroiliitis. There is a strong association with the class I HLA-B27. In most series, well over 80% of white patients with ankylosing spondylitis are HLA-B27–positive, in comparison with 8% of the general white population. There is also a strong association in males between onset of disease symptoms and age (second and third decades). For a complete discussion of diagnosis, pathogenesis, and prognosis, see Kelley and coauthors, Chapter 56.[1]

The natural history of ankylosing spondylitis is somewhat controversial. Cheret and associates[2] described a population of 150 war veterans who were monitored prospectively for more than 30 years. In this group, the mean age at onset of symptoms was 24 years, the duration of symptoms was 38 years, and the average age at follow-up was 62 years. At follow-up, one third of the patients denied having any pain. Thirty-eight percent described their axial pain as mild, 28% as moderate, and 4% as severe. More than 70% of the patients stated that their symptoms had not changed in the preceding 10 years. Spinal restriction was graded as mild (41%), moderate (18%), or severe (41%); peripheral joint involvement believed to be related to ankylosing spondylitis was present in 36% of this group of patients. Peripheral joints that were involved, in order of decreasing frequency, were the hips, shoulders, knees, ankles, metatarsal joints, and interphalangeal joints. Of patients who were tested, 89% were HLA-B27–positive. Sixty-one deaths occurred in this series. Eight of these deaths were considered to be disease related: two were caused by cervical subluxations, three patients died of aortic insufficiency, two died of respiratory failure as a result of severe spinal involvement, and one died of amyloidosis. Six of the eight patients who died had peripheral joint disease at onset, and six were believed to have severe spinal restriction or deformity. The conclusions of these authors included the following:

1. Ankylosing spondylitis can have a benign course.
2. In most patients a predictable pattern of disease emerges within the first 10 years.

Radford and colleagues[3] described age-specific mortality rates among 836 patients with ankylosing spondylitis who did not receive radiation therapy and found that there was excess mortality from ulcerative colitis, nephritis, and tuberculosis. In addition, mortality risks in relation to those in the general population were increased for all gastrointestinal and circulatory diseases. Smith and Doll[4] reported a mortality study of more than 14,000 patients with ankylosing spondylitis who had received radiation therapy; they found excess risk of leukemia and other malignancies that became apparent 9 or more years after the radiation exposure.

Gran and Skomsvoll[5] found that loss of functional outcome in 100 patients with ankylosing spondylitis most frequently occurred within the first 10 years of disease. Poor outcome was most frequently associated with the development of peripheral arthritis or radiographic evidence of severe spinal involvement (bamboo spine).

## Nonarticular Manifestations of Disease

ACUTE ANTERIOR UVEITIS. Up to 40% of patients with ankylosing spondylitis have one or more episodes of acute anterior uveitis. Eye pain, photophobia, injection, excess tearing, and impaired vision are common presenting manifestations. Early symptoms may be ignored if patients with ankylosing spondylitis are not specifically warned to expect them. Prompt diagnosis and management with the help of an ophthalmologist are important for a good outcome. Therapy is directed at topical pupillary dilation and instillation of steroid solutions.

PULMONARY MANIFESTATIONS OF ANKYLOSING SPONDYLITIS. Mechanical problems, such as severe thoracic kyphosis, can lead to ventilation/perfusion mismatching and restrictive pulmonary disease, but these mechanical problems are usually of minimal clinical significance. Apical pulmonary fibrosis is a specific but uncommon pulmonary process associated with ankylosing spondylitis, the diagnosis of which requires that coexistent pulmonary tuberculosis be excluded. Patients with ankylosing spondylitis should be strongly counseled against smoking in order to avoid concurrent obstructive lung disease that can complicate possible restrictive disease.[6]

MECHANICAL SPINE DISEASE. The rigid spine seen in patients with advanced, aggressive ankylosing spondylitis can present a number of clinically challenging complications. Minor trauma can result in spinal fracture. The most common site of fracture is the C5–6 region, and instability can lead to paraplegia. Fracture may occur in the thoracic and lumbar spine as well.[7]

Nondisplaced fractures generally do well with external fixation, whereas spinal instability generally necessitates internal fixation and surgical fusion.

There have been numerous reports of cauda equina syndrome in patients with advanced ankylosing spondylitis. The onset is generally insidious, making diagnosis very challenging. A high index of suspicion is necessary for patients with lower extremity symptoms. Evaluation with magnetic resonance imaging is often necessary for documenting the diagnosis.

Spinal surgery in patients with ankylosing spondylitis is problematic. Patients are often osteoporotic, which makes fixation difficult. Prolonged bed rest and inactivity are often difficult to achieve, as is rehabilitation when movement can be reinstituted. Thus surgery should be given thoughtful, deliberate consideration by the patient, the rheumatologist, the physical therapist, and an experienced orthopedic surgeon.

## Treatment

Although the majority of this section details the medical treatment of ankylosing spondylitis, it should be noted that before medications are instituted, patient education about the disease process and course, along with physical therapy intervention and instruction, should be an integral part of the management of patients with ankylosing spondylitis, as well as the other spondyloarthropathies. The goals of patient education should include instructions about the natural history of the disease, the prognosis, and the importance of maintaining an upright posture that will also allow function in the patient's vocation. Patients should be counseled to avoid smoking and other activities that may impair pulmonary function and may be additive to either the restrictive pulmonary diseases that can be seen secondary to fusion of the thoracic spine or the less common interstitial pulmonary fibrosis. Other extra-articular complications, including iritis/iridocyclitis, aortitis, and cardiac involvement, should be discussed with the patient and reviewed regularly on follow-up visits.

Physical therapy should address maintenance of good posture, spine mobility and function, muscle strengthening, general conditioning, and exercise. Consistent, moderate physical exercise improved function and lessened disease activity in patients with ankylosing spondylitis.[8] Kraag and associates[9] reported a randomized controlled trial of 53 patients with ankylosing spondylitis, in which 26 patients received extensive education about their disease and instruction in physical therapy, and the remaining 27 patients received neither of these interventions. The results of the study showed significant improvement in fingertip-to-floor distance, the primary outcome measure of this study, as well as in a functional assessment among the patients who received the interventions. O'Driscoll and colleagues[10] reported improvement in cervical spine mobility with physical therapy.

### Nonsteroidal Anti-inflammatory Drugs

Nonsteroidal anti-inflammatory drugs (NSAIDs) are used almost universally in the medical treatment of ankylosing spondylitis. More than 80% of patients with ankylosing spondylitis[11] in the United Kingdom take one of the NSAIDs for control of the symptoms related to the disease. Numerous comparative studies have been undertaken to evaluate the efficacy and safety of NSAIDs in the management of this disease. Table 22–1 summarizes the results of some of the larger trials.[12] The methods of these trials were so variable that it is difficult to conclude that any single nonsteroidal agent is either more efficacious or less toxic than any other, and thus it is difficult to establish clear preferences. Standard textbooks state that indomethacin may offer increased efficacy in these diseases,[13] and that has been our clinical experience. In the United States, the following NSAIDs have received approval from the US Food and Drug Administration for use in ankylosing spondylitis: indomethacin, sulindac, naproxen, diclofenac, and phenylbutazone. Because of the potential for bone marrow suppression as an adverse drug reaction, phenylbutazone should not be used unless other nonsteroidal agents have failed. Because of its safety profile,

phenylbutazone is no longer marketed in the United States.

Patients with ankylosing spondylitis are no more susceptible to the adverse drug effects associated with NSAIDs than is any other group of rheumatology patients. Patients should be carefully questioned about any evidence of previous gastrointestinal problems or predisposition to develop renal insufficiency, so that appropriate accommodations can be made for those at increased risk of adverse drug reactions. Otherwise, it is recommended that patients in whom NSAID treatment is newly instituted have a complete blood cell count and determination of creatinine at baseline. Complete blood counts annually and creatinine and transaminase determinations as indicated are recommended in clinically treated patients.[14]

The release of selective cyclooxygenase-2 (COX-2) inhibitors raises the likelihood of additional therapeutic anti-inflammatory options. To date, no reports documenting experience with COX-2 selective agents in the management of seronegative spondyloarthropathies have been published.

In summary, NSAIDs are effective in ameliorating many of the clinical symptoms associated with ankylosing spondylitis. None has documented superiority in terms of efficacy or safety, except that phenylbutazone has more potential for bone marrow suppression. Selection of the most appropriate agent in any given patient often requires balancing between more clinical benefit and less toxicity. Patients on these regimens should be monitored for adverse reactions, be monitored clinically for disease progression, receive continued education about their disease process, and receive physical therapy instruction with the objectives of maintaining function and quality of life. For a more comprehensive discussion of the individual agents, see Kelley and coauthors.[1]

### Amitriptyline

Koh and colleagues reported a 2-week trial of low-dose amitriptyline treatment in ankylosing spondylitis.[15] One hundred patients took up to 30 mg of amitriptyline nightly or placebo. The patients who took amitriptyline noted significantly more restful sleep, and trends toward functional improvement were seen.

### Pamidronate

In an open-label study, 16 patients with refractory ankylosing spondylitis received intravenous pamidronate.[16] Improvement was noted in some of the outcome measures, and further evaluation in a controlled setting was recommended.

### Potentially Disease Modifying Antirheumatic Drugs

D-PENICILLAMINE. D-Penicillamine has been used in ankylosing spondylitis in a number of open-label trials. The largest series was reported in a letter detailing clinical experience with D-penicillamine in 49 patients

**TABLE 22–1**
## Some Double-Blind Trials of Nonsteroidal Anti-inflammatory Drugs in Ankylosing Spondylitis

| STUDY DRUG | COMPARATOR DRUG | NO. OF PATIENTS | RESULTS |
|---|---|---|---|
| Dic | Sul | 62 | Dic > Sul |
| Eto | Indo | 99 | Eto = Indo |
|  | Nap/Pl | 128 | Eto > Pl |
| Fen | Pbz | 30 | Fen < Pbz |
|  | Indo | 19 | Fen = Indo |
| Flu | Indo | 57 | Flu = Indo |
|  | Indo | 26 | Flu = Indo |
|  | Pbz |  | Flu = Pbz |
| Ibu | Open study | 65 | Effective |
| Indo | Pl |  | Indo > Pl |
|  | Nap | 27 | Indo > Nap |
|  | Dic | 262 | Indo > Dic |
| Keto | Pl | 13 | Keto > Pl |
|  | Pbz |  | Keto = Pbz |
| Nap | Indo | 35 | Nap = Indo |
|  | Flu | 30 | Nap = Flu |
| Pbz | Nap | 20 | Pbz = Nap |
|  | Nap | 25 | Pbz = Nap |
|  | Keto | 25 | Pbz > Keto |
| Pir | Indo | 55 | Pir = Indo |
|  | Indo | 87 | Pir = Indo |
| Sul | Pbz | 120 | Sul < Pbz |
|  | Pbz | 24 | Sul = Pbz |
|  | Pl | 83 | Sul > Pl |
|  | Indo | 23 | Sul < Indo |
| Ten | Dic | 57 | Ten = Dic |
| Tol | Indo | 60 | Tol = Indo |
|  | Nap | 34 | Tol = Nap |

Dic = diclofenac; Eto = etodolac; Fen = fenoprofen; Flu = flurbiprofen; Ibu = ibuprofen; Indo = indomethacin; Keto = ketoprofen; Nap = naproxen; Pbz = phenylbutazone; Pir = piroxicam; Pl = placebo; Sul = sulindac; Ten = tenoxicam; Tol = tolmetin. Symbols: > indicates superior efficacy; < indicates inferior efficacy; = indicates equivalent efficacy.

Reprinted from *Drugs* 1992; 44(4):585–603 with permission. © Adis International, Inc.

with ankylosing spondylitis.[17] The D-penicillamine was titrated to a total dose of 500 mg/day. Tytman and coworkers[17] noted an improvement in Schober's test results and the fingertip-to-floor test within the first 4 weeks of therapy. This improvement was at a time when the patients were taking a very low dose of D-penicillamine, and improvement was seen much earlier than an antirheumatic effect from D-penicillamine would be anticipated. Steven and associates[18] reported a double-blind, placebo-controlled trial of D-penicillamine in 17 patients over a 6-month period in which no clinical improvement was seen.

AURANOFIN. Grasedyck and colleagues[19] reported a series of patients in whom auranofin produced no improvement in the disease manifestations of ankylosing spondylitis.

SULFASALAZINE. In 1984, Amor and associates[20] suggested that sulfasalazine may be effective against ankylosing spondylitis, particularly in patients with peripheral arthritis. Since that time, at least 10 other double-blind placebo-controlled trials with mixed results have been published.[21–23] It appears likely that sulfasalazine has a beneficial effect on lowering erythrocyte sedimentation rates and C-reactive protein levels. Data regarding the potential benefit of sulfasalazine on clinical symptoms or signs of disease are less clear. For example, morning stiffness was ameliorated in two of the studies but did not change in six and was not reported in two; night pain was improved in one, did not change in four, and was not reported in four; chest expansion was improved in three, did not change in four, and was not reported in three; spinal mobility was not improved in seven and not reported in three. Ferraz and colleagues[24] reported a meta-analysis of five randomized controlled trials. The results of this analysis indicated that sulfasalazine had clinical benefit over placebo in duration of morning stiffness, severity of morning stiffness, severity of pain, general well-being, erythrocyte sedimentation rate, and serum immunoglobulin A values. Taggart and coworkers[25] reported a trial of 90 patients with ankylosing spondylitis who took sulfasalazine or one of its moieties, 5-aminosalicylic acid or sulfapyridine. They noted a fall in plasma viscosity, a fall in serum levels of immunoglobulins G and A, and improvement in spine and night pain in the patients taking sulfasalazine and sulfapyridine but not in those taking 5-aminosalicylic acid; this suggests that sulfapyridine may be the active moiety in treating ankylosing spondylitis.

Conceptually, it is possible that the most beneficial effect associated with sulfasalazine in ankylosing spondylitis might be seen in patients who have peripheral arthritis in association with axial disease. Mielants and Veys[26] discussed the increased incidence of histologic changes suggestive of subclinical inflammatory bowel disease in patients with ankylosing spondylitis and peripheral arthritis. Anecdotally, those patients seemed particularly responsive to sulfasalazine therapy. They may represent a subgroup of patients with subclinical inflammatory bowel disease, sacroiliitis, and peripheral arthritis rather than true ankylosing spondylitis.

Although the efficacy data regarding sulfasalazine in ankylosing spondylitis are somewhat unclear, the medication is well tolerated. Mild gastrointestinal intolerance, including nausea and anorexia, is the most commonly reported symptom. In addition, minor rashes are reported with some frequency. Much less frequently reported abnormalities include liver function aberrations, hematologic abnormalities, such as agranulocytosis, hemolytic anemia, and thrombocytopenia, and neurologic effects, including dizziness, headache, and vertigo. Sulfasalazine has been studied in divided doses of 2 to 3 g/day. Blood counts and chemistry profiles should initially be monitored at twice-monthly intervals to detect cytopenias; however, once a patient is successfully tolerating the medications, toxicity surveillance can be modified after several months.

In summary, sulfasalazine may have a role in the treatment of ankylosing spondylitis. It appears likely that the potentially beneficial effects of sulfasalazine are in the treatment of the peripheral arthritis associated with ankylosing spondylitis.[27] There have been no studies to evaluate its long-term potential as a disease-modifying agent. The recommended daily dose is 30 to 40 mg/kg/day. Sulfasalazine was discussed in detail by Kelley and coauthors.[1]

There are anecdotal reports of methotrexate use in ankylosing spondylitis in which studies involved fewer than five patients. However, to the best of our knowledge, there have been no controlled trials evaluating methotrexate, antimalarials, parenteral gold, or cyclosporine in ankylosing spondylitis.

RADIOTHERAPY. Radiotherapy was used empirically in treating the symptoms of ankylosing spondylitis in the 1940s. A sham-controlled trial using various radiation dosages suggested improvement in patients with ankylosing spondylitis who underwent radiation, compared with controls who had rheumatoid arthritis.[28]

The use of radiotherapy declined with the introduction of effective therapy with the NSAIDs, initially phenylbutazone and then others. Subsequently, toxicity studies demonstrated an increased incidence of leukemia and other neoplasms in patients who had undergone irradiation. Although studies have not been done with radiation approaches that employ smaller, well-localized fields and lower total radiation dosages, consideration of any patient for radiotherapy would be exceptional.

## Approach to Management

After a careful diagnostic evaluation, the patient with ankylosing spondylitis should first receive education about the disease and the importance of a physical therapy program aimed at good posture and maintenance of motion and muscle strength. NSAIDs should be used for symptomatic relief of the discomfort associated with inflammatory musculoskeletal complaints. Indomethacin may be more effective than other NSAIDs; however, there are few controlled data to support this position. Sulfasalazine is likely a beneficial adjunct for patients with peripheral joint involvement. There is little published clinical evidence to suggest that any of the other second-line agents have any beneficial activity in the management of ankylosing spondylitis.

## REACTIVE ARTHRITIS

### Definition and Natural History

Hans Reiter first reported the association of arthritis, nongonococcal urethritis, and conjunctivitis in 1916.[29] In the early 1970s the association between Reiter's syndrome and HLA-B27 positivity was made, and from that association arose the concept of "incomplete" Reiter's syndrome,[30] which consisted of asymmetric oligoarthritis and HLA-B27 positivity. Because of the frequent association between venereal and enteric infections and the subsequent development of Reiter's syndrome, the term *reactive arthritis*[31] was proposed in 1969. It now seems clear that fully manifest Reiter's syndrome is seen in a subset of patients with reactive arthritis. Thus the term *reactive arthritis* seems more appropriate to describe the condition in this unique group of patients whose main clinical manifestations include asymmetric oligoarthritis, an increased prevalence of HLA-B27 positivity, nongonococcal urethritis, conjunctivitis, distinct rashes (including circinate balanitis and keratoderma blennorrhagicum), oral ulcers, uveitis, subclinical enterocolitis, carditis, and nephritis.[32] Aspects of differential diagnosis, pathogenesis, and clinical features were discussed by Kelley and coauthors.[1]

The natural history of reactive arthritis is extremely variable; most patients experience exacerbations and remissions, which can last from several weeks to several months.[33] Although a few patients have only a single episode of the disease, the rule is multiple flares of disease activity. Fox and associates[34] reported that 83% of 122 patients with reactive arthritis had persistent disease at 5.6 years. Approximately one fourth of those patients were unable to work or had changed vocations because of the disease. Inman and colleagues found that at 1-year follow-up, 7 of 15 patients with postenteric infection-induced reactive arthritis continued to have persistent joint symptoms.[35]

REACTIVE ARTHRITIS AND HUMAN IMMUNODEFICIENCY VIRUS DISEASE. There have been several reports of reactive arthritis in association with human immunodeficiency virus (HIV) infection. Although reactive arthritis can occur after the patient becomes seropositive for HIV, clinical features of reactive arthritis frequently precede the recognition of clinical HIV-associated diseases. Therefore, a high index of suspicion for HIV infection in patients with reactive arthritis is warranted.[36] HIV infection does not appear to alter the course of the reactive arthritis per se; however, there have been reports in which the use of immunosuppressive medications in this patient population resulted in abrupt clinical deterioration and the onset of other manifestations of the acquired immunodeficiency syndrome.[37]

## Treatment

Patients with reactive arthritis are, in general, relatively young and geographically mobile. As has already been mentioned, reactive arthritis has a highly variable course that is punctuated by remissions and exacerbations. These factors, combined with the relatively low incidence of the disease, make it extremely difficult to conduct controlled trials with a follow-up period that is adequate for assessing response and with sufficient numbers of patients to obtain clinical and statistical meaning. Therefore, rather than report on uncontrolled and controlled experience, this section is subdivided by drug class.

NONSTEROIDAL ANTI-INFLAMMATORY DRUGS. The NSAIDs are widely used in treating the musculoskeletal manifestations of reactive arthritis. Indomethacin has probably had the most extensive use,[38] but there are no published data to suggest that any nonsteroidal agent is either more effective or less toxic in patients with reactive arthritis. At this time there is no published experience with the selective COX-2 agents in reactive arthritis. To our knowledge, there are no studies to suggest that patients with reactive arthritis have any unique susceptibility or resistance to the adverse drug reactions that are commonly associated with NSAIDs. As with other inflammatory arthropathies, NSAIDs seem to ameliorate the articular complaints associated with reactive arthritis. Choice of any given agent often requires balancing clinical response against the potential for medication toxicity.

SULFASALAZINE. Sulfasalazine was shown to be well tolerated and effective in the treatment of reactive arthritis in a 9-month double-blind, placebo-controlled trial of 134 patients with reactive arthritis from the United States and Canada.[39] The toxicity of sulfasalazine in reactive arthritis appears comparable with the toxicity seen in patients with other spondyloarthropathies.

As has been seen with ankylosing spondylitis patients, some patients with reactive arthritis appear to have histologic enterocolitis that also improves with sulfasalazine therapy. The causal association of these findings with a clinical response to sulfasalazine remains unclear.[40]

IMMUNOSUPPRESSIVE DRUGS. Methotrexate, azathioprine, and cyclosporine have been used empirically to treat patients with recalcitrant reactive arthritis. Some improvement has been reported, although the results are not striking and published anecdotal reports are obviously biased in favor of positive results. Use of either methotrexate or azathioprine in patients with reactive arthritis and HIV seropositivity may hasten the manifestations of acquired immunodeficiency syndrome.[41] Thus the use of these medicines should be carefully considered in patients at risk of HIV positivity.

ANTIBIOTICS. The demonstration of bacterial cell wall components in the synovium of patients with reactive arthritis[42, 43] makes the concept of long-term antibiotic therapy intriguing. In an early report,[44] 10 patients with peripheral arthritis after *Chlamydia trachomatis* infection were treated for 3 months with methacycline and showed improvement in morning stiffness and number of active joints. Subsequently, a controlled trial of 40 patients who received either 2 weeks' worth of antibiotics appropriate for their cultured infections (*Salmonella, Yersinia,* or *Campylobacter*) or placebo did not reveal a difference between the two groups.[45] Finally, in a double-blind, placebo-controlled trial of 3 months of treatment with a tetracycline derivative, a group of patients with primarily postchlamydial arthritis showed some improvement in comparison with the placebo group.[46] These data, along with others, suggest that antibiotics do not seem to affect the course of enteropathic reactive arthritis. The course of urogenital reactive arthritis may be affected by antibiotic therapy,[47] as may the course of the primary insult, and thus antibiotic treatment should be considered in this subset of patients with reactive arthritis. Longer term antibiotic treatment may have some role, although additional trials with patients with disease defined by urogenital cultures and other appropriate additional studies are necessary for better determining such a role.[48] The mechanism of response to antibiotics remains undefined.

## Approach to Management

It is difficult to base recommendations for treatment of reactive arthritis on clinical data alone. Patient education and physical therapy goals as outlined in the section on ankylosing spondylitis are important in patients with chronic disease. In conventional medical therapy, an NSAID or corticosteroid injection would be administered in an attempt to control the articular manifestations. Sulfasalazine ameliorates chronic peripheral arthritis. It should probably be tried before either methotrexate or azathioprine is considered. Therapy with antibiotics for articular complaints remains controversial. If antibiotic therapy is useful, prolonged (3 months or longer) oral tetracycline may be the medication of choice in patients with urogenital reactive arthritis. Immunosuppressive drugs such as methotrexate or azathioprine may produce some benefit in chronic, unrelenting articular disease. The data on treatment of established chronic reactive arthritis with either methotrexate or azathioprine are empirical; a rationale for recommending one over the other cannot be substantiated. The experience and comfort level of the treating physician with the use of these agents and with the necessary monitoring for potential toxicity play an important role in agent choice. Drug side effects and recommended monitoring have been covered in previous sections of this chapter. Except for the caveat that HIV-positive patients may have untoward reactions to immunosuppressive medications, no particular drug interactions are seen in patients with reactive arthritis.

## Future Directions

The reactive arthritides comprise a spectrum of fascinating rheumatologic disorders with a genetic basis (HLA-B27 positivity) and an environmental component (postenteric or postvenereal infections). Basic research aimed at further elucidating the complex interactions between these factors is ongoing and will likely provide answers to the pathophysiology of not only the reactive arthritides but also the other seronegative spondyloarthropathies and, perhaps, other rheumatologic disorders in the future. Clinical research in reactive arthritis is problematic because the number of new cases seems to be diminishing both in the United States and abroad. This may be the result of changes in sexual practices, related to the HIV epidemic, as well as improved safety of the world's food supply. Thus, it is difficult to conduct controlled clinical trials in the reactive arthritides because of the low incidence and diminishing prevalence of the disease, its variable natural history, and the mobility of the young population that it most frequently affects. Thus current therapy is empirical and anecdotal and must be highly individualized.

## PSORIATIC ARTHRITIS

### Definition and Natural History

The term *psoriatic arthritis* describes a spectrum of inflammatory joint disease that occurs in association with psoriasis. Musculoskeletal complaints are not uncommon in the psoriatic population; however, the prevalence of actual inflammatory disease is about 5%. The skin disease is usually, but not uniformly, present before the development of arthritis, but neither the pattern nor the extent of skin disease is predictive of the eventual development or severity of the arthritis. Genetics, pathogenesis, and clinical features of psoriatic arthritis are discussed by Kelley and coauthors.[1]

Psoriatic arthritis may involve both appendicular and axial skeletons; five characteristic clinical presentations have been described: (1) asymmetric oligoarticular, (2) predominantly distal interphalangeal, (3) arthritis mutilans, (4) symmetric polyarticular, and (5) spondylitis. The asymmetric oligoarticular pattern is most common and is seen in 50% to 60% of patients, whereas the predominantly distal interphalangeal presentation occurs in 5% to 10%, arthritis mutilans in 5%, and the symmetric polyarticular pattern in approximately 25%. The activity of peripheral psoriatic arthritis is typically episodic in that relatively asymptomatic periods are usually followed by periods of flare; synchronous skin/arthritis flares may occur, but asynchronous flares appear to be more common. Spondylitis without peripheral arthritis accounts for approximately 5% of psoriatic arthritis; however, radiographic changes of sacroiliitis and spondylitis may be seen in up to 40% of the psoriatic arthritis population. Sacroiliac involvement is usually seen in HLA-B27–positive patients.

These presentations are not always distinct, and many patients exhibit features of two or more patterns at a given time, or the disease may evolve from one pattern to another over the course of time. This heterogeneity has made it difficult to establish specific prognoses for each subtype; however, the oligoarticular presentation seems to be the least aggressive. Although the course of psoriatic arthritis is, in general, more favorable than is that of rheumatoid arthritis, the destructive potential of psoriatic arthritis has been adequately demonstrated by a prospective study showing that the number of patients with psoriatic arthritis who had five or more damaged joints more than doubled (from 19% to 41%) over a 5-year period despite treatment that produced improvement in both the erythrocyte sedimentation rate and the number of tender/swollen joints.[49]

Evaluation of the efficacy of therapeutic interventions in psoriatic arthritis is made difficult by (1) the wide spectrum and variable activity of the arthritis, (2) the uncertain correlation between present measures of response and eventual functional outcome, and (3) the uncertain contribution of concurrent therapy directed at the skin disease. The importance of well-designed prospective studies that are carefully controlled, have an adequate number of patients and an adequate period of observation, and employ appropriate efficacy and toxicity measures cannot be overemphasized.

## Treatment

Because the cause of psoriasis and psoriatic arthritis is unknown and pathologic mechanisms are only partially understood, treatment remains empirical. Most of the agents and therapeutic regimens currently in use or under investigation are (1) those that have been used with demonstrated benefit in the treatment of other inflammatory arthropathies and (2) those that have been used in the treatment of cutaneous psoriasis and have possible articular benefit.[50] The efficacy of nearly all treatment regimens in psoriatic arthritis has yet to be unequivocally established.

### NSAIDs

NSAIDs are widely believed to be efficacious in psoriatic arthritis and are the most common initial therapy prescribed by most clinicians for both peripheral and axial disease. However, no controlled studies exist to document their efficacy, and no NSAID at present has formal approval from the US Food and Drug Administration for use in psoriatic arthritis. Many rheumatologists prefer to use nonsalicylate NSAIDs on the basis of a clinical impression of better efficacy; no controlled data exist to either refute or substantiate that position. Arachidonic acid metabolites are known to influence the activity of cutaneous psoriasis, and worsening of the skin disease with initiation of NSAID therapy has been observed, perhaps resulting from cyclooxygenase blockade with increased use of the lipoxygenase pathway. No other unusual toxic effect associated with the use of NSAIDs in psoriatic arthritis has been reported. A complete blood cell count (CBC) and creatinine and serum transaminase levels should be attained when NSAID treatment is instituted.[51] In chronically treated patients, an annual CBC and creatinine and transaminase determinations as indicated are recommended.[14]

### Glucocorticoids

Intra-articular injection of glucocorticoids can produce marked improvement in joint pain and swelling. Periodic injections can be of particular value in the management of patients with oligoarticular disease or those with controlled polyarticular disease but persistently active disease in one or two joints. In general, systemic use of glucocorticoids should be avoided because of the possibility of provoking a pustular flare in the skin disease on withdrawal.

### Other Antirheumatic Drugs

If a patient does not respond to an adequate NSAID trial or has evidence of destructive disease, the institution of additional therapy should be considered. As in other inflammatory arthropathies, these agents are sometimes referred to as "disease-modifying." However, because no true disease modification in either the peripheral arthritis or the spondylitis has yet been shown, *second-line agents* may be a preferable term.

ORAL AND PARENTERAL GOLD. A beneficial response with both oral and parenteral gold in psoriatic arthritis has been observed. In a 6-month double-blind, placebo-controlled study of auranofin (6 mg/day) involving 238 patients, the auranofin-treated group showed a modest but significant improvement in physician's global assessment and occupational/daily function scores in comparison with the placebo recipients, but no significant difference in morning stiffness or joint tenderness/swelling scores was seen.[52] The rate of withdrawal from auranofin because of adverse drug reactions was 10%. An uncontrolled study involving 14 patients treated with injectable gold showed either remission or improvement (50% reduction in number of inflamed joints) in 71% of the patients.[53] Toxic effects were similar to those observed with parenteral gold in rheumatoid arthritis. A double-blind comparison of auranofin (6 mg/day), intramuscular gold sodium thiomalate (50 mg/week), and placebo showed significant improvement in the Ritchie articular index, the visual analog pain score, and the erythrocyte sedimentation rate (ESR) over 24 weeks in patients receiving parenteral gold but no significant difference between those receiving auranofin and those receiving placebo.[54] Neither significant flare nor improvement in cutaneous psoriasis with oral or parenteral gold has been observed. Appropriate monitoring consists of a CBC and a urinalysis before each injection for parenteral gold and a CBC and a urinalysis every 4 weeks for oral gold.

METHOTREXATE. The efficacy of methotrexate in psoriatic arthritis was first demonstrated in 1964 with a double-blind, placebo-controlled study of 21 patients who had active skin disease and peripheral arthritis.[55] This study design compared parenteral methotrexate (1 to 3 mg/kg in three doses at 10-day intervals) with placebo during an observation period of approximately 3 months. Significant improvements in joint tenderness and joint range of motion, in extent of skin involvement, and in erythrocyte sedimentation rate were seen. After completion of therapy, however, the majority of patients experienced a recurrence of skin and joint disease within 1 to 4 months. Although adverse effects were common (anorexia/nausea in 62%; paresthesias in 48%; transient leukopenia in 33%; oral ulcerations in 10%; and alopecia in 5%), they did not necessitate cessation of therapy in any patient. This study and additional experience with similar dosages (25 mg/week) documented the beneficial effect of methotrexate for both cutaneous and synovial disease; however, the transient nature of the response and the frequency of adverse reactions suggested that more sustained therapy with lower dosages might be of greater benefit. A randomized, double-blind, placebo-controlled trial comparing oral low-dose pulse methotrexate, 7.5 to 15 mg/week, with placebo over 12 weeks did show better patient tolerance; however, efficacy of this regimen was not established, inasmuch as the only response measure to attain statistical significance was the physician's assessment of arthritis activity.[56] A larger study of longer duration might have shown greater benefit, and the clinical experience of some investigators is consistent with this possibility. According to a retrospective report of 40 patients over 12 years of treatment with a mean methotrexate dose of 11.2 mg/week, 38 patients had an excellent or good articular response, 36 had cutaneous resolution, and only 2 patients withdrew because of toxic effects (leukopenia and stomatitis).[57] In seven patients who underwent 11 liver biopsies during the study, one patient was found to have micronodular cirrhosis at a cumulative methotrexate dose of 400 mg (with an unchanged biopsy finding at a cumulative dose of 1080 mg). Otherwise, no inflammation or disruption of hepatic architecture was seen on initial or serial biopsy specimens.

Methotrexate-induced liver disease and bone marrow suppression continue, appropriately, to be major clinical concerns. Whether the use of methotrexate in psoriasis and psoriatic arthritis is associated with more frequent or severe adverse drug effects than with its use in rheumatoid arthritis is unknown. Less methotrexate toxicity has been observed with its current use in rheumatoid arthritis than would have been predicted from the early experience in psoriasis and psoriatic arthritis. However, this apparent decrease in toxicity may be better explained by improved patient selection, administration of lower dosages in pulse fashion, and more careful monitoring rather than by postulating that psoriatic patients have a predilection for toxic effects. Adverse events involving methotrexate in the two studies just described were similar to those in the current experience with rheumatoid arthritis. Recommended monitoring consists of a monthly CBC and monthly liver enzyme studies. Drug withdrawal should be considered if frequent, persistent, or severe transaminase elevations are seen. No consensus exists as to the indications for liver biopsy either before treatment or at specified intervals during treatment. However, most rheumatologists would agree that a

biopsy should be considered if transaminase abnormalities are recurrent or persist after drug withdrawal; discontinuation of therapy is mandatory if any clinical evidence of hepatic dysfunction appears.[14]

AZATHIOPRINE AND 6-MERCAPTOPURINE. Both 6-mercaptopurine and its derivative, azathioprine, are purine analogs that have been used in the treatment of psoriasis and psoriatic arthritis. Although favorable results have been reported, the study populations are very small, and no placebo-controlled data are available. Of 13 patients treated with 6-mercaptopurine (20 to 50 mg/kg/day), 11 showed improvement in both joint and skin disease within 3 weeks of initiation of therapy and maintenance of this improvement on a dose of 1 mg/kg/day with minimal adverse effects.[58] A 12-month double-blind crossover study of azathioprine (3 mg/kg/day) in six patients reported moderate or marked joint improvement in all six patients and cutaneous improvement in four; however, the dose of azathioprine had to be reduced in five patients because of leukopenia.[59] In view of the known toxic effects of these agents, most rheumatologists reserve their use for severe and refractory disease. Regular laboratory monitoring with a monthly CBC and monthly hepatic transaminase determinations is imperative.

SULFASALAZINE. The effectiveness of sulfasalazine in rheumatoid arthritis and other seronegative arthritides has led to trials with psoriatic arthritis as well. Apparent efficacy was suggested in pilot studies and was subsequently confirmed in a 24-week double-blind, placebo-controlled study of 30 patients with a dosage of 2 g/day.[60] There were significant improvements in morning stiffness, number of painful joints, articular index, clinical score, and pain score; the favorable response was more pronounced in the patients with polyarticular disease. The drug was well tolerated, and no exacerbation or remission of cutaneous psoriasis was seen.

CYCLOSPORINE. Cyclosporine has been used with success in cutaneous psoriasis, and preliminary experience also suggests a beneficial effect in psoriatic arthritis. Representative of this preliminary experience is a 6-month open study of eight patients (seven of whom had disease refractory to methotrexate) with a starting dosage of 3.5 mg/kg/day, which produced marked improvement in joint and skin disease in seven of the eight patients after 2 months.[61] There was one withdrawal from the study because of lack of efficacy, and three patients required a 25% reduction in the cyclosporine dosage because of a 50% increase in serum creatinine. Further controlled study is warranted to confirm efficacy and to determine the extent to which toxic renal effects will limit long-term therapy.

ANTIMALARIAL AGENTS. The use of antimalarial agents in the treatment of psoriatic arthritis has been controversial. Reports of favorable response to both chloroquine (250 mg/day) and hydroxychloroquine (200 to 400 mg/day) in approximately 75% of patients have been offset by concerns that antimalarial drugs may have an adverse effect on skin disease. The spectrum of suspected cutaneous toxicity includes exacerbation of plaques, photosensitivity, generalized erythroderma, evolution to pustular psoriasis, and the development of an exfoliative dermatitis. Although the reported incidence of these reactions ranges from 0% to 100%, it is important to note that more frequent reactions were observed in early trials that had few patients and primarily used regimens with quinacrine; much less toxicity has been seen in the more recent experience involving larger numbers of patients and using chloroquine or hydroxychloroquine.[62] Further experience would suggest that hydroxychloroquine may be safer than chloroquine. Appropriate monitoring of antimalarial agents requires baseline and periodic ophthalmologic examinations to include visual acuity, slit-lamp, funduscopic, and visual field testing. The package insert for hydroxychloroquine stipulates that such examinations be performed every 3 months, whereas according to a more recent recommendation, examinations every 6 months are adequate.[50] In addition, a CBC should be obtained every 6 months. A prospective, controlled trial is needed to establish the efficacy and safety of these agents in the treatment of psoriatic arthritis.

D-PENICILLAMINE. A favorable effect on psoriatic arthritis has been observed with the use of D-penicillamine, but the available information is anecdotal and very limited. Eleven patients (two with spondylitis, four with asymmetric oligoarthritis, and five with symmetric polyarthritis) were randomly assigned to an initial phase consisting of treatment with either D-penicillamine or placebo for 4 months,[63] followed by 4 months of treatment with D-penicillamine for all patients. The maximum dosage of D-penicillamine was 750 mg/day, and no unusual toxic effect was observed. Clinical benefit was seen only during D-penicillamine treatment; however, no efficacy measure attained statistically significant improvement.

COLCHICINE. Colchicine is an alkaloid that is known to attenuate the inflammatory response by interfering with intracellular microtubule formation; this interference, in turn, impairs neutrophil chemotaxis. The presence of neutrophils in early psoriatic lesions suggested that colchicine might have a beneficial effect. A pilot study showed that of 22 patients treated with colchicine (0.02 mg/kg/day), 11 had significant cutaneous clearing, and 4 of 8 patients with arthralgias were symptomatically improved.[64] A subsequent 16-week double-blind crossover study of 15 patients compared colchicine, 1.5 mg/day, with placebo.[65] With the patient global assessment as the primary efficacy measure, colchicine was judged more effective than placebo by 10 (83%) of the 12 patients who completed the study, and significant improvement was seen in grip strength, Ritchie index, joint pain, and joint swelling during colchicine treatment. Gastrointestinal symptoms necessitated the withdrawal of two patients from the study and a temporary dose reduction in five other patients. No unanticipated clinical or laboratory toxic effects were seen. Larger studies of longer duration are needed to establish the role of colchicine in the management of psoriatic arthritis.

RETINOIDS. Etretinate, a vitamin A derivative, is the most commonly used retinoid in the treatment of psori-

asis, and initial experience with this agent in psoriatic arthritis suggests a beneficial effect. In one pilot study, 40 patients treated with etretinate (50 mg/day) for a mean of 21.9 weeks experienced significant improvement in the number of tender joints, the duration of morning stiffness, and the erythrocyte sedimentation rate.[66] Maximal improvement for most efficacy measurements was seen between 12 and 16 weeks. Mucocutaneous reactions consisting of dried and cracked lips, mouth soreness, and nosebleeds were seen in 39 of the 40 patients and necessitated cessation of treatment in 9 patients. Other relatively frequent adverse effects were alopecia, hyperlipidemia, myalgias, and elevated transaminase levels. Etretinate is a teratogen and should not be administered to women of childbearing potential.

PHOTOCHEMOTHERAPY. The most commonly used form of photochemotherapy involves the oral administration of 8-methoxypsoralen, followed by exposure to long-wave ultraviolet-A light (PUVA). A prospective study of 27 patients treated with PUVA found a favorable response in 49% of patients with peripheral arthritis, whereas no benefit was seen in patients with spondylitis.[67] In responders, improvement in the peripheral arthritis seemed to correlate with clearing of the skin disease, whereas no such relationship was observed in patients with axial disease. Extracorporeal photochemotherapy, also known as photopheresis, has been shown to diminish the in vitro viability, proliferation, and mitogen response of lymphocytes, but clinical improvement in arthritis symptoms appears modest, and no effect on skin lesions has been observed.[68]

SOMATOSTATIN. Somatostatin may benefit some psoriatic arthritis patients, but prolonged intravenous infusion (48 hours) is required, and the drug is poorly tolerated because of nausea. In one study, patients with extensive skin lesions and polyarticular involvement seemed more responsive.[69]

INTERFERON GAMMA. A placebo-controlled, double-blind trial of recombinant interferon gamma in 24 patients over a period of 4 weeks showed a modest improvement in arthritis activity; however, the effect may be transient: Over a 6-month period of observation, improvement that was present at 1 month was not sustained despite continued treatment.[70] The putative efficacy of interferon gamma is further clouded by reports from trials of interferon in cutaneous psoriasis in which arthritis developed during interferon treatment and subsided after termination of therapy.[71]

DIETARY SUPPLEMENTS. In a small 6-month open-label trial of oral 1,25-hydroxyvitamin $D_3$, 7 of 10 patients with active arthritis experienced either substantial or moderate improvement. Hypercalciuria precluded the use of therapeutic doses in 2 patients.[72] Dietary supplementation with polyunsaturated ethyl ester lipids resulted in subjective articular benefit for 18 of 34 patients in an uncontrolled study.[73] Controlled trials of these agents are needed to confirm efficacy.

MISCELLANEOUS. Other agents that have been reported to have activity in psoriatic arthritis include bromocriptine, cimetidine, fumaric acid, parenteral nitrogen mustard, peptide T, radiation synovectomy with yttrium 90, and total lymph node irradiation. Further study is needed to define which role, if any, these regimens might have in patient management.

## Approach to Management

The selection of an appropriate therapeutic regimen can be made only after careful clinical, laboratory, and, in most cases, radiographic evaluations. These evaluations should (1) determine the activity and extent of the skin disease; (2) ascertain whether joint symptoms are caused by structural damage, inflammatory disease, both, or neither; (3) identify, in the case of inflammatory disease, whether peripheral and/or axial involvement is present; and (4) document the presence of any coexisting condition or disease that could either contribute to the patient's symptoms or affect the selection of therapy. Concurrent dermatologic care is strongly recommended in nearly all cases, and some patients may experience marked improvement in joint symptoms with treatment and control of their skin disease. As is true with all inflammatory arthropathies, both patient education and the involvement of physical and occupational therapists can have a significant impact on functional capacity, especially for spondylitic patients.

Although occasional patients with oligoarticular disease benefit from intra-articular steroid injection, NSAIDs should be the initial therapeutic agent. An adequate trial of a particular NSAID should be at least 2 to 3 weeks in duration and should entail maximal dosage; the efficacy of the trial is established on clinical grounds. Patients unresponsive to one NSAID may benefit from another; the initial and subsequent selection of the particular NSAID is empirical, but in our experience indomethacin may be more efficacious for spondylitic patients.

For most patients with asymmetric oligoarticular disease, treatment with NSAIDs is usually sufficient. In unresponsive patients, particularly those with a symmetric polyarthritis or evidence of destructive disease, a second-line agent should be considered. The selection of the particular second-line agent is empirical. Nonetheless, regimens with more predictable efficacy and relatively less toxicity should be considered before those that are more experimental and potentially more toxic. It has been our experience that of the treatment regimens reviewed, low-dose pulse methotrexate is the most consistently useful second-line agent currently available for NSAID-refractory psoriatic arthritis. If methotrexate is not effective or tolerated, a trial of gold salt therapy or sulfasalazine should be initiated in most patients. Azathioprine, with controlled data documenting its efficacy, might next be considered in patients in whom methotrexate and gold have failed. However, azathioprine toxicity is such that, at present, we most often first favor a trial of sulfasalazine over azathioprine. It is important to note that no single regimen is efficacious or suitable for every patient; even ideal clinical trials cannot predict individual response or toxic effects; therefore, optimal treatment for each patient depends on thoughtful evaluation, careful monitoring, and sound clinical judgment.

## REFERENCES

1. Kelley WN, Harris ED, Ruddy S, et al (eds): Textbook of Rheumatology, 6th ed. Philadelphia: WB Saunders, 2000.
2. Cheret S, Graham D, Little H, et al: The natural disease course of ankylosing spondylitis. Arthritis Rheum 1983; 26:186.
3. Radford EP, Doll R, Smith PG: Mortality among patients with ankylosing spondylitis not given x-ray therapy. N Engl J Med 1977; 297:572.
4. Smith PG, Doll R: Mortality among patients with ankylosing spondylitis after a single treatment course with x-rays. BMJ 1982; 284:449.
5. Gran JT, Skomsvoll JF: The outcome of ankylosing spondylitis: A study of 100 patients. Br J Rheumatol 1997; 36:766–771.
6. Averns HL, Oxtoby J, Taylor HG, et al: Smoking and outcome in ankylosing spondylitis. Scand J Rheumatol 1996; 25:138–142.
7. Olerud C, Frost A, Bring J: Spinal fractures in patients with ankylosing spondylitis. Eur Spine J 1996; 5(1):51–55.
8. Santos H, Brophy S, Calin A: Exercise in ankylosing spondylitis: How much is optimum? J Rheumatol 1998; 25:11.
9. Kraag G, Stokes B, Groh J, et al: The effects of comprehensive home physiotherapy and supervision on patients with ankylosing spondylitis. J Rheumatol 1990; 17:228.
10. O'Driscoll SL, Hayson MIV, Baddeley H: Neck movements in ankylosing spondylitis and their responses to physiotherapy. Ann Rheum Dis 1978; 37:64.
11. Clain A, Elswood J: A prospective nationwide cross-sectional study of NSAID usage in 1331 patients with ankylosing spondylitis. J Rheumatol 1990; 17:801.
12. Gran JT, Husby G: Ankylosing spondylitis: Current drug treatment. Drugs 1992; 44:585–603.
13. Harrison TR, Wilson JD: Ankylosing spondylitis and reactive arthritis. *In* Jeffers HD, Boynton SD (eds): Principles of Internal Medicine, 12th ed. New York: McGraw-Hill, 1991:1453.
14. American College of Rheumatology Ad Hoc Committee on Clinical Guidelines: Guidelines for monitoring drug therapy in rheumatoid arthritis. Arthritis Rheum 1996; 39:723–731.
15. Koh WH, Pande I, Samuels A, et al: Low dose amitriptyline in ankylosing spondylitis: A short term, double blind, placebo controlled study. J Rheumatol 1997; 24:11.
16. Maksymowych WP, Jhangri G, Leclercq S, et al: An open study of pamidronate in the treatment of refractory ankylosing spondylitis. J Rheumatol 1998; 25:4.
17. Tytman K, Bernacka K, Sierakowski S: D-Penicillamine in the therapy of ankylosing spondylitis. Clin Rheumatol 1989; 8:419.
18. Steven MM, Morrison M, Sturrock R: Penicillamine in ankylosing spondylitis: A double blind placebo controlled trial. J Rheumatol 1985; 12:735.
19. Grasedyck K, Schattenkirchner M, Bandilla K: Treatment of ankylosing spondylitis with auranofin. J Rheumatol 1990; 49:98.
20. Amor B, Kahan A, Dougados M, et al: Sulfasalazine and ankylosing spondylitis. Ann Intern Med 1984; 101:878.
21. Dougados M, Boumier P, Amor B: Sulphasalazine in ankylosing spondylitis: A double blind controlled study in 60 patients. BMJ 1986; 293:911.
22. Dougados M, vam der Linden S, Leirisalo-Repo M, et al: Sulfasalazine in the treatment of spondylarthropathy. A randomized, multicenter, double-blind, placebo-controlled study. Arthritis Rheum 1995; 38:618–627.
23. Clegg DO, Reda DJ, Weisman MH, et al: Comparison of sulfasalazine and placebo in the treatment of ankylosing spondylitis. Arthritis Rheum 1996; 39:2004–2012.
24. Ferraz MB, Tugwell P, Goldsmith CH, et al: Meta-analysis of sulfasalazine in ankylosing spondylitis. J Rheumatol 1990; 17:1482.
25. Taggart A, Gardiner P, McEvoy F, et al: Which is the active moiety of sulfasalazine in ankylosing spondylitis? Arthritis Rheum 1996; 39(8):1400–1405.
26. Mielants H, Veys EM: The gut in the spondyloarthropathies. J Rheumatol 1990; 17:7.

27. Clegg DO, Reda DJ, Abdellatif M, et al: Comparison of sulfasalazine and placebo for the treatment of axial and peripheral articular manifestations of the seronegative spondyloarthropathies. Arthritis Rheum 1999; 11:2325–2329.

28. Des Maris HCL: Radiotherapy in arthritis. Ann Rheum Dis 1953; 12:25–28.

29. Reiter H: Über eine bisher unerkannte Spirochanteninfektion (spirochaetosis arthritica). Dtsch Med Wochenschr 1916; 42:1535.

30. Arnett FC, McClusky OE, Schacter BZ, et al: Incomplete Reiter's syndrome: discriminating features and HL-A W27 in diagnosis. Ann Intern Med 1976; 84:8.

31. Ahvonen P, Sievers K, Aho K: Arthritis associated with *Yersinia enterocolitica* infection. Acta Rheum Scand 1969; 15:232.

32. Lahesmanaa-Rantala R, Toivanen A: Clinical spectrum of reactive arthritis. *In* Toivanen A, Toivanen P (eds): Reactive Arthritis. Boca Raton, FL: CRC Press, 1988:1.

33. Keat A: Reiter's syndrome and reactive arthritis in perspective. N Engl J Med 1983; 309:1606.

34. Fox R, Calin A, Gerber RC, et al: The chronicity of symptoms and disability in Reiter's syndrome. Ann Intern Med 1979; 91:190.

35. Inman RD, Johnston MAE, Hodge M, et al: Postdysenteric reactive arthritis. Arthritis Rheum 1988; 31:1377.

36. Keat A, Rowe I: Reiter's syndrome and associated arthritides. Rheum Dis Clin North Am 1991; 17:25.

37. Winchester R, Bernstein DH, Fischer HD, et al: The co-occurrence of Reiter's syndrome and acquired immunodeficiency. Ann Intern Med 1987; 106:19.

38. Thim Fan P, Yu DTY: Reiter's syndrome. *In* Kelley WN, Harris ED, Ruddy S, et al (eds): Textbook of Rheumatology, 4th ed, vol 1. Philadelphia: WB Saunders, 1993:961.

39. Clegg DO, Reda DJ, Weisman MH, et al; Comparison of sulfasalazine and placebo in the treatment of reactive arthritis (Reiter's syndrome). Arthritis Rheum 1996, 39:2021–2027.

40. Mielants H, Veys EM: The gut in the spondyloarthropathies. J Rheumatol 1990; 17:7.

41. Winchester R, Bernstein DH, Fischer HD, et al: The co-occurrence of Reiter's syndrome and acquired immunodeficiency. Ann Intern Med 1987; 106:19.

42. Granfors K, Jalkanen S, von Essen R, et al: *Yersinia* antigens in synovial fluid cells from patients with reactive arthritis. N Engl J Med 1989; 320:216.

43. Granfors K, Jalkanen S, Lindberg AA, et al: *Salmonella* lipopolysaccharide in synovial cells from patients with reactive arthritis. Lancet 1990; 335:685.

44. Panayi GS, Clark B: Minocycline in the treatment of patients with Reiter's syndrome. Clin Exp Rheumatol 1989; 7:100.

45. Foyden A, Bengtsson A, Foberg U, et al: Early antibiotic treatment of reactive arthritis associated with enteric infection, clinical and serological study. BMJ 1990; 301:1299.

46. Lauhio A, Leirisalo-Repo M, Lahdevirta J, et al: Double-blind, placebo-controlled study of three-month treatment with lymecycline in reactive arthritis, with special reference to chlamydia arthritis. Arthritis Rheum 1991; 34:6.

47. Leirisalo-Repo M: Are antibiotics of any use in reactive arthritis? APMIS 1993; 101:575–581.

48. Sièper J, Braun J: Treatment of reactive arthritis with antibiotics. Br J Rheumatol 1990; 37:717–719.

49. Gladman DD, Stafford-Brady F, Chang C, et al: Longitudinal study of clinical and radiological progression in psoriatic arthritis. J Rheumatol 1990; 17:809.

50. Goupille P, Soutif D, Valat J: Treatment of psoriatic arthropathy. Semin Arthritis Rheum 1992; 21:355.

51. Campbell RM, Wilske K: Drug monitoring schedules. *In* Weaver AL (ed): Guidelines for Reviewers of Rheumatic Disease Care, 2nd ed. Atlanta: The American Rheumatism Association, 1989:24.

52. Carette S, Calin A, McCafferty JP, et al: A double-blind placebo-controlled study of auranofin in patients with psoriatic arthritis. Arthritis Rheum 1989; 32:158.

53. Dorwart BB, Gall EP, Schumacher HR, et al: Chrysotherapy in psoriatic arthritis. Arthritis Rheum 1978; 21:513.

54. Palit J, Hill J, Capell HA, et al: A multicentre double-blind comparison of auranofin, intramuscular gold thiomalate and placebo in patients with psoriatic arthritis. Br J Rheumatol 1990; 29:280.

55. Black RL, O'Brien WM, Van Scott EJ, et al: Methotrexate therapy in psoriatic arthritis. JAMA 1964; 189(10):141.

56. Willkens RF, Williams HJ, Ward JR, et al: Randomized, double-blind placebo-controlled trial of low-dose pulse methotrexate in psoriatic arthritis. Arthritis Rheum 1984; 27:376.

57. Espinoza LR, Zakraui L, Espinoza CG, et al: Psoriatic arthritis: Clinical response and side effects to methotrexate therapy. J Rheumatol 1992; 19:872.

58. Baum J, Hurd E, Lewis D, et al: Treatment of psoriatic arthritis with 6-mercaptopurine. Arthritis Rheum 1973; 16:139.

59. Levy J, Paulus HE, Barnett EV, et al: A double-blind controlled evaluation of azathioprine treatment in rheumatoid arthritis and psoriatic arthritis. Arthritis Rheum 1972; 15:116.

60. Farr M, Kitas GD, Waterhouse L, et al: Sulphasalazine in psoriatic arthritis: A double-blind placebo-controlled study. Br J Rheumatol 1990; 29:46.

61. Steinsson K, Jonsdottir I, Valdimarsson H: Cyclosporin A in psoriatic arthritis: An open study. Ann Rheum Dis 1990; 49:603.

62. Gladman DD, Blake R, Brubacher B, et al: Chloroquine therapy in psoriatic arthritis. J Rheumatol 1992; 19:1724.

63. Price R, Gibson T: d-Penicillamine and psoriatic arthritis [Letter]. Br J Rheumatol 1986; 25:228.

64. Wahba A, Cohen H: Therapeutic trials with oral colchicine in psoriasis. Acta Derm Venereol (Stockh) 1980; 60:515.

65. Seideman P, Fjellner B, Johannesson A: Psoriatic arthritis treated with oral colchicine. J Rheumatol 1987; 14:777.

66. Klinkhoff AV, Gertner E, Chalmers A, et al: Pilot study of etretinate in psoriatic arthritis. J Rheumatol 1989; 16:789.

67. Perlman SG, Gerber LH, Roberts RM, et al: Photochemotherapy and psoriatic arthritis. A prospective study. Ann Intern Med 1979; 91(5):717–722.

68. Wilfert J, Honigsmann H, Steiner G: Treatment of psoriatic arthritis by extracorporeal photochemotherapy. Br J Dermatol 1990; 122:225.

69. Matucci-Cerinic M, Lotti T, Cappugi P, et al: Somatostatin treatment of psoriatic arthritis. Int J Dermatol 1988; 27:56.

70. Fierlbeck G, Rassner G: Treatment of psoriasis and psoriatic arthritis with interferon gamma. J Invest Dermatol 1990; 95:138S.

71. O'Connell PG, Gerber LH, Digiovanna JJ, et al: Arthritis in patients with psoriasis treated with gamma-interferon. J Rheumatol 1992; 19:80.

72. Huckins D, Felson DT, Holick M. Treatment of psoriatic arthritis with oral 1,25-dihydroxyvitamin $D_3$: A pilot study. Arthritis Rheum 1990; 33:1723.

73. Lassus A, Dahlgren AL, Halpern MJ, et al: Effects of dietary supplementation with polyunsaturated ethyl ester lipids (angiosan) in patients with psoriasis and psoriatic arthritis. J Int Med Res 1990; 18:68.

# 23 | Systemic Lupus Erythematosus (Including Pregnancy and Antiphospholipid Antibody Syndrome)

*Michelle Petri*

## NATURAL HISTORY

The prognosis of systemic lupus erythematosus (SLE) has improved dramatically in the last 40 years. Of 55 patients monitored by Bywaters and Bauer, 52% died within 2 years after onset.[1] A similar poor outcome with a mean survival time of 2 years without treatment was reported by Posnick.[2] Jessar and associates[3] reported the prognosis of 103 patients (44 of their own patients from the 15 years before 1952 and 59 from 279 reported in the literature in the years 1948 to 1952): Only 38% survived 4 years after onset.

Harvey and coworkers[4] reported the outcome of 99 cases diagnosed from 1949 to 1953. This case series, which included both outpatients and inpatients, reflected two major clinical advances: the evolution of the lupus erythematosus (LE) cell test and the use of adrenocorticotropic hormone (ACTH) and cortisone in treatment. The LE test was positive in 29 of 33 clinically doubtful cases that were then included in the series. ACTH or cortisone was used in the treatment of 75 of the 99 patients. The steepest decline in survivorship occurred during the first 3 months after diagnosis, with 13% of the patients dying in this period. The 1-year survival rate was 78%, and the 4-year rate was 52%. Of the survivors to any year, about 10% died in the following year. This much more favorable experience probably represented both the inclusion of milder or earlier cases confirmed by the LE cell test and the beneficial effect of ACTH and corticosteroid therapy.

Some improvement in survival resulted from factors other than better diagnosis and corticosteroid treatment. Ropes[5] reported a 4-year survival rate of 24% for the years 1932 to 1944, increasing to 55% for the years 1945 to 1963. She attributed much of this improved survival to antibiotic therapy.

Recent studies have continued to show improved 5- and 10-year survival. Among middle-class, privately insured SLE patients, 97% 5-year and 93% 10-year survival rates have been reported.[6] Inner-city academic centers in the United States report lower but still greatly improved 10-year survival rates.[7] However, in the most recent American epidemiologic study, the 10-year survival rate in Rochester, Minnesota, was less than 80%.[8]

In the years before widespread use of corticosteroid therapy, it was recognized that some disease flares improved spontaneously or with bed rest.[9] The evolution of the disease over time could not be ascertained in these early studies because of the high mortality rate. We have shown that new disease manifestations of lupus continue to evolve more than 5 years after diagnosis.[10] Flares of lupus occur with a median time of 12 months, even in patients with long-standing disease and treatment.[11] Therefore the understanding of treated SLE continues to expand. A general discussion of the management of SLE was provided by Kelley and colleagues, *Textbook of Rheumatology,*[12] Chapter 62. Clinical features of the disease are discussed in Kelley and colleagues, Chapter 61, and pathogenesis in Chapter 60 of that book.

## OPEN-LABEL TRIALS

### Nonsteroidal Anti-inflammatory Drugs

Aspirin is the best-studied nonsteroidal anti-inflammatory drug (NSAID) in open-label trials of large numbers of patients with lupus[4, 9] (Table 23–1). Both ibuprofen and indomethacin have been effective in open-label trials, especially for arthritis and pleurisy[13] and in combination with corticosteroids and antimalarials.[14] Long-term efficacy was demonstrated for indomethacin in a 9-month trial.[14] Open-label trials differ, however, in whether NSAIDs have a corticosteroid-sparing effect; indomethacin, for example, was corticosteroid-sparing in one trial,[15] but ibuprofen was steroid-sparing in only 18% in another.[13] In an open-label trial of ibuprofen, the median time to improvement was 14 days.[13] Cyclooxygenase-2 (Cox-2)–specific NSAIDs have not yet been studied in SLE.

### Antimalarials

Important open-label trials of the two antimalarial drugs in common use, chloroquine and hydroxychlor-

## TABLE 23–1
## Nonsteroidal Anti-inflammatory Drugs (NSAIDs): Open-label Trials

| NSAID | STUDY, YEAR (REFERENCE) | N | OUTCOME |
|-------|-------------------------|---|---------|
| Aspirin | Harvey et al., 1955 (4) | 19 | Overall: 58% improved |
| | Dubois, 1956 (9) | 163 | |
| Ibuprofen | Dubois, 1975 (13) | 17 | Arthritis: 69% improved |
| Indomethacin | Marmont et al., 1965 (15) | 10 | |
| | Dubois, 1966 (14) | 22 | Overall: 82% improved |

NSAID, nonsteroidal anti-inflammatory drug.

oquine, are summarized in Table 23–2. Clinical manifestations of patients in these open-label trials included predominantly discoid lupus, although a few trials contained patients with other forms of cutaneous lupus.[16–18] The early open-label trials used higher doses of chloroquine (up to 750 mg/day[9]) and hydroxychloroquine (up to 1600 mg/day in one study[19] and up to 2000 mg/day in another[17]) than are used today. Side effects were more common in the trials that used higher doses[9, 19] and included some rarely seen today, such as graying of the skin or bleaching of hair pigment.

## Corticosteroids

TOPICAL CORTICOSTEROIDS. Open-label trials of topical corticosteroids for cutaneous lupus (usually discoid) have reached conflicting results. In one study of 59 patients with discoid lupus, 73% were controlled with topical fluocinolone.[20] In contrast, only 26% of patients with discoid lupus had a good or better response to topical corticosteroids in a second study.[21]

INTRALESIONAL CORTICOSTEROIDS. In two large open-label trials of intralesional corticosteroids for the treatment of chronic discoid lesions, 93% of 28 patients treated[22] and 88% of 40 patients treated[21] responded.

ORAL CORTICOSTEROIDS. Early open-label trials of corticosteroids demonstrated their effectiveness in the critically ill lupus patient. For example, of 119 patients who received corticosteroids (or ACTH) for at least 48 hours, 90% achieved benefit.[9] Doses of cortisone ranged from 200 to 4000 mg/day. In an early study, the disease was well controlled in 20 of 22 patients treated with prednisone and 13 of 18 treated with prednisolone.[23] Fever responded in 24 to 48 hours, arthritis within several days, and pleural effusions and cutaneous lupus in 1 to 2 weeks.

Of 62 patients treated with ACTH or cortisone in another early series, 39 had an excellent immediate response, 5 had a slower but satisfactory response, 8 eventually responded to escalating doses, 6 had little or no response, and 4 were withdrawn from the study because of hypertension.[4] In later follow-up, 17 of the 42 living patients still required maintenance corticosteroid treatment.

In a series of 82 patients seen in 1949 or later, 72% at some point required corticosteroid therapy. The importance of slow reduction of dose was recognized; two patients in the series died within 2 weeks after rapid withdrawal.[24]

ALTERNATE-DAY CORTICOSTEROIDS. A prospective study of intravenous methylprednisolone therapy, followed by alternate-day corticosteroid therapy, was prematurely terminated because only 4 of 11 patients could be maintained on alternate-day corticosteroids.[25] Three patients had worsening of presenting nonrenal symptoms, and four had worsening renal disease. However, the benefit of alternate-day administration in reducing undesirable catabolic effects of corticosteroids remains an impetus for this dosing regimen.[26]

INTRAVENOUS "PULSE" METHYLPREDNISOLONE. Many case reports have demonstrated the utility of intravenous pulse methylprednisolone therapy (usually 1000 mg/day for 3 days) in severe cases of neurologic lupus,[27] thrombocytopenia,[28] and life-threatening multisystem disease[29] refractory to previous treatments, including high-dose oral corticosteroids, azathioprine, and cyclophosphamide. Multiple open-label trials (Table 23–3) have confirmed improvement, usually rapid, in extrarenal manifestations of lupus. How-

## TABLE 23–2
## Antimalarial Agents: Open-label Trials

| DRUG | STUDY, YEAR (REFERENCE) | N | OUTCOME |
|------|-------------------------|---|---------|
| Chloroquine | Dubois, 1956 (9) | 14 | 86% improved |
| | | 28 (with corticosteroids) | 53% improved |
| | Goldman et al., 1953 (16) | 21 | 76% improved |
| | Rogers and Finn, 1954 (127) | 43 | 91% improved |
| | Pillsbury and Jacobson, 1954 (128) | 16 | 94% improved |
| | Ziff et al., 1958 (18) | 4 | 50% improved |
| | | 12 (with corticosteroids) | 92% reduced corticosteroids |
| Hydroxychloroquine | Cornbleet, 1956 (129) | 7 | 100% improved |
| | Callen, 1982 (21) | 34 | 88% improved |
| | Lewis and Frumess, 1956 (19) | 22 | 77% improved |
| | Mullins et al., 1956 (17) | 40 | 88% improved |

**TABLE 23–3**
**Intravenous Methyl Prednisolone Pulse Therapy: Open-label Trials**

| STUDY, YEAR (REFERENCE) | N | NONRENAL MANIFESTATIONS | OUTCOME |
|---|---|---|---|
| Ponticelli et al., 1977 (130) | 6 | Fever, arthritis, rash | Improvement: fever, arthritis, rash |
| Dosa et al., 1978 (131) | 4 | Leukopenia, thrombocytopenia, rash | Improvement |
| Eyanson et al., 1980 (132) | 2 | Neurologic, thrombocytopenia, anemia | Improvement |
| Fessel, 1980 (133) | 11 | Neurologic, pulmonary, thrombocytopenia, cutaneous | Improvement: 64% |
| Isenberg et al., 1982 (30) | 20 | Arthritis, pleurisy, vasculitis, fever, lymphadenopathy | Improvement: fever, arthritis, pleurisy, vasculitis, lymphadenopathy Occasional response: thrombocytopenia |
| Goldberg and Lidsky, 1984 (134) | 2 | Subacute cutaneous lupus | Rapid improvement |
| Ballou et al., 1985 (25) | 11 | Fever, arthritis, rash thrombocytopenia, pneumonitis | Rapid improvement: 73% |

ever, the response of thrombocytopenia can be variable.[30]

## Azathioprine

Azathioprine, in doses of 100 to 200 mg daily, has been widely used in the control of lupus nephritis.[31–35] Its use has been beneficial for refractory discoid lupus.[36, 37]

## Cyclophosphamide

The majority of trials of cyclophosphamide have been for the treatment of lupus nephritis. However, cyclophosphamide has been successfully used for the treatment of autoimmune thrombocytopenia refractory to high-dose corticosteroids,[38] discoid and subacute cutaneous lupus refractory to corticosteroids and antimalarials,[39] neuropsychiatric lupus,[40] and myositis.[41]

Synchronization of plasmapheresis and subsequent high-dose pulse cyclophosphamide therapy, followed by 6 months of oral cyclophosphamide, led to long-term remission in 8 of 14 treated SLE patients in one study.[42] However, a later randomized, controlled trial of the addition of pulse/synchronization apheresis to cyclophosphamide did not find added benefit in renal outcome.[43]

The use of low-dose intravenous pulse cyclophosphamide therapy has been reported in 43 SLE patients, with fewer adverse effects than full-dose intravenous cyclophosphamide (750 to 1000 mg/m$^2$ body surface area) and no cases of premature ovarian failure.[44] We have reported high-dose intravenous cyclophosphamide, 50 mg/kg for 4 days, without stem cell rescue, as an alternative to stem cell transplantation for severe SLE.[45]

## Methotrexate

Methotrexate has been used in patients with corticosteroid-resistant lupus. Ten patients with fever, arthritis, and cutaneous lupus treated with weekly intravenous or daily oral methotrexate improved rapidly.[46] Of 10 patients with multiple nonrenal lupus manifestations treated with 7.5 mg weekly, seven showed benefit.[47] In an open-label prospective trial, 13 of 16 SLE patients

improved with methotrexate, but secondary relapse occurred in 4.[48] In another series, 12 of 21 SLE patients improved with methotrexate therapy, with responses largely found in those with cutaneous or musculoskeletal lupus.[49] In an open-label trial of methotrexate in 22 SLE patients, disease activity and prednisolone dose significantly decreased.[50] A life table analysis study of SLE patients receiving methotrexate predominantly for arthritis showed that 68% were still taking the drug at 12 months and 61% at 24 months. Only 36% reduced their corticosteroid dose, and the reduction was not significant.[51] In a trial of 12 patients with cutaneous lupus, 10 improved with low-dose weekly methotrexate[52] (Table 23–4).

## Cyclosporine

In one open-label trial of cyclosporine in 30 SLE patients, a decrease in disease activity and reduction in prednisone dose was found, but side effects were common.[53] In a second open-label trial in 16 patients, 2 patients had no benefit, 4 had flares, 3 discontinued the drug because of side effects, 2 discontinued because of pregnancy, and 4 remained taking the drug. In this study, the most benefit was observed in the 10 patients with proteinuria.[54]

## Plasmapheresis

Most case series and open-label trials of plasmapheresis have been for renal lupus.[55] One open-label trial of plasmapheresis alone in four SLE patients (one with central nervous system lupus, two with arthritis, and one with thrombocytopenia) resulted in poor clinical outcome in all patients.[56] A second open-label trial of 14 SLE patients treated with plasmapheresis and concurrent conventional therapy resulted in improvement in 8, with joint and cutaneous symptoms responding best.[57] Concurrent immunosuppressive therapy may prevent or ameliorate the increased antibody production after removal of serum antibody and circulating immune complexes. A combination of lymphapheresis and plasmapheresis was beneficial in an open-label trial in 16 of 19 SLE patients receiving concurrent immunosuppression.[58]

TABLE 23–4
Methotrexate: Open-label Trials

| STUDY, YEAR (REFERENCE) | N | NONRENAL MANIFESTATIONS | OUTCOME |
| --- | --- | --- | --- |
| Miescher and Riethmüller, 1965 (46) | 10 | Fever, arthritis, cutaneous | Rapid improvement |
| Rothenberg et al., 1988 (47) | 10 | Nonrenal | Improvement: 70% |
| Arfi et al., 1995 (48) | 16 | | Improvement: 81% but relapse in 25% |
| Wise et al., 1996 (49) | 21 | Cutaneous, musculoskeletal | Improvement: 57% |
| Gansauge et al., 1997 (50) | 22 | | Improvement: disease activity Prednisolone reduction |
| Kipen et al., 1997 (51) | 24 | Arthritis | 61% remained on drug at 24 mo 36% reduced corticosteroid dose |
| Boehm et al., 1998 (52) | 12 | Cutaneous | Improvement: 83% |

Plasmapheresis has also been used to remove maternal anti-Ro (SS-A)[59] and in patients with antiphospholipid antibody syndrome resistant to conventional therapies.[60]

## Intravenous Immune Globulin

Intravenous immune globulin (IVIG), at usual doses of 400 mg/kg, daily for up to 5 days, may be helpful in some SLE patients with severe thrombocytopenia.[61–64] IVIG has been used (with other therapies) for pregnancy loss in antiphospholipid antibody syndrome.[65, 66] IVIG has been used for multiple nonrenal manifestations of lupus, including cutaneous vasculitis,[63, 67] pancytopenia,[68] arthritis,[61, 69] neurologic lupus,[69] and pericarditis.[70]

## Dehydroepiandrosterone

Long-term (up to 1 year) treatment with dehydroepiandrosterone (DHEA) was evaluated in 50 patients in a prospective, open-label trial. Patients were treated with oral DHEA, 50 to 200 mg/day. Thirty-four SLE patients (68%) completed 6 months of treatment, and 21 (42%) completed 12 months. Those that remained taking the drug had significant decreases (vs. baseline) in SLE Disease Activity Index (SLEDAI) patient and physician global assessment.[71]

## Bromocriptine

An open-label trial of bromocriptine in seven patients with active but not life-threatening lupus, for 6 to 9 months, showed a reduction in disease activity as measured by Systemic Lupus Activity Measure (SLAM) and SLEDAI indices. After bromocriptine was discontinued, all patients had an increase in prolactin levels and in disease activity. However, the mechanism of action of bromocriptine in SLE is probably complex, with effects not just on prolactin but also on T cells.[72]

## Stem Cell Transplantation

Multiple case reports of remission of SLE after stem cell transplantation exist,[73, 74] but the numbers of patients were small, the follow-up periods were short, and the morbidity and mortality rates were not been adequately evaluated.

## CONTROLLED CLINICAL TRIALS

## Nonsteroidal Anti-inflammatory Drugs

A 10-day randomized, double-blind trial of ibuprofen versus aspirin demonstrated improvement in number of swollen joints, joint pain, and global assessment of arthritis only in the aspirin group.[75] However, ibuprofen was shown to be efficacious for lupus arthritis in an open trial[13] with a longer treatment period.

## Antimalarials

In two retrospective studies, before and after withdrawal of atabrine, patients were more likely to relapse after withdrawal of medication.[76, 77] In a study of five patients taking amodiaquine, with a placebo crossover design, the placebo group relapsed within 1 to 3 months.[9] In a large retrospective study matching years on and off antimalarial drugs (predominantly chloroquine, although hydroxychloroquine, quinacrine, and triquin were also used), antimalarials reduced flares and were corticosteroid-sparing. In addition, chloroquine reduced fever, fatigue, weight loss, and cutaneous lupus (Table 23–5).[78, 79] In the Canadian Hydroxychloroquine Study, which was a randomized, double-blind placebo-controlled withdrawal study, the relative risk of disease flare was 2.5 times higher in the placebo group, and the time to a flare was shorter ($P = .02$). However, no significant difference in prednisone dose was found.[80] In a later, unblinded follow-up study, severe flares appeared to be reduced in the hydroxychloroquine group.[81] A randomized trial of hydroxychloroquine in lupus pregnancy suggested not just safety but better pregnancy outcome in the hydroxychloroquine group.[82] There were fewer flares, less toxemia, and a decrease in prednisone dose in this group.

## Intravenous Methylprednisolone

One randomized, double-blind trial of 1000-mg versus 100-mg doses of intravenous methylprednisolone

**TABLE 23–5**
**Antimalarial Drugs: Controlled Trials**

| STUDY (REFERENCE) | TREATMENT GROUP (N) | COMPARISON GROUPS (N) | STUDY DESIGN | OUTCOME |
|---|---|---|---|---|
| Rothfield, 1988 (79) | Antimalarial (43) | Postwithdrawal (43) | Retrospective withdrawal study | Antimalarial use reduced corticosteroid dose and disease flares |
| Canadian Hydroxychloroquine Study Group, 1991 (80) | Hydroxychloroquine (25) | Placebo (22) | 6-Month randomized double-blind placebo-controlled withdrawal study | Antimalarial use reduced disease flares and increased time to flare |
| Ruzicka et al., 1992 (135) | Hydroxychloroquine (25) | Acitretin (22) | 8-Week randomized double-blind | 46% improved in acitretin group; 50% improved in antimalarial group |
| Levy et al., 1998 (82) | Hydroxychloroquine (10) | Placebo (10) | Randomized controlled | There were no flares in hydroxychloroquine group vs. four flares in placebo |

found no difference in response (Table 23–6).[83] A second randomized, double-blind trial of 1000 mg intravenous methylprednisolone versus placebo in patients who were also treated with high doses of oral prednisolone found greater improvement in the methylprednisolone group at 14 days but not at 28 days.[84] Cutaneous and arthritis manifestations improved faster in the treatment group, but the difference did not reach statistical significance.

## Azathioprine

Because most controlled trials of azathioprine have included only patients with lupus nephritis, information on extrarenal manifestations is usually lacking. Three controlled trials that included data on nonrenal lupus reached conflicting conclusions (Table 23–7), with two studies finding that azathioprine reduced flares and corticosteroid requirements[85, 86] and one finding no difference.[87]

## Methotrexate

In a case control study, 15 to 17 patients with lupus arthritis improved when given methotrexate, compared with only 2 of 17 in the control group.[88]

## Cyclophosphamide

The National Institutes of Health prospective controlled trials clearly showed significantly greater benefit of cyclophosphamide compared with corticosteroids in the treatment of lupus nephritis but lacked data on nonrenal manifestations of lupus. One controlled trial of cyclophosphamide versus prednisone alone included four patients with nonrenal lupus (two in each group). In this trial, there were no responders in the group treated with cyclophosphamide alone.[89]

## Dehydroepiandrosterone

The first double-blind, placebo-controlled, randomized clinical trial of DHEA in SLE compared 200 mg of DHEA with placebo for 3 months in 28 female patients with mild to moderate SLE. There were significant differences in patients' assessments and flares (which were more common in the placebo group). Although disease activity (SLEDAI) improved in the DHEA group, the difference failed to reach statistical significance.[90] A second double-blind, placebo-controlled trial of two doses of DHEA (100 mg and 200 mg) versus placebo was carried out in 191 women with steroid-dependent SLE to determine whether DHEA could be steroid-sparing. Responders were de-

**TABLE 23–6**
**Intravenous Methylprednisolone (IV MP): Controlled Trials**

| STUDY (REFERENCE) | TREATMENT GROUP (N) | COMPARISON | STUDY DESIGN | OUTCOME |
|---|---|---|---|---|
| Edwards et al., 1987 (83) | 1000 mg IV MP for 3 d (11), other medications as needed | 100 mg IV MP for 3 d (10), other medications as needed | Randomized double-blind | 45% 1000 mg IV MP vs. 60% 100 mg IV MP responded |
| Mackworth-Young et al., 1988 (84) | 1000 mg IV MP for 3 d (12), oral prednisolone 40–60 mg | Placebo (13), oral prednisolone 40–60 mg | Randomized double-blind | Greater improvement in IV MP group (83%) at 14 d, but no difference at 28 d |

**TABLE 23-7**
## Azathioprine: Controlled Trials

| STUDY (REFERENCE) | TREATMENT GROUP (N) | COMPARISON GROUPS (N) | STUDY DESIGN | OUTCOME |
|---|---|---|---|---|
| Sztejnbok et al., 1971 (85) | Prednisone and azathioprine (16) | Prednisone (19) | Nonblinded | Azathioprine use decreased morbidity, mortality, prednisone dose, and flares |
| Sharon et al., 1973 (86) | Prednisone and azathioprine (7) | Prednisone (9) | Randomized withdrawal | Azathioprine reduced flares |
| Hahn et al., 1975 (87) | Prednisone and azathioprine (11) | Prednisone (13) | Randomized trial | No reduction in mortality, flares, or prednisone dose in the azathioprine group |

fined as SLE patients who achieved a sustained reduction of prednisone to physiologic doses of 7.5 mg or less for 2 or more months. Although the results were not significant in the entire patient group, 200 mg/day of DHEA was able to "steroid spare" in those patients who began the trial with active lupus, defined as a SLEDAI score greater than 2.[91]

## AUTHORS' APPROACH TO MANAGEMENT

Routine screening of the patient with SLE should be performed at least every 3 months and should include an interval history, a directed physical examination, and laboratory monitoring including complete blood cell count, creatinine and cholesterol determinations, urinalysis, and, in patients in whom they have proven clinically useful, serum C3, C4, and anti-dsDNA. Monitoring of lifestyle factors and guidance in coronary artery disease risk factors, including smoking, obesity, hyperlipidemia, hypertension, and homocysteine, are an integral part of the quarterly visits. Hypertension should be aggressively managed by both nonpharmacologic and pharmacologic means. Hypertension is one of the major predictive variables for both renal failure and mortality in SLE.[7, 92, 93] Except for the avoidance of β-blocking agents in patients with Raynaud's phenomenon, antihypertensive agents of all classes can be used. There is special interest in the use of angiotensin-converting enzyme inhibitors, given their role in renal protection in other diseases such as diabetes mellitus.

All SLE patients undergoing corticosteroid or immunosuppressive treatment should receive the pneumococcal pneumonia vaccine and yearly influenza vaccination. Patients should be counseled that infections, including bronchitis and urinary tract infections, should be brought to the physician's attention promptly. If possible, sulfa antibiotics should be avoided because of their propensity to cause allergy or disease flares in SLE.[94]

Because of the increased risk of cancer (even without exposure to alkylating agents), screening for malignant change should be instituted whenever appropriate. In adult female SLE patients, this includes yearly pelvic examination and mammography (beginning at age 35

to 40 years). Sunscreens should be used routinely, not just in photosensitive patients, to reduce cutaneous cancers.

Ongoing dental care is important to avoid a potential source of systemic infection and to avoid unnecessary caries due to secondary Sjögren's syndrome. Yearly ophthalmologic consultation is essential, not just to monitor antimalarial therapy but also to screen for and treat glaucoma and posterior subcapsular cataracts resulting from corticosteroid therapy.

For purposes of the discussion to follow, three dosage forms of oral daily corticosteroids are used in prednisone equivalents, mild, 5 to 10 mg/day; moderate, 15 to 30 mg/day; and high, 40 to 60 mg/day.

## Cutaneous Lupus

Malar rash, photosensitive rash elsewhere, and discoid lupus are approached in a similar manner. The patient is cautioned against ultraviolet (UV) light exposure, but not to the point of excessive paranoia. However, some patients have extreme sun sensitivity. Reducing UV light exposure represents a major challenge to all caregivers and patient support systems. Sunscreens should be used not just to help cutaneous lupus but to prevent skin cancer and to retard aging. Topical corticosteroid lotions and creams may have limited benefit. The use of topical corticosteroids should not delay the institution of systemic therapy. Fluorinated compounds should not be used on the face because of cutaneous atrophy.

Antimalarial agents remain the mainstay of treatment. Because of difficulty in obtaining quinacrine and concern about retinopathy with chloroquine, the agent of choice is hydroxychloroquine, with an average adult dose of 400 mg/day. Side effects are unusual when hydroxychloroquine is given at a dose of less than 6 mg/kg. Response usually begins within 1 month, and the full effect of treatment can be assessed at 3 months.

In many patients, antimalarial therapy is sufficient for cutaneous lupus. In some cases of cutaneous lupus with incomplete response to hydroxychloroquine at 400 mg/day, quinacrine at 100 mg/day may be added with some success. In the rare patient with allergic rash, severe gastrointestinal intolerance, or one of the unusual nervous system side effects (e.g., nightmares) of antimalarial therapy, it may be necessary to try alternative therapies. Retinoids, including isotretinon or etretinate (for patients practicing effective birth control) or dapsone (for patients who are not glucose-6-phosphate dehydrogenase deficient) may be helpful. Dapsone, starting at 50 mg/day with gradual, careful increases, usually not exceeding 200 mg/day, may be the agent of choice for a rare form of cutaneous lupus, bullous lupus.

For very severe discoid lesions, intralesional corticosteroid injection may be necessary. Waiting weeks (or months) for control of disease by antimalarial therapy might allow irreversible scarring to occur. Therefore, low to moderate doses of corticosteroids (prednisone in doses of 5 to 20 mg/day) may be necessary for initial control of moderate cutaneous lupus, with rapid taper being the goal. Severe cutaneous vasculitis or severe discoid lupus (especially on areas such as the soles of the feet) may require intravenous pulse methylprednisolone (1000 mg/day for 3 days) to achieve initial control.

In the rare patient who requires a high maintenance dose of corticosteroid for severe vasculitic or other forms of cutaneous lupus, methotrexate (initially 7.5 mg orally once a week), mycophenolate mofetil (500 to 3000 mg/day) or azathioprine (100 to 200 mg/day) may play a corticosteroid-sparing role.

Raynaud's phenomenon is often seasonal and usually not very severe in SLE patients. Patients with more severe symptoms benefit from the calcium channel blockers nifedipine and diltiazem. Purchase of battery-operated warming gloves and socks is a worthwhile investment.

## Musculoskeletal Lupus

NSAIDs are used in the initial management of polyarthralgias or polyarthritis. COX-2–specific NSAIDs, because of their greater gastrointestinal safety, are of great interest but have not yet been tested. Many patients require the addition of antimalarial therapy for adequate control.

Although corticosteroids in moderate to high doses are very effective for lupus arthritis, the long-term side effects do not justify their use for arthritis. If steroids are to be used at all, the lowest dose (usually 5 to 10 mg/day of prednisone) should be employed, keeping the dosage just above the threshold for symptoms. A severe, incapacitating polyarthritis or myositis flare may require intravenous pulse methylprednisolone therapy (1000 mg/day for 3 days). Patients who require unacceptably high daily corticosteroid doses may do well with the addition of azathioprine or methotrexate (initially 7.5 mg orally once a week) as a corticosteroid-sparing agent. Lupus patients with features that overlap with rheumatoid arthritis ("rhupus") are good candidates for methotrexate therapy. Newly introduced therapies for rheumatoid arthritis, including leflunomide (Arava) and the recombinant tumor necrosis factor (TNF) receptor etanercept (Enbrel), have not been adequately tested in SLE. In the case of TNF-specific therapies, there are case reports of patients with rheumatoid arthritis who developed the new onset of lupus autoantibodies.

## Cardiopulmonary Lupus (Including Serositis)

The initial management of severe serositis, either pericarditis or pleurisy with pleural effusion, may require intravenous pulse methylprednisolone therapy (1000 mg/day for 3 days) followed by oral prednisone at moderate or high dosage depending on the clinical severity. Milder forms of serositis can be managed with NSAIDs, supplemented by low-dose prednisone as necessary. In a patient already taking a maintenance dose of an NSAID and low-dose prednisone, a mild exacerbation may be managed by temporarily increasing the prednisone dose to moderate levels, followed by a slow reduction back to the maintenance dose.

Interstitial lung disease can occur in an acute or chronic form in SLE. In a patient already taking immunosuppressive therapy, the initial differential diagnosis requires a work-up for bacterial or opportunistic infection. Often a lung biopsy is required to ascertain whether the condition is caused by SLE and to assess the degree of active inflammation. In many patients, high-dose corticosteroid therapy is required in the initial phases. The addition of azathioprine or alkylating agents is frequently necessary in patients with the chronic form. Serial monitoring of chest roentgenogram, pulmonary function tests (including single-breath diffusion capacity and helium lung volumes), arterial blood gases, and high-resolution chest computed tomography is used to evaluate response.

Pulmonary hypertension in a mild, stable form may be detected by noninvasive cardiac Doppler echocardiography in as many as 10% of SLE patients.[95] In the rare patient who progresses to severe pulmonary hypertension, the differential diagnosis includes recurrent pulmonary emboli or the presence of a hypercoagulable state. Management of idiopathic pulmonary hypertension with pulmonary artery pressures greater than 50 mm usually requires an initial right-sided heart catheterization to monitor response to therapy, including calcium channel blockers and prostacyclin (if available as an investigational agent). Long-term anticoagulation is the rule. For follow-up, noninvasive monitoring with Doppler echocardiography correlates well with catheterization.[95]

Libman-Sacks endocarditis is extremely rare in the poststeroid era. In many patients, antiphospholipid antibodies are found. If accompanied by embolic events, anticoagulation is necessary. Small lesions can be monitored by serial transesophageal echocardiography, and treatment with corticosteroids and anticoagulation can be instituted if they enlarge. Warfarin is usually adjusted to an international normalized ratio (INR) of 3 to 4, as long as the patient is not profoundly thrombocytopenic.

Myocarditis or congestive heart failure is a very rare cardiac presentation or manifestation. Treatment with high-dose corticosteroids, usually initially pulse methylprednisolone (1000 mg/day for 3 days), is essential. The addition of intravenous monthly cyclophosphamide is usually necessary. Coronary arteritis is also rare. Most cases of angina pectoris or myocardial infarction are caused by premature atherosclerosis.

## Hematologic Lupus

SLE patients with severe cytopenia require periodic laboratory monitoring to detect life-threatening declines in their blood counts.

Anemia in SLE can be caused by bleeding in the gut, hemolysis, chronic disease, iron deficiency, low erythropoietin, or immunosuppressive therapy. When the cause is unclear, a bone marrow biopsy may be helpful. Hemolytic anemia can be managed with corticosteroids. If unacceptably high doses of daily prednisone are required, the addition of azathioprine as a steroid-sparing agent can be tried. In a few patients, danocrine may be a useful adjunct. A severe hemolytic anemia may require intravenous pulse methylprednisolone, 1000 mg/day for 3 days, followed by a maintenance dose of prednisone.

Mild stable thrombocytopenia can be tolerated. Severe thrombocytopenia (platelet counts lower than 35,000) is treated with corticosteroids. For life-threatening thrombocytopenia, intravenous pulse methylprednisolone, 1000 mg/day for 3 days, is given initially. Refractory thrombocytopenia may require IVIG (contraindicated for persons deficient in immunoglobulin A) or Rho (D) immunoglobulin (Win Rho) if Rh-positive. Danocrine may be tried, although it is variably successful. The patient who has had severe, persistent thrombocytopenia for longer than 6 months, for whom alternative therapies have failed, and who has developed complications from high-dose corticosteroids, is a candidate for splenectomy of primary and accessory spleens. Although such surgery is not curative, many patients require lower doses of medication for control of cytopenia after splenectomy. In rare cases, thrombocytopenia is a manifestation of thrombotic thrombocytopenia purpura, and should be managed with plasmapheresis.

## Constitutional Features

Occasionally a patient with SLE has weight loss. Often this responds to a very small maintenance dose of prednisone in the range of 5 to 10 mg/day. Generalized lymphadenopathy is rare in the adult patient with SLE but usually responds rapidly to low-dose prednisone. Lymphadenopathy that is local or that does not respond to low-dose corticosteroid therapy should instigate a search for infection or malignancy.

Fever in a lupus patient is always a diagnostic and sometimes a therapeutic challenge. In an untreated patient, after a routine search for infection, fever can be attributed to SLE with some security, particularly if the leukocyte count is decreased or the concentration anti-DNA antibody is elevated.[96] NSAIDs can be used, but usually a low dose of corticosteroids is necessary to suppress fever. Patients should be counseled that mild elevations of temperature can be tolerated.

Fever in a lupus patient treated with corticosteroids or with immunosuppressive agents should be assumed to be caused by infection until proved otherwise. Persistent high temperatures should be evaluated in the hospital setting. After appropriate bacterial cultures (and often opportunistic organisms must be considered), an empirical course of antibiotic treatment may be necessary. If infection is ruled out, an increase in corticosteroid dose should control fever resulting from an underlying SLE flare. If fever occurs in the setting of activation of lupus in other organs, control of lupus activity elsewhere usually leads to resolution of fever as well.

## Cystitis

Acute interstitial cystitis may be a manifestation of SLE. Management consists of ruling out infection, performing imaging studies to confirm the presence of a thickened bladder wall, and prescribing mild to moderate doses of corticosteroids.

## Gastrointestinal Lupus

Rarely, a patient requires corticosteroid therapy for abdominal serositis or protein-losing enteropathy. The more serious, but still rare, manifestation of abdominal vasculitis requires therapy with high-dose corticosteroids (intravenous methylprednisolone, 1000 mg/day for 3 days, followed by 40 to 80 mg/day until the patient can absorb oral prednisone).

## Pregnancy

Prepregnancy counseling is important, but all too often the patient announces an unplanned pregnancy. It is optimum to have control of disease activity for at least 6 months before embarking on pregnancy, but successful pregnancies are the rule even if lupus is active at conception. However, there are certain stringent contraindications to pregnancy. First, women receiving cyclophosphamide (orally or intravenously) should not become pregnant because of the substantial risk of congenital defects. Methotrexate must be stopped for at least 3 months before a woman becomes pregnant because it is an abortifacient and a teratogen. Second, women receiving warfarin should not become pregnant. Women who require anticoagulation should receive extensive counseling about the increased risk of thrombosis to themselves during pregnancy; if they remain adamant about pregnancy, they should be switched to therapeutic doses of subcutaneous heparin or low-molecular-weight heparin while trying to conceive or as soon as the pregnancy is recognized.

Before pregnancy, the risks of pregnancy to both the fetus and the mother should be assessed and reviewed with the patient (and, optimally, with the obstetrician). The risk of lupus flare in our Lupus Pregnancy Center is 60%, although most flares are mild or moderate in severity. The risk of preterm birth is 45%, and the risk of pregnancy loss is 15%.[94] Women with anti-Ro antibodies (SS-A), especially if accompanied by anti-La (SS-B), need to have fetal four-chamber echocardiograms performed during pregnancy to detect congenital heart block (or myocarditis) at an early and, presumably, treatable stage. Women with a history of pregnancy loss (two consecutive first-trimester spontaneous abortions or any late loss without known cause) should be tested for both anticardiolipin antibody and lupus anticoagulant. Women with severe renal insufficiency or with nephrotic syndrome are at increased risk of renal and pregnancy complications but may be able to have a successful pregnancy. Women with a history of preeclamptic toxemia or toxemia are candidates for daily low-dose aspirin (81 mg) therapy.[97] Maternal diastolic hypertension (90 mm Hg or higher) is a risk factor for preterm birth.[94] $\alpha$-Methyldopa, hydralazine, and labetolol are the antihypertensive agents most widely used in pregnancy.

Management of medications during lupus pregnancy involves weighing of risk-benefit ratios and should be done on an individual basis, with the following guidelines. If azathioprine is necessary to control disease activity in crucial organs, it can be continued. NSAIDs should be avoided during the second and third trimesters because of potential adverse effects on labor and on the fetus.[98] Use of an NSAID for a very short period, however, might be permissible to treat a severe serositis or arthritis flare. Hydroxychloroquine use in pregnancy is a complex issue.[99] The theoretical concern is the potential for deposition in the fetal eye and ear. It is, of course, widely used in Africa and did not appear to cause any adverse effects during lupus pregnancies in one series.[100] It is illogical to stop hydroxychloroquine once pregnancy is recognized, because it is stored in tissues and, in any case, the fetus was already exposed during the first trimester. If hydroxychloroquine has been shown to be necessary to control disease activity, a good case can be made in the individual patient for continuing its use during pregnancy. Documentation of discussion of these issues with the patient and obstetrician is important.

Women with two or more first-trimester losses, or one or more midtrimester or late intrauterine losses without known cause, should be evaluated for antiphospholipid antibodies. Women with pregnancy loss due to antiphospholipid antibody syndrome have a choice of regimens. In a clinical trial that did not include lupus patients, prednisone, 40 mg/day, with low-dose aspirin had efficacy equal that of subcutaneous heparin, 10,000 units twice a day, with low-dose aspirin. However, maternal morbidity was higher in the prednisone-treated group.[101] It is not necessary to use 40 mg of prednisone; 20 mg or less appears to be efficacious and less likely to cause maternal morbidity. If a woman with lupus and recurrent pregnancy loss already requires prednisone in the range of 20 mg to control her SLE, low-dose aspirin can be added while she is trying to conceive. If a woman requires only low doses of prednisone, aspirin can be added while she is trying to conceive, and when she becomes pregnant,

subcutaneous heparin can be added. Low-molecular-weight heparin can be used instead of unfractionated heparin, especially for women with thrombocytopenia and/or osteoporosis.

Monthly rheumatology visits for all pregnant women with SLE to monitor and treat disease activity are important. Lupus flares that are mild or moderate may be managed with appropriate doses of oral prednisone. NSAIDs are usually avoided in the late second or third trimester. Severe lupus flares may require intravenous pulse methylprednisolone therapy or the addition of azathioprine. Cyclophosphamide, including intravenous pulse cyclophosphamide, must be avoided in the first trimester. Its use later in pregnancy can be justified only for life-threatening disease. Termination of pregnancy is not necessary to treat severe lupus flares and may, in fact, aggravate lupus activity. Referral to an obstetrician who specializes in high-risk cases is best, not just because of the increased frequency of fetal loss but, more important, because of the increased frequency of preterm birth (40%), which is caused largely by preterm premature rupture of membranes and preeclamptic toxemia.

## Antiphospholipid Syndrome

As many as 50% of patients with SLE manifest the ability to make antiphospholipid antibodies (lupus anticoagulant or anticardiolipin antibody), often intermittently, when observed sequentially over time. Prophylactic therapy for SLE patients who produce antiphospholipid antibodies but have not had venous or arterial thrombosis (or vasculopathy) is not currently recommended.

Patients with venous thrombosis (usually deep venous thrombosis of the lower extremities) and either the lupus anticoagulant or anticardiolipin antibody can be treated initially with heparin or with thrombolytic therapy, as appropriate. Long-term anticoagulation with warfarin is strongly recommended because of the high rate of recurrent thrombosis.[102–104]

Initial management of arterial thrombosis or vasculopathy is dictated by the site and severity of the thrombotic event. Ischemic strokes may be treated initially with heparin, provided that there is no hemorrhagic complication. Myocardial infarction due to thrombosis may be treated initially with heparin, thrombolytic therapy, or angioplasty, as appropriate. Peripheral arterial emboli or thrombi may require emergency embolectomy/thrombectomy, thrombolytic therapy, angioplasty, or heparin. Long-term anticoagulation with warfarin appears to be preferable to antiplatelet therapy.[102]

In most cases, full anticoagulation, achieving an INR of 3 to 4, is recommended,[102] so long as the platelet count remains higher than 50,000/$\mu$L. Close monitoring of the prothrombin time is necessary to reduce bleeding complications. Patients are switched to either intravenous heparin or subcutaneous heparin/low-molecular-weight heparin before elective surgical procedures.

# DRUG SIDE EFFECTS AND RECOMMENDED MONITORING SCHEDULES

## Nonsteroidal Anti-inflammatory Agents

For an in-depth discussion of NSAIDs, see Kelley and colleagues, *Textbook of Rheumatology*, Chapter 43.[12] Of 99 SLE patients exposed to an NSAID (including aspirin), 49.5% reported epigastric distress at some time; 7.1%, peptic ulcer disease; 9.1%, stomatitis; 4.0%, worsening renal insufficiency; 5.1%, bronchospasm; and 5.1%, urticaria/angioedema. Tinnitus was reported in 21.2%, vertigo in 7.1%, and an increase in ecchymoses in 34.3%.[105] Mild epigastric distress can be managed initially with the introduction of a histamine-2 ($H_2$)–blocker. Patients with past peptic ulcer disease secondary to or aggravated by NSAIDs are candidates for misoprostol therapy or a proton-pump inhibitor. Although COX-2–specific NSAIDs have not yet been tested for SLE, their use could be considered in a patient with gastrointestinal complications from NSAIDs. However, there is a theoretical concern that COX-2–specific NSAIDs might increase hypercoagulability through reduction in prostacyclin.

## Antimalarial Drugs (Hydroxychloroquine)

Reported side effects of antimalarial drugs include ocular toxicity (corneal deposits or retinopathy), cutaneous eruptions, gastrointestinal intolerance, and rare nervous system complaints, including myopathy. Of 104 SLE patients exposed to one or more antimalarial drugs, 22.1% had nausea, 15.4% had abdominal cramps, 12.5% had anorexia, and 9.6% had diarrhea. Only 5% (five patients) had any evidence of retinopathy (reversible in every case). One of these five patients had renal insufficiency.

The risk of retinopathy from hydroxychloroquine is so low—only one patient in one series,[106] no patients among 73 in a second series,[107] and 3% to 4% in a third series[108]—that ophthalmologic monitoring every 6 months should be more than sufficient. In fact, it can be argued that ophthalmologic monitoring is not cost-effective for hydroxychloroquine alone and that it is more important to monitor for ocular effects of lupus itself or of corticosteroid therapy. This subject is reviewed in-depth in Kelley and colleagues, *Textbook of Rheumatology*, Chapter 44.[12]

## Corticosteroids

Major side effects attributed to corticosteroid therapy include avascular necrosis of bone, osteoporosis (with or without fractures), steroid myopathy, diabetes mellitus, and increased frequency of infections. Corticosteroid therapy also increases the level of several cardiovascular risk factors, including cholesterol, hypertension, and obesity; this is one explanation of the association of corticosteroid use with premature atherosclerotic disease.[109] Of 170 SLE patients receiving corticosteroids, 21% developed avascular necrosis, 8% had recognized osteoporosis, 8% had steroid myopathy, 7% had vertebral compression fractures, and 7% had diabetes mellitus. Cutaneous fungal infections occurred in 18%, oral candida in 29%, and herpes zoster in 7%.[105]

Minor side effects of corticosteroid use include the cushingoid habitus, dermatologic toxicity, and neurologic symptoms. In the same group of 170 patients, 26% had a buffalo hump, 62% had moon facies, and 49% had truncal obesity. Dermatologic side effects included spontaneous ecchymoses (44%), impaired wound healing (32%), increased sweating (30%), new-onset acne (28%), and striae (22%). Other minor side effects included insomnia (31%) and steroid mood change or psychosis (18%). Corticosteroids are discussed in Kelley and colleagues, *Textbook of Rheumatology*, Chapter 48.[12]

If avascular necrosis of the hip (the most frequently involved joint) is detected at an early stage before collapse of the femoral head, core decompression of bone may prevent or delay the need for total joint replacement. Shoulder and knee avascular necrosis are less likely to require total joint replacement. Some cases of avascular necrosis may be asymptomatic, and some regress spontaneously.

All patients taking corticosteroids should receive supplemental calcium to achieve an intake of 1200 mg daily and vitamin D (as part of a daily multiple-vitamin regimen). Although it is not currently available, deflazacort may engender less osteoporosis. For the postmenopausal patient, estrogen replacement (with progesterone, if the uterus is intact) may be considered. The safety of estrogen replacement in SLE is the focus of the ongoing Safety of Estrogens in Lupus Erythematosus National Assessment (SELENA) trial. Estrogen replacement after menopause was not associated with lupus flares in retrospective series.[110] Estrogen replacement may also decrease the risk of coronary artery disease. Bisphosphonates, either alendronate or cyclic etidronate, can also be used. In the premenopausal patient, calcitonin and, probably, biphosphonates may be useful. Whether oral contraceptive therapy can be considered as a therapy for premenopausal osteoporosis awaits safety data from the ongoing SELENA trial.

In the patient who is hypercholesterolemic and who either already has atherosclerotic disease or has other major risk factors for atherosclerotic disease, referral to a registered dietician for instruction in the step II American Heart Association diet[110a] is recommended. For the patient with atherosclerotic disease who fails to achieve dietary control of hyperlipidemia, pharmacologic management can be instituted. We have found that lupus patients have a higher frequency of increased creatine phosphokinase (CPK) concentration, usually asymptomatic, with both lovastatin and gemfibrozil than the general population; initial monthly monitoring of CPK level is recommended.

## Intravenous Pulse Methylprednisolone

Pulse methylprednisolone therapy may lead to fluid overload, hypertension, and hyperglycemia. In rare cases, it has been associated with cardiac arrhythmias, seizures, or steroid psychosis. Attention to fluid and electrolyte balance before and during therapy is important.

## Immunosuppressive Drugs

Major side effects of cytotoxic drugs include premature ovarian failure, hemorrhagic cystitis and bladder fibrosis, malignancy, bone marrow suppression, and infection. SLE patients taking oral or intravenous cyclophosphamide should be monitored monthly with interval history, directed physical examination, complete blood cell count, chemistry panel, and urinalysis. Pneumovax 23 and yearly influenza vaccination are recommended. Intravenous cyclophosphamide appears to be as efficacious as oral cyclophosphamide and at the present time is the preferred cytotoxic drug for severe SLE manifestations. It can be given with mesna to avoid the risk of hemorrhagic cystitis that occurs with oral cyclophosphamide use. Appropriate maintenance therapy with intravenous cyclophosphamide (dosage, timing, duration) remains unclear and needs further study.

Premature ovarian failure is more common in women older than 30 years of age and after longer courses of cyclophosphamide (either oral or intravenous). Oral contraceptive pills or leuprolide acetate (Lupron), a luteinizing hormone–releasing hormone agonist, have been considered as possible means to preserve fertility, but data are lacking in terms of both efficacy and safety.

Both cutaneous and gynecologic cancers can occur in cytotoxically treated patients. Cervical carcinoma is increased in African-American patients with lupus, patients without renal disease, and azathioprine-treated patients.[111] Use of sunscreens and yearly gynecologic examinations (including mammograms in women older than 40 years of age) are important. Leukemias and lymphomas, which occur in SLE patients treated with oral cyclophosphamide, appear to be rarer in patients exposed to intravenous cyclophosphamide. The mechanism of action and the immunoregulatory effects of the drugs are discussed in Kelley and colleagues, *Textbook of Rheumatology,* Chapter 49.[12]

## CLINICAL PHARMACOLOGY AND DRUG INTERACTIONS

### Nonsteroidal Anti-inflammatory Drugs

PHARMACOLOGY. NSAIDs can be divided into those with short elimination half-times (ibuprofen, indomethacin, tolmetin, ketoprofen), those with intermediate half-times of 12 to 18 hours (naproxen, sulindac, diflunisal), and those with long half-times (piroxicam, nabumetone). Biotransformation includes hepatic metabolism to inactive metabolites, which are excreted renally. Indomethacin and sulindac have an enterohepatic circulation with fecal excretion.

MECHANISM OF ACTION. Although NSAIDs reversibly inactivate platelet cyclooxygenase, their in vivo action is also mediated through neutrophil function.[112] COX-2–specific NSAIDs inhibit the inducible inflammatory actions rather than the constitutive gastroprotective functions.

DRUG INTERACTIONS. Potential renal effects of NSAIDs, including sodium retention, hyperkalemia,[113] reduction in glomerular filtration rate, interstitial nephritis, and papillary necrosis, among others, can occur in SLE patients. A rare SLE patient may have fever and aseptic meningitis while taking ibuprofen, sulindac, or tolmetin. NSAID use may inhibit renal excretion of chlorpropamide, methotrexate, and lithium, and it may potentiate sulfonylurea hypoglycemics and warfarin because of protein-binding changes. Use of NSAIDs (other than nonacetylated salicylates) is considered high-risk therapy in anticoagulated patients because of the increased chance of bleeding. The COX-2–specific NSAID celecoxib has significantly less gastrointestinal toxicity, does not affect platelet function, and does not affect warfarin metabolism. However, it has not yet been studied in SLE. NSAIDs, in addition to aspirin, can also cause a drug hepatitis.

## Antimalarials

PHARMACOLOGY. Chloroquine and hydroxychloroquine are water-soluble 4-aminoquinolones. They are rapidly absorbed in 2 to 4 hours, reaching a peak in 8 to 12 hours, with 50% transported by binding to serum proteins. Biotransformation of hydroxychloroquine results in two first-stage metabolites (chloroquine has one) that lead to a primary amine with a short half-life. The second stage of elimination has a half-life of 18 days. The clinical half-life is 50 to 52 hours.[114, 115] The plasma concentration rises rapidly during the first week and then more slowly until equilibrium is reached by the fourth week. Fifty percent to 60% is excreted in the urine, with 8% to 10% of chloroquine and 15% to 24% of hydroxychloroquine excreted in the feces.[116] Hydroxychloroquine is also excreted in the bile.[117] Plasma concentrations are related to the daily dosage. Tissue levels are highest in melanin-containing tissues (choroid, ciliary body, inner ear), with most distributed in adrenals, spleen, lung, liver, and kidneys.[117] The concentration of antimalarial drug in leukocytes is 100 to 200 times that in plasma. It is concentrated in the epidermis of the skin, with an epidermis-to-corium ratio of 5 to 15.[118] Chloroquine may persist in the retina for months to years.[119]

MECHANISM OF ACTION. Antimalarial drugs raise the pH within lysosomes, thereby interrupting the generation and presentation of antigenic peptides.[120] Other potential effects include a reduction of light absorption, inhibition of antigen-antibody complexes, anti-inflammatory actions, and nucleoprotein binding (reviewed in reference 121).

## Corticosteroids

PHARMACOLOGY. Corticosteroids bind to transcortin (corticosteroid-binding globulin) and to albumin, with only the unbound corticosteroid having biologic activity. Corticosteroids are inactivated by several pathways, including 11-dehydrogenation, which is accelerated by hyperthyroidism. Dihydro and tetrahydro corticosteroid derivatives are conjugated in the liver and excreted. Drugs (e.g., phenobarbital) that activate hepatic microsomal enzymes increase corticosteroid inactivation. Corticosteroids are classified into short-acting (hydrocortisone, prednisone, prednisolone, methylprednisolone), intermediate-acting (triamcinolone), and long-acting (betamethasone, dexamethasone) types according to duration of ACTH suppression. Doses of prednisone greater than 15 mg/day cause adrenal suppression within 1 week. Doses of 5 mg/day or less of prednisone are not adrenally suppressive.[122]

PHARMACOLOGIC EFFECTS. Corticosteroids bind to cytoplasmic receptors and then to DNA regions in target cells. Changes in the rate of DNA transcription, reflected in protein synthesis, explain the effects of corticosteroids. Anti-inflammatory effects include inhibition of leukocyte recruitment at inflammatory sites, decreased bactericidal activity, and reduced phagocytic activity.[123, 124] Glucocorticoids also decrease the release of arachidonic acid, inhibiting prostaglandin synthesis. Immunosuppressive actions of corticosteroids include lymphopenia, with a reduction in the T-inducer/helper subset. Corticosteroids inhibit antibody production and production of interleukin and other cytokines. They also affect cell-mediated immunity by decreasing proliferation in response to mitogens, inhibiting interleukin-2 production, and suppressing cutaneous delayed hypersensitivity. Some of these effects are dose- and time-dependent.

DRUG INTERACTIONS. Corticosteroids can aggravate diabetes mellitus, congestive heart failure, and glaucoma. Corticosteroid-induced hypokalemia can predispose to digoxin toxicity and cardiac arrhythmias. Drugs that affect hepatic microsomal enzymes, such as phenobarbital, accelerate corticosteroid metabolism. Corticosteroids can reduce serum salicylate levels.

# INVESTIGATIONAL DRUGS AND FUTURE DIRECTIONS

Future directions in the treatment of lupus include refinement of the use of currently available immunosuppressive drugs, the introduction of biologics into the treatment of SLE, and the study of stem cell transplantation for the most severe cases.

We have introduced the use of immunoablative doses of intravenous cyclophosphamide (50 mg/kg for 4 days) for severe SLE. In early experience, this treatment has led to both immediate (through immunosuppresion) and long-term (through achievement of tolerance) remission in SLE patients.[45] For moderate lupus, other immunosuppressive drugs, including mycophenolate mofetil,[125] will play an increasing role.

Several biologics are under study for active lupus, especially renal disease. The investigational drug LJP 394, a B-cell tolerogen for anti-dsDNA,[126] did not reduce renal lupus flares. Studies of anti-CD40 ligand,

which blocks a costimulatory pathway of B and T cells, will be undertaken for both renal lupus and moderate to severe nonrenal lupus.

Stem cell transplantation for severe lupus is under study at multiple institutions. Long-term follow-up is not available. Comparison of results from different centers will be difficult, because multiple different preparatory regimens are in use.

Although discovery of the cause and cure of lupus may be decades away, therapies to reintroduce tolerance, including high-dose cyclophosphamide and stem cell transplantation, are an exciting and more immediate goal. Although these therapies may seem aggressive, the current "status quo," in which the major damage sustained by SLE patients derives from their chronic treatment with corticosteroids and alkylating drugs rather than from the disease directly, is unacceptable.

# REFERENCES

1. Pickering G, Bywaters EGL, Damielli JF, et al: Treatment of systemic lupus erythematosus with steroids. Report to the Medical Research Council by the Collagen Diseases and Hypersensitivity Panel. BMJ 1961; 5257:915–920.
2. Posnick J: Systemic lupus erythematosus: The effect of corticotropin and adrenocorticoid therapy on survival rate. CA Med 1963; 98:308–312.
3. Jessar RA, Lamont-Havers W, Ragan C: Natural history of lupus erythematosus disseminatus. Ann Intern Med 1953; 38:717–731.
4. Harvey AM, Shulman LE, Tumulty PA, et al: Systemic lupus erythematosus: Review of the literature and clinical analysis of 138 cases. Medicine (Baltimore) 1954; 33:291–437.
5. Ropes MW: Observations on the natural course of disseminated lupus erythematosus. Medicine (Baltimore) 1964; 43:387–391.
6. Wallace DJ, Dubois EL: Dubois' Lupus Erythematosus, 3rd ed. Philadelphia: Lea & Febiger, 1987.
7. Reveille JS, Bartolucci A, Alarcón GS: Prognosis in systemic lupus erythematosus: Negative impact of increasing age at onset, black race, and thrombocytopenia, as well as causes of death. Arthritis Rheum 1990; 33:37–48.
8. Uramoto KM, Michet CJJ, Thumboo J, et al: Trends in the incidence and mortality of systemic lupus erythematosus, 1950–1992. Arthritis Rheum 1999; 42:46–50.
9. Dubois EL: Systemic lupus erythematosus: Recent advances in its diagnosis and treatment. Ann Intern Med 1956; 45:163–184.
10. Petri M, Conroy M, Caffentzis E, et al: The evolution of systemic lupus erythematosus (SLE) [Abstract]. Arthritis Rheum 1993; 36(suppl 9):S274.
11. Petri M, Genovese M, Engle E, et al: Definition, incidence and clinical description of flare in systemic lupus erythematosus: A prospective cohort study. Arthritis Rheum 1991; 34:937–944.
12. Kelley WN, Harris ED, Ruddy S, et al: Textbook of Rheumatology, 4th ed. Philadelphia: WB Saunders, 1993.
13. Dubois EL: Ibuprofen for systemic lupus erythematosus [Letter]. N Eng J Med 1975; 293:779.
14. Dubois EL: Management of systemic lupus erythematosus. Modern Treatment 1966; 3:1245–1279.
15. Marmont AM, Damasio E: The place of indomethacin in the treatment of SLE. Atti del Simposio Internazionale su Recenti Acquisizioni nella Terapia Antireumatica nonsteroidea. Minerva Med 1965; 219–258.
16. Goldman L, Cole DP, Preston RH: Chloroquine diphosphate in treatment of discoid lupus erythematosus. JAMA 1953; 152:1428–1429.
17. Mullins JF, Watts FL, Wilson CJ: Plaquenil in the treatment of lupus erythematosus. JAMA 1956; 161:879–881.
18. Ziff M, Esserman P, McEwen C: Observations on the course and treatment of systemic lupus erythematosus. Arthritis Rheum 1958; 1:332–350.

19. Lewis HM, Frumess GM: Plaquenil in the treatment of discoid lupus erythematosus. Arch Dermatol 1956; 73:576–581.

20. Jansen GT, Dillaha CJ, Honeycutt WM: Discoid lupus erythematosus: Is systemic treatment necessary. Arch Dermatol 1965; 92:283–285.

21. Callen JP: Chronic cutaneous lupus erythematosus. Arch Dermatol 1982; 118:412–416.

22. Rowell NR: Treatment of chronic discoid lupus erythematosus with intralesional triamcinolone. Br J Dermatol 1962; 74:354–357.

23. Dubois EL: Prednisone and prednisolone in the treatment of systemic lupus erythematosus. JAMA 1956; 161:427–433.

24. Ropes MW: Systemic Lupus Erythematosus. Cambridge, MA: Harvard University Press, 1976.

25. Ballou SP, Kahn MA, Kushner I: Intravenous pulse methylprednisolone followed by alternate day corticosteroid therapy in lupus erythematosus: A prospective evaluation. J Rheumatol 1985; 12:944–948.

26. Walton J, Watson BS, Ney RL: Alternate-day vs shorter-interval steroid administration. Arch Intern Med 1970; 126:601–607.

27. Davies UM, Ansell BM: Central nervous system manifestations in juvenile systemic lupus erythematosus: A problem of management. J Rheumatol 1988; 15:1720–1721.

28. Lurie DP, Kahaleh MB: Pulse corticosteroid therapy for refractory thrombocytopenia in systemic lupus erythematosus. J Rheumatol 1982; 9:311–314.

29. Oto A, Sozen T, Boyacioglu S: Pulsed methylprednisolone [Letter]. Ann Rheum Dis 1981; 40:630–631.

30. Isenberg DA, Morrow WJW, Snaith ML: Methylprednisolone pulse therapy in the treatment of systemic lupus erythematosus. Ann Rheum Dis 1982; 41:347–351.

31. Levitt JI: Deterioration of renal function after discontinuation of long-term prednisone-azathioprine therapy in primary renal disease. N Engl J Med 1970; 282:1125–1127.

32. Drinkard JP, Stanley TM, Dornfeld L, et al: Azathioprine and prednisone in the treatment of adults with lupus nephritis. Medicine (Baltimore) 1970; 49:411–432.

33. Cade R, Spooner G, Schlein E, et al: Comparison of azathioprine, prednisone, and heparin alone or combined in treating lupus nephritis. Nephron 1973; 10:37–56.

34. Donadio Jr JV, Holley KE, Wagoner RD, et al: Treatment of lupus nephritis with prednisone and combined prednisone and azathioprine. Ann Intern Med 1972; 77:829–835.

35. Carette S, Klippel JH, Decker JL, et al: Controlled studies on oral immunosuppressive drugs in lupus nephritis: A long term follow-up. Ann Intern Med 1983; 99:1–8.

36. Tsokos GC, Caughman SW, Klippel JH: Successful treatment of generalized discoid skin lesions with azathioprine. Arch Dermatol 1985; 121:1323–1325.

37. Shehade S: Successful treatment of generalized discoid skin lesions with azathioprine [Letter]. Arch Dermatol 1986; 122:376–377.

38. Boumpas DT, Barez S, Klippel JH, et al: Intermittent cyclophosphamide for the treatment of autoimmune thrombocytopenia in systemic lupus erythematosus. Ann Intern Med 1990; 112:674–677.

39. Schulz EJ, Menter MA: Treatment of discoid and subacute lupus erythematosus with cyclophosphamide. Br J Dermatol 1971; 86 (suppl 7):60–65.

40. Fricchione GL, Kaufman LD, Gruber BL, et al: Electroconvulsive therapy and cyclophosphamide in combination for severe neuropsychiatric lupus with catatonia. Am J Med 1990; 88:442–443.

41. Kono DH, Klashman DJ, Gilbert RC: Successful IV pulse cyclophosphamide in refractory PM in 3 patients with SLE [Letter]. J Rheumatol 1990; 17:982–983.

42. Euler HH, Schroeder JO, Harten P, et al: Treatment-free remission in severe systemic lupus erythematosus following synchronization of plasmapheresis with subsequent pulse cyclophosphamide. Arthritis Rheum 1994; 37:1784–1794.

43. Wallace DJ, Goldfinger D, Pepkowitz SH, et al: Randomized controlled trial of pulse/synchronization cyclophosphamide/apheresis for proliferative lupus nephritis. J Clin Apheresis 1998; 13:163–166.

44. Martin-Suarez I, D'Cruz D, Mansoor M, et al: Immunosuppressive treatment in severe connective tissue diseases: Effects of low dose intravenous cyclophosphamide. Ann Rheum Dis 1997; 56:481–487.

45. Brodsky RA, Petri M, Smith BD, et al: Immunoblative high-dose cyclophosphamide without stem cell rescue for refractory, severe autoimmune disease. Ann Intern Med 1998; 129:1031–1035.

46. Miescher PA, Riethmüller D: Diagnosis and treatment of systemic lupus erythematosus. Semin Hematol 1965; 2:1–28.

47. Rothenberg RJ, Graziano GM, Grandone JT, et al: The use of methotrexate in steroid-resistant systemic lupus erythematosus. Arthritis Rheum 1988; 31:612–615.

48. Arfi S, Numeric P, Grollier L, et al: [Treatment of corticodependent systemic lupus erythematosus with low-dose methotrexate]. Rev Med Interne 1995; 16:885–890.

49. Wise CM, Vuyyuru S, Roberts WN: Methotrexate in nonrenal lupus and undifferentiated connective tissue disease—A review of 36 patients. J Rheumatol 1996; 23:1005–1010.

50. Gansauge S, Breitbart A, Rinaldi N, et al: Methotrexate in patients with moderate systemic lupus erythematosus (exclusion of renal and central nervous system disease). Ann Rheum Dis 1997; 56:382–385.

51. Kipen Y, Littlejohn GO, Morand EF: Methotrexate use in systemic lupus erythematosus. Lupus 1997; 6:385–389.

52. Boehm IB, Boehm GA, Bauer R: Management of cutaneous lupus erythematosus with low-dose methotrexate: indication for modulation of inflammatory mechanisms. Rheumatol Int 1998; 18:59–62.

53. Caccavo D, Lagana B, Mitterhofer AP, et al: Long-term treatment of systemic lupus erythematosus with cyclosporin A. Arthritis Rheum 1997; 40:27–35.

54. Manager K, Kalden JR, Manger B: Cyclosporin A in the treatment of systemic lupus erythematosus: Results of an open clinical study. Br J Rheumatol 1996; 35:669–675.

55. Wallace DJ, Goldfinger D, Nichols S, et al: A controlled study on the use of plasmapheresis in steroid/immunosuppressive resistant systemic lupus erythematosus with nephrotic syndrome. In Uda T, Shiokawa Y, Inoue N (eds). Proceedings of the First International Congress of the World Apheresis Association. Cleveland: ISAO Press, 1987; 91–102.

56. Schlansky R, Dettoratius RJ, Pincus T, et al: Plasmapheresis in systemic lupus erythematosus: A cautionary note. Arthritis Rheum 1981; 24:49–53.

57. Verrier-Jones J, Cumming RH, Bacon PA, et al: Evidence for a therapeutic effect of plasmapheresis in patients with SLE. Q J Med 1979; 48:535–576.

58. Spiva DA, Cecere FA: The use of combination plasmapheresis/leukocytapheresis in the treatment of refractory systemic lupus erythematosus. Plasma Ther Trans Tech 1983; 4:151–164.

59. Buyon JP, Swersky SH, Fox HE, et al: Intrauterine therapy for presumptive fetal myocarditis with acquired heart block due to systemic lupus erythematosus: Experience in a mother with a predominance of SS-B (La) antibodies. Arthritis Rheum 1987; 30:44–49.

60. Fullcher D, Stewart G, Exner T, et al: Plasma exchange and the anticardiolipin syndrome in pregnancy. Lancet 1989; 2:171.

61. Kater L, Derksen RHWM, Houwert DA, et al: Effect of plasmapheresis in active systemic lupus erythematosus. Neth J Med 1981; 24:209–216.

62. Howard RF, Maier WP, Gordon DS, et al: Clinical and immunological investigation of intravenous human immunoglobulin (IVIG) therapy in SLE-associated thrombocytopenia [Abstract]. Arthritis Rheum 1989; 32:S75.

63. Gaedicke G, Teller WM, Kohne E, et al: IgG therapy in systemic lupus erythematosus: Two case reports. Blut 1984; 48:387–390.

64. Maier WP, Gordon DS, Howard RF, et al: Intravenous immunoglobulin therapy in systemic lupus erythematosus-associated thrombocytopenia. Arthritis Rheum 1990; 33:1233–1239.

65. Katz VL, Thorp JM Jr, Watson WJ, et al: Human immunoglobulin therapy for preeclampsia associated with lupus anticoagulant and anticardiolipin antibody. Obstet Gynecol 1990; 76:986–988.

66. Carreras LO, Pérez GN, Vega HR, et al: Lupus anticoagulant and recurrent fetal loss: Successful treatment with gammaglobulin. Lancet 1988; 2:393–394.

67. Ballow M, Parke A: The uses of intravenous immune globulin in collagen vascular disorders. J Allergy Clin Immunol 1989; 84:608–612.

68. Akashi K, Nagasawa K, Mayumi T, et al: Successful treatment of refractory systemic lupus erythematosus with intravenous immunoglobulins. J Rheumatol 1990; 17:375–379.

69. Lin RY, Racis SP: In vivo reduction of circulating C1q binding immune complexes by intravenous gammaglobulin administration. Int Arch Allergy Appl Immunol 1986; 79:286–290.

70. Petersen HH, Nielsen H, Hansen M, et al: High-dose immunoglobulin therapy in pericarditis caused by SLE [Letter]. Scand J Rheumatol 1990; 19:91–93.

71. Van Vollenhoven RF, Morabito LM, Engleman EG, et al: Treatment of systemic lupus erythematosus with dehydroepiandrosterone: 50 patients treated up to 12 months. J Rheumatol 1998; 25:285–289.

72. McMurray RW, Weidensaul D, Allen SH, et al: Efficacy of bromocriptine in an open label therapeutic trial for systemic lupus erythematosus. J Rheumatol 1995; 22:2084–2091.

73. Schachna L, Ryan PF, Schwarer AP: Malignancy-associated remission of systemic lupus erythematosus maintained by autologous peripheral blood stem cell transplantation. Arthritis Rheum 1998; 41:2271–2272.

74. Burt RK, Traynor AE, Pope R, et al: Treatment of autoimmune disease by intense immunosuppressive conditioning and autologous hematopoietic stem cell transplantation. Blood 1998; 92:3505–3514.

75. Karsh J, Kimberly RA, Stahl NI, et al: Comparative effects of aspirin and ibuprofen in the management of systemic lupus erythematosus. Arthritis Rheum 1980; 23:1401–1404.

76. Christiansen JV, Nielsen JP: Treatment of lupus erythematosus with mepacrine: Results and relapses during a long observation. Br J Dermatol 1956; 65:73–87.

77. Buchanan R Jr, King H, Hamilton CM: Quinacrine in discoid lupus erythematosus. South Med J 1954; 47:678–683.

78. Rudnicki RD, Gresham GE, Rothfield NF: The efficacy of antimalarials in systemic lupus erythematosus. J Rheumatol 1975; 2:323–330.

79. Rothfield N: Efficacy of antimalarials in systemic lupus erythematosus. Am J Med 1988; 85 (suppl 4A):53–56.

80. Canadian Hydroxychloroquine Study Group: A randomized study of the effect of withdrawing hydroxychloroquine sulfate in systemic lupus erythematosus. N Engl J Med 1991; 324:150–154.

81. Tsakonas E, Joseph L, Esdaile JM, et al: A long-term study of hydroxychloroquine withdrawal on exacerbations in systemic lupus erythematosus. The Canadian Hydroxychloroquine Study Group. Lupus 1998; 7:80–85.

82. Levy RA, Jesus NR, Vilela V, et al: Hydroxychloroquine (HCQ) in lupus pregnancy: Double-blind placebo controlled study. Arthritis Rheum 1998; 41:S241.

83. Edwards JCW, Snaith ML, Isenberg DA: A double blind controlled trial of methylprednisolone infusions in systemic lupus erythematosus using individualized outcome assessment. Ann Rheum Dis 1987; 46:773–776.

84. Mackworth-Young CG, David J, Morgan SH, et al: A double blind, placebo controlled trial of intravenous methylprednisolone in systemic lupus erythematosus. Ann Rheum Dis 1988; 47:496–502.

85. Sztejnbok M, Stewart A, Diamond H, et al: Azathioprine in the treatment of systemic lupus erythematosus: A controlled study. Arthritis Rheum 1971; 14:639–645.

86. Sharon E, Kaplan D, Diamond HS: Exacerbation of systemic lupus erythematosus after withdrawal of azathioprine therapy. N Engl J Med 1973; 288:122–124.

87. Hahn BH, Kantor OS, Osterland CK: Azathioprine plus prednisone compared with prednisone alone in the treatment of systemic lupus erythematosus. Ann Intern Med 1975; 83:597–605.

88. Rahman P, Humphrey-Murto S, Gladman DD, et al: Efficacy and tolerability of methotrexate in antimalarial resistant lupus arthritis. J Rheumatol 1998; 25:243–246.

89. Fries JF, Sharp GC, McDevitt HO, et al: Cyclophosphamide therapy in systemic lupus erythematosus and polymyositis. Arthritis Rheum 1973; 16:154–162.

90. van Vollenhoven RF, Engleman EG, McGuire JL: Dehydroepiandrosterone in systemic lupus erythematosus: Results of a double-blind, placebo-controlled, randomized clinical trial. Arthritis Rheum 1995; 38:1826–1831.

91. Petri M, Lahita R, McGuire J, et al: Results of the GL701 (DHEA) multicenter steroid-sparing SLE study. Arthritis Rheum 1997; 40(suppl 9):S327.

92. Studenski S, Allen NB, Caldwell DS, et al: Survival in systemic lupus erythematosus: A multivariate analysis of demographic factors. Arthritis Rheum 1987; 30:1326–1332.

93. Ginzler EM, Diamond HS, Weiner M, et al: A multicenter study of outcome in systemic lupus erythematosus: I. Entry variables as predictors of prognosis. Arthritis Rheum 1982; 25:601–611.

94. Petri M, Howard D, Repke J, et al: The Hopkins Lupus Pregnancy Center: 1987–1991 update. Am J Reprod Immunol 1992; 28:188–191.

95. Simonson JS, Schiller NB, Petri M, et al: Pulmonary hypertension in systemic lupus erythematosus. J Rheumatol 1989; 16:918–925.

96. Stahl NI, Klippel JH, Decker JL: Fever in systemic lupus erythematosus. Am J Med 1979; 67:935–940.

97. Sibai BM, Caritis SN, Thom E, et al: Prevention of preeclampsia with low-dose aspirin in healthy, nulliparous pregnant women. The National Institute of Child Health and Human Development Network of Maternal-Fetal Medicine Units. N Engl J Med 1993; 329:1213–1218.

98. Norton ME, Merrill J, Cooper BAB, et al: Neonatal complications after the administration of indomethacin for preterm labor. N Engl J Med 1993; 329:1602–1607.

99. Levy M, Buskila D, Gladman DD, et al: Pregnancy outcome following first trimester exposure to chloroquine. Am J Perinatol 1991; 8:174–178.

100. Parke AL: Antimalarial drugs, systemic lupus erythematosus and pregnancy. J Rheumatol 1988; 15:607–610.

101. Cowchock FS, Reece EA, Balaban D, et al: Repeated fetal losses associated with antiphospholipid antibodies: A collaborative randomized trial comparing prednisone with low-dose heparin treatment. Am J Obstet Gynecol 1992; 166:1318–1323.

102. Rosove MH, Brewer PMC: Antiphospholipid thrombosis: Clinical course after the first thrombotic event in 70 patients. Ann Intern Med 1992; 117:303–308.

103. Derksen RHWM, de Groot PG, Kater L, et al: Patients with antiphospholipid antibodies and venous thrombosis should receive long term anticoagulant treatment. Ann Rheum Dis 1993; 52:689–692.

104. Khamashta MA, Cuadrado MJ, Mujic F, et al: The management of thrombosis in the antiphospholipid antibody syndrome. N Engl J Med 1995; 332:993–997.

105. Petri M, Howard D, Goldman DW: Side-effects of medications prescribed for systemic lupus erythematosus [Abstract]. Arthritis Rheum 1992; 35:S358.

106. Easterbrook M: Useful and diagnostic tests in the detection of early chloroquine retinopathy [Abstract]. Arthritis Rheum 1989; 32:R8.

107. Morsman CD, Livesey SJ, Richards IM, et al: Screening for hydroxychloroquine retinal toxicity: Is it necessary? Eye 1990; 4:572–576.

108. Bernstein HN: Ophthalmologic considerations and testing in patients receiving long-term antimalarial therapy. Am J Med 1983; 75 (suppl 1A):25–34.

109. Petri M, Lakatta C, Magder L, et al: Effect of prednisone and hydroxychloroquine on coronary artery disease risk factors in systemic lupus erythematosus: A longitudinal data analysis. Am J Med 1994; 96:254–259.

110. Arden NK, Lloyd M, Spector TD, et al: The safety of estrogen replacement therapy (ERT) in systemic lupus erythematosus [Abstract]. Arthritis Rheum 1993; 36(suppl 9):S64.

110a. Krauss RM, Deckelbaum RJ, Ernst D, et al: Dietary guidelines for healthy American adults. Circulation 1996; 94:1795–1800.

111. Ginzler E, Feldman D, Giovaniello G, et al: The association of cervical neoplasia (CN) and SLE [Abstract]. Arthritis Rheum 1989; 32(suppl 4):S30.

112. Abramson S, Weissmann G: The mechanisms of action of nonsteroidal antiinflammatory drugs. Clin Exp Rheumatol 1989; 7:S163–S170.

113. Kimberly RF, Bowden RE, Keiser HR, et al: Reduction of renal function by newer nonsteroidal antiinflammatory drugs. Am J Med 1978; 64:804.

114. Carr RE, Gouras P, Gunkel RD: Chloroquine retinopathy: Early detection by retinal threshold test. Arch Ophthalmol 1966; 75:171–178.

115. MacKenzie A: Dose refinements in long-term therapy of rheumatoid arthritis with antimalarials. Am J Med 1983; 75: 40–45.

116. Legros J, Rosner I, Berger C: Influence du niveau d'eclairement ambiant sur les modifications oculaires induites par l'hydroxychloroquine chez le rat. Arch Ophthalmol 1973; 33:417–424.

117. McChesney EW: Animal toxicity and pharmacokinetics of hydroxychloroquine sulfate. Am J Med 1983; 75:11–18.

118. Shaffer B, Cahn MM, Levy EJ: Absorption of antimalarial drugs in human skin: Spectroscopic and chemical analysis in epidermis and corium. J Invest Dermatol 1958; 30:341–345.

119. Tuffanelli DL, Abraham RK, Dubois EL: Pigmentation associated with antimalarial therapy: Its possible relation to ocular lesions. Arch Dermatol 1963; 88:419–426.

120. Fox RI, Kang H-I: Mechanism of action of antimalarial drugs: Inhibition of antigen processing and presentation. Lupus 1993; 2(suppl 1):S9–S12.

121. Dubois EL: Antimalarials in the management of discoid and systemic lupus erythematosus. Semin Arthritis Rheum 1978; 8:33–51.

122. Danowski TS, Bonessi JV, Sabeh G, et al: Probabilities of pituitary adrenal responsiveness after steroid therapy. Ann Intern Med 1964; 61:11–26.

123. Jones CJP, Morris KJ, Jayson MIV: Prednisolone inhibits phagocytosis by polymorphonuclear leukocytes via steroid receptor-mediated events. Ann Rheum Dis 1983; 42:56–62.

124. Rinehart JJ, Sagone AL, Balcerzak SP, et al: Effects of corticosteroid therapy on human monocyte function. N Engl J Med 1975; 292:236–241.

125. Glicklich D, Acharya A: Mycophenolate mofetil therapy for lupus nephritis refractory to intravenous cyclophosphamide. Am J Kidney Dis 1998; 32:318–322.

126. Weisman MH, Bluestein HG, Berner CM, et al: Reduction in circulating dsDNA antibody titer after administration of LJP 394. J Rheumatol 1997; 24:314–318.

127. Rogers J, Finn OA: Synthetic antimalarial drugs in chronic discoid lupus erythematosus and light eruptions. Arch Dermatol Syphilol 1954; 70:61–66.

128. Pillsbury DM, Jacobson C: Treatment of chronic discoid lupus erythematosus with chloroquine (Aralen). J Am Med Assoc 1954; 154:1330–1333.

129. Cornbleet T: Discoid lupus erythematosus treatment with Plaquenil. Arch Dermatol 1956; 73:572–575.

130. Ponticelli C, Tarantino A, Pioltelli P, et al: High-dose methylprednisolone pulses in active lupus nephritis [Letter]. Lancet 1977; 1:1063.

131. Dosa S, Cairns SA, Lawler W, et al: The treatment of lupus nephritis by methylprednisolone pulse therapy. Postgrad Med J 1978; 54:628–632.

132. Eyanson S, Passo MH, Aldo-Benson MA, et al: Methylprednisolone pulse therapy for nonrenal lupus erythematosus. Ann Rheum Dis 1980; 39:377–380.

133. Fessel JW: Megadose corticosteroid therapy in systemic lupus erythematosus. J Rheumatol 1980; 7:486–500.

134. Goldberg JW, Lidsky MD: Pulse methylprednisolone therapy for persistent subacute cutaneous lupus [Letter]. Arthritis Rheum 1984; 27:837–838.

135. Ruzicka T, Sommerburg C, Goerz G, et al: Treatment of cutaneous lupus erythematosus with acitretin and hydroxychloroquine. Br J Dermatol 1992; 127:513–518.

CHAPTER

# 24 | Antiphospholipid Syndrome

*Ann L. Parke*

## INTRODUCTION AND NATURAL HISTORY

*Antiphospholipid* (APL) *syndrome,* like its predecessor, the lupus anticoagulant, is something of a misnomer. In 1952 Conley and Hartman recognized a phenomenon occurring in patients with systemic lupus erythematosus (SLE) that resulted in the prolongation of normal tests of coagulation, an apparent anticoagulant.[1] In 1977, Feinstein and Rapaport called this factor *lupus anticoagulant,*[2] and it was subsequently shown that these anticoagulants (1) were associated with a biologically falsely positive test for syphilis,[3] (2) were caused by an antibody directed at phospholipids,[4] (3) occurred frequently in patients who did not have SLE,[5] and (4) paradoxically predisposed patients to thrombosis.[6,7]

The APL syndrome may occur in patients who also fulfill criteria for well-defined connective tissue diseases such as SLE, rheumatoid arthritis, or systemic sclerosis, or it may occur alone, in which case it is known as *primary antiphospholipid syndrome.*[8,9] The current definition of APL syndrome includes the presence of antibodies to negatively charged phospholipids (antibodies to cardiolipin, a lupus anticoagulant, or both) and clinical complaints that include venous or arterial thromboses, recurrent fetal loss, and/or thrombocytopenia.[10,11]

Venous and arterial thromboses manifest in a variety of ways (Table 24–1), and in some patients with APL they appear to be triggered by pathologic and physiologic events, resulting in what has become known as the *second hit phenomenon*[12,13] (Table 24–2). Thrombocytopenia does not prevent thrombosis in these patients, and therefore the disease can be extremely difficult to manage.

The APL syndrome is a misnomer because these antibodies are not directed only at negatively charged phospholipids; rather, they are primarily directed at protein-phospholipid complexes.[14,15] $\beta_2$-glycoprotein I (Apolipoprotein H), a natural anticoagulant, appears to be a protein cofactor necessary for enhancing antigen binding for some of these phospholipid antibodies.[14,15] Immunization of animals with $\beta_2$-glycoprotein I has resulted in the production of antibodies to $\beta_2$-glycoprotein I, antibodies to negatively charged phospholipids, and a constellation of clinical manifestations that mirror the human disease.[16,17]

Since the publication of the first reports identifying the association between antibodies to negatively charged phospholipids and a prothrombotic state, the precise nature of this thrombotic diathesis has still not been determined. Animal studies reproducing human clinical disease after active immunization with $\beta_2$-glycoprotein I[16,17] or passive immunization with phospholipid antibodies[18,19] suggest that the antibodies themselves are directly involved in the pathogenesis of the thrombotic events. However, even though APL may occur in patients with systemic autoimmune inflammatory diseases (e.g., SLE), the pathology of the APL syndrome is a noninflammatory, widespread, bland thrombotic process.[20,21] Epidemiologic studies have suggested that APL occurs rarely in "normal" individuals,[22–24] whereas approximately 30% of SLE patients produce these antibodies.[25,26] The level of APL may vary in SLE patients,[27] but it has been our experience that APL levels are fairly consistent in patients with primary disease.

The natural history of APL-positive patients is that only some develop clinical thromboses, thereby fulfilling criteria for the syndrome. It has been shown that fewer than 50% of APL-positive SLE patients and 31% of all APL patients ever experience thrombosis.[28] Several other studies have suggested that only about 50% of patients with a history of a previous thrombosis and known APL syndrome experience rethrombosis[29,30]; furthermore, approximately 76% of those patients who initially experienced a venous thrombosis sustain another, and 93% of those who have had an arterial event have another arterial event if rethrombosis occurs.[29] The reason for this selective pattern of thrombosis is unknown. The factors that determine which patients undergo rethrombose and the triggers for clinical thrombotic events need to be elucidated further, but they may be personal to each patient. Current evidence suggests that genetic variations of factor V or prothrombin are not more common in APL patients.[31]

The first reports of fetal wastage in mothers who had circulating anticoagulants appeared in the mid-1950s and have been confirmed by many subsequent reports.[32–35] Recurrent fetal loss is one of the most emotionally distressing aspects of the APL syndrome, because these are frequently late fetal losses and pathologic studies have revealed that the fetuses are usually normal. It appears that fetal wastage is a consequence

289

## TABLE 24–1
## Clinical Manifestations of APL Syndrome

Recurrent fetal loss
Thrombocytopenia
Hemolytic anemia
Central nervous system involvement
    Multifocal infarct dementia
    Seizures
    Sudden vision loss
    Chorea
    Demyelinating syndromes
Other organ involvement
    Multiple organ ischemia and infarction including leg ulcers and
        livido reticularis
    Venous thrombosis and embolism
    Mitral valve prolapse
    Toxemia of pregnancy

of an inadequate, thrombosed placenta that can sustain the pregnancy only for a limited time.[36, 37] To make matters worse, these patients experience *recurrent* fetal wastage[38] and some never successfully complete a pregnancy.

This chapter addresses several aspects of the management of APL syndrome, including recurrent fetal wastage and recurrent clinical thrombotic events in the arterial and venous systems. Patients who also have a systemic inflammatory connective tissue disease (i.e., SLE) appear to be at risk for rethromboses during flares of their disease,[39, 40] so controlling SLE disease is an important factor in preventing thrombosis in these patients. Other prothrombotic states, such as elective surgery, infection, pregnancy, and exogenous estrogens, are triggers that frequently result in clinical thrombosis in APL patients[13, 40–42] (see Table 24–2) and therefore need to be avoided or managed appropriately (e.g., no exogenous estrogens, perioperative and antepartum or postpartum anticoagulation).

## Open Trials

In 1983, Lubbe and associates published a report describing six women, each with recurrent fetal wastage and a lupus anticoagulant. None had successfully completed pregnancy, but five of the six produced a live infant after they were treated with aspirin and high-dose prednisone to suppress the production of lupus

## TABLE 24–2
## Pathologic and Physiologic States Capable of Triggering Clinical Thrombosis in Patients with APL Syndrome

Pregnancy
Postpartum status
Exogenous estrogens
Elective surgery
Infections
Flares of inflammatory disease (i.e., systemic lupus
    erythematosus)

anticoagulant.[35] This paper set the stage for a treatment regimen for recurrent fetal wastage in patients with APL. Subsequent reports addressed combinations of immunosuppressive therapy and anticoagulation,[43–46] confirming the benefits of some of these therapies[45] but also concluding that fetal loss still occurred despite treatment and that pre-eclampsia, impaired fetal growth, and premature delivery occurred commonly in APL patients.[46] Aspirin alone was shown to be an effective therapy,[47] with the added benefit that it can be started prophylactically when pregnancy is anticipated.[48] The use of subcutaneous heparin in 14 APL-positive women with a total of 28 previous fetal losses was found to reduce placental infarcts, and 14 of 15 subsequent pregnancies with heparin therapy resulted in live births.[49]

It has been concluded that steroids alone are not effective at preventing thrombosis in APL-positive patients,[50] but, even so, high-dose prednisone became the "standard of care" for APL-positive patients with fetal wastage. Several reports addressing the benefits of corticosteroids and oral anticoagulants in preventing cerebral ischemic attacks have demonstrated that recurrent strokes still occur.[51, 52]

## Controlled Clinical Trials

There have been virtually no prospective, randomized, controlled trials addressing the management of APL syndrome. This oversight can probably be attributed to the early retrospective case studies that suggested that the risk of recurrent cerebral ischemic events in young, untreated patients with APL syndrome was 14% per year[53] and that recurrent fetal wastage could be prevented by treatments that combined some form of anticoagulation with prednisone.[35, 45] These reports gave rise to a great reluctance to enroll patients in placebo-controlled studies, so that the prospective studies that have been done have compared different treatment regimens.

Some of the earliest controlled studies addressed the use of prednisone in patients with recurrent fetal wastage and concluded that, because these patients were at particular risk for preterm birth and toxemia of pregnancy, high doses of prednisone only made a bad situation worse.[54, 55] It was also demonstrated that APL comprised a family of antibodies that could be suppressed at different rates by the use of prednisone,[56, 57] and it is now known that some patients can successfully complete pregnancy despite high levels of APL.[57, 58]

Two studies have compared aspirin alone versus aspirin and heparin in APL syndrome patients with recurrent fetal wastage. Rai and colleagues conducted a randomized, controlled trial to compare aspirin (75 mg) and aspirin with heparin (5000 units twice daily) in APL-positive women with three or more consecutive losses. This study excluded women who had had a previous clinical thrombotic event, because of their requirement for full-dose heparin throughout pregnancy. Seventy-one percent of the pregnancies treated with aspirin and heparin resulted in a live birth, compared with 42% of those receiving only aspirin (odds ratio, 3.37).[59] More than 90% of the miscarriages in this study occurred in the first trimester, which is not typical for APL fetal wastage; of the 45 women in each treatment group, 31 of those receiving aspirin alone and 29 of those receiving aspirin and heparin had experienced *only* first-trimester losses, raising the question of alternative reasons for recurrent fetal wastage in these subjects. An earlier study by Kutteh had reached a similar conclusion, with 44% of subjects given aspirin alone and 80% of these given aspirin and heparin successfully completing pregnancy ($P < .05$). In that study, women with lupus anticoagulant were excluded and heparin dosages were adjusted to maintain the partial thromboplastin time (PTT) at 1.5 times baseline, with the maximum heparin dosage being 20,000 units twice daily.[60]

## Long-Term Experience

Several retrospective studies addressing long-term thrombosis-free survival in APL-positive patients have concluded that the only adequate therapy is lifelong high-dose oral anticoagulation producing International Normalized Ratios (INRs) of 3 or higher.[29, 30, 61, 62] In 1991, Asherson and colleagues reported a 5-year follow-up study of 19 APL syndrome patients who had sustained clinical thrombotic events (10 arterial, 7 venous, and 2 both venous and arterial); they concluded that only INRs greater than 3 were effective at preventing rethrombosis.[61] One year later, Rosove and Brewer retrospectively studied 70 APL syndrome patients who had experienced a clinical thrombotic event (39 venous, 31 arterial). Thirty-seven patients had 54 recurrent thrombotic events. The mean follow-up period was 5.2 years, and a comparison of treatment regimens (i.e., no treatment, aspirin, high-dose and low-dose anticoagulation) revealed that only high-dose anticoagulation was effective at preventing rethrombosis.[29]

In another retrospective, long-term follow-up study (median, 93 months) Derksen and associates, studying 19 patients with an initial venous thrombotic event, determined that 12 patients (63%) experienced a second clinical thrombosis and concluded that the probability for recurrence of thrombosis was zero with anticoagulation but rose to 50% in 2 years and 78% in 5 years for those not taking anticoagulants.[62]

In 1995, a retrospective study of 147 APL syndrome patients, with a median follow-up period of 6.0 years, revealed that 69% had a recurrent thrombotic event. This paper by Khamashta and coworkers also revealed that high-dose anticoagulation (INR greater than 3) was significantly more effective at preventing recurrent thrombosis than low-dose warfarin, and patients were at greatest risk for rethrombosis in the first 6 months after discontinuing oral anticoagulation.[30] An editorial in the same issue stated that high-dose oral anticoagulation should be considered the "standard of treatment" for APL syndrome patients who had experienced a major clinical thrombosis.[63]

The problem with this management strategy is that it considers all APL syndrome patients to be at equal risk for thrombosis and does not address the effect of "second hit" or prothrombotic triggers. It also assumes that the benefits of high-dose oral anticoagulation outweigh the complications, which are predominately abnormal bleeding.

## University of Connecticut Health Center Experience

At the University of Connecticut Health Center, we have a large collection of APL syndrome patients, including many who have experienced recurrent fetal wastage. A retrospective review was undertaken and was limited to 44 patients who had been monitored consistently at our institution for a minimum of 3 years, some for more than 20 years, none of whom had been routinely given high-dose anticoagulants. In this study, we divided treatment into five regimens: no treatment, low-dose aspirin, aspirin plus oral anticoagulants, oral anticoagulants alone, and aspirin with heparin. Patients receiving aspirin and heparin were usually pregnant. We analyzed these five treatment regimens with respect to the occurrence of either a thrombotic event or significant bleeding (i.e., life-threatening or requiring therapeutic intervention). Our study revealed that low-dose aspirin was equivalent to no treatment and that oral anticoagulation (INR less than 3) was effective at preventing rethrombosis in APL syndrome patients ($P < .003$). Even more significantly, only 54% of these patients ever experienced rethrombosis, and patients were at greater risk for a significant bleeding event than for a recurrent thrombosis if they received long-term anticoagulation ($P < .0001$).[64] The rate of significant bleeding events in these APL syndrome patients was 20.2% per year, which is considerably higher than is found in routine anticoagulant clinics.[64–66]

## AUTHOR'S PREFERENCE FOR MANAGEMENT

### Diagnosis of Antiphospholipid Syndrome

A patient with a clinically significant event (see Table 24–1) and more than one positive APL test probably has APL syndrome. The laboratory tests that need to be done to establish the diagnosis of APL syndrome include determination of cardiolipin antibodies and one of the many tests for detecting lupus anticoagulants. It has been suggested that the cardiolipin antibodies should be $\beta_2$-glycoprotein–dependent for patients to fulfill preliminary criteria for APL syndrome. Because this syndrome is part of the spectrum of autoimmune disease, other laboratory tests, including other antibody determinations, may help to delineate the extent of the problem (i.e., antinuclear antibody, extractable nuclear antibodies, anticentromere antibodies, direct and indirect Coombs' tests). It has also been our experience that other nonspecific tests may be useful, such as erythrocyte sedimentation rate, complement levels, and a platelet count. Two of our most severely affected patients, one with recurrent emboli and severe pulmonary hypertension and one with multifocal infarct dementia, have only a positive lupus anticoagulant result and an elevated erythrocyte sedimentation rate.

## Management for Pregnancy

### Primigravidas

For *primigravidas* who have never experienced a clinical thrombotic event and have a significantly elevated APL concentration, management usually consists of low-dose aspirin alone. Primigravidas with APL who have had a previous clinical thrombotic event are given full-dose anticoagulation (i.e., subcutaneous heparin at 10,000 units twice a day to increase the PTT to 1.5 times baseline and low-dose aspirin). If the PTT is prolonged as a result of the presence of a lupus anticoagulant, the patient is monitored by measuring levels of activated X, which is the equivalent of plasma heparin levels.[67]

### Multiparous Patients

Patients who have had previous fetal wastage that is considered to be significant for the APL syndrome (i.e., at more than 10 weeks' gestation)[68] and are positive for APL are given 5000 units of subcutaneous heparin twice a day if they have not had a previous clinical thrombotic event or 10,000 units twice a day if they have. These patients also take low-dose aspirin (Fig. 24–1). If these patients have had recurrent fetal wastage, then the dosage of heparin is increased to prolong the PPT to 1.5 times baseline. We routinely try to obtain previous placentas in order to examine the placental pathology; if this demonstrates significant thrombosis, the patient is given therapeutic doses of heparin (i.e., 10,000 units twice daily) rather than prophylactic doses (5000 units twice daily).

None of these patients is routinely treated with prednisone unless she also has SLE that is active and requires management with corticosteroids to control the underlying inflammatory disease. Heparin and corticosteroids are not a good combination and should be avoided if possible, because both drugs cause osteoporosis. Some patients taking this combination therapy may complain of muscle cramps and need calcium supplementation. In those multiparous patients for whom previous full-dose anticoagulation with subcutaneous heparin and low-dose aspirin has failed, we have tried other therapeutic parameters, including intravenous immune globulin (IVIG).[69] This is difficult to justify because of the expense and the results of our previous studies, which demonstrated that placental changes are still evident in patients despite the use of IVIG.[69, 70] However, IVIG should be considered as a treatment option in patients for whom other therapies have failed.

Some patients who fail to meet revised American Rheumatism Association criteria for SLE but who have

a lupus-like disease (LLD) may demonstrate inflammation in their placentas.[37] We have treated some of these patients with prednisone, but such patients are the exception rather than the rule.

## Management of Antiphospholipid Syndrome

Patients at the University of Connecticut Health Center are not routinely managed with high-dose anticoagulation, and patients with APL syndrome who have had a clinical thrombotic event are managed routinely with anticoagulation at the time of the thrombotic event. Patients with venous thromboses have Doppler studies done before anticoagulation is discontinued. Long-term management of these patients is then dictated by their previous history of thrombotic events and the association of a known triggering pathologic or physiologic event that may have precipitated the clinical thrombosis. If such a event can be identified and is a known trigger for this particular patient, then everything possible is done to avoid the same trigger. For example, patients are advised not to take oral contraceptives or exogenous estrogens, are told not to smoke, are anticoagulated perioperatively, or are anticoagulated for 6 weeks after delivery. Patients with APL syndrome who are planning vascular intervention studies (e.g., cardiac catheterization) or are scheduled for elective surgical procedures are advised to have periprocedure anticoagulation.

Patients who have had only one clinical thrombotic event and in whom a triggering factor can be identified are advised to take low-dose aspirin after the appropriate length of anticoagulation for their clinical event and given advice about avoiding triggering events. If they subsequently experience rethrombosis, the problem is discussed with the patient. It is explained that they have antibodies in their blood that could predispose them to rethrombosis and that it may be necessary to consider long-term anticoagulation (see Fig. 24–1). Patients with a history of an arterial thrombosis and an anatomic abnormality such as mitral valve prolapse, with an inherent risk for arterial embolization, are usually prescribed long-term anticoagulation and advised with regard to the potential for complications of this therapy. We routinely provide long-term anticoagulation sufficient to achieve an INR of 2.5 to 3. In the few cases in which this level has appeared to be inadequate, we have increased the INR and added low-dose aspirin. However, our more recent studies suggest that low-dose aspirin does not add any benefit.[64]

In patients who have catastrophic APL syndrome with thrombosis in multiple organs, treatment is very difficult.[71, 72] In such patients, if anticoagulation appears to fail, immune-modulating therapies (i.e., plasmapheresis and intravenous Cytoxan) have been used with some success.[71, 73] We have had very few of these patients. One patient with a flare of SLE as an initiating prothrombotic trigger eventually came under control with high-dose pulse corticosteroids.[40] A second patient with primary APL syndrome was eventually

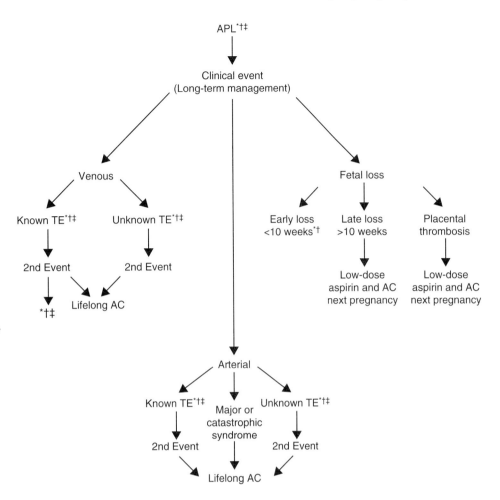

**FIGURE 24–1**
Management of antiphospholipid (APL) syndrome. TE = triggering events; AC = anticoagulation; APL = antiphospholipid. *Advise patient about avoiding triggering events (see Table 24–2). †Low-dose aspirin. (Although our recent data have suggested that low-dose aspirin may be no more effective than placebo, other reports suggest that it may be useful for patients with recurrent fetal wastage, even in the absence of APL syndrome.) ‡Hydroxychloroquine. (Whenever possible, we treat all patients with systemic lupus erythematosus who have APL syndrome with hydroxychloroquine.) Some variation from this scheme should be made based on (1) patient's wishes and (2) site of thrombotic event.

treated empirically with pulse steroids and subsequently improved.

Hydroxychloroquine may be of some benefit in that it is useful in preventing platelet aggregation,[74, 75] as well as controlling some aspects of disease activity in patients who have SLE.[76, 77] It therefore has dual benefit for patients with SLE and APL syndrome, in that it may prevent mild flares of SLE disease, which we now know can be a trigger for thrombosis in APL syndrome (see Table 24–2). We have even used this antimalarial drug in APL syndrome patients who did not meet criteria for SLE when control was difficult.

## Drug Side Effects and Monitoring

Several studies have addressed the risks of bleeding in patients given anticoagulants; rates have varied between 0.14 and 13.4 per 100 patient-years of treatment.[65, 66, 78–80] The problem of bleeding with high-dose anticoagulants has not been well studied in APL syndrome patients. Several of the retrospective studies of such patients have reported rates of major bleeding episodes,[30, 62] but this problem is quite complex because (1) some of these patients are demented from their multifocal cerebral infarctions and are at significant risk for falling, (2) many of these patients are young women who complain bitterly about the excessive bleeding they experience during their menses, and

(3) some of these patients are difficult to anticoagulate and require high doses of warfarin (Coumadin).

Khamashta and coworkers reported that bleeding occurred in 29 patients and was severe in 7. The rate of occurrence of bleeding for high-dose anticoagulation was 0.071 per patient-year of treatment; for low-dose anticoagulation it was 0.017 per patient-year.[30] A separate study addressing only the hemorrhagic complications of long-term anticoagulation in seven patients with SLE and APL syndrome described six episodes of subdural hematoma in five patients, one of pericarditis with tamponade, one of hemoptysis, and of ovarian hemorrhage. The INR was abnormally elevated in six of the nine bleeding episodes.[81] Our study showed that the risk of a hemorrhagic event was greater than the risk of a thrombotic event in patients given oral anticoagulants.[64] This finding is even more significant considering that it is our policy not to anticoagulate with INRs more than 3, and it suggests that, just as some APL patients appear to be predisposed to recurrent thrombosis, some may be predisposed to bleeding while anticoagulated. It is therefore important to monitor these patients closely and the educate them about the many drug interactions that can occur in patients taking anticoagulants.

Oral anticoagulation is the mainstay of treatment except during pregnancy. Coumadin derivatives can be safely given up to 6 weeks of gestation, but continued use during pregnancy has been associated with the fetal warfarin syndrome, which manifests with nasal hypoplasia and central nervous system defects.[82]

Some APL syndrome patients have protein S deficiency contributing to the pathogenesis of their thrombotic state.[83, 84] Protein C and protein S are natural vitamin K–dependent anticoagulant factors, and treatment with oral anticoagulation, which inhibits vitamin K, may lower the levels of these proteins still further, predisposing such patients to development of clinical thromboses. For this reason it is important that the level of free protein S be checked before commencement of oral anticoagulation, or that treatment with heparin be initiated first. Accurate levels of protein S cannot be obtained after a recent thrombotic event, because such an event lowers the protein S level; a more accurate result will be obtained 6 weeks after the thrombosis. Bleeding events occur less frequently with low-molecular-weight heparin that has to be given only once a day, which suggests that these preparations may be more useful than standard heparin in pregnant APL syndrome patients.[85] There is restricted use for low-molecular-weight heparin as a long-term therapy, because osteoporosis remains a major problem.[86]

### Clinical Pharmacology and Drug Interactions

Anticoagulation is the main therapeutic choice for patients with APL syndrome. How much anticoagulation and for how long are questions for debate, as explained earlier. Drug interactions with oral anticoagulants are numerous.[87]

Oral anticoagulants are vitamin K antagonists, so supplementation with vitamin K negates their effects. This means that patients must be warned not only about drug interactions but also about vitamin interactions and the effects of ''health food'' supplements, particularly *Ginkgo biloba,* which inhibits platelet aggregation.

### Investigational Drugs and Future Directions

IVIG has been shown to be very useful in the management of thrombocytopenia, and, because thrombocytopenia is a feature of the APL syndrome, IVIG has also been used in its management.[69, 88, 89] Several papers have suggested that it may be particularly useful during pregnancy for APL-positive mothers,[88, 89] although we have been disappointed by the persistence of typical APL placental pathology in some patients despite the use of IVIG.[70] We have found IVIG to be most useful for the APL syndrome patients who have a clinical thrombosis and thrombocytopenia simultaneously. Continued high doses of corticosteroids, IVIG, and cautious anticoagulation have worked well in these difficult cases.

Our most recent studies have suggested that low-dose aspirin is equivalent to no therapy in APL syndrome patients. There appears to be no benefit from other antiplatelet therapies, because they are no more efficacious than aspirin (except for hydroxychloroquine).[69] Other experimental treatments of APL syndrome that have been tried include the use of fish oils in humans[90] and recombinant interleukin-3 in animal models.[91]

Preliminary criteria for the diagnosis of definite APL syndrome have been established.[92] Validation of these criteria have determined a sensitivity of 0.71, specificity of 0.98, and positive predicted value and negative predicted value of 0.95 and 0.88, respectively.[93]

## SUMMARY

It has become increasingly clear that all APL-positive patients are not the same. Some appear to be predisposed to recurrent thrombosis, whereas others may never experience a clinical thrombosis. Similarly, some patients are predisposed to recurrent bleeding events when anticoagulated. Large numbers of randomized, controlled prospective studies need to be carried out. The conclusions from previous retrospective studies are that lifelong high-dose anticoagulation is essential to prevent rethrombosis in patients with APL. Our studies do not concur with these findings. We believe that high-dose lifelong anticoagulation is sometimes required but that therapy for each APL patient should be unique, determined by known triggering factors for thrombosis and the history of previous thrombotic events.

## REFERENCES

1. Conley CL, Hartman RC: A hemorrhagic disorder caused by circulating anticoagulant in patients with disseminated lupus erythematosus. J Lab Clin Invest 1952; 31:621–622.
2. Feinstein DI, Rapaport SI: Acquired inhibitors of blood coagulation. Prog Hemost Thromb 1972; 1:75–95.
3. Laurell AB, Nilsson IM: Hypergammaglobulinaemia, circulating anticoagulant, and biological false positive Wasserman reaction: A study of two cases. J Lab Clin Med 1957; 49:694–707.
4. Lee SL, Sanders MA: A disorder of blood coagulation in systemic lupus erythematosus. J Clin Invest 1955; 34;1814–1822.
5. Johansson EA, Lassus A: The occurrence of circulating anticoagulants in patients with syphilitic and biologically false positive antilipoidal antibodies. Ann Clin Res 1974; 6:105–108.
6. Bowie EJ, Thompson JH Jr, Pascuzzi CA, et al: Thrombosis in systemic lupus erythematosus despite circulating anticoagulants. J Lab Clin Med 1963; 62:416–430.
7. Mueh JR, Herbst KD, Rapaport SI: Thrombosis in patients with the lupus anticoagulant. Ann Intern Med 1980; 92:156–159.
8. Asherson RA, Khamashta MA, Ordi-Ros J, et al: The ''primary'' antiphospholipid antibody syndrome: Major clinical and serologic features. Medicine (Baltimore) 1989; 68:366–374.
9. Alarcon-Segovia D, Sanches-Guerrero J: Primary antiphospholipid syndrome. J Reumatol 1989; 16:482–488.
10. Asherson RA, Cervera R, Piette JC, et al: The antiphospholipid syndrome: History, definition, classification, and differential diagnosis. *In* Asherson RA, Cervera R, Piette JC, et al (eds): The Antiphospholipid Syndrome. Boca Raton, Florida: CRC Press, 1996:3–12.
11. Alarcon-Segovia D, Perez-Vasquez ME, Villa AR, et al: Preliminary classification criteria for the antiphospholipid syndrome within systemic lupus erythematosus. Semin Arthritis Rheum 1992; 21:275–285.
12. Lockshin MD: Editorial: Why do patients with antiphospholipid antibody clot? Lupus 1997; 6:351–352.
13. Nasr S, Parke AL. Letter to the editor. N Engl J Med 1995; 333:666.
14. McNeil HD, Simpson RJ, Chesterman CN, et al: Antiphospholipid antibodies are directed against a complex antigen

that included a lipid-binding inhibitor of coagulation: Beta-2-glucoprotein I (apolipoprotein H). Proc Natl Acad Sci USA 1990; 87:4120–4124.

15. Galli M, Confurius P, Massau C, et al: Anticardiolipin antibodies (ACA) directed not to cardiolipin but to a plasma protein cofactor. Lancet 1990; 335:1544–1547.

16. Blank M, Faden D, Tincani A, et al: Immunization with anticardiolipin cofactor β (beta 2-glycoprotein I) induces experimental antiphospholipid syndrome in naïve mice. J Autoimmunity 1994; 7:441–445.

17. Gharavi AE, Sammaritano LR, Wen J, et al: Induction of antiphospholipid autoantibodies by immunization with β2 glycoprotein I (apolipoprotein H). J Clin Invest 1992; 90:1105–1109.

18. Branch DW, Dudley DJ, Mitchell MD, et al: Immunoglobulin G fractions from patients with antiphospholipid antibodies cause fetal death in BALB/c mice: A model for autoimmune fetal loss. Am J Obstet Gynecol 1990; 163:210–216.

19. Blank M, Cohen J, Toder V, et al: Induction of antiphospholipid syndrome by passive transfer of anticardiolipin antibodies. Proc Nat Acad Sci U S A 1991; 88:3069–3073.

20. Lie JT: Vasculitis in the antiphospholipid syndrome: Culprit or consort? J Rheumatol 1994; 21:397–399.

21. Lie JT: Pathology of the antiphospholipid syndrome. In Asherson RA, Cervera R, Piette JC, et al (eds): The Antiphospholipid Syndrome. Boca Raton, Florida: CRC Press, 1996:89–104.

22. Shi W, Krilis SA, Chong BH, et al: Prevalence of lupus anticoagulant and anticardiolipin antibodies in a healthy population. Aust N Z J Med 1990; 20:231–236.

23. Harris EN, Spinnato JA: Should anticardiolipin tests be performed in otherwise healthy pregnant women? Am J Obstet Gynecol 1991; 165:1272–1277.

24. Perez MC, Wilson WA, Brown HL, et al: Anticardiolipin antibodies in unselected pregnant women in relationship to fetal outcome. J Perinatol 1991; 11:33–36.

25. Alarcon-Segovia D, Deleze M, Oria CV, et al: Antiphospholipid antibodies and the antiphospholipid syndrome in systemic lupus erythematosus: A prospective analysis of 500 consecutive patients. Medicine (Baltimore) 1989; 68:353–374.

26. Cervera R, Khamashta MA, Fond J, et al: Systemic lupus erythematosus: Clinical and immunologic patterns of disease expression in a cohort of 1,000 patients. Medicine (Baltimore) 1993; 72:113–124.

27. Drenkard C, Sánchez-Guerrero J, Alarcón-Segovia D: Fall in antiphospholipid a antibody at time of thrombocclusive episodes in systemic lupus erythematosus. J Rheumatol 1989; 16:614–617.

28. McNeil HP, Hunt JE, Krilis SA: Antiphospholipid antibodies: New insights into their specificity and clinical importance. Scand J Immunol 1992; 36:647–652.

29. Rosove MH, Brewer P: Antiphospholipid thrombosis: Clinical course after the first thrombotic event in 70 patients. Ann Intern Med 1992; 117:303–308.

30. Khamashta MA, Cuadrado MJ, Mujic F, et al: The management of thrombosis in the antiphospholipid antibody syndrome. N Engl J Med 1995; 332:993–997.

31. Bengtsson A, Zoller B, de Frutos PG, et al: Factor V:Q$^{506}$ mutation and anticardiolipin in systemic lupus erythematosus. Lupus 1996; 5:598–601.

32. Beaumont JL: Syndrome hemorrhagique acquis du a un anticoagulant. Sang 1954; 25:1–5.

33. Nilsson IM, Astedt B, Hedner U, et al: Intrauterine death and circulating anticoagulant "antithromboplastin." Acta Med Scand 1975; 197:153–159.

34. Carreras LO, Defreyn G, Machin SJ, et al: Arterial thrombosis, intrauterine death and "lupus" anticoagulant: Detection of immunoglobulin interfering with prostacyclin formation. Lancet 1981; 1:244–246.

35. Lubbe WF, Butler WS, Palmer SJ, et al: Fetal survival after prednisone suppression of maternal lupus anticoagulant. Lancet 1983; 1:1361–1363.

36. Abramowsky CR, Vegas ME, Swinehart G, et al: Decidual vasculopathy of the placenta in systemic lupus erythematosus. Ann Rheum Dis 1979; 37:129–134.

37. Salafia CM, Parke AL: Placental pathology in systemic lupus erythematosus and phospholipid antibody syndrome. Clin Rheum Dis 1997; 23:85–97.

38. Ramsey Goldman R, Kutzer JE, Kuller LH, et al: Previous pregnancy outcome is an important determinant of subsequent pregnancy outcome in women with systemic lupus erythematosus. Am J Reprod Immunol 1992; 28:195–198.

39. Ginsberg JS, Demers C, Brill-Edwards P, et al: Increased thrombin generation and activity in patients with systemic lupus erythematosus and anticardiolipin antibodies: Evidence for a prothrombotic state. Blood 1993; 81:2958–2963.

40. Amante E, Sanders MM, Parke AL: "Second hit" phenomenon triggering thrombosis in a patient with SLE and APL syndrome: A case report. J Rheum, submitted.

41. Lockshin MD: New perspectives in the study and treatment of antiphospholipid syndrome. In Asherson RA, Cervera R, Piette JC, et al (eds): The Antiphospholipid Syndrome. Boca Raton, Florida: CRC Press, 1996:323–329.

42. Jouhikainen T, Stephansson E, Leirisalo-Repo M: Lupus anticoagulant as a prognostic marker in SLE. Br J Rheum 1993; 32:568–573.

43. Many A, Pauzner H, Carp H, et al: Treatment of patients with antiphospholipid antibodies during pregnancy. Am J Reprod Immunol 1992; 28:216–218.

44. Cowchock FS, Reece EA, Balaban D, et al: Repeated fetal losses associated with antiphospholipid antibodies: A collaborative randomized trial comparing prednisone with low-dose heparin treatment. Am J Obstet Gynecol 1992; 166:318–323.

45. Silveira LH, Hubble CL, Jara LJ, et al: Prevention of anticardiolipin antibody-related pregnancy losses with prednisone and aspirin. Am J Med 1992; 93:403–411.

46. Branch WA, Silver RM, Blackwell JA, et al: Outcome of treated pregnancies in women with antiphospholipid syndrome: An update of the Utah experience. Obstet Gynecol 1992; 80:614–620.

47. Balasch J, Carmona F, Lopez-Soto A, et al: Low-dose aspirin for prevention of pregnancy losses in women with primary antiphospholipid syndrome. Hum Reprod 1993; 8:2234–2239.

48. Kwak JYH, Gilman-Sachs A, Beaman KD, et al: Reproductive outcome in women with recurrent spontaneous abortions of alloimmune and autoimmune causes: Preconception versus postconception treatment. Am J Obstet Gynecol 1992; 166:1787–1789.

49. Rosove MH, Tabsh K, Wasserstrum N, et al: Heparin therapy for pregnant women with lupus anticoagulant or anticardiolipin antibodies. Obstet Gynecol 1990; 75:660–634.

50. Triplett DA, Brandt JT. Lupus anticoagulants: Misnomer, paradox, riddle, epiphenomenon. Hematol Pathol 1988; 2:121–143.

51. Antiphospholipid Antibodies in Stroke Study Group: Recurrent thromboembolic and stroke risk in patients with neurological events and antibodies [Abstract]. Ann Neurol 1990; 28:226.

52. Babikian VL, Levin AR: Therapeutic consideration for stroke patients with antiphospholipid antibodies. Stroke 1992; 23(suppl I):I33–I37.

53. Brey RL, Hart RG, Sherman DG, et al: Antiphospholipid antibodies and cerebral ischemia in young people. Neurology 1990; 40:1190–1196.

54. Lockshin MD, Druzin ML, Qamar T: Prednisone does not prevent recurrent fetal death in women with antiphospholipid antibody. Am J Obstet Gynecol 1989; 160:439–443.

55. Silver RK, MacGregor SN, Sholl JS, et al: Comparative trial of prednisone plus aspirin versus aspirin alone in treatment of anticardiolipin antibody-positive obstetric patients. Am J Obstet Gynecol 1993; 169:1411–1417.

56. Parke A, Maier D, Hakim C, et al: Subclinical autoimmune disease and recurrent spontaneous abortion. J Rheumatol 1986; 13:1178–1180.

57. Out HJ, Bruinse HW, Christiaens GCML, et al: A prospective controlled multicenter study on the obstetric risks of pregnant women with antiphospholipid antibodies. Am J Obs Gynecol 1992; 167:26–32.

58. Stafford-Brady FJ, Gladman DD, Urowitz MB: Successful pregnancy in SLE with an untreated lupus anticoagulant. Arch Intern Med 1988; 148:1647–1648.

59. Rai R, Cohen H, Dave M, et al: Randomized controlled trial of aspirin and aspirin plus heparin in pregnant women with recurrent miscarriage associated with phospholipid antibodies (or antiphospholipid antibodies). BMJ 1997; 314:253–257.

60. Kutteh MD: Antiphospholipid antibody-associated recurrent pregnancy loss: Treatment with heparin and low-dose aspirin is superior to low-dose aspirin alone. Am J Obstet Gynecol 1996; 174:1584–1589.

61. Asherson RA, Baguley E, Pal C, et al: Antiphospholipid syndrome: Five year follow up. Ann Rheum Dis 1991; 50:805–810.

62. Derksen RHWM, de Groot Ph G, Kater L, et al: Patients with antiphospholipid antibodies and venous thrombosis should receive long term anticoagulant treatment. Ann Rheum Dis 1993; 52:689–692.

63. Lockshin MD: Answers to the antiphospholipid antibody syndrome? N Engl J Med 1995; 332:1025–1027.

64. Amante EJB, Nasr S, Walsh SJ, et al: Long term follow-up of different therapeutic interventions in patients with the phospholipid antibody syndrome. Submitted.

65. Palareti G, Leali N, Coccheri S, et al: Bleeding complications of oral anticoagulant treatment: An inception-cohort, prospective collaborative study (ISCOAT). Lancet 1996; 338:423–428.

66. ASPECT Research Group: Effect of long-term oral anticoagulant treatment on mortality and cardiovascular morbidity after myocardial infarction. Lancet 1994; 343:499–503.

67. Barbour LA, Smith JM, Marlar RA, et al: Heparin levels to guide thromboembolism prophylaxis during pregnancy. Am J Obstet Gynecol 1995; 173:1869–1873.

68. Branch WD: Thoughts on the mechanism of pregnancy loss associated with antiphospholipid syndrome. Lupus 1994; 3:275–280.

69. Parke A: The role of IVIG in the management of patients with antiphospholipid antibodies and recurrent pregnancy losses. *In* Ballow M (ed): IVIG Therapy Today. Totowa, NJ: Humana Press, 1992:105–118.

70. Parke AL: Intravenous gammaglobulin in pregnancy: The Connecticut experience. Scand J Rheumatol 1998; 27(suppl 107):103–104.

71. Asherson RA: The catastrophic antiphospholipid syndrome. J Rheumatol 1992; 19:508–512.

72. Asherson RA, Cervera R, Font J: Multiorgan thrombotic disorders in systemic lupus erythematosus: A common link? Lupus 1992; 1:119–203.

73. Frances C, Tribout B, Boisnic S, et al: Cutaneous necrosis associated with the lupus anticoagulant. Dermatologica 1989; 178:194–201.

74. Christman OD, Snook GA, Wilson TC, et al: Prevention of venous thromboembolism by administration of hydroxychloroquine: A preliminary report. J Bone Joint Surg Am 1976; 58:918–920.

75. Johnson R, Loudon JR: Hydroxychloroquine sulfate prophylaxis for pulmonary embolism for patients with low-friction arthroplasty. Clin Orthop 1986; 211:151–153.

76. Rudnicki RD, Gresham GE, Rothfield NF: The efficacy of antimalarials in systemic lupus erythematosus. J Rheumatol 1975; 2:323–330.

77. The Canadian Hydroxychloroquine Study Group: A randomized study of the effect of withdrawing hydroxychloroquine sulfate in systemic lupus erythematosus. N Engl J Med 1991; 342:150–154.

78. Levin MN, Raskob G, Hirsh J, et al: Hemorrhagic complications of long-term anticoagulant therapy. Chest 1989; 95(suppl):26S–36S.

79. The Boston Area Anticoagulation Trial for Atrial Fibrillation (BAATAF) investigators: The effect of low-dose warfarin on the risk of stroke in patients with nonrheumatic atrial fibrillation. N Engl J Med 1990; 323:1505–1511.

80. Fihn SD, McDonell M, Martin D, et al: Risk factors for complications of chronic anticoagulation. Ann Intern Med 1993; 118:511–520.

81. Al-Sayegh FA, Ensworth S, Huang S, et al: Hemorrhagic complications of longterm anticoagulant therapy in 7 patients with systemic lupus erythematosus and antiphospholipid syndrome. J Rheumatol 1997; 24:1716–1718.

82. Hall JG, Pauli RM, Wilson KM: Maternal and fetal sequelae of anticoagulation during pregnancy. Am J Med 1980; 68:120–140.

83. Parke AL, Weinstein RE, Bona RD, et al: The thrombotic diathesis associated with the presence of phospholipid antibodies may be due to low levels of free protein S. Am J Med 1992; 93:49–56.

84. Atsumi T, Khamasta MA, Ames PRJ, et al: Effect of $\beta2$ glycoprotein-1 and human monoclonal anticardiolipin antibody on the protein-S/C4b-binding protein system. Lupus 1996; 6:358–364.

85. Lorber M, Blumenfeld Z: Low molecular heparin (Clexane): Promising treatment in women with recurrent abortions in SLE and antiphospholipid antibody syndrome. Lupus 1992; 1(suppl 1):162.

86. Dahlman TC, Sjobert HE, Rigertz H: Bone mineral density during long-term prophylaxis with heparin in pregnancy. Am J Obstet Gynecol 1994; 170:1315–1320.

87. Physicians' Desk Reference, vol 53. Montvale, NJ: Medical Economics Company, 1999:929–933.

88. Spinnato JA, Clark AL, Pierangeli SS, et al: Intravenous immunoglobulin therapy for the antiphospholipid syndrome in pregnancy. Am J Obstet Gynecol 1995: 166:690–694.

89. Valensis H, Vaquero E, DeCarolis C, et al: Normal fetal growth in women with antiphospholipid syndrome treated with high-dose intravenous immunoglobulin. Prenat Diagn 1995; 15:509–517.

90. Rossi E, Costa M: Fish oil derivatives as a prophylaxis of recurrent miscarriage associated with antiphospholipid antibodies (APL): A pilot study. Lupus 1993; 2:319–323.

91. Fishman P, Falach-Vaknine E, Zigelman R, et al: Prevention of fetal loss in experimental antiphospholipid syndrome by in vivo administration of recombinant interleukin-3. J Clin Invest 1993; 91:1834–1837.

92. Wilson WA, Gharavi AE, Koike T, et al: International consensus statement on preliminary classification criteria for definite antiphospholipid syndrome. Arthritis Rheum 1999; 42:1309–1311.

93. Lockshin MD, Sammaritano LR, Schwartzman S: Validation of the Sapporo criteria for antiphospholipid syndrome. Arthritis Rheum 2000; 40:440–443.

# 25 | Renal Disease in Systemic Lupus Erythematosus

*Ellen M. Ginzler*

The diagnosis, routine follow-up, and treatment of nephritis in patients with systemic lupus erythematosus (SLE) is based on knowledge of the renal histologic changes, serologic and clinical correlations with renal disease, and the natural history of the disease, as well as on the expected response to therapeutic interventions. Our understanding of these various factors is derived from anecdotal reports in individual patients, from both small and large retrospective and prospective cohort studies, and from both uncontrolled and randomized controlled therapeutic intervention trials. Statistical techniques have also been applied to use data from small studies or to correct for multiple factors that could have an influence on outcome. This chapter reviews what is generally accepted with regard to the clinical features and prognosis of lupus nephritis, as well as what remains controversial, in order to provide an approach to the management of patients with this disease. In so doing, specific issues are considered:

- What are the clinical correlations and the natural history of the various histologic forms of lupus nephritis?
- What is the role of renal biopsy in predicting outcome or in making therapeutic decisions?
- How should patients with SLE be monitored in order to predict an exacerbation of nephritis at any early stage?
- Should patients with abnormal serologic or other immunologic abnormalities that occur alone (without renal exacerbation) be treated?
- Which therapeutic modalities have demonstrated efficacy in controlled trials versus anecdotal reports?
- How should outcome be monitored? What are the criteria for therapeutic success?
- Which ancillary measures other than treatment of the acute exacerbation of nephritis should be considered in order to preserve renal function and prevent other, especially cardiovascular, features of morbidity?
- When progression to end-stage renal disease occurs, what is the expected course with chronic dialysis and/or renal transplantation?

## HISTOLOGIC CLASSIFICATION OF LUPUS NEPHRITIS

The histologic classification of lupus nephritis is based on glomerular pathology, as described initially by Baldwin and associates in 1970[1a] and in a subsequent modification by the World Health Organization (WHO), which includes immunofluorescent and electron microscopic findings.[2] Class I, an unusual finding in patients with SLE, represents a renal biopsy specimen that is normal on light microscopy and demonstrates no immune complex deposition on either immunofluorescence or electron microscopy. The scenario of normal findings of light microscopy that are coincident with immune deposits, usually limited to the mesangium, is designated WHO class IIA. The scenario of mesangial immune deposits accompanied by histologic change, including either increased mesangial matrix or areas of increased mesangial cellularity in some or all glomeruli sampled, is designated class IIB, or mesangial lupus nephritis (Fig. 25–1A).

Focal proliferative lupus nephritis, generally corresponding to WHO class III, may include mesangial disease as well as more severe histologic abnormalities, such as capillary endothelial cell proliferation, necrosis, and polymorphonuclear leukocyte infiltration (see Fig. 25–1B). These changes are limited to some lobules of the glomerulus, whereas other glomeruli may be entirely unaffected. Immune complex deposition frequently extends beyond the mesangium to the subendothelial surface of the capillary basement membrane of some or all glomeruli.

Diffuse proliferative lupus nephritis, as originally described by Baldwin and associates,[1a] includes disease within all lobules of the glomerulus, and essentially all glomeruli are affected (see Fig. 25–1C). The membranoproliferative variant may show a predominance of capillary basement membrane thickening. However, proliferative changes, polymorphonuclear leukocyte infiltration, and subendothelial immune deposits are also characteristic. Epithelial crescents and totally sclerotic glomeruli are also well described but less frequent features of class IV lupus nephritis.

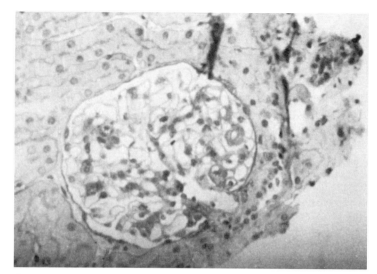

A

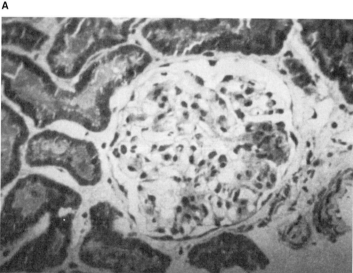

B

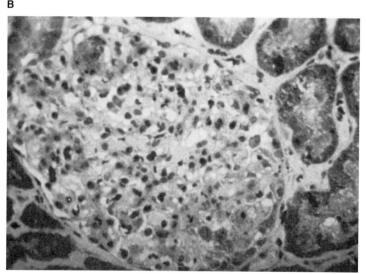

C

**FIGURE 25–1**

*A,* High-power light microscopic appearance of World Health Organization (WHO) class IIB (mesangial) lupus nephritis, showing mesangial thickening and mild mesangial hypercellularity with normal, patent capillary loops. *B,* High-power light microscopic appearance of WHO class III (focal proliferative) lupus nephritis, showing segmental proliferation and basement membrane thickening of capillary tufts; other lobules of the glomerulus remain normal. *C,* High-power light microscopic appearance of WHO class IV (diffuse proliferative) lupus nephritis, showing generalized basement membrane thickening, endothelial cell proliferation, and infiltration with inflammatory cells.

Although it was originally believed that the various proliferative forms of lupus nephritis were distinct entities, it is now well accepted that progression from the milder to the more severe histologic forms occurs with time.[3-5] The nature of a continuum of severity of glomerular disease is also reflected in the WHO definition of class IV nephritis, according to which more than 50%, but not all, of the glomeruli have light microscopic changes as described earlier. In fact, the three glomeruli shown in Figure 25–1 were all found in the same biopsy specimen from a young woman in whom lupus nephritis had been clinically apparent for less than 1 year. Several years later, during an exacerbation of her renal disease, a repeat renal biopsy showed diffuse proliferative changes in 100% of the glomeruli in the biopsy specimen.

Membranous lupus nephritis, designated WHO class V, is characterized by diffusely thickened glomerular capillary walls (Fig. 25–2). This histologic pattern, in which endothelial cell proliferation and polymorphonuclear leukocyte infiltration are absent, may represent a pathophysiologic process different from the one that results in the proliferative forms of lupus nephritis. Furthermore, immune complexes are identified by immunofluorescence and electron microscopy only in the mesangium and the subepithelial, but not subendothelial, surface of the glomerular basement membrane in true membranous lupus nephritis. With treatment and healing of the proliferative forms of nephritis, the histologic appearance may resemble a membranous lesion, but some cellular proliferation and immune complex deposition generally remain.

Nonglomerular pathology may also be present in lupus renal disease, generally as tubular fatty change or tubular atrophy in areas adjacent to glomerular abnormalities. Interstitial infiltration with mononuclear cells is generally a mild, scattered phenomenon, but dense generalized infiltration is occasionally the predominant histologic abnormality.

## CLINICAL CORRELATIONS AND NATURAL HISTORY OF THE HISTOLOGIC LESIONS OF LUPUS NEPHRITIS

The severity of serologic abnormalities (hypocomplementemia and anti–double-stranded DNA [anti-dsDNA] antibodies) and clinical abnormalities (active urinary sediment, proteinuria, azotemia, and hypertension) in patients with active lupus nephritis generally parallels the severity of histologic change.[6] A random renal biopsy in a patient with SLE who has no clinical or serologic abnormalities might show class IIA or IIB lesions; however, this histologic appearance would also be characteristic of a few leukocytes or red blood cells in the urinary sediment and with minimal proteinuria (200 to 500 mg/24 hours). Hypocomplementemia, an active urinary sediment containing cellular casts, and proteinuria with protein levels of 1 to 2 g/24 hours typically accompany class III lesions during active disease; a modest increase in serum creatinine to the range of 1.2 to 1.5 mg/dL is not incompatible. Active class IV lupus nephritis is characterized by the presence of antibodies to dsDNA and hypocomplementemia, as measured by C3, C4, and $CH_{50}$, in addition to the frequent findings of red blood cell casts and protein casts in the urine and nephrotic-range proteinuria. The development of azotemia is to be expected in more than 50% of patients with this lesion. Even with treatment and reversal of serologic abnormalities, some degree of persistent proteinuria and azotemia may be observed. Hypertension may be present initially, or it may be the consequence of treatment.

Differing clinically from the proliferative lesions, the hallmark of membranous lupus nephritis is severe proteinuria, in which protein levels may reach the range of 10 to 15 g/24 hours. Moderate hypocomplementemia is present in up to 50% of patients, but antibodies to dsDNA are rare, as is significant azotemia, especially

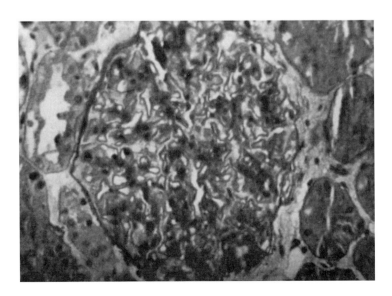

**FIGURE 25–2**
High-power light microscopic appearance of World Health Organization class V (membranous) lupus nephritis, showing diffuse basement membrane thickening without cellular proliferation or necrosis.

early in the disease course. Hypertension is common, and the development of renal vein thrombosis, probably secondary to a general hypercoagulable state, is well described. Massive proteinuria, often accompanied by defects in renal tubular function such as renal tubular acidosis, may also be a marker for severe interstitial nephritis, even in the absence of significant glomerular damage.[7]

In considering the individual patient with lupus nephritis, however, it must be remembered that the variation from patient to patient in serologic parameters and degree of proteinuria or azotemia may be large, and a particular combination of clinical and serologic abnormalities may be characteristic of more than one type of lesion. Similarly, it must be remembered that not all derangements in renal function can be attributed to active nephritis. Cardiovascular disease may result in hemodynamic changes that diminish glomerular filtration rate. The use of nonsteroidal anti-inflammatory drugs (NSAIDs) for nonrenal disease manifestations may result in a rising serum creatinine level that is secondary to an ischemic nephropathy induced by inhibition of prostaglandins or to an active interstitial nephritis without evidence of immune complex deposition.[8]

Just as the severity of clinical disease manifestations is generally directly related to the severity of the histologic lesions, the overall prognosis for preservation of renal function and patient survival is inversely related to the severity of the pathologic findings. The natural history of lupus nephritis—that is, a measure of survival and/or a determination of renal function in untreated patients—is difficult to establish. The series reported by Estes and Christian[9] in 1971 does, however, reflect an era before the general use of high-dose corticosteroids and immunosuppressive drugs and a time when dialysis was not generally available. From the first appearance of overt renal disease, the rate of 5-year survival was only about 50%; among patients with renal biopsy evidence of diffuse proliferative or membranous nephritis, the rate of 5-year survival was less than 30%.[9] Other early series observed patients with mesangial and focal lesions on biopsy to have survival rates similar to that of patients without clinical renal disease. Diffuse proliferative nephritis, on the other hand, was associated with survival rates as poor as 47% at 2 years and 29% at 5 years after biopsy.[5] This is in contrast with the 1992 report by Moroni and colleagues,[10] who documented a major improvement in outcome. Of 34 patients with lupus nephritis first seen between 1964 and 1980, 6 died within 1 to 62 months and 3 progressed to end-stage renal disease. Among the remaining 25, 18 had diffuse proliferative nephritis on initial renal biopsy; 13 of those 18 had normal renal function, and 15 had proteinuria with levels of less than 1 g/per 24 hours at last observation 11 to 27 years later. Furthermore, the incidence of disease exacerbations fell significantly after the 10th year of follow-up.

There is controversy concerning the natural history of the membranous form of lupus nephritis, especially in the absence of adherence to the strict criteria for its designation, as outlined earlier. Early studies suggested that maintenance of normal renal function and overall survival were generally good in pure membranous disease, even among patients with persistent nephrotic syndrome.[11] In a 1993 series reported by Pasquali and coworkers,[12] 2 of 26 patients with pure class V disease died of cerebrovascular accidents, 2 progressed to end-stage renal disease more than 10 years after biopsy, and 3 others developed renal insufficiency 3.5 to 10.9 years after biopsy. Survival rates to death or end-stage renal disease were 96% at 5 years and 92% at 10 years.[12] A meta-analysis of 11 studies of membranous lupus nephropathy published between 1965 to 1998, with follow-up ranging from 30 to 114 months, points to a more guarded prognosis.[13] In four studies with available information regarding proteinuria, treatment resulted in complete resolution in 27 (29.7%) of 91 patients, improvement in 38 (41.8%) of 91, no change in 19 (20.9%) of 91, and worsening in 7 (7.7%) of 91. Overall renal function remained stable in 94 (52.8%) of 178, deteriorated in 17 (16.8%) of 101, and dialysis was required in 44 (21.3%) of 207. Death by any cause occurred in 23 (13.2%) of 174 reported cases. Of patients with any features of proliferative histology on biopsy, 33.3% developed end-stage renal disease, and 17.7% died.

## IMMUNOLOGIC PREDICTORS OF DISEASE ACTIVITY

If the premise that treatment can alter the natural history of lupus renal disease is accepted, it becomes increasingly important to identify disease activity at an early stage, before irreversible pathologic changes associated with permanent functional impairment ensue. The notion that immunochemical measures were predictive of disease activity was first proposed by Schur and Sandson[14] in 1968. They found elevated anti-dsDNA titers in 57% of patients in association with active nephritis. Among 32 patients tested serially, 22 had a 50% or greater fall in serum $CH_{50}$ level; 19 of the 22 subsequently had an exacerbation of nephritis. Other investigators subsequently noted similar correlations between hypocomplementemia and increased evidence of dsDNA binding with active renal disease; however, a number of discrepancies between serologic and clinical activity have also been documented. Lightfoot and Hughes[15] followed 16 patients with serial serum samples; in 21 of 28 instances in which anti-dsDNA antibodies became elevated, the titers remained abnormal until a clinical flare occurred after 60 to 450 days; however, only 10 instances included an exacerbation of renal disease.[15] In three instances anti-dsDNA titer reverted to normal spontaneously, and in four it remained abnormal without a clinical flare at the end of the study. Among the same patients, low levels of $CH_{50}$ resolved spontaneously in 16 of 35 instances, most of which occurred in patients with prior renal disease. Gladman and associates[16] also identified 14 patients with persistently low C3 and $CH_{50}$

levels who remained untreated and free of clinical renal manifestations for a mean of 4.25 years.

Since these early studies were published, many other investigators have attempted with varying degrees of success to correlate specific complement components and both anti-dsDNA antibodies and circulating immune complexes by various immunochemical techniques with clinical manifestations of active nephritis.[17-21] Several long-term prospective studies have been reported. In one, which stressed the predictive value of anti-dsDNA antibodies, measurement by the Farr assay was generally superior to enzyme-linked immunosorbent assay or *Crithidia luciliae* methods.[22] All renal flares were accompanied by increases in anti-dsDNA titer, which were frequently characterized by a biphasic pattern, with a gradual increase in antibody level during the first phase followed by a rapid increase a few months to weeks before clinical disease exacerbation. Interestingly, 23% of the renal flares in this series were not accompanied by a fall in C3 or C4 levels.

In 1991 the Lupus Nephritis Collaborative Study Group reported their observations on 12 patients with severe nephritis studied serially over 12 to 77 months through 25 renal and 16 nonrenal relapses with SLE.[23] C3 and C4 were measured by both nephelometry and radial immunodiffusion. During remission, C3 levels tended to be normal by both methods, whereas C4 levels showed no such tendency. Decreases in C3 levels by both methods were predictive of relapse with 95% sensitivity and 85% specificity, in comparison with 56% sensitivity and 54% specificity for decreases in C4 levels. This appears to be due to the much broader range of normal C4 levels, which is characterized by a high prevalence of at least one null allele in normal subjects (up to 40%) as well as in patients with SLE (up to 80%).

Discordance between levels of complement components and clinical evidence of active nephritis may be related not only to congenital and acquired complement deficiencies but also to increases in complement components as acute-phase reactants. Buyon and colleagues[24] suggested that levels of complement split products better reflect disease activity and impending flares than do traditional complement components. They serially measured Ba, Bb, SC5b-9, and C4d in 86 patients, whose clinical status was subclassified initially as inactive, moderately active, or severely active (acute renal disease with rising serum creatinine, cellular sediment, or increasing proteinuria). The mean values of all complement split products were highest in the group with the most severe disease; an elevated C4d level had the highest degree of sensitivity for an exacerbation within the next 3.5 months, occurring in 86% of such patients, in comparison with increased Ba or SC5b-9 levels in 73% of the patients with a subsequent flare. Bb, on the other hand, was the most specific for active disease; 81% of patients who did not experience flares had normal levels, whereas 60% had normal Ba levels, 67% had normal SC5b-9 levels, and 69% had normal C4d levels. In comparison, fewer than 50% of the patients with low C3, C4, or $CH_{50}$ levels had a subsequent disease flare.

Is it possible to reach a consensus from the disparate results of these numerous studies that will enable a logical approach to management of the individual patient with SLE and either no previous renal disease or established prior clinical nephritis? It appears that no single measure is a reliable predictor of impending or even currently active nephritis. A specific parameter may, however, be consistently associated with disease activity in a given patient, so that a pattern emerges over time. In the patient with newly diagnosed SLE, frequent monitoring may increase the likelihood of identifying that pattern of serologic abnormalities. Furthermore, the absolute value of each parameter may be less important than the appearance of changes in level or titer. On a practical basis, technical and financial considerations make C3 and anti-dsDNA the most useful predictors of active nephritis in most patients. Should monitoring of complement split products become more cost effective, they may replace conventional complement components as the parameters of choice to monitor.

Investigators continue to seek new immunochemical measures that will serve as better predictors of disease activity and will distinguish between activity in different organ systems. For example, activated T lymphocytes produce the cytokine interleukin-2 (IL-2) and are induced to secrete IL-2 receptors on their cell surface, which can then be measured as a soluble form in the serum (sIL-2R). sIL-2R has been shown to be elevated in a number of autoimmune conditions, with increased levels in patients with SLE and even higher mean levels during active disease.[25-27] One study found that sIL-2R levels were highest among patients with SLE and active nephritis and that 9 of 10 patients undergoing a renal flare had a significant increase in sIL-2R, whereas only 6 of 10 had either increased anti-dsDNA antibodies or decreased $CH_{50}$; this suggests that sIL-2R may be a more reliable marker than are conventional measures.[28]

Similar attempts have been made to identify products of immune activation in the urine of patients with SLE, which would provide a simple and less invasive means of frequent monitoring. Anti-RNA polymerase I antibodies and neopterin have been measured, but neither marker has been shown to distinguish between renal and nonrenal involvement.[29, 30] Perhaps a more promising approach, albeit not yet accepted commercially, is the measurement of urinary cytokines such as interleukin-6 or interleukin-10. Both serum and urine interleukin-10 levels have been shown to be elevated in patients with active lupus nephritis in comparison with the levels in patients without nephritis or in healthy controls.[31] Urinary, but not serum, interleukin-6 levels are also elevated in patients with active lupus nephritis[32] and have been shown to be correlated with general measures of lupus activity, indices of active renal disease, active urinary sediment, and severity of the renal lesion on biopsy.[32]

Regardless of which immunochemical markers are chosen to monitor disease activity, changes in these levels should signal the clinician that a therapeutic decision is in order. Treating serologic abnormalities in the absence of clinical disease features might prevent serious manifestations, irreversible organ damage, or both; however, such treatment may subject the patient to potentially toxic therapy despite the possibility of spontaneous remission of immunologic activity. My own approach, especially in patients whose disease is newly diagnosed or who had no prior evidence of clinical renal disease, is to increase the frequency of monitoring of clinical parameters such as urinalysis, degree of proteinuria, serum creatinine level, and blood pressure, as well as nonrenal features of activity, but not to treat abnormal serologic conditions alone in the absence of change in clinical parameters. In patients with well-established disease and a clear pattern of serologic abnormalities preceding clinical manifestations, early treatment may abort subsequent disease activity.

## THE ROLE OF RENAL BIOPSY IN MANAGEMENT OF PATIENTS WITH LUPUS NEPHRITIS

Despite the fact that much of our understanding of the natural history of lupus nephritis is based on renal biopsy studies, some investigators have suggested that renal biopsy is an invasive and expensive procedure in which the information regarding glomerular class yields no marginal predictive value regarding outcome beyond that provided by clinical data.[33] Investigators at the National Institutes of Health (NIH) have, however, proposed that more specific features of glomerular and tubulointerstitial disease reflecting histologic activity and chronicity are both predictive of outcome and beneficial in identifying subsets of patients with lupus nephritis who are most likely to respond to aggressive therapy.[34, 35] In a large retrospective study examining demographic and clinical variables as well as renal biopsy activity and chronicity indexes, Nossent and coworkers[36] found that only a chronicity index greater than 3 was predictive of survival without renal transplantation/treatment. Although neither Esdaile and associates[37] nor Schwartz and colleagues[38] were able to show a marginal contribution to the prediction of renal failure when chronicity index scores were added to clinical information, Goulet and associates commented that it is necessary to classify patients on the basis of renal severity in order to demonstrate the relationship of disease activity to outcome.[39] The ongoing controversy may be explained by an analysis by the Lupus Nephritis Collaborative Study Group, which failed to demonstrate reproducibility of the activity and chronicity indexes by different pathologists, concluding that these measures are too subjective to be used as prognosticators or therapeutic guides.[40]

Considering the foregoing caveats, it remains important to establish guidelines regarding the decision to perform a renal biopsy. When immunochemical and clinical parameters clearly indicate active disease and the pattern of abnormalities is consistent with a particular histologic type, it is reasonable to initiate therapy without a biopsy. When the pattern of abnormal results is inconsistent or the possibility of non–lupus-related abnormalities such as diabetes mellitus or NSAID-induced nephropathy is a consideration, renal biopsy is appropriate before a course of therapy is initiated. When clinical features such as advanced azotemia or hypertension suggest the possibility of irreversible disease, review of the pathologic changes may enable the clinician to devise a rational approach to treatment. Statistical considerations aside, it may not be necessary to compute the actual value of the activity or chronicity index to become more comfortable with the probability of therapeutic response in the individual patient.

## CORTICOSTEROID THERAPY FOR LUPUS NEPHRITIS

For more than three decades, the use of corticosteroids has been accepted as appropriate initial therapy for active lupus nephritis. Pollak and coworkers[41] showed that prednisone in a dose of 15 to 20 mg/day did not alter survival in patients with nephritis, but when high-dose oral prednisone (60 to 100 mg/day) was given for 6 months in an uncontrolled trial, longer survival and reduction in azotemia were observed. Other anecdotal reports supporting this finding followed.[1, 42, 43] In fact, these early observations rendered the conducting of randomized placebo-controlled clinical trials of corticosteroids as essentially unethical. Recognizing the significant short- and long-term morbidity attributed to high-dose oral steroids—including cushingoid features, hyperglycemia or frank diabetes, myopathy, hypertension, an increase in pyogenic and opportunistic infections, and avascular necrosis—investigators have sought to devise steroid regimens that minimize toxicity. Ackerman[44] reported improvement in renal function in five of seven patients with lupus nephritis treated with 100 to 120 mg of prednisone every other day. Cushingoid changes were avoided, and stabilization of renal function was maintained with subsequent tapering of the steroid dose. In my experience, an alternate-day steroid regimen is rarely successful in suppressing constitutional symptoms, azotemia, or proteinuria associated with active disease but may minimize toxicity as a maintenance regimen in steroid-dependent patients whose disease flares with tapering of medication.

A regimen of intravenous pulse methylprednisolone (1 g/day for 3 consecutive days) for severe lupus nephritis was first advocated in 1976 by Cathcart and colleagues,[45] who hypothesized that this extremely high dose of steroids would rapidly reverse the pathologic findings of inflammation and clinical deterioration in renal function, allowing for subsequent treatment with steroids in a dose necessary only to control extrarenal disease manifestations. Indeed, in five of seven patients so treated, renal function returned to baseline within 1 month, and all patients demonstrated reversal of immunologic abnormalities. Subsequent larger, uncontrolled series with longer follow-up have confirmed an initial response to pulse methylprednisolone therapy in about 50% of instances; responders were characterized by more recent deterioration in renal function and more profound abnormalities of immunochemical measures.[46, 47] Even among patients with an initial response, however, improvement was neither complete nor sustained in most.[47] A quasi-randomized, unblinded study of pulse methylprednisolone in comparison with high-dose prednisone in pediatric patients with diffuse nephritis concluded that long-term effects on renal function were similar in both groups, although there was more rapid improvement in glomerular filtration rate (GFR) with pulse therapy.[48] One small, double-blind, controlled study examined the efficacy of 1 year of monthly pulse methylprednisolone in comparison with placebo.[49] The five patients in the treatment group showed a significant improvement in serum creatinine levels, whereas the four patients in the placebo group did not. After an additional 2 years of follow-up, renal function remained stable in the treatment group but deteriorated further in the placebo group. In a randomized NIH trial comparing one year of serial monthly pulse methylprednisolone with regimens containing cyclophosphamide, remission of active nephritis occurred in only 7 (29%) of 24 patients in the methylprednisolone group, and 4 of 11 (36%) who eventually achieved remission had a subsequent relapse.[50]

There is no doubt that pulse methylprednisolone therapy is useful for initial treatment of acute lupus nephritis, especially in the presence of recent deterioration in renal function. It is unlikely, however, that this regimen can be successfully followed immediately by treatment with zero- or low-dose prednisone. It is generally necessary to continue conventional high-dose steroids for at least several weeks, as well as to consider addition of another immunosuppressive agent as a maintenance regimen. Furthermore, it is essential that attention be paid to preexisting hypertension and edema, because a single course of pulse methylprednisolone may result in marked salt and fluid retention.

## IMMUNOSUPPRESSIVE AGENTS IN THE TREATMENT OF LUPUS NEPHRITIS

Immunosuppressive agents other than corticosteroids have for many years been added to the therapeutic regimen of patients with lupus nephritis in order to reverse acute clinical and immunologic abnormalities and to maintain remission. In considering the efficacy of these agents, it is important to keep in mind that these two goals are different and that various drugs may be appropriate for one or both goals. In several early uncontrolled studies, azathioprine, a purine analog, appeared to be associated with improvement in azotemia and proteinuria in 50% to 100% of patients with severe lupus nephritis.[51–54] Among the series of 47 azathioprine-treated patients with diffuse proliferative and membranous nephritis reported by Barnett and associates,[54] survival rates were 82% at 5 years and 74% at 10 years. In a prospective randomized trial that included 35 patients, Sztejnbok and coworkers[55] observed, among azathioprine-treated patients, de-

creased mortality and morbidity, lower steroid requirements, and better maintenance of renal function after 1 to 4 years.[55] These findings were confirmed at the same institution in a larger, uncontrolled, retrospective comparison study.[56] Survival was not improved in the azathioprine group during the first 6 months of therapy; however, a subsequent survival benefit and steroid sparing were observed. Other studies failed to show a survival benefit with azathioprine; this included two controlled trials of 2 and 3 years' duration in 24 and 16 patients, respectively.[57, 58]

As with azathioprine, early experience with the nitrogen mustard derivative cyclophosphamide in patients with SLE began in the 1960s and 1970s. Feng and colleagues[59] treated 42 patients, 31 of whom had evidence of nephritis, with oral cyclophosphamide for periods of 6 months to 7 years.[59] Responses ranged from sustained clinical remission in 16 patients to death in 5, along with the common toxic effects of amenorrhea and infection. Donadio and associates[60] reported the results of a controlled trial of oral cyclophosphamide plus prednisone in comparison with prednisone alone; no difference in outcome was seen between the two groups at the end of 6 months, and improvement was observed in 84% of the patients. During a 4-year follow-up, recurrent nephritis occurred more often in the group treated with prednisone only; however, survival and the prevalence of stable or improved renal function were similar in both groups.[61] In a series of reports from NIH with increasingly longer duration of follow-up, in which patients with diffuse proliferative or membranous nephritis were randomly assigned to receive prednisone alone or low-dose prednisone in combination with oral cyclophosphamide or azathioprine, no substantial benefit with either immunosuppressive agent was noted with regard to patient survival or renal function.[62–64]

In addition to the obvious problems with drawing conclusions from anecdotal series, most of the controlled trials of immunosuppressive therapy for lupus nephritis conducted in the 1970s and early 1980s suffered from methodologic difficulties, including small numbers of patients, noncomparable groups, and short follow-up. Potential trends in the direction of a positive association with a treatment regimen were likely to be missed. Felson and Anderson[65] performed a meta-analysis of all published randomized trials comparing prednisone alone with prednisone plus azathioprine or cyclophosphamide (Table 25–1). They found that patients who received an immunosuppressive drug had significantly less renal deterioration or progression to end-stage renal disease and were significantly less likely to die of renal disease. Rates of overall mortality and death from nonrenal causes were not different in the two groups.

To avoid hemorrhagic cystitis in patients receiving cyclophosphamide, NIH added to the randomized trial of lupus nephritis a group of patients receiving intravenous cyclophosphamide (IVC), given monthly in incremental doses (0.5 to 1.0 g/m² body surface area) for three successive doses, followed by a maintenance dose of up to 1.0 g/m² every 3 months.[63] Toxicity in

**TABLE 25–1**
**Results of Pooled Analysis Comparing Immunosuppressive Therapy Plus Steroids with Steroids Alone in the Treatment of Lupus Nephritis**

| | NO. OF PATIENTS | | OUTCOME RATE | | |
| --- | --- | --- | --- | --- | --- |
| | Steroids Alone | Combined Therapy | Steroids Alone | Combined Therapy | P Value |
| **All Studies** | 113 | 137 | — | — | — |
| Renal deterioration | 37 | 27 | 0.0096 | 0.0048 | .006 |
| ESRD | 24 | 16 | 0.0058 | 0.0028 | .023 |
| Nephritis-related death | 19 | 12 | 0.0049 | 0.0022 | .024 |
| All deaths | 32 | 29 | 0.0083 | 0.0052 | .066 |
| **Studies Using Cyclophosphamide** | 60 | 59 | — | — | — |
| Renal deterioration | 18 | 11 | 0.0070 | 0.0043 | .190 |
| ESRD | 10 | 7 | 0.0035 | 0.0027 | .561 |
| Nephritis-related death | 5 | 4 | 0.0019 | 0.0015 | .739 |
| All deaths | 11 | 12 | 0.0043 | 0.0047 | .835 |
| **Studies Using Azathioprine** | 68 | 62 | — | — | — |
| Renal deterioration | 27 | 15 | 0.0115 | 0.0061 | .047 |
| ESRD | 18 | 9 | 0.0068 | 0.0036 | .102 |
| Nephritis-related death | 15 | 8 | 0.0062 | 0.0033 | .135 |
| All deaths | 26 | 16 | 0.0111 | 0.0068 | .095 |
| **Patients with DPGN** | 72 | 91 | — | — | — |
| Renal deterioration | 28 | 19 | 0.0097 | 0.0045 | .008 |
| ESRD | 19 | 10 | 0.0060 | 0.0023 | .012 |
| Nephritis-related death | 14 | 7 | 0.0048 | 0.0016 | .017 |
| All deaths | 21 | 21 | 0.0073 | 0.0050 | .207 |
| **Patients Without DPGN on Biopsy** | 9 | 14 | — | — | — |
| Renal deterioration | 3 | 3 | 0.0079 | 0.0040 | .416 |
| ESRD | 1 | 2 | 0.0026 | 0.0026 | .986 |
| Nephritis-related death | 1 | 1 | 0.0026 | 0.0013 | .642 |
| All deaths | 2 | 2 | 0.0052 | 0.0027 | .506 |

DPGN = diffuse proliferative glomerulonephritis; ESRD = end-stage renal disease.
From Felson DT, Anderson J: Evidence for the superiority of immunosuppressive drugs and prednisone over prednisone alone in lupus nephritis: Results of a pooled analysis. N Engl J Med 1984; 311:1528. Copyright © 1984 Massachusetts Medical Society. All rights reserved.

the early phases of the study was minimal; however, this regimen had no clear therapeutic advantage over prednisone alone or in combination with oral immunosuppressive agents. Improved preservation of renal function associated with IVC plus low-dose prednisone, in comparison with high-dose prednisone alone, became apparent only after 5 years of follow-up.[66] The most recent report from this randomized study, in which the duration of follow-up extended beyond 15 years for some patients, indicated better preservation of renal function for all patient groups receiving cyclophosphamide, with the most significant benefit in the IVC group (Fig. 25–3).[67] Although the original intention of the investigators was to continue the study protocol indefinitely, study drugs were discontinued if clinical remission was sustained for at least 18 months. In all treatment groups, progression to renal failure was significantly more frequent among patients with a high chronicity score on renal biopsy.

Despite the general acceptance of IVC as the standard of care for treating severe forms of lupus nephritis, many reports have documented a considerable proportion of patients who fail to respond or who experience relapse during maintenance therapy after

achieving remission. In the New York University experience with 45 patients treated with a mean of nine courses of IVC from 1987 to 1993 for severe lupus nephritis, 9 progressed to end-stage renal disease, 3 experienced a doubling of serum creatinine level, and 2 had persistent nephrotic syndrome during a mean follow-up of 52 months.[68] The overall experience of Dooley and coworkers[69] at the University of North Carolina at Chapel Hill was similar: Of 89 patients treated with the NIH IVC protocol, 19 progressed to end-stage renal disease; in 8 cases, this occurred within 8 months of the beginning of therapy.[69] Significant racial differences were noted, in that 95% of white patients retained renal function at 5 years, whereas among African-American patients, the rate of survival with renal function declined progressively from 85% at 1 year to 58% at 5 years. These differences in renal outcome were independent of age, duration of SLE, history or control of hypertension, and activity and chronicity indices on renal biopsy. Other academic centers, which might also be expected to observe a more severe spectrum of disease, reported rates of failure of IVC as high as 46% when failure was represented by deterioration of renal function and 69% with persistent

**FIGURE 25–3**

Probability of progression to end-stage renal disease in the study population by treatment group: prednisone only (PRED); azathioprine (AZ); oral cyclophosphamide (POCY); oral azathioprine plus oral cyclophosphamide (AZCY); and intravenous cyclophosphamide (IVCY). Survival curves are shown, with end-stage renal disease as the outcome. The number of patients at risk in each group is shown for each 20-month time point. The curves for the AZCY, IVCY, and POCY groups were significantly different from that of the control (PRED) group ($P = .0011$, $P = .0025$, and $P = .032$, respectively). The AZ group did not differ significantly from the PRED group ($P = .09$). The Mantel statistic from which the $P$ values (versus PRED) were obtained were 2.872 (AZ), 4.619 (POCY), 10.571 (AZCY), and 9.169 (IVCY). The 95% confidence intervals at the 120-month (10-year) point were 0.67 to 0.23 (PRED), 0.93 to 0.49 (AZ), 0.97 to 0.53 (POCY), 1.00 to 0.78 (AZCY), and 1.00 to 0.74 (IVCY). (From Steinberg AD, Steinberg SC: Long-term preservation of renal function in patients with lupus nephritis receiving treatment that includes cyclophosphamide versus those treated with prednisone only. Arthritis Rheum 1991; 34:945.)

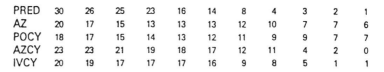

| | | | | | | | | | | | |
|------|----|----|----|----|----|----|----|----|----|----|----|
| PRED | 30 | 26 | 25 | 23 | 16 | 14 | 8  | 4  | 3  | 2  | 1  |
| AZ   | 20 | 17 | 15 | 13 | 13 | 13 | 12 | 10 | 7  | 7  | 6  |
| POCY | 18 | 17 | 15 | 14 | 13 | 12 | 11 | 9  | 9  | 7  | 7  |
| AZCY | 23 | 23 | 21 | 19 | 18 | 17 | 12 | 11 | 4  | 2  | 0  |
| IVCY | 20 | 19 | 17 | 17 | 17 | 16 | 9  | 8  | 5  | 1  | 1  |

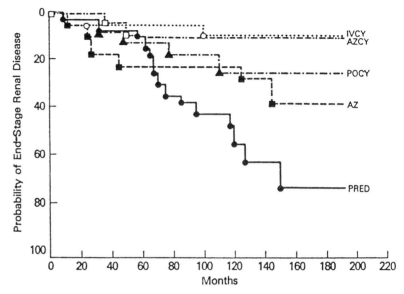

nephrotic-range proteinuria.[70, 71] Even data from the NIH reveal a discouraging rate of failure to achieve renal remission with IVC therapy; 40 of 92 patients did not meet criteria for remission.[72] Furthermore, of the 52 responders, 12 subsequently experienced relapse. In a randomized study of 52 Chinese patients, the authors suggested that increasing the frequency of IVC to every 2 weeks, with a reduction to half of each intravenous dose, may result in an improvement in overall remission rate and the time to remission, without increasing the frequency of adverse events.[73]

Among patients who do achieve remission with cyclophosphamide, prediction of subsequent relapse is difficult. In a study of 48 such patients at three university hospitals in Spain, 11 had a relapse of nephritis during a mean follow-up of 33 months from the time of cyclophosphamide discontinuation, with cumulative relapse rates of 25% at 5 years and 46% at 10 years.[74] The time to relapse was associated with age less than 29 years and duration from onset of nephritis to initiation of cyclophosphamide therapy but not to onset of hypertension, serum creatinine level, urinary protein excretion, WHO classification, chronicity index, activity index, tubulointerstitial damage, use of high-dose steroids, or the route or duration of cyclophosphamide therapy.

The toxic effects of IVC are numerous and vary widely in frequency. Nausea during administration and occasionally lasting several days thereafter may limit patients' willingness to continue therapy. Pretreatment with antiemetics is essential. Another less common gastrointestinal side effect is diarrhea. Hyponatremia with seizures secondary to vigorous hydration has been reported as an acute side effect.[75] Both short- and long-term therapy may be associated with

bone marrow suppression and an increased risk of infection and reactivation of herpes zoster. As the cumulative dose of cyclophosphamide increases with time, the development of subtle or obvious alopecia is noted. Similarly, the risk of secondary amenorrhea is increased, in relation not only to the number of doses of cyclophosphamide received but also to the age of the patient at initiation of therapy.[76] Hemorrhagic cystitis may occur, even with hydration, and bladder cancer has been reported.[77] The increased risk of lymphoproliferative malignancies that has been documented with prolonged oral cyclophosphamide therapy has so far not been reported with the intravenous regimen.

## GOALS IN THE MONITORING OF THERAPEUTIC EFFICACY

If the reader accepts the conclusions of the studies just described that initial treatment of active nephritis with corticosteroids is indicated, supplemented in some patients with an immunosuppressive agent, it is still necessary to outline a plan for decision making with regard to the appropriate regimen and for monitoring of the immunologic and clinical responses. As stated previously, my approach is not to treat immunochemical abnormalities in the absence of clinical manifestations unless a pattern of exacerbations after changes in serologic findings has already been established in a given patient. I also believe that therapy must be tailored to the individual, taking into account the patient's lifestyle and personal wishes. Treatment for proteinuria or active urinary sediment, in the absence of the nephrotic syndrome, azotemia, or serious nonrenal manifestations can usually be managed with prednisone in moderate doses (40 to 60 mg/day), and renal biopsy is not essential. Serologic and clinical parameters should be monitored weekly to biweekly, with upward adjustments in steroid dose if significant worsening of clinical markers ensues. If azotemia or the nephrotic syndrome is present, I prefer to obtain a renal biopsy before deciding on a supplemental immunosuppressive regimen for acute therapy; however, I am comfortable with institution of intravenous pulse methylprednisolone for deteriorating renal function, even if a biopsy is contraindicated or the patient refuses it. In the absence of biopsy documentation of class IV nephritis with histologic evidence of active lesions, I am likely to err on the side of aggressive treatment (i.e., institution of IVC).

Renal function and proteinuria should improve within 1 to 2 weeks after the institution of therapy, whereas amelioration of hypocomplementemia (especially improvement in C3 levels) and anti-dsDNA titers may lag behind by several weeks.[78] Tapering of prednisone may begin when a therapeutic response is sustained and clinical parameters have stabilized for at least 2 weeks, unless significant toxicity (hyperglycemia, intractable edema or hypertension, steroid psychosis) necessitates more urgent reduction in dose. It is important to be aware that a partial response may occur, either with improvement in immunochemical parameters but failure to reverse azotemia or proteinuria or with improvement in clinical markers with persistent serologic abnormalities. The goal of normalization of serum complement levels is laudatory but not always possible. Laitman and associates[79] reported the results of an ongoing study of 39 patients with lupus nephritis in whom an attempt was made to maintain normal $CH_{50}$ levels with prednisone and the addition of azathioprine in nonresponders. Twenty-five patients achieved normal $CH_{50}$ levels within 6 months, and immunosuppressive therapy was then tapered but continuously readjusted to the lowest dose that preserved normal $CH_{50}$ and maintained clinical remission. Of the 25 responders, 17 patients had continuous control of $CH_{50}$ and 8 became persistently hypocomplementemic; the 14 nonresponders failed to achieve normal $CH_{50}$ within the first 6 months, and they were subsequently treated on the basis of clinical considerations only. No differences were observed in clinical or histologic features during the first 6 months between patients with complement-controlled disease and those with complement-uncontrolled disease. After a mean 10-year follow-up, however, patients in the normal $CH_{50}$ group had significantly better renal function, less diastolic hypertension, and better rates of overall survival than did either group of complement-uncontrolled patients.

I favor institution of IVC for patients with documented class IV nephritis and active lesions, as well as for patients with azotemia and/or membranous nephropathy with steroid-resistant nephrotic syndrome. In general, my approach is to continue monthly intravenous administration of cyclophosphamide for 6 months, followed by maintenance doses every 3 months. I follow serologic parameters and renal function at least monthly, especially just after beginning the maintenance schedule. If there is a deterioration in either laboratory or clinical status, I decrease the interval between doses to 6 to 8 weeks, until a stable status is maintained. Unless significant toxicity develops, I usually continue maintenance IVC during at least 1 year of sustained remission and 2 years if azotemia has developed during a prior exacerbation.

Cyclophosphamide is excreted almost completely by the kidneys as an active metabolite, and so impaired renal function results in a prolonged half-life and a potential for increased bone marrow suppression. In mild renal insufficiency (GFR >50 mL/min), no reduction in dose is generally necessary, whereas reductions to 75% of the usual dose for moderate renal insufficiency (GFR = 10 to 50 mL/min) and 50% for severe renal insufficiency (GFR < 10 mL/min) are recommended.[80]

I find azathioprine to be especially useful as a steroid-sparing agent in patients whose disease, although nonazotemic and non-nephrotic, flares with tapering or in whom exacerbations are frequent. It is also appropriate to treat patients with azathioprine when they are no longer willing to tolerate the side effects of cyclophosphamide or to administer it initially in young patients who wish to preserve ovarian function.

When conventional therapy fails and life-threatening disease manifestations are present, the use of new, experimental therapies is warranted, but only if the patient understands the potential for toxicity and the possible lack of efficacy. With the ready availability of chronic dialysis, the withdrawal of steroids, immunosuppressive agents, or both may also be appropriate, allowing for progression to end-stage renal disease. This option may preserve patient survival at the expense of renal function.

## UNPROVEN, ANECDOTAL, AND EXPERIMENTAL THERAPIES

There are several reasons to consider therapies other than those outlined; the most obvious is that a substantial proportion of patients fail to respond completely, and progression to end-stage renal disease continues to occur. In addition, therapeutic manipulations based on pathophysiologic mechanisms other than glomerular immune complex deposition have been proposed. Plasmapheresis, designed to remove antigen-antibody complexes from the circulation, was advocated in the late 1970s in patients with severe nephritis, especially when unresponsive to steroids. Verrier Jones and colleagues[81] treated eight patients who demonstrated a fall in circulating immune complexes and anti-dsDNA titers. In five patients, cessation of plasmapheresis was followed by a rapid rebound in immune complexes and antibody to pretreatment levels. In subsequent anecdotal reports, several investigators suggested synchronization of plasmapheresis with pulse cyclophosphamide in order to take advantage of the plasmapheresis-induced proliferation of pathogenetic clones, with subsequent clonal deletion by large doses of cytotoxic drugs during a period of increased B-cell vulnerability.[82, 83] Even before the results of a large-scale, controlled trial by the Lupus Nephritis Collaborative Study Group with 86 patients were reported, the initial enthusiasm for this therapeutic modality was dampened because of its invasive nature and considerable cost. It has since been shown that treatment with plasmapheresis plus a standard regimen of prednisone and cyclophosphamide does not result in more significant clinical improvement of severe lupus nephritis than does the standard regimen alone.[84]

High-dose intravenous immunoglobulins have been used to treat patients with SLE who have drug-resistant, life-threatening disease manifestations, especially profound thrombocytopenia. Lin and associates[85] reported the use of this aggressive therapeutic modality in nine patients who had lupus nephritis with azotemia and nephrotic syndrome unresponsive to methylprednisolone pulse therapy and cyclophosphamide. All were treated with 400 mg of human gamma globulin per kilogram of body weight for 5 consecutive days.[85] Creatinine clearance, proteinuria, and anti-dsDNA titers improved in all nine patients; in all seven who had a second renal biopsy 2 months after the course of treatment, there was a dramatic decrease in intensity of immune complex deposition. Two subsequent anecdotal reports describe an additional three patients with severe unresponsive lupus nephritis whose condition improved with intravenous immunoglobulin; one of these patients had a prolonged remission in association with monthly therapy over 20 months.[86, 87]

Cyclosporine, a fungal polypeptide with immunosuppressive activity, has become the most common agent used to suppress rejection of renal transplants. It has also been used with varying efficacy in the treatment of patients with active lupus. Isenberg and co-workers[88] treated five patients at a dose of 10 mg/kg/day; no patient was able to tolerate more than 7 weeks of therapy because of side effects, including nephrotoxicity and angioedema. Subsequently, a number of anecdotal studies have reported better success in pediatric and adult patients with steroid- and/or cytotoxic agent–resistant nephritis.[89–92] Most of these series have used cyclosporine in an average dose of 5 mg/kg/day along with corticosteroids, in trials generally lasting 1 year. Results have been variable: About 50% of patients have demonstrated suppression of extrarenal and renal activity, whereas others have had some evidence of steroid-sparing on the basis of clinical symptoms but no serologic improvement. The most promising results were reported by Favre and associates[90] in 26 patients, all of whom exhibited improvement in global disease activity and decrease in proteinuria. Nephrotic-range proteinuria, originally present in 19 patients, was reduced below 1 g/24 hours at 9 months in all 19. Serum creatinine levels increased somewhat during the first 6 months of therapy and then returned to baseline or better. Nephrotoxicity was generally managed by lowering the dose of cyclosporine; however, elevated blood pressure required control with antihypertensive medications in a significant proportion of patients. Despite this positive anecdotal experience, clinicians appear reluctant to enter patients in a randomized double-blind trial of cyclosporine, given its potential nephrotoxicity.

Mycophenolate mofetil (MMF), another immunosuppressive agent approved for prevention of renal allograft rejection, has been used with increasing frequency for the management of steroid and cyclophosphamide-resistant nephritis. MMF is metabolized to mycophenolic acid, a reversible inhibitor of the enzyme inosine monophosphate dehydrogenase, a critical rate-limiting enzyme in the synthesis of purines. It has a relatively selective effect on lymphocytes, blocking proliferation of both B and T cells, causing the inhibition of antibody formation and generation of toxic T cells and decreasing the expression of adhesion molecules on lymphocytes, impairing their ability to bind to endothelial cells.[93] It differs from azathioprine by its lack of effect on neutrophils and platelets, and it differs from cyclosporine by a lack of effects on cytokine production.[93]

Studies of MMF in the New Zealand black/New Zealand white murine model of human SLE have demonstrated its ability to prevent or retard the development of proteinuria and anti-dsDNA antibodies, as well as to prolong survival and prevent renal histologic damage.[94, 95] These favorable results are paralleled by anecdotal reports of small series of patients with various forms of autoimmune nephritis who have been treated successfully with MMF. Most have had relapsing or steroid and immunosuppressive drug resistant disease. Twenty-two patients with lupus nephritis and persistent nephrosis and/or azotemia have been described, all with benefits observed within 2 months of starting therapy.[95–100] The experience at the State University of New York with five patients with SLE has been associated with significant improvement in proteinuria in three patients and stabilization of serum creatinine in another. Furthermore, the safety profile of MMF is encouraging. Dose-related gastrointestinal side effects such as nausea, vomiting, and diarrhea occur in about 30% of patients. Leukopenia and its associated increased risk of infection may occur; however, nephrotoxicity, hypertension, and hepatotoxicity have not been reported.[93] At this time, neither the duration nor the appropriate dose of therapy necessary to maintain therapeutic benefits is known. Controlled trials of MMF in lupus nephritis are clearly warranted, both as a substitute for IVC in initial induction therapy and for IVC-resistant or relapsing disease.

Achieving immunosuppression via total lymphoid irradiation had been suggested as an alternative to cytotoxic therapy. The largest series, which was not randomized, was reported by Strober and colleagues,[101] who treated 15 patients with SLE who had diffuse nephritis that was unresponsive to steroids and azathioprine, as well as a high chronicity index on renal biopsy, with a total dose of 2000 rad over a 4- to 6-week period. There was significant improvement in serum creatinine level, urinary protein excretion, and anti-dsDNA antibody titer, with a significant reduction in the mean prednisone requirement. With post-treatment follow-up as long as 6 years, 13 of the 15 patients remained alive with stable renal function. One died of a nonrenal cause at 13 months, and one progressed to renal failure at 24 months. Infection was the most common complication in this series; its potential catastrophic nature was stressed in another anecdotal report on two patients who received total lymphoid irradiation without clinical benefit.[102]

Immunosuppressive therapy has been directed at reversing the abnormal immunologic events that lead to inflammation and secondary tissue injury and dysfunction. Treatment designed to prevent the inflammatory process through the use of dietary supplementation with fish oil, which contains naturally occurring marine lipids rich in the n-3 fatty acids eicosapentaenoic acid and docosahexaenoic acid, has been suggested. These substances substitute for arachidonic acid in the cyclooxygenase and lipoxygenase pathways and have been shown to retard the development of nephritis in murine models of SLE. Results from preliminary trials in humans have been inconsistent.[103, 104] Clark and associates[105] completed a 1-year double-blind, crossover study of dietary fish oil supplementation in 21 patients with stable lupus nephritis. They found no improvement in renal function or reduction in disease activity, as reflected by C3, C4, and anti-dsDNA antibody levels. Serum levels of very low density lipoprotein cholesterol were markedly decreased. Preexisting renal disease may not be reversed, and immunochemical measures of disease activity may remain unaffected. Because fish oil suppresses the inflammatory response elicited by immune complex deposition, it may merely prevent tissue damage without changing the underlying immunologic dysfunction. Its usefulness, therefore, might be in preventing further damage, rather than reversing existing abnormalities. It is likely that a much larger series of patients, treated for a significantly longer period of time, would be required in order to show a benefit of this generally inexpensive and nontoxic intervention.

Conventional immunosuppressive therapy has general effects on the immune system. One anecdotal report employing the concept of specific immunotherapy documented the use of anti-CD4 monoclonal antibody in a man with steroid and immunosuppressive refractory SLE, including azotemia and nephrosis.[106] Clinical improvement lasted for 1 month. The number of CD4 cells fell by 50% within 1 day and remained decreased for a month. In vitro studies showed that production of anti-dsDNA antibodies by the patient's cultured peripheral blood mononuclear cells was significantly inhibited after treatment.

A number of other potential therapeutic modalities have been based on nonimmunologic pathophysiologic mechanisms. In 1973 Kincaid-Smith[107] suggested that obliteration of glomerular capillaries in lupus nephritis might result not only from immunoglobulin deposition but also from fibrin deposition, which has been identified by immunofluorescence in renal biopsy specimens. Several uncontrolled series subsequently reported clinical improvement in manifestations of nephritis in patients treated with intravenous hepa-

rin.[108, 109] Reversal of glomerular thrombosis with the defibrinating agent ancrod (the venom of the Malayan pit viper) has been described in a series of 22 patients with SLE, most of whom had deteriorating renal function. Long-term follow-up (mean, 58 months) noted 3 deaths from nonrenal causes, progression to end-stage renal disease in 11 patients (a mean of 27 months after therapy), and stabilization of renal function in 8 patients.[110] With increasing attention to the antiphospholipid syndrome and its associated thrombotic manifestations, interest may be renewed in the use of anticoagulation as a treatment for patients with SLE, such as those described in a report with the insidious development of renal insufficiency in the presence of anticardiolipin antibodies or the lupus circulating anticoagulant.[111]

The clinical manifestations of renal disease in SLE may be mediated in part by hemodynamic mechanisms, as suggested by beneficial results of treatment with thromboxane antagonists in a small, randomized, double-blind crossover study[112] and by the improvement observed in eight patients treated with intravenous prostaglandin $E_1$.[113]

A number of other therapeutic modalities targeted to specific immunologic functions or dysfunction are currently being evaluated in controlled clinical trials. These include LJP394, an agent designed to induce tolerance to DNA and thereby reduce the production of anti-dsDNA antibodies. Another such agent is a monoclonal antibody to CD40 ligand (CD40L) on T lymphocytes. The interaction between B cell CD40 and T cell CD40L is essential for antigen-driven antibody production. Interference with the complement cascade is also a potential mechanism for decreasing tissue damage; an anti-C5 monoclonal antibody has been designed to prevent the activation of C5 and the resulting formation of C5a, a proinflammatory molecule. Data regarding the safety and efficacy of these agents is not yet complete; however, phase II and phase III clinical trials are in progress.

## THE RELATIONSHIP OF HYPERTENSION TO OUTCOME

In addition to modalities designed to treat active manifestations of lupus renal disease, it is now well accepted that other conservative measures may protect renal function, decrease morbidity, and prolong survival. Attention to the maintenance of normal blood pressure is probably the most important of these measures. Budman and Steinberg[114] demonstrated the independence of hypertension and active nephritis with their observations in 36 patients that hypertension was not correlated with the degrees of proteinuria, hematuria, or serum complement; with urinary casts; or with biopsy findings of necrosis or interstitial inflammation. Studies in several large lupus cohorts have documented that hypertension early in the course of disease is an important predictor of mortality. Reveille and coworkers[115] found that both systolic and diastolic hypertension present within 6 months of SLE diagnosis were associated with decreased survival. Seleznick and

Fries[116] similarly identified systolic hypertension as the only significant risk factor for mortality, when statistical corrections were made for the multiple variables under study. Ward and Studenski[117] showed the association between diastolic hypertension at the onset of nephritis with the development of end-stage renal disease: Of 160 patients studied, 41 progressed to renal failure; the median times were more than 273 months, 146 months, and only 7 months among patients with normal blood pressure, mild hypertension, and severe hypertension, respectively.[117] Ginzler and associates[118] reported a long-term retrospective study of a cohort of 685 patients, which was designed to examine the continuous effect of hypertension at any time in the course of the disease on subsequent renal deterioration, end-stage renal disease, and mortality. They found that, independent of measures of active nephritis, hypertension is a potent risk factor for adverse renal outcomes, as well as for death from any cause.[118]

## MANAGEMENT OF END-STAGE RENAL DISEASE

Some patients may have renal failure as a consequence of unresponsive active nephritis, even with the many therapeutic modalities currently available. Others may slowly progress to end-stage renal disease in the absence of immunochemical measures of disease activity, presumably secondary to irreversible renal damage that leads to a combination of progressive glomerulosclerosis, vascular disease, interstitial fibrosis, and/or tubular atrophy.[119] It is important to recognize this subset of patients so that they are not put at increased risk of toxic manifestations of immunosuppressive therapy, such as infection, in a futile attempt to reverse azote-

mia. The most critical period with regard to morbidity and mortality appears to be the first several months on dialysis, especially for patients who have progressed to renal failure during an acute episode of SLE and who continue to have disease manifestations. As remission is achieved, maintenance dialysis may continue to be complicated by an increased incidence of infection, in comparison with that in patients with other causes of renal failure.[120] Furthermore, although it is true that the frequency and severity of extrarenal disease manifestations decrease with end-stage renal disease, SLE exacerbations do occur and should be treated accordingly. Occasionally, in fact, patients receiving long-term maintenance dialysis develop new organ system manifestations that were not present before the onset of renal failure.

An initial reluctance to perform renal transplantation in patients with SLE appears to have been overcome. As of the early 1990s, patients with SLE accounted for 4% of all renal transplantation procedures in the United States.[121] Numerous centers have reported their experience with both live donor and cadaver transplants,[122, 123] with general agreement that the prognosis for both allograft and patient survival has increased significantly with the availability of potent immunosuppressive agents such as cyclosporine. In a comprehensive review of end-stage renal disease in SLE published in 1996, Mojcik and Klippel[124] found that the rate of recurrence of lupus in transplanted allografts was 2.7% to 3.8%, which was comparable with that for all allograft transplantation failures. In the series of 16 transplantations in 14 patients reported by Goss and colleagues,[122] the overall survival rate was 95% after a mean follow-up period of 44 months, and the mean serum creatinine level was 1.4 mg/dL. They found that graft survival rates were similar in patients

### TABLE 25–2
### Predictors of Renal Allograft Survival in Patients with Systemic Lupus Erythematosus

| PREDICTOR | GRAFT SURVIVAL | GRAFT FAILURE |
|---|---|---|
| Transplantations (no.) | 10 | 6 |
| Mean duration of dialysis before transplantation (months) | 27.9 | 47.8 |
| Mean duration of graft survival (months) | 43.6 | 9.2 |
| Mean serum creatinine level at last follow-up or at graft failure (mg/dL) | 1.4 | Data not given |
| **Pretreatment Serologic Findings** | | |
| Patients positive for ANAs (no.) | 2 | 2 |
| Patients positive for anti-dsDNA (no.) | 2 | 1 |
| Patients with hypocomplementemia (no.) | 1 | 0 |
| **Post-treatment Serologic Findings** | | |
| Patients positive for ANAs (no.) | 4 | 2 |
| Patients positive for anti-dsDNA (no.) | 1 | 1 |
| Patients with hypocomplementemia (no.) | 1 | 0 |

ANAs = antinuclear antibodies.
Based on data from Goss JA, Cole BR, Jendrisak MD, et al: Renal transplantation for systemic lupus erythematosus and recurrent lupus nephritis: A single-center experience and a review of the literature. Transplantation 1991; 52:805.
From Ginzler EM, Antoniadis I: Clinical manifestations of systemic lupus erythematosus, measures of disease activity and long-term complications. Curr Opin Rheumatol 1992; 4:672.

undergoing short- or long-term dialysis before transplantation and suggested that the development of recurrent nephritis in the transplanted kidney may be related to the presence of antinuclear antibodies and anti-dsDNA antibodies both before and after transplantation (Table 25–2).[122]

A 1998 report comparing the course of 97 patients with SLE who underwent 106 renal transplantations with that of control patients who had other forms of renal failure concluded that the outcome in SLE may not, in fact, be as benign.[125] Controls were matched for age, gender, race, type of allograft (cadaveric vs. living related), number of previous transplantations, and year of transplantation. Patient survival in the two groups did not differ, but the relative hazard of allograft loss in patients with SLE was 2.1 ($P = 0.031$).[125] Thrombotic complications of antiphospholipid antibodies contributed significantly to eight allograft losses among the patients with SLE. It is therefore important to continue frequent monitoring of the serologic as well as the clinical status of patients who have received renal transplants. Although it may be difficult at times to distinguish between mild transplant rejection and recurrent nephritis, treatment with increased doses of immunosuppression (steroids and/or other immunosuppressive drugs) should have a beneficial effect on both and may prevent loss of the transplanted kidney.

# REFERENCES

1. Kelley WN, Harris ED, Ruddy S, et al (eds): Textbook of Rheumatology, 4th ed. Philadelphia: WB Saunders, 1993.
1a. Baldwin DS, Lowenstein J, Rothfield NF, et al: The clinical course of the proliferative and membranous forms of lupus nephritis. Ann Intern Med 1970; 73:929.
2. McCluskey RT: Lupus nephritis. *In* Sommers SC (ed): Kidney Pathology Decennial 1966–1975. New York: Appleton-Century-Crofts, 1975:437.
3. Ginzler EM, Nicastri AD, Chen C-K, et al: Progression of mesangial and focal to diffuse lupus nephritis. N Engl J Med 1975; 291:693.
4. Zimmerman SW, Jenkins PG, Shelp WD, et al: Progression from minimal or focal to diffuse proliferative lupus nephritis. Lab Invest 1975; 32:665.
5. Baldwin DS, Gluck MC, Lowenstein J, et al: Lupus nephritis: Clinical course as related to morphologic forms and their transitions. Am J Med 1977; 62:12.
6. Appel GB, Silva FG, Pirani CL, et al: Renal involvement in systemic lupus erythematosus (SLE): A study of 56 patients emphasizing histologic classification. Medicine 1978; 57:371.
7. Brentjens JR, Sepulveda M, Baliah T, et al: Interstitial immune complex nephritis in patients with systemic lupus erythematosus. Kidney Int 1975; 7:342.
8. Ling BN, Bourke E, Campbell WG Jr, et al: Naproxen-induced nephropathy in systemic lupus erythematosus. Nephron 1990; 54:249.
9. Estes D, Christian CL: The natural history of systemic lupus erythematosus by prospective analysis. Medicine 1971; 50:85.
10. Moroni G, Banfi G, Ponticelli C: Clinical status of patients after 10 years of lupus nephritis. Q J Med 1992; 84:681.
11. Donadio JV Jr, Burgess JH, Holley KE: Membranous lupus nephropathy: A clinicopathologic study. Medicine 1977; 56:527.
12. Pasquali S, Banfi G, Zucchelli A, et al: Lupus membranous nephropathy: Long-term outcome. Clin Nephrol 1993; 39:173.
13. Kolasinski SL, Chung JB, Albert DA: What do we know about lupus membranous nephropathy? A meta-analytic approach. Arthritis Rheum 1998; 41(suppl):S280.
14. Schur P, Sandson J: Immunologic factors and clinical activity in SLE. N Engl J Med 1968; 278:533.
15. Lightfoot RW, Hughes GRV: Significance of persisting serologic abnormalities in SLE. Arthritis Rheum 1976; 19:837.
16. Gladman DD, Urowitz MB, Keystone EC: Serologically active clinically quiescent systemic lupus erythematosus: A discordance between clinical and serologic features. Am J Med 1979; 66:210.
17. Bardana EJ Jr, Harbeck RJ, Hoffman AA, et al: The prognostic and therapeutic implications of DNA:anti-DNA immune complexes in systemic lupus erythematosus (SLE). Am J Med 1975; 59:515.
18. Harkiss GD, Hazleman BL, Brown DL: A longitudinal study of circulating immune complexes, DNA antibodies and complement in patients with systemic lupus erythematosus: An analysis of their relationship to disease activity. J Lab Clin Med 1979; 2:275.
19. Abrass CK, Nies KM, Louie JS, et al: Correlation and predictive accuracy of circulating immune complexes with disease activity in patients with systemic lupus erythematosus. Arthritis Rheum 1980; 23:273.
20. Swaak AJG, Groenwold J, Aarden LA, et al: Prognostic value of anti-dsDNA in SLE. Ann Rheum Dis 1982; 41:388.
21. Valentijn RM, van Overhagen H, Hazevoet HM, et al: The value of complement and immune complex determinations in monitoring disease activity in patients with systemic lupus erythematosus. Arthritis Rheum 1985; 28:904.
22. ter Borg EJ, Horst G, Hummel EJ, et al: Measurement of increases in anti-double stranded DNA antibody levels as a predictor of disease exacerbations in systemic lupus erythematosus: A long-term prospective study. Arthritis Rheum 1990; 33:634.
23. Ricker DM, Hebert LA, Rohde R, et al: Serum C3 levels are diagnostically more sensitive and specific for systemic lupus erythematosus activity than are serum C4 levels. Am J Kidney Dis 1991; 18:678.
24. Buyon JP, Tamerius J, Belmont HM, et al: Assessment of disease activity and impending flare in patients with systemic lupus erythematosus: Comparison of the use of complement split products and conventional measurements of complement. Arthritis Rheum 1992; 35:1028.
25. Campen DH, Horwitz DA, Quismorio FP, et al: Serum levels of interleukin-2 receptor and activity of rheumatic diseases characterized by immune system activation. Arthritis Rheum 1988; 31:1358.
26. Ward MM, Dooley MA, Christenson VD, et al: The relationship between soluble interleukin 2 receptor levels and antidouble stranded DNA antibody levels in patients with systemic lupus erythematosus. J Rheumatol 1991; 18:235.
27. Wong KL, Wong RPO: Serum soluble interleukin 2 receptor in systemic lupus erythematosus: Effects of disease activity and infection. Ann Rheum Dis 1991; 50:706.
28. Laut J, Senitzer D, Petrucci R, et al: Soluble interleukin-2 receptor levels in lupus nephritis. Clin Nephrol 1992; 35:179.
29. Picking WL, Smith C, Petrucci R, et al: Anti-RNA polymerase I antibodies in the urine of patients with systemic lupus erythematosus. J Rheumatol 1990; 17:1308.
30. Lim KL, Jones AC, Brown NS, et al: Urine neopterin as a parameter of disease activity in patients with systemic lupus erythematosus: Comparisons with serum sIL-2R and antibodies to dsDNA, erythrocyte sedimentation rate, and plasma C3, C4, and C3 degradation products. Ann Rheum Dis 1993; 52:429.
31. Gourley M, Segal K, Stewart M, et al: Urine cytokines in patients with SLE. Arthritis Rheum 1998; 41(suppl):S281.
32. Peterson E, Robertson AD, Emlen W: Serum and urinary interleukin-6 levels in SLE. Lupus 1996; 5:571.
33. Fries JF, Porta J, Liang MH: Marginal benefit of renal biopsy in systemic lupus erythematosus. Arch Intern Med 1978; 138:1386.
34. Austin HA III, Muenz LR, Joyce KM, et al: Prognostic factors in lupus nephritis: contribution of renal histologic data. Am J Med 1983; 75:382.
35. Austin HA III, Muenz LR, Joyce KM, et al: Diffuse proliferative lupus nephritis: identification of specific pathologic features effecting renal outcome. Kidney Int 1984; 25:689.

36. Nossent HC, Henzen-Logmans SC, Vroom TM, et al: Contribution of renal biopsy data in predicting outcome in lupus nephritis: Analysis of 116 patients. Arthritis Rheum 1990; 33:970.

37. Esdaile JM, Levinton C, Federgreen W, et al: The clinical and renal biopsy predictors of long-term outcome in lupus nephritis: A study of 87 patients and review of the literature. Q J Med 1989; 72:779.

38. Schwartz MM, Bernstein J, Hill GS, et al: Predictive value or renal pathology in diffuse proliferative lupus glomerulonephritis. Lupus Collaborative Study Group. Kidney Int 1989; 35:891.

39. Goulet J-R, Mackenzie T, Levinton C, et al: The long-term prognosis of lupus nephritis: The impact of disease activity. J Rheumatol 1993; 20:59.

40. Schwartz MM, Lan S-P, Bernstein J, et al: Irreproducibility of the activity and chronicity indices limits their utility in the management of lupus nephritis. Am J Kidney Dis 1993; 21:374.

41. Pollak VE, Pirani CL, Schwartz FD: The natural history of the renal manifestations of systemic lupus erythematosus. J Lab Clin Med 1964; 63:537.

42. Mackay IR, Chan D, Robson G: Prednisolone treatment of lupus nephritis: Effect of high doses on course of disease, renal function, histological lesions, and immunological reactions. Aust Ann Med 1970; 2:123.

43. Boelaert J, Morel-Maroger L, Mery J-P: Renal insufficiency in lupus nephritis. Adv Nephrol 1974; 4:249.

44. Ackerman GL: Alternate-day steroid therapy in lupus nephritis. Ann Intern Med 1970; 72:511.

45. Cathcart ES, Idelson BA, Scheinberg MA, et al: Beneficial effects of methylprednisolone "pulse" therapy in diffuse proliferative lupus nephritis. Lancet 1976; 1:163.

46. Kimberly RP, Lockshin MD, Sherman RL, et al: High-dose intravenous methylprednisolone pulse therapy in systemic lupus erythematosus. Am J Med 1981; 70:817.

47. Isenberg DA, Morrow WJW, Snaith ML: Methylprednisolone pulse therapy in the treatment of systemic lupus erythematosus. Ann Rheum Dis 1982; 41:347.

48. Barron KS, Person DA, Brewer EJ Jr, et al: Pulse methylprednisolone therapy in diffuse proliferative nephritis. J Pediatr 1982; 101:137.

49. Liebling MR, McLaughlin K, Boonsue S, et al: Monthly pulses of methylprednisolone in SLE nephritis. J Rheumatol 1982; 9:543.

50. Gourley MF, Austin HA III, Scott D, et al: Methylprednisolone and cyclophosphamide, alone or in combination, in patients with lupus nephritis. A randomized, controlled trial. Ann Intern Med 1996; 125:549.

51. Hayslett JP, Kashgarian M, Cook CD, et al: The effect of azathioprine on lupus glomerulonephritis. Medicine 1972; 51:393.

52. Drinkard JP, Stanley TM, Dornfeld L, et al: Azathioprine and prednisone in the treatment of adults with lupus nephritis. Medicine 1970; 49:411.

53. Shelp WD, Bloodworth JMB Jr, Rieselbach RE: Effect of azathioprine on renal histology and function in lupus nephritis. Arch Intern Med 1971; 128:566.

54. Barnett EV, Dornfeld L, Lee DBN, et al: Long-term survival of lupus nephritis patients treated with azathioprine and prednisone. J Rheumatol 1978; 5:275.

55. Sztejnbok M, Stewart A, Diamond H, et al: Azathioprine in the treatment of systemic lupus erythematosus: A controlled study. Arthritis Rheum 1971; 14:639.

56. Ginzler E, Sharon E, Diamond H, et al: Long-term maintenance therapy with azathioprine in systemic lupus erythematosus. Arthritis Rheum 1975; 18:25.

57. Hahn B, Kantor O, Osterland K: Azathioprine plus prednisone compared with prednisone alone in the treatment of SLE. Ann Intern Med 1975; 83:592.

58. Donadio JV Jr, Holley KE, Wagoner RD, et al: Further observations in the treatment of lupus nephritis with prednisone and combined prednisone and azathioprine. Arthritis Rheum 1974; 17:573.

59. Feng PH, Jayaratnam FJ, Tock EPC, et al: Cyclophosphamide in treatment of systemic lupus erythematosus: 7 years' experience. BMJ 1973; 2:450.

60. Donadio JV Jr, Holley KE, Ferguson RH, et al: Progressive lupus glomerulonephritis: Treatment with prednisone and combined prednisone and cyclophosphamide. Mayo Clin Proc 1976; 51:484.

61. Donadio JV Jr, Holley KE, Ferguson RH, et al: Treatment of diffuse proliferative lupus nephritis with prednisone and combined prednisone and cyclophosphamide. N Engl J Med 1978; 299:1151.

62. Decker JL, Klippel JH, Plotz PH, et al: Cyclophosphamide or azathioprine in lupus glomerulonephritis. A controlled trial: Results at 28 months. Ann Intern Med 1975; 83:606.

63. Dinant HJ, Decker JL, Klippel JH, et al: Alternative modes of cyclophosphamide and azathioprine therapy in lupus nephritis. Ann Intern Med 1982; 96:728.

64. Carette S, Klippel JH, Decker JL, et al: Controlled studies of oral immunosuppressive drugs in lupus nephritis. Ann Intern Med 1983; 99:1.

65. Felson DT, Anderson J: Evidence for the superiority of immunosuppressive drugs and prednisone over prednisone alone in lupus nephritis: Results of a pooled analysis. N Engl J Med 1984; 311:1528.

66. Austin HA III, Klippel JH, Balow JE, et al: Therapy of lupus nephritis: Controlled trial of prednisone and cytotoxic drugs. N Engl J Med 1986; 314:614.

67. Steinberg AD, Steinberg SC: Long-term preservation of renal function in patients with lupus nephritis receiving treatment that includes cyclophosphamide versus those treated with prednisone only. Arthritis Rheum 1991; 34:945.

68. Belmont HM, Storch M, Buyon J, et al: New York University/ Hospital for Joint Diseases experience with intravenous cyclophosphamide treatment: Efficacy in steroid unresponsive lupus nephritis. Lupus 1995; 4:104.

69. Dooley MA, Hogan S, Jennette CJ, et al: Cyclophosphamide therapy for lupus nephritis: Poor renal survival in black Americans. Kidney Int 1997; 31:1188.

70. Schwartzman S, Delguidice-Asch G, Kimberly R. Intravenous cyclophosphamide (IVCY) for the treatment of lupus nephritis (LN). Arthritis Rheum 1995; 38(suppl):S304.

71. Garcia C, Gutierrez S, Molina JF, et al: Intravenous pulse cyclophosphamide (IVCY) therapy of severe lupus nephritis. Arthritis Rheum 1995; 38(suppl):S347.

72. Pando JA, Gourley MF, Boumpas DT, et al: Rates of renal remission and relapse in patients with lupus nephritis (LN) treated with bolus cyclophosphamide (CY). Arthritis Rheum 1994; 37(suppl):S179.

73. Yang X, Yin P, Gao X: A study on interval of intravenous cyclophosphamide pulse in the treatment of severe systemic lupus erythematosus. Chung Hua Nei Ko Tsa Chih 1996; 35:257.

74. Ciruela F, de la Cruz J, Lopez I, et al: Cumulative rate of relapse of lupus nephritis after successful treatment with cyclophosphamide. Arthritis Rheum 1996; 39:2028.

75. Lehman TJA, Sherry DD, Wagner-Weiner L, et al: Intermittent intravenous cyclophosphamide therapy for lupus nephritis. J Pediatr 1989; 114:1055.

76. Boumpas DT, Austin HA III, Vaughan EM, et al: Risk for sustained amenorrhea in patients with systemic lupus erythematosus receiving intermittent pulse cyclophosphamide therapy. Ann Intern Med 1993; 119:366.

77. Ortiz A, Gonzalez-Parra E, Alvarez-Costa G, et al: Bladder cancer after cyclophosphamide therapy for lupus nephritis. Nephron 1992; 60:378.

78. Lloyd W, Schur PH: Immune complexes, complement, and anti-DNA in exacerbations of systemic lupus erythematosus (SLE). Medicine 1981; 60:208.

79. Laitman RS, Glicklich D, Sablay LB, et al: Effect of long-term normalization of serum complement levels on the course of lupus nephritis. Am J Med 1989; 87:132.

80. Seyffart G: Drug dosage in renal insufficiency. Dordrecht, The Netherlands: Kluwers Academic Publishers, 1991:167.

81. Verrier Jones J, Robinson MF, Parciany RK, et al: Therapeutic plasmapheresis in systemic lupus erythematosus: Effect on immune complexes and antibodies to DNA. Arthritis Rheum 1981; 24:1113.

82. Schroeder JO, Euler HH, Loffler H: Synchronization of plasmapheresis and pulse cyclophosphamide in severe systemic lupus erythematosus. Ann Intern Med 1987; 107:344.

83. Dau PC, Callahan J, Parker R, et al: Immunologic effects of plasmapheresis synchronized with pulse cyclophosphamide in systemic lupus erythematosus. J Rheumatol 1991; 18:270.

84. Lewis EJ, Hunsicker LG, Lan S-P, et al: A controlled trial of plasmapheresis therapy in severe lupus nephritis. N Engl J Med 1992; 326:1373.

85. Lin C-Y, Hsu H-C, Cliang H: Improvement of histological and immunological change in steroid and immunosuppressive drug-resistant lupus nephritis by high-dose intravenous gamma globulin. Nephron 1989; 53:303.

86. Akashi K, Nagasawa K, Mayumi, et al: Successful treatment of refractory systemic lupus erythematosus with intravenous immunoglobulins. J Rheumatol 1990; 17:375.

87. Winder A, Molad Y, Ostfeld I, et al: Treatment of systemic lupus erythematosus by prolonged administration of high dose intravenous immunoglobulin: Report of 2 cases. J Rheumatol 1993; 20:495.

88. Isenberg DA, Snaith ML, Morrow WJW, et al: Cyclosporin A for the treatment of systemic lupus erythematosus. Int J Immunopharmacol 1981; 3:163.

89. Feutren G, Querin S, Noel LH, et al: Effects of cyclosporine in severe systemic lupus erythematosus. J Pediatr 1987; 111:1063.

90. Favre H, Miescher PA, Huang YP, et al: Cyclosporine in the treatment of lupus nephritis. Am J Nephrol 1989; 9(suppl 1):57.

91. Dostal C, Tesai V, Rychlik I, et al: Effect of 1 year cyclosporin A treatment on the activity and renal involvement of systemic lupus erythematosus: A pilot study. Lupus 1998; 7:29.

92. Caccavo D, Lagana B, Mitterhofer AP, et al: Long-term treatment of systemic lupus erythematosus with cyclosporin A. Arthritis Rheum 1997; 40:27.

93. Hood KA, Zarembski DG: Mycophenolate mofetil: A unique immunosuppressive agent. Am J Health Syst Pharm 1997; 54:285.

94. McMurray RW, Elbourne KB, Lai S: Mycophenolate mofetil prevents lupus nephritis and mortality in the female B/W mouse model of SLE. Arthritis Rheum 1997; 40(suppl):S324.

95. Corna D, Morigi M, Facchinetti D, et al: Mycophenolate mofetil limits renal damage and prolongs life in murine lupus autoimmune disease. Kidney Int 1997; 51:1583.

96. Hebert LA, Losio FG, Bay, WH, et al: Mycophenolate mofetil (CellCept, MMF) therapy of systemic lupus erythematosus (SLE) and ANCA vasculitis (V) [Abstract]. J Am Soc Nephrol 1997; 8:87A.

97. Briggs WA, Choi MJ, Scheel PJ Jr: Successful mycophenolate mofetil treatment of glomerular disease. Am J Kidney Dis 1998; 31:213.

98. Dooley MA, Cosio FG, Nachman PH, et al: Mycophenolate mofetil therapy in lupus nephritis: Clinical observations. J Am Soc Nephrol 1999; 10:833.

99. Glicklich D, Acharya A: Mycophenolate mofetil therapy for lupus nephritis refractory to intravenous cyclophosphamide. Am J Kidney Dis 1998; 32:318.

100. Pashinian N, Wallace DJ, Klinenberg JR: Mycophenolate mofetil for systemic lupus erythematosus. Arthritis Rheum 1998; 41(suppl):S110.

101. Strober S, Farinas C, Field EH, et al: Lupus nephritis after total lymphoid irradiation: Persistent improvement and reduction of steroid therapy. Ann Intern Med 1987; 107:689.

102. Ben-Chetrit E, Gross DJ, Braverman A, et al: Total lymphoid irradiation in refractory systemic lupus erythematosus. Ann Intern Med 1986; 105:58.

103. Westberg G, Tarkowski A: Effect of MaxEPA in patients with SLE. Scand J Rheumatol 1990; 19:137.

104. Walton AJE, Snaith ML, Locniskar M, et al: Dietary fish oil and the severity of symptoms in patients with systemic lupus erythematosus. Ann Rheum Dis 1991; 50:463.

105. Clark WF, Parbtani A, Naylor CD, et al: Fish oil in lupus nephritis: Clinical findings and methodological implications. Kidney Int 1993; 44:75.

106. Hiepe F, Volk H-D, Apostoloff E, et al: Treatment of severe systemic lupus erythematosus with anti-CD4 monoclonal antibody [Letter]. Lancet 1991; 338:1529.

107. Kincaid-Smith P: The role of coagulation in the obliteration of glomerular capillaries. *In* Kincaid-Smith P, Mathew TH, Lovell Becker D (eds): Glomerulonephritis. New York: Wiley, 1973:871.

108. Suc JM, Conte J, Mignon-Conte M: Treatment of glomerulonephritis with indomethacin and heparin. *In* Kincaid-Smith P, Mathew TH, Lovell Becker D (eds): Glomerulonephritis. New York: Wiley, 1973:927.

109. Cade R, Spooner F, Schlein E, et al: Comparison of azathioprine, prednisone, and heparin alone or combined in treating lupus nephritis. Nephron 1973; 10:37.

110. Hariharan S, Pollak VE, Kant KS, et al: Diffuse lupus nephritis: Long-term observations in patients treated with ancrod. Clin Nephrol 1990; 34:61.

111. Leaker B, McGregor A, Griffiths M, et al: Insidious loss of renal function in patients with anticardiolipin antibodies and absence of overt nephritis. Br J Rheumatol 1991; 30:422.

112. Pierucci A, Simonetti BM, Pecci G, et al: Improvement of renal function with selective thromboxane antagonism in lupus nephritis. N Engl J Med 1989; 320:421.

113. Lin C-Y: Improvement in steroid and immunosuppressive drug resistant lupus nephritis by intravenous prostaglandin E1 therapy. Nephron 1990; 55:258.

114. Budman DR, Steinberg AD: Hypertension and renal disease in systemic lupus erythematosus. Arch Intern Med 1976; 136:1003.

115. Reveille JD, Bartolucci A, Alarcon GS: Prognosis in systemic lupus erythematosus: Negative impact of increasing age at onset, black race, and thrombocytopenia, as well as causes of death. Arthritis Rheum 1990; 33:37.

116. Seleznick MJ, Fries JF: Variables associated with decreased survival in systemic lupus erythematosus. Semin Arthritis Rheum 1991; 21:73.

117. Ward MM, Studenski S: Clinical prognostic factors in lupus nephritis: The importance of hypertension and smoking. Arch Intern Med 1992; 152:2082.

118. Ginzler EM, Felson DT, Anthony JM, et al: Hypertension increased the risk of renal deterioration in systemic lupus erythematosus. J Rheumatol 1993; 20:1694.

119. Fries JF, Powers R, Kempson RL: Late-stage lupus nephropathy. J Rheumatol 1974; 1:166.

120. Cheigh JS, Stenzel KH: End-stage renal disease in systemic lupus erythematosus. Am J Kidney Dis 1993; 21:2.

121. US Renal Data System: USRDS 1991 Annual data report: The National Institutes of Health, National Institute of Diabetes and Digestive and Kidney Diseases, Bethesda, MD, August 1991. Am J Kidney Dis 1991; 18(suppl 2):1.

122. Goss JA, Cole BR, Jendrisak MD, et al: Renal transplantation for systemic lupus erythematosus and recurrent lupus nephritis: A single-center experience and a review of the literature. Transplantation 1991; 52:805.

123. Sumrani N, Miles AM, Delaney V, et al: Renal transplantation in cyclosporine-treated patients with end-stage lupus nephropathy. Transplant Proc 1992; 24:1785.

124. Mojcik CF, Klippel JH: End-stage renal disease and systemic lupus erythematosus. Am J Med 1996; 101:100.

125. Stone JH, Amend WC, Criswell LA: Outcome of renal transplantation in ninety-seven cyclosporine-era patients with systemic lupus erythematosus and matched controls. Arthritis Rheum 1998; 41:1438.

# 26 | Treatment of Neuropsychiatric Systemic Lupus Erythematosus

*Joan Marie Von Feldt*

In 1872, Kaposi first described lupus as a systemic disease, but the clinical spectrum of neuropsychiatric manifestations of systemic lupus erythematosus (SLE) was not well delineated until the writings of Harvey and Dubois in the 1950s.[1] Neuropsychiatric manifestations occur in 30% of patients with SLE and continue to be a cause of significant morbidity and mortality in the lupus population. The mortality rate for neuropsychiatric systemic lupus erythematosus (NP-SLE) appears to be diminishing. In the first half of the 20th century, nervous system disease was reportedly responsible for 25% of the deaths in SLE patients.[1-3] Since the 1970s that figure has dropped to approximately 10%.[4, 5] The change coincided with the availability of aggressive immunotherapeutic modalities as well as improvement in overall SLE survival.

Despite improved understanding of the immunopathologic processes in SLE, rheumatologists continue to define the disease descriptively using a list of criteria. The 1982 revised American College of Rheumatology classification criteria for SLE include two neuropsychiatric manifestations: seizure and psychosis. However, numerous other manifestations of NP-SLE occur in SLE patients. Committees comprising the experts in the medical community have tried to establish a similar list of criteria for the myriad manifestations of NP-SLE and have published case definitions for 19 neuropsychiatric syndromes.[6] A working definition for NP-SLE, first described by Kassan and Lockshin, that has been used in case reports is the following: a neuropsychiatric disturbance, with a significant and unequivocal change in baseline neurologic or psychiatric function, identified by history and physical examination.[7] This definition would include most if not all of the neuropsychiatric manifestations of SLE, including organic brain syndrome (organic mood disorder, delirium, dementia), psychiatric disorder, stroke syndrome (hemiparesis or upper motor neuron signs), cranial neuropathy, and cognitive disorders.

In discussing the treatment of NP-SLE, it is helpful to review the major clinical manifestations, because treatment is usually directed toward the specific manifestation. It is also helpful to review neuropathologic studies and their contribution to what is known about disease pathogenesis in NP-SLE. Because treatment regimens for NP-SLE have wide variation and are frequently empiric, a review of the basis for this variation—proposed theories of etiopathogenesis—can be helpful.

## MAJOR CLINICAL MANIFESTATIONS

Diffuse manifestations (acute global dysfunction), including psychosis, delirium, and dementia, are the most common presentation in NP-SLE. Organic brain syndrome can be the most devastating of central nervous system (CNS) manifestations and is seen in 30% to 55% of NP-SLE patients. Frank psychosis is seen in 5% to 15% of patients and can be the presenting sign of the disease. Major depression can be a manifestation of the disease secondary to NP-SLE activity, and there also can be a reactive depression to a chronic devastating illness. Delirium can be seen in SLE patients, frequently in association with multisystem failure, and may be a manifestation of NP-SLE or secondary to metabolic abnormalities from other organ dysfunction. Dementia can be a presentation of acute global dysfunction in SLE patients. Onset of SLE occurs after the age of 65 years in 10% of patients with SLE. In a subset of these patients, dementia can be the initial manifestation of NP-SLE.[8]

The importance of distinguishing secondary causes of acute global dysfunction in patients who present with neuropsychiatric manifestations cannot be overstressed. In addition to clues from the history, physical examination, and laboratory studies, serum and cerebrospinal fluid (CSF) antibodies have been useful in distinguishing NP-SLE from neuropsychiatric manifestations due to secondary causes. There is a strong association between the diffuse neuropsychiatric manifestations, especially psychosis, and antineuronal antibodies in the CSF. Serum and CSF antiribosomal P antibodies have been associated with psychosis and can be helpful, if present, in distinguishing NP-SLE from other causes of psychosis.[9]

Focal manifestations (e.g., strokes) occur in a minority of patients with SLE affecting the CNS, about 10% to 35%. These stroke syndromes can affect any area of the brain and are frequently caused by thrombosis from vasculopathy or emboli from cardiac valvular lesions. Most focal neurologic events are associated with antiphospholipid antibodies (aPL Ab), and management of focal manifestations has evolved as the aPL Ab syndrome has become better described.[10]

Seizures are a common manifestation of both NP-SLE and secondary causes of CNS events in SLE patients. Grand mal seizures are the most common type, although focal, petit mal, and temporal lobe seizures, as well as status epilepticus, have been described. A number of factors can contribute to seizures, including focal infarction or ischemia caused by vasculitis or the aPL Ab syndrome, embolic phenomena (perhaps from Libman-Sacks cardiac valvular lesions), hemorrhage by various mechanisms, and brain-reactive antibodies.

Transverse myelitis is an infrequent but devastating manifestation of NP-SLE; it has been associated with aPL Ab in some, but not all, studies. The cervical cord is the most common site of involvement, and patients frequently have characteristic CSF abnormalities. Abnormal T2 signals on magnetic resonance imaging (MRI) of the spinal cord may also be present. In a review by Mok and colleagues,[11] 10 cases of transverse myelitis were identified in a lupus cohort of 315 patients. In five of these patients, transverse myelitis was the initial manifestation of SLE. If the myelitis is not aggressively treated at the time of presentation, significant neurologic compromise can result.

Peripheral neuropathies include mononeuropathy and polyneuropathy and can be sensory, motor, or mixed. Antineuronal antibodies, aPL Ab, and vasculitis have all been implicated in causing these neuropathies. Cranial neuropathies can be transient or permanent. Sensorineural hearing loss (SNHL) is occasionally seen in SLE, and sudden SNHL has been reported to occur in association with the aPL Ab.[12–15] Movement disorders such as chorea are rare. All of these neuropathies and chorea are frequently associated with aPL Ab, and the mechanism of nerve damage is presumed to be thrombotic.

Headaches are one of the most common maladies in SLE, occurring in 30% to 50% of patients. Some have intractable headache, the so-called "lupus headache." Common migraine headache is reported to occur more frequently than classical migraine in this population.[16, 17] However, headache is not a common manifestation of NP-SLE; more often it occurs secondary to other causes, including fatigue, anxiety, and depression. Two studies looked at headache in SLE patients, and their conclusions were similar. Sfikakis and coworkers[18] compared 78 SLE patients with 89 healthy control subjects and observed that the prevalence of headache did not differ between the two groups (28% vs 32%). Only one SLE patient with headache refractory to analgesics responded to corticosteroids. Migraine occurred in a quarter of the SLE patients.[18] Rozell and associates[19] looked at 40 SLE patients—10 without headache, 11 with nonmigraine headache, and 20 with migraine—and found that migraine was not associated with increased disease activity, severity, other neuropsychiatric manifestations, or more frequent MRI abnormalities. Therefore, even SLE patients with migraine should be evaluated for secondary causes of headache, because headache is rarely a harbinger of more serious neuropsychiatric manifestations. SLE patients with frequent headache should be treated with prophylactic regimens in common use, including low-dose tricyclic antidepressants, $\beta$ blockers, calcium channel blockers, and serotonin reuptake antagonists. Serotonin agonists such as sumatriptan and rizatriptan can also be effective when used at the time of migraine onset.

Impairment of cognitive function is a frequent consequence of overt NP-SLE. However, cognitive impairment is also common in patients who have never manifested overt NP-SLE. Numerous groups have documented and quantified cognitive dysfunction in this group of patients, which often goes unrecognized and untreated.[20–23] The "lupus personality" that is occasionally used to describe some SLE patients may ultimately be determined to be a combination of cognitive dysfunction, frequently seen in lupus, plus the anxiety and depression that result from having an unpredictable chronic illness.

## NEUROPATHOLOGIC STUDIES

Johnson and Richardson[24] in 1968 and, a decade later, Ellis and Verity[25] determined from their neuropathologic studies (from autopsies of SLE patients) that true vasculitis of the CNS was rare. The most common finding was a vasculopathy of small arterioles and capillaries. Sixty-five percent of patients had vasculopathy; 54% had vascular hyalinization, 28% had perivascular inflammation, and 21% had endothelial proliferation.[25] This vasculopathy was seen in patients who never demonstrated CNS symptoms as well as those with overt neuropsychiatric manifestations. Only occasionally did the anatomy of the vasculopathy correlate with neuropsychiatric manifestations. These important studies highlight two major features of NP-SLE. The first is that the vasculopathy of brain vessels is pervasive and occurs in significant numbers of SLE patients, symptomatic or not. The second is that many of the patients' CNS manifestations of SLE cannot be explained by vascular changes.

Because vasculopathy alone cannot account for the clinical manifestations, at least one other mechanism must be invoked to describe the more diffuse symptoms of psychosis, cognitive impairment, and dementia. Since these two neuropathologic studies were published, evidence has accumulated implicating several different immunopathogenic mechanisms. Autoantibodies reacting with neuronal membrane molecules as measured in CSF have been associated with the active NP-SLE,[26, 27] suggesting that these autoantibodies may be pathogenic. Studies demonstrating immunohistochemical staining of these autoantibodies in neuronal tissue are lacking, however. In addition, there are no animal models for NP-SLE, in contrast to the numerous murine models of lupus nephritis.

Other autoantibodies in addition to antineuronal antibodies are associated with neurologic events in NP-

SLE. Focal ischemic events frequently correlate with anticardiolipin and other aPL Ab and are thought to represent thrombotic events.[28, 29] In addition, aPL Ab and associated antibodies to $\beta_2$-glycoprotein-I may not solely cause thrombotic events but also may act directly on neuronal tissue.[30] Jara and colleagues reported elevations of prolactin and interleukin-6 (IL-6) in patients with active NP-SLE, confirming earlier reports of increased IL-6 in the CSF of patients with active CNS disease.[31] They found that the majority of NP-SLE patients with increased concentrations of prolactin and IL-6 had seizures. These findings suggest that intrathecal synthesis of IL-6 occurs, but it is unclear whether increased IL-6 in NP-SLE is a marker of NP-SLE and acute inflammation as an epiphenomenon, or whether IL-6 is directly involved in pathogenesis. Therefore, NP-SLE cannot be viewed as a monolithic entity. Rather, it is a collection of a variety of clinical manifestations of one or a combination of pathologic events, which could include neuron-reactive autoantibodies, the sequelae of the aPL Ab syndrome, or immune complex–mediated vasculitis.

## DIFFERENTIAL DIAGNOSIS

Just as a single pathogenetic process cannot account for the multiplicity of neuropsychiatric manifestations of SLE, no single clinical sign or diagnostic test is abnormal in all NP-SLE presentations. As discussed earlier, NP-SLE is probably caused by a variety of immunopathologic mechanisms, and diagnosis is hampered by the lack of characteristic histologic changes. Even if a brain biopsy were easily available, neuropathologic studies have demonstrated that no pathognomonic lesions analogous to the "wire loop" lesion of lupus nephritis or "onion skin" vascular changes of SLE in the spleen exist in the brain. Therefore, the clinician makes the diagnosis by first excluding other causes and then using clues in the history, physical examination, and serologic studies.

The most important investigative process in the evaluation of a patient with neuropsychiatric manifestations is to exclude secondary causes of the presenting symptoms. Most reviews of SLE patients with neuropsychiatric manifestations note that a third of these patients have neuropsychiatric manifestations that are caused by secondary causes of CNS dysfunction rather than NP-SLE.[8, 32, 33] These other causes of CNS events include infection, severe hypertension, uremia, fluid and electrolyte imbalances, and medication effects and should be excluded by history and routine laboratory testing. Other peripheral stigmata of SLE disease activity accompany NP-SLE at least 50% of the time. This means that in about 50% of cases, a neuropsychiatric symptom can be the sole presenting sign of SLE disease activity. In West and associates' review of NP-SLE patients, 58% of patients with neuropsychiatric manifestations secondary to SLE had evidence of increased disease activity, whereas only 14% of those with neuropsychiatric manifestations secondary to other causes had increased disease activity.[34] Clinical manifestations, however, were similar in both groups. Patients with severe neuropsychiatric disease caused by SLE frequently have more than one NP-SLE manifestation. In West and associates' cohort, 19% had complex presentations (i.e., more than one neuropsychiatric manifestation). In Neuwelt and coworkers' cohort of patients with refractory NP-SLE, 80% had more than one neuropsychiatric manifestation.[35] In summary, the diagnosis of NP-SLE involves eliminating secondary causes of neuropsychiatric manifestations, searching for concurrent lupus disease activity in other organ systems, and garnering evidence of active disease in the CNS.

## TREATMENT

Recommendations for treatment of CNS manifestations of SLE suffer from the absence of randomized, controlled trials. Current therapeutic regimens have been distilled from case reports, retrospective reviews of outcomes in patients treated with various therapeutic regimens, and clinical experience.

## Corticosteroids

The mainstay of therapy for the neuropsychiatric manifestations of SLE remains corticosteroids. The use of corticosteroids evolved primarily from the 1950s writings of DuBois. He recommended an aggressive regimen of corticosteroids, initiating therapy with the equivalent of 1 mg/kg/day of prednisone and doubling it each day until the patient responded.[36] Follow-up studies some years later documented decreased mortality from CNS disease after the initiation of that therapeutic program.[2] DuBois's work had a profound impact and resulted in the widespread use of high corticosteroid dosages which, in turn, led to increasing complications. Enthusiasm for high-dose steroids was tempered considerably by a study published in the mid-1970s that documented a high death rate from infection in patients treated with more than 100 mg of prednisone equivalent per day for longer than 2 weeks.[37] Current practice includes initiation of therapy at a daily dose of 1 to 1.5 mg/kg/day of prednisone equivalent. Alternatively, intravenous daily pulses of 1 g of methylprednisolone for 3 days may be given, followed by a daily dose in the range of 0.6 to 1 mg/kg/day of prednisone equivalent given intravenously or orally.[38, 39]

Corticosteroids are used for almost every manifestation of NP-SLE. An international survey of rheumatologists to assess how clinicians manage various clinical manifestations of NP-SLE was published in 1996.[40] Corticosteroids were the most common immunosuppressive regimen, and the use of intravenous cyclophosphamide was rare. Similarly, I distributed a survey to members of a loosely knit rheumatology clinical cooperative in the Philadelphia region to ascertain the standard of care for NP-SLE in our area. This group included rheumatologists from academic and private practices. This survey also found that rheumatologists used corticosteroids most commonly to manage NP-SLE and that intravenous cyclophosphamide was infrequently used even in critically ill patients. Unfortunately, corticosteroids do not always effectively treat the manifestations of NP-SLE, and infection is not the only side effect of high-dose corticosteroid use.

### Corticosteroid Side Effects

Side effects of corticosteroids are protean, and most rheumatologists are acutely aware of the double-edged sword of corticosteroid treatment in SLE patients. Susceptibility to infections is one of the most serious side effects. Although high doses of corticosteroids magnify the risk, lower doses of 0.25 to 0.5 mg/kg/day can also predispose to infection. The morbidity associated with use of corticosteroids in the SLE population is well recognized. A widely accepted index for measuring cumulative organ damage in SLE patients was put together by the Systemic Lupus International Clinic Cooperative (SLICC). The SLICC Disease Damage Index includes not only damage from the disease but also organ damage from chronic steroid use.[41] Bone loss from even low-dose steroids has been well documented in the literature, and resultant osteoporosis in young women has grave long-term risks.[42, 43] Cataracts occur in patients with chronic steroid use. Weight gain is an extremely common side effect of chronic steroid use, and with it many related side effects occur, including hypertension, hypercholesterolemia, and hyperglycemia. Patients receiving chronic steroid therapy can develop insulin resistance and not infrequently require hypoglycemic or insulin therapy. Steroid myopathy can be seen in patients receiving chronic corticosteroid therapy as well. Premature atherosclerotic cardiovascular disease is seen in SLE patients, and corticosteroid use may contribute to it.

### "Steroid Psychosis"

No discussion of steroid side effects is complete without addressing "steroid psychosis," an entity that is well recognized and is frequently placed high on the list of differential diagnoses of lupus patients with a psychotic presentation.[44, 45] However, virtually all large clinical studies of NP-SLE have emphasized that steroid psychosis is uncommon.[1, 46–48] Reports in the literature vary between 1.3% and 50%, the variability explained by dose and definition of neuropsychiatric dysfunction. Corticosteroid therapy has been associated with prominent disturbances in memory, attention, and concentration and poor performance in intelligence quotient (IQ) testing.[49] It was also associated with improvement in cognition in a small group of SLE patients.[20] However, collective review of these series and my own experience implicate steroids as causing fewer than 10% of true psychotic events that occur in patients with lupus. Steroid psychosis should be considered if a significant change in corticosteroid dose preceded the onset of the psychiatric manifestations. There are clinical features that can help to distinguish between the steroid and lupus causes of psychoses.

Steroid psychosis tends not to be accompanied by the classical features of organic brain syndrome, such as diminished consciousness, concurrent focal neurologic signs, or the presence of visual, tactile, or olfactory hallucinations, or by other signs of organic neurologic dysfunction. Almost all patients with psychosis due to lupus have accompanying organic brain syndrome. If any signs of organicity are present, or if the psychosis occurs in the setting of increased systemic activity of the SLE, the event is most likely lupus induced.

### Corticosteroid Toxicity Monitoring

Patients taking corticosteroids need to be counseled about the risk of infection, as well as the other known side effects. All patients receiving corticosteroids should also take calcium, 1500 mg/day, and 800 units/day of vitamin D. If the patient is known to be osteoporotic or osteopenic, she should be prescribed an antiresorptive agent at the time of institution of corticosteroid therapy. In a premenopausal woman with normal bone mineral density, it is controversial whether to use an antiresorptive drug, but this is routinely done in my practice. If the patient is hospitalized, pamidronate (30, 45, or 60 mg, depending on weight) can be given intravenously and obviates the need for further antiresorptive therapy for 3 to 4 months.[50–52]

## Cyclophosphamide

In the 1990s, after the documented successful use of intermittent pulse intravenous cyclophosphamide therapy in the treatment of lupus nephritis, several small, uncontrolled, retrospective studies and anecdotal case reports appeared suggesting an important therapeutic role for cyclophosphamide as an immunosuppressive regimen in the treatment of steroid-resistant NP-SLE.[35, 53–57] I and others have reported the benefit of pulse intravenous cyclophosphamide in steroid-resistant neuropsychiatric disease. These studies have established a basis for what has become general practice in treating refractory NP-SLE despite the lack of prospective, randomized, controlled trials. The initial dose of cyclophosphamide is 500 to 1000 mg/m² body surface area as a single intravenous dose, with subsequent monthly intravenous treatments modified depending on the nadir of the white blood cell (WBC) count. Other methods of administration can be used as well. Ramos and colleagues[58] reported their use of cyclophosphamide as 500 mg intravenously each week for at least 3 weeks, then 500 mg intravenously each month if necessary. In their study, patients responded favorably to this regimen with few adverse side effects. Cyclophosphamide can also be given orally in doses of 2 to 5 mg/kg/day, but this increases the total cumulative dose of cyclophosphamide and increases toxicity as well.

Cyclophosphamide is an inactive precursor that requires hepatic activation. It is an indiscriminate alkylator of DNA, making it a relative B cell–specific toxin. However, all cell lines are affected by cyclophosphamide, contributing to its toxicity. When given in a single intravenous pulse dose of 500 to 1000 mg/m$^2$, cyclophosphamide causes a WBC nadir at 7 to 14 days. Studies of patients with lupus nephritis suggest that cyclophosphamide is more effective in patients in whom the WBC nadir is at least 3000 cells/mm$^3$. Therefore, subsequent doses of intravenous cyclophosphamide are adjusted to reduce the WBC count down to that range. If the nadir WBC count is too low or too prolonged, granulocyte colony-stimulating factor (G-CSF, Neupogen) can be given for "rescue," to stimulate a more rapid recovery by the bone marrow. The G-CSF dose of 5 $\mu$g/kg/day subcutaneously or intravenously is given until bone marrow recovery. Although cyclophosphamide is not free of serious side effects, especially infection, it is the most effective modality for corticosteroid-resistant disease. The appropriate clinical settings for its use are discussed in a later section.

## Cyclophosphamide Side Effects

Although cyclophosphamide has been associated with improvement in NP-SLE, it carries with it potentially serious side effects. Acutely it can cause hemorrhagic cystitis, which can largely be avoided with the administration of 2-mercaptoethane sulfonate (mesna). Nausea and vomiting are usually controlled with ondansetron. There is an increased risk of infection, not only at the WBC nadir but chronically, while the patient is receiving monthly cyclophosphamide. In addition to a much greater risk of infection, cumulative doses increase the risk of numerous malignancies, including lymphoma, bladder cancer, and cervical cancer. In men and women of child-bearing age sterility may result, because cyclophosphamide can cause premature ovarian failure as well as testicular toxicity. In a review of the National Institutes of Health experience in SLE patients treated for lupus nephritis under the standard 2-year protocol, women aged 20 to 30 years became infertile 50% of the time, and all women older than 30 years of age became infertile.[59] Studies are under way to evaluate the effectiveness of using birth control pills or drugs that induce reversible menopause to reduce some of the ovarian toxicity. Cyclophosphamide is also a potent teratogen and should not be used during pregnancy. Most especially because of the side effects to women of child-bearing age compounded by the high prevalence of SLE in women aged 15 to 45 years, there is continued investigation into alternative therapeutic regimens.

## Cyclophosphamide Toxicity Monitoring

Patients taking cyclophosphamide should be counseled regarding the risks of cyclophosphamide just outlined. Even after cyclophosphamide administration is complete, routine urinalyses should be done regularly to look for hematuria as an indicator of bladder cancer. Women should have a pelvic examination and Papanicolaou smear done yearly.

## Plasmapheresis

After a number of reports of successful treatment of lupus nephritis appeared in the 1980s, plasmapheresis was applied to patients with steroid-resistant neuropsychiatric manifestations.[60-63] Several anecdotal studies described a good outcome.[64-66] Some studies reported on the use of synchronous plasmapheresis, or plasmapheresis administered for three cycles followed by intravenous cyclophosphamide.[67] Theoretically, plasmapheresis should induce proliferation of pathogenic B-cell clones (termed *antibody rebound*), which are subsequently ablated by cyclophosphamide during this period of vulnerability. More recently, controlled trials of plasmapheresis in lupus nephritis have shown no statistically significant therapeutic benefit, and enthusiasm for this mode of treatment has waned. No controlled studies for neuropsychiatric disease have been done.[68, 69]

## Plasmapheresis Side Effects

Plasmapheresis can cause significant intravascular volume shifts and is therefore risky in patients who are not hemodynamically stable. In addition, plasmapheresis requires a large-bore needle and central venous access. More importantly, plasmapheresis increases the risk of infection. A retrospective review of patients treated with plasmapheresis and intravenous cyclophosphamide compared with patients treated with cyclophosphamide alone has been published.[70] The patients treated with plasmapheresis plus intravenous cyclophosphamide had a higher incidence of serious bacterial or viral infections: 7 of 9 patients, compared with 2 of 12 in the group treated with intravenous cyclophosphamide alone. These side effects, in addition to the lack of proven efficacy of plasmapheresis in neuropsychiatric disease, make plasmapheresis a rare therapeutic option. It should be reserved only for patients with severe, refractory disease for whom all other treatment options have failed, with the caveat that it may have no benefit.

## Refractory Neuropsychiatric Systemic Lupus Erythematosus

The largest review to date of treatment for catastrophic NP-SLE included 31 patients treated with intravenous cyclophosphamide.[35] These SLE patients had various presentations including diffuse and focal disease. Most patients had multiple neuropsychiatric manifestations, with a median of two. Eight patients had anticardiolipin antibodies with focal stroke syndromes and were treated with anticoagulation as well. The patients were subclassified as group I, those who substantially improved after pulse intravenous cyclophosphamide (61%); group S, those who stabilized with this treatment (29%); and group P, those who progressively deteriorated (10%). Eight patients received adjunct plasmapheresis when they failed to improve or stabilize with intravenous cyclophosphamide. One patient received plasmapheresis at the same time as cyclophosphamide; with the other seven patients, plasmapheresis was begun only after a mean of 9 monthly cyclophosphamide infusions. The NP-SLE stabilized in one patient and improved in five. Two patients died while receiving plasmapheresis, neither of whom had received synchronous plasmapheresis and cyclophosphamide.

Plasmapheresis is still used to treat refractory disease unresponsive to conventional therapeutic modalities. Because of reports of increased morbidity and mortality associated with plasmapheresis (usually from infection), it should be reserved for the very ill patient, and great precautions should be used with regard to infection.

Other unconventional treatments for refractory disease have been reported, and their utility in the management of NP-SLE is questionable. They include the combination of electroconvulsive therapy with intravenous cyclophosphamide for catatonia and the use of intrathecal methotrexate.[71, 71a]

## THERAPY DIRECTED BY SPECIFIC MANIFESTATIONS

The treatment of NP-SLE is summarized in Table 26–1.

### Acute Global Dysfunction: Psychosis, Delirium, and Dementia

Acute onset of diffuse neuropsychiatric manifestations of lupus requires a two-pronged therapeutic approach: control of the acute neuropsychiatric manifestation with neuroactive drugs and suppression of the immunopathogenic mechanisms responsible for the CNS dysfunction. Control of agitation or panic is an important early therapeutic goal for patients with acute or chronic organic mental dysfunction and/or psychosis. Neuroleptic agents such as haloperidol or chlorpromazine are the most common medications used. Because the agitation eventually resolves in most patients, long-term use is not often required and the long-term consequences, such as extrapyramidal or parkinsonian side effects, are rare.

Acute cerebral dysfunction, with or without psychosis, should also be treated with an immunosuppressive regimen. The patient is usually hospitalized, and parenteral therapy with approximately 1 to 2 mg/kg/day of methylprednisolone is given intravenously in divided doses. If the patient does not respond within 5 to 7 days or if there is further deterioration in neurologic dysfunction, methylprednisolone, 1 g/day for 3 days, is usually administered.[38, 71b] Although randomized trials supporting this regimen are lacking, disease that remains refractory is then often treated with intravenous cyclophosphamide.

### Subacute Global Manifestations

In less life-threatening presentations, the patient may be treated with oral prednisone in a dose that is signifi-

cantly higher than that given before the onset of the neuropsychiatric problem. However, other causes of mood disorder or organic brain syndrome should be excluded before empiric therapy is initiated.

### Focal Manifestations

As discussed earlier, the incidence of vasculitis of the CNS in NP-SLE is rare, occurring only 10% of the time. Most vascular events are not caused by vasculitis but more probably by thromboembolic disease. With better understanding of the role of aPL Ab in SLE patients, there has been a paradigm shift in the management of focal neurologic events over the past decade.

The presence of aPL Ab in an SLE patient does not imply that the patient will have a thrombotic event. The frequency of aPL Ab is high but thromboembolic events are rare.[28, 29, 72, 73] However, when a patient with known aPL Ab status presents with a focal neurologic event, the likely cause is a thrombotic event promoted by aPL Ab. Therefore, the treatment of these patients is directed at preventing further neurologic events with anticoagulation.[10, 74]

### Seizures

Management of seizures depends on their cause. As emphasized previously, secondary causes of seizures must be excluded. Seizures can occur in conjunction with other neurologic events (e.g., stroke) or psychosis, or they can occur in isolation. Initial management of seizures is with anticonvulsants, such as diphenylhydantoin. If seizures occur in association with a focal neurologic event, the patient may require anticoagulation and anticonvulsants. Grand mal seizures in isolation are usually treated as acute global dysfunction, with parenteral corticosteroids together with antiseizure medications. Management of petit mal and temporal lobe seizures varies depending on the presumed cause.

A seizure focus resulting from a previous acute focal neurologic event may cause seizures later in the course of illness. These patients need to be thoughtfully evaluated and may not require acute immunosuppression at the time of presentation. Seizure management should involve the expertise of a neurologist.

### Transverse Myelitis

Most reports of transverse myelitis emphasize that early treatment is critical to good outcome. Uniformly, patients who are not diagnosed promptly fare poorly. Corticosteroid therapy alone is frequently inadequate to ameliorate transverse myelitis, and there are numerous studies that report much better outcome with the use of early aggressive therapy with corticosteroids plus intravenous cyclophosphamide.[11, 75–77, 77a] In patients with aPL Ab, anticoagulation should be seriously considered as well, because numerous reports suggest that the myelopathy can be mediated in part by vaso-occlusive phenomena.[72, 78, 79]

**TABLE 26–1**
**Treatment of Neuropsychiatric Systemic Lupus Erythematosus**

| NP MANIFESTATION | PRESUMED PATHOGENETIC MECHANISM | OBJECTIVE DATA THAT HELP DIRECT TREATMENT | INITIAL MANAGEMENT | INITIAL MANAGEMENT ADJUNCT NEUROLEPTICS | REFRACTORY DISEASE |
|---|---|---|---|---|---|
| Acute global dysfunction: psychosis, delirium, and dementia | Neuron reactive antibodies, cytokine effects | Antineuronal Ab (CSF) Antiribosomal P Ab (CSF, serum) IL-6 (CSF) | Parenteral corticosteroids 1–2 mg/kg/d or pulse IV steroids 1 g/d for 3 d followed by PO corticosteroids, 1 mg/kg | Haloperidol, chlorpromazine to control psychotic features; benzodiazepines to control agitation and panic | Pulse IV cyc, monthly for 3–6 mo Consider synchronous plasmapheresis if pulse IV cyc fails |
| Acute focal neurologic event | Antiphospholipid antibody vasculitis (rare) | Neuroimaging studies such as MRI | Anticoagulation +/− parenteral corticosteroids 1–2 mg/kg/d | — | Pulse IV cyc monthly for 3–6 mo |
| Seizures | Multiple mechanisms; vasculitis (rare), vaso-occlusive disease, neuron reactive | Neuroimaging study such as MRI | Parenteral corticosteroids or pulse IV steroids: 1 g/d for 3 d | Antiseizure medications such as diphenylhydantoin | Pulse IV cyc monthly for 3–6 mo |
| Transverse myelitis | Multiple mechanisms | MRI of the spinal cord with gadolinium enhancement | Pulse IV steroids: 1 g/d for 3 d or pulse IV cyc monthly for 3–6 mo | — | Synchronous plasmapheresis |
| Cranial neuropathies | Multiple mechanisms | — | Oral corticosteroids 0.5–1 mg/kg/d | — | Parenteral corticosteroids Pulse IV cyc |
| Cognitive deficits | Multiple mechanisms | Neurocognitive testing | No treatment recommendations at this time | Treat possible confounding illnesses such as depression | — |
| Headache | Usually not due to NP-SLE | — | No immunosuppressive treatment | Analgesics, prophylaxis with β blockers or tricyclics or sumatriptan | — |

Ab = antibody; CSF = cerebrospinal fluid; cyc = cyclophosphamide; IL = interleukin; MRI = magnetic resonance imaging; NP = neuropsychiatric; SLE = systemic lupus erythematosus.
Parenteral steroids = parenteral (IV) corticosteroids @ 1 mg/kg; IV pulse steroids = parenteral (IV) corticosteroids @ 1 g/d for 3 d; IV cyc = parenteral (IV) cyclophosphamide @ 500–1000 mg/m$^2$; synchronous plasmapheresis = plasma exchange followed by IV cyclophosphamide.

## Cranial Neuropathies

Cranial neuropathies are seen infrequently and usually respond to corticosteroids. The most common cranial nerves affected are the third and sixth, but neuropathies of the fifth and seventh have also been reported. Optic neuropathy is a rare complication, seen in 1% of SLE patients, and can result in blindness. Refractory optic neuritis may require more aggressive immunosuppression (e.g., intravenous cyclophosphamide).[13]

## Sensorineural Hearing Loss

SNHL continues to be described in patients with collagen vascular diseases, including SLE. The presentation varies from an insidious decline to an acute-onset loss of hearing in one or both ears. Historically, when the hearing loss is acute or subacute, treatment has been with corticosteroids in doses of 1 mg/kg/day. If the patient does not respond, treatment with pulse-dose corticosteroids at 1 g/day for 3 days is given. Use of pulse intravenous cyclophosphamide has been anecdotally described for the treatment of refractory disease, and I have used cyclophosphamide for SNHL, with variable success. If the patient responds to corticosteroids or intravenous cyclophosphamide and hearing is stabilized, then a corticosteroid-sparing (or cyclophosphamide-sparing) agent is considered, most commonly azathioprine or methotrexate, both of which have been used with anecdotal success.[12, 14]

Although the pathogenesis of sudden SNHL in patients with SLE is not clear, several reports suggest an association with the aPL Ab. Naarendorp and Spiera[15] reported on six patients with SLE or a lupus-like syndrome who had sudden SNHL and increased levels of anticardiolipin antibodies or the lupus anticoagulant. The authors suggested that acute SNHL in patients with SLE who have aPL Ab may be a manifestation of the aPL Ab syndrome and recommended anticoagulation treatment of these patients. Although this view is not universally shared, treatment regimens continue to evolve.

## Cognitive Impairment

The only randomized, double-blind, controlled trial of treatment of NP-SLE is Denburg and colleagues' N-of-1 trial for the treatment of mild NP-SLE with prednisone at 0.5 mg/kg/day.[20] Ten women participated in the study, and outcome measures included symptom ratings by questionnaire, cognition by a 1-hour test battery, and mood by a self-report adjective scale. These women completed three cycles of two treatment regimens. Each regimen was composed of three stages: a 21-day full medication (or placebo) stage, a 7-day tapering-dosage stage, and a 7-day drug-free washout stage. A completed trial of three cycles lasted a total of 30 weeks. Analysis of variance on the group data yielded significant positive drug effects for cognition, mood, and SLE symptomatology. Denburg and colleagues' conclusion was that steroids improve cognition in a selected group of SLE pa-

tients.[20] This study raises significant issues for the clinician who has SLE patients who complain of dysphoria and/or cognitive deficits that they attribute to their SLE. The dose of 0.5 mg/kg is a significant dose of steroids with potential side effects. Further trials are necessary before blanket recommendations can be made for management of SLE patients with cognitive deficits.

## CONCLUSIONS

Management of NP-SLE is dependent on making the correct diagnosis. Secondary causes of neuropsychiatric dysfunction must be excluded. Anecdotal reports currently guide treatment decisions and the management of the myriad manifestations of NP-SLE. Prospective clinical trials of therapeutic regimens in SLE patients stratified by presentation are needed.

*Acknowledgments*

*The author gratefully acknowledges the editorial assistance of Dr. Sharon L. Kolasinski and the secretarial assistance of Wanda Foster Massey and Agnes R. Robideaux.*

## REFERENCES

1. Dubois EL, Tuffanelli DL: Clinical manifestations of systemic lupus erythematosus. JAMA 1964; 190:104–111.
2. DuBois EL, Wierzchowiecki M, Cox MB, et al: Duration and death in systemic lupus erythematosus: An analysis of 249 cases. JAMA 1974; 227:1399.
3. Klemperer P, Pollack D, Baehr G: Pathology of disseminated lupus erythematosus. Arch Pathol 1941; 32:569.
4. Wallace D, Podell T, Weiner J: Systemic lupus erythematosus survivial patterns: Experience with 609 patients. JAMA 1981; 245:934.
5. Rosner S, Ginzler E, Hs D: A multicenter study of outcome in systemic lupus erythematosus: II. Causes of death. Arthritis Rheum 1982; 25:612.
6. ACR Ad Hoc Committee on Neuropsychiatric Lupus Nomenclature: The American College of Rheumatology nomenclature and case definitions for neuropsychiatric lupus syndromes. Arthritis Rheum 1999; 42:599–608.
7. Kassan S, Lockshin M: Central nervous system lupus: The need for classification. Arthritis Rheum 1979; 22:1382–1385.
8. West S: Neuropsychiatric lupus. Rheum Dis Clin North Am 1994; 20:129–159.
9. Schneebaum A, Singleton JD, West SG, et al: Association of psychiatric manifestations with antibodies to ribosomal P proteins in systemic lupus erythematosus. Am J Med 1991; 90:54–62.
10. Asherson RA, Cervera R, Piette JC, et al: *In* Asherson RA, Cervera R, Piette JC, et al (eds): The Antiphospholipid Syndrome. Boca Raton: CRC Press, 1996:249–257.
11. Mok CC, Lau CS, Chan EY, et al: Acute transverse myelopathy in systemic lupus erythematosus: Clinical presentation, treatment, and outcome. J Rheumatol 1998; 25:467–473.
12. Andonopoulos AP, Naxakis S, Goumas P, et al: Sensorineural hearing disorders in systemic lupus erythematosus: A controlled study. Clin Exp Rheumatol 1995; 13:137–141.
13. Galindo-Rodriguez G, Avina-Zubieta JA, Diaz de Leon V, et al: Treatment and outcome of otoneurologic manifestations in systemic lupus erythematosus. Arthritis Rheum 1997; 40 (suppl):256.

14. Kataoka H, Takeda T, Nakatani H, et al: Sensorineural hearing loss of suspected autoimmune etiology: A report of three cases. Auris Nasus Larynx 1995; 22:53–58.

15. Naarendorp M, Spiera H: Sudden sensorineural hearing loss in patients with systemic lupus erythematosus or lupus-like syndromes and antiphospholipid antibodies. J Rheumatol 1998; 25:589–592.

16. Brandt KD, Lessel S: Migrainous phenomenon in systemic lupus erythematosus. Arthritis Rheum 1978; 21:7.

17. Isenberg DA, Meyrick-Thomas D, Snaith ML, et al: A study of migraine in systemic lupus erythematosus. Ann Rheum Dis 1982; 41:30.

18. Sfikakis PP, Mitsikostas DD, Manoussakis MN, et al: Headache in systemic lupus erythematosus: A controlled study. Br J Rheumatol 1998; 37:300–303.

19. Rozell C, Sibbitt WJ, Brooks W: Structural and neurochemical markers of brain injury in the migraine diathesis of systemic lupus erythematosus. Cephalalgia 1998; 18:209–215.

20. Denburg SD, Carbotte RM, Denburg JA: Corticosteroids and neuropsychological functioning in patients with systemic lupus erythematosus. Arthritis Rheum 1994; 37:1311–1320.

21. Hay EM, Black D, Huddy A, et al: Psychiatric disorder and cognitive impairment in systemic lupus erythematosus. Arthritis Rheum 1992; 35:411–416.

22. Ginsburg KS, Wright EA, Larson MG, et al: A controlled study of the prevalence of cognitive dysfunction in randomly selected patients with systemic lupus erythematosus. Arthritis Rheum 1992; 35:776–782.

23. Hanly JG, Liang MH: Cognitive disorders in systemic lupus erythematosus: Epidemiologic and clinical issues. Ann N Y Acad Sci 1997; 832:60–68.

24. Johnson RT, Richardson EP: The neurological manifestations of systemic lupus erythematosus: A clinical-pathological study of 24 cases and review of the literature. Medicine (Baltimore) 1968; 47:337.

25. Ellis SG, Verity MA: Central nervous system involvement in systemic lupus erythematosus: A review of neuropathologic findings in 57 cases, 1955–1957. Semin Arthritis Rheum 1979; 8:212.

26. Bluestein HG: Antibodies to neurons I. *In* Wallace DJ, Hahn BH (eds): Dubois Lupus Erythematosus, 4th ed. Philadelphia: Lea & Febiger, 1993:260.

27. Bluestein HG, Williams GW, Steinberg AD: Cerebrospinal fluid antibodies to neuronal cells: Association with neuropsychiatric manifestations of systemic lupus erythematosus. Am J Med 1981; 70:240.

28. Asherson RA: Antiphospholipid antibodies and syndromes. *In* Lahita RG (ed): Systemic Lupus Erythematosus: An Analysis of 249 Cases, 2nd ed. New York: Churchill Livingstone, 1992:587.

29. Petri M: Thrombosis and systemic lupus erythematosus: The Hopkins Lupus Cohort perspective [Editorial]. Scand J Rheumatol 1996; 25:191–193.

30. McLean BN: Neurological involvement in systemic lupus erythematosus. Curr Opin Neurol 1998; 11:247–251.

31. Jara L, Irigoyen L, Ortiz Mde J, et al: Prolactin and interleukin-6 in neuropsychiatric lupus erythematosus. Clin Rheumatol 1998; 17:110–114.

32. Stimmler M, Coletti P, Quismorio FJ: Magnetic resonance imaging of the brain in neuropsychiatric systemic lupus erythematosus. Semin Arthritis Rheum 1993; 22:335–349.

33. West S: Lupus and the central nervous system. Curr Opin Rheumatol 1996; 8:408–414.

34. West S, Emlen W, Wener M, et al: Neuropsychiatric lupus erythematosus: A 10 year prospective study of the value of diagnostic tests. Am J Med 1995; 99:153–163.

35. Neuwelt CM, Lacks S, Kaye BR, et al: Role of intravenous cyclophosphamide in the treatment of severe neuropsychiatric systemic lupus erythematosus. Am J Med 1995; 98:32–41.

36. DuBois E: Systemic lupus erythematosus: Recent advances in its diagnosis and treatment. Ann Intern Med 1956; 45:163.

37. Sergent JS, Lockshin MD, Klempner MS, et al: Central nervous system disease in systemic lupus erythematosus. Am J Med 1975; 58:644–654.

38. Kimberly RP, Lockshin MD, Sherman RL, et al: High-dose intravenous methylprednisolone pulse therapy in systemic lupus erythematosus. Am J Med 1981; 70:817–824.

39. Price J, Klestov A, Beacham B, et al: A case of cerebral systemic lupus erythematosus treated with methylprednisolone pulse therapy. Aust N Z J Psychiatry 1985; 19:184–188.

40. Tincani A, Brey R, Balestrieri G, et al: International survey on the management of patients with SLE: II. The results of a questionnaire regarding neuropsychiatric manifestations. Clin Exp Rheumatol 1996; 14:S23–S29.

41. Gladman D, Ginzler E, Goldsmith C, et al: Systemic lupus international collaborative clinics: Development of a damage index in systemic lupus erythematosus. J Rheumatol 1992; 19:1820–1821.

42. Hansen M, Halberg P, Kollerup G, et al: Bone metabolism in patients with systemic lupus erythematosus: Effect of disease activity and glucocorticoid treatment. Scand J Rheumatol 1998; 27:197–206.

43. Li EK, Tam LS, Young RP, et al: Loss of bone mineral density in Chinese pre-menopausal women with systemic lupus erythematosus treated with corticosteroids. Br J Rheumatol 1998; 37:405–410.

44. Hall RCW, Popkin MK, Stickney SK, et al: Presentation of the steroid psychoses. J Nerv Ment Dis 1979; 167:229.

45. Lewis D, Smith R: Steroid-induced psychiatric syndromes: A report of 14 cases and a review of the literature. J Affect Disord 1983; 5:319.

46. O'Connor J: Psychoses association with systemic lupus erythematosus. Ann Intern Med 1959; 5:526.

47. Stern M, Robbins E: Psychoses in systemic lupus erythematosus. Arch Gen Psychiatry 1960; 3:205.

48. Fessel WJ, Solomon GF: Psychosis and systemic lupus erythematosus: Review of the literature and case report. Calif Med 1960; 92:266.

49. Varney NR, Alexander B, MacIndoe JH: Reversible steroid dementia in patients without steroid psychosis. Am J Psychiatry 1984; 141:369–372.

50. Boutsen Y, Jamart J, Esselinckx W, et al: Primary prevention of glucocorticoid-induced osteoporosis with intermittent intravenous pamidronate: A randomized trial. Calcif Tissue Int 1997; 61:266–271.

51. Reid IR: Steroid-induced osteoporosis. Osteoporos Int 1997; 7:S213–S216.

52. Reid IR: Glucocorticoid osteoporosis: Mechanisms and management. Eur J Endocrinol 1997; 137:209–217.

53. Boumpas DT, Yamada H, Patrones NJ, et al: Pulse cyclophosphamide for severe neuropsychiatric lupus. Q J Med 1991; 81:975.

54. LaRochelle G, Lacks S, Borenstein D: IV cyclophosphamide therapy of steroid resistant neuropsychiatric SLE (NPSLE) [Abstract]. Arthritis Rheum 1990; 33:R21.

55. Von Feldt J, Ostrov B: The use of cyclophosphamide in the treatment of CNS lupus [Abstract]. Arthritis Rheum 1990; 33:R21.

56. Barile L, Lavalle C: Transverse myelitis in systemic lupus erythematosus: The effect of IV pulse methylprednisolone and cyclophosphamide. J Rheum 1992; 19:370.

57. Klaiman M, Miller S: Transverse myelitis complicating systemic lupus erythematosus: Treatment including hydroxychloroquine. Am J Phys Med Rehab 1993; 72:158.

58. Ramos PC, Mendez MJ, Ames PR, et al: Pulse cyclophosphamide in the treatment of neuropsychiatric systemic lupus erythematosus. Clin Exp Rheumatol 1996; 14:295–299.

59. Klippel J: Is aggressive therapy effective for lupus? Rheum Dis Clin North Am 1993; 19:249–261.

60. Jones JV, Cumming RH, Bacon PA, et al: Evidence for a therapeutic effect of plasmapheresis in patients with systemic lupus erythematosus. Q J Med 1979; 48:555–576.

61. Sharon Z, Roberts J, Fennel J, et al: Plasmapheresis in lupus nephritis. Plasma Therapy 1982; 3:165.

62. Lockwood CM, Pussell B, Wilson CB, et al: Plasma exchange in nephritis. Adv Nephrol Necker Hosp 1979; 8:383–418.

63. Leaker BR, Becker GJ, Dowling JP, et al: Rapid improvement in severe lupus glomerular lesions following intensive plasma exchange associated with immunosuppression. Clin Nephrol 1986; 25:236–244.

64. Smith G, Leyland M: Plasma exchange for cerebral lupus erythematosus. Lancet 1987; 1:103.

65. Unterweger B, Klein G, Fleischacker W: Plasma exchange for cerebral lupus erythematosus [Letter]. Biol Psychiatry 1988; 24:946–947.

66. Couillault G, Gouyon JB, Chalopin JM, et al: [Value of plasma exchange in neurologic complications of acute disseminated lupus erythematosus in children]. Arch Fr Pediatr 1985; 42:41–43.
67. Schroeder JO, Euler HH, Loffler H: Synchronization of plasmapheresis and pulse cyclophosphamide in severe systemic lupus erythematosus. Ann Intern Med 1987; 107:344–346.
68. Hebert L, Nielsen E, Pohl M, et al: Clinical course of severe lupus nephritis during the controlled trial of plasmapheresis therapy. Kidney Int 1987; 31:207.
69. Lewis E, Lachin J: Primary outcomes in the ontrolled trial of plasmapheresis therapy in severe lupus nephritis. Kidney Int 1987; 31:208.
70. Aringer M, Smolen JS, Graninger WB: Severe infections in plasmapheresis-treated systemic lupus erythematosus. Arthritis Rheum 1998; 41:414–420.
71. Fricchione G, Kaufman LD, Gruber B, et al: Electroconvulsive therapy and cyclophosphamide in combination for severe neuropsychiatric lupus with catatonia. Am J Med 1990; 88:442–443.
71a. Xuan Z, Yi D, Fu-Lin T, et al: Central nervous system involvement in systemic lupus erythematosus—A hospital based study of 171 patients. J Clin Rheumatol 1999; 5:314–319.
71b. Ballou SP, Khan MA, Kushner I: Intravenous pulse methylprednisolone followed by alternate day corticosteroid therapy in lupus erythematosus: A prospective evaluation. J Rheumatol 1985; 12:944–948.
72. Piette JC: Towards improved criteria for the antiphospholipid syndrome. Lupus 1998; 7:S149–S157.
73. Petri M: Epidemiology of the antiphospholipid syndrome. *In* Asherson RA, Cervera R, Piette JC, et al (eds): The Antiphospholipid Syndrome. Boca Raton: CRC Press, 1996: 13–28.
74. Rosove M, Brewer P: Antiphospholipid thrombosis: Clinical course after the first thrombotic event in 70 patients. Ann Intern Med 1992; 117:303.
75. Boumpas DT, Patronas NJ, Dalakas MC, et al: Acute transverse myelitis in systemic lupus erythematosus: Magnetic resonance imaging and review of the literature. J Rheumatol 1990; 17:89–92.
76. Misteli M, Conen D: [Acute transverse myelitis in systemic lupus erythematosus: Successful therapy with cyclophosphamide and prednisone]. Schweiz Med Wochenschr 1991; 121:77–80.
77. Barile L, Lavalle C: Transverse myelitis in systemic lupus erythematosus: The effect of IV pulse methylprednisolone and cyclophosphamide. J Rheumatol 1992; 19:370–372.
77a. Kovacs B, Lafferty TL, Brent LH, et al: Transverse myelopathy in systemic lupus erythematosus: An analysis of 14 cases and review of the literature. Ann Rheum Dis 2000; 59:120–124.
78. Lavalle C, Pizarro S, Drenkard C, et al: Transverse myelitis: A manifestation of systemic lupus erythematosus strongly associated with antiphospholipid antibodies [see comments]. J Rheumatol 1990; 17:34–37.
79. Ito H, Nagasato K, Nakamura T, et al: [Transverse myelopathy in a patient with systemic lupus erythematosus associated with positive anticardiolipin antibody: A case report]. Rinsho Shinkeigaku 1992; 32:639–641.

# CHAPTER

# 27 | Vasculitis

### E. William St. Clair

The major vasculitic syndromes encompass a broad spectrum of clinical disorders (see Table 27–1 for a partial listing of the recognized syndromes).[1, 2] These diagnostic categories have many overlapping clinical, laboratory, and histopathologic features, a fact that has created much nosologic confusion and impeded the acceptance of a standard nomenclature. Disease definitions have been updated to reflect our increased knowledge of systemic vasculitis. A consensus conference held in Chapel Hill, North Carolina (CHCC, or Chapel Hill Consensus Conference) partially revised the current scheme; of most note it created a subgroup within the major polyarteritis nodosa (PAN) group called microscopic polyangiitis.[3] In addition, the American College of Rheumatology (ACR) has developed criteria for classifying patients with systemic vasculitis in clinical studies.[4]

The heterogeneity of the systemic vasculitides not only poses diagnostic challenges but also shapes management. Appropriate treatment of these complex diseases requires a comprehensive assessment of each patient in order to determine the extent and severity of organ system involvement and to exclude other diagnoses that may be confused with vasculitis (e.g., infection, neoplasm). Continual reevaluation of disease activity and close monitoring for possible treatment-related complications are essential for attaining the best possible outcomes.

This chapter reviews the treatment of systemic vasculitis. It aims to characterize the natural history of each of the disorders, to critically review the clinical studies, and to provide guidelines for their management on the basis of expert opinion and the best clinical evidence. The specific types of vasculitis discussed in this chapter are PAN, microscopic polyangiitis (MPA), Churg-Strauss syndrome (CSS), Wegener's granulomatosis (WG), essential type II mixed cryoglobulinemia, Henoch-Schönlein purpura (HSP), hypersensitivity vasculitis, and Cogan's syndrome.

## POLYARTERITIS NODOSA, MICROSCOPIC POLYARTERITIS, AND CHURG-STRAUSS SYNDROME

The pathologic hallmark of PAN is a small or medium-sized necrotizing arteritis. Its clinical features include fever, weight loss, cutaneous ulcers, livedo reticularis, muscle pain and weakness, arthralgias and arthritis, neuropathy, abdominal pain, ischemic bowel, testicular pain or tenderness, hypertension, and renal failure. Although PAN classically spares the lung, a polyangiitis overlap syndrome with PAN-like features and pulmonary involvement has been described.[5] Many of these overlap cases fit current definitions of CSS and MPA.

A focal segmental necrotizing glomerulonephritis without interlobar or intralobar artery involvement has been termed *microscopic polyarteritis*.[6] It is often accompanied by a small or medium-sized vessel vasculitis in other organ systems.[6] Microscopic polyarteritis, originally a pathologic designation, has been renamed *microscopic polyangiitis* (MPA), a necrotizing, pauci-immune vasculitis affecting small vessels (capillaries, venules, or arterioles).[3] By definition, MPA may also target small and medium-sized arteries. The dominant clinical and pathologic features of MPA are glomerulonephritis and pulmonary capillaritis with alveolar hemorrhage. Other clinical features of MPA are similar to those of classic PAN except that PAN entails a lower frequency of peripheral neuropathy.[7, 8] Although angiography has not been performed uniformly in patients with MPA, abnormal angiograms with microaneurysms and vessel stenosis have been only rarely observed in this disease subgroup.[7] Unlike PAN, MPA has not been associated with hepatitis B virus infection. Serologically, serum from about 60% of patients with MPA contain antineutrophil cytoplasmic antibodies (ANCA) with a perinuclear staining pattern.[7, 8] More than 90% of these sera are positive for reactivity with myeloperoxidase (MPO).[7]

Classic PAN was redefined at the CHCC as a necrotizing vasculitis of medium-sized or small arteries without glomerulonephritis and without vasculitis in arterioles, capillaries, or venules. Most authorities believe that this definition is too restrictive because small-vessel involvement occurs commonly in patients with classic PAN.[9] No cases of classic PAN as defined by the CHCC were identified in a 6-year epidemiologic study of systemic vasculitis in Norwich, United Kingdom, in comparison with 13 patients who met criteria for MPA.[10] Of the 13 patients with MPA, 8 also met ACR criteria for PAN. Thus, the CHCC definition of classic PAN should be revised to include patients with

## TABLE 27–1
## Classification of the Vasculitic Syndromes

**Polyarteritis Group**

| | |
|---|---|
| Classic polyarteritis nodosa | Medium- and small-vessel vasculitis<br>Necrotizing vasculitis of small and medium-sized arteries |
| Microscopic polyangiitis | Necrotizing vasculitis affecting capillaries, venules, and arterioles |
| Churg-Strauss syndrome | Eosinophilic and granulomatous inflammation of the respiratory tract and necrotizing vasculitis affecting small and medium-sized vessels |
| Polyangiitis overlap syndrome | Overlapping features of specific types of vasculitis |
| **Wegner's Granulomatosis** | Granulomatous vasculitis affecting small to medium-sized vessels |
| **Small-Vessel Vasculitis** | Inflammation affecting capillaries, venules, or arterioles |
| Cutaneous leukocytoclastic vasculitis | Small-vessel vasculitis limited to the skin (no systemic involvement) |
| Essential mixed cryoglobulinemia | Small-vessel vasculitis with serum cryoglobulins (usually skin and glomeruli) |
| Henoch-Schönlein purpura | Small-vessel vasculitis with IgA-dominant immune deposits (usually skin, gut, and glomeruli) and arthritis |
| Serum sickness | Small-vessel vasculitis resulting from repeated injections of a foreign antigen |
| Vasculitis associated with malignancies | Small-vessel vasculitis associated with cancer (hairy cell leukemia, lymphoma, solid tumors) |
| Vasculitis associated with other primary disorders | Small-vessel vasculitis associated with rheumatoid arthritis, systemic lupus erythematosus, other connective tissue diseases |
| **Primary Angiitis of the Central Nervous System Vasculitis** | Small- and medium-vessel vasculitis of the central nervous system |
| **Kawasaki's Disease** | Small-, medium-, and large-vessel arteritis associated with mucocutaneous lymph node syndrome (usually occurs in children and commonly results in coronary artery involvement) |
| **Giant Cell Arteritides** | Granulomatous inflammation of the large vessels |
| Temporal arteritis | Granulomatous inflammation of the extracranial branches of the carotid artery (may also involve the aorta and its major branches); occurs in patients more than 50 years of age |
| Takayasu's arteritis | Granulomatous inflammation of the aorta and its major branches; occurs in patients less than 50 years of age |
| **Miscellaneous Vasculitides (Cogan's Syndrome, Behçet's Syndrome)** | Medium- and large-vessel vasculitis<br>Small-, medium-, and large-vessel vasculitis |

IgA = immunoglobulin A.

small-vessel involvement whose disease otherwise fits the clinical picture. Patients with classic PAN are characterized by renal vasculitis with hypertension, the absence of glomerulonephritis, abnormal angiograms, a high prevalence of multiple mononeuropathies, and a lack of lung involvement.[8] Classic PAN is further distinguished from MPA by its association with hepatitis B infection[11, 12] and the usual absence of serum ANCA. Not to be confused with microscopic polyarteritis or MPA, cutaneous PAN is a clinical variant of necrotizing vasculitis that predominantly targets the skin and subcutaneous tissue and does not usually progress to systemic involvement.

Separating PAN into two subsets, classic PAN and MPA, may provide useful prognostic information. Guillevin and Lhote suggested that classic PAN is a monophasic disease with relatively few relapses, im-

plying that treatment of this subset may be limited to a defined time period (e.g., 1 year).[9] In comparison, MPA is characterized by a high probability of relapse and often necessitates more prolonged therapy to control the intermittent flares of disease. The outcome of MPA appears to be similar to that of the other systemic necrotizing vasculitides.[7]

CSS, also called *allergic angiitis and granulomatosis*, is characterized by asthma, pulmonary vasculitis, and peak eosinophil counts exceeding $1.5 \times 10^9/L$.[13, 14] The heart, nervous system, gastrointestinal and urinary tracts, and joints as well as the lungs are the principal targets of this vasculitis. A minority of affected patients exhibit severe renal disease. CSS must be differentiated from other clinical disorders associated with marked eosinophilia, such as eosinophilic leukemia, hypereosinophilic syndrome, Löffler's syndrome, chronic eosinophilic pneumonia, eosinophilic gastroenteritis, parasitic infections, and bronchopulmonary aspergillosis.

Laboratory studies in patients with PAN, MPA, and CSS reflect the heightened inflammatory state (e.g., increased levels of acute-phase reactants) and ischemic injury to affected organ systems. These findings are nonspecific. ANCA are associated with certain forms of vasculitis and may provide clues to the diagnosis. Finding the typical arteriographic abnormalities[15] and histopathologic changes of necrotizing vasculitis[16] remains the gold standards for the diagnosis of vasculitis.

## Natural History of Disease

Our understanding of the natural history of PAN (and MPA) and CSS derives from clinical observations made before the introduction of glucocorticoids. These clinical and histopathologic descriptions did not take into account the major subdivisions of systemic vasculitis or distinguish classic PAN from MPA. Instead, PAN, CSS, and other vasculitic syndromes were grouped into the broader category of "periarteritis nodosa." Patients with periarteritis nodosa who were seen between 1946 and 1962 at the Mayo Clinic and left untreated had 1- and 5-year survival rates of 35% and 13%, respectively.[17] Initial presentation with renal or gastrointestinal disease was associated with a worse outcome; most early deaths were caused by active vasculitis.

Before the introduction of antiviral therapy, outcomes of patients with PAN were not substantially worsened by concomitant hepatitis B virus (HBV) infection. In one study, the 5-year survival rates among patients with systemic necrotizing vasculitis with and without HBV markers were 61% and 58%, respectively.[18] However, the HBV-positive group had a significantly higher mortality rate (30%) during the first year of disease than did the HBV-negative group (15%).[18] The most common causes of death in the patients with PAN and HBV infection were gastrointestinal bleeding and bowel perforation.[18]

Patients with CSS seemingly fare no better without therapy than does the periarteritis nodosa group as a whole. A retrospective analysis showed that untreated patients with CSS have a 1-year survival rate of 4%.[19] Allergic rhinitis and asthma, the prodrome to CSS, were found to precede the onset of vasculitis by as long as 7 years.[14] Deaths in patients with CSS have commonly resulted from pulmonary compromise, cardiac failure, renal failure, and cerebral hemorrhage.[14, 19]

## Uncontrolled Treatment Studies

Glucocorticoids became widely accepted as efficacious therapy for systemic necrotizing vasculitis on the basis of uncontrolled data from retrospective studies. Patients with PAN who were treated with glucocorticoids had survival rates of 60% to 71% at 1 year and 48% to 55% at 5 years.[17, 20] Further improvement in the prognosis of PAN and CSS came with the use of cytotoxic therapy. Fauci and associates[21] reported in 1979 that

treatment with 2 mg/kg/day of oral cyclophosphamide produced a high rate of remissions in 17 patients with PAN in whom disease had been previously refractory to glucocorticoid therapy. Although 3 of the patients in this study died, the other 14 patients achieved a complete or partial remission and within a few months were able to tolerate a reduction in glucocorticoid doses to a less toxic, alternate-day regimen. Because the patients in this study had had disease of more than 2 years' duration when cytotoxic therapy was initiated, the outcomes observed during follow-up may have been affected by the natural history of disease and previous glucocorticoid therapy as well as by the addition of cytotoxic agents.

The experience at the Mayo Clinic, however, did not yield improved outcomes with cytotoxic therapy.[20] In a retrospective study, Nachman and colleagues[22] assessed treatment outcomes in 107 patients with ANCA-associated MPA and necrotizing, crescentic glomerulonephritis. None of the patients in that study had WG. All of the patients initially received 7 mg/kg/day of methylprednisolone for the first 3 days, which was followed by nonrandom assignment to one of three treatment regimens: prednisone (1 mg/kg/day); prednisone (1 mg/kg/day) plus oral cyclophosphamide (2 mg/kg/day); or prednisone (1 mg/kg/day) plus 6 monthly intravenous pulses of cyclophosphamide (0.5 to 1.0 mg/m$^2$). The remission rate was significantly higher in the two cyclophosphamide-treated groups (84%) than among the patients receiving glucocorticoids alone (56%). Much of the mortality in these retrospective studies occurred in the first 2 years of disease. The results of these studies must be interpreted with caution because nonrandom allocation of patients at various stages of disease into different treatment groups may bias the survival analysis. For example, a bias against glucocorticoid therapy would occur if the most severely affected patients treated initially with glucocorticoids alone died before they had an opportunity to receive cytotoxic therapy.

The treatment of hepatitis B virus (HBV)-related PAN is complicated by the fact that immunosuppressive therapy may interfere with the body's immune response to the virus and actually worsen disease outcomes. The exacerbating effects of immunosuppressive therapy are reflected in the negative impact of glucocorticoid therapy on the survival of patients with HBV-associated liver disease. Also, sudden cessation of immunosuppressive therapy may reconstitute cellular immunity and provoke fulminant hepatitis.[23]

The treatment of HBV-related PAN has evolved with advances in antiviral therapy. The most widely studied agents for HBV-related PAN are vidarabine and interferon-alpha (IFN-alpha). A retrospective analysis of 66 patients with HBV-related PAN monitored for a mean of 50 ± 46 months showed that treatment with glucocorticoids, plasma exchange, and cyclophosphamide was associated with a higher mortality rate (46%) than was treatment with vidarabine, plasma exchange, and a short initial course of prednisone therapy (18%).[24] In another series, a mortality rate was 19.5% among 41 patients with HBV-related PAN who had been monitored for a mean of 70 ± 45 months after receiving either vidarabine or IFN-alpha coupled with a short course of prednisone and plasma exchange to achieve initial disease control.[25] These results suggest that immunosuppressive therapy should be minimized in HBV-positive patients.

Glucocorticoids and cytotoxic agents have also been employed in the treatment of CSS. Patients with CSS who received 40 to 60 mg of prednisone or its equivalent had 1- and 5-year survival rates of 90% and 62%, respectively.[26] Most deaths in this group resulted from myocardial infarction and cardiac failure. Clinical disease unresponsive to glucocorticoids could often be brought under control with azathioprine[26] or cyclophosphamide.[26]

## Prospective Clinical Trials

The French Vasculitis Study Group has conducted several prospective treatment trials in systemic vasculitis. In their first trial, 71 patients with PAN or CSS were randomly assigned to receive initial treatment either with prednisone plus plasma exchange or with prednisone, plasma exchange, and oral cyclophosphamide.[27] Both treatment groups achieved similar remission and survival rates, although the group receiving oral cyclophosphamide suffered fewer relapses during followup. Only two patients receiving prednisone plus plasma exchange deteriorated during the first 6 months of treatment. Age over 55 years and an elevated serum creatinine level at presentation were predictive of a worse outcome. Although initiation of therapy with oral cyclophosphamide did not enhance overall survival in patients with PAN and CSS, this approach was still favored by the trial's investigators because it prolonged the disease-free interval.

Plasma exchange has been used as initial therapy in systemic vasculitis to afford rapid disease control. The incremental therapeutic value of plasma exchange was examined in a clinical trial in which patients with PAN and CSS were randomly assigned to receive either prednisone plus plasma exchange or prednisone alone. The two treatments produced nearly identical remission rates (83%) and 7-year survival rates (79%).[28] The potential efficacy of plasma exchange was further tested in a randomized, controlled trial of 62 patients with severe PAN and CSS. To be eligible, patients with PAN and CSS had to have at least one factor indicative of a poor prognosis (e.g., renal disease, gastrointestinal tract involvement, cardiomyopathy, central nervous system involvement, loss of >10% of body weight, or age of >50 years). Eligible patients were randomly assigned to receive plasma exchange or placebo and then treated with glucocorticoids and intravenous (IV) pulse cyclophosphamide.[29] Plasma exchange was associated with only three complications: local hematoma, transient hypotension, and sepsis resulting from catheter infection with Staphylococcus. The trial was stopped after 5 years because the two treatment arms showed similar 5-year cumulative survival rates. Together, these results argue that plasma exchange should not be routinely prescribed as initial treatment for systemic vasculitis.

The toxic effects of long-term treatment with oral cyclophosphamide has caused investigators to evaluate other immunosuppressive regimens with potentially less toxicity. Monthly IV cyclophosphamide therapy is one example of a potentially less toxic approach. In a small, randomized trial of 25 patients with PAN or CSS, 1 year of treatment with oral cyclophosphamide, 2 mg/kg/day, was compared with 1 year of monthly IV cyclophosphamide (0.6 mg/m²) pulses.[30] There were no significant differences in clinical efficacy between the two regimens.[30] However, the frequency of side effects was significantly higher with oral cyclophosphamide. Similar results were observed in another small, randomized trial comparing outcomes of intermittent pulse and daily oral cyclophosphamide therapy in 47 patients with WG and MPA.[31] The small sample sizes in these studies preclude any conclusions about the possible equivalence of daily oral and IV monthly cyclophosphamide therapy despite the similarity in response rates.

The concept of induction and maintenance therapy was examined by Adu and associates[32] in a 1-year randomized trial of 54 patients with PAN, CSS, and WG. In one of the treatment arms, daily oral cyclophosphamide served as induction therapy and was followed by a maintenance regimen of azathioprine. In the other arm, repeated cyclophosphamide pulses at progressively greater time intervals were used to first induce and then maintain remission. There were no significant differences between the two groups in survival or frequency of relapses. The rate of toxic effects was slightly higher in the patients receiving the daily oral dosage than in those receiving intermittent pulse cyclophosphamide, but this difference was not statistically significant.

These prospective clinical trials are informative because they provide a contemporary prognostic view of PAN and CSS. The 7- and 10-year survival rates of patients treated with glucocorticoids alone in two of these trials were 72% and 83%,[27, 28] exceeding the 50% long-term survival rates of glucocorticoid-treated patients of prior studies. Earlier diagnosis, differences in case severity, improved use of glucocorticoids, and closer monitoring of patients may explain the superior outcomes in these prospective trials. These survival data also reveal that large sample sizes are necessary for a clinical trial to show that oral cyclophosphamide or another treatment strategy is superior to glucocorticoids alone. None of the clinical trials involving PAN and CSS had sufficient numbers of subjects to yield any definite conclusions about the superiority of a particular treatment strategy over glucocorticoids alone with survival rate as the primary endpoint.

Uncontrolled, prospective trials suggest that antiviral therapy may afford salutary effects in patients with HBV-related PAN. The French Vasculitis Study Group performed an uncontrolled, open-label trial of glucocorticoids, plasma exchange, and vidarabine A therapy in 33 patients with PAN and HBV infection.[33] After a 2-week course of prednisone, patients were treated with plasma exchange for several months and vidarabine for 3 weeks. Circulating hepatitis B early antigen (HB$_e$Ag) and surface antigen (HBsAg) cleared after the first cycle of vidarabine in 12 (36%) and 5 (15%) patients, respectively. A second cycle of vidarabine produced HB$_e$Ag clearance in 3 additional patients. Of the patients treated by this protocol, 24 recovered completely from vasculitis. Eight patients died: three from uncontrolled vasculitis, one from fulminant hepatitis, and four from other causes. Although these results are somewhat encouraging, vidarabine therapy is no longer used for the treatment of HBV infection because of its neuromuscular toxic effects and its failure to sustain long-term benefits.

More recently, IFN-alpha has been shown to be effective for the treatment of chronic hepatitis B. The results of a meta-analysis involving more than 800 patients with chronic hepatitis B show that IFN-alpha treatment was associated with disappearance of serum Hb$_e$Ag and serum HBV DNA in 33% and 37% of patients, respectively.[46] Among the placebo recipients, Hb$_e$Ag seroconversion occurred in 12%, and serum HBV DNA disappeared in 17%. The immunomodulatory effects of IFN-alpha are complex and may theoretically hasten the progression of vasculitis. In fact, treatment with IFN-alpha can provoke various autoimmune phenomena, including vasculitis. The results from a small prospective trial involving six patients with HBV-related PAN suggested that plasma exchange combined with 3 MU of IFN-alpha administered three times a week can control the vasculitic manifestations of PAN.[34] In this open-label study, HB$_e$Ag and HbsAg cleared in four and three patients, respectively. The recommended IFN-alpha dose for the treatment of chronic hepatitis B is 5 MU/day for 16 weeks, higher than that used in the cited studies.

Lamivudine and famciclovir, oral nucleoside analogs, have been shown to inhibit HBV replication in vitro and in vivo. The use of lamivudine in HBV-related PAN has not yet been reported. In one patient with HBV-related PAN who was treated with a combination of IFN-alpha and famciclovir, HBV DNA and Hb$_e$Ag were cleared from the circulation, and the patient showed clinical resolution of PAN.[35]

## Long-Term Experience

Certain clinical features of PAN and CSS are associated with a worse prognosis. The French Vasculitis Study Group prospectively studied 342 patients in five different clinical trials. The investigators found that proteinuria of more than 1 g/day, a serum creatinine level exceeding 1.6 mg/dL, and gastrointestinal tract involvement were associated with a significantly higher mortality rate than patients without these risk factors.[36] Fortin and colleagues[37] also found in 45 patients with PAN that renal and cardiac involvement are independent predictors of increased mortality. Older studies suggested that HBV infection in patients with PAN confers an increased risk of chronic liver failure.[11, 12, 18]

Relapses occur in approximately one third of patients with PAN who achieve initial disease control with a variety of treatment regimens.[28, 29, 38] Relapses have been documented in 26% of patients with CSS.[39] In most cases, these relapses have been preceded by a rise in the eosinophil count.[39] Despite aggressive therapy, about 10% to 20% of patients with PAN and CSS die 5 to 10 years after disease onset from active disease or from a disease- or treatment-related complication.[17, 20, 21, 27–29] Most early deaths result from a perforated viscus, massive gastrointestinal hemorrhage, myocardial infarction, cerebrovascular accident, or renal failure caused by active disease. Cardiac insufficiency, sudden cardiac death, and respiratory failure are frequent causes of death in patients with CSS.[39] A minority die of infections during treatment.

PAN, MPA, and, in rare cases, CSS can lead to end-stage renal disease (ESRD). Patients who become dialysis-dependent at the outset of treatment may nonetheless recover renal function and exhibit favorable renal outcomes.[40] Proteinuria in the range of 3 to 5 g/day has been associated with the development of chronic renal failure. ESRD developed in 61 (20%) of 308 patients with ANCA-associated systemic vasculitis (WG, MPA, isolated necrotizing glomerulonephritis). These patients later received either chronic dialysis or a kidney transplant and had survival rates of 74% at 1 year and 40% at 5 years,[41] which were similar to the survival rates of the general dialysis population in a U.S. national registry. In this group of vasculitis-induced ESRD patients, vasculitic relapses occurred in 2 of the 22 patients with a renal transplant who were receiving maintenance immunosuppressive therapy and in 7 of 37 patients undergoing dialysis. The flares in these instances generally responded to increased doses of glucocorticoids or reinstitution of cyclophosphamide. Other small series show that patients with ANCA-associated MPA can undergo successful renal transplantation with a low rate of subsequent vasculitic relapse.[42, 43]

## Management

The treatment of PAN and MPA was reviewed by Guillevin and Lhote.[44] Patients with active PAN, MPA, or CSS are treated with high doses of glucocorticoids. Some judgment can be exercised in deciding whether to initially combine these drugs with a cytotoxic agent. In my view, serious visceral organ system disease—such as mononeuritis multiplex, central nervous system deficits, congestive heart failure, renal involvement, or evidence of mesenteric ischemia—justifies the addition of oral cyclophosphamide to the initial treatment regimen. Patients with PAN who lack serious visceral organ involvement can be managed initially with glucocorticoids alone and, if immediate improvement does not occur, subsequently treated with oral cyclophosphamide.

Certain factors may modify this treatment approach. For example, a concurrent diabetic state may support the initial use of cytotoxic therapy to allow more rapid reduction in the glucocorticoid dose and better control of hyperglycemia. Conversely, other considerations, such as diagnostic uncertainty, compliance issues, or a patient's concern about drug side effects, may militate against use of a cytotoxic agent.

The glucocorticoids most commonly prescribed are prednisone and methylprednisolone (orally or intravenously) in starting doses of 1 to 2 mg/kg/day. A protocol for initiating glucocorticoid therapy without concomitant cytotoxic agents in systemic vasculitis is shown in Table 27–2. Treatment is begun in rapidly progressing disease with divided daily doses of glucocorticoids, which are more immunosuppressive and potentially toxic than equivalent doses of the same preparation given once a day. A 70-kg person, for example, would be treated initially with prednisone or methylprednisolone in dosages of 15 to 30 mg four times/day. Administration of glucocorticoids is then converted from divided daily doses to a single morning dose over the next 7 to 10 days. With clinical improvement, the prednisone dose can be tapered over the first 2 weeks of therapy to a single morning dose of 60 to 80 mg and over the next 3 to 4 months to 20 mg. The daily prednisone dose may then be converted to an alternate-day schedule, an approach I favor, or reduced further in small decrements (e.g., 2.5 mg) until reaching the lowest dose that effectively controls the disease. Concomitant cytotoxic therapy usually allows both a more rapid reduction in prednisone dose, starting about 4 weeks after initiation of therapy, and an earlier conversion of the prednisone regimen from a daily dose to an alternate-day schedule (e.g., at 3 to 4 months).

The initial dosage of cyclophosphamide for treatment of systemic vasculitis is 2 mg/kg/day (usually given orally); this dose is later adjusted, depending on the peripheral leukocyte count (to be described). More fulminant vasculitis may warrant initiation of cyclophosphamide at a dose of 4 mg/kg/day for 3 days, followed by a dosage reduction within 7 days to 2 mg/kg/day. Azathioprine (2 mg/kg/day) is far less effective than cyclophosphamide in inducing remission but may serve as an alternative in this situation.[21]

Disease refractory to cyclophosphamide therapy may be managed by increasing the daily dose of cyclophosphamide in 25-mg increments until the peripheral leukocyte and neutrophil counts approach $3000/mm^3$ and $1500/mm^3$, respectively (to be discussed). Sometimes higher doses of cyclophosphamide are tolerated when the prednisone dose is increased, preferably on the alternate-day schedule. A second option is alternative or experimental therapy (to be described).

The tolerance of the myeloid compartment to cyclophosphamide usually wanes with prolonged treatment because of diminishing bone marrow reserves. The cyclophosphamide dose is reduced only if the peripheral leukocyte count drops below $3000/3 \times 10^9/L$ or the absolute neutrophil count falls below $1500/1.5 \times 10^9/L$. Azathioprine may sustain remission if unacceptable side effects result from oral cyclophosphamide therapy.[38, 45] The patient should receive oral cyclophosphamide for 12 months after a complete remission, followed by a gradual withdrawal of the drug over 2 to 3 months.

Cutaneous PAN generally necessitates less immunosuppression because of its lack of systemic manifestations and favorable long-term prognosis. Local measures and high-potency topical or intralesional glucocorticoids may be tried as the first approach. Salicylates, dipyridamole, sulfapyridine, pentoxifylline, and dapsone are only variably effective in the treatment of cutaneous PAN,[46] but they may be useful in individual cases. Severe, rapidly progressive skin disease can respond to prednisone in doses of up to 1 mg/kg/day.

Some patients with chronic skin lesions may not improve with glucocorticoids or may suffer excessive complications from the prolonged use of these drugs. In this situation, low-dose weekly oral methotrexate (7.5 to 20 mg/week) may promote healing of skin lesions and act as a steroid-sparing agent.[47] Although oral cyclophosphamide is effective in the treatment of systemic vasculitis, it less consistently induces remissions of cutaneous PAN. Moreover, combining oral

### TABLE 27–2
### A Protocol for Initiating Glucocorticoid Therapy Without Concomitant Cytotoxic Agents in Systemic Necrotizing Vasculitis

| GLUCOCORTICOID PREPARATION | ROUTE | DOSE AND FREQUENCY | TIME FROM ONSET OF THERAPY |
|---|---|---|---|
| Methylprednisolone | IV | 20 mg q6h | Day 1 |
| Methylprednisolone | IV | 40 mg q12h | Day 5 |
| Prednisone | Oral | 60 mg/d | Day 10 |
| Prednisone | Oral | 60 mg/d | Week 4 |
| Prednisone | Oral | 40 mg/d | Week 8 |
| Prednisone | Oral | 20 mg/d | Week 12 |
| Prednisone | Oral | 40 mg, alt w/30 mg/d | Week 17 |
| Prednisone | Oral | 40 mg, alt w/20 mg/d | Week 18 |
| Prednisone | Oral | 40 mg, alt w/10 mg/d | Week 19 |
| Prednisone | Oral | 40 mg QOD | Week 20 |

alt w/ = Alternating with; IV = intravenous.

cyclophosphamide with daily doses of glucocorticoids can predispose the patient to bacterial infections of nonhealing skin lesions. Thus cytotoxic agents are used with caution in cutaneous PAN. Because the major clinical manifestations of cutaneous PAN are painful skin ulcers, local therapy aimed at protecting the wound, decreasing superficial infection, and promoting healing is often the most productive avenue of therapy.

The treatment approach must be modified in cases of HBV-related PAN because excessive immunosuppression may worsen outcomes. The vasculitic manifestations may be brought under initial control with a short course of prednisone. According to published studies, successful outcomes have been achieved by starting prednisone at a dose of 1 mg/kg/day for 1 week and stopping it by the end of the second week after a rapid taper. The treatment of HBV-related PAN should include an antiviral agent. IFN-alpha has emerged as the drug of choice for HBV infection. The recommended dose of IFN-alpha is 5 MU every day for 16 weeks. However, IFN-alpha has only been used in patients with HBV-related PAN at doses of 3 to 5 MU three times a week, the usual doses for treating hepatitis C. The treatment duration depends on the clearance of serum $HB_eAg$. IFN-alpha injections are discontinued after loss of serum $Hb_eAg$, whereas persistent $HB_e$ antigenemia calls for continuation of the IFN-alpha treatments for up to 1 year. There does not appear to be a rationale for using less than the recommended dosage unless the patient has difficulty tolerating that dosage.

IFN-alpha should be considered as first-line therapy in patients with low HBV loads (e.g., low HBV DNA levels), in whom the cure rate has been the highest. IFN-alpha treatment offers a low probability of cure in patients with high pretreatment HBV DNA levels. In such cases, lamivudine, 100 mg/day, would be a reasonable alternative despite the lack of published studies in which it is administered to patients with HBV-related PAN. Lamivudine has been well tolerated by most patients and significantly reduces serum HBV DNA levels in almost all cases of chronic hepatitis B infection. However, treatment with lamivudine has little effect on the cure rate in chronic hepatitis B regardless of viral load.

Another treatment option for HBV-related PAN is plasma exchange. The therapeutic value of plasma exchange has not been shown in controlled trials. Plasma exchange may serve to control the acute and subacute manifestations of vasculitis, and the antiviral agent acts to eliminate the triggering antigen (e.g., HBV). Plasma exchange may be initiated after tapering of the prednisone therapy, beginning three times weekly for the first 6 weeks, followed by twice weekly for 3 weeks and then once or twice every week according to the clinical response. One plasma volume (30 mL/kg $\times$ [100 − hematocrit]) is removed per session and replaced with lactated Ringer's solution and albumin. Fresh-frozen plasma is used as needed to replenish coagulation factors.

## Clinical Pharmacology and Drug Interactions

Glucocorticoids produce a myriad of biologic effects. After moving across the cell membrane, they complex with high-affinity receptors and enter the nucleus, where they change the transcription of specific genes. The products of these genes regulate diverse intracellular and extracellular events associated with cellular activation and inflammation. Glucocorticoids interfere with endothelial cell function, inhibit recruitment of circulating leukocytes to sites of tissue inflammation, and block proinflammatory mediator production. Pharmacologic doses of glucocorticoids suppress the hypothalamic-pituitary-adrenal axis, reducing endogenous cortisol production.

Glucocorticoid preparations differ in relative potency, sodium-retaining properties, and biologic half-life. Those most commonly used to treat vasculitis are the short-acting preparations: prednisone and methylprednisolone. Because of their longer biologic half-life, the longer-acting preparations, such as dexamethasone, exhibit a much greater "steroid effect" than do equivalent doses of shorter-acting agents. A single daily dose of dexamethasone, for example, suppresses cortisol production for more than 48 hours, and thus dexamethasone is not suitable for long-term daily administration.

Because glucocorticoids are inactivated in the liver, drugs that induce hepatic microsomal enzyme activity, such as phenytoin, barbiturates, and rifampin, may accelerate the elimination of glucocorticoids.[48] Glucocorticoids may also speed the metabolism of salicylates in the liver, lowering the serum salicylate levels.[48] Pharmacologic doses of glucocorticoids can accentuate the need for antihypertensive medications or increase the insulin requirements of patients with diabetes mellitus.

Cyclophosphamide is a potent immunosuppressive drug. It inhibits cellular activity by alkylating DNA, which crosslinks the DNA coil and introduces coding errors during DNA synthesis and transcription. Thus rapidly dividing cells are its principal target. In doses used to treat vasculitis, cyclophosphamide inhibits lymphocyte proliferation more strongly than neutrophil proliferation, resulting in a greater degree of lymphopenia than neutropenia. Cyclophosphamide also down-regulates both B cell and T cell function.

Hepatic microsomal enzymes are involved in the activation of cyclophosphamide. Drugs that induce these enzymes may alter the conversion of cyclophosphamide from its inactive to its active form. Of more importance is that the elimination and detoxification of cyclophosphamide may be prolonged in patients with liver or renal dysfunction.

## Drug Side Effects and Recommended Monitoring

Glucocorticoid complications are more pronounced with longer acting preparations, more frequent administration, and prolonged use. Physicians should be alert for the occurrence of these toxic effects. The initiation of high-dose glucocorticoids may produce sudden and dramatic hyperglycemia in susceptible persons. Patients should be warned about polyuria and polydipsia. An intervening serious illness or a surgical procedure may warrant temporary administration of "stress doses" of glucocorticoids because of hypothalamic-pituitary-adrenal suppression. Unless contraindicated, 400 IU of vitamin D and 1000 to 1500 mg of elemental calcium can be given daily to retard the development of glucocorticoid-induced osteoporosis. Alendronate sodium or calcitonin may also be indicated for prevention of glucocorticoid-induced osteoporosis.

Cyclophosphamide therapy is associated with substantial toxicity. The most common side effects are dose related and include gastrointestinal intolerance, hair loss, and myelosuppression.[49] Its myelosuppressive actions can be a major factor in the development of serious infections. Patients receiving cyclophosphamide have frequent infections from common bacterial pathogens, opportunistic organisms, and herpes zoster; these infections occur most often in patients who are receiving concurrent daily dosages of prednisone.[50, 51] Keeping the prednisone dosage on an alternate-day schedule appreciably lowers the risk of infection.

The cyclophosphamide dosage must be adjusted on an individual basis to avoid excessive myelosuppression. With renal impairment (e.g., serum creatinine level >2 mg/dL), the initial dosage can be reduced by 25% to 50%, although the level of renal function does not reliably correlate with the maximum tolerated dose. The cyclophosphamide dose is held constant for the first 10 to 14 days of therapy, with subsequent dosage adjustments to keep the total leukocyte count above $3000/3 \times 10^9/L$ and the neutrophil count above $1500/1.5 \times 10^9/L$. The peripheral leukocyte count begins to drop 8 to 14 days after cyclophosphamide is initiated or its dosage is increased. Thus measured counts in peripheral blood reflect suppression of the marrow, not from the current dose, but rather from the dose taken 1 to 2 weeks earlier. Waiting until the leukocyte counts drop below safe limits almost invariably results in prolonged myelosuppression. Such unwanted toxicity can be avoided by monitoring the rate of decline in the peripheral leukocyte count, anticipating its nadir, and making the appropriate dosage adjustment before the full myelosuppressive effects of the current dose are realized. Recovery from myelosuppression takes 18 to 25 days.

Glucocorticoids influence the numbers of circulating neutrophils by stimulating their release from the bone marrow and inhibiting their adhesion to vascular endothelium. Treatment with high doses of glucocorticoids often increases the peripheral leukocyte count to the range of $10,000$ to $20,000/10-20 \times 10^9/L$. About 2 weeks into the treatment of systemic vasculitis, the usual practice of consolidating the glucocorticoid dose to once a day, combined with the delayed myelosuppressive effects of cyclophosphamide, can result in a rapid fall in the leukocyte count that must be closely monitored to avoid excessive immunosuppression. Cyclophosphamide overdosage can be averted by checking the peripheral leukocyte count at least twice weekly for the first 3 weeks of therapy (or possibly longer until the counts level off in a safe range) and making prompt dosage adjustments. Subsequently, the peripheral leukocyte counts can be monitored on a weekly basis and every 2 weeks after 2 months of constant dosing.

The teratogenicity of cyclophosphamide mandates that effective birth control practices be maintained during the treatment period. Cyclophosphamide interferes with the development of oocytes and spermatocytes and can promote gonadal fibrosis and clinical sterility. These gonadal effects frequently produce oligomenorrhea and amenorrhea in women and decreased libido, impotence, and azoospermia in men. The risk of permanent sterility appears to be dose related and higher in women over 30 years of age.[52] Concomitant use of oral contraceptives by women during cyclophosphamide therapy may reduce the incidence of sterility.[53] Before initiation of treatment with cyclophosphamide, male patients should be advised about banking sperm to aid future conception.

Acrolein, a toxic metabolite of cyclophosphamide, can irritate the bladder and promote hemorrhagic cystitis, bladder fibrosis, and transitional and squamous cell carcinoma.[49] Two preventive measures may lessen the frequency of bladder complications. One widely accepted approach is maintenance of a liberal fluid intake of several liters daily. Mesna (2-mercaptoethanesulfonate) has also been advocated for prophylaxis[54] and is available for intravenous use. The parenteral solution can be taken orally because it is 29% to 81% bioavailable by this route and stable for up to 24 hours in a variety of beverages.[55]

The urine should be examined every month during cyclophosphamide therapy to monitor for signs of bladder toxicity. Unexplained hematuria, unless it clears rapidly, mandates an immediate diagnostic evaluation, including urology consultation and cystoscopy. The occurrence of severe cystitis usually necessitates discontinuation of oral cyclophosphamide. On the other hand, mild cystitis that resolves quickly can be managed by reemphasizing the need for good hydration and resuming the cyclophosphamide at a 25- to 50-mg lower dosage. Hematuria also can signal a neoplastic change in the bladder mucosa. To screen for bladder cancer, a urine cytologic examination is performed yearly in patients whose total cyclophosphamide dose exceeds 10 g. Neoplastic changes have been detected in the bladder mucosa up to 11 years after the completion of cyclophosphamide therapy.[54] Thus, after cyclophosphamide therapy, patients must have annual surveillance for the potential development of bladder neoplasms. An overall scheme for monitoring oral cyclophosphamide therapy is outlined in Table 27–3.

A major concern of long-term cyclophosphamide therapy is delayed appearance of malignant disease, mostly leukemias and lymphomas.[56] Because the risk of these secondary malignant conditions is greater with higher total doses of cyclophosphamide, the need for this drug should be reexamined in patients who have received it for more than 2 years.

**TABLE 27–3**
**Recommended Monitoring of Patients Receiving Oral**
**Cyclophosphamide for the Treatment of Systemic**
**Necrotizing Vasculitis**

| TIME PERIOD* | MONITORING TESTS | COMMENTS |
|---|---|---|
| Weeks 1–3 | CBC twice a week | Carefully note the rate of decline in peripheral leukocyte count; adjust cyclophosphamide dose to keep leukocyte count >3000/3 × 10⁹/L and neutrophil count >1500/1.5 × 10⁹/L |
| Weeks 3–8 | CBC every week | As for weeks 1–3 |
|  | Urinalysis every month | Hematuria may indicate cystitis |
| Week 9 until end of therapy | CBC every 2 weeks | As above |
|  | Urinalysis every month | As above |
|  | Urine cytology study every year | Screen for bladder cancer |
| After therapy | Urine cytology study every year | Maintain surveillance for bladder cancer indefinitely |

* CBC = complete blood cell count. The period after initiation of cyclophosphamide therapy.

## Investigational Drugs and Future Directions

Alternative approaches have been used frequently in patients with systemic vasculitis. Intravenous pulse glucocorticoid therapy (e.g., methylprednisolone, 0.5 to 1 g/day for 3 days) has shown efficacy in the treatment of PAN and CSS[57, 58] and may be useful as a therapeutic alternative in certain clinical situations (e.g., for patients receiving anticoagulation therapy) or in refractory disease. Pulse cyclophosphamide therapy (500 to 750 mg/m² given IV every month for 6 months) may produce therapeutic benefits in PAN and CSS.[30–32, 59, 60] Pulse cyclophosphamide therapy can be administered as a single intravenous bolus, as routinely done in the management of lupus nephritis, or as multiple oral doses over a 3-day period.[38] Whether pulse cyclophosphamide can substitute for daily oral cyclophosphamide in the treatment of systemic vasculitis remains controversial.

Cyclosporine is a powerful immunoregulatory agent that can effectively suppress active systemic vasculitis, although it may be frequently toxic at the dosages necessary to control disease.[61] Treatment with cyclosporine has been initiated at dosages of 5 mg/kg/day and, depending on the clinical response and tolerability, gradually reduced to doses of 1 to 3 mg/kg/day for long-term maintenance.

Treatment with a combination of two monoclonal antibodies transiently reduced the number of circulating T cells and improved clinical disease manifestations in four patients with refractory systemic vasculitis.[62, 63] Innovative therapies such as this will undoubtedly be the focus of more research in the future. The approval by the US Food and Drug Administration of etanercept, a p75-soluble tumor necrosis receptor fusion protein (TNFR:Fc), will almost certainly stimulate future studies of tumor necrosis factor-alpha blockade therapy for PAN, MPA, and CSS.

## WEGENER'S GRANULOMATOSIS

WG is a necrotizing vasculitis with a predilection for the upper and lower respiratory tracts and kidneys. Otitis media, mucosal ulceration, nasal perforation and deformity, and sinusitis dominate the manifestations of upper airway involvement. The most common symptoms of lower airway disease are cough and hemoptysis. In addition, symptoms of subglottic stenosis occurred in 43 (23%) of 189 patients with WG followed at the National Institutes of Health (NIH).[64] Chest radiographs of patients with symptoms as well as of those who have no symptoms may show bilateral nodular infiltrates and cavities. Other features of WG include ocular inflammation, retroorbital masses, arthritis, multiple mononeuropathies, cerebral arteritis, and vasculitic skin lesions.

WG has a variable course, depending on the sites of clinical involvement. The presence of both respiratory and renal disease has been termed *generalized WG*, which, without aggressive immunosuppressive therapy, augurs a poor prognosis. A less ominous course is taken by patients with *limited WG*, a subgroup with respiratory disease and no clinical evidence of renal or other serious organ system disease.[65]

The erythrocyte sedimentation rate (ESR) is positively correlated in WG with clinical disease activity. However, caution must be exercised in interpreting this test result because concomitant infection, such as sinusitis, may also elevate the ESR. ANCA with a granular cytoplasmic staining pattern (c-ANCA) have diagnostic significance in WG. They occur in sera from 88% to 96% of patients with active, generalized WG.[66, 67] The frequency of a positive c-ANCA test result drops to 67% among patients with locally active disease[67] and to 41% to 43% among patients with inactive disease.[66] c-ANCA occur infrequently in association with MPA, idiopathic rapidly progressive glomerulonephritis, autoimmune hepatitis, uveitis, amebiasis, fungal infection, and human immunodeficiency virus (HIV) infection and must not be used as the only criterion for diagnosis.[66, 68] Proteinase 3 (PR3), a major autoantigen in WG, is a constituent of azurophilic granules in neutrophils. The presence of serum antibody to PR3 is highly specific for the diagnosis of WG. The c-ANCA titer and levels of serum PR3 antibodies have been used to monitor disease activity in WG. Some studies have shown that a rise in the c-ANCA titer or level of anti-PR3 antibodies over time may correlate with increased clinical activity or may be the harbinger of a relapse.[69] However, the evidence to date does not support the use of this serologic marker as a sole basis for initiating or increasing immunosuppressive therapy.[69]

Depending on the biopsy site, areas of disease involvement in WG may exhibit histologic evidence of necrotizing granulomatous vasculitis, necrotizing granuloma without vasculitis, or acute and chronic inflammation. The diagnosis is most often confirmed by the pathologic findings from an open-lung biopsy, which are also valuable for ruling out infection and other conditions that may resemble WG such as lymphomatoid granulomatosis or lymphoma. Other biopsy sites may be equally informative, although biopsy specimens from upper airways are notorious for yielding nondiagnostic material. Brochoscopy with tracheobronchial mucosal biopsy may be useful in evaluating lower airway symptoms such as cough, dyspnea, wheezing, or hoarseness. Of 21 transbronchial biopsies from 17 patients with WG and airway symptoms, results of 3 specimens from 3 patients were diagnostic for WG and results of 9 specimens from 7 patients were compatible with WG.[70] Renal biopsies show histologic evidence of a pauci-immune focal, segmental, necrotizing glomerulonephritis.

Nearly all patients with WG and upper airway involvement suffer from recalcitrant sinus infections. Patients with WG are predisposed to chronic sinus infections because of the damage to the nasal mucosa from acute and chronic inflammation. The organism to infect the paranasal sinuses most frequently is *Staphylococcus aureus*. The nasal carriage of *S. aureus* is considered to be a risk factor for the development of *S. aureus* infections, and chronic nasal carriage of *S. aureus* in patients with WG may define a subgroup who are at high risk for disease relapse.[71] The role of *S. aureus* and other microbial pathogens in triggering disease relapse is unclear.

## Natural History of Disease

The initial clinical and histopathologic descriptions of patients with WG portray a rapidly fatal course without therapy. Such patients survive a mean of 5 months and die of uremia, respiratory failure, or disseminated vasculitis. Some patients with limited WG survive longer and die later of respiratory complications or progression to renal failure.

## Uncontrolled Treatment Studies and Long-Term Experience

Although treatment with glucocorticoids extends the mean survival of WG patients to 12 months, vastly improved outcomes followed the adoption of oral cyclophosphamide as standard therapy.[72] Researchers from the NIH summarized their experience in treating 158 patients with WG who had been monitored for 1229 patient-years.[72, 73] Nearly all the patients in this group had received initial treatment with 1 mg/kg/day of prednisone and 2 mg/kg/day of oral cyclophosphamide, with subsequent reduction of the prednisone dose to an alternate-day schedule and maintenance of daily oral cyclophosphamide for 12 months after a complete remission. With this therapy, 91% of the patients showed clinical improvement, and 75% attained a complete remission.[66] About half of the group had at least one relapse, and nearly the same number sustained a remission that lasted more than 5 years.[66]

Disease- and treatment-related morbidity were common in this patient population and included chronic sinus dysfunction (47%), chronic renal insufficiency (42%), hearing loss (35%), nasal deformities (28%), pulmonary insufficiency (17%), tracheal stenosis (13%), and visual loss (8%). Complications attributed to cyclophosphamide were cystitis (43%), hair loss (17%), bladder cancer (2.8%), and myelodysplasia (2%).[66] Overall, the rate of bladder cancer was 33 times higher than in the general population. Non-Hodgkin's lymphoma developed in two patients; this rate represented an 11-fold increase in overall risk. Glucocorticoid therapy was associated with transient cushingoid features (in most patients), cataracts (21%), fractures (11%), diabetes mellitus (8%), and avascular necrosis (3%).[66] Slightly more than half of the women of childbearing age could not become pregnant or had ovarian failure after more than 1 year of cyclophosphamide therapy.[66] Nearly half of the patients required at least one hospitalization for treatment of a serious infection, usually bacterial.[66] Eight fungal, six *Pneumocystis carinii*, and two mycobacterial infections, as well as 34 episodes of herpes zoster, occurred during follow-up.[66]

Of the patients in this study, 20% died.[66] Death was caused by active WG or a disease- or treatment-related complication in 13% of the patients; other deaths resulted from renal disease (3%), pulmonary disease (3%), a combination of pulmonary and renal disease (1%), infection (3%), and cancer (2.5%).[66]

Progression to ESRD occurred in 11% of the NIH patients.[66] ESRD developed in 27 (22%) of 123 patients in a selected group with renal involvement secondary to WG or MPA.[73] Extrarenal relapses of disease occur in a minority of patients during dialysis. The relapses have been readily treated with high doses of glucocorticoids but, in some cases, have necessitated addition of cyclophosphamide.[74] The experience with renal transplantation in WG has been generally favorable, with only rare recurrences of disease in the transplanted organ and maintenance of graft function at a rate comparable with that of the total transplant population.[74, 75]

WG may manifest during pregnancy and may necessitate aggressive immunsuppressive therapy. According to case reports, excellent outcomes have been achieved during pregnancy despite the need to treat active disease with glucocorticoids and cyclophosphamide.[76] The mothers have usually improved clinically with an aggressive treatment approach, and their infants have had relatively few complications.

## Prospective Clinical Trials

The high rate of treatment-related complications from daily oral cyclophosphamide therapy has stimulated a search for less toxic immunosuppressive regimens. In an open-level, prospective trial, 14 patients with WG were treated with IV monthly pulses of cyclophosphamide, 1 g/m$^2$.[77] Of the 14 patients, 12 had previously received glucocorticoids and oral cyclophosphamide. In this study, pulse cyclophosphamide therapy was associated with a rate of relapse higher than that in historical controls who had been treated with daily oral cyclophosphamide. These results are similar to those of other prospective and retrospective studies.[78,79]

The relative benefits of pulse cyclophosphamide over daily oral cyclophosphamide were evaluated in a randomized, controlled trial involving 50 patients with newly diagnosed WG.[80] After 6 months, 24 (90%) of the patients receiving pulse cyclophosphamide therapy achieved remission, as opposed to 18 (78%) patients receiving oral cyclophosphamide; this difference was not statistically significant. However, the relapse rate was significantly higher among patients receiving pulse cyclophosphamide than among those receiving oral cyclophosphamide (52% vs. 18%; P <.05). Infectious complications were more frequent in those receiving daily oral cyclophosphamide than in those receiving pulse cyclophosphamide. In particular, P. carinii pneumonia was diagnosed in 30% of patients receiving oral cyclophosphamide but in only 11% of pulse cyclophosphamide-treated patients, which prompted the investigators to institute routine prophylaxis with trimethoprim-sulfamethoxazole (T/S) during the trial. Deaths were more common in this prospective study than in previous uncontrolled studies. After more than 2 years of follow-up, the mortality rates were 33% (9 deaths) and 44% (10 deaths) in the pulse and oral cyclophosphamide arms, respectively. These rates are much higher than the 20% mortality rate noted in the NIH series. Some of the excessive deaths in the clinical trial resulted from serious infections, which caused 3 (33%) of the deaths in the pulse cyclophosphamide recipients and 6 (60%) of the deaths in the oral cyclophosphamide recipients.

A few points about this trial deserve further comment. Although treatment with pulse and oral cyclophosphamide in this trial produced similar survival rates, the two therapies should not be judged equivalent, because of the high probability of type II error. The unusually high rate of serious infectious may have come from the use of relatively high dosages of glucocorticoids.[81] According to the protocol, the patients were treated initially with methylprednisolone, 15 mg/kg/day for 3 days, then 1 mg/kg/day on day 4 for 6 weeks, followed by a 2.5-mg dose reduction every 10 days, which translates to a dose of 15 mg/day at 6 months after initiation of therapy. In comparison, the NIH group reduced the prednisone dosage in their patients to alternate-day therapy (e.g., 60 mg every other day) within a mean of 3.2 months. These data provide further support for the concept that an expedient reduction of the prednisone dose to alternate-day therapy significantly lowers the incidence of infectious complications. Further studies are required before pulse cyclophosphamide therapy can be accepted as an initial standard treatment for WG.

More promising results have been obtained with methotrexate in a subset of WG patients without immediately life-threatening disease. In an open-label prospective study, oral weekly methotrexate, combined with standard glucocorticoid therapy, produced remission in 30 of 42 patients with WG fitting this clinical profile.[82] Of the 42 patients, 26 had had prior therapy with glucocorticoids, T/S, or daily oral cyclophosphamide. The dosage of methotrexate was begun at 0.3 mg/kg/week (not exceeding 15 mg/week) and increased to 20 to 25 mg/week as tolerated. Although the majority sustained remission, 11 (36%) of the 30 patients achieving remission with methotrexate therapy subsequently suffered relapse. Seven patients developed serious toxic effects that necessitated discontinuation of the methotrexate therapy, including four cases of P. carinii pneumonia and three cases of methotrexate pneumonitis. These results suggest that weekly methotrexate therapy may play a role in the treatment of patients with non–life-threatening manifestations of WG (e.g., limited WG).

Considerable interest has focused on the role of T/S in the treatment of WG.[83–85] Because infection has long been suspected to trigger WG, any beneficial effects from T/S could stem from its antimicrobial properties. De Groot and coworkers[86] compared the clinical efficacy of methotrexate alone, T/S alone, methotrexate plus prednisone, and T/S plus prednisone in 65 patients with WG who had achieved remission with conventional therapy. Approximately 85% to 90% of the patients maintained remission in the two groups receiving methotrexate, whereas nearly 50% of the patients taking T/S suffered relapse. Although methotrexate was superior to T/S in this study for maintaining remission, the strength of the evidence is relatively weak because of the nonrandomized study design, the inclusion of some patients in the trial who had not attained a complete remission, and the unknown effects of previous induction therapy.

The therapeutic value of T/S was further investigated in a 24-month, prospective, randomized, placebo-controlled trial involving 81 patients with WG whose disease had been brought into complete remission through standard therapy. T/S (160 mg of trimethoprim, 800 mg of sulfamethoxazole) given twice daily significantly reduced the rate of relapse, in comparison with placebo.[87] Eight patients (20%) withdrew from the trial in the T/S group because of side effects. The difference in relapse rate between the two treatment groups was significant only for recurrent disease in the nasal and upper airways and did not obviate the need for subsequent immunosuppressive therapy.

## Management

Most authorities stage the initial treatment of WG on the basis of the severity of disease. Glucocorticoids and another immunosuppressive drug are initially required for virtually all patients with active WG. Patients with severe WG should receive initial treatment with 1 mg/kg/day of prednisone (or its equivalent) and 2 mg/kg/day of oral cyclophosphamide. The prednisone dose is usually tapered to 20 mg/day by 2 months, to alternate-day therapy by 3 to 4 months, and stopped after 6 months. Oral cyclophosphamide therapy is maintained for 1 year after the patients have achieved disease remission. Many authorities have begun to shorten the course of oral cyclophosphamide therapy to minimize treatment-related complications. Patients who achieve remission in 3 to 6 months with daily oral cyclophosphamide may be switched to weekly methotrexate therapy (described next). The methotrexate is continued until the disease has been in complete remission for 1 year, and the dose is then tapered by 2.5 mg/month. Patients with a complete remission and a serum creatinine level exceeding 2.0 mg/dL switch to azathioprine, 2 mg/kg/day, and are likewise treated for 1 year. The azathioprine may be subsequently tapered every 2 months in 50-mg dose decrements.

Methotrexate may substitute for oral cyclophosphamide in patients with limited WG. In such cases, the methotrexate dose is initiated at 0.25 mg/kg/week (maximum of 15 mg/week) and increased by 2.5 mg/week increments every week up to 0.35 mg/kg week (maximum dose, 25 mg/week) as tolerated. The methotrexate should be continued until the disease has been in complete remission for 1 year, and then the dosage should be tapered by 2.5 mg/month. Pulse cyclophosphamide, 500 to 750 mg/m$^2$, may be considered for initial or maintenance treatment of patients with WG who have contraindications to oral cyclophosphamide and methotrexate. Patients receiving glucocorticoids in combination with methotrexate or cyclophosphamide should be treated with T/S three times weekly to reduce the risk for *P. carinii* pneumonia. Alternatively, sulfa-allergic patients may be given dapsone, 100 mg/day, or inhaled pentamidine, once a month.

Patients receiving methotrexate therapy should take concomitant folic acid, 1 mg/day, or folinic acid, 5 mg/week, to reduce the risk of methotrexate toxicity. Methotrexate should not be combined with therapeutic doses of T/S because together they may increase hematologic toxicity. Because methotrexate is excreted through the kidneys, its use should be avoided by patients with a serum creatinine level above 2 to 2.5 mg/dL. Patients with mild renal insufficiency who are treated with methotrexate should receive this agent

in lower than usual doses (5–10 mg/week) and be closely monitored for possible toxicity.

A disease flare necessitates intensification of immunosuppressive therapy. Patients with severe disease and a major flare who are receiving methotrexate or azathioprine may require reinduction with high dosages of prednisone and with oral cyclophosphamide therapy. Those with limited disease who develop severe flares are treated with increased doses of prednisone and may be switched from methotrexate to oral cyclophosphamide. Less severe flares in the context of limited disease may be managed by higher doses of methotrexate. Alternatively, mild-to-moderate flares of WG may be treated for 1 month with an increased dose of prednisone, followed by resumption of a taper.

Integral to the treatment of WG is aggressive treatment of sinus disease. Chronic sinus inflammation in WG impairs mucosal immunity and increases susceptibility to infection, usually from *S. aureus*. Frequent irrigation to relieve nasal crusting and blocked airways, surgical procedures to drain impacted sinuses, and prompt initiation of antibiotics at the earliest signs of infection are the cornerstones of managing chronic nasal and sinus disease. Worsening nasal or sinus disease that is unresponsive to local measures and antibiotic therapy may necessitate tissue biopsy for diagnosis. T/S in therapeutic doses may have a role in managing patients with smoldering sinus disease who are otherwise in remission.

Subglottic stenosis may mandate additional therapy if the patient is symptomatic. Intratracheal dilation and instillation of corticosteroids has been shown to be a safe and effective option.[64] Alternatively, successful repair of stenotic segments has been achieved with surgical reconstruction.[88]

Conjunctivitis, episcleritis, and anterior uveitis in WG are treated with topical glucocorticoid preparations. In contrast, active scleritis and optic nerve vasculitis threaten vision and mandate immediate ophthalmologic evaluation to assess the need for systemic immunosuppressive therapy. A retroorbital mass, another worrisome ocular manifestation, can also jeopardize vision and may warrant emergency orbital decompression.

## Investigational Drugs and Future Directions

Several other therapies have been tried successfully in WG, including intravenous pulse methylprednisolone,[89] cyclosporine,[61] intravenous gamma globulin,[90] etoposide,[91] and monoclonal antibodies to CD52 or CD4 T cell antigens.[92] Clinical trials are now under way with etanercept (soluble TNFR:Fc) in patients with WG because of the possible role of TNF-$\alpha$ in the pathogenesis of this disease.

## TYPE II MIXED CRYOGLOBULINEMIA (CRYOGLOBULINEMIA WITH VASCULITIS)

Type II mixed cryoglobulinemia (MC) is characterized by recurrent purpura, arthralgias/arthritis, weakness, peripheral neuropathy, hepatomegaly, splenomegaly, Raynaud's syndrome, Sjögren's syndrome, and glomerulonephritis.[93, 94] The immunochemical composition of the cryoprecipitate defines the type of cryoglobulinemia. Type I cryoglobulins consist of a single monoclonal immunoglobulin and are found predominantly in patients with malignancies of the immune system. Type II cryoglobulins are composed of a monoclonal immunoglobulin M (IgM) rheumatoid factor and polyclonal immunoglobulin G (IgG), whereas type III cryoglobulins contain polyclonal IgM rheumatoid factor and polyclonal IgG. Most of the type II cryoglobulinemias are essential, or primary. Secondary type II cryoglobulinemia has been associated with lymphoid malignancies, and secondary type III cryoglobulinemia may occur with infections, autoimmune disease, and chronic liver disease.

There is evidence indicating that hepatitis C virus (HCV) plays a major role in the pathogenesis of type II MC. Early series of trials with first-generation assays found a high prevalence of HBV infection in patients with type II MC,[95] but later studies failed to confirm this association.[96] More than 80% of cases of type II MC appear to be caused by HCV infection.[97, 98] Many patients with type II MC have no biochemical or clinical evidence of liver damage.

Histopathologic examination of skin lesions in type II MC reveals perivascular inflammation with varying degrees of leukocytoclasis. A study of lesional skin has shown by in situ hybridization that HCV as well as IgM and IgG localize in the epidermis, dermis, and the vessel wall.[99] The glomerular pathologic process is characterized by focal or diffuse proliferative changes with intraglomerular thrombi. IgG, IgM, and C3, the most prevalent immunoreactants, produce intense granular staining of peripheral capillary loops and massive staining of intraluminal thrombi.[98] Electron microscopy shows electron-dense subendothelial deposits with a peculiar fibrillar or crystalloid structure. These morphologic patterns are also found in the serum cryoprecipitate and presumably represent high-molecular-weight aggregates of antigen-antibody complexes. Other involved organ systems show histopathologic evidence of small-vessel vasculitis.

## Natural History of Disease and Long-Term Experience

The natural history of type II MC is poorly understood because virtually all patients with this condition have been treated with glucocorticoids and immunosuppressive therapy. Type II MC typically exhibits a chronic course and has a high probability of relapse. Episodes of purpura last 3 to 10 days and may recur sporadically over a period of years. Confluent purpura on the lower legs may evolve into deep skin ulcers, which are susceptible to infection and may progress to osteomyelitis.

Focal or diffuse proliferative glomerulonephritis develops in 8% to 54% of patients with type II MC. It may accompany the first episode of purpura or, more frequently, appear several years after the onset of skin and joint disease.[96, 100, 101] The renal lesion pursues a variable course.[96, 100, 101] A partial or complete remission of renal disease occurs in nearly one third of affected patients, whereas in the others the disease typically progresses in an indolent manner or acute, reversible exacerbations occur. Earlier studies suggested that chronic renal failure develops commonly in type II MC; however, more recent studies have found that chronic renal failure develops in only about 10% of cases.[102]

Most deaths in type II MC result from cardiovascular disease, cerebral hemorrhage, or infection.[98, 101] Cardiovascular deaths have occurred in patients with severe hypertension. Autopsies in two cases revealed evidence of coronary arteritis.[98] Hypertension and cerebral arteritis are contributing factors in most cerebrovascular deaths.[98, 101] Infections of chronic, deep skin ulcers have led to death from sepsis.[98, 101]

Some investigators have postulated that HCV-related type II MC is a benign or low-grade B-cell lymphoproliferative disease. Bone marrow biopsy specimens from patients with type II MC have shown B-cell monoclonality as well as focal lymphoplasmacytoid infiltrates suggestive of non-Hodgkin's lymphoma.[102] In one study of type II MC, bone marrow biopsy revealed findings diagnostic or suggestive of non-Hodgkin's lymphoma in 9 of 16 cases.[103] Follow-up of 200 patients with type II MC in another series disclosed 14 cases of non-Hodgkin's lymphoma that had developed on average 5.6 years (SD, ±3.8 years) after the original diagnosis.[104] Four of these patients died of the malignancies. The rate of progression was even more striking in another group, in which non-Hodgkin's lymphoma developed in 12 (39%) of 31 patients with type II MC after long-term follow-up.[102] The results from these studies confirm the presence of occult lymphoproliferative disorders in patients with HCV-related type II MC and show that some cases may progress to overt lymphoma.

## Uncontrolled Treatment Studies

The treatment of type II MC has evolved with our growing understanding of the pathogenesis of this disease. Initial therapies focused on the evidence that type II MC was an immune complex–mediated disease. Glucocorticoids and other immunosuppressive drug such as cyclophosphamide were the mainstays of therapy.[96, 98, 101] Plasma exchange and cryofiltration have been used to rapidly remove cryoprecipitable immune complexes from the circulation, and they typically produce transient clinical responses.[105–107] Disease manifestations usually rebound when plasma exchange is stopped without concurrent immunosuppressive therapy.[105] Despite the diagnostic value of serum cryoglobulins in type II MC, uncontrolled observations show that improvement in disease activity after treatment does not always correlate with a reduction in the cryocrit.[105]

Outcomes are relatively poor in patients with type II MC treated with a combination of plasma exchange, glucocorticoids, and cyclophosphamide. In 1980, Popp and associates[96] reported 18 deaths among 40 patients with type II MC despite aggressive combination therapy. Of the 20 patients with renal disease in this study, 14 died after an average of 7.4 years of follow-up.

Evidence that type II MC is probably caused by HCV infection has dramatically altered the management of this disorder. The first available antiviral drug for HCV infection was IFN-alpha.[108] IFN-alpha treatment of chronic hepatitis B for 48 weeks produces a sustained virologic response in 15% to 20% of patients.[109] Initial case reports suggested that IFN-alpha therapy for HCV-positive patients with type II MC decreased serum cryoglobulin levels and improved clinical disease activity.[110] Longer term studies of patients with type II MC treated with IFN-alpha showed sustained decreases in the level of viremia, reductions in cryocrit, and favorable clinical responses.[111]

Casato and colleagues[111] prospectively analyzed the outcomes of 31 patients with HCV-positive type II MC who had received 3 MU of recombinant IFN-alpha daily for the first 3 months and then every other day for at least 9 additional months. Of the 31 patients, 17 (62%) achieved a complete remission after treatment with IFN-alpha. Only the presence of antibodies to C22 (which is an HCV structural protein antigen) and low levels of HCV RNA before treatment were predictive of a complete response. Clinical responses were correlated with the disappearance of serum HCV RNA and of cryoglobulins and a decrease in the titer of anti-C22 antibodies. Relapses also occurred in 5 of the 31 patients during IFN-alpha therapy. In 3 of the 4 patients monitored during follow-up, relapse was accompanied by the detection of serum antibodies to IFN-alpha. These 4 patients were then successfully treated with natural IFN-alpha, which suggests that treatment resistance may have resulted from the development of antibodies to recombinant IFN-alpha.

## Prospective Trials

The efficacy of IFN-alpha therapy has been examined in a randomized, crossover trial of 26 patients with type II MC.[112] Patients were eligible for this trial only if they had hepatic or neurologic involvement and had no clinical evidence of renal disease. Most of the patients had been receiving low doses of prednisolone. HCV infection was documented in 25 of the 26 patients who entered this trial. IFN-alpha therapy was administered for 6 months (2 MU/day for 1 month, then every other day for 5 months). Treatment with IFN-alpha was associated with statistically significant reductions in the purpura score, liver enzyme values, and cryocrit.[112] Upon stopping INF-alpha therapy, patients often experienced a rebound in disease manifestations.

A randomized, placebo-controlled, parallel trial was performed in 53 patients with HCV-related type II MC.[113] In this study, patients were randomly assigned to receive treatment with placebo or IFN-alpha, 1.5 MU three times a week for 1 week and then 3 MU three times a week for the next 23 weeks. At the start of treatment, all 25 patients who received IFN-alpha and 25 of 26 patients who received placebo had

detectable serum HCV RNA. The analysis was performed on only patients who completed the treatment course. IFN-alpha treatment significantly reduced the levels of viremia. Serum HCV RNA levels became undetectable in 15 of the 25 patients who received IFN-alpha, in comparison with none of the 24 patients who received placebo. All of the patients in whom HCV RNA disappeared from the serum showed clinical improvement and a markedly decreased level of serum cryoglobulins. Viremia recurred between 24 and 48 weeks after discontinuation of therapy in 13 of the 15 INF-alpha recipients and 1 year after discontinuation of therapy in the other 2 patients. In some cases, retreatment with IFN-alpha induced a disease remission. Treatment-related side effects observed during the trial included flu-like symptoms after the first few injections (most patients), mild leukopenia and thrombocytopenia, loss of appetite, alopecia, depression, and insomnia. The dose of IFN-alpha had to be reduced in two cases because of thrombocytopenia. These data provide strong evidence that eradicating HCV infection may cure HCV-related type II MC.

The results of randomized, controlled trials involving patients with chronic hepatitis C indicate that treatment with the combination of IFN-alpha and ribavirin produces a higher rate of cure than does treatment with IFN-alpha alone.[114, 115] Ribavirin, a synthetic guanosine nucleoside analog, has antiviral activity in vitro against a wide range of RNA and DNA viruses. In these trials, IFN-$\alpha$2b was administered at a dosage of 3 MU three times a week, and ribavirin was given orally at 1000 or 1200 mg/day. As initial treatment, sustained virologic and biochemical responses were observed in 35% to 43% of patients treated with the combination therapy for 24 to 48 weeks, in comparison with 18% to 19% of patients receiving IFN-alpha alone.[114, 115] The combination therapy also yielded higher rates of virologic and biochemical responses than did IFN-alpha alone in patients with chronic hepatitis B who suffered relapse after IFN-alpha treatment.[116] The main side effect of ribavirin in these trials was hemolytic anemia (hemoglobin <10 g/dL), which was observed in 10% of patients receiving the combination therapy in clinical trials and may necessitate a decrease in the ribavirin dose.

There are no published studies of the combination therapy in patients with HCV-associated type II MC. However, five patients with HCV-positive type II MC have been treated in an open-label trial with 1000 to 1200 mg/day of ribavirin as monotherapy for 10 to 36 months.[117] The virologic and clinical responses were transient in the five treated patients; thus, ribavirin therapy alone does not produce a sustained therapeutic effect in patients with HCV-positive type II MC. Other agents may hold promise. For example, treatment with a novel purine analog, 2-chlorodeoxyadenosine, produced a remission in a patient with type II MC previously refractory to glucocorticoids, cyclophosphamide, plasma exchange, and IFN-alpha.[118]

## Management

The cornerstone of management is antiviral therapy, and the goal is to eradicate HCV from the body. Patients with moderate or severe clinical manifestations of small-vessel vasculitis may be treated initially with plasma exchange and low dosages of glucocorticoids to bring the disease quickly under control. However, the dosage of glucocorticoids should be tapered as rapidly as possible after the introduction of antiviral therapy. Local measures such as compressive stockings or Unna boots may be indicated for the management of purpura and skin ulcers. Immunosuppressive drugs such as cyclophosphamide should be strictly avoided in patients with chronic HCV infection.

Studies have shown that most patients with HCV-related type II MC benefit clinically from IFN-alpha therapy. The treatment protocols typically call for 3 MU of IFN-alpha (Intron A), given three times a week for 6 to 12 months. Although clinical responses to IFN-alpha monotherapy have been favorable, the cure rate appears to be only 15% to 20% with this approach. Higher cure rates may be possible through the combination of IFN-alpha and ribavirin for 24 to 48 weeks. However, no published experience with the combination therapy in patients with HCV-related type II MC is available. In view of the goal of antiviral therapy, the combination therapy would probably produce superior long-term outcomes in comparison with IFN-alpha alone and should be considered in patients with HCV-related type II MC, especially those with chronic hepatitis.

IFN-alpha therapy has been associated with severe depression and suicidal behavior and should be used with extreme caution in patients with a history of previous psychiatric illness. Because ribavirin often causes significant hemolytic anemia, all patients receiving the combination therapy should have a complete blood count at weeks, 1, 2, and 4 after starting treatment and monthly thereafter. A liver biopsy should be considered for any patient with HCV infection and biochemical evidence of hepatic injury to monitor the response to antiviral therapy.

## HENOCH-SCHÖNLEIN PURPURA (ANAPHYLACTOID PURPURA)

HSP is a multisystem disease that affects primarily the skin, joints, gastrointestinal tract, and kidneys. The ACR has developed criteria for the classification of HSP.[119] This illness is most common in children. The key clinical feature is a purpuric rash that involves the lower extremities and buttocks. The majority of patients experience joint pain and swelling. Abdominal pain commonly occurs in HSP and may be complicated by gastrointestinal hemorrhage or, in rare cases, intussusception. Some degree of renal involvement, ranging from microscopic hematuria to acute nephritis and nephrotic syndrome, develops in approximately 40% of patients.

In addition to the urinary findings, laboratory studies may reveal mild leukocytosis and an elevated ESR. A characteristic clinical picture with a normal platelet count is usually sufficient for a clinical diagnosis. Biopsy of the purpuric skin lesions reveals a leukocytoclastic vasculitis and prominent immunoglobulin A deposition in the vessel walls, which confirm its vasculitic nature.

## Natural History of Disease

The acute illness usually lasts about 4 weeks, but more than one third of the cases persist longer.[120] Recurrent episodes of HSP occur in 12% to 40% of children and are reminiscent of the initial clinical presentation, although milder.[120] Age greater than 5 years at presentation has been associated with increased severity of renal disease.[121]

Kidney involvement accounts solely for the long-term morbidity and mortality in HSP. Most studies of unselected HSP cases suggest that progression to chronic renal failure occurs in fewer than 5%.[122, 123] Kobayashi and coworkers[123] retrospectively classified 203 Japanese children with HSP according to renal findings at presentation. They found no abnormalities in 80 (39%), minimal hematuria or proteinuria in 83 (41%), and severe proteinuria or hematuria in 40 (20%). Many children in the third group suffered multiple recurrences of nephritis for more than 1 year. Only four cases (2%) showed progressive deterioration in renal function. HSP has been reported in adults with both higher[124] and similar[125] frequencies of renal disease as in children with HSP. A retrospective analysis of 162 children and adults with HSP showed more frequent and severe renal involvement in adults.[126]

The extent of hematuria, proteinuria, and renal dysfunction at presentation has been shown to correlate with greater morphologic severity of glomerular disease,[121, 127] which in turn has been associated with worse long-term renal outcomes.[121, 128] Despite these clinicopathologic correlations, extended follow-up has revealed unexpected deterioration in several HSP patients who had only mild renal manifestations at the initial assessment.[128] Furthermore, the predictive value of an initial biopsy is poor because many patients with severe glomerular changes recover completely from the illness.[128] For these reasons, a renal biopsy is not recommended in the routine initial evaluation of HSP patients.

## Treatment Studies

The evidence to date does not show that immunosuppressive therapy alters the natural history of HSP. Glucocorticoids play only a limited role in the treatment of HSP. Adults require drug therapy more frequently than do children.[126] In the acute illness, glucocorticoids can promptly relieve severe abdominal pain and arrest gastrointestinal hemorrhage.[120] Glucocorticoids and cytotoxic agents have been prescribed during the acute illness to prevent serious renal disease, but they do not appear to change long-term outcomes.[120, 129] An uncontrolled study of low-dose immunoglobulin therapy has also been performed in patients with HSP and renal disease, but the outcomes, although favorable, are difficult to interpret without a control group.[130] In contrast, other investigators have reported a case of

HSP in which renal function deteriorated after immunoglobulin therapy.[131]

In a prospective trial, 168 children with HSP who lacked renal abnormalities at presentation were assigned to receive either no treatment or 1 mg/kg/day of prednisone for 2 weeks.[132] None of the prednisone-treated patients developed clinical signs of nephropathy. Microscopic hematuria, proteinuria, or both appeared within 2 to 6 weeks after recovery from the acute illness in 10 of the untreated patients. These abnormalities resolved within 1 year in 8 of these children, whereas in the other 2 children the urinary findings persisted without decline in renal function. Although this study suggests that prednisone therapy may reduce the incidence of early HSP renal disease, it does not address the critical question of whether glucocorticoids prevent progression to chronic renal failure.

Patients with HSP and severe nephritis have usually been treated with aggressive glucocorticoid therapy, often in combination with other immunosuppressive drugs. Twelve children aged 6 to 14 years with rapidly progressive glomerulonephritis were treated with pulse methylprednisolone for 3 days, followed by oral prednisolone for 3 months, oral cyclophosphamide for 2 months, and oral dipyridamole for 6 months.[133] The serum creatinine normalized in all but one patient by the end of therapy. Seven patients achieved a complete remission with no urinary sediment abnormalities. Four patients had persistent urine sediment abnormalities. The remaining patient developed chronic renal insufficiency with continued hematuria and proteinuria. Other studies have shown regression of glomerulonephritis with intensive immunosuppressive therapy.[134]

## Management

Most children and adults with HSP can be managed conservatively as outpatients during the acute illness. Antibiotics may be necessary to treat an infection. Salicylates and other nonsteroidal anti-inflammatory drugs (NSAIDs) can alleviate symptoms from purpura and joint manifestations. Patients with severe abdominal pain or other gastrointestinal complications require hospitalization. Severe abdominal pain, melena, or hematemesis usually responds promptly to 1 mg/kg/day of prednisone, which should not be continued longer than 2 weeks. Persistence of abdominal pain beyond 24 hours or a tender abdominal mass may be a sign of intussusception. Such findings mandate further diagnostic evaluation and surgical consultation.

Patients with rapidly progressive glomerulonephritis should be treated with high dosages of glucocorticoids in combination with cyclophosphamide. Treatment should be initiated with IV methylprednisolone, 0.5 mg/kg/day for 3 days, and oral cyclophosphamide, 2 mg/kg/day. After the methylprednisolone pulses, the patient is switched to oral prednisone, 1 mg/kg/day for 1 month, followed by tapering of the dose as described earlier. The appropriate duration of oral cyclophosphamide therapy is unclear, but it probably should be continued for at least 3 to 6 months, depending on the treatment response.

# HYPERSENSITIVITY VASCULITIS

The term *hypersensitivity vasculitis* defines a heterogenous group of vasculitic disorders in which the predominant pathologic lesion is inflammation of arterioles, capillaries, and venules. Although virtually any organ system or vessel size can be attacked in this condition, skin manifestations and biopsy evidence of leukocytoclastic vasculitis dominate the clinical and histopathologic picture. The ACR has developed criteria for the classification of hypersensitivity vasculitis.[135] The cutaneous disease can variously appear as purpura, urticaria-like lesions, bullous lesions, ulcers, erythematous plaques, or nodules.[136] Less frequently, hypersensitivity vasculitis may produce vessel inflammation outside the skin, leading to joint, kidney, liver, lung, heart, or nervous system involvement.[136, 137]

As the name implies, hypersensitivity vasculitis is thought to represent an immune response to an antigenic stimulus resulting from exposure to an environmental toxin, foreign protein, drug, tumor antigen, infectious agent, or self-antigen. Historically, several clinical syndromes have been included under the general heading of hypersensitivity vasculitis: drug-induced vasculitis, serum sickness, HSP, type II MC, vasculitis associated with malignancies, and vasculitis associated with other primary disorders.[137] Hypersensitivity vasculitis is a diagnosis usually reserved for patients with a small-vessel vasculitis apart from HSP, type II MC, and the secondary causes of small-vessel vasculitis.

## Natural History of Disease

The heterogeneity of hypersensitivity vasculitis as a diagnostic category has obscured our understanding of its natural history. Several subgroups of hypersensitivity vasculitis have been described. Serum sickness occurs after exposure to a foreign antigen (e.g., heterologous horse serum) and typically produces a 2- to 4-week self-limited bout of fever, urticaria, arthralgias, and lymphadenopathy. The clinical course of patients with hypersensitivity vasculitis of unknown cause is more variable than that of serum sickness. In one study of 82 patients with this condition, the clinical course was characterized as acute (56%), chronic (28%), or relapsing (16%), with recurring episodes of skin disease separated by intervals of months to years.[136] The subgroup of patients with drug-related hypersensitivity vasculitis also has a highly variable course. Often lacking in studies is convincing proof that the drug actually caused the vasculitis.

## Treatment Studies

Discontinuation of a potentially inciting drug has been shown to be effective therapy for most cases of drug-related hypersensitivity vasculitis. Skin involvement has been reported to respond to treatment with topical glucocorticoids, antihistamines, and NSAIDs.[136] For patients with chronic or relapsing disease, Callen[138] reported success with oral colchicine in a dosage of 0.6 mg twice daily. However, the results of a small, randomized, controlled trial did not find that colchicine, 0.5 mg twice daily, was more effective than topical emollients in preventing relapses of cutaneous leukocytoclastic vasculitis.[139] Other agents, including hydroxychloroquine, dapsone, and azathioprine, have also been reported to produce favorable responses in refractory cases. A retrospective analysis of 95 patients from a university hospital suggests that hypersensitivity vasculitis has an excellent outcome regardless of therapy.[140] Only two of the patients in this study failed to recover completely.

## Management

The first step in treating hypersensitivity vasculitis is removal of the offending antigen. Because the vasculitic process is often self-limited, it is treated conservatively with local measures, including topical glucocorticoids, protective dressings, and Unna boots, as well as antihistamines and NSAIDs. Treatment with colchicine, hydroxychloroquine, dapsone, or azathioprine may be considered in patients with chronic or relapsing disease. A short course of prednisone (<20 mg/day) may be warranted in selected patients with severe skin or joint manifestations. Although systemic glucocorticoids can suppress the development of new skin lesions, their withdrawal is often followed by the appearance of new eruptions. Evidence does not support the prolonged use of glucocorticoids or cytotoxic agents for treating hypersensitivity vasculitis. However, in rare cases, such as severe bullous or ulcerative disease, this approach may be undertaken with caution. The occasional patient with serious or life-threatening systemic involvement may require treatment with 40 to 60 mg/day of prednisone, followed by a 2- to 3-month taper to the lowest dosage that effectively controls the disease.

## COGAN'S SYNDROME

Cogan's syndrome is a rare disorder characterized by recurrent episodes of bilateral ocular inflammation and vestibuloauditory dysfunction.[141, 142] The hallmark of the ocular involvement is interstitial keratitis, a patchy mononuclear cell infiltrate in the cornea that causes eye discomfort, redness, and photophobia. Other types of ocular inflammation, including conjunctivitis, iritis, episcleritis/scleritis, posterior uveitis, vitritis, choroiditis, and retinal vasculitis, may accompany interstitial keratitis.[141] Vestibuloauditory disease, the other major feature of Cogan's syndrome, provokes sudden and debilitating attacks resembling Ménière's disease. These attacks may be characterized by nausea, vomiting, hearing impairment, and severe vertigo. In about half of the cases, onsets of ocular and vestibuloauditory symptoms are simultaneous; in the remainder, the disease unfolds as isolated ocular and vestibuloauditory events occurring within months of each other.[143]

Systemic inflammatory disease arises commonly in Cogan's syndrome and may produce constitutional symptoms, central nervous system manifestations, cutaneous lesions, and systemic necrotizing vasculitis.[141, 143, 144] Widespread vasculitis develops in about 10% of patients and can affect either large vessels (resembling Takayasu's disease) or medium-sized vessels (PAN-like).[143] Aortic insufficiency with aortitis has been reported in up to 10% of patients with Cogan's syndrome.[144]

## Natural History of Disease

The ocular outcomes in Cogan's syndrome are excellent unless the course is complicated by posterior segment inflammation (e.g., scleritis, vitritis, posterior uveitis). Interstitial keratitis, conjunctivitis, and iritis target the anterior segment of the eye and only rarely cause visual loss. In contrast, ocular inflammation of the posterior segment, if left unchecked, can rapidly destroy ocular tissue and cause permanent visual loss. Blindness has been reported in about 5% of patients with Cogan's syndrome and results from ocular inflammation beyond the anterior segment.[141, 144]

Hearing loss, sometimes asymmetric, is the major cause of disability in Cogan's syndrome. Deafness was noted in 21 of 78 ears in one series[143] and in 78 of 156 ears in another previous review.[144] Vestibular symptoms usually resolve, although mild oscillopsia may persist in the minority of cases. Cochlear hydrops can develop as a consequence of prolonged disease and produce hearing fluctuations as a result of hormonal changes (e.g., the menstrual cycle in women), ingestion of salty foods, allergic conditions, or an upper respiratory illness. Such hearing fluctuations are clinically indistinguishable from those of inflammatory origin.

## Treatment Studies

Prompt treatment of interstitial keratitis with topical glucocorticoids usually prevents corneal scarring and vascularization.[143] The rare occurrence of severe visual loss from corneal scarring has been treated with corneal transplantation. Posterior segment ocular disease has responded variably to treatment with systemic glucocorticoids, cyclophosphamide, and cyclosporine.[61, 141, 145, 146]

Acute hearing loss may be at least partially reversed by systemic prednisone therapy, 1 to 2 mg/kg/day.[145] Some evidence suggests that prompt therapy with systemic glucocorticoids can reduce hearing loss.[147] Acute hearing loss resistant to glucocorticoid therapy has been managed successfully with oral cyclophosphamide, methotrexate, and azathioprine therapy[145]; however, the true efficacy of these agents is uncertain, in view of the variable nature of the disease.

Aortic insufficiency resulting from aortitis has been ameliorated after treatment with glucocorticoids and cytotoxic agents.[141] Other patients have required aortic valve replacement.[141-144, 148] Large- and medium-vessel vasculitis in Cogan's syndrome can be controlled with prednisone, oral cyclophosphamide, and cyclosporine.[61, 141, 143] Occlusive vascular disease caused by coronary[141] and mesenteric[149] arteritis has necessitated surgical bypass to correct end-organ ischemia.

## Management

Interstitial keratitis and iritis are satisfactorily managed with mydriatics and topical glucocorticoid therapy. Ocular signs and symptoms generally improve within 3 to 7 days after the start of therapy. A poor treatment response may signal the presence of another disease process such as chlamydial infection, which can mimic the ocular manifestations of Cogan's syndrome.[150] Episcleritis and scleritis also usually resolve with topical glucocorticoid therapy. In contrast, nodular scleritis, posterior uveitis, and retinal artery disease often mandate systemic therapy, consisting initially of 1 to 2 mg/kg/day of prednisone for 1 month, followed by a gradual dosage taper over the next 2 to 3 months (see Table 27–2). Serious ocular inflammation that progresses despite glucocorticoid therapy can be treated with oral cyclophosphamide or cyclosporine.[146] Because such cytotoxic therapy is potentially hazardous, end points must be set to define the period of therapy.

Audiograms are obtained routinely to quantify hearing loss and monitor the response to therapy. Patients with acute hearing loss are initially given a 2-week trial of prednisone at a dosage of 1 mg/kg/day. This dosage is usually maintained for an additional 2 weeks with a favorable treatment response and tapered within 6 to 8 weeks to an alternate-day regimen as long as auditory acuity is preserved. Some patients require continuous low doses of prednisone on a daily or alternate-day schedule to prevent further deterioration in hearing, whereas others can stop taking prednisone for variable periods and maintain their hearing. Patients whose auditory acuity does not improve with glucocorticoids may be treated with oral cyclophosphamide (1 to 2 mg/kg/day), methotrexate (7.5 to 20 mg/week), or azathioprine (2 mg/kg/day). Because the benefits of these agents are uncertain, therapeutic response criteria are mandatory for defining the period of treatment. Patients with complete deafness may benefit from a cochlear implant.

The heart should be periodically examined for signs of aortic insufficiency. Cardiac symptoms, signs of heart failure, or clinical evidence of a valvular abnormality merits further diagnostic evaluation with two-dimensional echocardiography or cardiac catheterization. The treatment of systemic inflammatory vascular disease in Cogan's syndrome parallels that described for PAN.

## CONCLUDING REMARKS

The management of the major vasculitic syndromes is summarized in Table 27–4. These recommendations serve as treatment guides; it is recognized that the standard approach can entail modification in individual cases. Beyond current therapy, future progress in the management of vasculitis will probably result from new insights into disease pathogenesis.

*Acknowledgments*

*The author thanks David Pisetsky, Rex McCallum, Nancy Allen, and Barton Haynes for reviewing this chapter and*

## TABLE 27–4
## Guidelines for Initial Therapy of the Major Vasculitic Syndromes

| DISEASE CATEGORY | INITIAL THERAPY | INITIAL REMISSION RATE WITH STANDARD THERAPY |
|---|---|---|
| PAN, MPA, and CSS | Mild disease: prednisone, 1 mg/kg/d<br>Serious disease: prednisone, 1 mg/kg/d, + oral cyclophosphamide, 1–2 mg/kg/d | More than 80% |
| Hepatitis B virus–related PAN | Interferon-alpha, 5 MU/d | |
| Wegener's granulomatosis | Severe disease: prednisone, 1 mg/kg/d, + oral cyclophosphamide, 2 mg/kg/d<br>Limited disease: prednisone, 1 mg/kg/d, + methotrexate, 0.3 mg/kg/week | 75% |
| Hepatitis C virus–related type II mixed cryoglobulinemia | Interferon-alpha, 3 million U thrice weekly, + short course of prednisone (optional) + plasma exchange (optional) | 60%–70% |

CSS = Churg-Strauss syndrome; MPA = microscopic polyarteritis; PAN = polyarteritis nodosa.

*providing needed advice and criticism. Appreciation is also extended to my other valued colleagues, John Rice and David Caldwell, who have taught me much about vasculitis and its treatment.*

# REFERENCES

1. Haynes BF: Vasculitis: Pathogenic mechanisms of vessel damage. *In* Gallin JI, Goldstein IM, Snyderman R (eds): Inflammation: Basic Principles and Clinical Correlates, 2nd ed. New York: Raven Press, 1992:921–941.
2. Fauci AS, Haynes BF, Katz P: The spectrum of vasculitis: Clinical, pathologic, immunologic, and therapeutic considerations. Ann Intern Med 1978; 89:660.
3. Jennette JC, Falk RJ, Andrassy K, et al: Nomenclature of systemic vasculitis. Proposal of an international consensus conference. Arthritis Rheum 1994; 37:187.
4. Hunder GG, Arends WP, Bloch DA, et al: The American College of Rheumatology 1990 criteria for the classification of vasculitis. Arthritis Rheum 1990; 33:1065.
5. Leavitt RY, Fauci AS: Polyangiitis overlap syndrome: Classification and prospective clinical experience. Am J Med 1986; 81:79.
6. Savage COS, Winearls CG, Evans DJ, et al: Microscopic polyarteritis: Presentation, pathology, and prognosis. Q J Med 1985; 56:467.
7. Guillevin L, Durand-Gasselin B, Cevallos R, et al: Microscopic polyangiitis. Clinical and laboratory findings in eighty-five patients. Arthritis Rheum 1999; 42:421.
8. Guillevin L, Lhote F, Gherardi R: Polyarteritis nodosa, microscopic polyangiitis, and Churg-Strauss syndrome: Clinical aspects, neurologic manifestations, and treatment. Neurol Clin 1997; 15:865.
9. Guillevin L, Lhote F: Distinguishing polyarteritis nodosa from microscopic polyangiitis and implications for treatment. Curr Opin Rheumatol 1995; 7:20.
10. Watts RA, Jolliffe VA, Carruthers DM, et al: Effect of classification on the incidence of polyarteritis nodosa and microscopic polyangiitis. Arthritis Rheum 1996; 39:1208.
11. Sergent JS, Lockshin MD, Christian CL, et al: Vasculitis with hepatitis B antigenemia: Long-term observations in nine patients. Medicine 1976; 55:1.
12. McMahon BJ, Heyward WL, Templin DW, et al: Hepatitis B–associated polyarteritis nodosa in Alaskan Eskimos: Clinical and epidemiologic features and long-term follow-up. Hepatology 1989; 9:97.
13. Valente RM, Hall S, O'Duffy JD, Conn DL: Vasculitis and related disorders. *In* Kelley WN, Ruddy S, Harris ED Jr, Sledge CB (eds): Textbook of Rheumatology, 5th ed. Philadelphia: WB Saunders, 1997:1079.
14. Churg J, Strauss L: Allergic granulomatosis, allergic angiitis, and periarteritis nodosa. Am J Pathol 1951; 27:277.
15. Ewald EA, Griffin D, McCune WJ: Correlation of angiographic abnormalities with disease manifestations and disease severity in polyarteritis nodosa. J Rheumatol 1987; 14:952.
16. Lie JT: Diagnostic histopathology of major systemic and pulmonary vasculitic syndromes. Rheum Dis Clin North Am 1990; 16:269.
17. Frohnert PP, Sheps SG: Long-term follow-up study of periarteritis nodosa. Am J Med 1967; 43:8.
18. Guillevin L, Le Thi Huong D, Gayraud M: Systemic vasculitis of the polyarteritis nodosa group and infections with hepatitis B virus: A study in 98 patients. Eur J Intern Med 1989; 1:97.
19. Rose GA, Spencer H: Polyarteritis nodosa. Q J Med 1957; 26:43.
20. Cohen RD, Conn DL, Ilstrup DM: Clinical features, prognosis, and response to treatment in polyarteritis. Mayo Clin Proc 1980; 55:146.
21. Fauci AS, Katz P, Haynes BF, et al: Cyclophosphamide therapy of severe systemic necrotizing vasculitis. N Engl J Med 1979; 301:235.
22. Nachman PH, Hogan SL, Jennette JC, et al: Treatment responses and relapse in antineutrophil cytoplasmic autoantibody–

associated microscopic polyangiitis and glomerulonephritis. J Am Soc Nephrol 1996; 7:33.
23. Lam KC, Lai CL, Ng RP, et al: Deleterious effect of prednisolone in HBsAg-positive chronic active hepatitis. N Engl J Med 1981; 304:380.
24. Guillevin L, Lhote F, Jarrousse B, et al: Polyarteritis nodosa related to hepatitis B virus. A retrospective study of 66 patients. Ann Med Interne 1992; 143:63.
25. Guillevin L, Lhote F, Cohen P, et al: Polyarteritis nodosa related to hepatitis B virus. A prospective study with long-term observation of 41 patients. Medicine (Baltimore) 1995; 74:238.
26. Chumbley LC, Harrison EG, DeRemee RA: Allergic granulomatosis and angiitis (Churg-Strauss syndrome): Report and analysis of 30 cases. Mayo Clin Proc 1977; 52:477.
27. Guillevin L, Jarrousse B, Lok C, et al: Long-term follow-up after treatment of polyarteritis nodosa and Churg-Strauss angiitis with comparison of steroids, plasma exchange and cyclophosphamide to steroids and plasma exchange: A prospective randomized trial of 71 patients. J Rheumatol 1991; 18:567.
28. Guillevin L, Fain O, Lhote F, et al: Lack of superiority of steroids plus plasma exchange to steroids alone in the treatment of polyarteritis nodosa and Churg-Strauss syndrome. Arthritis Rheum 1992; 35:208.
29. Guillevin L, Lhote F, Cohen P, et al: Corticosteroids plus pulse cyclophosphamide and plasma exchange versus corticosteroids plus pulse cyclophosphamide alone in the treatment of polyarteritis nodosa and Churg-Strauss syndrome patients with factors predicting poor prognosis. A prospective, randomized trial in 62 patients. Arthritis Rheum 1995; 38:1638.
30. Gayraud M, Guillevin L, Cohen P, et al: Treatment of good-prognosis polyarteritis and Churg-Strauss syndrome: Comparison of steroids and oral or pulse cyclophosphamide in 25 patients. French Cooperative Study Group for Vasculitides. Br J Rheumatol 1997; 36:1290.
31. Haubitz M, Schellong S, Gobel U, et al: Intravenous pulse administration of cyclophosphamide versus daily oral treatment in patients with antineutrophil cytoplasmic antibody–associated vasculitis and renal involvement: A prospective, randomized study. Arthritis Rheum 1998; 41:1835.
32. Adu D, Pall A, Lugmani RA, et al: Controlled trial of pulse versus continuous prednisone and cyclophosphamide in the treatment of systemic vasculitis. Q J Med 1997; 90:401.
33. Guillevin L, Lhote F, Leon A, et al: Treatment of polyarteritis nodosa related to hepatitis B virus with short term steroid therapy associated with antiviral agents and plasma exchanges. A prospective trial in 33 patients. J Rheumatol 1993; 20:289.
34. Guillevin L, Lhote F, Sauvaget F, et al: Treatment of polyarteritis nodosa related to hepatitis B virus with interferon-alpha and plasma exchange. Ann Rheum Dis 1994; 53:334.
35. Kruger M, Boker KH, Zeidler H, et al: Treatment of hepatitis B–related polyarteritis nodosa with famciclovir and interferon alfa-2b. J Hepatol 1997; 26:935.
36. Guillevin L, Lhote F, Gayraud M, et al: Prognostic factors in polyarteritis nodosa and Churg-Strauss syndrome. A prospective study in 342 patients. Medicine (Baltimore) 1996; 75:17.
37. Fortin PR, Larson MG, Watters AK, et al: Prognostic factors in systemic necrotizing vasculitis of the polyarteritis nodosa group—A review of 45 cases. J Rheumatol 1995; 22:78.
38. Gordon M, Luqmani RA, Adu D, et al: Relapses in patients with a systemic vasculitis. Q J Med 1993; 86:779.
39. Guillevin L, Cohen P, Gayraud M, et al: Churg-Strauss syndrome. Clinical study and long-term follow-up of 96 patients. Medicine (Baltimore) 1999; 78:26.
40. Franssen CFM, Stegeman CA, Oost-Kort WW, et al: Determinants of renal outcome in anti-myeloperoxidase–associated necrotizing crescentic glomerulonephritis. J Am Soc Nephrol 1998; 9:1915.
41. Allen A, Pusey C, Gaskin G: Outcome of renal replacement therapy in antineutrophil cytoplasmic antibody–associated systemic vasculitis. J Am Soc Nephrol 1998; 9:1258.
42. Frasca GM, Neri L, Martello M, et al: Renal transplantation in patients with microscopic polyarteritis and antimyeloperoxidase antibodies: Report of 3 cases. Nephron 1996; 72:82.
43. Rostaing L, Modesto A, Oksman F, et al: Outcome of patients with antineutrophil cytoplasmic autoantibody–associated vas-

culitis following cadaveric kidney transplantation. Am J Kidney Dis 1997; 29:96.

44. Guillevin L, Lhote F: Treatment of polyarteritis nodosa and microscopic polyangiitis. Arthritis Rheum 1998; 41:2100.

45. Haynes BF, Allen NB, Fauci AS: Diagnostic and therapeutic approach to the patient with vasculitis. Med Clin North Am 1986; 70:355.

46. Cupps TR, Fauci AS: The Vasculitides. Philadelphia: WB Saunders, 1981:42.

47. Jorizzo JL, White WL, Wise CM, et al: Low-dose weekly methotrexate for unusual neutrophilic vascular reactions: Cutaneous polyarteritis nodosa and Behçet's disease. J Am Acad Dermatol 1991; 24:973.

48. Stein CM Pincus T: Glucocorticoids. *In* Kelley WN, Ruddy S, Harris ED Jr, Sledge CB (eds): Textbook of Rheumatology, 5th ed. Philadelphia: WB Saunders, 1997:787.

49. Fraiser LH, Kanekal S, Kehrer JP: Cyclophosphamide toxicity. Characterizing and avoiding the problem. Drugs 1991; 42:781.

50. Bradley JD, Brandt KD, Katz BP: Infectious complications of cyclophosphamide treatment for vasculitis. Arthritis Rheum 1989; 32:45.

51. Sen RP, Walsh TE, Fisher W, et al: Pulmonary complication of combination therapy with cyclophosphamide and prednisone. Chest 1991; 99:143.

52. Boumpas DT, Austin HA, Vaughn EM, et al: Risk for sustained amenorrhea in patients with systemic lupus erythematosus receiving intermittent pulse cyclophosphamide therapy. Ann Intern Med 1993; 119:366.

53. Chapman RM, Sutcliffe SB: Protection of ovarian function by oral contraceptives in women receiving chemotherapy for Hodgkin's disease. Blood 1981; 58:849.

54. Shepherd JD, Pringle LE, Barnett MJ, et al: Mesna versus hyperhydration for the prevention of cyclophosphamide-induced hemorrhagic cystitis in bone marrow transplantation J Clin Oncol 1991; 9:2016.

55. Goren MP, Lyman BA, Li JT: The stability of mesna in beverages and syrup for oral administration. Cancer Chemother Pharmacol 1991; 28:298.

56. Escalante A, Kaufman RL, Beardmore TD: Acute myelocytic leukemia after the use of cyclophosphamide in the treatment of polyarteritis nodosa. J Rheumatol 1989; 16:1147.

57. Guillevin L, Rosser J, Cacoub P, et al: Methylprednisolone in the treatment of Wegener's granulomatosis, polyarteritis nodosa and Churg-Strauss angiitis. APMIS Suppl 1990; 19:98.

58. MacFayden R, Tron V, Keshmiri M, et al: Allergic angiitis of Churg and Strauss syndrome: Response to pulse methylprednisolone. Chest 1987; 91:629.

59. De Vita S, Neri R, Bombardieri S: Cyclophosphamide pulses in the treatment of rheumatic diseases: An update. Clin Exp Rheumatol 1991; 9:179.

60. Chow C, Li EKM, Lai FM: Allergic granulomatosis and angiitis (Churg-Strauss syndrome): Response to pulse intravenous cyclophosphamide. Ann Rheum Dis 1989; 48: 605.

61. Allen NB, Caldwell DS, Rice JR, et al: Cyclosporin A therapy for Wegener's granulomatosis. *In* Gross WL (ed): ANCA-Associated Vasculitides: Immunological and Clinical Aspects. New York: Plenum Press, 1993:473.

62. Mathieson PW, Cobbold SP, Hale G, et al: Monoclonal antibody therapy in systemic vasculitis. N Engl J Med 1990; 323:250.

63. Lockwood CM, Thiru S, Issacs JD, et al: Long-term remission of intractable systemic vasculitis with monoclonal antibody therapy. Lancet 1993; 341:1620.

64. Langford CL, Sneller MC, Hallahan CW, et al: Clinical features and therapeutic management of subglottic stenosis in patients with Wegener's granulomatosis. Arthritis Rheum 1996; 39:1754.

65. Carrington CB, Liebow AA: Limited forms of angiitis and granulomatosis of Wegener's type. Am J Med 1966; 41:497.

66. Hoffman GS, Kerr GS, Leavitt RY, et al: Wegener granulomatosis: An analysis of 158 patients. Ann Intern Med 1992; 116:488.

67. Cohen Trevaert JW, van der Woude FJ, Fauci AS, et al: Association between active Wegener's granulomatosis and anticytoplasmic antibodies. Arch Intern Med 1989; 149:2461.

68. Homer RJ: Antineutrophil cytoplasmic antibodies as markers for systemic autoimmune disease. Clin Chest Med 1998; 19:627.

69. Kerr GS, Fleisher TA, Hallahan CW, et al: Limited prognostic value of changes in antineutrophil cytoplasmic antibody titer in patients with Wegener's granulomatosis. Arthritis Rheum 1993; 36:365.

70. Daum TE, Specks U, Colby TV, et al: Tracheobronchial involvement in Wegener's granulomatosis. Am J Respir Crit Care Med 1995; 151:522.

71. Stegman CA, Cohen Tervaert JW, Sluiter WJ, et al: Association of chronic nasal carriage of *Staphylococcus aureus* and higher relapse rates in Wegener granulomatosis. Ann Intern Med 1994; 120:12.

72. Fauci AS, Haynes BF, Katz P, et al: Wegener's granulomatosis: Prospective clinical and therapeutic experience with 85 patients for 21 years. Ann Intern Med 1983; 98:76.

73. Westman KWA, Bygren PG, Olsson H, et al: Relapse rate, renal survival, and cancer morbidity in patients with Wegener's granulomatosis or microscopic polyangiitis with renal involvement. J Am Soc Nephrol 1998; 9:842.

74. Schmitt WH, Haubitz M, Mistry N, et al: Renal transplantation in Wegener's granulomatosis. Lancet 1993; 342.860.

75. Wrenger E, Pirsch JD, Cangro CB, et al: Single-center experience with renal transplantation in patients with Wegener's granulomatosis. Transpl Int 1997; 10:152.

76. Luisir P, Lance NJ, Curran JJ: Wegener's granulomatosis in pregnancy. Arthritis Rheum 1997; 40:1354.

77. Hoffman GS, Leavitt RY, Fleisher TA, et al: Treatment of Wegener's granulomatosis with intermittent high-dose intravenous cyclophosphamide. Am J Med 1990; 89:403.

78. Reinhold-Keller E, Kekow J, Schnabel A, et al: Influence of disease manifestation and antineutrophil antibody titer on the response to pulse cyclophosphamide therapy in patients with Wegener's granulomatosis. Arthritis Rheum 1994; 37:919.

79. Koldingsnes W, Gran JT, Omdal R, et al: Wegener's granulomatosis: Long term follow-up of patients treated with pulse cyclophosphamide. Br J Rheumatol 1998; 37:659.

80. Guillevin L, Cordier JF, Lhote F, et al: A prospective, multicenter, randomized trial comparing steroids and pulse cyclophosphamide versus steroids and oral cyclophosphamide in the treatment of generalized Wegener's granulomatosis. Arthrirtis Rheum 1997; 40:2187.

81. Hoffman GS: Treatment of Wegener's granulomatosis: Time to change the standard of care? Arthritis Rheum 1997; 40:2099.

82. Sheller MC, Hoffman GS, Talar-Williams C, et al: An analysis of forty-two Wegener's granulomatosis patients treated with methotrexate and prednisone. Arthritis Rheum 1995; 38:608.

83. DeRemee RA, McDonlad TJ, Weiland LH: Wegener's granulomatosis: Observations on treatment with antimicrobial agents. Mayo Clin Proc 1985; 60:27.

84. West BC, Todd JR, King JW: Wegener granulomatosis and trimethoprim-sulfamethoxazole. Ann Intern Med 1987; 106:840.

85. Leavitt RY, Hoffman GS, Fauci AS: Response: The role of trimethoprim/sulfamethoxazole in the treatment of Wegener's granulomatosis. Arthritis Rheum 1988; 31:1073.

86. de Groot K, Reinhold-Keller E, Tatsis E, et al: Therapy for the maintenance of remission in sixty-five patients with generalized Wegener's granulomatosis. Methotrexate versus trimethoprim-sulfamethoxazole. Arthritis Rheum 1996; 39:2052.

87. Stegeman CA, Cohen Tervaert JW, de Jong PE, et al: Trimethoprim-sulfamethoxazole (co-trimazole) for the prevention of relapses of Wegener's granulomatosis. Dutch Co-Trimazole Wegener Study Group. N Engl J Med 1996; 335:16.

88. Herridge MS, Pearson FG, Downey GP: Subglottic stenosis complicating Wegener's granulomatosis: Surgical repair as a viable treatment option. J Thorac Cardiovasc Surg 1996; 111:961.

89. Chapman PT, O'Donnell JL: Respiratory failure in Wegener's granulomatosis: Response to pulse intravenous methylprednisolone and cyclophosphamide. J Rheumatol 1993; 20:504.

90. Tuso P, Moudgil A, Hay J, et al: Treatment of antineutrophil cytoplasmic autoantibody–positive systemic vasculitis and glomerulonephritis with pooled intravenous gammaglobulin. Am J Kidney Dis 1992; 20:504.

91. D'Cruz D, Payne H, Timothy A, et al: Response of cyclophosphamide-resistant Wegener's granulomatosis to etoposide. Lancet 1992; 340:425.

92. Lockwood CM, Thiru S, Stewart S, et al: Treatment of refractory Wegener's granulomatosis with humanized monoclonal antibodies. Q J Med 1996; 89:903.

93. Meltzer M, Franklin EC, Elias K, et al: Cryoglobulinemia: A clinical and laboratory study: II. Cryoglobulins and rheumatoid factor activity. Am J Med 1966; 40:837.

94. Agnello V, Romain PL: Mixed cryoglobulinemia secondary to hepatitis C infection. Rheum Dis Clin North Am 1996; 22:1.

95. Gorevic PD, Kassar HJ, Levo Y, et al: Mixed cryoglobulinemia: clinical aspects and long-term follow-up of 40 patients. Am J Med 1980; 69:287.

96. Popp JW Jr, Dienstag JL, Wands JR, et al: Essential mixed cryoglobulinemia without evidence for hepatitis B infection. Ann Intern Med 1980; 92:379.

97. Agnello V, Chung RT, Kaplan LM: A role for hepatitis C virus infection in type II cryoglobulinemia. N Engl J Med 1992; 327:1490.

98. Misiani R, Bellavita P, Fenili D, et al: Hepatitis C virus infection in patients with essential mixed cryoglobulinemia. Ann Intern Med 1992; 117:573.

99. Agnello V, Abel G: Localization of hepatitis C virus in cutaneous vasculitic lesions in patients with type II cryoglobulinemia. Arthritis Rheum 1997; 40:2007.

100. D'Amico G, Colasanti G, Ferrario F, et al: Renal involvement in essential mixed cryoglobulinemia. Kidney Int 1989; 35:1004.

101. Tarantino A, De Vecchi A, Montagnino G, et al: Renal disease in essential mixed cryoglobulinemia: Long-term follow-up of 44 patients. Q J Med 1981; 197:1.

102. Pozzato G, Mazzaro C, Crovatto M, et al: Low-grade malignant lymphoma, hepatitis C virus infection, and mixed cryoglobulinemia. Blood 1994; 84:3047.

103. Rasul I, Shepherd FA, Kamel-Reid S, et al: Detection of occult low-grade non-Hodgkin's lymphoma in patients with chronic hepatitis C infection and mixed cryoglobulinemia. Hepatology 1999; 29:543.

104. La Civita L, Zignego AL, Monti M, et al: Mixed cryoglobulinemia as a possible preneoplastic disorder. Arthritis Rheum 1995; 38:1859.

105. Ferri C, Moriconi L, Gremignai G, et al: Treatment of the renal involvement in mixed cryoglobulinemia with prolonged plasma exchange. Nephron 1986; 43:246.

106. McLeod BC, Sassetti RJ: Plasmapheresis with return of cryoglobulin-depleted autologous plasma (cryoglobulinpheresis) in cryoglobulinemia. Blood 1980; 55:866.

107. Sawada K, Segal AM, Malchesky PS, et al: Rapid improvement in a patient with leukocytoclastic vasculitis with secondary mixed cryoglobulinemia treated with cryofiltration. J Rheumatol 1991; 18:91.

108. Hoofnagle JH, Muller KD, Jones B, et al: Treatment of chronic non-A, non-B hepatitis with recombinant human alpha-interferon. N Engl J Med 1986; 315:1575.

109. Poynard T, Leroy V, Cohard M, et al: Meta-analysis of interferon randomized trials in the treatment of viral hepatitis C: Effects of dose and duration. Hepatology 1996; 24:778.

110. Knox TA, Hillyer CD, Kaplan MM, et al: Mixed cryoglobulinemia responsive to interferon-α. Am J Med 1991; 91:554.

111. Casato M, Agnello V, Pucillo LP, et al: Predictors of long-term response to high-dose interferon therapy in type II cryoglobulinemia associated with hepatitis C infection. Blood 1997; 90:3865.

112. Ferric C, Marzo E, Longombardo G, et al: Interferon-α in mixed cryoglobulinemia patients: A randomized, crossover-controlled trial. Blood 1993; 81:1132.

113. Misiani R, Bellavita P, Fenili D, et al: Interferon alfa-2a therapy in cryoglobulinemia associated with hepatitis C virus. N Engl J Med 1994; 330:751.

114. Reichard O, Norkrans G, Frydén A, et al: Randomised, double-blind, placebo-controlled trial of interferon alpha-2b with and without ribavirin for chronic hepatitis C. Lancet 1998; 351:83.

115. McHutchison JG, Gordon SC, Schiff ER, et al: Interferon alfa-2b alone or in combination with ribavirin as initial treatment for chronic hepatitis C. N Engl J Med 1998; 339:1485.

116. Davis GL, Esteban-Mur R, Rustgi V, et al: Interferon alfa-2b alone or in combination with ribavirin for the treatment of relapse of chronic hepatitis C. N Engl J Med 1998; 339:1493.

117. Durand J, Cacoub P, Lunel-Fabiani F, et al: Ribavirin in hepatitis C related cryoglobulinemia. J Rheumatol 1998; 25:1115.

118. Lee TC, Miller WE, Curd JG, et al: Prolonged, complete remission after 2-chlorodeoxyadenosine therapy in a patient with refractory essential mixed cryoglobulinemia. Mayo Clin Proc 1996; 71:966.

119. Mills JA, Michel BA, Bloch DA, et al: The American College of Rheumatology 1990 criteria for the classification of Henoch-Schönlein purpura. Arthritis Rheum 1990; 33:1114.

120. Allen DM, Diamond LK, Howell DA: Anaphylactoid purpura in children (Schönlein-Henoch syndrome). Am J Dis Child 1960; 99:833.

121. Meadow SR: The prognosis of Henoch-Schönlein nephritis. Clin Nephrol 1978; 9:87.

122. Koskimies O, Mir S, Rapola J, et al: Henoch-Schönlein nephritis: Long-term prognosis of unselected patients. Arch Dis Child 1981; 56:482.

123. Kobayashi O, Wada H, Okawa K, et al: Schönlein-Henoch's syndrome in children. Contrib Nephrol 1977; 4:48.

124. Fogazzi GB, Pasquali S, Moriggi M, et al: Long-term outcome of Schönlein-Henoch nephritis in the adult. Clin Nephrol 1989; 31:60.

125. Cream JJ, Gumpel JM, Peachey RDG: Schönlein-Henoch purpura in the adult: A study of 77 adults with anaphylactoid or Schönlein-Henoch purpura. Q J Med 1970; 39:461.

126. Blanco R, Martinez-Taboada VM, Rodriguez-Valverde V, et al: Henoch-Schönlein purpura in adulthood and childhood. Two different expressions of the same syndrome. Arthritis Rheum 1997; 40:859.

127. Niaudet P, Levy M, Broyer M, et al: Clinicopathologic correlations in severe forms of Henoch-Schönlein purpura nephritis based on repeat biopsies. Contrib Nephrol 1984; 40:250.

128. Goldstein AR, White RHR, Akuse R, et al: Long-term follow-up of childhood Henoch-Schönlein nephritis. Lancet 1992; 339:280.

129. Saulsbury FT: Corticosteroid therapy does not prevent nephritis in Henoch-Schönlein purpura. Pediatr Nephrol 1993; 7:69.

130. Rostoker G, Desvaux-Belghiti D, Pilatte Y, et al: Immunomodulation with low-dose immunoglobulins for moderate IgA nephropathy and Henoch-Schönlein purpura. Preliminary results of a prospective uncontroed trial. Nephron 1995; 69:327.

131. Blanco R, Gonzalez-Gay MA, Ibanez D, et al: Paradoxical and persistent renal impairment in Henoch-Schönlein purpura after high-dose immunoglobulin therapy. Nephron 1997; 76:247.

132. Mollica F, Li Volti S, Garozzo R, et al: Effectiveness of early prednisone treatment in preventing the development of nephropathy in anaphylactoid purpura. Eur J Pediatr 1992; 151:140.

133. Oner A, Tinaztepe K, Erdogan O: The effect of triple therapy on rapidly progressive type of Henoch-Schönlein nephritis. Pediatr Nephrol 1995; 9:6.

134. Faedda R, Pirisi M, Satta A, et al: Regression of Henoch-Schönlein disease with intensive immunosuppressive treatment. Clin Pharmacol Ther 1996; 60:576.

135. Calabrese LH, Michel BA, Bloch DA, et al: The American College of Rheumatology 1990 criteria for the classification of hypersensitivity vasculitis. Arthritis Rheum 1990; 33:1108.

136. Ekenstam E, Callen JP: Cutaneous leukocytoclastic vasculitis: Clinical and laboratory features of 82 patients seen in private practice. Arch Dermatol 1984; 120:484.

137. Cupps TR, Fauci AS: The Vasculitides. Philadelphia: WB Saunders, 1981:50.

138. Callen JP: Colchicine is effective in controlling chronic cutaneous leukocytoclastic vasculitis. J Am Acad Dermatol 1985; 13:193.

139. Sais G, Vidaller A, Jucgla A, et al: Colchicine in the treatment of cutaneous leukocytoclastic vasculitis. Results of a prospective, randomized controlled trial. Arch Dermatol 1995; 131:1399.

140. Martinez-Taboada VM, Blanco R, Garcia-Fuentes M, et al: Clinical features and outcome of 95 patients with hypersensitivity vasculitis. Am J Med 1997; 102:186.

141. Haynes BF, Kaiser-Kupfer MI, Mason P, et al: Cogan's syndrome: Studies in thirteen patients, long-term follow-up, and a review of the literature. Medicine 1980; 59:426.

142. St. Clair EW, McCallum RM: Cogan's syndrome. Curr Opin Rheumatol 1999; 11:47.

143. McCallum RM, Haynes BF: Cogan's syndrome. *In* Pepose JS, Holland GN, Wilhelmus KR (eds): Ocular Infection and Immunity. St. Louis: Mosby–Year Book, 1996:446.

144. Vollersten RS, McDonald TJ, Younge BR, et al: Cogan's syndrome: 18 Cases and a review of the literature. Mayo Clin Proc 1986; 61:344.

145. McCallum RM: Cogan's syndrome. *In* Franunfelder FT, Roy EH, Grove J (eds): Current Ocular Therapy, 4th ed. Philadelphia: WB Saunders, 1995:410.

146. Allen NB, Cox CC, Cobo M, et al: Use of immunosuppressive agents in the treatment of severe ocular and vascular manifestations of Cogan's syndrome. Am J Med 1990; 88:296.

147. McCallum RM: Cogan's syndrome: Clinical features and outcomes. Arthritis Rheum 1992; 35(suppl):S51.

148. Bielory L, Conti J, Frohman L: Cogan's syndrome. J Allergy Clin Immunol 1990; 85:808.

149. LaRaja RD: Cogan syndrome associated with mesenteric vascular insufficiency. Arch Surg 1976; 111:1028.

150. Darougar S, John AC, Viswalingam M, et al: Isolation of *Chlamydia psittaci* from a patient with interstitial keratitis and uveitis associated with otological and cardiovascular lesions. Br J Ophthalmol 1978; 62:709.

# 28 | Vasculitis of the Central Nervous System

*Leonard H. Calabrese and George F. Duna*

Vasculitis of the central nervous system (CNS) may be classified as primary or secondary.[1, 2] Vasculitis affecting the CNS that is not associated with systemic disease or vasculitis outside of the CNS is referred to as *primary angiitis of the central nervous system* (PACNS). This disorder was once considered quite rare and inexorably fatal, but in recent years has become more frequently diagnosed and understood to be more clinically heterogeneous. *Secondary vasculitis of the CNS* is found in association with a wide variety of conditions including systemic vasculitides and connective tissue diseases, infections, other inflammatory disorders, and malignancies. In both types of disorders there are limited data on pathophysiologic mechanisms and treatment.

Hampering the clinical approach to these disorders are several factors. First, the diagnosis of CNS vasculitis is often problematic, there currently being no noninvasive test of sufficient predictive value to secure the diagnosis. Second, these diseases, particularly PACNS, are clinically rare, so that no single clinician or center has extensive experience in evaluating or treating such patients. As a result, virtually all therapeutic decisions in the diagnosis or treatment of these disorders are made on the basis of consensus derived from expert opinions and a limited medical literature absent controlled clinical trials. This review attempts to summarize a rational therapeutic approach based on the best available evidence supplemented by the authors' clinical experience.

## PRIMARY ANGIITIS OF THE CENTRAL NERVOUS SYSTEM

### Historical Perspective and Definition

The modern era of CNS vasculitis investigation began in the 1950s with a small but elegantly described series of patients with a chronic progressive and fatal form of CNS vasculitis limited to the brain and its meninges with granulomatous pathology.[3] The disease was considered genuinely rare until the 1970s, when the increasing utility of cerebral angiography led to an increased frequency of this diagnosis. As of 1988, only 46 cases had been described in the world literature.[4] At that time, Calabrese and Mallek proposed three criteria for a diagnosis of PACNS[4]:

1. A history or clinical finding of an acquired neurologic deficit that remained unexplained after a thorough initial basic evaluation.
2. Either classical (high-probability) angiographic evidence or histopathologic demonstration of angiitis within the CNS.
3. No evidence of systemic vasculitis or any other condition to which the angiographic or pathologic features could be secondary (Table 28–1).

At the time these criteria were proposed, there was little evidence to suggest that PACNS was anything other than a homogeneous, highly progressive and fatal illness. Based on a preliminary report of successful therapy with a combination of glucocorticoids and cyclophosphamide by Cupps and associates in 1981,[5] it became standard practice for patients diagnosed either by biopsy or solely on angiographic grounds to be treated with such therapy for prolonged periods.[6, 7] However, it has become increasingly clear that within the spectrum of PACNS there is considerable clinical heterogeneity. In support of this concept was first the identification of cases with benign outcome and later the establishment of criteria to identify such.[8–10] Furthermore, although neurodiagnostic techniques have become progressively more sensitive at defining CNS ischemia, there are no reliable tests that differentiate inflammatory from noninflammatory vascular disease, hence compromising the specificity of angiography as well as other imaging studies.[10, 11] Therefore, the starting point of all therapeutic recommendations regarding PACNS lies with a methodical attempt to identify groups with relatively benign outcomes who do not require high-intensity immunosuppressive therapy or, at times, any immunosuppressive therapy at all.

### Clinical Subsets

It is clinically useful to categorize PACNS as being either pathologically or angiographically documented (i.e., in the absence of histologic confirmation). Patients in the former category may be further classified as

**TABLE 28–1**
**Conditions Resembling PACNS Excluded by the Preliminary Diagnostic Criteria**

Systemic vasculitis
  Polyarteritis nodosa
  Allergic granulomatosis
  Hypersensitivity vasculitis group disorders
  Vasculitis with connective tissue disease
  Wegener's granulomatosis
  Temporal arteritis
  Takayasu's arteritis
  Behçet's disease
  Lymphomatoid granulomatosis
  Cogan's syndrome
Infection
  Viral, bacterial, fungal, rickettsial
Neoplasm
  Angioimmunoproliferative disorders
  Carcinomatous meningitis
  Infiltrating glioma
  Malignant angioendotheliomatosis
Drug use
  Amphetamines
  Ephedrine
  Phenylpropanolamine
  Cocaine
  Ergotamine
Vasospastic disorders
  Postpartum angiopathy
  Eclampsia
  Pheochromocytoma
  Subarachnoid hemorrhage
  Migraine and exertional headache
Other vasculopathies and mimicking conditions
  Fibromuscular dysplasia
  Moyamoya disease
  Thrombotic thrombocytopenic purpura
  Sickle cell anemia
  Neurofibromatosis
  Cerebrovascular atherosclerosis
  Demyelinating disease
  Sarcoidosis
  Emboli (i.e., subacute bacterial endocarditis, cardiac myxoma, paradoxical emboli)
  Acute posterior placoid pigment epitheliopathy and cerebral vasculitis
  Antiphospholipid syndrome and other hypercoagulable states
  Radicular vasculopathy
  Traumatic dissection

having either granulomatous or nongranulomatous pathology. We believe that within the pathologically defined subset is a single group deserving nosologic distinction. This entity is commonly referred to as *granulomatous angiitis of the CNS* (GACNS). This diagnosis should be restricted to those patients with pathologically documented angiitis, with granulomatous features, affecting the small and medium-sized arteries and, rarely, the veins of the brain and or meninges.[12] Clinical features of GACNS include a long prodrome of 6 months or longer and a clinically progressive course. A cerebrospinal fluid (CSF) analysis consistent with a chronic meningitis is characteristic of this syndrome. The remainder of pathologically documented cases, in which the underlying histology is nongranulomatous (estimated to be in excess of 50%), are even less well understood.[1] The literature on PACNS regarding

these pathologic issues and terms is confusing. The term GACNS has frequently been loosely applied to any case of PACNS regardless of whether there are compatible histologic and/or clinical findings. As a result, inferences drawn from case reports and series not scrutinized for such details may be misleading.

Today, most patients are diagnosed by angiography, often without even an attempt to confirm the diagnosis by biopsy. Reluctance to proceed to brain biopsy is often contributed to by overconcern for excessive morbidity of the procedure or lack of a cooperative neurosurgeon. In our experience, such a decision often leads to a dangerous degree of diagnostic uncertainty if the patient fails to improve with therapy. Another common scenario is for CNS vasculitis to be diagnosed unexpectedly on the basis of a high-probability angiogram obtained in a situation of low clinical probability for vasculitis. We believe strongly that in this group of patients the highest degree of clinical caution must be exerted. Studies by Duna and coworkers,[11] confirmed by others,[13] have demonstrated the lack of specificity of angiography in the diagnosis of CNS angiitis. Even a high-probability angiogram (defined as alternating areas of stenosis and ectasia in multiple vessels in more than a single vascular bed) can be mimicked by atherosclerotic, neoplastic, or reversible vasoconstrictive disorders.[14, 15] Furthermore, the vascular changes induced by infection cannot be differentiated from those found in PACNS, and thus the clinical correlation is vital. In summary, the angiogram can readily detect intraluminal vascular irregularities in medium- and large-caliber vessels, but by itself is not capable of securing a diagnosis of PACNS.

Among the subsets of PACNS defined partially by angiography is that of *benign angiopathy of the central nervous system* (BACNS). This term was proposed to define a subset of patients with PACNS characterized by a predominance in young women who clinically present with an acute neurologic event such as severe headache and/or focal neurologic deficit. Diagnostic testing in such patients often reveals a normal or near-normal CSF and a high-probability angiogram.[9] The course of BACNS is generally monophasic and often resolves with rather minimal therapy in comparison to GACNS. The pathophysiology of BACNS is unknown, but it is believed by some[1] to be caused by reversible vasoconstriction rather than true angiitis. Because histologic confirmation is usually lacking and the majority of biopsies reported in this setting have been normal, this latter point remains speculative.

The nosologic distinction of BACNS has been justifiably questioned by some based on clinical and epidemiologic grounds.[16] The rationale for proposing BACNS as a distinct subset of PACNS was an attempt to define a patient population who have a better prognosis and require far less, and possibly fundamentally different, therapy from those with GACNS.[9] We agree that the term "benign" is probably unfortunate and does not reflect the fact that some patients present with fulminate disease resulting in significant neurologic deficits or even death. Another point of practical importance regarding this syndrome is that merely diagnosing BACNS by angiography alone should not imply benignity, because 40% to 50% of patients with GACNS display similar angiographic findings.[10] A reported series of patients with angiographically defined BACNS who presented to a stroke service documented a high incidence of morbidity and clinical courses that were often progressive as opposed to monophasic.[16] Such reports underscore the importance of the combined clinical and angiographic criteria suggested for diagnosis.[16] Clearly, prospective studies designed to test the operating definitions of BACNS and GACNS are needed.

Aside from the subsets of GACNS and BACNS, the remainder of PACNS cases are less clearly defined. Approximately 15% of all patients present with mass lesions (usually single, occasionally multiple), which should always be considered neoplastic or infective in origin until proven otherwise.[1] The natural history of such lesions, even when proven to be vasculitic on biopsy, is highly variable. Reports of cure by resection have been described,[17] whereas other patients have required combination immunosuppressive therapy. PACNS can also manifest with spinal cord involvement; the majority of these cases probably represent GACNS.[17] Cases of histologically proven PACNS with nongranulomatous pathology are of great interest but are poorly understood at present.

The clinical diagnosis of PACNS is complex and requires a team approach. This team must recognize that no single specialist can be expert in every condition (e.g., autoimmune, inflammatory, infective, neoplastic, thrombo-occlusive) within the differential diagnosis of PACNS. Another point of practical importance is that the majority of patients in whom PACNS is even highly suspected ultimately are found to have another condition.[18] The team should include an expert in autoimmune diseases associated with CNS vasculitis and in the use of immunosuppressive drugs, a neurologist expert in the noninflammatory diseases capable of mimicking CNS angiitis, a capable neurosurgeon willing to tailor the appropriate biopsy, and a knowledgeable neuroradiologist and neuropathologist.

## Rational Therapeutic Approach

The initial evaluation of possible CNS vasculitis should determine whether the patient definitely had the GACNS or BACNS variant of PACNS (Fig. 28–1). For the patient presenting with a chronic progressive CNS disorder associated with a chronic meningitis CSF formula, a detailed evaluation for systemic infections and malignancies is the foremost priority (Table 28–2). The details of this differential diagnosis and its evaluation are beyond the scope of this chapter, but the subject has been well reviewed in recent years.[19] For patients in whom a distinct cause of chronic meningitis is not found, a biopsy of CNS tissues, including leptomeninges and underlying cortex, is often required. Rarely is angiographic investigation of such patients of diagnostic value. The methodologic issues surrounding biopsy have been reviewed elsewhere,[20] and the yield has been demonstrated to be increased when there is meningeal

enhancement detected by magnetic resonance imaging (MRI).[21] We believe that virtually all patients with suspected or presumed GACNS should undergo CNS biopsy before the initiation of intense and prolonged immunosuppressive therapy. The rationale for this recommendation is based as much on diagnosing mimicking conditions of PACNS as on confirming the underlying diagnosis of PACNS. All such patients should be screened for human immunodeficiency virus (HIV) infection by serum antibody testing. We also recommend that all patients with suspected PACNS undergo screening by polymerase chain reaction for varicella-zoster virus (VZV) infection in the CSF.

For the patient presenting with an acute focal event or severe and unexplained headache, a somewhat different differential diagnosis should be entertained Table 28–3. In most of these patients the CSF analysis is either normal or near-normal; in addition, the MRI would not be expected to display evidence of meningeal inflammation and may be entirely normal. In the absence of meningeal changes on MRI or CSF abnormalities, the yield of a CNS biopsy would be expected to be exceedingly low.[20, 21] If CNS angiitis is still suspected after a detailed search for emboli and hypercoagulability, angiography may be of value even in the presence of a normal MRI. As mentioned previously, even a high-probability angiogram is incapable in itself of securing a definite diagnosis of PACNS, and it clearly is unable to differentiate inflammatory from noninflammatory disease.[14, 15]

In our experience, only 50% to 60% of patients ultimately found to have PACNS can readily be classified as having the GACNS or BACNS variant; thus there is a sizable portion of patients with less well-defined disease. Common examples of such ill-defined presentations are mass lesions, high-probability angiogram but clinically not either BACNS or GACNS, nongranulomatous pathology, spinal cord involvement, and cerebral hemorrhage. In patients with these presentations, a more global evaluation is in order, one that encompasses all of the disorders found in Table 28–1. Further work is clearly needed to better define this patient population.

## Specific Therapy

There are no controlled trials of any therapeutic agents in PACNS; therefore, all recommendations are made on the basis of uncontrolled observations and the authors' experience. The report of successful therapy of PACNS by Cupps and colleagues[5] in the early 1980s suggested that all patients with PACNS should be treated with combined glucocorticoids and cyclophosphamide. Others, including our own group,[4] were initially impressed by outcome analysis of historical cases documenting a frequently fatal course if the disease is left untreated, a partial response to glucocorticoids alone, and a good response to combination therapy. However, these early investigations were heavily influenced by historical bias and did not recognize the heterogeneity within the PACNS spectrum.

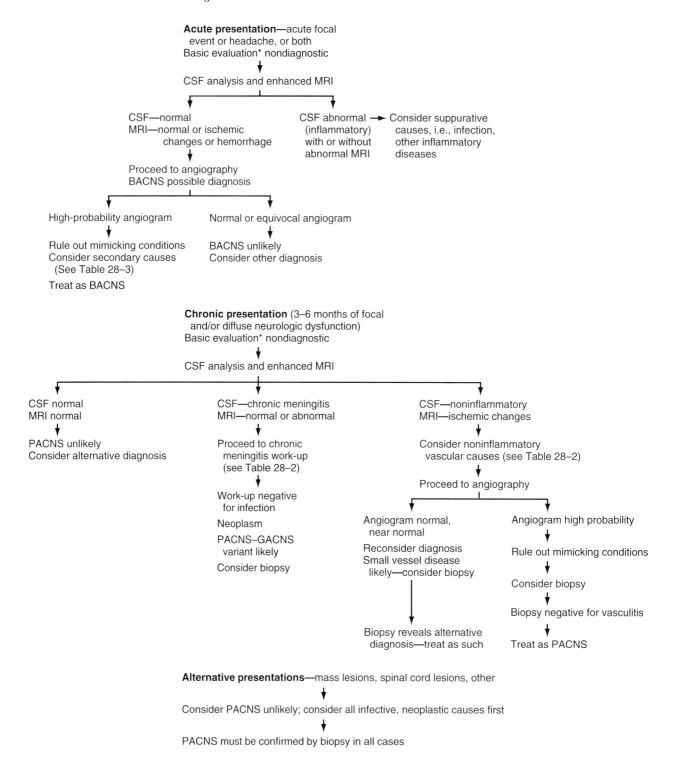

*Basic evaluation: complete history and physical examination, chest radiography, screening chemistry panels of hepatic and renal function. Acute-phase reactants, appropriate cultures, and other tests as indicated by initial evaluation.

**FIGURE 28–1**

Clinical approach to primary angiitis of the central nervous system. Basic evaluation consists of complete history and physical examination; chest radiography; screening chemistry panels of hepatic and renal function; and acute phase reactants, appropriate cultures, and other tests as indicated by initial evaluation. BACNS = benign angiopathy of the central nervous system; CSF = cerebrospinal fluid; GACNS = granulomatous angiitis of the central nervous system; MRI = magnetic resonance imaging.

**TABLE 28–2**

## Differential Diagnosis* and Suggested Basic Evaluation of Patients with Chronic Meningitis Presentations

Infectious diseases
  Mycobacterial infections
  Fungal infections
  Spirochete infections including *Borrelia burgdorferi* and syphilis
  Viral infections including human immunodeficiency virus, herpes simplex, and varicella-zoster
    virus
Neoplasms
  Primary and metastatic hematologic and solid tumors
  Primary brain tumors involving the meninges
Inflammatory diseases
  Primary angiitis of the central nervous system (PACNS)
  Behçet's disease†
  Sarcoidosis
  Parameningeal focus of infection or tumor†
  Systemic lupus erythematosus†
  Mollaret's meningitis†
  Uveomeningoencephalitis
Basic investigations
  Complete history and physical examination
  Complete blood count, acute phase reactants, liver and renal function assessment, purified
    protein derivative tuberculin and anergy battery, chest radiography, blood and urine culture
    for mycobacterial and fungal pathogens, serology for human immunodeficiency virus, Lyme
    disease, syphilis, hepatitis C, cryptococcal antigen, antinuclear antigens
  Cerebrospinal fluid analysis and culture and stain for mycobacteria, fungi, syphilis (Venereal
    Disease Research Laboratory), cryptococcal antigen, cytology; preserve extra fluid for special
    studies including polymerase chain reaction for mycobacteria, varicella-zoster virus, others
    when indicated

* Major categories and diagnoses.
† May present as recurrent meningitis.
From Gripshover BM, Ellner JJ: Chronic meningitis. *In* Mandell GL, Bennett JE, Dolin R (eds): Principles and Practice of Infectious Diseases, 4th ed. Philadelphia: Churchill Livingstone, 1995:865.

**TABLE 28–3**

## Differential Diagnosis and Standard Diagnostic Tests for Patients with Acute Focal Neurologic Presentations Suggesting the Clinical Picture of BACNS

Clinical variants of BACNS or reversible vasoconstrictive disease
  Postpartum angiopathy
  Drug induced (sympathomimetics)
  Pheochromocytoma
  Post–carotid embolectomy
  Complex exertional and/or migraine headache
  Idiopathic BACNS
Angiographic mimics of PACNS that may manifest with acute focal presentations
  Atherosclerosis
  Emboli
  Anticardiolipin antibody syndrome or other hypercoagulable states
  Fibromuscular disease with secondary dissection and emboli
  Moyamoya disease
Recommended basic work-up
  History and physical examination including detailed drug history, toxic screening panel, chest
    radiography, electrocardiography, and basic renal and hepatic function tests
  Hypercoagulability screening panels including anticardiolipin antibodies
  Transesophageal echocardiography
  Blood cultures

BACNS = benign angiitis of the central nervous system; PACNS = primary angiitis of the central nervous system.

We currently recommend that, for patients presumed to have the GACNS variant of PACNS, aggressive therapy is warranted from the outset. We favor high-dose glucocorticoid therapy with prednisone at a dose of 1 mg/kg/day and oral cyclophosphamide at a dose of approximately 2 mg/kg/day. The usual precautions of administering these drugs clearly apply in terms of adequate hydration to minimize the risks of toxic effects on the bladder, osteoporosis prophylaxis and treatment, and appropriate monitoring.[22] All such patients should be given prophylactic drugs for *Pneumocystis carinii* pneumonia. The treatment is tapered in a similar fashion to its use in patients with Wegener's granulomatosis; it is continued for approximately 1 year after the disease is controlled, after which it is tapered and discontinued. Because late relapses have been observed, careful follow-up is necessary.

The follow-up of such patients is complicated. Fixed neurologic deficits present at the outset of therapy are unlikely to completely or even partially resolve. Headache alone is also problematic, because many patients, in our experience, develop chronic vascular-type headaches after successful treatment of PACNS that may persist indefinitely. Serial MRI investigations at 3- to 6-month intervals are usually needed even while the patient is clinically stable, in an effort to detect new areas of ischemia and/or infarction. If the CSF is abnormal at the outset, it should be re-examined in 8 to 12 weeks to ensure its improvement. These studies may need to be repeated if a question of disease reactivation arises during or after treatment.

For patients with classic BACNS, there are fewer firm therapeutic recommendations. It is our practice to use a brief course of high-dose prednisone (i.e., prednisone, 1 mg/kg/day orally) for a period of 3 to 6 weeks, depending on the severity of the presentation.[1, 2] The rationale for such therapy is the efficacy of glucocorticoids in experimental forms of cerebral vasospasm[23] and their common use in refractory headaches of presumed vascular origin. In addition, we employ calcium channel blockers in maximally tolerated doses and maintain them indefinitely. Whether any specific agent in this class of drugs is therapeutically superior is unknown, but we commonly use verapamil in a dose of 240 mg/day as a starting point and reserve agents such as nimodipine for patients failing to respond adequately. All such patients need to be counseled on avoiding sympathomimetic drugs in any form.[24, 25] We believe that nicotine should be avoided as well. A follow-up angiogram performed approximately 12 weeks into such therapy demonstrating complete or near-complete resolution serves to secure the diagnosis. Failure to clear or angiographic progression should prompt a complete re-evaluation of this diagnosis.

For the considerable number of patients who present with variants of PACNS, as noted previously, therapy is applied individually based on the clinical picture. For patients with fulminate or progressive disease, regardless of the pathology or other clinical features, we usually advocate combined therapy as described for GACNS. For patients with a more indolent presentation and course, glucocorticoids alone may suffice. In patients with solitary mass lesions, cure by resection has been reported, though it is difficult to make definitive recommendations in this setting. All patients require careful serial monitoring, which relies heavily on baseline abnormalities in the CSF or MRI as barometers.

Finally, the complex issue of the relationship of varicella-zoster virus (VZV) to GACNS needs to be mentioned. A small percentage of patients develop a syndrome of contralateral hemiplegia 1 week to several months after VZV infection of cranial nerve V or the syndrome of herpes zoster ophthalmicus (HZO).[26, 27] The disease has been demonstrated to be the result of a vasculitis of the ipsilateral carotid artery and middle cerebral artery branches.[28] Viral particles have been demonstrated in vascular tissues and are presumed to have spread from the trigeminal ganglion to adjacent tissues.[29, 30] In the setting of altered host defenses, vasculitis after HZO or VZV in more distant tissues may be clinically and histologically indistinguishable from GACNS.[31] Using molecular techniques, Gilden and colleagues[32] have demonstrated VZV particles, but not herpes simplex or cytomegalovirus, in segments of vascular tissues of a man dying from GACNS without a preceding zosteriform rash. Based on these data, we advocate the routine search for such pathogens in all of these patients. We also believe that these data[32–35] raise the question of empiric therapy and prophylaxis for herpes virus infections, especially VZV, in any patient with PACNS and a history of recent or remote VZV infection. This may be of particular importance in those patients with evidence of underlying alterations of host defenses.

## TREATMENT OF SECONDARY SYSTEMIC VASCULITIS

Cerebral vasculitis may be associated with a variety of conditions including infections, drugs, lymphoproliferative diseases, systemic vasculitides, and connective tissue diseases[1] (see Table 28–2). Although the evidence for a direct cause-and-effect mechanism is generally lacking, removal of the exogenous inciting agent or control of the associated systemic disease may result in amelioration of the *secondary* CNS vasculitis. Therefore, a diligent search for associated conditions is essential in the approach to the patient with suspected cerebral arteritis.

### Infections

In the evaluation of CNS vasculitis, the importance of searching for infection through microbiologic analysis of CSF and biopsy material cannot be overemphasized, because the clinical and angiographic presentations of infection-related cerebral arteritis mimic those of PACNS.[1, 36] Furthermore, the underlying infection may be occult when the neurovascular complication occurs. Suspicion of specific pathogens should be guided by epidemiologic features and individual risk factors. The possibility of infection with HIV-1, VZV, or syphilis should be actively ascertained (see Table 28–2). Whether hepatitis C virus can cause CNS vasculitis remains unclear.

The clinical outcome is variable even when appropriate antimicrobial drugs are given. This reflects the diverse pathophysiologic mechanisms of infection-associated CNS vasculitis, which may include a direct cytopathic effect of an angioinvasive pathogen, injury to endothelial cells via induction of neoantigen formation, or immune complex–mediated damage.[37] Adjunctive anti-inflammatory or immunosuppressive therapy may be beneficial for patients who do not respond to antimicrobial therapy, although such an approach remains to be tested.

## Drugs

A variety of drugs, particularly those with sympathomimetic properties, have been associated with a myriad of neurologic complications including cerebral infarcts, intracerebral bleeding, and subarachnoid hemorrhage. The most commonly implicated drugs are oral and intravenous amphetamines, cocaine, heroin, ephedrine, and phenylpropanolamine (see Table 28–2). Most reported cases of "drug-induced" CNS vasculitis have been diagnosed on the basis of cerebral angiography alone, in the absence of pathologic confirmation.[1, 25] Because the implicated drugs are capable of inducing vasospasm, some of the cases may have represented CNS angiopathy rather than true angiitis. Ascertaining the relationship between a particular drug exposure and CNS vasculitis is further complicated by numerous other pitfalls[25] (see Table 28–3). Nonetheless, pathologically documented cases of drug-associated CNS vasculitis do exist, with findings ranging from perivascular cuffing to frank vasculitis with or without necrosis.[25, 38–40]

Recognition and withdrawal of the offending drug is obviously the cornerstone of treatment. For drugs of abuse, the risk profile dictates the need to ascertain associated infections. When present, hypertension should be controlled effectively. For most angiographically defined cases, we recommend the use of calcium channel blockers and a limited course of corticosteroids. The use of long-term steroid therapy or the addition of cytotoxic drugs, or both, should be reserved for pathologically documented cases of CNS arteritis.

## Lymphoproliferative Diseases

Vasculitis of the CNS has been reported in association with Hodgkin's lymphoma, non-Hodgkin's lymphoma, and angioimmunolymphoproliferative lesions (AIL).[1] The anatomic location of the lymphoproliferative disease may be either outside or within the CNS. Although the clinical presentation is generally similar to that of PACNS, the presence of mass lesions, spinal cord involvement, and CNS hemorrhage should raise the index of suspicion for an underlying lymphoproliferative disease.[1, 17] A biopsy of the CNS lesions or masses may reveal only the angiitis without evidence of the malignancy itself.[2] On the other hand, a lymphocytic angiitis may itself be the malignant lesion of AIL, a diagnosis then established by detailed immunohistochemistry, T-cell receptor analysis, and B-cell immunoglobulin studies. Finally, one should also search for concomitant infections, particularly with VZV.

Treatment directed at the underlying lymphoproliferative disease usually consists of combination chemotherapy or irradiation, or both. Favorable neurologic outcomes have been reported.[41–42]

## Systemic Vasculitides

Vasculitis of the CNS may occur with any of the systemic vasculitides, but is most commonly reported in polyarteritis nodosa, microscopic polyangiitis, Behçet's disease, Wegener's granulomatosis, and Churg-Strauss syndrome.[1, 43–45] The true prevalence of CNS arteritis is difficult to estimate, because the diagnosis is most often presumed on clinical grounds when neurologic events occur in the setting of systemic disease (i.e., angiographic and/or pathologic evidence of CNS vasculitis is rarely sought). Alternative explanations for CNS dysfunction should be considered in patients with systemic vasculitis, including infections (CNS and systemic), toxic effects of the drug (e.g., steroid-induced CNS effects, cyclophosphamide-induced hyponatremia), extracranial end-organ damage (e.g., hypoxic or uremic encephalopathy), and accelerated hypertension.[1]

Treatment is directed at the underlying systemic vasculitis and usually consists of high-dose corticosteroids. The use of cytotoxic drugs, particularly cyclophosphamide, appears necessary in microscopic polyangiitis and Wegener's granulomatosis as well as other systemic vasculitides that threaten life or permanent CNS damage.

## Connective Tissue Diseases

CNS involvement is not uncommon in connective tissue diseases, mainly systemic lupus erythematosus (SLE) and Sjögren's syndrome. In SLE, brain pathology most often represents a vasculopathy, with small-vessel hyalinization, thickening, intramural platelet deposition, and thrombus formation.[46] Frank CNS vasculitis occurs in fewer than 7% of cases.[47] When SLE patients present with CNS symptoms and signs, it is important to consider mechanisms other than CNS vasculitis. Such mechanisms include antiphospholipid antibody–associated thrombosis, cardiac emboli, thrombotic thrombocytopenic purpura, CNS hemorrhage related to immune thrombocytopenia or acquired coagulation factor deficiency, CNS infection, and side effects of medications. Treatment of CNS vasculitis in SLE generally consists of high-dose intravenous corticosteroids as well as cyclophosphamide in patients who are critically ill or progressively deteriorating. The use of intravenous immunoglobulins remains anecdotal, but they may be considered as adjunctive therapy.

In Sjögren's syndrome, CNS manifestations may be caused by a mononuclear inflammatory vasculopathy involving the small vessels of the cortex and meninges.[48] Angiographic abnormalities consistent with vasculitis are uncommonly seen. Treatment issues remain unresolved.

# REFERENCES

1. Calabrese LH, Duna GF, Lie JT: Vasculitis in the central nervous system. Arthritis Rheum 1997; 40:1189.
2. Calabrese LH: Vasculitis of the central nervous system. Rheum Dis Clin North Am 1995; 21:1059.
3. Cravioto M, Feigin I: Noninfectious granulomatous angiitis with a predilection for the nervous system. Neurology 1959; 9:599.
4. Calabrese LH, Mallek JA: Primary angiitis of the central nervous system: Report of eight new cases, review of the literature and proposal for diagnostic criteria. Medicine (Baltimore) 1988; 67:20.
5. Cupps TR, Moore PM, Fauci AS: Isolated angiitis of the central nervous system. Am J Med 1983; 74:97.
6. Moore PM: Vasculitis of the central nervous system. Semin Neurol 1994; 14:307.
7. Younger DS, Hays AP, Burst JCM, et al: Granulomatous angiitis of brain: An inflammatory reaction of diverse etiology. Arch Neurol 1988; 45:514.
8. Hankey GJ: Isolated angiitis/angiopathy of the central nervous system. Cerebrovasc Dis 1991; 1:2.
9. Calabrese L, Gragg LA, Furlan AJ: Benign angiopathy: A distinct subset of angiographically defined primary angiitis of the central nervous system. J Rheumatol 1993; 20:2046.
10. Calabrese LH, Furlan AJ, Gragg LA, et al: Primary angiitis of the central nervous system: Diagnostic criteria and clinical approach. Cleveland Clin J Med 1992; 59:293.
11. Duna G, Calabrese L: Limitations in the diagnostic modalities in the diagnosis of primary angiitis of the central nervous system (PACNS). J Rheumatol 1995; 22:662.
12. Younger DS, Calabrese LH, Hays AP: Granulomatous angiitis of the nervous system. Neurol Clin 1997; 15:821.
13. Chu C, Gray L, Goldstein LB, et al: Diagnosis of intracranial vasculitis: A multidisciplinary approach. J Neuropathol Exp Neurol 1998; 57:30.
14. Hurst RW, Grossman RI: Neuroradiology of central nervous system vasculitis. Semin Neurol 1994; 14:320.
15. Berlit P: The spectrum of vasculopathies in the differential diagnosis of vasculitis. Semin Neurol 1994; 14:370.
16. Woolfenden AR, Tang DC, Marks MP, et al: Angiographically defined primary angiitis of the CNS: Is it really benign? Neurology 1998; 51:183.
17. Duna GF, George T, Rybicki L, et al: Primary angiitis of the central nervous system: An analysis of unusual presentations [Abstract]. Arthritis Rheum 1995; 38(suppl 9):S340.
18. Villa Forte A, Vassilopoulos D, Calabrese LH: What is not primary angiitis of the CNS (PACNS) [Abstract]? Arthritis Rheum 1998; 41:S124.
19. Gripshover BM, Ellner JJ: Chronic meningitis. *In* Mandell GL, Bennett JE, Dolin R (eds): Principles and Practice of Infectious Diseases, 4th ed. Philadelphia: Churchill Livingstone, 1995;865.
20. Parisi JE, Moore PM: The role of biopsy in vasculitis of the central nervous system. Semin Neurol 1994; 14:341.
21. Cheng TM, O'Neill BP, Schechthauer BW, et al: Chronic meningitis: The role of meningeal or cortical biopsy. Neurosurgery 1994; 34:S90.
22. Calabrese LH: Therapy of systemic vasculitis. Neurol Clin 1997; 15:973.
23. Chyatte O, Sundt TM: Response of chronic experimental vasospasm to methylprednisolone and dexamethasone. J Neurosurg 1984; 60:923.
24. Lake CR, Gallant H, Masson E, et al: Adverse drug effects attributed to phenylpropanolamine: A review of 142 cases. Am J Med 1990; 89:195.
25. Calabrese LH, Duna GT: Drug induced vasculitis. Curr Opin Rheumatol 1996; 8:34.
26. Sigal LH: The neurologic presentation of vasculitis and rheumatologic syndromes: A review. Medicine (Baltimore) 1987; 66:157.
27. Martin JR, Mitchell WJ, Henken DB: Neurotropic herpes viruses, neural mechanisms and arteritis. Brain Pathol 1990; 1:6.
28. MacKenzie RA, Forbes GS, Karnes WE: Angiographic findings in herpes zoster arteritis. Ann Neurol 1981; 10:458.
29. Doyle PW, Gibson G, Dolman CL: Herpes zoster ophthalmicus with contralateral hemiplegia: Identification of cause. Ann Neurol 1983; 14:85.
30. Linneman C, Alvira M: Pathogenesis of varicella-zoster angiitis of the CNS. Arch Neurol 1980; 37:239.
31. Lie JT: Primary (granulomatous) angiitis of the central nervous system: A clinical pathologic analysis of 15 new cases and a review of the literature. Hum Pathol 1992; 23:164.
32. Gilden DH, Kleinschmidt-DeMasters BK, Wellish M, et al: Varicella zoster virus, a cause of waxing and waning vasculitis. Neurology 1996; 47:1441.
33. Younger DS, Hays AP, Brust JCM, et al: Granulomatous angiitis of the brain: An inflammatory reaction of diverse etiology. Arch Neurol 1988; 45:514.
34. Rosenblum WI, Hadfield MG, Young HF: Granulomatous angiitis with preceding varicella-zoster. Ann Neurol 1978; 3:374.
35. DeReuck J, Crevitus L, Sieben G, et al: Granulomatous angiitis of the nervous systems: A CPC of one case. J Neurol 1982; 277:49.
36. Grang DW: Central nervous system vasculitis secondary to infections, toxins and neoplasms. Semin Neurol 1994; 14:313.
37. Jenette JP, Falk RJ, Milling DM: Pathogenesis of vasculitis. Semin Neurol 1994; 14:291.
39. Citron BP, Halpern M, McCarron M, et al: Necrotizing angiitis associated with drug abuse. N Engl J Med 1970; 283:1003.
40. Fredericks RK, Lefkowitz DS, Challa CR, et al: Cerebral vasculitis associated with cocaine abuse. Stroke 1991; 22:1437.
41. Morrow PL, McQuillen JB: Cerebral vasculitis associated with cocaine abuse. J Forensic Sci 1993; 38:732.
42. Kleinschmidt-DeMasters GK, Filley CM, Bitter MA: Central nervous system angiocentric, angiodestructive T-cell lymphoma. Surg Neurol 1992; 37:130.
43. Greco FA, Kolins J, Rajjoub RK, et al: Hodgkin's disease and granulomatous angiitis of the central nervous system. Cancer 1976; 38:2027.
44. Moore P, Calabrese LH: Neurologic manifestations of systemic vasculitides. Semin Neurol 1994; 14:300.
45. Nishino H, Rubino FA, DeRemee RA, et al: Neurological involvement in Wegener's granulomatosis: An analysis of 324 consecutive patients at the Mayo Clinic. Ann Neurol 1993; 33:4.
46. Tervaert JWC, Kallenberg C: Neurologic manifestations of systemic vasculitides. Rheum Dis Clin North Am 1993; 19:913.
47. Ellis SG, Verity MA: Central nervous system involvement in systemic lupus erythematosus: A review of neuropathologic findings in 57 cases. Semin Arthritis Rheum 1979; 8:212.
48. Alexander EL: Neurologic disease in Sjögren's syndrome: Mononuclear inflammatory vasculopathy affecting the central/peripheral nervous system and muscles: A clinical review and update of immunopathogenesis. Rheum Dis Clin North Am 1993; 19:869.

# 29 | Takayasu's Arteritis, Giant Cell Arteritis, and Polymyalgia Rheumatica*

*Carol A. Langford*

Giant cell arteritis and Takayasu's arteritis are primary systemic vasculitides that have a similar histologic appearance but vary with regard to patterns of vascular distribution and affected population. Polymyalgia rheumatica, in contrast, is not a vasculitis, but it has prominent associations with giant cell arteritis that are relevant to the discussion of its treatment.

One issue that is common to all three diseases is that the assessment of optimal therapy has been complicated by difficulties in the currently existing literature. Because these illnesses are uncommon, most therapeutic studies to date have been retrospective series in which patients did not receive a standardized treatment regimen. Another significant factor has been that for all these illnesses, there exists no reliable means of assessing disease activity and thus defining outcome. This limitation affects not only the interpretation and planning of studies but also treatment of the individual patient.

This chapter focuses on factors critical to therapeutic management, including natural history, assessment of disease activity, the data for different treatment regimens, and strategies to monitor for and prevent drug toxicity (for a more general discussion of these diseases, see Kelley et al, Chapters 68 and 69[1, 2]).

## TAKAYASU'S ARTERITIS

### Natural History

Takayasu's arteritis (TKA) is an idiopathic vasculitis that affects the aorta, its main branches, and the pulmonary arteries.[3–5] The blood vessel changes that occur in these sites are typically those of inflammation, followed by stenosis or occlusion, although aortic aneurysms can also develop.[3, 6, 7] Although TKA is reported to affect young women of Asian origin, the disease is not exclusive for any age, race, or gender.

TKA has historically been viewed as a triphasic process characterized by an initial systemic phase, an active vessel inflammatory phase, and a final "burnt-out"

or pulseless phase. Increasing evidence has suggested that such a view is of limited use in management because it does not accurately depict the status of blood vessel inflammation and does not reflect the course that many patients experience. The systemic symptoms observed in TKA frequently include fatigue, malaise, weight loss, night sweats, fever, arthralgias, and myalgias.[3] However, some series have found systemic features to be absent in up to 80% of affected patients.[3, 6–9] Furthermore, TKA has been found to be a chronic and relapsing disease in many instances. In one study, regardless of treatment, 45% of patients were found to experience at least one disease relapse, and 23% of patients never achieved a remission.[3]

The long-term outcome in TKA has varied between studies. Although two North American reports found the overall survival rate to be 94% or greater,[3, 4] the 5-year mortality rate from other series has ranged from 0% to 35%.[10–13] The cause for this variability is probably multifactorial, reflecting differences in disease severity, rapidity of diagnosis, access to medical care, and potential impact of medical and surgical treatment. Disease-related mortality is usually caused by congestive heart failure, cerebrovascular events, myocardial infarction, aneurysm rupture, or renal failure.[6, 10–14] In a 1994 study, Ishikawa and Maetani found that statistically significant predictors of poor outcome included a progressive disease course and the presence of major complications defined as Takayasu's retinopathy, secondary hypertension, aortic valve insufficiency, and aneurysms.[10, 14] The overall 15-year survival rate was 83%, but when analyzed by predictors, the rate of 15-year survival was 100% among patients who had neither a major complication nor a progressive course, in comparison with 43% among those who had both.[10] Even in the absence of life-threatening disease, TKA can be associated with substantial morbidity. In one series, 74% of patients were found to have some compromise in activities of daily living, and 47% were permanently disabled.[3]

### Assessment of Disease Activity

The inability to accurately assess disease activity in TKA has been a critical limitation both in managing

---

* This chapter is in the public domain.

the individual patient and in evaluating the efficacy of therapeutic regimens. Although clinical features have typically been used to define disease activity, active arteritis has been observed in 44% of surgical bypass specimens taken from patients in whom disease was judged to be quiescent by current methods.[3] Some investigators have found the erythrocyte sedimentation rate (ESR) to be a useful marker by which to assess active inflammatory disease,[4, 10, 15, 16] whereas others have not found it to be uniformly reliable.[3, 6, 17] Kerr and colleagues found a normal ESR to be present in one third of patients who were thought to have clinically active disease, whereas elevated values were demonstrated in up to 56% of patients in remission.[3]

Interpretation of arteriography is complicated by the fact that progression of vascular disease may result from either acute vasculitis or noninflammatory fibrosis of healing lesions. In one study, although 88% of patients with active disease had new lesions on follow-up arteriography, 61% of patients in clinical remission also had progressive changes.[3] Thus, arteriography demonstrates luminal patency but does not necessarily provide information on the degree of inflammation present in the arterial wall. Repeat arteriographic studies should be obtained for new or progressive ischemic symptoms. In the absence of new symptoms, the necessity for obtaining arteriograms must be determined on an individual basis because these procedures are invasive and involve significant contrast and radiation exposure. Patients with lesions affecting cerebral blood flow may require closer monitoring because the availability of collateral circulation may be limited and resultant ischemia is potentially catastrophic. Some reports suggest that noninvasive techniques such as ultrasonography,[18] computed tomography, or magnetic resonance imaging[19, 20] may provide alternative means for serial evaluation. To date, however, none of these modalities have reproducibly provided information on whether vascular changes are related to active disease.[5, 19]

Because no single clinical feature has proved useful in identifying active disease, one method of assessment has been to combine information from multiple parameters (Table 29–1). Although such guidelines are useful, individual factors must also be considered when therapeutic decisions are made. These include the location and severity of lesions, the availability of collateral circulation, the nature and intensity of symptoms, past correlation of a patient's laboratory parameters and symptoms with disease activity, and the risks of medication toxicity.

## Treatment

### General Principles

At the time of diagnosis, approximately 20% of patients with TKA are clinically asymptomatic; the disease is detected from abnormal findings on physical examination, such as vascular bruits, asymmetric blood pressures, or absence of pulses.[3] Although these patients require regular follow-up and education regarding the illness, for the most part they do not require medical treatment.

The remaining 80% of patients have features of active disease that necessitate treatment. Immunosuppressive therapy is usually effective in treating the systemic symptoms of TKA. Although the natural history data suggest that interruption of active inflammation before the development of significant vessel stenosis will lessen the development of disease complications and improve prognosis, the role of immunosuppressive treatment in the preservation of organ function and improvement of survival has been difficult to assess.

Overall patient management must take into consideration the long-term risks and benefits of disease versus treatment and the potential for TKA to be a chronic and relapsing disease that has the capacity to remit spontaneously. Because TKA frequently affects a young female population, the potential for pregnancy and the impact of treatment on child bearing must also be remembered.

Treatment of TKA includes managing both the active inflammatory disease and the chronic fixed vascular lesions, for which nonmedical therapeutic modalities play an important role. Establishing a multidisciplinary team of physicians skilled in the administration of immunosuppressive regimens, cardiovascular surgeons, and imaging/interventional radiologists early in the course of patient care is helpful.

### Glucocorticoids

Glucocorticoids are considered the mainstay of treatment in TKA, although the data regarding their efficacy have varied widely; 25% to 100% of patients have experienced a prompt improvement in systemic symptoms.[3, 4, 15, 16, 21, 22] Objectively, selected reports have demonstrated an improvement in arteriographic blood flow[23, 24] and a return of previously absent pulses[4, 15, 16, 22] in glucocorticoid-treated patients.

The optimal dose and length of glucocorticoid treatment has not been specifically defined because there have been no comparative trials of dosage and duration. Retrospective series have investigated a broad spectrum of initial prednisone doses ranging from 20 to

## TABLE 29–1
## Criteria for Active Disease in Patients with Takayasu's Arteritis*

| CLINICAL CRITERIA | LIMITATION |
| --- | --- |
| Elevated erythrocyte sedimentation rate | Poor correlation in some series |
| Systemic symptoms | Absent in up to 80% |
| New or progressive features of vascular ischemia | May result from noninflammatory vessel stenosis related to healing |
| New or progressive arteriographic changes | May result from noninflammatory vessel stenosis related to healing |

*Active disease is said to be defined by the presence of two of the four criteria.

100 mg/day.[4, 13–15, 22, 23] The Systemic Vascular Disorders Research Committee of the Ministry of Health and Welfare of Japan recommended that patients with evidence of active arteritis be treated initially with prednisolone, 30 mg/day.[22] In a retrospective analysis of 150 patients who had received glucocorticoids at doses similar to those used in this regimen, 51% of patients experienced improvement in quality of life, whereas 37% experienced no change, and 12% experienced worsening, although the definitions of these outcome measures were not stated.[22]

The largest prospective standardized experience with glucocorticoids in TKA comes from the National Institutes of Health (NIH).[3] Of 48 patients judged to have active disease, 52% experienced remission after first-time therapy with glucocorticoids and 60% achieved remission at least once. The median time to remission was 22 months (confidence interval, 11 to 35 months). In the NIH study, patients initially received prednisone, 1 mg/kg/day (60 mg daily for most patients), for the first 1 to 3 months with careful observation for adverse effects and response.[3, 25] Over the next 2 to 3 months, when disease activity decreased, the prednisone dosage was tapered to an alternate-day schedule (60 mg alternating with 0 mg). Once alternate-day therapy was achieved, the glucocorticoid dosages were then slowly tapered toward discontinuation. The use of alternate-day therapy has the advantage of lessening glucocorticoid toxicity. Although these time estimates should be pursued, it is often necessary to temporarily halt or slow the prednisone tapering because signs of active disease develop.

Although the NIH series remains the only studied regimen from which prospective, standardized data have been obtained, a lower starting dose may be considered in selected individuals at high risk for steroid toxicity, if there is no threat of immediate tissue ischemia[3, 25] (Table 29–2).

## Cytotoxic Therapy

The addition of a cytotoxic agent to glucocorticoids is of less proven benefit in TKA than in other forms of systemic vasculitis. Cytotoxic therapy is considered primarily for patients who have persistent disease activity despite daily glucocorticoid treatment or when remission cannot be maintained on an alternate-day glucocorticoid regimen. Using these criteria, Kerr and colleagues observed that 52% of patients required the addition of a cytotoxic agent during the course of their disease; 40% of these patients achieved remission at least once.[3] In a similar treatment-resistant group, the Systemic Vascular Disorders Research Committee of the Ministry of Health and Welfare of Japan retrospectively found that among 28 patients treated with adjunctive azathioprine, cyclophosphamide, or mercaptopurine, results of treatment were judged to be excellent in none, good in 29%, fair in 33%, and ineffective in 29%.[22] In considering the choice of cytotoxic agent, the greatest experience has been with the use of methotrexate[26–28] and, to a lesser degree, cyclophosphamide.[25] Data regarding the efficacy of other cytotoxic agents in the treatment of TKA is confined solely to case reports.[22, 29]

Although cyclophosphamide was the first studied cytotoxic agent for TKA, the data regarding its use are limited. Shelhamer and coworkers treated seven patients with cyclophosphamide, all of whom had active arteritis despite 3 months of daily glucocorticoids.[25] In all seven patients, cyclophosphamide allowed the glucocorticoid dose to be decreased, and the progression of vascular lesions ceased in four patients, all of whom had experienced progression on prednisone alone. The regimen used in this study was similar to the NIH protocol used for Wegener's granulomatosis, whereby cyclophosphamide is initiated at a dose of 2 mg/kg/day and given for 1 year after the beginning of remission, after which time it is tapered and discontinued.[30]

The utility of methotrexate in TKA was prospectively evaluated at the NIH with a standardized protocol in a glucocorticoid-resistant population.[26] In this regimen, methotrexate was initiated orally at a dose of 0.3 mg/kg (not to exceed 15 mg) once a week and increased by 2.5 mg every 1 to 2 weeks, up to a maxi-

## TABLE 29–2
## Suggested Treatment Approaches

|  | TAKAYASU'S ARTERITIS | GIANT CELL ARTERITIS | POLYMYALGIA RHEUMATICA |
|---|---|---|---|
| Glucocorticoids (GC) | | | |
| Initial dose | 1 mg/kg/day (60 mg/day) for 1–3 months | 40–60 mg/day for ~1 month (consider pulse therapy for acute visual impairment) | 15–20 mg/day for 2–4 weeks |
| Tapering | Over 2–3 months, taper to alternate day (60 mg QOD); then continue to taper by 5 mg every 1–2 weeks | Taper on daily schedule by 5 mg every 2–4 weeks until 10 mg/day, then by 1 mg every 4 weeks | Taper on daily schedule by 2.5 mg every 2–4 weeks until 10 mg/day, then by 1 mg every 4–6 weeks |
| Cytotoxic agents | Consider for GC-resistant disease, GC toxicity | Rarely used Consider in selected cases of GC-resistant disease, GC toxicity | Not indicated |
| Other treatments | Hypertension management Surgery or percutaneous transluminal angioplasty | | Nonsteroidal anti-inflammatory drugs |

mum dose of 25 mg once a week. This was administered together with prednisone, 1 mg/kg/day, which was tapered after 1 month to an alternate-day regimen within 3 to 6 months. If, within 6 months of starting methotrexate, the symptoms and signs of active disease had resolved and the prednisone dose could be reduced, the methotrexate was continued for an additional 6 months, after which time it was tapered until discontinuation. Among 16 patients, this regimen led to remission in 81%; 25% of the 16 patients experienced a sustained remission for approximately 1 year in the absence of immunosuppressive medications. However, remission was followed by relapse in 54%, and 19% of patients had progressive disease. Approximately half of the patients who suffered relapse were reinduced into remission on the same protocol. The toxic effects of therapy in this population included reversible elevated hepatic transaminase levels (28%), nausea (22%), and stomatitis (6%) and one episode of *Pneumocystis carinii* pneumonia, which was successfully treated.

When a cytotoxic agent is indicated in TKA, methotrexate is the preferred choice. Although the NIH study has limitations, these data provide evidence that methotrexate may be an effective means of inducing remission and minimizing glucocorticoid toxicity in difficult-to-treat TKA. Additional factors to consider include the potential for TKA to relapse and the significant toxic effects of cyclophosphamide. Cyclophosphamide should be reserved for patients who have clear evidence of active inflammatory disease in which glucocorticoids are effective but cannot be tapered and for patients who are unresponsive to, intolerant of, or unable to take methotrexate.

### Other Medical Therapies

Hypertension occurs in 32% to 93% of TKA patients[3, 4, 6, 8, 12, 13, 21] and contributes to renal, cardiac, and cerebral injury. Because the subclavian arteries are frequently a site of vessel stenosis, blood pressure measurements in one or both arms may not be representative of aortic root pressure. Renovascular hypertension can be treated with either medical or nonmedical management. In either setting, the level of blood pressure control must be balanced against the risk of worsening ischemia across stenotic sites that require high pressure to maintain blood flow.

Thrombosis of vessels is uncommon in TKA, and the routine use of anticoagulants is not recommended. Antiplatelet agents such as aspirin and dipyridamole were used in some retrospective reports, but their potential benefit remains unclear.[10, 14, 16, 22]

### Surgery and Percutaneous Transluminal Angioplasty

Surgical therapy plays an important role in revascularization of stenosed or occluded vessels that produce significant ischemia. The most frequent indications for surgery include cerebral hypoperfusion, renovascular hypertension, limb claudication, aneurysms, and valvular insufficiency. In carefully selected patients, the safety and potential benefits of surgery have been favorable, although the graft patency and complication rates have varied greatly.[3, 4, 9, 10, 14, 17, 31, 32] Ideally, vascular reconstruction should be deferred until acute inflammation is medically controlled, because aneurysm formation, graft dehiscence, or graft occlusion may be more likely in the setting of active arteritis.[4, 32, 33] However, surgery to prevent imminent ischemia of a vital organ should not be delayed because of acute inflammation or ongoing immunosuppressive therapy. The role of perioperative glucocorticoid in clinically quiescent disease remains unclear. Although it is possible that glucocorticoids may have a beneficial role if active arteritis is present, authors caution that this must be tempered against the concern for delayed wound healing, susceptibility to infection, and possible long-term effects on suture line weakening.[17, 31]

Percutaneous transluminal angioplasty (PTCA) can be an effective procedure in TKA to control hypertension related to renal artery stenosis. The ability of PTCA to reduce stenosis has ranged from 56% to 100%.[3, 34–36] In three large series, improved blood pressure control was achieved in more than 85% of patients after successful PTCA.[34–36] The longevity of results was variable; the risk of restenosis was highest within the first year.[3, 35] Several reports have also found PTCA to be beneficial in treating short stenotic segments of other aortic branches as well as the aorta, although less is known about its efficacy in these settings.[34, 37]

## GIANT CELL ARTERITIS

### Natural History

Giant cell (temporal) arteritis (GCA) is the most common form of systemic vasculitis, with an incidence of 17.8 new cases per 100,000 person-years in Olmstead County, Minnesota.[1] It occurs predominantly in women over 50 years of age who are of European ancestry.

Frequent clinical manifestations of GCA include headache, jaw or tongue claudication, scalp tenderness, constitutional features, fever, and associated polymyalgia rheumatica.[1] The most dreaded complication is visual loss, which results from involvement of the ocular circulation. Anterior ischemic optic neuropathy, the predominant ocular manifestation of GCA, is caused by ischemia of the optic nerve head, which is supplied mainly by the posterior ciliary arteries. GCA is rarely directly responsible for acute patient mortality, although there have been reports of deaths from coronary and cerebral vasculitis.[38–40] In addition, thoracic aortic aneurysms have been found to occur as a late complication of disease and may be associated with mortality.[41]

### Assessing Disease Activity

Disease activity in GCA has often been evaluated by considering multiple factors, including symptoms, clinical examination findings, and laboratory test results. Acute-phase reactants, the ESR in particular, are often used as parameters by which to assess inflammation. However, they can become abnormal in other settings and do not always predict or concur with clinical relapse.[42]

## Treatment

### General Principles

Glucocorticoids were first used to manage GCA in 1950[43] and have since become the foundation of treatment for this disease. Glucocorticoids rapidly improve cranial and systemic symptoms[42, 44, 45] and reduce acute mortality from vasculitis. Of more importance, glucocorticoids prevent visual complications in GCA. Since the 1950s, the frequency of blindness in GCA has decreased from 60%[46, 47] to more recent estimates of 7% to 25%.[48–50] Although there is little published preglucocorticoid data, R. W. Ross Russell found that visual failure occurred in one third of patients treated with salicylates, in comparison with none who received glucocorticoids.[47] Birkhead and associates found that the frequency of bilateral blindness was 9% among steroid-treated patients, in comparison with 17% among patients seen in their clinic before the time of glucocorticoid use and 22% in a group of 250 patients described in the literature.[46] Since the advent of glucocorticoid use, in almost all reported cases, visual impairment has occurred before steroids were started.[47, 51, 52] Aiello and colleagues found that the probability of loss of vision after starting glucocorticoids was calculated to be only 1% according Kaplan-Meier estimates.[48]

### Glucocorticoids

Although most authors agree that glucocorticoids are mandatory in the treatment of active GCA, there are differing opinions regarding the initial dosage and tapering schedule. Because of difficulties in the available literature, many of the questions regarding the optimal regimen in GCA cannot be unequivocally answered.[42] In most instances, the therapeutic data in GCA come from retrospective, nonstandardized studies in which in many patients disease was not biopsy proven.

In literature from the 1950 to the 1960s, prednisone doses of more than 40 mg/day were used, in response to concern about anecdotal reports in which patients had not responded to lower doses.[43, 46, 47] The retrospective series published in the 1970s to the 1980s investigated doses of 40 to 60 mg/day, and it has been from these collective studies that the majority of experience regarding glucocorticoid efficacy has been gained[38–40, 51, 53, 54] (Table 29–3).

Unfortunately, these doses of glucocorticoids are not without associated toxicity. Furthermore, steroid-related side effects are a particular concern in the older population affected by GCA. In studies that have specifically examined the risk of glucocorticoid toxicity in GCA, 36% to 65% of patients experience one or more side effects related to treatment.[55–57] This risk has in some instances been found to be associated with increased age at the time of diagnosis,[56] female sex,[56] a cumulative dose of prednisone of 1800 mg or more,[56] and an initial prednisone dose of more than 30 mg.[55, 57]

Initial dosages of prednisone of less than 30 mg/day have been suggested by some authors to be effective in preventing blindness and associated with a lower risk of side effects.[44, 58] Others, however, have argued that higher initial doses were necessary to prevent blindness. Supportive of this have been reports of visual complications and symptom unresponsiveness with lower doses.[39, 45, 47] In a prospective study of 96 patients, 48 of whom had biopsy-proven disease, Myles and associates found that dosage increases were required in 5%, 5%, and 46% of GCA patients who received a daily initial prednisolone dose of more than 20 mg, 20 mg, or less than 20 mg, respectively.[45] In another prospective study, Kyle and Hazleman observed that disease was inadequately controlled in 40% of patients in whom the prednisolone dosage was reduced to 20 mg/day after they had received 40 mg/day for 5 days.[59] The remaining studies are retrospective,

## TABLE 29–3
## Selected Retrospective Series in the Treatment of Giant Cell Arteritis

| REFERENCE | NO. OF PATIENTS | NO. OF BIOPSY-PROVEN CASES | INITIAL GC DOSAGE (mg/day) | DURATION OF GC (MEAN MONTHS) | RELAPSE RATE* (%) |
|---|---|---|---|---|---|
| Fauchald et al[53] | 61 | 61 | PD: 40–60 | 23 | 26 |
| Sorensen and Lorenzen[52] | 46 | 46 | PD: 30–60 | 24 | NR |
| Huston et al[39] | 42 | 42 | NR | 7 | 26 |
| von Knorring[61]† | 10 | NR | PN: 30–40 | 26 | 35 |
| Fernandez-Herlihy[54] | 29 | 20 | PD: 40–80 | 72 | 90 |
| Graham et al[38] | 90 | 90 | PD: 80 | NR | 31 |
| Bengtsson and Malmvall[51]† | 73 | 50 | PN: <20–60 | 43 | 73 |
| Lundberg and Hedfors[58] | 51 | 31 | PN: 15–60 | 23 | 57 |

GC = glucocorticoid; NR = not reported; PD = prednisone; PN = prednisolone.
* Where disease activity parameters were not specifically stated, relapse has been defined as improvement on initial glucocorticoid dosage, with worsened disease occurring at a later point and necessitating a therapeutic intervention.
† Population includes patients with isolated polymyalgia rheumatica.

which raises concern that patients with less severe disease may have received lower dosages.[44, 50, 58, 60, 61] No firm conclusions can currently be reached with regard to the safety and efficacy of lower dosages of glucocorticoids in GCA, and the majority of data continue to support the initial use of prednisone at 40 to 60 mg/day (see Table 29–2).

Once the disease has been controlled, the duration of glucocorticoid treatment in GCA remains unestablished. In retrospective series, none of which used a standardized tapering schedule, most patients required glucocorticoids for more than 2 years, and many received such treatment for more than 4 years.[39, 52–54, 58, 61] Relapses were reported to occur within 2 years of diagnosis at a frequency that ranged from 26% to 90%.[38, 39, 51, 53, 54, 58, 61] Ideally, the glucocorticoid dosage should be decreased and discontinued as directed by the status of disease activity. In the absence of uniformly reliable indicators, the rate of tapering is usually individualized to the patient and is based on clinical parameters and the presence of glucocorticoid toxicity.

In GCA, glucocorticoids have historically been tapered on a daily schedule. Only two studies have addressed whether an alternate-day regimen could be used for this disease, although neither employed a schedule similar to that used successfully for other vasculitides. Bengtsson and Malmvall prospectively treated 27 patients with 40 mg/day, which was tapered to 15 mg/day and then to 30 mg every other day according to a staggered schedule.[62] On this regimen, 67% remained stable and 33% described symptoms on the days that they did not receive glucocorticoids. In an another study by Hunder and colleagues, 60 patients received 20 mg three times a day for 5 days and were then randomly assigned to receive 15 mg three times a day, 45 mg/day, or 90 mg every other day.[63] After 1 month, the arteritis was suppressed in 90% of patients on the three-times-a-day regimen and in 80% of those on the daily regimen but in only 30% of patients on the alternate-day regimen. Although this study provided evidence that alternate-day glucocorticoids are not effective early in the course of disease, it remains an interesting question for future investigation as to whether a more gradual alternate-day taper might be effective and less toxic.

### Treatment of Acute Visual Impairment

High-dose pulse steroids, given as methylprednisolone (Solu-Medrol), 1 g/day for 3 to 5 days are frequently administered to patients with acute visual disease, but no studies have directly addressed their efficacy. Some authors query whether pulse steroids offer any benefits and raise concerns about the associated risks,[64] whereas others[48, 65, 66] recommend the use of pulse doses for the preeminent reason of protecting remaining vision. A secondary reason is the possibility of ameliorating acute visual loss. In patients with visual impairment short of blindness, several studies reported an improvement in vision in 15% to 34% of patients, although there was variability in how these patients were

treated.[48, 66, 67] Although there are rare published reports of patients with complete visual loss who regained their sight after the use of pulse steroids,[48, 65–67] such cases are unusual, and patients should be counseled that once blindness has occurred, vision is unlikely to return.[39, 46–48, 52, 66] Because the duration of arterial occlusion may be a critical factor, pulse glucocorticoids should be started immediately if they are to be used.[65]

### Cytotoxic Therapy

To diminish glucocorticoid toxicity, several anecdotal reports describe the use of azathioprine (50 to 150 mg/day),[68] dapsone (100 mg/day),[69] and methotrexate (7.5 to 10 mg/week)[70, 71] for steroid-sparing effects. Evidence to date remains insufficient to support the use of these agents for this purpose.[1, 42]

Glucocorticoid-resistant GCA is another setting in which cytotoxic agents have been used.[42] The issue of glucocorticoid resistance remains controversial and is further complicated by lack of a universally accepted definition. Some authors have considered glucocorticoid resistance to be present when the prednisone dosage cannot be tapered to less than 15 mg/day or when the patient does not respond to initial high-dosage treatment. The latter scenario is distinctly unusual, and if treatment with prednisone, 40 to 60 mg/day, does not dramatically reduce symptoms within a week, the diagnosis should be questioned. There have been brief reports on the use of dapsone (100 mg/day),[72] methotrexate (7.5 to 12.5 mg/week),[73] and cyclophosphamide (given as low-dose weekly pulses: 0.5 g/week intravenously for 3 weeks)[74] in the setting of glucocorticoid-resistant GCA, but none of these studies allows definitive conclusions to be reached.

When a cytotoxic agent is being contemplated for GCA for reasons of either resistant disease or glucocorticoid toxicity, methotrexate, 5 to 15 mg/week, has often been the preferred agent despite the absence of direct data. This preference has been based largely on the experience with this agent in TKA and Wegener's granulomatosis and its favorable side effect profile in comparison with other cytotoxic agents.

## POLYMYALGIA RHEUMATICA

### Natural History

Polymyalgia rheumatica (PMR) is a nonvasculitic disease entity symptomatically characterized by aching and morning stiffness in the proximal muscles of the shoulder and hip girdles. In Olmstead County, Minnesota, PMR occurs with an annual incidence rate of 52.5 per 100,000 persons aged 50 and older.[1] PMR occurs in isolation or as part of GCA; it affects 40% to 60% of patients with GCA. In addition to the clinical association between PMR and GCA, pathogenetic links have been found from human leukocyte antigen sequencing[75] and temporal artery cytokine analyses.[1, 76]

Early reports of patients who did not receive glucocorticoids described PMR as a self-limited condition that lasted 2 to 5 years.[77–80] Although PMR occurring in the absence of GCA can cause significant pain and debilitation, it is not associated with joint destruction or other evidence of organ injury. Systemic inflammation, however, can be present in PMR and may have deleterious effects on bone mass[81] and red blood cell production.

The link between PMR and GCA has raised concerns about whether PMR should be thought of as a heralding event in GCA.[40, 51, 53, 82] In one series, positive temporal artery biopsy specimens were obtained in 16% of patients with PMR,[83] although other authors have demonstrated this rate to be higher.[1, 40, 53, 82] Clinically, several reports have found progression of PMR to GCA to occur infrequently,[44, 50, 84–86] particularly with regard to the development of visual sequelae.

## Assessment of Active Disease

Assessment of disease activity in PMR is based on clinical symptoms, physical examination, and elevated levels of acute-phase reactants, of which the ESR is measured most frequently. In PMR, this assessment can be further complicated by the similarities between disease symptoms and glucocorticoid withdrawal.

## Treatment

### General Principles

The goal of treatment in PMR should be to use the least toxic regimen that is effective at relieving symptoms and controlling inflammation. Symptom severity is variable, and some patients experience discomfort to the point of incapacitation, which can cause morbidity. However, because treatment carries its own risk of morbidity, the appropriate management of PMR must always carefully weigh the therapeutic benefits and risks.

### Glucocorticoids

PMR typically responds in a rapid and dramatic manner to prednisone at dosages of 10 to 20 mg/day. This is such a characteristic feature that the failure to respond to low doses of glucocorticoids within 5 days should prompt reconsideration of the underlying diagnosis. The degree of therapeutic responsiveness, together with the lack of standard measures of disease activity, has restricted the ability to conduct prospective trials to delineate the optimal initial prednisone dose or subsequent tapering schedule. In most retrospective series, initial prednisone doses of 10 to 20 mg/day were administered[44, 58, 61, 83–85, 87] (Table 29–4). When Delecoeuillerie and associates retrospectively examined the use of lower dosages, they found no difference in the rate of remission or relapse between patients who received prednisone at an initial dosage of 7 to 12 mg/day and those who received 15 to 30 mg/day.[50] However, two other studies have demonstrated inadequate control of symptoms when 10 mg/day or less was used.[59, 87] At the other end of the dosage spectrum, some authors have suggested that PMR should be treated with high initial glucocorticoid dosages similar to those for GCA.[40, 51, 53, 82] Although this remains controversial, the effectiveness of low-dosage treatment, the lack of progression to GCA in most patients, and the toxic effects of high-dosage glucocorticoid therapy appear to support the notion that initial dosages of 15 to 20 mg/day can be used to treat isolated PMR (see Table 29–2).

Several studies have demonstrated that PMR patients experience significant toxic effects related to treatment.[55, 84] In one retrospective study, Gabriel and coworkers found that 65% of patients treated with glucocorticoids alone experienced at least one adverse event, in comparison with 67% of the patients treated with nonsteroidal anti-inflammatory drugs (NSAIDs) alone and 80% of the patients treated with both.[56] For

## TABLE 29–4
### Selected Retrospective Series in the Treatment of Polymyalgia Rheumatica

| REFERENCE | NO. OF PATIENTS | INITIAL GC DOSAGE (mg/day) | DURATION OF GC (MEAN OR MEDIAN MONTHS) | RELAPSE RATE* (%) |
|---|---|---|---|---|
| Ayoub et al[84] | 76 | PD: 22.8 | 37.3 (40% required >4 years) | 56 |
| Myles[87†] | 52 | PN: 10 | 21 (33% required >4 years) | 31 |
| von Knorring[61†] | 43 | PN: 10–20 | 26 (64% required a mean of 3 years) | 35 |
| Delecoeuillerie et al[50] | 132 | PD: 13.9 | 25.7 | 12 |
| Behn et al[44†] | 114 | PN: 10 | 31 (range, 3–103) | 47 |
| Lundberg and Hedfors[58] | 40 | PN: 10–20 | 17 | 68 |
| Bahlas et al[86†] | 133 | PD: 20–30 | 28 (54% required >3 years) | 18 |
| Coomes et al[88†] | 92 | PN: 15 | NR (84% required 5 years) | NR |
| Spiera and Davison[85] | 56 | PD: 10 | NR | NR |
| Chuang et al[83†] | 96 | PD: 20 | NR (>80% able to stop treatment in 2 years) | 63 |

GC = glucocorticoid; NR = not reported; PN = prednisolone. PD = prednisone.
* Where disease activity parameters were not specifically stated, relapse has been defined as improvement on initial glucocorticoid dosage, with worsened disease occurring at a later point and necessitating a therapeutic intervention.
† Population includes patients with giant cell arteritis.

this reason, it is desirable to taper the prednisone to as low a dosage as is effective in managing symptoms. Retrospective series have demonstrated wide variability in the mean length of glucocorticoid treatment.[61, 84, 86-88] Several studies have provided supportive evidence that patients with PMR may in fact be divided into two populations: One can discontinue glucocorticoids within 2 years, and the other requires longer term treatment.[61, 83, 84] Relapse in PMR should be determined primarily by the presence of increased clinical symptoms. A rise in ESR alone should not be used as the basis for increasing or restarting treatment. The rate of disease relapse has ranged from 15% to 70%, according to the literature[50, 58, 61, 83, 84, 86]; however, these studies often did not employ standardized methods of treatment or definitions of relapse.

A variation of glucocorticoid treatment that has been examined is the use of intermittent long-acting glucocorticoid injections. In 60 patients, Dasgupta and associates found similar rates of remission in patients who received intramuscular methylprednisolone, 120 mg every 3 weeks, and in patients who received oral prednisolone, 15 mg/day.[89] Although potentially promising, further study of this regimen is needed on a larger number of patients to fully determine its long-term toxicity and efficacy. The use of deflazacort as an alternative glucocorticoid preparation was also examined but was not found to have any advantage over prednisolone with regard to bone toxicity.[90]

### Nonsteroidal Anti-inflammatory Agents

NSAIDs and salicylates were the first medications used to treat PMR and continue to have a potential role in disease management.[77-80] These agents have been found to be effective in some patients, particularly those with milder symptoms.[83] Whether to consider a trial of NSAIDs before glucocorticoids in a patient thought to have PMR should be based largely on individual patient factors, including severity of disease and potential for toxicity. The side effects of NSAIDs in an older population are often underappreciated, and the risks of gastrointestinal and renal toxicity should be considered carefully.[56] One disadvantage of using NSAIDs as initial treatment is that the rapid response to glucocorticoids, which is often used to support the diagnosis, is not usually observed with NSAIDs.

### Cytotoxic Therapy

Cytotoxic agents currently appear to play no role in the treatment of PMR. Studies of methotrexate, 7.5 to 12.5 mg/week, have yielded conflicting results; one study found it to be useful in reducing the total glucocorticoid dose,[91] whereas others have found it to be of no benefit.[70, 92]

## DRUG TOXICITY: MONITORING AND PREVENTION

### General Concepts: Infection

Infection remains the complication of greater concern in any patient receiving immunosuppressive therapy.

Depending on the degree of host defense suppression, patients may be at increased risk of infection from both bacterial and opportunistic organisms.[93] In particular, an increased frequency of *P. carinii* pneumonia was described in patients with vasculitis who received daily glucocorticoids in combination with a cytotoxic agent.[93, 94] Because a mortality rate of 35% has been observed in some series, *P. carinii* pneumonia prophylaxis with trimethoprim 160 mg/sulfamethoxazole 800 mg three times a week[95] is recommended for any non–sulfa-allergic patient with vasculitis who is receiving high-dosage daily glucocorticoids together with a cytotoxic agent.

### Glucocorticoids

Glucocorticoids have a broad range of toxic effects that includes infection, hyperglycemia, hypertension, osteoporosis, avascular necrosis, cataracts, myopathy, psychosis, poor wound healing, growth disturbance, acne, striae, weight gain, and change in fat distribution. Dividing the glucocorticoid dose throughout the day appears to be more anti-inflammatory but is associated with a higher risk of side effects. Therefore, the use of split-dose glucocorticoids should be reserved for acute settings, and consolidation to a single morning dose should be made as soon as possible. For diseases in which a single daily dose is possible, tapering of glucocorticoids to an alternate-day schedule is associated with a lower risk of toxicity, particularly infection. In all patients, a plan for monitoring and minimizing glucocorticoid-induced osteoporosis should be actively pursued.[96]

### Methotrexate

The toxicity profile observed with methotrexate treatment in vasculitis has to date been similar to the experience in rheumatoid arthritis.[26, 97] Rash, mucositis, gastrointestinal intolerance, and alopecia may develop.[98, 99] Some of these toxic effects may be lessened or prevented by the use of calcium leucovorin, 2.5 to 10 mg once a week given 24 hours after methotrexate, or folic acid, 1 mg/day.[100] Because methotrexate can be teratogenic, effective contraception should be used by both male and female patients; this is particularly important for younger patients receiving methotrexate for TKA. Bone marrow suppression has been observed in up to 30% of patients receiving methotrexate for nonneoplastic diseases. In protocols in which methotrexate has been used to treat vasculitis, complete blood counts were obtained weekly while the dose was being adjusted and monthly after a stable dose was reached for as long as the patient was taking the drug.

Methotrexate pneumonitis has been observed in up to 7% of patients and can be life-threatening.[101] The main presenting symptoms include a nonproductive cough, dyspnea, headache, and fever. Clinical findings include hypoxia, decreased diffusion capacity, and bilateral radiographic interstitial infiltrates. Although pneumonitis is usually reversible with drug discontinuation, glucocorticoid treatment with split-dose methylprednisolone (Solu-Medrol), 60 to 160 mg/day, has been used in the majority of reported cases and is thought to be beneficial.

Hepatic fibrosis and cirrhosis are potential complications of methotrexate treatment. To date, in series in which methotrexate has been used to treat vasculitis, surveillance monitoring of liver function tests and liver biopsies have been performed according to the standards for rheumatoid arthritis.[102]

## Cyclophosphamide

Daily cyclophosphamide has significant potential for both short- and long-term toxicity, and as such, it should rarely if ever be used for the diseases discussed in this chapter. Although some of the toxic effects of cyclophosphamide can be lessened by intermittent administration, there have been no data concerning an intermittent schedule for these vasculitic diseases. Bone marrow suppression should be anticipated with cyclophosphamide treatment, especially during glucocorticoid tapering and as a progressive event over time.[30] With daily therapy, complete blood counts should be performed every 1 to 2 weeks. Leukopenia is not a goal of therapy, and the dose of cyclophosphamide should be reduced to maintain the leukocyte count at a level over $3000/\mu L$.[30, 99, 103] Long-term effects can be seen on the bone marrow; the development of myeloproliferative diseases has been reported in 1% to 2% of patients.[103, 104]

Urothelial toxicity is believed to be caused by mucosal injury from the cyclophosphamide metabolite acrolein. Approximately 50% of patients taking daily cyclophosphamide experience cyclophosphamide-induced bladder injury, which in severe cases causes life-threatening hemorrhage.[105] In any patient in whom gross hematuria develops, cyclophosphamide should be withheld and cystoscopy promptly performed. In order to minimize cyclophosphamide-induced bladder injury, the daily dosage of cyclophosphamide should be taken all at once in the morning with a large amount of fluid. With intermittent therapy, sodium 2-mercaptoethanesulfonate (mesna), given concurrently with cyclophosphamide in three intravenous infusions of 20% of the cyclophosphamide dose every 4 hours (the initial dose is given at the time of cyclophosphamide administration with subsequent doses 4 and 8 hours after cyclophosphamide), may protect the bladder by the mechanism of binding to acrolein. However, this is not currently an option with daily treatment. Transitional-cell carcinoma of the bladder has developed in 6% of the patients with Wegener's granulomatosis monitored at the NIH who were treated with daily cyclophosphamide. Fifteen years after the first exposure to cyclophosphamide, this frequency may reach as high as 16%, according to Kaplan-Meier analysis.[105] The risk for bladder cancer and the need for monitoring should be considered lifelong because cancers have been detected 17 years after drug discontinuation. Urine cytologic study is useful if results are abnormal, but it has poor sensitivity for detecting low-grade cancers. Nonglomerular hematuria has been found to be the most useful marker in identifying

patients at risk for developing bladder cancer. For this reason, a urinalysis with microscopic examination should be performed every 3 to 6 months indefinitely in all patients who have received cyclophosphamide.[105] In patients who are found to have nonglomerular hematuria, cystoscopy every 1 to 2 years is recommended.

Permanent infertility has been reported to occur in 10% to 100% of cyclophosphamide-treated men and women.[105a, 105b] This is a particular consideration for patients with TKA who are young and hope to have children. In men, cyclophosphamide damages the germinal epithelium, whereas in women, sterility appears to be caused by primary ovarian failure from premature follicle depletion.[106, 107] On the basis of these patterns of injury, hormonal manipulation is hypothesized to be of benefit; however, this has thus far not been proved in large series.[107] Although ova or sperm banking is not an option in an acutely life-threatening vasculitis, there may be time to consider this possibility in TKA. Cyclophosphamide is potentially teratogenic, making effective contraception critical.

## REFERENCES

1. Hunder GG: Giant cell arteritis and polymyalgia rheumatica. *In* Kelley WM, Harris ED, Ruddy S, et al (eds): Textbook of Rheumatology, 5th ed. Philadelphia: WB Saunders, 1997:1123.
2. Valente RM, Hall S, O'Duffy JD, et al: Vasculitis and related disorders. *In* Kelley WM, Harris ED, Ruddy S, et al (eds): Textbook of Rheumatology, 5th ed. Philadelphia: WB Saunders, 1997:1079.
3. Kerr GS, Hallahan CW, Giordano J, et al: Takayasu's arteritis. Ann Intern Med 1994; 120:919.
4. Hall S, Barr W, Lie JT, et al: Takayasu's arteritis: A study of 32 North American patients. Medicine 1986; 64:89.
5. Wilke WS: Large vessel vasculitis (giant cell arteritis, Takayasu's arteritis). Baillière's Clin Rheumatol 1997; 11:285.
6. Sharma BK, Sagar S, Singh AP, et al: Takayasu arteritis in India. Heart Vessels 1992; 7(suppl):37.
7. Lande A, Rossi P: The value of total aortography in the diagnosis of Takayasu's arteritis. Radiology 1975; 114:287.
8. Chugh KS, Sakhuja V: Takayasu's arteritis as a cause of renovascular hypertension in Asian countries. Am J Nephrol 1992; 12:1.
9. Lagneau P, Michel JB, Vuong PN: Surgical treatment of Takayasu's disease. Ann Surg 1987; 205:157.
10. Ishikawa K, Maetani S: Long-term outcome for 120 Japanese patients with Takayasu's disease: Clinical and statistical analyses of related prognostic factors. Circulation 1994; 90:1855.
11. Subramanyan R, Joy J, Balakrishnan KG: Natural history of aortoarteritis (Takayasu's disease). Circulation 1989; 80:429.
12. Morales E, Pineda C, Martinez-Lavin M: Takayasu's arteritis in children. J Rheumatol 1991; 18:1081.
13. Deyu Z, Dijun F, Lisheng L: Takayasu arteritis in China: A report of 530 cases. Heart Vessels 1992; 7(suppl):32.
14. Ishikawa K: Survival and morbidity after diagnosis of occlusive thromboaortopathy (Takayasu's disease). Am J Cardiol 1981; 47:1026.
15. Fraga A, Mintz, Valle L, et al: Takayasu's arteritis: Frequency of systemic manifestations (study of 22 patients) and favorable response to maintenance steroid therapy with adrenocorticosteroids (12 patients). Arthritis Rheum 1972; 15:617.
16. Nakao K, Ikeda M, Kimata SI, et al: Takayasu's arteritis: Clinical report of eighty-four cases and immunological studies of seven cases. Circulation 1967; 35:1141.
17. Weaver FA, Yellin AE, Campen DH, et al: Surgical procedures in the management of Takayasu's arteritis. J Vasc Surg 1990; 12:429.

18. Maeda H, Handa N, Matsumoto M, et al: Carotid lesions detected by B-mode ultrasonography in Takayasu's arteritis. Ultrasound Med Biol 1991; 17:695.
19. Miller DL, Reinig JW, Volkman DJ: Vascular imaging with MRI: Inadequacy in Takayasu's arteritis compared with angiography. Am J Radiol 1986; 146:949.
20. Matsunaga N, Hayashi K, Sakamoto I, et al: Takayasu arteritis: MR manifestations and diagnosis of acute and chronic phase. J Magn Reson Imaging 1998; 8:406.
21. Lupi-Herrera E, Sanchez-Torres G, Marcushamer J, et al: Takayasu's arteritis: Clinical study of 107 cases. Am Heart J 1977; 93:94.
22. Ito I: Medical treatment of Takayasu arteritis. Heart Vessels 1992; 7(suppl):48.
23. Ishikawa K: Effects of prednisolone therapy in arterial angiographic features in Takayasu's disease. Am J Cardiol 1991; 68:410.
24. Ishikawa K, Yonekawa Y: Regression of carotid stenoses after corticosteroid therapy in occlusive thromboaortopathy (Takayasu's disease). Stroke 1987; 18:677.
25. Shelhamer JH, Volkman DJ, Parrillo JE, et al: Takayasu's arteritis and its therapy. Ann Intern Med 1985; 103:121.
26. Hoffman GS, Leavitt RY, Kerr GS, et al: Treatment of glucocorticoid-resistant or relapsing Takayasu's arteritis with methotrexate. Arthritis Rheum 1994; 37:578.
27. Liang GC, Nemickas R, Madayag M: Multiple percutaneous transluminal angioplasties and low dose pulse methotrexate for Takayasu's arteritis. J Rheumatol 1989; 16:1370.
28. Mevorach D, Leibowitz G, Brezis M, et al: Induction of remission in a patient with Takayasu's arteritis by low dose pulses of methotrexate. Ann Rheum Dis 1992; 51:904.
29. Waern AU, Andersson P, Hemmingsson A: Takayasu's arteritis: A hospital-region based study on occurrence, treatment, and prognosis. Angiology 1983; 34:311.
30. Fauci AS, Haynes BF, Katz P, et al: Wegener's granulomatosis: Prospective clinical and therapeutic experience with 85 patients for 21 years. Ann Intern Med 1983; 98:76.
31. Tada Y, Sato O, Ohshima A, et al: Surgical treatment of Takayasu arteritis. Heart Vessels 1992; 7(suppl):159.
32. Giordano JM, Leavitt RY, Hoffman GS, et al: Experience with surgical treatment of Takayasu's disease. Surgery 1991; 109:252.
33. Pajari R, Hekali P, Harjola PT: Treatment of Takayasu's arteritis: An analysis of 29 operated patients. Thorac Cardiovasc Surg 1986; 34:176.
34. Khalilullah M, Tyagi S: Percutaneous transluminal angioplasty in Takayasu's arteritis. Heart Vessels 1992; 7(suppl):146.
35. Tyagi S, Singh B, Kaul UA, et al: Balloon angioplasty for renovascular hypertension in Takayasu's arteritis. Am Heart J 1993; 125:1386.
36. Dong Z, Li S, Lu X: Percutaneous transluminal angioplasty for renovascular hypertension in arteritis: Experience in China. Radiology 1987; 162:477.
37. Rao SA, Mandalam KR, Rao VR, et al: Takayasu arteritis: Initial and long-term follow-up in 16 patients after percutaneous transluminal angioplasty of the descending thoracic and abdominal aorta. Radiology 1993; 189:173.
38. Graham E, Holland A, Avery A, et al: Prognosis in giant cell arteritis. BMJ 1981; 282:269.
39. Huston KA, Hunder GG, Lie JT, et al: Temporal arteritis: A 25 year epidemiologic, clinical, and pathological study. Ann Intern Med 1978; 88:162.
40. Hamilton CR, Shelley WM, Tumulty PA: Giant cell arteritis: Including temporal arteritis and polymyalgia rheumatica. Medicine 1971; 50:1.
41. Evans JM, O'Fallon M, Hunder GG: Increased incidence of aortic aneurysm and dissection in giant cell (temporal) arteritis. Ann Intern Med 1995; 122:502.
42. Wilke WW, Hoffman GS: Treatment of corticosteroid-resistant giant cell arteritis. Rheum Dis Clin North Am 1995; 21:59.
43. Shick RM, Baggenstoss AH, Fuller BF, et al: Effects of cortisone and ACTH on periarteritis nodosa and cranial arteritis. Mayo Clin Proc 1950; 25:492.
44. Behn AR, Perara T, Myles AB: Polymyalgia rheumatica and corticosteroids: How much for how long? Ann Rheum Dis 1983; 42:374.
45. Myles AB, Perara T, Ridley MG: Prevention of blindness in giant cell arteritis by corticosteroid treatment. Br J Rheumatol 1992; 31:103.
46. Birkhead NC, Wagener HP, Shick RM: Treatment of temporal arteritis with adrenal corticosteroids. JAMA 1957; 163:821.
47. Ross Russell RW: Giant cell arteritis. Q J Med 1959; 112:471.
48. Aiello PD, Trautman JC, McPhee TJ, et al: Visual prognosis in giant cell arteritis. Ophthalmology 1993; 100:550.
49. Bengtsson BA, Malmvall BE: The epidemiology of giant cell arteritis including temporal arteritis and polymyalgia rheumatica: Incidences of different clinical presentations and eye complications. Arthritis Rheum 1981; 24:899.
50. Delecoeuillerie G, Joly P, Cohen de Lara A, et al: Polymyalgia rheumatica and temporal arteritis: A retrospective analysis of prognostic features and different corticosteroid regimens. Ann Rheum Dis 1988; 47:733.
51. Bengtsson BA, Malmvall BE: Prognosis of giant cell arteritis including temporal arteritis and polymyalgia rheumatica. Acta Med Scand 1981; 209:337.
52. Sorensen PS, Lorenzen I: Giant cell arteritis, temporal arteritis, and polymyalgia rheumatica: A retrospective study of 63 patients. Acta Med Scand 1977; 201:207.
53. Fauchald P, Rygvold O, Oystese B: Temporal arteritis and polymyalgia rheumatica: Clinical and biopsy findings. Ann Intern Med 1972; 77:845.
54. Fernandez-Herlihy L: Duration of corticosteroid therapy in giant cell arteritis. J Rheumatol 1980; 7:361.
55. Kyle V, Hazleman BL: Treatment of polymyalgia rheumatica and giant cell arteritis: II. Relation between steroid dose and side effects. Ann Rheum Dis 1989; 48:662.
56. Gabriel SE, Sunku J, Salvarani C, et al: Adverse outcomes of antiinflammatory therapy among patients with polymyalgia rheumatica. Arthritis Rheum 1997; 40:1873.
57. Nesher G, Sonnenblick M, Friedlander Y: Analysis of steroid related complications and mortality in temporal arteritis: A 15-year survey of 43 patients. J Rheumatol 1994; 21:1283.
58. Lundberg I, Hedfors E: Restricted dose and duration of corticosteroid treatment in patients with polymyalgia rheumatica and temporal arteritis. J Rheumatol 1990; 17:1340.
59. Kyle V, Hazleman BL: Treatment of polymyalgia rheumatica and giant cell arteritis: I. Steroid regimens in the first two months. Ann Rheum Dis 1989; 48:658.
60. Nesher G, Rubinow A, Sonnenblick M: Efficacy and adverse effects of different corticosteroid dose regimens in temporal arteritis: A retrospective study. Clin Exp Rheumatol 1997; 15:303.
61. von Knorring J: Treatment and prognosis in polymyalgia rheumatica and temporal arteritis. Acta Med Scand 1979; 205:429.
62. Bengtsson BA, Malmvall BE: An alternate-day corticosteroid regimen in maintenance therapy of giant cell arteritis. Acta Med Scand 1981; 209:347.
63. Hunder GG, Sheps SG, Allen GL, et al: Daily and alternate-day corticosteroid regimens in treatment for giant cell arteritis. Ann Intern Med 1975; 82:613.
64. Cornblath WT, Eggenberger ER: Progressive visual loss from giant cell arteritis despite high-dose intravenous methylprednisolone. Ophthalmology 1997; 104:854–858.
65. Matzkin DC, Slamovits TL, Sachs R, et al: Visual recovery in two patients after intravenous methylprednisolone treatment of central retinal artery occlusion secondary to giant cell arteritis. Ophthalmology 1992; 99:68.
66. Liu GT, Glaser JS, Schatz NJ, et al: Visual morbidity in giant cell arteritis. Ophthalmology 1994; 101:1779.
67. Schneider HA, Weber AA, Ballen PH: The visual prognosis in temporal arteritis. Ann Ophthalmol 1971; 3:1215.
68. De Silva M, Hazleman BL: Azathioprine in giant cell arteritis/polymyalgia rheumatica: A double-blind study. Ann Rheum Dis 1986; 45:136.
69. Boesen P, Dideriksen K, Stentoft J, et al: Dapsone in temporal arteritis and polymyalgia rheumatica. J Rheumatol 1988; 15:879.
70. Van der Veen MJ, Dinant HJ, van Booma-Frankfort C, et al: Can methotrexate be used as a steroid sparing agent in the treatment of polymyalgia rheumatica and giant cell arteritis? Ann Rheum Dis 1996; 55:218.

71. Hernandez-Garcia C, Soriano C, Morado C, et al: Methotrexate treatment in the management of giant cell arteritis. Scand J Rheumatol 1994; 23:295.
72. Doury P, Pattin S, Eulry F, et al: The use of dapsone in the treatment of giant cell arteritis and polymyalgia rheumatica. Arthritis Rheum 1983; 30:689.
73. Krall PL, Mazanec DJ, Wilke WS: Methotrexate for corticosteroid-resistant polymyalgia rheumatica and giant cell arteritis. Cleve Clin J Med 1989; 56:253.
74. DeVita S, Tavoni A, Jeracitano G, et al: Treatment of giant cell arteritis with cyclophosphamide pulses. J Intern Med 1992; 232:373.
75. Weyand CM, Hunder GG, Hicok KC, et al: HLA-DRB1 alleles in polymyalgia rheumatica, giant cell arteritis, and rheumatoid arthritis. Arthritis Rheum 1994; 37:514.
76. Weyand CM, Hicok KC, Hunder GG, et al: Tissue cytokine patterns in patients with polymyalgia rheumatica and giant cell arteritis. Ann Intern Med 1994; 121:484.
77. Barber HS: Myalgic syndrome with constitutional effects: Polymyalgia rheumatica. Ann Rheum Dis 1957; 16:230.
78. Gordon I: Polymyalgia rheumatica: A clinical study of 21 cases. Q J Med 1960; 116:473.
79. Bagratuni L: Prognosis in the anarthritic rheumatoid syndrome. BMJ 1963; 1:513.
80. Hunder GG, Disney TF, Ward LE: Polymyalgia rheumatica. Mayo Clin Proc 1969; 44:849.
81. Dolan AL, Moniz C, Dasgupta B, et al: Effects of inflammation and treatment on bone turnover and bone mass in polymyalgia rheumatica. Arthritis Rheum 1998; 40:2022.
82. Jones JC, Hazleman BL: Prognosis and management of polymyalgia rheumatica. Ann Rheum Dis 1981; 40:1.
83. Chuang TY, Hunder GG, Ilstrup DM, et al: Polymyalgia rheumatica: A 10-year epidemiologic and clinical study. Ann Intern Med 1982; 97:672.
84. Ayoub WT, Franklin CM, Torretti D: Polymyalgia rheumatica: Duration of therapy and long-term outcome. Am J Med 1985; 79:309.
85. Spiera H, Davison S: Long-term follow-up of polymyalgia rheumatica. Mt Sinai J Med 1978; 45:225.
86. Bahlas S, Ramos-Remus C, Davis P: Clinical outcome of 149 patients with polymyalgia rheumatica and giant cell arteritis. J Rheumatol 1998; 25:99.
87. Myles AB: Polymyalgia rheumatica and giant cell arteritis: A seven-year survey. Rheumatol Rehab 1975; 14:231.
88. Coomes EN, Ellis RM, Kay AG: A prospective study of 102 patients with the polymyalgia rheumatica syndrome. Rheumatol Rehab 1976; 15:270.
89. Dasgupta B, Dolan, Panayi GS, et al: An initially double-blind controlled 96 week trial of depot methylprednisolone against oral prednisolone in the treatment of polymyalgia rheumatica. Br J Rheumatol 1998; 37:189.
90. Krogsgaard MR, Thamsborg G, Lund B: Changes in bone mass during low dose corticosteroid treatment in patients with polymyalgia rheumatica: A double blind, prospective comparison between prednisolone and deflazacort. Ann Rheum Dis 1996; 55:143.
91. Ferraccioli, Salaffi F, de Vita S, et al: Methotrexate in polymyalgia rheumatica: Preliminary results of an open, randomized study. J Rheumatol 1996; 23:624.
92. Feinberg HL, Sherman JD, Schrepferman CG, et al: The use of methotrexate in polymyalgia rheumatica. J Rheumatol 1996; 23:1550.
93. Segal BH, Sneller MC: Infectious complications of immunosuppressive therapy in patients with rheumatic diseases. Rheum Dis Clin North Am 1997; 23:219.
94. Langford CA: Chronic immunosuppressive therapy for systemic vasculitis. Curr Opin Rheumatol 1997; 9:41.
95. Masur H: Prevention and treatment of pneumocystis pneumonia. N Engl J Med 1992; 327:1853.
96. Dale DC, Fauci AS, Wolff SM: Alternate-day prednisone: Leukocyte kinetics and susceptibility to infections. N Engl J Med 1974; 291:1154.
97. Langford CA, Sneller MC, Hoffman GS: Methotrexate use in systemic vasculitis. Rheum Dis Clin North Am 1997; 23:841.
98. Goodman TA, Polisson RP: Methotrexate: Adverse reactions and major toxicities. Rheum Dis Clin North Am 1994; 20:513.
99. Langford CA, Klippel JH, Balow JE, et al: Use of cytotoxic agents and cyclosporine in the treatment of autoimmune disease: Part 2. Inflammatory bowel disease, systemic vasculitis, and therapeutic toxicity. Ann Intern Med 1998; 129:49.
100. Shiroky JB: The use of folates concomitantly with low-dose pulse methotrexate. Rheum Dis Clin North Am 1997; 23:969.
101. Cannon GW: Methotrexate pulmonary toxicity. Rheum Dis Clin North Am 1997; 23:917.
102. Kremer JM, Alarcan GS, Lightfoot RW, et al: Methotrexate for rheumatoid arthritis: Suggested guidelines for monitoring liver biopsy. Arthritis Rheum 1994; 37:316.
103. Hoffman GS, Kerr GS, Leavitt RY, et al: Wegener granulomatosis: An analysis of 158 patients. Ann Intern Med 1992; 116:488.
104. Radis CD, Kahl LE, Baker GL, et al: Effects of cyclophosphamide on the development of malignancy and on long-term survival of patients with rheumatoid arthritis. A 20-year followup study. Arthritis Rheum 1995; 38:1120.
105. Talar-Williams C, Hijazi TM, Walther MM, et al: Cyclophosphamide-induced cystitis and bladder cancer in patients with Wegener granulomatosis. Ann Intern Med 1996; 124:477.
105a. Fairley KF, Barrie JR, Johnson W: Sterility and testicular atrophy related to cyclophosphamide therapy. Lancet 1972; 1:568.
105b. Warne GL, Fairley KF, Hobbs JB, et al: Cyclophosphamide-induced ovarian failure. N Engl J Med 1973; 289:1159.
106. Boumpas DT, Austin HA, Vaughan EM, et al: Risk for sustained amenorrhea in patients with systemic lupus erythematosus receiving intermittent pulse cyclophosphamide therapy. Ann Intern Med 1993; 119:366.
107. Masala A, Faedda R, Alagna S, et al: Use of testosterone to prevent cyclophosphamide-induced azoospermia. Ann Intern Med 1997; 126:292.

# 30 | Scleroderma

*Fredrick M. Wigley and Alan K. Matsumoto*

Scleroderma is a chronic disfiguring disease that can change every aspect of a person's life. The skin involvement of scleroderma is often the most distressing manifestation, because it not only alters the patient's appearance but frequently causes major disability of the hands and limbs. Scleroderma is a multisystem disease that can threaten a patient's life or limit the ability to function normally in family or profession. Patients must also cope with fatigue, cold intolerance, pain, decreased exercise tolerance, and a general inability to fully perform their usual role in life. As a consequence, emotional problems such as fear, anxiety, misconceptions, and depression are common among patients with scleroderma.[1]

Scleroderma can be equally frustrating for the physician. Because scleroderma is an uncommon rheumatic disease, physicians have less experience with the problems of these patients. Although several features of the disease are seemingly monotonous, the course of scleroderma is highly variable and the overall outcome cannot be completely predicted. Visceral involvement is frequently relatively silent until an irreversible stage develops. At the same time, no treatment has proved uniformly successful in either prevention or reversal of the *overall* disease process.

Effective management of the patient with scleroderma begins with a solid patient-doctor relationship. Patients must feel comfortable and have confidence that their care is well directed. Physicians must be sensitive to patients' needs, both physical and emotional. This usually requires frequent and regular contact. Careful education is important so that the patient and the family understand the rationale and limitations of the treatment. The patient must understand that although the course of scleroderma is a chronic one, it is also quite variable in expression and not uniformly "progressive." Designing a management program frequently involves a team of subspecialists and health professionals. Consultation with an experienced expert in the management of scleroderma is helpful, especially in early disease when decisions about treatment options are especially critical. Experimental treatments should be done with *informed consent* and in conjunction with an academic center that is experienced in conducting clinical trials in scleroderma.

At first encounter a comprehensive evaluation and baseline studies (Table 30–1) provide an important frame of reference for future management, and early detection of organ involvement provides an opportunity to prevent irreversible damage. Every patient with a diagnosis of scleroderma should have a baseline chest radiograph, electrocardiogram, and pulmonary function test in addition to a complete physical examination. A baseline two-dimensional echocardiogram is recommended for all patients, especially if they have either cardiopulmonary symptoms or abnormal pulmonary function tests. Several scleroderma-specific measurements are helpful in assessing status over time. These include the degree of skin thickening by measurement of total body skin score, size of maximal oral aperture, and a patient global evaluation of current status. In addition to a complete blood cell count, electrolytes, urinalysis, and general chemistry determinations, the laboratory assessment should include measurement of muscle enzymes (creatine phosphokinase, aldolase) and thyroid function testing. Active myositis and hypothyroidism are common and may not be clinically obvious. Specific autoantibodies are useful in defining disease subsets and predicting outcome. (For more detail see Kelley et al., *Textbook of Rheumatology*, Chapter 66.[1a]) Other special testing is dictated by the clinical situation.

## NATURAL HISTORY

The natural history of scleroderma differs among the various subsets of the disease. Patients with *limited scleroderma* have an indolent course with little change in visceral involvement over their lifetime. Skin changes are limited and, therefore, aggressive treatment directed at the skin is inappropriate. Treatment should be directed at the vascular complications, including severe digital ischemia and isolated pulmonary hypertension. It is prudent to periodically reevaluate these patients with special attention to emerging cardiopulmonary disease. No drug has been shown to alter the disease course in limited disease; however, there are drugs that improve organ function or help alleviate the complications of tissue injury.

In *diffuse cutaneous scleroderma*, the natural course of disease is generally aggressive in the early years, with rapidly changing skin involvement and development of significant visceral disease, particularly in the gas-

**TABLE 30–1**
**Baseline Evaluation of the**
**Scleroderma Patient**

Complete history and physical examination with special attention to cardiopulmonary symptoms
Measurement of total body skin score, size of maximal oral aperture, patient global assessment
Routine laboratory work, including complete blood cell count, chemistries, urinalysis, muscle enzymes and thyroid function testing
Chest radiograph, electrocardiogram, complete pulmonary function testing with diffusing capacity, 2-D echocardiography

trointestinal tract, lung, heart, and kidney. (For more detail, see Kelley et al., *Textbook of Rheumatology*, Chapter 66.[1a]) After approximately 1 to 3 years, the patient may "stabilize" to a very indolent course and gradual deterioration of a damaged organ. In some patients the disease seems to wax and wane, and some patients improve. Improvement of the skin changes is common during this period of stabilization. In the active or early stage of diffuse disease, it is appropriate to consider treatment with "disease-modifying" drugs. Patients with advanced skin thickening may or may not be treatable; patients who have begun a spontaneous regression of the skin symptoms can be monitored without specific drug treatment. It is a major challenge in scleroderma to differentiate active, progressive disease from stable damage and loss of function. Scleroderma experts are developing activity and severity scores along with methods to determine functional status. These tools will provide methods to guide and assess management. Currently, there are no scleroderma-specific laboratory measurements that are available to clearly define disease activity. All patients should be sequentially evaluated for visceral involvement and then considered for organ-specific treatment.

## RATIONALE FOR TREATMENT APPROACH

The current understanding of scleroderma suggests that there is a complex interplay among at least four different biologic processes that are prominent in the disease: inflammation, an autoimmune process, fibrosis, and a chronic noninflammatory small-vessel vasculopathy. (For more detail, see Kelley et al., *Textbook of Rheumatology*, Chapter 66.[1a]) Each of these processes is a potential target for therapeutic intervention. Current therapy has focused primarily on preventing or reversing fibrosis or controlling the immune system. Numerous drugs have been tried in the treatment of scleroderma, mostly in small numbers of patients or in open and uncontrolled trials. There is no drug that is generally accepted as helpful, and none has proved useful in a rigorous controlled trial. Therefore the risks and benefits of almost all of the drugs that have been used

as disease modifying agents in scleroderma remain unknown.

For several reasons, research into the drug treatment of scleroderma has been less than ideal.[2] First, the pathogenesis of scleroderma is yet unsolved; therefore, the rationale for medications currently used is often theoretical rather than proven. Most academic research centers do not treat a large enough number of patients for a definitive clinical trial. There are also different subsets of scleroderma, each with its own unique clinical course and probably unique response to treatment. In addition, the course of the disease is highly variable, with periods of waxing and waning activity. Fibrosis and tissue atrophy dominate the final stages of scleroderma and may not respond to treatment. Many trials have chosen an inappropriate outcome variable or have not lasted long enough to determine the usefulness of the agent being tested. Therefore clinical trials in scleroderma need to select a large enough uniform population of patients who have the potential for recovery. Combination therapy with agents that address more than one of the known biologic processes in scleroderma may ultimately be necessary.

From a practical standpoint, many of the distressing symptoms of scleroderma can be improved with organ-specific therapy, including Raynaud's phenomenon, cardiopulmonary disease, musculoskeletal pain, symptoms of gastrointestinal disease, and emotional stress.

## DRUGS USED AS DISEASE-MODIFYING AGENTS IN SCLERODERMA

Excellent reviews of the drugs used in the treatment of scleroderma have been published.[2–4] This section highlights agents that are currently used in the treatment of scleroderma, recognizing that no drug has been proven to change the natural course of the disease.

### D-Penicillamine

(For more detail see Kelley et al., *Textbook of Rheumatology*, Chapter 46.[1a])

D-Penicillamine was first thought to be useful in scleroderma because of its ability to alter maturation of collagen by decreasing intermolecular cross-linking of collagen, increasing soluble collagen, and inhibiting collagen biosynthesis, thus thinning the skin. It continues to be used in the treatment of scleroderma despite the lack of a randomized, placebo-controlled trial to prove its efficacy or to define the appropriate dose and duration of therapy.

A trial involving 134 patients with early (less than 18 months) diffuse scleroderma compared low-dose (62.5 mg/day) with high-dose (750–1000 mg/day) D-penicillamine. The modified Rodnan skin score was not different at 24 months between the two treatment groups. The incidence of scleroderma renal crisis and mortality also was not different.[5] Eighty percent of the adverse reactions occurred in the high-dose group.

Most of the data supporting the use of D-penicillamine suggest that it primarily improves the skin. However, if benefit is to be expected, it may not be noted for at least 6 months after the start of therapy, and therefore treatment should be directed toward early active disease. During this 6-month period, severe skin changes may occur, particularly facial changes and irreversible finger and hand contractures. Approximately two thirds of patients are reported to improve. Some investigators have suggested that this long interval before improvement is secondary to the long time necessary for skin remodeling to occur[3]; others have countered that the natural course in untreated patients shows the same gradual improvement.

Steen and colleagues[6] reported a retrospective review, one of the first large, uncontrolled experiences with D-penicillamine in which only patients with diffuse disease were treated. Seventy-three patients who had received the drug for at least 6 months (mean, 24 months; range, 6 to 68 months) were compared with 45 patients who for various reasons were not treated with the drug. The patients treated with D-penicillamine had a greater decrease in skin thickness, less new visceral involvement (primarily renal disease), and a greater 5-year survival rate than the untreated group (88% atrophic or inactive disease). Some may consider D-penicillamine for treatment of active scleroderma lung disease or other internal organ involvement, but the data as to whether it has any significant role for visceral disease are inconclusive.

D-Penicillamine should be started at 125 or 250 mg/day. The daily dose can be increased at intervals of 6 weeks to 3 months by increments of 250 mg. The maximal dose is 1000 mg/day. The dose should not be increased if the patient shows improvement or if potential toxicity is suspected. The maximal dose should be maintained for a minimum of 6 months after there is no further improvement and then tapered. Although specific data are not available to determine the maintenance dose or duration, it is recommended that a dose of 250 mg/day be continued unless toxicity occurs or a long remission is established.

D-Penicillamine should be carefully monitored for toxicity. Not all toxicity is related to dose; some toxic effects occur early in therapy (rash, proteinuria) and others late in the course of treatment (autoimmune disease). It is recommended that clinical and laboratory parameters be monitored, first at 2-week intervals and then monthly until a stable maximum dose is established. Once a stable dose is established, the patient should be seen and laboratory data should be obtained at intervals of 1 to 2 months. A complete blood cell count looking for leukopenia and thrombocytopenia and a urinalysis should be done at each safety visit. If protein or abnormal sediment is detected on urinalysis, then the drug should be stopped and a 24-hour urine sample collected to quantitate the total protein excretion. Mild proteinuria of less than 500 mg/24 hours can be tolerated and the drug can be continued with careful serial assessment of renal function and proteinuria. Any worsening would dictate discontinuation of drug, with no rechallenge. Proteinuria usually occurs

after 3 months of therapy; it most commonly is secondary to an immune complex–mediated membranous nephropathy and is reversible with discontinuation of the drug. In rare cases, rapidly progressive glomerulonephritis occurs.[9] Long-term monitoring should be done to detect proteinuria, cytopenias, and the late onset of autoimmune diseases such as myasthenia gravis, pemphigus, myositis, and lupus-like reactions.

In summary, some scleroderma experts are currently using D-penicillamine in early disease when cutaneous disease is the dominant clinical problem. Although it has been suggested that D-penicillamine may be helpful for internal organ involvement and may improve survival, the data are not conclusive. The controlled trial of low-dose versus high-dose D-penicillamine[5] has dampened enthusiasm for this drug as a treatment option in scleroderma, and, given its significant toxicity, we can no longer recommend it.

## Colchicine

Initial uncontrolled trials of colchicine reported disappointing results.[10, 11] However, a randomized, double-blind, crossover trial of 1 mg/day of colchicine versus placebo for 3 months was conducted in 1979 and suggested some benefit.[12] Despite the lack of objective measurable changes, 9 of the 14 patients who completed the trial believed they had improved while taking colchicine. These same investigators then entered patients into a long-term, uncontrolled trial of colchicine.[13] Nineteen patients took an average dose of 10.1 mg of colchicine per week for an average of 39 months. Patients who were less than 5 years into the course of their disease showed improvement or stability in subjective measures of skin elasticity, measures of grip strength, fingertip-to-palm distance, mouth opening, dysphagia, and pulmonary function testing. A placebo-controlled crossover trial of 28 patients treated with 2 mg/day of colchicine versus placebo for 9 months failed to confirm that colchicine was beneficial to skin or visceral involvement.[14] All studies to date have had major study design problems, and therefore the role of colchicine in the treatment of scleroderma is unknown. We do not recommend the use of colchicine.

## Potassium Para-aminobenzoic Acid

In both normal and scleroderma dermal fibroblasts, potassium para-aminobenzoic acid (PABA) inhibits glycoaminoglycan production.[15] However, there has been no evidence that PABA inhibits collagen synthesis. Zarafonetis and associates[16] reported their uncontrolled experience with PABA in 224 patients with scleroderma. Of the patients treated with PABA, 90% showed a mild to moderate improvement while taking PABA, 8 to 12 g/day for 8 to 24 months, whereas of 96 patients who were not treated with PABA, only 19% showed similar improvement. PABA-treated patients had less progression of lung involvement and increased survival when compared with the untreated group. The first large, double-blind, placebo-controlled trial found no improvement in skin mobility or skin thickening in patients treated with PABA compared with those given placebo.[17] PABA cannot be recommended in the treatment of scleroderma.

## Dimethyl Sulfoxide

Dimethyl sulfoxide (DMSO) has been reported to be an analgesic, a vasodilator, an anti-inflammatory agent, and a cytoprotective agent. Although there are a number of uncontrolled studies suggesting some benefit of topical DMSO, the overall experience is controversial, and therefore the use of DMSO cannot be recommended in the treatment of scleroderma. Scherbel[18] reported some modest benefit in terms of grip strength and skin softening after the application of 50% to 70% topical DMSO, whereas Binnick and colleagues[19] found no benefit in skin induration, ischemic ulcers, or range of motion in 20 patients treated for 3 to 15 months. The largest double-blind study found no benefit for healing of digital ulcers, and no study has demonstrated any benefit for visceral involvement.[19] Some analgesic effect on painful digital ulcers may occur with topical DMSO; however, a number of severe skin reactions were reported with the use of the 70% solution.[20] DMSO cannot be recommended for the treatment of scleroderma.

## Interferon

In vitro studies demonstrate that interferon gamma and interferon alpha can inhibit collagen production by fibroblasts, and they may have important effects on the immune system.[21] Uncontrolled open-label studies in small numbers of patients suggested that interferon gamma given subcutaneously improved skin score.[22] Renal crisis and significant flu-like symptoms were associated with interferon therapy. A small (n = 8), controlled trial of interferon gamma found no difference between active drug and placebo.[23] Interferon alpha was used in 19 patients with diffuse scleroderma.[24] This study reported unimpressive (10%) improvement in skin score and a sense of overall improvement in 50%. The results of a randomized, double-blind, placebo-controlled trial of 35 patients with diffuse scleroderma found greater improvement in skin score and less deterioration in lung function in the placebo-treated group compared with those given interferon.[25] Although the data are limited, we do not recommend interferon therapy in scleroderma and have major concern about the potential vascular toxicity of these agents.

## Relaxin

Relaxin is a polypeptide that inhibits collagen and increases collagenase production by dermal and scleroderma fibroblasts. In animal models it decreases fibrosis of the skin and lung.[26, 27] A open-label study of a continuous subcutaneous infusion of recombinant relaxin found improved skin scores over 6 months of treatment.[28] A controlled trial of recombinant relaxin at 25 µg/kg/day in 68 patients with diffuse scleroderma

found a significant improvement in skin score (−8.7 ± 1.0) compared with placebo (−4.9 ± 1.4).[29] Relaxin is still an investigational agent, and more studies are planned to pursue its role in the treatment of scleroderma.

## Immunosuppressive Agents

Autoantibody production and the presence of inflammatory cellular infiltrates suggest that scleroderma is an autoimmune inflammatory disease. A number of therapies have been designed to target components of the immune system. Most of these studies have been uncontrolled trials and have mixed patients with both limited and diffuse disease or patients at various stages of disease. It is difficult to make a judgment about immunosuppressive therapy, but in general these agents have been disappointing for the treatment of progressive skin disease.

The use of corticosteroids has not been completely studied. However, it is the general impression that corticosteroids do not influence the course of scleroderma. A case control study discouraged the use of high-dose corticosteroids (15 mg or more per day of prednisone) in early diffuse scleroderma because of an associated increased risk of developing scleroderma renal crisis.[30] Corticosteroids should be used only when patients have a specific organ problem that may be responsive, such as inflammatory myositis or an unresponsive polyarthritis (see later discussion). Topical corticosteroids have been used on the skin for localized scleroderma (e.g., morphea) or during the early edematous, pruritic stage of scleroderma when skin is rapidly worsening.

Chlorambucil is an alkylating agent with immunosuppressive properties. An unblinded trial of chlorambucil in 11 patients with scleroderma suggested some benefit,[31] whereas another trial in 21 patients reported no effect.[32] Furst and colleagues[33] conducted a 3-year parallel, double-blind, placebo-controlled trial of chlorambucil in 65 patients with scleroderma. Although the chlorambucil-treated group had evidence of immunosuppression manifested by decreases in leukocyte, lymphocyte, and platelet counts compared with the control group, the drug had no clinical advantage over placebo in terms of skin score or internal organ involvement.

Azathioprine was studied in an open, uncontrolled trial involving 21 patients with various forms and stages of scleroderma for an average of 14 months' follow-up.[34] A starting dose of 150 mg/day was used and was adjusted during the trial to a maximum of 250 mg/day. Eight patients were subjectively improved, seven were judged unchanged, two progressed, and one was lost to follow-up. Judgment on the role of azathioprine cannot be made on the basis of this study, and azathioprine is not recommended.

5-Fluorouracil (5-FU) was found to soften fibrotic skin when applied topically and to improve the skin in a patient with scleroderma when used as part of a chemotherapeutic program for breast cancer. Twelve patients with scleroderma, in an open-label, uncontrolled trial of 5-FU, demonstrated improvement in skin scores (mean total score increased from 36 to 22) and in visceral involvement.[35] An additional international collaborative study randomly assigned patients with scleroderma to receive either 5-FU or placebo.[36] The 5-FU was given in a dose of 12 mg/kg/day for 4 days, then 6 mg/kg for 2 days, followed by weekly doses of 12.5 mg/kg for a total of 6 months. Mild improvement in skin score was found in those receiving 5-FU compared with the placebo group, but there was no effect on internal organ involvement. It does not appear that 5-FU is very helpful in scleroderma, and it cannot be recommended.

Methotrexate (MTX) has been used in uncontrolled trials in the treatment of scleroderma. The rationale is the potential anti-inflammatory and immunosuppressive effects of MTX and the success of this agent in the management of other autoimmune diseases. (For more detail see Kelley et al., *Textbook of Rheumatology,* Chapter 47.[1a]) One unblinded study used a dosage of MTX of 15 mg/week given intramuscularly for the first 6 months and then orally thereafter.[37] Seven of the eight patients had a 25% improvement in skin score but no significant visceral improvement. A placebo-controlled, double-blind trial was reported in patients with early or progressive disease.[38] Seventeen patients were assigned to receive MTX 15 mg intramuscularly per week and 12 to receive placebo. After 24 weeks, 53% of patients receiving MTX had improved, compared with 10% of the placebo group. Another multicenter, placebo-controlled trial of MTX in early diffuse scleroderma reported some trends in favor of MTX, but none reached statistical significance.[39] The differences between the groups were not clinically impressive. The role of MTX in the treatment of scleroderma is unresolved, but MTX probably should be limited to the treatment of steroid-resistant active polymyositis or difficult-to-treat polyarthritis.

Cyclosporine was reported to be helpful in an open study of eight patients with scleroderma.[40] Skin score improved at 6 months, and four patients had improvement in baseline hypoxia. However, a reduction of renal function was reported in four patients in the trial. It has also been reported that a patient with scleroderma and a renal transplant developed rapid renal failure during immunosuppressive therapy that included cyclosporine.[41] In a 48-week open safety study of cyclosporine in 10 scleroderma patients, Clements and associates[42] found that skin score improved in all of the 10 patients and significantly improved (greater than 35%) in 6, whereas cardiac and pulmonary organ involvement remained stable. This improvement in the skin was significant in comparison with an historical control group. However, there was frequent dose-related and usually transient renal toxicity. FK 506, a drug with properties similar to cyclosporine, is also being used in the treatment of scleroderma. Steen reported benefit in 10 patients, but there was significant toxicity.[43] We hesitate to recommend cyclosporine or FK 506 because of potential renal toxicity, but we recognize that in difficult situations low-dose cyclosporine

can be used with very careful monitoring of blood pressure and renal function.

Total lymphoid irradiation (TLI) has been used in immunosuppressive therapy for scleroderma.[44] The rationale for using TLI has been supported by its reported use in rheumatoid arthritis and systemic lupus erythematosus. Six scleroderma patients were randomly assigned to receive either TLI or no therapy. Despite good evidence of immunosuppression, there was no clinical benefit. Of note was the fact that severe pulmonary and gastrointestinal progression was reported in the patients treated with TLI.

Antithymocyte globulin has been used because of the postulated central role of T cells in the pathogenesis of scleroderma. One patient with aplastic anemia and scleroderma-like syndrome was treated daily for 10 days with 15 mg/kg body weight.[45] The skin sclerosis improved and remained better after 5 months of follow-up. The same investigators treated two patients with scleroderma and reported a decrease in palpable skin induration and improvement in pulmonary function in both patients.[46] A randomized trial of intravenous saline solution versus antithymocyte globulin was reported in abstract.[47] Six months after treatment skin score and lung function were not altered by treatment. Significant side effects, including fever and serum sickness, occurred during antithymocyte treatment.

Extracorporeal photopheresis (ECP) has been used to treat T cell–dependent disorders, including cutaneous T-cell lymphoma, pemphigus, and graft-versus-host disease. Its use in scleroderma is based on the hypothesis that the inflammation and subsequent fibrosis in scleroderma are mediated by T cells. A multicenter, single-blind trial of ECP versus D-penicillamine in early diffuse scleroderma was reported in 1992.[48] The investigators reported that ECP was marginally more beneficial than D-penicillamine at 6 months but there was no difference at 10 months. The reported benefit of ECP was limited to the skin, without significant effects in other organ systems. Extracorporeal photopheresis is costly, and there were a number of study design flaws (including an unexplained differential drop-out rate in the two treatment arms) that do not permit conclusions to be drawn from the report. We do not recommend photopheresis in the treatment of scleroderma.

Autologous stem cell transplantation is being studied in both the United States and Europe. The rationale is that bone marrow ablation will eliminate autoreactive cells and the marrow will reconstitute without autoimmunity.[49] We believe that any patient who might be considered for this type of treatment (i.e., patients with aggressive, diffuse disease with evidence of reversible visceral involvement) should be referred to experienced academic centers doing this research.

## Other Agents

Several additional agents and therapeutic approaches have been reported in the treatment of scleroderma. However, the data, although of interest, are inconclusive and the use of these therapies cannot be recommended. Some of these agents are minocycline,[50] factor XIII,[51, 52] isotretinoin,[53] griseofulvin,[54] plasma exchange,[55, 56] disodium edetate (EDTA),[57, 58] N-acetylcysteine,[59] cyclofenil,[60] dextran infusion,[61] and ketotifen.[62]

## FUTURE APPROACHES

The future is exciting for the development of new therapies for scleroderma. Investigations into the pathogenesis of scleroderma have suggested that specific cytokines are important mediators of fibrosis. Therapy that inhibits the production or interferes with the function of specific cytokines may target a key factor that provokes the fibroblast and promotes the propagation of tissue fibrosis. Inhibitors of transforming growth factor-$\beta$ is one example of this type of approach.[63] Understanding of the molecular mechanisms of gene regulation, cytokine production, and collagen production by fibroblasts may reveal methods to control the activation of the tissue fibroblast.

Rather than using global immunosuppressive drugs, targeting of specific immune cells or targeting of the ability of inflammatory and immune cells to traffic into target tissues may be an effective approach. Examples of this approach include inhibitors of key adhesion molecules that are upregulated in the tissues and on the vascular endothelium of scleroderma patients, inhibition of specific autoreactive T-cell clones, and regulation of antigen-processing cells.

A fundamental understanding of the chronic vasculopathy that is so widespread and prominent in scleroderma is a major key to developing effective new treatments. Control of abnormal vascular reactivity and vascular occlusion is difficult without reversing the basic pathologic process and fibrosis of the blood vessel. Prevention of tissue ischemia and reperfusion tissue injury is yet another major puzzle to unravel in scleroderma. Potential approaches include vasodilator therapy, prevention of coagulation, fibrinolysis therapy, interference with cell trafficking by blockade of important adhesion molecules, and the use of antioxidants to reduce tissue damage.

## THE AUTHORS' APPROACH

Most of the drugs that have been studied as disease-modifying agents in scleroderma have focused on the skin as the major important outcome variable. Certainly, skin involvement is the most obvious problem to the scleroderma patient, particularly early in the disease. However, the systemic-visceral disease often dominates later treatment decisions, as these effects emerge as clinically important and potential life-threatening problems. One should also recognize that the placebo arm of several studies has demonstrated that the skin (and visceral) effects can remain quite stable or improve after the initial insult of active disease.[64] The treatment approach must be comprehensive without focusing solely on the skin. It must also

recognize both the shortcomings and the toxicity of currently available drugs. Aggressive use of experimental therapies in the stable patient or the patient with limited disease is not indicated.

The fact that no available drug has been proven to alter the natural course of the disease makes us choose carefully whom we consider for a therapeutic trial. First, we use potential disease-modifying drugs only in patients with diffuse skin disease who are in an active phase and demonstrate significant progression over a 1- to 2-month period of observation. We recognize that therapy directed toward specific organ dysfunction (see later discussion) can improve the quality of the patient's life and be more important than potentially toxic or experimental drugs of unknown benefit. If the patient has significant joint or muscle disease, then low-dose weekly MTX is used. In the patient with active alveolitis (see later discussion), we use daily oral cyclophosphamide. Patients who only have continued evidence of skin progression and who do not have treatment programs dictated by specific organ involvement (see later discussion) are considered for experimental treatment on either an open or controlled protocol. Some patients do not want to enter into a formal study. These patients are offered treatment with minocycline, D-penicillamine, low-dose MTX, or daily cyclophosphamide, depending on the situation. Corticosteroids are used as an adjunct only if there is a situation such as active myositis that warrants steroid use. We start an angiotensin-converting enzyme (ACE) inhibitor whenever possible in active diffuse scleroderma, because it may prevent a renal crisis and is likely to provide benefit by reducing fibroblast collagen production. All patients are treated for any specific organ disease, and almost every patient is treated aggressively to control Raynaud's phenomenon and, presumably, the vascular disease in other organs.

## ORGAN-SPECIFIC TREATMENT

### Management of Scleroderma Lung

Lung involvement is a major cause of morbidity and in recent years has replaced scleroderma renal crisis as the leading cause of mortality in scleroderma. Although the entities are not completely distinct, there are two major pulmonary processes (Fig. 30–1). Interstitial lung disease occurs predominantly in patients with diffuse scleroderma, and pulmonary vascular disease is seen in all subsets of scleroderma. Pulmonary hypertension is a consequence of severe interstitial fibrosis due to advanced vascular disease. Isolated pulmonary hypertension manifests in approximately 10% of patients with limited scleroderma. On initial evaluation and subsequent visits, scleroderma patients should be asked specifically about cardiopulmonary complaints: cough, exertional dyspnea, pedal edema, chest pain, orthopnea. At baseline, all patients regardless of symptoms should undergo chest radiography, complete pulmonary function testing (PFT), and two-dimensional echocardiography. Mild to moderate re-

**FIGURE 30–1**
Pulmonary symptoms or documented decline, or both, in pulmonary function tests.

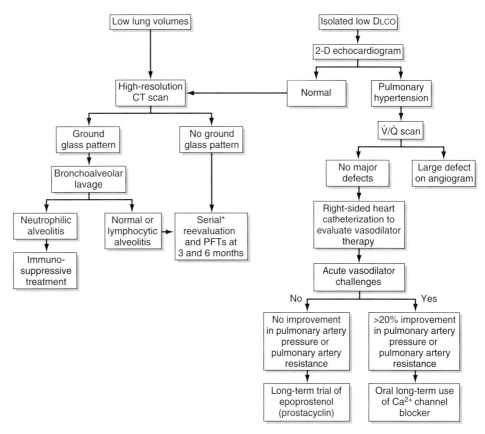

*Patients with normal two-dimensional (2-D) echocardiogram and severe symptoms with lung diffusing capacity for carbon monoxide (DLCO) less than 50% predicted who do not have evidence of alveolitis should be considered for right-sided heart catherization.

duction in total lung capacity (TLC), forced vital capacity (FVC), or diffusing capacity ($DL_{CO}$) may indicate active alveolitis even in the absence of symptoms. Echocardiography may be useful in detecting pulmonary hypertension.

Patients with severe interstitial lung disease complain of dyspnea on exertion and a nonproductive cough. Dry rales are heard on ascultation of the lung. Chest radiographs show diffuse fibrotic changes, and pulmonary function testing reveals a restrictive pattern with reduced FVC and reduction in $DL_{CO}$. Evidence correlating gallium scanning, bronchoalveolar lavage (BAL), and open lung biopsy has demonstrated that the pulmonary fibrosis is often preceded by a persistent inflammatory alveolitis.[65] The presence of an alveolitis correlates with progressive dyspnea and reductions in lung volume and $DL_{CO}$.[66] Patients with an active alveolitis should be considered for anti-inflammatory treatment and should be distinguished from patients who have stable, chronic, fibrotic lung changes.

Patients who have progressive pulmonary symptoms or progressive declines of greater than 10% in lung function on serial PFTs at 3-month intervals, suggestive of an active process, should undergo a high-resolution computed tomography (HRCT) scan. If a "ground-glass" pattern indicative of an alveolitis is seen on the HRCT scan,[67] BAL is then used as safe

and sensitive means to confirm and characterize the alveolitis.[68] If HRCT does not demonstrate an alveolitis, patients with progressive symptoms or declining PFTs should then undergo BAL despite the negative HRCT.

Although there is no uniformly agreed-upon therapeutic approach to the interstitial fibrosis of the lung in scleroderma, patients with deteriorating lung function and objective evidence by BAL of an active, neutrophilic alveolitis should be considered for aggressive treatment. An alveolitis is considered to be present if the number of cells in the BAL fluid exceeds the normal control values established for the reporting laboratory. Treatment in patients with a predominantly lymphocytic infiltrate is controversial; some suggest that the disease may follow a benign course in this subset of patients.[69] These patients, as well as those with normal BAL results, can be monitored by PFT at 3- to 6-month intervals.

One treatment approach has been the use of anti-inflammatory or immunosuppressive agents in the subset of patients with alveolitis. Corticosteroids have been used without clinical benefit[65] except in isolated case reports.[70, 71] Corticosteroids did not suppress the alveolitis in four scleroderma patients treated with prednisone 1 mg/kg/day for 1 to 1.5 months, tapering by 5 mg every 10 days to a baseline of 0.25 mg/kg/day.[65] Similarly, corticosteroids alone have had little effect in suppressing the neutrophilic alveolitis seen in idiopathic pulmonary fibrosis.[72, 73] The use of cyclophosphamide in addition to corticosteroids has been promising in both idiopathic pulmonary fibrosis[73] and scleroderma.[74] Prospectively, 14 scleroderma patients with moderately severe restrictive lung disease and evidence of alveolitis were treated with oral cyclophosphamide, 1 to 2 mg/kg/day, together with less than 10 mg/day of prednisone. Twelve patients showed either a stable or improved FVC and a stable $DL_{CO}$ at 18 to 24 months of follow-up.[74] An additional study of 18 patients treated with oral cyclophosphamide also showed benefit, particularly in those patients with elevated acute phase serum proteins.[75] Monthly intravenous cyclophosphamide (1 g) was found to be disappointing in a pilot study of five patients.[76] Although another study found no clinical benefit from chlorambucil, the investigators did not select for treatment patients who had an active alveolitis.[33]

It is recommended that the subset of patients with evidence on BAL of an active neutrophilic alveolitis be treated with a combination of prednisone and cyclophosphamide. Treatment is initiated with cyclophosphamide, 2 mg/kg/day orally, together with a dose of prednisone starting at 0.5 mg/kg/day and tapering to less than 10 mg daily within the first 6 to 8 weeks. Therapy is reevaluated with a repeal BAL and PFT at 6 months. If patients respond by an improvement in BAL and improvement or stabilization on PFT, treatment is continued for 1 year. The patient is then monitored by symptoms and PFT every 3 months. Should there be deterioration in PFT and recurrent symptoms associated with active alveolitis, therapy is reinstituted for an additional year. Other immunosuppressive regimens can be tried, but there are few data to give guidance. Patients need to understand that immunosuppressive therapy is not proven to be effective and is associated with significant potential risk. Patients treated with cyclophosphamide need to be monitored frequently, initially every 2 weeks, with a complete blood count and urinalysis and need to understand the risk of cyclophosphamide therapy.

Two studies limited by their retrospective designs showed modest benefit of D-penicillamine in scleroderma lung.[77, 78] However, the difference between treated and untreated groups was probably not clinically significant, nor were there any data on the subset of patients with active alveolitis and declining lung function. A recent double-blind, prospective study of low- and high-dose D-penicillamine showed no benefit for the lung.[5]

Although pulmonary artery hypertension is a frequent complication of the interstitial parenchymal lung changes, it is usually indolent in nature and less worrisome than the isolated pulmonary hypertension seen primarily in patients with limited scleroderma. Isolated pulmonary hypertension should be suspected in patients whose pulmonary complaints appear in the absence of evidence of interstitial fibrosis. All patients with pulmonary hypertension should also undergo an HRCT to evaluate for concomitant interstitial lung disease. It is difficult to detect mild-to-moderate pulmo-

nary hypertension by physical findings. Isolated pulmonary hypertension may be predicted by a $DL_{CO}$ lower than 55% of predicted and a ratio of FVC (% predicted) to $DL_{CO}$ (% predicted) greater than 1.4.[79] It is recommended that all patients with scleroderma who have cardiopulmonary symptoms or pulmonary function abnormalities have a Doppler echocardiogram to look for evidence of pulmonary hypertension. If significant pulmonary hypertension is present, a ventilation perfusion scan or spiral computed tomogram should be done to rule out pulmonary embolism, and a positive result should be confirmed by pulmonary angiography. Although pulmonary hypertension can result in indeterminate ventilation-perfusion abnormalities, defects causing significant pulmonary hypertension would be expected to be large. Thromboarterectomy has been used successfully in patients with pulmonary hypertension resulting from large pulmonary emboli.

Treatment of primary pulmonary hypertension (PPH) and pulmonary hypertension secondary to scleroderma is controversial, with no universally accepted regimens. Like patients with PPH, patients with pulmonary hypertension secondary to scleroderma should be treated with supplemental oxygen, diuretics, anticoagulation, vasodilator therapy, and, if medical therapy fails, heart-lung transplantation.[80]

Hypoxic pulmonary vasoconstriction occurs in both PPH and scleroderma,[81] and patients should undergo testing to look for resting and exercise-induced oxygen desaturation. In cases of significant desaturation, supplemental resting or ambulatory oxygen should be used. Anticoagulation, although not formally studied in the scleroderma population, has been demonstrated to significantly increase the survival rate in patients with PPH.[82] It is recommended that scleroderma patients with severe pulmonary hypertension and no contraindication for anticoagulation be treated with warfarin. Diuretics are used to treat the edema associated with right-sided heart failure.

Vasodilator therapy with calcium channel blockers, ACE inhibitors, and, more recently, intravenous prostacyclin analogs have been used for both scleroderma and PPH. In PPH, high doses of calcium channel blockers (mean daily dose of nifedipine, 172 mg; diltiazem, 720 mg) improved pulmonary artery pressures and survival.[83] Both acute and chronic administration of nifedipine (10 to 30 mg every 8 hours) to patients with CREST syndrome produced a significant reduction of pulmonary artery pressures.[84] The ACE inhibitor captopril has been disappointing in the treatment of PPH. High doses of ACE inhibitors can lower systemic blood pressure and thereby limit the doses of calcium channel blockers when used concomitantly. However, captopril reverses the renovascular complications of scleroderma, and in a small study of eight CREST patients with mild to moderate pulmonary hypertension captopril, 12.5 to 50 mg, reduced pulmonary artery pressures.[85] ACE inhibitors may benefit by improving secondary right-sided heart failure. Therefore, captopril should not be totally excluded from future studies on pulmonary hypertension secondary to scleroderma.

Treatment of PPH with the intravenous prostacyclin (epoprostenol, prostaglandin $I_2$), chronically infused through a portable pump, improves the hemodynamic and symptomatic responses,[86, 87] improves survival,[88] and has sustained efficacy.[89] It is currently approved in the United States for use in PPH. However, acute administration of a synthetic, more stable prostacylin analog, iloprost, failed to improve $DL_{CO}$ in patients with scleroderma.[90] Additional studies of limited numbers of patients showed an improvement in exercise tolerance in PPH[91] and scleroderma.[92] A study of 111 scleroderma patients with pulmonary hypertension showed improvement in exercise tolerance, hemodynamics, dyspena, and Raynaud's severity when treated with continuous intravenous epoprostenol compared with conventional therapy.[93]

Symptomatic patients with evidence of pulmonary hypertension and pulmonary artery pressures of 40 mm Hg are considered eligible for a trial of vasodilator therapy. They should be hospitalized for monitoring and right-sided heart catheterization. During catherization a vasodilator is administered (e.g., calcium channel blocker, epoprostenol, nitric oxide, adenosine). If benefit is seen, with 20% fall in pulmonary artery pressure or pulmonary artery resistance, therapy is instituted with short-acting preparations of nifedipine, with doses titrated according to systemic blood pressure, pulmonary artery pressure, and cardiac output. Systemic hypotension, increased right-sided heart failure, and negative inotropy are frequent complications limiting therapy. Patients who respond are maintained on nifedipine over a long term and are monitored clinically. Other calcium channel blockers such as diltiazem, nicardipine, and amlodipine may also be tried. Patients failing acute administration of calcium channel blockers are given a trial of intravenous prostacyclin and considered for long-term continous infusion. However, unlike therapy with calcium channel blockers, lack of hemodynamic improvement with acute administration of prostacyclin does not predict lack of long-term response. We do not recommend corticosteroids or immunosuppressive therapy for pulmonary hypertension in the absence of an active alveolitis. It should also be noted that in the subset of patients with pulmonary hypertension secondary to interstitial lung disease, vasodilator therapy may worsen lung function because of the reversal of shunting from poorly ventilated lung. Lung transplantation has been undertaken successfully in patients with scleroderma and appears to be as efficacious as in those patients with diseases limited to the lung.[94]

Pleural reactions are a common finding but are usually clinically silent. When active pleuritis is present, other causes should be considered. A short course of a nonsteroidal anti-inflammatory drug is usually effective. All scleroderma patients with lung involvement should be given both influenza and pneumococcal vaccines. They should be treated with antibiotics at the first signs of purulent bronchitis or pulmonary infection.

In the long term, aspiration may be clinically important, even in patients without severe myositis and pharyngeal muscle involvement. Patients with reflux symptoms should be treated aggressively (see Management of the Gastrointestinal Tract). Nocturnal wakenings caused by choking or shortness of breath, recurrent pneumonias, recent onset of hoarseness, and unexplained bronchospasm are suggestive of chronic aspiration. The incidence of carcinoma of the lung has been reported to be increased in patients with scleroderma. However, the risk is not sufficient to recommend increased surveillance in the absence of clinical suspicion and other risk factors.

## Management of the Gastrointestinal Tract

Involvement of the gastrointestinal tract in scleroderma is almost universal, but the severity of the clinical problem is highly variable and generally unpredictable. A vasculopathy or muscular atrophy with fibrosis causes neuromuscular dysfunction throughout the gastrointestinal tract and, as a consequence, a loss of normal coordinated motility. No therapeutic intervention has been shown to prevent or alter the natural course of the gastrointestinal involvement.

Facial scleroderma can make chewing difficult, and a small oral aperture often precludes normal dental care. In addition, hand deformities, muscle weakness, and disease of the temporomandibular joint may all complicate care of the mouth and accelerate caries and loss of teeth. Adaptive devices such as an electric toothbrush are helpful, and more frequent dental visits for cleaning and surveillance are prudent. Dry mucous membranes (the sicca syndrome) are frequent in scleroderma and may dampen normal taste and appetite and complicate dental care (see Chapter 21). Frequent small meals and avoidance of large, difficult-to-chew foods are wise. Some patients require liquid supplements to maintain adequate caloric intake.

Dysphagia is caused by distal esophageal dysmotility. Patients who have difficulty initiating a swallow or who have regurgitation of food into the upper airway may have a superimposed neuromuscular disease such as D-penicillamine–induced myasthenia gravis or polymyositis affecting the striated muscles of the oral pharynx.

A high prevalence of esophagitis is present in patients with scleroderma as a result of abnormal motility and decreased acid clearance from the esophagus.[95] Esophageal disease may be associated with ulceration, blood loss, stricture, and, in rare cases, Barrett's esophagus (predisposing to carcinoma). Therefore, patients with a diagnosis of scleroderma should be evaluated aggressively for esophageal disease. Treatment is directed at symptomatic disease or the complications of abnormal esophageal motility. However, patients may be without symptoms and yet develop significant esophageal disease. Patients with normal motility studies rarely have esophagitis.[95] A barium swallow is useful to rule out esophageal stricture but is insensitive as a measurement of dysmotility. Ideally, every patient with a diagnosis of scleroderma should have a motility study by either cine-esophagography or manometry. If these studies are abnormal, then endoscopy should be done, even if the patient does not have symptoms. In practice, patients may be treated empirically as long as symptoms of reflux or dysphagia are controlled. Those who fail a therapeutic trial or have signs of gastrointestinal blood loss should have motility studies or endoscopy. The presence of esophagitis warrants aggressive therapy and careful follow-up to document healing. Because symptoms may not correlate directly with the degree of reflux or with resolution of the esophagitis, the decision to do gastrointestinal studies is based on the overall status of the patient and on laboratory parameters.

The treatment of gastrointestinal reflux disease (GERD) and esophagitis in scleroderma is the same as in idiopathic GERD. Nondrug treatment should include avoidance of meals before bedtime, elevation of the head of the bed, eating small frequent meals, avoidance of tightly fitting clothing, discontinuation of smoking, and avoidance of certain foods such as fatty meals or chocolate. Calcium channel blockers, often used for Raynaud's phenomenon, can aggravate gastrointestinal reflux by decreasing lower esophageal sphincter tone. Medications that can cause esophagitis (e.g., alendronate, nonsteroidal anti-inflammatory drugs) should be avoided.

Drug therapy for GERD includes neutralizing the gastric acid and improving esophageal and gastric motility with a prokinetic drug. Antacids or histamine (H$_2$) receptor blockers[96] are not recommended as sole therapy because they are not as effective as the proton pump inhibitors. Most patients benefit from the use of omeprazole (20 to 80 mg daily) or lansoprazole (15 to 60 mg) alone. Omeprazole or lansoprazole inhibits the activity of H$^+$, K$^+$-ATPase and dramatically inhibits gastric acid, thus promoting healing of refractory esophagitis. Although it is recommended that patients rest from omeprazole or lansoprazole periodically, most patients with scleroderma require continuous therapy. Long-term use greatly improves the quality of life in scleroderma patients and thus far there has been no evidence for an increase in gastric tumors in humans. Careful follow-up analysis documenting resolved symptoms or repeat endoscopic examination is recommended because the esophagitis of scleroderma may be resistant to treatment.

Studies show that promotility drugs improve esophageal and gastric emptying if used early in scleroderma, before advanced fibrosis and muscle atrophy occur. Metoclopramide and cisapride have been reported to be helpful in scleroderma.[97–100] Cisapride had been preferable to metoclopramide because it has less central nervous system toxicity, increases esophageal contractions, and improves gastric emptying. The effect of cisapride on lower esophageal sphincter pressure in scleroderma is controversial.[99, 100] Horowitz and coworkers reported significant improvement in gastric emptying after 10 mg by mouth four times daily but no definite effect on esophageal emptying.[98] Cisapride can be tried by starting at 10 to 20 mg 30 to 60 minutes before meals and at bedtime. Although objective documentation of improved motility would be ideal, improvement of symptoms is generally reasonable

as a measure of drug effectiveness. Serious cardiac arrhythmias have been associated with the use of cisapride, particularly if it is used with other drugs that inhibit the cytochrome P450 enzyme (erythromycin, clarithromycin, ketoconazole, fluconazole, and other drugs of the imidazole class). Caution should be taken if the patient has scleroderma, heart disease, and arrhythmias. Metoclopramide should not be continued without clear evidence of clinical benefit. (Editors Note: Cisapride was withdrawn from the US market in April 2000 by the Food and Drug Administration due to cardiac arrhythmias.)

Patients who with combination therapy continue to have reflux symptoms, dysphagia, or weight loss should be restudied to assess whether esophagitis or stricture is present and to determine whether the motility problem is reversible. Another prokinetic drug is erythromycin, a motilin receptor agonist. Intravenous erythromycin (150 mg) has been shown in scleroderma patients to lower esophageal pressure and improve gastric (fundi) waves, suggesting that it may be helpful in reflux disease or gastroparesis.[101] It is recommended that a small dose of erythromycin (25 mg 1 hour before meals) be tried if metoclopramide is not helpful. It should not be added to metoclopramide.

Feeding tubes bypassing esophageal strictures or severe gastroparesis can be tried. However, scleroderma patients with severe gastrointestinal disease often have significant small-bowel aperistalsis, and tube feeding usually is not successful. Surgical repair has been reported to be successful in the treatment of esophageal strictures,[102] but patients with scleroderma have less success from surgical therapy of GERD because of the profound loss of distal esophagus peristalsis. Patients can be managed with periodic endoscope-guided dilatation. Barrett's esophagus is best treated with aggressive treatment of reflux. Laser therapy for Barrett's esophagus is now under study.

Delayed gastric emptying is frequently present and aggravates GERD, causes bloating and may lead to early satiety and weight loss. This problem is handled in the same way that GERD is managed, with the use of the prokinetic drug metoclopramide. A watermelon stomach secondary to ectasia of mucosal vessels occurs in scleroderma and can cause gastrointestinal bleeding. Treatment is best done by laser coagulation therapy during endoscopy.

Small-bowel involvement causes abnormal peristalsis that manifests itself clinically as intermittent distention and pain, alternating diarrhea and constipation, bouts of pseudo-obstruction, and, rarely, malnutrition from malabsorption secondary to bacterial overgrowth. Most patients tolerate mild symptoms and, in the absence of weight loss, need no specific therapy except a sensible diet and appropriate natural fiber intake. The prokinetic drugs metoclopramide or erythromycin may also improve intestinal transit and small-bowel motility in patients with pseudo-obstruction. Calcium channel blockers and narcotics may aggravate small-bowel motility problems and should be avoided in the problematic patient. If weight loss or signs of malnutrition are present despite a reasonable caloric intake, then an evaluation for malabsorption should be done. A comprehensive work-up may include fecal fat collection, a breath test to determine whether there is bacterial overgrowth, cultures of duodenal contents, and motility studies. However, a trial of cyclic intermittent antibiotics (2 to 3 weeks of each month) such as ampicillin, tetracycline, trimethoprim, ciprofloxacin, or metronidazole is reasonable in the patient with suspected or proven malabsorption. Caloric intake, number of bowel movements, and weight can be monitored. Proper replacement of calcium, iron, fat-soluble vitamins, vitamin $B_{12}$, and supplemental protein or medium-chain triglycerides may be necessary.

Octreotide, a synthetic octapeptide analog of somatostatin, has been reported in several cases to help patients with scleroderma-related intestinal pseudo-obstruction.[103] Octreotide is given as subcutaneous injections, 50 to 100 $\mu$g daily. Side effects include depression of normal feeding responses (therefore it should be given at nighttime) and hypoglycemia. The experience thus far has been limited to a few cases.[103] Our experience has been disappointing, without any long-term or consistent success.

Severe malabsorption or pseudo-obstruction that is unresponsive to medical management is treated with total parenteral nutrition (TPN).[104] These patients can be cycled onto feeding for 12 hours at night so that they are free for other activities during the day. Although long-term TPN may be necessary, some patients have significant improvement in bowel function after relatively short-term TPN. TPN should be continued until the patient has reached normal weight and nutritional status and can demonstrate adequate oral intake.

Acute episodes of pseudo-obstruction are best treated with bowel rest and decompression. Surgical resection of atonic sections of bowel has reportedly been successful in individual cases, but in general surgical resection is not helpful because of the widespread nature of the bowel disease. The rare complication of pneumatosis cystoides intestinalis and pneumoperitoneum is best treated conservatively with bowel decompression, oxygen therapy (70% to 100% inhaled oxygen), and antibiotics (metronidazole).[105, 106]

Colonic involvement is also common but usually asymptomatic.[107, 108] However, wide-mouthed diverticula may rupture, causing a bowel crisis and peritonitis. Colonic volvulus with or without stricture can mimic pseudo-obstruction. Endoscopic decompression of the volvulus or surgical repair of a stricture can be lifesaving. Scleroderma involving the colon or anorectal area may cause distention, constipation, diarrhea, or incontinence. Most cases can be managed with administration of a synthetic fiber such as Metamucil to increase the stool bulk and yet maintain a soft stool. Low doses of diphenoxylate hydrochloride with atropine sulfate (Lomotil) or loperamide hydrochloride (Imodium) may be used to control diarrhea. Caution should be taken with these agents or narcotics that can precipitate atonic bowel or pseudo-obstruction. Surgical correction of rectal prolapse has been reported to improve incontinence, but the surgery may be difficult because of local tissue fibrosis.

Primary biliary cirrhosis is the main hepatic disease that is found in a small subset of patients with limited scleroderma. The associated pruritus may respond to cholestyramine or colestipol. Ursodeoxycholic acid may slow the progressive cirrhosis.[109] Scleroderma patients are candidates for liver transplantation if necessary.

## Management of Kidney Involvement

Since the first description of the use of captopril to treat renal crisis in 1979,[110, 111] ACE inhibitors have revolutionized the management of scleroderma kidney. The use of captopril or the long-acting ACE inhibitor enalapril rapidly controls blood pressure and stabilizes renal function.[112, 113] Efficacy of the other ACE inhibitors (lisinopril, ramipril, fosinopril, and benazepril) and of the angiotension II receptor antagonists, losartan and candesartan, has not been reported except for one case report of a failure with losartan.[114] Hypertension in scleroderma, particularly new-onset hypertension in patients with diffuse scleroderma, should be considered a medical emergency. Patients suspected of a renal crisis should have laboratory checkup including urinalysis, electrolytes, serum creatinine, complete blood count, and blood smear to determine if there is evidence of a renal crisis. Rapid control of blood pressure is best done in the hospital setting if scleroderma renal crisis is evident. Therapy with ACE inhibitors should be instituted in all patients who have any hypertension (blood pressure higher than 140/90), particularly in the presence of renal insufficiency. Because the onset of hypertension and renal insufficiency can be rapidly progressive, particularly in patients with diffuse skin involvement, patients should be told to purchase a home blood pressure monitor and to monitor blood pressure on a weekly basis. It is the general impression that early treatment of mild or modest hypertension with ACE inhibitors has dramatically reduced the incidence of renal crisis. Hypertension in the absence of a renal crisis should be treated with small doses of either captopril (12.5 mg three times a day) or enalapril (2.5 mg daily). Patients with evidence of scleroderma renal crisis should be hospitalized and treated aggressively with the short-acting agent, captopril (Table 30–2). Patients with hypertension who cannot take an ACE inhibitor should be treated with a calcium channel blocker either alone or in combination with other antihypertensive medications.

Patients who are intravascularly volume depleted are particularly susceptible to ACE inhibitor–induced hypotension. Therefore, patients taking diuretics and other vasodilators should be monitored carefully for hypotension. Blood pressure, renal function, and potassium level should be monitored carefully during therapy in all patients.

Helfrich and associates[115] reviewed the records of 131 patients encountered over 33 years who presented with acute renal failure thought to be caused by scleroderma. Of these patients, 11% had normal recorded

**TABLE 30–2**
**Treatment of Scleroderma Renal Crisis**

Definition of renal crisis: Diastolic pressure of 110 mm Hg or greater with at least two of the following: hemolytic anemia, or rapidly changing renal function
Patients should be hospitalized emergently and monitored closely
Start a short-acting angiotensin-converting enzyme inhibitor, captopril, at 25 mg every hour until blood pressure is controlled; maximum dosage of captopril is 450 mg daily
Toxicities: hypotension, proteinuria, neutropenia, agranulocytosis, anemia, pancytopenia, dysgeusia, dermatitis, cough, angioedema, and hyperkalemia

blood pressure, atypical for scleroderma renal crisis. The normotensive group had more microangiopathic hemolytic anemia, thrombocytopenia, pulmonary hemorrhage, and recent prior corticosteroid use than the hypertensive group. Although the mechanism in normotensive renal failure is unclear, some postulate that administration of ACE inhibitors improves outcome. In patients with scleroderma who present with increasing renal dysfunction and normal blood pressure, other causes of renal insufficiency should be investigated, particularly drug toxicities and prerenal causes. Nonsteroidal medications should be stopped and corticosteroid use curtailed if possible. If no other cause of the renal insufficiency is found, then judicious use of ACE inhibitors can be tried with careful monitoring of renal function and systemic blood pressure.

## Management of Raynaud's Phenomenon in Scleroderma

Calcium channel blockers are the drugs most commonly used for the management of Raynaud's phenomenon, but they can be disappointing in patients with scleroderma. Despite the lack of objective improvement, most scleroderma patients subjectively benefit and report fewer and less intense Raynaud's attacks. There has been no evidence to suggest that vasodilator therapy improves the primary vessel disease in scleroderma, but calcium channel blockers have been shown to improve blood flow to the lung and heart in patients with scleroderma.[83, 116, 117]

Patients with scleroderma who develop ischemic fingertip ulcers may benefit from vasodilator therapy, and all the recommendations in the general section on treatment of Raynaud's phenomenon can be followed (see Chapter 31). In addition, all patients with new ischemic ulcerations or evidence of demarcation of a digit from ischemia should be put at rest and kept warm. Hospitalization may be necessary. The digital circulation in scleroderma, in fact, has some reserve and the capacity to vasodilate if external provoking stimuli are eliminated. When scleroderma patients are at rest in a warm ambient temperature, their skin surface temperature may return to normal without other therapy.[118]

All scleroderma patients, particularly those with digital ischemia, should be given low-dose aspirin (81 mg/day), inasmuch as platelet activation, fibrin deposition, and local thrombosis occur in these patients. The calcium channel blockers have been shown to inhibit platelet activation in scleroderma.[119] Although fibrinolytic therapy has been suggested for the treatment of Raynaud's phenomenon and digital occlusion in scleroderma,[120] there are no good clinical trials to define the role for these agents. Chronic anticoagulation is not recommended; however, the precise role of anticoagulation has not been studied, and it can be considered in an acute ischemic crisis. Patients with scleroderma and severe Raynaud's phenomenon or digital ischemic ulcers may benefit from prostaglandin (PG) therapy. These agents are currently given by the intravenous route. $PGE_1$ is available but requires placement of a central intravenous line for administration (see Raynaud's section). Prostacyclin and its analog, iloprost, have been shown to be of benefit to patients with scleroderma but are not available for use in the United States.[121, 122] Oral prostaglandins are now being tested. Misoprostol is an oral $PGE_1$ analog marketed for the prevention of peptic ulceration secondary to use of nonsteroidal anti-inflammatory drugs. It has not been tested in scleroderma but was no better than placebo in reversing cold-induced Raynaud's phenomenon in patients with primary Raynaud's phenomenon.[123] Pentoxifylline (Trental) has frequently been used in scleroderma patients with ischemia.[124–126] However, there are no convincing studies to show that it improves local blood flow in these patients, and its use cannot be recommended. Antioxidant therapy makes sense, but no studies are available to provide guidance.

Anti-inflammatory or immunosuppressive therapy for ischemic ulcerations secondary to scleroderma is not recommended. There is no evidence of a vasculitis, and these agents may be counterproductive by inhibiting tissue healing. This is particularly true of corticosteroids.

Patients with scleroderma may develop occlusion of a major blood vessel, which could be reversed by surgical correction. Ulnar artery disease was reported to be common in scleroderma.[127] One must consider other causes of major vessel disease, such as atherosclerosis in more proximal vessels. Relief of these lesions may improve peripheral blood flow. However, the most common situation involves severe peripheral vascular changes alone that do not provide surgical options. Noninvasive vascular studies should be considered in scleroderma patients who have evidence of larger-vessel disease. Angiographic studies are not recommended unless the diagnosis of the vascular lesion is unclear or noninvasive studies show evidence of a surgically correctable lesion.

## Management of Skin in Scleroderma

In early stages of scleroderma there is an inflammatory process in the skin and other organs. The cutaneous signs are thickened skin with nonpitting edema and, on occasion, impressive erythema. The symptoms of early active skin involvement are intense pruritus, loss of flexibility, pain, and stiffness. It is during this phase of scleroderma that a disease-modifying drug (see previous discussion) has the best chance of preventing fibrosis and damage. This inflammatory phase continues for weeks to months and is seemingly unresponsive to conventional anti-inflammatory therapy or antihistamines. Topical corticosteroid (1% hydrocortisone or 0.1% triamcinolone cream applied one to two times daily) has been used with some success but should be limited to short-term treatment. The intense pruritus and inflammatory signs spontaneously decrease independent of treatment.

The natural lubrication of the skin is abnormal in scleroderma because of damage to sweat and exocrine glands. Drying causes pruritus, which leads to scratching, skin excoriation, and more skin damage. Topical care is essential. Frequent use of topical lubricants and emollients containing lanolin, silicone, or petroleum derivatives (Aquaphor, Eucerin, Lubriderm, Vaseline Dermatology lotion, Theraplex, or Lac-Hydrin 12% lotion) is helpful. Patients need to avoid excessive exposure to sun and water. Less frequent bathing, use of protective gloves, and avoidance of detergents and soaps that can dry the skin are important measures.

Patients may have telangiectasis over the face (not on the fingers or palms) removed by phototherapy (laser) for cosmetic reasons. Some patients benefit from education about the use of cosmetic products that can cover areas of hypopigmentation or telangiectasis.

There are several types of digital lesions in scleroderma. Although all are aggravated by vascular disease, not all the lesions are ischemic in nature. Drying of the skin with fissuring and scaling is common, and the skin may ulcerate. Fissuring and drying of the fingertips can be decreased by nighttime application of petrolatum followed by the use of cotton gloves to cover the treated fingers. Paronychia can occur and can be complicated by secondary soft-tissue infection or ulceration. Traumatic ulcerations over the proximal interphalangeal joints of the fingers or other sites, such as the elbow or ankle, are most problematic because these sites usually have thin, atrophic overlying skin. Secondary infection of these traumatic ulcers can be severe and can threaten the viability of the digit. Digital ischemic ulcerations occur at the fingertip; they can be superficial or deep infarctions with associated gangrene.

Theoretically, improving local blood flow with vasodilator therapy should improve healing of ischemic and other lesions (see Management of Raynaud's Phenomenon). Ulcerations are best treated with a topical antibiotic such as bacitracin and periodic cleansing by whirlpooling (two times daily) of the skin with soap and water or a warm povidone-iodine (Betadine) solution. Colloid dressings (Mitraflex) that reduce skin maceration caused by dressing tapes are now available, but patients usually prefer a simple light bandage. Signs of cellulitis or soft-tissue infection should be treated aggressively with systemic antibiotics. Débridement may be necessary, but allowing the lesion to naturally demarcate generally prevents further loss of healthy tissue. Prevention of repeated trauma to an active lesion is helpful and can be accomplished by local padding or protective cages designed by the occupational therapist.

Pain control should be liberal during the acute phase of ischemic lesions, because uncontrolled pain may potentiate vasospasm. However, narcotics are also vasoconstrictors and therefore should be discontinued as soon as possible.

Surgical management of ulcerations in lesions of scleroderma should be conservative. However, digital gangrene usually requires surgical amputation. Surgical correction of finger contractures improves digital function and prevents repeated trauma of the flexion contracture. Large ankle ulcers have been successfully treated with skin grafting.

Subcutaneous calcinosis occurs in all subsets of scleroderma but is more prominent in limited scleroderma. It is caused by the deposition of amphorous calcium hydroxyapatite in connective tissue and tends to occur at sites of trauma (around the elbow or forearm) or in the tissues of the finger, probably as a consequence of ischemia. The calcinosis may become superficial and rupture through the skin, leading to ulceration and secondary infection. Deposits may just become bothersome lumps, or they can be associated with recurrent local inflammatory episodes induced by the crystalline material. Crystal-induced inflammation can be treated with a nonsteroidal anti-inflammatory drug or low doses of colchicine (0.6 mg twice daily).

Medical management of subcutaneous calcinosis has been disappointing. Treatment with low-dose warfarin (1 to 2 mg/day),[128] chelation therapy,[129] bisphosphonates,[130] diltiazem,[131] and probenecid[132] has been reported. However, there is no convincing evidence that any of these agents are effective. Management is limited to protection of these sites from trauma, aggressive treatment of infection, and, if technically possible, surgical removal. Lesions on the fingers are usually associated with poor blood flow, and therefore there may be no surgical options other than amputation. Sites that have formed skin ulcerations or fistulas are particularly difficult to manage because the local skin thickening and calcinosis usually does not allow for surgical maneuvers and closure of the wound. Local padding and bandages may be the only option.

Localized scleroderma has been managed with a variety of agents, but the natural history of these lesions is spontaneous resolution. We and others have used psoralen with ultraviolet-A (PUVA) therapy.[133, 134]

## Management of the Musculoskeletal System

Although the musculoskeletal pain in scleroderma is usually present during the early inflammatory phase of the disease, it is often not very responsive to anti-inflammatory drugs. This is particularly true when the signs of an inflammatory arthritis are not present. "Tendon friction rubs" around the ankle, knee, elbow, wrist, or shoulder are likewise difficult to treat; usually not even responding to local corticosteroid injection.

It is reasonable to use a nonsteroidal anti-inflammatory drug or low doses of corticosteroid (prednisone, 5 to 10 mg daily) in patients with pain, but their use should be carefully monitored. Low doses of narcotics may be necessary in some cases. Patients with an inflammatory polyarthritis can be treated with the same drugs used for rheumatoid arthritis (see Chapter 18).

In the late stages of diffuse scleroderma, muscle wasting and joint contractures caused by inflexible fibrosis of the skin are best managed with the help of comprehensive physical and occupational therapy. Almost every patient benefits from a management program that includes exercise and, especially, hand therapy. Early consultation with an experienced physical or occupational therapist is recommended. Although not well studied, it is the general impression that digits or limbs that are immobilized are more likely to develop serious contracture and worse scleroderma. At the same time, range of motion may be limited by the overlying skin sclerosis; therefore, forced exercise may be painful and counterproductive. Patients find that massage, local heat, and gentle stretching are soothing and reduce pain. An appropriate cardiovascular conditioning exercise program is always helpful. Activities of daily living, such as dressing, personal hygiene, preparing meals, and mobilization, can be difficult for the patient and the family. A variety of devices are available to help improve the patient's ability to perform independent activities. Most scleroderma patients lose a percentage of hand function secondary to joint contracture or painful skin ulcerations. Assessment of the home environment and family education can be most helpful for patients with severe musculoskeletal disability.

Surgery has a very limited role in management of the musculoskeletal problems of scleroderma. Finger contractures can be corrected by shortening the phalange and fusing the finger, but there is little gain in function from this procedure. Patients rarely require total joint replacement because the scleroderma process does not cause erosive joint disease.

Fatigue and a sense of weakness are common complaints of patients with scleroderma. The cause is multifactorial, including disease activity, the effects of drugs, malnutrition, and disuse from joint disease. A noninflammatory myopathy secondary to fibrosis of the connective tissue in muscle is a common cause of weakness in severe diffuse scleroderma. This process does not appear to respond to corticosteroid or immunosuppressive therapy and is best treated with exercise and supportive care. An inflammatory myositis can lead to rapid and profound weakness. Inflammatory myositis should be treated in the same manner as polymyositis or dermatomyositis alone (see Chapter 32).

## Management of Cardiovascular Disease

Serious cardiac disease is a late complication of scleroderma and is more common in diffuse scleroderma. Pericardial disease is usually clinically silent and requires no specific therapy unless it is associated with evidence of hemodynamic compromise. When it causes symptoms, pericarditis can be treated with nonsteroidal anti-inflammatory drugs or corticosteroids. A large pericardial effusion is uncommon but is associated with a poor overall outcome. When a large effusion is present the patient must be monitored closely for complications such as renal failure, heart failure, arrhythmias, or pericardial tamponade.

Myocardial injury in scleroderma is a consequence of microvascular disease and reperfusion injury after reversible vasospasm of myocardial vessels. Patchy tissue fibrosis leads to a cardiomyopathy, which can be complicated by arrhythmia or heart failure. Studies in scleroderma suggest that vasodilator therapy with a calcium channel blocker (nifedipine) reverses cold-induced cardiac vasospasm.[117] However, there are no data on which to make a judgment on the benefit of long-term vasodilator therapy. Coronary artery disease can be seen in scleroderma patients, but it is more likely a result of atherosclerosis and not the scleroderma process. Diastolic dysfunction is frequently detected by two-dimensional echocardiography, probably secondary to scleroderma myocardial fibrosis. Use of an ACE inhibitor may improve cardiac performance in this setting.

The heart in the patient with scleroderma may be secondarily affected by multiple factors, including severe lung disease (cor pulmonale), associated metabolic disease (hypothyroidism), malnutrition, hypertension, or medications. In particular, care should be taken not to overlook myocarditis associated with polymyositis. An endomyocardial biopsy may be helpful in a difficult diagnostic situation. Active immune-mediated myocarditis should be treated with corticosteroids or other immunosuppressive therapy.

All patients with symptoms of cardiac compromise should be evaluated with two-dimensional echocardiography to assess ventricular function and to noninvasively determine whether there is evidence of pulmonary hypertension. Because the presence of a cardiomyopathy is often underestimated and is a late complication in scleroderma, periodic objective testing to determine cardiac rhythm and function is prudent. Arrhythmias and heart failure are treated in the conventional manner, in conjunction with a cardiologist.

## Management of Psychosocial Issues in Scleroderma

A survey of patients with scleroderma found that almost half the patients had mild depressive symptoms and almost 20% had moderate to severe depression.[1] The degree of depression did not correlate with disease severity but was influenced by personality traits and the degree of supportive care available, both at home and professionally. Scleroderma can be demoralizing and both physically and emotionally stressful. Although it is frequently not mentioned by the patient to the physician, loss of usual sexual relationships is common. Each patient with scleroderma should be evaluated for depression or other emotionally distressful issues. These emotional issues are often very responsive if appropriate support and management are instituted. Treatment of serious depression is best managed in conjunction with a psychiatrist.

## Management of Other Issues

Impotence is a common problem among male patients with scleroderma. The cause is organic in most cases and is thought to be secondary to defects in neurovascular function. Patients can be helped by referral to a specialist in male dysfunction (urologist). Sildenafil (Viagra) has improved erectile dysfunction in several of our male patients. Surgical implantation of a penile prosthesis has also been used with success. Neuropathy from carpal tunnel syndrome or trigeminal neuralgia may occur. Carpal tunnel syndrome may require surgical release, whereas neuralgia may respond to a tricyclic antidepressants or neuroleptic drugs (Tegretol, Dilantin, and Neurontin). Anemia in scleroderma is a sign of active disease or some correctable cause; when it is present, careful assessment for chronic blood loss, malnutrition, and vitamin $B_{12}$ deficiency must be done. It should always be remembered that scleroderma belongs to the family of autoimmune diseases. Overlap syndromes, autoimmune hypothyroidism, autoimmune hepatitis, or full expression of another rheumatic disease may occur in patients with scleroderma.

## REFERENCES

1. Roca RP, Wigley FM, Needleman BW: Prevalence and correlates of depression in systemic sclerosis. Arthritis Rheum 1992; 35:S206.
1a. Kelley WN, Harris ED, Ruddy S, et al: Textbook of Rheumatology, 4th ed. Philadelphia: WB Saunders, 1993.
2. Pope JE: Treatment of systemic sclerosis. Rheum Dis Clin North Am 1996; 22:893.
3. Clements PJ, Furst DE (eds): Systemic Sclerosis. Baltimore: William & Wilkins, 1996.
4. Stone JH, Wigley FM: Management of systemic sclerosis: The art and science. Semin Cutan Med Surg 1998; 17:55–64.
5. Clements PJ, Wong WK, Seibold JR, et al: High-done (HI-DPA) vs low dose (LO-DPA) penicillamine in early diffuse systemic sclerosis (SSc) trial: Analysis of trial. Arthritis Rheum 1997; 854:S173.
6. Steen VD, Medsger TA Jr, Rodnan GP: D-Penicillamine therapy in progressive systemic sclerosis (scleroderma). Ann Intern Med 1982; 97:652.
7. Jimenez SA, Sigal SH: A 15-year prospective study of treatment of rapidly progressive systemic sclerosis with D-penicillamine. J Rheumatol 1991; 18:1496.
8. Steen VD, Blair S, Medsger TA Jr: The toxicity of D-penicillamine in systemic sclerosis. Ann Intern Med 1986; 104:699.
9. Ntoso KA, Tomaszewski JE, Jimenez SA, et al: Penicillamine-induced rapidly progressive glomerulonephritis in patients with progressive systemic sclerosis: Successful treatment of two patients and a review of the literature. Am J Kidney Dis 1986; 8:159.
10. Fernandez-Herlihy L: Skin elasticity and colchicine in scleroderma. Arthritis Rheum 1976; 19:832.
11. Guttadauria M, Diamond H, Kaplan D: Colchicine in the treatment of scleroderma. J Rheumatol 1977; 4:272.
12. Alarcon-Segovia D, Ibañez G, Kershenobich D, et al: Treatment of scleroderma by modification of collagen metabolism: A double-blind trial with colchicine vs placebo. J Rheumatol 1974; 1(suppl):97.
13. Alarcon-Segovia D, Ramos-Niembro F, Ibañez de Kasep G, et al: Long-term evaluation of colchicine in the treatment of scleroderma. J Rheumatol 1979; 6:705.
14. Steigarwald JC: Colchicine vs. placebo in the treatment of progressive systemic sclerosis. In Black CM, Myers AR (eds): Systemic Sclerosis (Scleroderma). New York: Gower Medical, 1985:415.
15. Priestley GC, Brown JC: Effects of potassium para-aminobenzoate on growth and macromolecule synthesis in fibroblasts cultured from normal and sclerodermatous human skin and human synovial cells. J Invest Dermatol 1979; 72:161.
16. Zarafonetis CJ, Dabich L, Shouronski JJ, et al: Retrospective studies in scleroderma: Skin response to potassium para-aminobenzoate therapy. Clin Exp Rheumatol 1988; 6:261.
17. Clegg DO for the Aminobenzoate Study Group: Comparison of aminobenzoate and placebo in the treatment of scleroderma. Arthritis Rheum 1992; 35:S205.
18. Scherbel AL: The effect of percutaneous dimethyl sulfoxide on cutaneous manifestations of systemic sclerosis. Ann N Y Acad Sci 1983; 411:120.
19. Binnick SA, Shore SS, Corman A, et al: Failure of dimethyl sulfoxide in the treatment of scleroderma. Arch Dermatol 1977; 113:1398.
20. William HJ, Furst DE, Dahl SL, et al: Double-blind, multicenter controlled trial comparing topical dimethyl sulfoxide and normal saline for treatment of hand ulcers in patients with systemic sclerosis. Arthritis Rheum 1985; 28:308.
21. Varga J: Recombinant cytokine treatment for scleroderma: Can the antibiotic potential of interferon-γ be realized clinically. Arch Dermatol 1997; 133:637–642.
22. Kahan A, Amor B, Menkes CJ, et al: Recombinant interferon-γ in the treatment of systemic sclerosis. Am J Med 1989; 87:273.
23. Luk AJ, Wong M, Lambert RE, et al: Treatment of scleroderma with interferon-γ. Arthritis Rheum 1996; 748:S152.
24. Stevens W, Vangheeswaren R, Black CM, et al: Alpha interferon-2a (Roferon-A) in the treatment of diffuse cutaneous systemic sclerosis: A pilot study. Br J Rheumatol 1992; 31:683.
25. Silman A, Herrick A, Denton C, et al: Raynaud's phenomenon and scleroderma: Therapy. Arthritis Rheum 1997; 556:S123.
26. Unemori EN, Pickford LB, Salles AL, et al: Relaxin induces an extracellular matrix-degrading phenotype in human lung fibroblasts in vitro and inhibits lung fibrosis in the murine model in vivo. J Clin Invest 1996; 98:2739.
27. Unemori EN, Beck LS, Lee WP, et al: Human relaxin decreases collagen accumulation in vivo in two rodent models of fibrosis. J Invest Dermatol 1993; 101:280.
28. Seibold JR, Clements PJ, Furst DE, et al: Safety and pharmacokinetics of recombinant human relaxin in systemic sclerosis. J Rheumatol 1998; 25:302.
29. Seibold JR, Korn J, Simms R, et al: Recombinant human relaxin in the treatment of scleroderma. A randomized, double-blind, placebo-controlled trial. Ann Intern Med 2000; 132:871.
30. Steen VD, Medsger TA: Case-control study of corticosteroid and other drugs that either precipitate or protect from the development of scleroderma renal crisis. Arthritis Rheum 1998; 41:1613.
31. MacKenzie AH: Prolonged alkylating drug therapy is beneficial in systemic sclerosis [Abstract]. Arthritis Rheum 1970; 13:334.
32. Steigerwald JC: Chlorambucil in the treatment of progressive systemic sclerosis. In Black CM, Myers AR (eds): Systemic Sclerosis (Scleroderma). New York: Gower Medical, 1985:423.
33. Furst DE, Clements PJ, Hillis S, et al: Immunosuppression with chlorambucil vs placebo, for scleroderma: Results of a three-year, parallel, randomized, double-blind study. Arthritis Rheum 1989; 32:584.
34. Jansen GT, Barraza DF, Ballard JL, et al: Generalized scleroderma: Treatment with an immunosuppressive agent. Arch Dermatol 1968; 97:690.
35. Casas JA, Subauste CP, Alarcon GS: A new promising treatment in systemic sclerosis: 5-Fluorouracil. Ann Rheum Dis 1987; 46:763.
36. Casas JA, Saway PA, Villarreal I, et al: 5-Fluorouracil in the treatment of scleroderma: A randomized, double-blind, placebo controlled international collaborative study. Ann Rheum Dis 1990; 49:926.

37. Van den Hoogen PH, Boerbooms AM, van de Putte LB, et al: Low dose methotrexate treatment in systemic sclerosis. J Rheumatol 1991; 18:1763.

38. Van den Hoogen FHJ, Boerbooms AMT, Henk JJ, et al: Methotrexate in systemic sclerosis: Preliminary 24 week results of a placebo controlled double blind trial. Arthritis Rheum 1993; 36:S217.

39. Pope J, Bellamy N, Seibold J, et al: A randomized controlled trial of methotrexate (MTX) versus placebo in early diffuse scleroderma: Preliminary analysis. Arthritis Rheum 1998; 420:S102.

40. Gisslinger H, Burghuber OC, Stacher G, et al: Efficacy of cyclosporin A in systemic sclerosis. Clin Exp Rheumatol 1991; 9:383.

41. Ruiz JO, Val F, de Francisco ALM, et al: Progressive systemic sclerosis and renal transplantation: A contraindication to the use of cyclosporin A? Transplant Proc 1991; 23:2211.

42. Clements PJ, Lachenbruch PA, Sterz M, et al: Cyclosporin in systemic sclerosis: Results of a 48-week open safety study in ten patients. Arthritis Rheum 1993; 36:75.

43. Steen V: An open trial of FK-506 in the treatment of early diffuse scleroderma. Arthritis Rheum 1998; 421:S103.

44. O'Dell JR, Steigerwald JC, Kennaugh RC, et al: Lack of clinical benefit after treatment of systemic sclerosis with total lymphoid irradiation. J Rheumatol 1989; 16:1050.

45. Balaban EP, Sheehan RG, Lipsky PE, et al: Treatment of cutaneous sclerosis and aplastic anemia with antithymocyte globulin. Ann Intern Med 1987; 106:56.

46. Balaban EP, Zashin SJ, Geppert TD, et al: Treatment of systemic sclerosis with antithymocyte globulin [Letter]. Arthritis Rheum 1991; 34:244.

47. Sinclair HD, Williams JD, Rahman MA, et al: Clinical efficacy of anti-thymocyte globulin in systemic sclerosis: Results of a placebo controlled trial. Arthritis Rheum 1993; 36:S217.

48. Rook AH, Freundlich B, Jegasothy BV, et al: Treatment of systemic sclerosis with extracorporeal photochemotherapy: Results of a multicenter trial. Arch Dermatol 1992; 128:337.

49. Clements PJ, Furst DE: Choosing appropriate patients with systemic sclerosis for treatment by autologous stem cell transplantation. J Rheum 1997; 24:85.

50. Le CH, Morales A, Trentham DE: Minocycline in early diffuse scleroderma. Lancet 1998; 352:1755.

51. Delbarre F, Godeau P, Thivolet J: Factor XIII treatment for scleroderma. Lancet 1981; 2:204.

52. Guillevin L, Chouvet B, Mery C, et al: Treatment of progressive systemic sclerosis using factor XIII. Pharmatherapeutica 1985; 4:76.

53. Maurice PDL, Bunker CB, Dowd PM: Isotretinoin in the treatment of systemic sclerosis. Br J Dermatol 1989; 121:367.

54. Ferri C, Bernini L, Bombardieri S, et al: Long-term griseofulvin treatment for progressive systemic sclerosis. Scand J Rheumatol 1986; 15:356.

55. Guillevin L, Leon A, Levy Y, et al: Treatment of progressive systemic sclerosis with plasma exchange: Seven cases. Int J Artif Organs 1983; 6:315.

56. Dau PC, Kahaleh MB, Sagebiel RW: Plasmapheresis and immunosuppressive drug therapy in scleroderma. Arthritis Rheum 1981; 24:1128.

57. Mongan ES: The treatment of progressive systemic sclerosis with disodium edetate. Arthritis Rheum 1965; 8:1145.

58. Fuleihan FJD, Kurban AK, Abboud RT, et al: An objective evaluation of the treatment of systemic scleroderma with disodium EDTA, pyridoxine and reserpine. Br J Dermatol 1968; 80:184.

59. Furst DE, Clements PJ, Harris R, et al: Measurement of clinical change in progressive systemic sclerosis: A 1-year double-blind placebo-controlled trial of N-acetylcysteine. Ann Rheum Dis 1979; 38:356.

60. Blom-Bülow B, Öberg K, Wollheim FA, et al: Cyclofenil vs placebo in progressive systemic sclerosis. Acta Med Scand 1981; 210:419.

61. Kirk A, Dixon ASJ: Failure of low molecular weight dextran infusions in scleroderma. Ann Rheum Dis 1969; 28:49.

62. Gruber BL, Kaufman LD: A double-blind randomized controlled trial of ketotifen vs placebo in early diffuse scleroderma. Arthritis Rheum 1991; 34:362.

63. Border WA, Noble NA, Yamamoto T, et al: Natural inhibitor of transforming growth factor-$\beta$ protects against scarring in experimental kidney disease. Nature 1992; 360:361.

64. Clements P, Lachenbruch P, Furst D, et al: The course of skin involvement in systemic sclerosis over three years in a trial of chlorambucil vs placebo. Arthritis Rheum 1993; 36:1575.

65. Giovanni AR, Bitterman PB, Rennard SI, et al: Evidence for chronic inflammation as a component of the interstitial lung disease associated with progressive systemic sclerosis. Am Rev Respir Dis 1985; 131:612.

66. Silver RM, Miller KS, Kinsella MB, et al: Evaluation and management of scleroderma lung disease using bronchoalveolar lavage. Am J Med 1990; 88:470.

67. Warrick JH, Bhalla M, Schabel SI, et al: High resolution computed tomography in early scleroderma lung disease. J Rheumatol 1991; 18:1520.

68. Strumpf JI, Feld MK, Cornelius MJ, et al: Safety of fiberoptic bronchoalveolar lavage in evaluation of interstitial lung disease. Chest 1981; 80:268.

69. Witt C, Romberg B, Brenke A, et al: Diagnostic and prognostic relevance of bronchoalveolar lavage in systemic sclerosis. Arthritis Rheum 1993; 36:5132.

70. Wallaert B, Hatron PY, Grosbois JM, et al: Subclinical pulmonary involvement in collagen-vascular diseases assessed by bronchoalveolar lavage. Am Rev Respir Dis 1986; 133:574.

71. Cess GM, Kallenberg MD, Henk MJ, et al: Steroid-responsive interstitial pulmonary disease in systemic sclerosis: Monitoring by bronchoalveolar lavage. Chest 1984; 86:489.

72. Keogh BA, Bernardo J, Hunninghake GW, et al: Effect of intermittent high dose parenteral corticosteroids on the alveolitis of idiopathic pulmonary fibrosis. Am Rev Respir Dis 1983; 127:18.

73. Johnson MA, Kwan S, Snell JN, et al: Randomized controlled trial comparing prednisone alone with cyclophosphamide and low dose prednisolone in combination in cryptogenic fibrosing alveolitis. Thorax 1989; 44:280.

74. Silver RM, Warrick JH, Kinsella MB, et al: Cyclophosphamide and low-dose prednisone therapy in patients with systemic sclerosis (scleroderma) with interstitial lung disease. J Rheumatol 1993; 20:838.

75. Akesson A, Scheja A, Lundin A, et al: Improved pulmonary function in systemic sclerosis after treatment with cyclophosphamide. Arthritis Rheum 1994; 37:729–735.

76. Varal G, Earle L, Jimenez SA, et al: A pilot study of intermittent intravenous cyclophosphamide for the treatment of systemic sclerosis interstitial lung disease. J Rheumatol 1998; 25:1325–1329.

77. Steen VD, Owens GR, Redmond C, et al: The effect of D-penicillamine on pulmonary findings in systemic sclerosis. Arthritis Rheum 1985; 28:882.

78. DeClerck LS, Dequeker J, Francx L, et al: D-Penicillamine therapy and interstitial lung disease in scleroderma. Arthritis Rheum 1987; 30:643.

79. Steen VD, Graham G, Conte C, et al: Isolated diffusing capacity reduction in systemic sclerosis. Arthritis Rheum 1992; 35:765.

80. Gaines SP, Rubin LJ: Primary pulmonary hypertension. Lancet 1998; 352:719–725.

81. Morgan JM, Griffiths M, Du Bois RM, et al: Hypoxic pulmonary vasoconstriction in systemic sclerosis and primary pulmonary hypertension. Chest 1991; 99:551.

82. Fuster V, Steele PM, Edwards WD, et al: Primary pulmonary hypertension: Natural history and the importance of thrombosis. Circulation 1984; 70:580.

83. Rich S, Kaufmann E, Levy PS: The effect of high doses of calcium-channel blockers on survival in primary pulmonary hypertension. N Engl J Med 1992; 327:76.

84. Alpert MA, Pressly TA, Mukerji V, et al: Short and long-term effect of nifedipine on pulmonary and systemic hemodynamics in patients with pulmonary hypertension associated with diffuse systemic sclerosis, the CREST syndrome and mixed connective tissue disease. Am J Cardiol 1991; 68:1687.

85. Alpert MA, Pressly TA, Mukerji W, et al: Short and long-term hemodynamic effects of captopril in patients with pulmonary hypertension and selected connective tissue disease. Chest 1992; 102:1407.

86. Rubin LJ, Mendoza J, Hood M, et al: Treatment of primary pulmonary hypertension with continuous intravenous prostacyclin (epoprostenol): Results of a randomized trial. Ann Intern Med 1990; 112:485.

87. Barst RJ, Rubin LJ, Long WA, et al: A comparison of continous intravenous epoprostenol (prostacyclin) with conventional therapy for primary pulmonary hypertension: The Primary Pulmonary Hypertension study group. N Engl J Med 1996; 334:296–302.

88. Barst RJ, Rubin LJ, McGoon MD, et al: Survival in primary pulmonary hypertension with long-term continuous infusion of prsotacyclin. Ann Intern Med 1994; 121:409–415.

89. McLaughlin VV, Genthner DE, Panella MM, et al: Reduction in pulmonary vascular resistance with long term epoprostenol (prostacyclin) therapy in primary pulmonary hypertension. N Engl J Med 1998; 338:273–277.

90. Thurm CA, Wigley FM, Dole WP, et al: Failure of vasodilator infusion to alter pulmonary diffusing capacity in systemic sclerosis. Am J Med 1991; 90:547.

91. Higenbottam TW, Butt AY, Dinh-Xaun AT, et al: Treatment of pulmonary hypertension with the continuous infusion of a prostacyclin analogue, iloprost. Heart 1998; 79:175–179.

92. De la Mata L, Gomez-Sanchez MA, Aranzana M, et al: Long-term iloprost infusion for severe pulmonary hypertension in patients with connective tissue disease. Arthritis Rheum 1994; 37:1528–1533.

93. Badesch DB, Brundage BH, McGoon MD, et al: Continous intraveonous epoprostenol versus conventional therapy in pulmonary hypertension due to the scleroderma spectrum of disease: A 12-week, multicenter, randomized, controlled trial. Circulation 1998; 1614:3226.

94. Pigula FA, Griffith BP, Zenati MA, et al: Lung transplantation for respiratory failure from systemic disease. Ann Thoracic Surg 1997; 64:1630–1634.

95. Zamost BJ, Hirschberg J, Ippoliti AF, et al: Esophagitis in scleroderma: Prevalence and risk factors. Gastroenterology 1987; 92:421.

96. Petrokubi RJ, Jeffries GH: Cimetidine vs antacid in scleroderma with reflux esophagitis: A randomized double-blind controlled study. Gastroenterology 1979; 77:691.

97. Johnson DA, Drane WE, Curran J: Metoclopramide response in patients with progressive systemic sclerosis. Arch Intern Med 1987; 147:1597.

98. Horowitz M, Maddern GJ, Maddox A, et al: Effects of cisapride on gastric and esophageal emptying in progressive systemic sclerosis. Gastroenterology 1987; 93:311.

99. Kahan A, Chaussade S, Gaudric M, et al: The effect of cisapride on gastroesophageal dysfunction in systemic sclerosis: A controlled manometric study. Br J Clin Pharmacol 1991; 31:683.

100. Limburg AJ, Smit AJ, Kleibeuker JH: Effects of cisapride on the esophageal motor function of patients with progressive systemic sclerosis or mixed connective tissue disease. Digestion 1991; 49:156.

101. Kahan A, Chaussade S, Michopoulos S, et al: Erythromycin and esophageal abnormalities in systemic sclerosis [Abstract]. Arthritis Rheum 1991; 34(suppl 52):116.

102. Mansour KA, Malone CE: Surgery for scleroderma of the esophagus: A 12-year experience. Ann Thorac Surg 1988; 46:513.

103. Soudah HC, Hasler WL, Owyang C: Effect of octreotide on intestinal motility and bacterial overgrowth in scleroderma. N Engl J Med 1991; 325:1461.

104. Ng SC, Clements PJ, Berquist WE, et al: Home central venous hyperalimentation in fifteen patients with severe scleroderma bowel disease. Arthritis Rheum 1989; 32:212.

105. Stafford-Brady FJ, Kahn HJ, Ross TM, et al: Advanced scleroderma bowel: Complications and management. J Rheumatol 1988; 15:869.

106. Sequeira W: Pneumatosis cystoides intestinalis in systemic sclerosis and other diseases. Semin Arthritis Rheum 1990; 19:269.

107. Battle WM, Snape WJ, Wright S, et al: Abnormal colonic motility in progressive systemic sclerosis. Ann Intern Med 1981; 94:749.

108. Whitehead WE, Taitelbaum G, Wigley FM, et al: Rectosigmoid mobility and myoelectric activity in progressive systemic sclerosis. Gastroenterology 1989; 32:428.

109. Bateson MC, Gedling P: Ursodeoxycholic acid therapy for primary biliary cirrhosis: A 10-year british single-centre population-based audit of efficacy and survival. Postgrad Med J 1998; 74:482.

110. Lopez-Ovejero JA, Saal SD, D'Angelo WA, et al: Reversal of vascular and renal crises of scleroderma by oral angiotensin-converting-enzyme blockade. N Engl J Med 1979; 300:1417.

111. Steen VD, Costantino JP, Shapiro AP: Outcome of renal crisis in systemic sclerosis: Relation to availability of angiotensin converting enzyme (ACE) inhibitors. Ann Intern Med 1990; 113:352.

112. Smith DC, Smith RD, Korn JH: Hypertensive crisis in systemic sclerosis: Treatment with the new oral angiotensin converting enzyme inhibitor MK 421 (enalapril) in captopril-intolerant patients. Arthritis Rheum 1984; 27:826.

113. Donohoe JF: Scleroderma and the kidney. Kidney Int 1992; 41:462.

114. Caskey FJ, Thacker EJ, Johnston PA, et al: Failure of losartan to control blood pressure in scleroderma renal crisis. Lancet 1997; 349:620.

115. Helfrich DJ, Banner B, Steen VD, et al: Normotensive renal failure in systemic sclerosis. Arthritis Rheum 1989; 32:1128.

116. Sfikakis PP, Pyriakidis MK, Vergos CG, et al: Cardiopulmonary hemodynamics in systemic sclerosis and response to nifedipine and captopril. Am J Med 1991; 90:541.

117. Kahan A, Devaux JY, Amor B, et al: Nifedipine and thallium-201 myocardial perfusion in progressive systemic sclerosis. N Engl J Med 1986; 314:1397.

118. Gelber AC, Wigley FM, White B: Continuous ambulatory skin temperature (CAST) in patients with Raynaud's phenomenon (RP). Arthritis Rheum 1993; 36:S217.

119. Rademaker M, Thomas RH, Kirby JD, et al: Anti-platelet effect of nifedipine in patients with systemic sclerosis. Clin Exp Rheumatol 1992; 10:57.

120. Fritzler MJ, Hart DA: Prolonged improvement of Raynaud's phenomenon and scleroderma after recombinant tissue plasminogen activator therapy. Arthritis Rheum 1990; 33:274.

121. Wigley FM, Seibold JR, Wise RA, et al: Intravenous iloprost treatment of Raynaud's phenomenon and ischemia ulcers secondary to systemic sclerosis. J Rheumatol 1992; 19:1407.

122. Wigley FM, Wise RA, Seibold JR, et al: Intravenous iloprost infusion in patients with Raynaud's phenomenon secondary to systemic sclerosis: A multi-center placebo-controlled double-blind study. Ann Intern Med 1994; 120:199.

123. Wise RA, Wigley FM: Acute effects of misoprostol on digital circulation in patients with Raynaud's phenomenon. J Rheumatol 1994; 21:80.

124. Neirotti M, Longo F, Molaschi M, et al: Functional vascular disorders: Treatment with pentoxifylline. Angiology J Vas Dis 1987; 38:575

125. Arosio E, Montesi G, Zannoni M, et al: Comparative efficacy of ketanserin and pentoxiphylline in treatment of Raynaud's phenomenon. Angiology 1989; 40:633.

126. Goodfield MJD, Rowell NR: Treatment of peripheral gangrene due to systemic sclerosis with intravenous pentoxifylline. Clin Exp Dermatol 1989; 14:161.

127. Taylor M, Bolster MB McFadden J, et al: Ulnar artery involvement in systemic sclerosis (scleroderma). Arthritis Rheum 1998; 1107:S217.

128. Berger RG, Hadler NM: Treatment of cutaneous calcinosis of dermatomyositis or scleroderma with low dose narfarin. Arthritis Rheum 1985; 28:539.

129. Klein R, Harris SB: Treatment of scleroderma, sclerodactylia and calcinosis by chelation (EDTA). Am J Med 1955; 19:798.

130. Metzger AL, Singer FR, Bluestone R, et al: Failure of disodium etidronate in calcinosis due to dermatomyositis and scleroderma. N Engl J Med 1974; 291:1294.

131. Farah MJ, Palmieri GMA, Sebes JI, et al: The effect of diltiazem on calcinosis in a patient with the crest syndrome. Arthritis Rheum 1990; 33:1287.

132. Dent CE, Stamp TCB: Treatment of calcinosis circumscripta with probenecid. Br Med J 1972; 1:216.

133. Morison WL: Psoralen UVA therapy for linear and generalized morphea. J Am Acad Dermatol 1997; 37:657.

134. Kanekura T, Fukumaru S, Matsushita S, et al: Successful treatment of scleroderma with PUVA therapy. J Dermatol 1996; 23:455.

# 31 | Raynaud's Phenomenon

*Fredrick M. Wigley*

## DEFINITIONS

Patients with Raynaud's phenomenon complain that their hands and feet are abnormally sensitive to cold temperatures. They also experience sudden episodes of sharply demarcated digital cutaneous color changes.[1] These episodes are caused by closure of the muscular digital arteries, precapillary arterioles, and arteriovenous shunts of the skin after exposure to cold temperatures or during periods of emotional stress. The key factor for making a definite diagnosis is a clinical history of cold-induced digital pallor and/or cyanosis. A color chart containing actual photographs of fingers during an attack has been used to validate the clinical history. Through the use of this method, it has been estimated that the prevalence of Raynaud's phenomenon is between 3% and 15% of the general population.[2] It is more common in women than in men (2:1 to 3:1). Unfortunately, laboratory testing that confirms a diagnosis of Raynaud's phenomenon uses complex research technology and is not available as a simple clinical test. Confirmation of the clinical history with laboratory testing such as a cold challenge with ice water is not recommended.

After a diagnosis of Raynaud's phenomenon has been made, it should be determined whether the patient has *primary* Raynaud's phenomenon or Raynaud's phenomenon *secondary* to another disease process. Patients with primary Raynaud's phenomenon are more likely to respond to treatment and less likely to have complications than patients with secondary forms of Raynaud's phenomenon. Patients with the primary form have the onset of Raynaud's phenomenon in their teens, are usually female, have mild episodes, deny ischemic damage to the tissues, have no evidence of a secondary process on physical examination, and have normal laboratory data, including a negative antinuclear antibody test result and Westergren sedimentation rate.[3] Although the natural history of primary Raynaud's phenomenon is not uniform in every patient, the episodes usually become less intense over time, particularly in women after menopause. In primary Raynaud's phenomenon, digital ulcerations do not occur, and the patient should have no systemic complications related to Raynaud's phenomenon. However, there is evidence that Raynaud's phenomenon may be the cutaneous manifestation of a generalized vasospastic disorder. For example, migraine headache, esophageal reflux, primary pulmonary hypertension, and atypical angina have all been associated with uncomplicated primary Raynaud's phenomenon.

The onset of secondary Raynaud's phenomenon almost always occurs after the second or third decades. The episodes are usually intense and painful, and digital ischemic lesions occasionally occur. The intensity of the Raynaud's attacks usually follows the course of the underlying cause. Secondary causes of Raynaud's phenomenon are frequently associated with vasospasm and either intrinsic vessel disease or abnormalities of the physical properties of the blood flowing in these vessels. Treatment should be directed at both the vasospasm and, if possible, the underlying disease process that is causing the vascular defect. For example, vasculitis can damage blood vessels, causing abnormal vascular reactivity and Raynaud's phenomenon. Controlling the vasculitis with immunosuppressive therapy may cure the associated secondary Raynaud's phenomenon.

## RECOMMENDED EVALUATION

The teenage patient who has cold sensitivity and typical Raynaud's episodes should have a thorough physical examination, including examination of the nailfold capillaries. If the examination findings are normal and the patient is otherwise in excellent health, careful follow-up is all that is necessary. Laboratory studies can confirm the diagnosis of primary Raynaud's phenomenon; the antinuclear antibody results and the Westergren sedimentation rate should be normal. Other special testing should be performed only if clinical clues suggest that they are necessary. The most common rheumatic diseases associated with Raynaud's phenomenon are scleroderma, systemic lupus erythematosus, Sjögren's syndrome, and dermatomyositis. Any of these diseases may manifest with Raynaud's phenomenon as the first symptom.

The cutaneous capillaries can be examined by placing a drop of grade B immersion oil on the skin at the base of a fingernail. The nailfold capillaries can then be viewed by means of a stereozoom microscope or an ordinary ophthalmoscope set at 40 diopters. Normal capillaries appear as orderly, delicate vascular loops

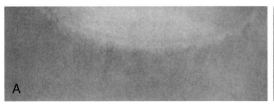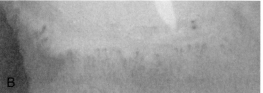

**FIGURE 31–1**
*A.* Normal capillaries at base of fingernail. *B.* Abnormal nailfold capillaries seen in secondary Raynaud's phenomenon.

(Fig. 31–1*A*). Patients with secondary Raynaud's phenomenon and a connective tissue disease frequently have abnormal nailfold capillaries characterized by enlargement of capillary loops, loss of capillaries, or distortion of normal capillary forms (see Fig. 31–1*B*). Approximately 80% of patients with scleroderma have abnormal nailfold capillaries, whereas fewer than 5% of systemic lupus erythematosus patients with Raynaud's phenomenon have abnormal capillary loops. Capillary loop abnormalities are also seen in dermatomyositis.

Patients with Raynaud's phenomenon may have abnormal nailfold capillaries or a positive antinuclear antibody test result or both, without any other systemic features of a connective tissue disease. Approximately 15% to 20% of these patients develop a definite connective tissue disease over the next few years of follow-up, usually scleroderma or a disease with sclerodermal features.[4] If a patient with Raynaud's phenomenon alone has abnormal nailfold capillaries or the presence of autoantibodies, an early stage of an autoimmune disorder should be suspected. Careful clinical follow-up monitoring is recommended. There is a significant association of parenchymal lung disease and/or evidence of pulmonary vascular abnormalities with Raynaud's phenomenon and abnormal nailfold capillaries. Therefore, affected patients should undergo pulmonary function testing and two-dimensional echocardiography to determine whether there is any evidence of emerging cardiopulmonary disease.

Patients over 30 years of age who have Raynaud's phenomenon for the first time are likely to have a defined secondary cause, particularly if the episodes are intense, painful, asymmetric, or associated with ischemic skin lesions. These patients should have a complete evaluation with appropriate special testing dictated by the clinical clues and situation. Special testing may include noninvasive vascular studies (e.g., arterial Doppler studies) to determine whether there is any evidence of large-vessel occlusive disease.

## NONDRUG MANAGEMENT OF RAYNAUD'S PHENOMENON

Primary Raynaud's phenomenon should be managed without drugs whenever possible. Some authorities argue that primary Raynaud's phenomenon is nothing more than an exaggeration of normal vascular response to changes in ambient temperature and is not associated with systemic disease or digital ischemic events. Drug therapy should be considered only if, despite the use of nondrug treatment, the patient has a poor quality of life because of frequent uncomfortable attacks and the annoying need to practice cold avoidance. Treatment begins in all cases with education. Raynaud's attacks are not only uncomfortable but sometimes also frightening. Fear (emotional stress) not only can trigger an attack but can also enhance cold sensitivity. Patients need to understand how attacks occur, what specifically triggers the attacks, how to prevent attacks, and what to expect in the future. The patient should be supplied with educational material that supplements the physician's explanation. Having the patient keep a diary that details the specific events and situations that provoke the attacks provides a useful tool to illustrate the factors that aggravate the particular patient's attacks of Raynaud's phenomenon. Patients also need to understand that in addition to cold exposure of the hands and feet, rapid shifts in the ambient temperature, core body temperature cooling, and a general body chill also provoke these attacks. Warm, loose-fitting clothing, warm stockings, warm headwear, and gloves or mittens are useful in preventing an attack during cold weather exposure. In fact, avoidance of cold temperatures is the best way to prevent an episode of Raynaud's phenomenon in any patient.

Some patients deny that emotional stress provokes a vasospastic episode in the absence of a cold stimulus. However, studies suggest that Raynaud's phenomenon is more likely to occur if a sympathetic stimulus is coupled with cold exposure. In fact, both observational and experimental studies have demonstrated that peripheral vasoconstriction can be affected by emotional and behavioral factors,[5] which suggests that behavioral interventions may be helpful in the treatment of Raynaud's phenomenon.

Temperature biofeedback has frequently been used in combination with different relaxation techniques in the treatment of Raynaud's phenomenon. Autogenic training (the use of relaxation-inducing self-statements that suggest warmth and heaviness) have been used alone or in combination with biofeedback.[6, 7] Results of a small, controlled trial of temperature biofeedback from one center suggested improvement in the number and intensity of Raynaud's symptoms over 1 year of follow-up.[7] A multicenter trial involving over 300 patients with primary Raynaud's phenomenon, however, compared temperature biofeedback with a control (electromyographic stimulation) procedure and found no benefit from biofeedback.[8] There remain questions about the role of temperature biofeedback in the treatment of Raynaud's phenomenon, but most authorities agree that it is not helpful for secondary forms of the condition.[9] Temperature biofeedback alone cannot be recommended as therapy for patients with either primary or secondary Raynaud's phenomenon.

Therapy that attempts to recondition the response to cold has been reported to be successful.[10, 11] One method involved pairing the unconditioned stimulus of warm water applied to the hands with a conditioned stimulus of exposure of the whole body to cold. After training, exposure to cold alone elicited vasodilatation in the hands (the conditioned response). Through this and similar techniques, patients with Raynaud's have been shown to have increases in digital temperatures in comparison with untreated controls.

## PHARMACOLOGIC TREATMENT OF RAYNAUD'S PHENOMENON

No drug is currently approved in the United States for the treatment of Raynaud's phenomenon. Many of the drugs used have not been tested scientifically. Several factors are pertinent in evaluation of the literature on therapeutic intervention in Raynaud's phenomenon. It is important that the drugs used for Raynaud's phenomenon be tested in a randomized, placebo-controlled clinical trial that accounts for the ambient temperature and patient activity. It is also important to determine whether the patient population studied has primary or secondary Raynaud's phenomenon. Primary patients are more likely to respond to vasodilators because of the absence of structural abnormalities of the blood vessels or other difficult-to-control factors.[12, 13] Investigators should distinguish between clinical self-reported measures and laboratory hemodynamic measures of response to treatment. Subjective improvement in the frequency, duration, or severity of Raynaud's attacks after drug treatment are generally considered a successful treatment outcome but may not correlate with laboratory-based measurements of digital blood flow.[13–18]

### Calcium Channel Blockers

Of the currently available drugs on the market, calcium channel blockers, because of their vasodilating properties, are the agents most frequently used for the treatment of Raynaud's phenomenon. Nifedipine has been the most widely studied of the available calcium channel blockers,[12, 14–17, 19–33] but nicardipine,[34, 35] diltiazem,[36–38] verapamil,[39] isradipine,[40] and nisoldipine[41] have also been investigated.

Three studies with nifedipine enrolled only patients with primary Raynaud's phenomenon,[21, 31, 33] and two studies enrolled only patients with scleroderma.[22, 32] The studies of patients with primary Raynaud's phenomenon reported a reduction of approximately 50% in frequency of attacks and a significant reduction in severity of attacks. In the two published studies on the evaluation of nifedipine for the treatment of Raynaud's phenomenon in patients with scleroderma, subjective improvement was documented with digital ulcer healing in one study[22] and improved finger temperature and finger blood flow in the other.[32] In contrast, other studies failed to show a response in the subset of patients with severe secondary Raynaud's phenomenon.[12, 19]

A multicenter study of patients with primary Raynaud's phenomenon investigated a slow-release preparation of nifedipine[8] (Procardia XL, Adalat CC). This placebo-controlled trial demonstrated the benefit of slow-release nifedipine over two winters of follow-up. Most physicians use the slow-release preparations because of the ease of administration and the reported lower frequency of side effects in comparison with the shorter-acting preparations. Nifedipine's side effects, although not serious, are frequent: 30% to 100% of patients have reported problems.[12, 19, 21, 33, 41] The most common side effects are headache, tachycardia, flushing, light-headedness, and edema.

There are few published studies about the other available calcium channel blockers of the dihydropyridine class. One study compared nicardipine and placebo therapy in 25 patients with primary and secondary Raynaud's phenomenon.[34] This study failed to show a difference between the two treatment groups with regard to number and severity of attacks, characteristics of the Raynaud's phenomenon, use of hands in the winter months, patient assessment of medication effectiveness, or objective measurements of finger systolic pressure and critical closing temperature.[34] Kahan and colleagues[35] reported that nicardipine reduced the frequency of attacks (mean $29.6 \pm 13.6$ attacks per 2 weeks on placebo vs. $23.1 \pm 17.0$ attacks per 2 weeks on nicardipine; $P < .05$) and the severity of Raynaud's phenomenon (mean score $2.2 \pm 0.4$ on placebo vs. $1.8 \pm 0.07$ on nicardipine; $P < .05$).[35] Felodipine and isradipine have been shown to be helpful in clinical trials conducted in Europe.

In the phenylalkylamine class of calcium channel blockers, verapamil failed to show clinical benefit in the one published study of 16 patients with Raynaud's phenomenon.[39] Diltiazem, a benzothiazepine, has been reported to reduce frequency and severity of Raynaud's attack in three placebo-controlled studies.[36–38] However, one study reported that although the improvement was striking in patients with primary Raynaud's phenomenon, it did not reach statistical significance in patients with associated systemic disease.[37]

### Other Drugs

Few controlled trials have scientifically defined the efficacy of other vasodilators in the treatment of Raynaud's phenomenon. In general, other agents have proved through experience to be disappointing in their clinical usefulness, or they are not currently available in the United States. New evidence suggests that Raynaud's phenomenon is mediated through provocation of $\alpha_2$-adrenergic receptors.[42]

Sympatholytic agents, including reserpine,[43, 44] guanethidine,[45] methyldopa,[46] prazosin,[47] phenoxybenzamine,[48] phentolamine,[49] indoramin,[50] and tolazoline,[51] have been reported to be useful. Reserpine was popular in the treatment of Raynaud's phenomenon until a controlled trial demonstrated that intra-arterial reserpine was no better than placebo.[44] Although the $\alpha_1$-adrenergic receptor blocker prazosin has been shown to reduce symptoms, it is less effective in secondary Raynaud's phenomenon, and the clinical improvement may not be sustained with prolonged treatment.

Other agents reported to work in the treatment of Raynaud's phenomenon include angiotensin-converting enzyme inhibitors,[52, 53] serotonin receptor blockers,[18, 54] thromboxane synthetase inhibitors,[19] evening primrose oil,[55] direct-acting vasodilating agents such as nitroglycerin[56] and hydralazine,[48] and calcitonin gene-related peptide.[57] The usefulness of most of these agents is hampered by the high frequency of side effects, the inconvenient route of administration, or the lack of demonstrated effectiveness in a placebo-controlled trial.

Prostaglandins that vasodilate, including prostaglandin (PG) $I_2$ (prostacyclin),[58] $PGE_1$,[59, 60] $PGE_2$,[61] and iloprost,[62, 63] are effective in treating severe Raynaud's phenomenon and critical ischemia. These agents are available in Europe but are still difficult to obtain in the United States. One study suggests that nifedipine is as effective as iloprost in the treatment of severe Raynaud's phenomenon.[22] Thus, nifedipine or another dihydropyridine calcium channel blocker remains the first choice in the treatment of Raynaud's phenomenon because of its availability, ease of administration, clinical benefit demonstrated in placebo-controlled studies, and reasonably low toxicity profile (Table 31–1).

## AUTHOR'S APPROACH TO DRUG TREATMENT

Patients should be considered candidates for drug therapy if management without drugs has failed or if there is evidence of ischemic tissue injury. Patients who have secondary Raynaud's phenomenon are more likely to need drug treatment, but they are also less likely to respond to treatment. A high number (up to 30%) of patients do show improvement when given a placebo, warm weather does reduce the attack rate, and subjective symptoms are more likely to improve than are objective measures of local blood flow. Therefore, careful assessment of the chosen drug treatment is prudent; if possible, treatment is usually stopped in the warm months. Although Raynaud's attacks can be uncomfortable and unattractive, most patients have little disability or significant consequences of the attacks, particularly if they have primary Raynaud's phenomenon.

In uncomplicated cases, it is reasonable to start therapy with the slow-release nifedipine or one of the newer dihydropyridines: isradipine, amlodipine, nicardipine, or felodipine. Evidence suggests these newer agents have less negative inotropic effects than do nifedipine and therefore may be safer. A dose of nifedipine XL, 30 mg/day, or of an equivalent dihydropyridine (e.g., amlodipine, 5 mg PO/day) is started. If there is no response in a 1- to 2-week period, the dose can be increased to 10 mg/day of amlodipine. Nifedipine can be increased by 30 mg at 1- to 4-week intervals until the maximal tolerated dose is reached. In general, patients who do not respond to nifedipine are unlikely to respond to other currently available vasodilators. However, if the extended-release nifedipine is not effective, it is reasonable either to try intermittent dosing with the shorter-acting nifedipine preparation or to try another calcium channel blocker. Amlodipine and the other dihydropyridines are well tolerated and are known to be effective. Diltiazem is another reasonable choice, whereas nicardipine and verapamil have been disappointing in the treatment of Raynaud's phenomenon. Combinations of calcium channel blockers have generally not been helpful.

Other classes of vasodilating drugs, including nitrates and sympatholytic agents, are usually of no greater value than the calcium channel blockers and may be poorly tolerated. However, patients with severe Raynaud's phenomenon and critical ischemia who fail to respond to a calcium channel blocker can try another vasodilator agent, either alone or in combination with a calcium channel blocker.

Topical nitrates are reported to be helpful. Patients can be started on ¼ to ½ inch of topical 2% nitroglycerin ointment applied two times daily: once in the morning on arising and repeated 6 hours later. A rest from nitrates for 10 to 12 hours is necessary to prevent a refractory state that can aggravate vasospasm. As in antianginal therapy, the dosage can be increased until a maximal tolerated dosage is reached (maximal recommended dosage, 2 inches). Alternatively, a nitrate patch can be used. Headaches are the most common reason that patients stop taking nitrates. Topical nitrates can be combined with a calcium channel blocker or with other vasodilators; however, the effects of combinations of these agents have not been studied in clinical trials.

Prazosin is the first choice among the sympatholytic agents. It can be started with a 1-mg test dose and then slowly increased to 2 to 5 mg by mouth three times daily (maximal daily dose, 20 mg). Most patients who benefit find prazosin less effective over time. Other $\alpha$-blocking agents are also not particularly useful for long-term therapy; however, uncontrolled experience has shown that intravenous phentolamine and phenoxybenzamine can be useful in reversing severe ischemia. These potent agents should be given only in an appropriate hospital setting for proper monitoring of cardiovascular parameters.

Intravenous prostaglandins can reduce the severity of Raynaud's phenomenon. This is true in scleroderma patients with severe Raynaud's and ischemic ulcers. $PGE_1$ (alprostadil) is available for maintaining a patent ductus arteriosus in neonates with congenital heart defects. It must be administered through a large vein (studies in Raynaud's phenomenon used a central vein), and the patient must be in the hospital and appropriately monitored. The drug is infused at a starting

**TABLE 31-1**
**Summary of Pharmacologic Treatment of Raynaud's Phenomenon (RP)**

| DRUG | CLINICALLY EFFECTIVE |
|------|---------------------|
| **Calcium Channel Blockers** | |
| Dihydropyridine | |
|   Nifedipine | Yes: multiple trials |
|   Nifedipine XL | Yes: one trial in primary RP |
|   Amlodipine | Yes: limited evidence |
|   Felodipine | Yes: limited evidence |
|   Nicardipine | Variable results in trials |
|   Isradipine | Yes: two trials |
|   Nimodipine | Not tested |
|   Nisoldipine | Not effective in one trial |
| Nondihydropyridine | |
|   Verapamil | Not effective in one trial |
|   Diltiazem | Yes: considered less potent than nifedipine |
|   Bepridil | Not tested |
|   Mibefradil | Not tested |
| **Sympatholytic Agents** | |
| Guanethidine | Yes: limited evidence |
| Methyldopa | No controlled studies |
| Phenoxybenzamine | Yes: limited evidence |
| Phentolamine | No controlled studies |
| Prazosin | Yes: less effective in secondary RP |
| Reserpine | Effect not sustained in controlled trial |
| Tolazoline | No controlled studies |
| **Angiotensin-Converting Enzyme Inhibitors** | |
| Captopril/enalapril (others not tested) | Controversy with overall mild benefit |
| **Vasodilators** | |
| Nitroglycerin | Yes: controlled trials |
| Hydralazine | Yes: limited studies |
| Niacin | Yes: limited studies |
| Isoxsuprine | No benefit |
| L-Arginine | No benefit |
| Minoxidil | Topically no benefit |
| **Other Vasoactive Drugs** | |
| Pentoxifylline | Yes: mild benefit |
| **Prostaglandins** | |
| Prostacyclin | Yes: intravenous (IV) administration |
| Prostaglandin E$_1$ | Yes: IV administration |
| Iloprost | Yes: IV administration |
| | No: orally |

dosage of 0.1 μg/kg/minute and increased if necessary to a maximum of 0.4 μg/kg/minute. Intravenous prostacyclin and its analog, iloprost, are effective in treating severe Raynaud's phenomenon but are not readily available. Epoprostenol (prostacyclin), approved for the treatment of primary pulmonary hypertension,[64] can also reduce Raynaud's attacks and reverse critical digital ischemia. Iloprost or epoprostenol can be given in a dosage starting at 0.5 ng/kg/minute and increased to a maximum of 2 ng/kg/minute in a 6- to 8-hour infusion each for 3 days. The benefit may continue for 6 to 10 weeks. Oral prostaglandins are now under study. Oral iloprost at 50 μg PO twice daily was not better than placebo in the treatment of Raynaud's phenomenon.[65] Misoprostol (oral PGE$_1$) is

available; however, one investigation found it to be no better than placebo in preventing vasospasm from an acute cold challenge in patients with Raynaud's phenomenon.[66]

Because the risk of ischemic tissue damage is minimal in primary uncomplicated Raynaud's phenomenon, every effort should be made to avoid potentially toxic medication. Secondary Raynaud's phenomenon often does not respond to currently available drug therapy. It is important to recognize that vasodilator therapy is successful if it reduces or stops new ischemic events, even if it does not stop every Raynaud's attack. In these difficult cases, warm temperature remains the best selective vasodilator, and it is therefore essential to maximize cold avoidance and nondrug therapy, including rest (hospitalization if necessary) during a crisis. All available vasodilators are nonselective and have the potential of dilating healthy vessels in preference to the diseased vessels directly involved in the ischemia. Aggressive care of ischemic ulcers with antibiotic ointments, periodic cleaning with soap and water, and appropriate use of systemic antibiotics help prevent complications and amputation.

## SURGICAL TREATMENT OF RAYNAUD'S PHENOMENON

Severe Raynaud's phenomenon may be refractory to any drug treatment, particularly if it is complicated by prolonged ischemia and tissue ulceration. Surgical sympathectomy has been reported to be helpful in these cases; however, few controlled data are available for assessing the role of these procedures. Cervical or lumbar sympathectomy may provide transient relief but is rarely curative. A temporary lumbar, cervical, or digital sympathetic block can be attempted in order to determine whether sympathectomy will reverse acute vasospasm. If a temporary chemical sympathectomy "breaks" the vasospasm, an oral vasodilator can be started to control new vasospastic events. I have successfully used digital sympathectomy by injecting either lidocaine or bupivacaine several times to maintain effective pain control and to provide maximum vasodilatation. Permanent sympathectomy should be considered if vasodilators fail to control the situation after there was clear evidence of a successful temporary chemical block. A permanent procedure by cervical sympathectomy for vasospasm in the upper extremities is not recommended. The long-term outcome of proximal sympathectomy is generally poor. A local digital sympathectomy procedure is more effective and may have the added benefit of releasing the vessel from local fibrosis that restricts good blood flow. Data suggest that patients with scleroderma often have significant obstructive disease in the ulnar artery that may be surgically repaired. It is our experience that the usefulness of these radical procedures is very limited and clearly should be done only by skilled and experienced surgeons after careful selection of appropriate cases. Unfortunately, patients often come to the physician's attention after the ischemic event has caused either ulceration or digital gangrene. In this situation, it is preferred to allow these areas to heal with topical care or self-amputation (either of which often minimizes loss of tissue in an area of poor blood flow) rather than perform surgical procedures.

## APPROACH TO CRITICAL ISCHEMIA

The key to successful management of an ischemic crisis is early and aggressive intervention. Delay in reversing vasospasm leads rapidly to vascular occlusion, irreversible disease, and tissue gangrene. Medical therapy should always be considered for the underlying associated disease process. It is important to investigate the possibility of larger vessel occlusive disease that may be surgically corrected. Every patient should be carefully examined and noninvasive vascular studies performed if needed. Arteriographic studies should be conducted if there is a possibility of a correctable lesion in larger vessels.

In an acute ischemic crisis, the following actions are recommended:

- Put the patient immediately to rest in a warm ambient temperature, and eliminate any definable stressful stimuli. Control of ischemic pain is most important. Narcotics are vasoconstrictors, so a chemical digital or limb sympathectomy may be used in difficult situations.
- Start vasodilator therapy immediately. An oral calcium channel blocker should be titrated to the maximal tolerated dose. I prefer amlodipine or short-acting nifedipine. Intravenous prostaglandins (PGE$_1$, epoprostenol, iloprost) are very effective in reversing an acute reversible ischemic event but may be difficult to obtain. Phentolamine or nitroprusside infusion can be helpful.
- Initiate antiplatelet therapy. Low-dose aspirin (81 mg/day) has been the traditional antiplatelet agent.
- I aggressively use temporary chemical digital sympathectomy. This provides both non-narcotic pain relief and is also a potent vasodilator. If the chemical block provides relief, repeated injections or performing a surgical digital sympathectomy is undertaken when persistent ischemia is present. In the lower extremity, lumbar sympathectomy is used.
- Anticoagulation or thrombolytic therapy can be considered during the acute phase of an ischemic event, but these treatments are best limited to embolic or vascular occlusive disease associated with new thrombosis. Anticoagulation with heparin may be used for short periods during a crisis. The use of chronic anticoagulation has not been studied and is generally not recommended. Patients with antiphospholipid antibodies with digital ischemia may require anticoagulation. Studies have suggested that thrombolytic therapy (e.g., urokinase and tissue plasminogen activator) may be helpful for patients with Raynaud's phenomenon and scleroderma. However, controlled studies are needed before it is known whether this approach reverses acute ischemia in severe Raynaud's phenomenon.
- Many patients are seen in later stages of ischemia, and some have severe structural disease without a capacity to vasodilate. In these patients, pain control and surgical amputation may be the only options.

## REFERENCES

1. Wigley FM, Flavahan N: Raynaud's phenomenon. Rheum Dis Clin North Am 1996; 22:765–781.
2. Maricq HR, Carpentier PH, Weinrich MC, et al: Geographic variation in the prevalence of Raynaud's phenomenon: Charleston, SC, USA, vs Tarentaise, Savoie, France. J Rheumatol 1993; 20:70.

3. LeRoy EC, Medsger TA Jr: Raynaud's phenomenon: A proposal for classification. Clin Exp Rheumatol 1992; 10:485.

4. Kallenberg CGM: Early detection of connective tissue disease in patients with Raynaud's phenomenon. Rheum Dis Clin North Am 1990; 16:11.

5. Freedman RR, Iaani P, Wenig P: Behavioral treatment of Raynaud's disease. J Consult Clin Psychol 1983; 51:539.

6. Surwit RS, Pilon RN, Fenton CH: Behavioral treatment of Raynaud's disease. J Behav Med 1978; 1:323.

7. Keefe FJ, Surwit RS, Pilon RN: A one-year follow-up of Raynaud's patients treated with behavioral therapy techniques. J Behav Med 1979; 2:385.

8. Medsger TA, Hill R, Kaufmann P, et al: The Raynaud's phenomenon (RP) treatment study (RTS): A comparison of pharmacologic and behavioral interventions. Arthritis Rheum 1997; 554:S123.

9. Freedman RR, Ianni P, Wenig P: Behavioral treatment of Raynaud's phenomenon in scleroderma. J Behav Med 1984; 7:343.

10. Jobe JB, Sampson JB, Roberts DE, et al: Comparison of behavioral treatments for Raynaud's disease. J Behav Med 1986; 9:89.

11. Melin H, Fagerstrom K: Treatment of peripheral vasospasm. Scand J Behav Ther 1981; 10:97–100.

12. Rodeheffer RJ, Rommer JA, Wigley FM, et al: Controlled double-blind trial of nifedipine in the treatment of Raynaud's phenomenon. N Engl J Med 1983; 308:880.

13. Wigley FM, Wise RA, Mikdashi J, et al: The post-occlusive hyperemic response in patients with systemic sclerosis. Arthritis Rheum 1990; 33:1620.

14. Aldoori M, Bruce W, Dieppe PA: Nifedipine in the treatment of Raynaud's syndrome. Cardiovasc Res 1986; 20:466.

15. Smith DC, McKendry RJR: Controlled trial of nifedipine in the treatment of Raynaud's phenomenon. Lancet 1982; 2:1299.

16. Sauza J, Kraus A, Gonzalez-Amaro R, et al: Effect of the calcium channel blocker nifedipine on Raynaud's phenomenon: A controlled double-blind trial. J. Rheumatol 1984; 11:362.

17. Kallenberg CG, Woundra AA, Kuitert JJ, et al: Nifedipine in Raynaud's phenomenon: relationship between short term and long term effects. J Rheumatol 1987; 14:284.

18. Coffman JD, Clement DL, Creager MA, et al: International study of ketanserin in Raynaud's phenomenon. Am J Med 1989; 87:264.

19. Ettinger WH, Wise RA, Schaffhausser DA, et al: Controlled double-blind trial of dazoxiben and nifedipine in the treatment of Raynaud's phenomenon. Am J Med 1984; 77:451.

20. White CJ, Phillips WA, Abrahams LA, et al: Objective benefit of nifedipine in the treatment of Raynaud's phenomenon: Double-blinded controlled study. Am J Med 1986; 80:623.

21. Sarzoki J, Blookman AM, Mahon W, et al: Nifedipine in the treatment of idiopathic Raynaud's syndrome. J Rheumatol 1986; 13:331.

22. Rademaker M, Cooke ED, Almond NE, et al: Comparison of intravenous infusions of iloprost and oral nifedipine in the treatment of Raynaud's phenomenon in patients with systemic sclerosis: A double-blind randomized study. B M J 1989; 298:561.

23. Vayssairat M, Capron L, Fiessinger JN, et al: Calcium channel blockers and Raynaud's disease. Ann Intern Med 1981; 95:243.

24. Dale J, Landmark KR, Myhre E, et al: The effects of nifedipine, a calcium antagonist, on platelet function. Am Heart J 1983; 105:103.

25. Kahan A, Weber S, Amor B, et al: Nifedipine and Raynaud's phenomenon. Ann Intern Med 1981; 94:546.

26. Winston EL, Pariser KM, Miller KB, et al: Nifedipine as a therapeutic modality for Raynaud's phenomenon. Arthritis Rheum 1983; 26:1177.

27. Nilsson H, Jonasson T, Ringqvist I, et al: Nifedipine in cold-induced vasospasm. Eur Heart J 1984; 33(Abstract suppl):5.

28. Nilsson H, Jonasson T, Ringqvist I, et al: Treatment of digital vasospastic disease with the calcium-entry blocker nifedipine. Acta Med Scand 1984; 215:135.

29. Wollersheim H, Thien TH, Van't Laar A, et al: Nifedipine in primary Raynaud's phenomenon and in scleroderma: Oral vs. sublingual hemodynamic effects. J Clin Pharmacol 1987; 27:907.

30. Kirch W, Linder HR, Hutt HJ, et al: Ketanserin vs. nifedipine in secondary Raynaud's phenomenon. Vasa 1987; 16:77.

31. Gjorup T, Kelbaek J, Hartling OJ, et al: Controlled double-blind trial of the clinical effect of nifedipine in the treatment of idiopathic Raynaud's phenomenon. Am Heart J 1986; 111:742.

32. Finch MB, Dawson J, Johnston GD, et al: The peripheral vascular effects of nifedipine in Raynaud's syndrome associated with scleroderma: A double-blind crossover study. Clin Rheumatol 1986; 5:493.

33. Corbin DOC, Wood DA, MacIntyre CC, et al: A randomized double-blind crossover trial of nifedipine in the treatment of primary Raynaud's phenomenon. Eur Heart J 1986; 7:165.

34. Wigley FM, Wise RA, Malamet R, et al: Nicardipine in the treatment of Raynaud's phenomenon: Dissociation of platelet activation from vasospasm. Arthritis Rheum 1987; 39:281.

35. Kahan A, Amor B, Menkes CJ, et al: Nicardipine in the treatment of Raynaud's phenomenon: A randomized double-blind trial. Angiology 1987; 38:333.

36. Rhedda A, McCans J, Willan AR, et al: A double-blind placebo controlled crossover randomized trial of diltiazem in Raynaud's phenomenon. J Rheumatol 1985; 12:720.

37. Kahan A, Amor B, Menkes C: A randomized double-blind trial of diltiazem in the treatment of Raynaud's phenomenon. Ann Rheum Dis 1985; 44:30.

38. Matoba T, Chiba M: Effects of diltiazem on occupational Raynaud's syndrome (vibration disease). Angiology 1985; 36:850.

39. Kinney EL, Nicholas G, Gallo J, et al: The treatment of severe Raynaud's phenomenon with verapamil. J Clin Pharmacol 1982; 22:74.

40. Leppert J, Jonasson T, Nilsson H, et al: The effect of isradipine, a new calcium-channel antagonist, in patients with primary Raynaud's phenomenon: A single-blind dose-response study. Cardiovasc Drugs Ther 1989; 3:397.

41. Gjorup T, Hartling O, Kelbaek H, et al: Controlled double-blind trial of nisoldipine in the treatment of idiopathic Raynaud's phenomenon. Eur J Clin Pharmacol 1986; 31:387.

42. Unemori EN, Pickford LB, Salles AL, et al: Relaxin induces an extracellular matrix-degrading phenotype in human lung fibroblasts in vitro and inhibits lung fibrosis in a murine model in vivo. J Clin Invest 1996; 98:2739.

43. Surwit RS, Gilgor RS, Duvic M, et al: Intra-arterial reserpine for Raynaud's syndrome. Arch Dermatol 1983; 119:733.

44. McFadyen IJ, Housley E, MacPherson AI: Intra-arterial reserpine administration in Raynaud's syndrome. Arch Intern Med 1973; 132:526.

45. LeRoy EC, Downey JA, Cannon PJ: Skin capillary blood flow in scleroderma. J Clin Invest 1971; 50:930.

46. Varadi DP, Lawrence AM: Suppression of Raynaud's phenomenon by methyldopa. Arch Intern Med 1969; 124:13.

47. Russell LJ, Lessard JA: Prazosin treatment of Raynaud's phenomenon: A double-blind single crossover study. J Rheumatol 1985; 12:94.

48. Russell IJ, Walsh RA: Selection of vasodilator therapy for severe Raynaud's phenomenon by sequential arterial infusion. Ann Rheum Dis 1985; 44(3):151.

49. Coffman JD, Cohen RA: Intra-arterial vasodilator agents to reverse finger vasoconstriction. Clin Pharmacol Ther 1987; 41:574.

50. Robson P, Pearce V, Antcliff AC, et al: Double-blind trial of indoramin in digital artery disease. Br J Clin Pharmacol 1978; 6:88.

51. Allegra C, Tonelli V, Ecari U, et al: Pharmacological treatment of Raynaud's phenomenon: A new therapeutic approach. Curr Ther Res 1986; 40:303.

52. Miyazaki S, Miura K, Kasai Y, et al: Relief of digital vasospasm by treatment with captopril and its complete inhibition by serine proteinase inhibitors in Raynaud's phenomenon. BMJ 1982; 284:310.

53. Tosi SA, Marchesoni A, Messina K, et al: Treatment of Raynaud's phenomenon with captopril. Drugs Exp Clin Res 1987; 13:37.

54. Seibold JR, Terregino CA: Selective antagonism of S₂-serotonergic receptors relieves but does not prevent cold-induced vasoconstriction in primary Raynaud's phenomenon. J Rheumatol 1986; 13:337.

55. Belch JJF, Shaw B, O'Dowd A, et al: Evening primrose oil (efamol) in the treatment of Raynaud's phenomenon: A double-blind study. Thromb Haemost 1985; 54:490.

56. Franks AG Jr: Topical glyceryl trinitrate as adjunctive treatment in Raynaud's disease. Lancet 1982; 1:76.

57. Bunker CB, Reavley C, O'Shaughnessy DJ, et al: Calcitonin gene–related peptide in treatment of severe peripheral vascular insufficiency in Raynaud's phenomenon. Lancet 1993; 342:80.

58. Belch JJF, Drury JK, Capell H, et al: Intermittent epoprostenol (prostacyclin) infusion in patients with Raynaud's phenomenon. Lancet 1983; 1:313.

59. Morhland JS, Porter JM, Smith EA, et al: A multicenter placebo-controlled, double-blind study of prostaglandin E$_1$ in Raynaud's syndrome. Ann Rheum Dis 1985; 44:754.

60. Langevitz P, Buskila D, Lee P, et al: Treatment of refractory ischemic skin ulcers in patients with Raynaud's phenomenon with PGE$_1$ infusions. J Rheum 1989; 16:1433.

61. Belch JJF, Shaw B, Sturrock RD, et al: Double-blind trial of CLII5,347, a transdermally absorbed prostaglandin E$_2$ analogue, in treatment of Raynaud's phenomenon. Lancet 1985; 1:1180.

62. Kyle MV, Belcher G, Hazelman B: Placebo controlled study showing therapeutic benefit of iloprost in the treatment of Raynaud's phenomenon. J Rheumatol 1992; 19:1403.

63. Wigley FM, Seibold JR, Wise RA, et al: Intravenous iloprost treatment of Raynaud's phenomenon and ischemic ulcers secondary to systemic sclerosis. J Rheumatol 1992; 19:1407.

64. Barst RJ, Rubin LJ, McGoon MD, et al: Survival in primary pulmonary hypertension with long-term continuous intravenous prostacyclin. Ann Intern Med 1994; 121:409.

65. Wigley FM, Korn JH, Csuka ME, et al: Oral iloprost in patients with Raynaud phenomenon secondary to systemic sclerosis: A multicenter, placebo-controlled, double-blind study. Arthritis Rheum 1998; 41:670.

66. Wise RA, Wigley FM: Acute effects of misoprostol on digital circulation in patients with Raynaud's phenomenon. J Rheumatol 1994; 21:80.

# 32 | Idiopathic Inflammatory Diseases of Muscle

*Robert L. Wortmann*

The idiopathic inflammatory diseases of muscle are uncommon and poorly understood conditions. Patients with one of these diseases generally have (1) proximal muscle weakness, (2) elevated serum levels of enzymes derived from skeletal muscle, (3) myopathic electromyographic changes, and (4) muscle biopsy evidence of inflammation. Over time, the inflammatory myopathies have been classified in a variety of ways.[1-7] Despite some more recent proposals,[6,7] the scheme proposed by Bohan and Peter[1] continued to be employed by most clinicians and investigators. Bohan and Peter proposed the first criteria for making a diagnosis of idiopathic myositis (Table 32-1) and divided the diseases that fulfilled those criteria into five groups: (1) primary idiopathic polymyositis, (2) primary idiopathic dermatomyositis, (3) dermatomyositis or polymyositis associated with cancer, (4) childhood dermatomyositis (or polymyositis) associated with vasculitis, and (5) polymyositis or dermatomyositis associated with another recognized collagen vascular disease. (For more information on pathogenesis and diagnosis, see Wortmann.[8])

More recently, additional types of myositis have been recognized. Those groups, such as inclusion body myositis and myopathy with circulating myositis-specific autoantibodies, have emerged from studies of patients whose diseases generally fulfill Bohan and Peter's criteria for polymyositis. Criteria for the diagnosis of inclusion body myositis have been proposed and employed for the investigation of these groups of patients (Table 32-2).[9] Discovery of myositis-specific autoantibodies has allowed further evolution of the classification of these diseases (Table 32-3). Most myositis-specific autoantibodies are directed against cytoplasmic ribonucleoproteins, bind to evolutionary conserved epitopes, and inhibit the functions of the target autoantigen.[10] Eight specific autoantibodies have been recognized to date; an individual patient has only one of these. In addition, a number of less specific autoantibodies are found to circulate in the blood in some other patients with myositis. These have been termed *myositis-associated autoantibodies* (Table 32-4). The presence of a particular autoantibody appears to define homogeneous groups of patients.[11]

Today it is therefore possible to apportion patients among six different groups and further subclassify them on the basis of absence or presence of a particular myositis-specific or myositis-associated autoantibody. The six groups are as follows:

1. Polymyositis
2. Dermatomyositis
3. Myositis with myositis-specific autoantibodies
4. Inclusion body myositis
5. Juvenile (childhood) dermatomyositis
6. Cancer-related myositis
7. Myositis with another recognized collagen vascular disease

It must be recognized that the differences among these groups are not always clear-cut. The initial approach to therapy for all patients with an idiopathic inflammatory muscle disease may be the same. Nevertheless, the diagnosis must be defined as accurately as possible because, despite similarities in initial therapeutic approach, the prognosis for each may differ significantly.

## NATURAL HISTORY AND LONG-TERM EXPERIENCE

The true natural history of the inflammatory myopathies is difficult to determine for several reasons. The diseases are relatively rare. Most series report small numbers of patients who were evaluated retrospectively over a period of many years. There exists much uncertainty concerning the accuracy of diagnoses in studies before the mid-1970s. Furthermore, the classification schemes applied have varied widely over time.[1-7, 9] Patients were not always divided among groups; when groups were identified, however, criteria were not employed consistently. Because of small numbers of patients studied, different groups were often combined for analysis. Serum enzymes, electrophysiologic studies, and autoantibody testing were less available, and the diagnosis and treatment of neoplastic diseases, hypertension, and infections were quite different, Finally, since the 1950s, almost every patient with a diagnosis of inflammatory muscle disease has

## TABLE 32–1
## Criteria to Define Polymyositis-Dermatomyositis Proposed by Bohan and Peter

1. Symmetric weakness of limb-girdle muscles and anterior neck flexors, progressing over weeks to months, with or without dysphagia or respiratory muscle involvement.
2. Skeletal muscle histology showing evidence of necrosis of type 1 and 2 muscle fibers, phagocytosis, regeneration with basophilia, large sarcolemmal nuclei and prominent nucleoli, atrophy in a perifascicular distribution, variation in fiber size, and an inflammatory exudate.
3. Elevation of serum skeletal muscle enzymes (CK, aldolase, AST, ALT, and LDH).
4. Electromyographic triad of short, small, polyphasic motor units; fibrillations, positive waves, and insertional irritability; and bizarre high-frequency discharges.
5. Dermatologic features, including lilac (heliotrope) discoloration of the eyelids with periorbital edema; scaly, erythematous dermatitis over the dorsa of the hands, especially over the metacarpophalangeal and proximal interphalangeal joints (Gottron's sign), and involvement of the knees, elbows, medial malleoli, face, neck, and upper torso.

ALT = alanine aminotransferase; AST = aspartate aminotransferase; CK = creatine kinase; LDH = lactate dehydrogenase.

Reprinted with permission from Bohan A, Peter JB: Polymyositis and dermatomyositis (first of two parts). N Engl J Med 1975; 292:344. Copyright 1975, Massachusetts Medical Society.

been treated with corticosteroids. Many of the problems that plagued earlier studies continue to be problems today. Physicians will continue to have difficulty defining the best treatment for these diseases until there is a truly accurate classification scheme and sufficient numbers of patients can be evaluated.

## TABLE 32–2
## Diagnostic Criteria Proposed for Inclusion Body Myositis

**Pathologic Criteria**

Electron microscopy
  1. Microtubular filaments in the inclusions
Light microscopy
  1. Lined vacuoles
  2. Intranuclear or intracytoplasmic inclusions or both

**Clinical Criteria**

1. Proximal muscle weakness (insidious onset)
2. Distal muscle weakness
3. Electromyographic evidence of a generalized myopathy (inflammatory myopathy)
4. Elevation of muscle enzymes (CK or aldolase or both)
5. Failure of muscle weakness to improve on a high-dose corticosteroid regimen (at least 40–60 mg/d for 3–4 months)

Definite IBM = pathologic electron microscopy criterion 1 and clinical criterion 1 plus one other clinical criterion. Probable IBM = pathologic light microscopy criterion 1 and clinical criterion 1 plus three other clinical criteria. Possible IBM = pathologic light microscopy criterion 2 plus any three clinical criteria.

CK = creatine kinase.

From Calabrese LH, Mitsumoto H, Chou SM: Inclusion body myositis presenting as treatment-resistant polymyositis. Arthritis Rheum 1987; 30:397.

Because of the difficulties of studying adequate numbers of patients and the lack of controlled clinical trials, treatment of the inflammatory myopathies is largely empirical.[8, 12–14] Corticosteroids have been the cornerstone of drug therapy for each of these diseases since their introduction to clinical medicine. Corticosteroid use has improved the prognosis for patients with idiopathic inflammatory myopathies, although some authorities argue about the amount of that improvement.[15, 16] Studies of adults indicate 5-year survival rates of 60% in the precorticosteroid era, 68% between 1947 and 1968,[17] and 80% to 90% in more recent reports.[11] Survival rate still varies among the different groups (Fig. 32–1). The reasons for the improvement in survival rate are not clear but may relate to earlier and more accurate diagnoses, better treatments for associated medical problems, and the earlier use of immunosuppressive agents. Today, determination of the appropriate clinical group and the time from disease onset to diagnosis of myositis provide the most useful information for predicted response to therapy.[11, 18–22] It appears that the presence of a circulating myositis-specific autoantibody is useful in this regard.[11, 23] Other poor prognostic factors include more severe weakness at the time therapy is initiated, pharyngeal muscle weakness, aspiration, and interstitial pulmonary fibrosis.[24–28] White patients generally have a better prognosis than do black patients.

Prognosis can be based on the classic clinical groups of Bohan and Peter[1] or on the presence or absence of a circulating myositis-specific autoantibody. Children have a better prognosis than do adults. Of the children with juvenile dermatomyositis who live 10 years, 90% lead normal lives. Mortality in children is attributable most often to myocarditis, perforation of a viscus, or infection. Adults with myositis and cancer fare the worst and almost always die of the neoplasm. However, some with a treatable or curable cancer may do quite well. The prognosis for patients with associated connective tissue diseases is determined by the other manifestations of the underlying diagnosis. The myositis of patients in that clinical group typically responds very well to corticosteroids, often at low doses. The actual prognosis for patients with inclusion body myositis appears to be good but is still unknown. In general, the course is slow and prolonged. In most persons the weakness becomes fixed or progresses slowly. Less commonly, progression is relentless, leading to severe incapacitation and death.

Identification of a circulating myositis-specific autoantibody seems to enable clinicians to predict the clinical characteristics and prognosis (see Fig. 32–1).[11, 23] According to the small number of observations to date, survival varies tremendously among the various autoantibody groups, with 5-year survival rates of 100% for patients with anti-Mi-2, 70% for those with antisynthetase, and 30% for persons with anti-SRP. Some caution should be exercised in accepting these data, because they were collected in a selected group of patients seen at the tertiary centers. Analysis of patients from rural community practices indicate that many may have a better prognosis.[29]

**TABLE 32–3**
**Myositis-Specific Autoantibodies**

| AUTOANTIBODY | ANTIGEN | CLINICAL FEATURES |
|---|---|---|
| Antisynthetases | Aminoacyl-tRNA synthetases | Myositis (polymyositis > dermatomyositis) with arthritis, fever, |
| Anti–Jo-1 | Histidyl-tRNA synthetase | interstitial lung disease, Raynaud's phenomenon, "mechanic's" hands, |
| Anti–PL-7 | Threonyl-tRNA synthetase | and poor response to therapy |
| Anti-EJ | Glycyl-tRNA synthetase | |
| Anti–PL-12 | Alanyl-tRNA synthetase | |
| Anti-OJ | Isoleucyl-tRNA synthetase | |
| Anti-KS | Asparaginyl-tRNA synthetase | |
| Anti-SRP | Signal recognition particle | Myositis, cardiomyopathy and treatment resistant to therapy |
| Anti–Mi-2 | Helicase proteins | Dermatomyositis, good response |

## CONTROLLED CLINICAL TRIALS

For the treatment of any idiopathic inflammatory myopathy, the information available from controlled clinical trials is extremely limited because only four studies have been published.[30–33] In addition, each of these studies involved low numbers of patients, and previous therapies had failed in all patients included.

The first blind, controlled trial evaluated the use of azathioprine.[30] Sixteen patients with polymyositis and dermatomyositis whose improvement had reached a plateau during treatment with prednisone alone were divided into two groups and randomly assigned to continue taking prednisone alone or to receive prednisone plus azathioprine. Although no difference between the groups was apparent at 3 months, the azathioprine recipients showed significant improvement with regard to functional abilities at 1 and 3 years. In addition, the azathioprine recipients required less prednisone.

Plasmapheresis and leukapheresis were studied in a double-blind manner and compared with a sham apheresis control group.[31] Corticosteroid therapy had failed in all 39 participants in that trial, and most of the patients had not responded to other agents. Patients who underwent plasma exchange did have significant reductions in serum levels of muscle enzymes, and those who had leukapheresis experienced significant decreases in lymphocyte counts. Nevertheless, only 3 of the 13 patients in each group showed improvement in strength and functional capacity. Deterioration oc-

curred in three patients treated with leukapheresis and in one treated with plasma exchange. At the conclusion of the study, there were no significant differences in muscle strength or functional capacity among the three treatment groups. This study suggests that leukapheresis and plasma exchange are not effective in patients with inflammatory myopathy. However, of the 39 patients, 26 (8 receiving plasma exchange, 11 leukapheresis, and 7 sham apheresis) had antisynthetase or anti-SRP antibodies in their sera. It is now recognized that patients with these serologic markers generally respond poorly to treatment.[11, 23] Consequently, it is difficult to extrapolate the results of this trial to patients with an inflammatory myopathy and no circulating myositis-specific antibody.

A double-blind, placebo-controlled trial of high-dose intravenous immune globulin has been performed in 15 adults with treatment-resistant dermatomyositis.[32] All patients had biopsy-proven disease and were unresponsive or poorly responsive to high-dose prednisone or therapeutic dosages of another immunosuppressive agent (azathioprine, methotrexate, or cyclophosphamide) for at least 4 months. The dosages of prednisone and other immunosuppressive agents were kept constant, and the patients were randomly assigned to receive one infusion of immune globulin (2 g/kg body weight) or placebo per month for 3 months, with the option of crossing over for 3 months. The eight patients assigned to receive immune globulin exhibited significant improvement in muscle strength and neuromuscular symptoms, whereas the seven who received pla-

**TABLE 32–4**
**Myositis-Associated Autoantibodies**

| AUTOANTIBODY | ANTIGEN | CLINICAL FEATURES |
|---|---|---|
| Anti–PM-Scl | Unidentified | Myositis, scleroderma, and arthritis |
| Anti-Ku | DNA-binding proteins | Myositis–scleroderma–systemic lupus erythematosus overlap |
| Anti-KJ | Unidentified translation factor | Polymyositis, interstitial lung disease, and Raynaud's phenomenon |
| Anti-Fer | Elongation factor 1$_\alpha$ | Myositis |
| Anti-MJ | Unidentified | Juvenile dermatomyositis |
| Anti-MAS | tRNA$^{ser}$ antigen-related | Myositis, hepatitis and alcoholic rhabdomyolysis |
| Anti-U1RNP | U1 small nuclear ribonuclear protein | Mixed connective tissue disease |
| Anti-snRNPs | U2–U6 small nuclear ribonuclear proteins | Polymyositis-scleroderma overlap |
| Anti-Ro/SSA | RNA protein | Myositis with Sjögren's syndrome or systemic lupus erythematosus |

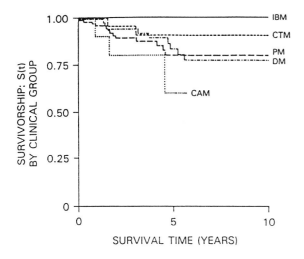

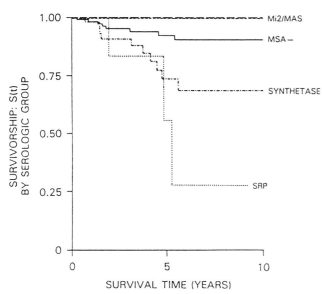

**FIGURE 32–1**

Classification of idiopathic inflammatory myopathy. Kaplan-Meier analysis of survival in the clinical (*top*) and serologic (*bottom*) groups of patients with idiopathic inflammatory myopathies. The data were analyzed by the Fisher exact test for significance with Bonferroni corrections for multiple comparisons. Patients with inclusion body myositis (IBM) had significantly prolonged survival from the time of diagnosis ($P < 3/4 .05$) in comparison with patients with polymyositis (PM) or dermatomyositis (DM). Although differences were noted between the patients with cancer-associated myositis (CAM) (all of whom died of cancer) and all the other clinical groups, they were not significant when corrected for multiple comparisons. Analysis of survival data in the serologic groups showed significantly increased mortality among patients with SRP autoantibodies in comparison with those without SRP autoantibodies and in the synthetase-positive patients in comparison with either patients with Mi-2 autoantibodies or those without myositis-specific autoantibodies (MSA). CTM = myositis with another connective tissue disease; Synthetase = autoantibodies to one of the five known aminoacyl-tRNA synthetases; SRP = autoantibodies to proteins of the signal recognition particle; Mi-2 = autoantibodies primarily directed against a 220-kd nuclear protein of unknown function; MAS = sera precipitating a common ~4S RNA of unknown function. (From Love LA, Leff RL, Fraser DD, et al: A new approach to the classification of idiopathic inflammatory myopathy: Myositis-specific autoantibodies define useful homogeneous patient groups. Medicine 1991; 70:360.)

cebo did not. With crossovers, a total of 12 patients received immune globulin. Of those, nine experienced major improvement to nearly normal function, two experienced mild improvement, and one experienced no change. Of 11 placebo-treated patients, none experienced major improvement, three experienced mild improvement, and five deteriorated. Thus high-dose intravenous immune globulin is effective for some patients with refractory dermatomyositis over a 3-month period. However, the positive effects of immune globulin remained for only 6 weeks. It appears that repeated treatment would be needed for long-term benefits.

A randomized crossover study comparing regimens of cytotoxic agents was performed in patients with refractory myositis.[33] Thirty patients were randomly assigned to receive the combination of weekly oral methotrexate (up to 25 mg/week) and daily azathioprine (up to 150 mg/day) or intravenous methotrexate (500 mg/m²) with oral leucovorin rescue (50 mg/m² every 6 hours for four doses beginning 24 hours after methotrexate injection) every 2 weeks for 6 months. Although the study lacked the power to directly compare both treatments and two thirds of the subjects were antisynthetase or anti-SRP antibody–positive, the results support the theory that the combination of oral methotrexate and azathioprine may benefit patients with treatment-resistant myositis, including those who previously had inadequate responses to either agent alone. Intravenous methotrexate with leucovorin rescue resulted in improvement in a smaller number of patients.

## AUTHOR'S APPROACH TO MANAGEMENT

### Pretreatment Decisions

The first steps in the management of any inflammatory myopathy include ensuring the accuracy of the diagnosis and assessing the patient's baseline status. Because there is no specific "diagnostic test" for these diseases, the diagnosis must be made by excluding other possible causes (Table 32–5). An objective baseline assessment is needed because the available outcome measures generally lack precision. It is difficult to determine the actual effects of therapy in some cases because some patients fail to respond to any treatment and others achieve only partial resolution of symptoms.

Muscle strength should be thoroughly evaluated before any medication is used. Objective testing of the strength of individual muscle groups provides valuable information. This can be done manually by a trained examiner (physician, nurse, physical therapist) or with isokinetic dynamometry.[34] A timed-stands test is also a simple and useful means of assessing lower extremity weakness (Fig. 32–2).[35] Baseline measurements should be compared with those obtained during the course of therapy to help determine the effects of treatment.

**TABLE 32–5**

**Causes of Muscle Weakness that Could Be Confused with Polymyositis**

**Other Rheumatic Diseases**

Giant cell arteritis/polymyalgia rheumatica
Wegener's granulomatosus
Polyarteritis nodosa
Systemic lupus erythematosus

**Neurologic Disorders**

Muscular dystrophies
　Becker's
　Limb-girdle
Myasthenia gravis
Amyotropic lateral sclerosis

**Infections**

Toxoplasmosis
Acquired immunodeficiency syndrome
Coxsackievirus
Influenza

**Metabolic/Nutritional Disorders**

Malabsorption
Electrolyte disorders
　Hyponatremia
　Hypokalemia
　Hypophosphatemia
　Hypomagnesemia
　Hypercalcemia

**Cancer-Related Diseases**

Carcinomatous neuromyopathy
Eaton-Lambert syndrome

**Toxins/Drugs**

Alcohol
Chloroquine/hydroxychloroquine
Clofibrate
Cimetidine
Cocaine
Corticosteroids
Colchicine
Cyclosporine
Gold salts
Lovastatin/dravastatin/simvastatin
Zidovudine (AZT)

**Inborn Errors of Metabolism**

Glycogen-storage diseases
　Myophosphorylase deficiency (McArdle's disease)
　Phosphofructokinase deficiency
Carnitine deficiency
Mitochondrial myopathies

---

Pretreatment assessment should also include measurements of serum levels of muscle enzymes, any tests that might be influenced by medications used in treatment, analysis of pulmonary status and swallowing, and screening for cancer. Muscle enzymes include the creatine kinase (CK), aldolase, alanine aminotransferase (ALT), aspartate aminotransferase (AST) and lactate dehydrogenase (LDH). Each should be measured at baseline, but only the most abnormal values need to be tested routinely. Such a value is almost always the CK. Blood cell counts, serum electrolytes,

creatinine, glucose, and other values that might be affected by therapeutic agents should be quantitated. Testing for antinuclear antibodies may prove useful if there is consideration of an associated collagen vascular disease. Today, testing for the presence or absence of a circulating myositis-specific autoantibody is of limited value. With the possible exception of testing for anti-Jo-1, most laboratories do not perform these tests. Furthermore, the presence of fever, interstitial lung disease, or arthritis provides the same information regarding therapy and prognosis as does the presence of an antisynthetase autoantibody. The practical value of testing for these antibodies is likely to improve in the future.

Blood pressure determination, chest examination, and chest radiography should be performed routinely. Pulmonary function testing, including diffusion capacity, may be indicated. Fluoroscopic swallowing studies with radiographic contrast material are important if the patient has difficulty swallowing, dysphagia, or dysphonia. Precautions that might prevent aspiration should be emphasized for patients at risk. These include swallowing education, elevation of the head of the bed on blocks, and use of antacids or $H_2$ blockers to neutralize gastric secretions. The recognized association between the inflammatory myopathies and cancer must always be considered. The clinician should therefore take a careful history; systems review, physical examination, and cancer-screening procedures are rec-

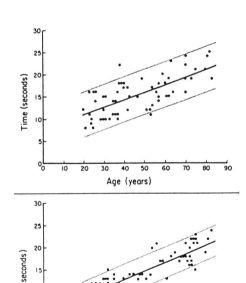

**FIGURE 32–2**

Timed-stands test as a function of age in 62 normal women (*top*) and in 77 normal men (*bottom*). The mean and limits of normal (90% prediction region) are shown. (From Csuka ME, McCarty DJ: Simple method for measurement of lower extremity muscle strength. Am J Med 1985; 78:77; with permission from Excerpta Medica Inc.)

ommended on the basis of the patient's age and sex. Because of the difficulty in diagnosing ovarian cancer, women of any age with dermatomyositis should undergo frequent gynecologic evaluations. Screening for nasopharyngeal carcinomas should be performed in patients with dermatomyositis who live in areas where that cancer is more prevalent.[36] Extensive, unfocused evaluations in search of an occult neoplasm are not warranted.[37, 38]

## Nonpharmacologic Considerations

Physical therapists can prove invaluable in the treatment of patients with myositis. Not only are they able to assist in testing muscle group strength, but they can also design, instruct, and assist in an exercise program. Although exercise programs may be unnecessary in very mild cases, they may be important in others. Physical therapy should be used to preserve function, avoid disuse atrophy, and prevent contractures.[34, 39] The patient's program must take into account the amount of inflammation. Initially, bed rest may be very important for severely affected persons. Anecdotally, muscle strength and CK levels have improved dramatically from a disabled to a functioning status with bed rest as the only intervention in some patients who refused to take any medication. Unfortunately, these remissions were transient and rarely lasted more than 2 months. Passive motion is encouraged during periods of maximal inflammation in an effort to maintain normal range of motion and prevent contractures. Contractures are more often a problem in juvenile dermatomyositis, in which residual contractures and calcinosis may contribute significantly to residual disability. However, these complications can occur in adults as well. With signs of improvement, the exercise program can include active-assisted exercises and then active exercises. Patients with active polymyositis and inclusion body myositis can perform resistive exercises without elevations in CK level and with improvement of muscle strength.[40, 41] With recovery, active isometric or isotonic exercises are clearly recommended to increase strength and endurance.

## Drug Therapies

Corticosteroids are the standard first-line medication for patients with any inflammatory myopathy. I prefer to begin with prednisone at a dosage of approximately 1 mg/kg taken orally in a single dose each morning. This preference is purely empirical, as are all programs proposed for treating inflammatory myopathies.[8, 11–14] Once instituted, daily high-dose prednisone is continued until strength improves. Clinical improvement may be noted in the first weeks or gradually over a period of 3 to 6 months. This variability is related, at least in part, to the timing of treatment initiation.[21] The earlier in the course of the disease the prednisone is given, the faster and more effectively it will work.[23] Evaluations of muscle strength are performed at 3- to 6-week intervals. Ideally, the initial steroid dosage is maintained until both strength and CK values have

returned to normal. Objective testing of strength is necessary to make certain that the patient's reported improvement is not simply a euphoric or "energizing" effect from the corticosteroids. Although it is reassuring to see strength improve and CK levels fall, strength is the more important measure.[20] Lowered CK values can be observed even when there is no improvement in strength because circulating CK inhibitors are present in some patients with active inflammation,[42] in some cases of myositis associated with cancer, or as a "nontherapeutic" result of treatments such as plasmapheresis or intravenous immune globulin. On the other hand, CK values may remain elevated after complete normalization of muscle strength because the disease process has resulted in damaged or "leaky" membranes.

At 6 weeks, a decision is made. If the patient is stronger or definitely improving, prednisone is continued at the initial dosage until strength and, it is hoped, CK values have returned to normal and have remained normal for 4 to 8 weeks. Once remission is apparent, the prednisone dosage is reduced by 10 mg/day each month. After a dosage of 10 mg/day has been taken for 1 month, the dosage is reduced to 5 mg/day. This dosage is maintained until the patient has remained in remission for 1 year. Control of a flare that occurs at any time during the tapering necessitates raising the prednisone dosage, often to the level that brought about the initial remission.

In view of the empirical nature of treatment for the inflammatory myopathies, other valid methods have been proposed for the use of corticosteroids. Starting doses range from a fixed dose of 60 mg/day up to 2 mg/kg/day.[43, 44] Some physicians begin with daily intravenous infusions of methylprednisolone.[45] Some physicians prefer to divide the initial daily dosage. Although a divided schedule may provide greater anti-inflammatory effect than does a single-dose schedule, it may prove more toxic. With improvement, some authors would taper as much as 25% each month. Others would employ an alternate-day schedule toward the end of the taper. Alternate-day steroid therapy does result in fewer side effects, but if initiated too soon, it may trigger a flare of the disease.

Corticosteroid therapy leads to improvement in up to 90% of patients and complete remission in 50% to 75%.[18] However, if improvement is not obvious at 6 weeks or if the improvement has reached a plateau before complete remission is achieved, I add a second agent. Invariably, the choice of second agents is between azathioprine and methotrexate. Azathioprine, which has been tested in a blind, controlled trial,[30] is favored as a second agent by some authorities.[44] Azathioprine, 2 to 3 mg/kg/day, is usually effective in a single oral dose. In adults, I begin with 50 mg/day and check for results and potential side effects, primarily bone marrow depression, after 3 weeks. If there is no response, the dose is increased to 100 mg/day, and the process is repeated. If response is still not adequate, the dose is increased again to a maximum of 150 mg/day.

Methotrexate, the other possible second agent, has been shown to be beneficial in adults and children with myositis.[46–48] Although oral methotrexate has not been tested in a blind or controlled manner, there is growing support for this agent.[14, 23] Methotrexate is given in a single weekly dose; the dosage is selected somewhat arbitrarily. I prefer to start with 7.5 mg orally in most patients and increase the dosage to 15 mg after 4 to 6 weeks if improvement has not occurred. Children are given oral methotrexate at a dosage of 20 mg/m². In sicker adults, or those in whom compliance may be questioned, I prefer a dosage of 25 mg, escalating to 50 mg, given by intramuscular or intravenous injection.

Once the patient is in remission (is free of symptoms, has a normal CK level, and has been off medication for 3 to 9 months), the serum enzyme levels are checked infrequently unless recurrence is suggested by symptoms or changes on physical examination. Before remission, the CK is monitored on a regular basis. If it becomes elevated but the patient has no symptoms, medication is not automatically prescribed. Rather, the patient is questioned about physical activity and other factors that might spuriously elevate the CK level, and the frequency of check-ups is increased. Therapy should be reinstituted at the first sign of weakness and must be considered if the enzyme levels continue to rise. As a general rule, however, the clinician should treat weakness, not laboratory results.

The general approach just outlined can be applied to all inflammatory myopathies. However, special consideration must be given to patients within certain clinical groups. The cutaneous lesions of dermatomyositis may respond to hydroxychloroquine at doses of up to 200 mg orally twice a day. This treatment may be effective even in patients with cancer.[49] Hydroxychloroquine, however, has no effect on the myositis. The primary focus of treatment for patients with myositis and cancer should be on the neoplasm. Removal (debulking) of the tumor or cure of the cancer may be accompanied by resolution of the myopathy. The myositis associated with another collagen vascular disease is often very sensitive to corticosteroid therapy. High dosages may be necessary for only short intervals, and dosages of 10 to 30 mg/day may suffice in many cases.

Inclusion body myositis and myopathy associated with certain myositis-specific autoantibodies represent the more challenging groups. When first described, inclusion body myositis was thought to be refractory to treatment.[9] However, a small number of affected patients have had excellent response to therapy, and there is now some evidence that treatment may retard progression in a percentage of patients.[50–52] Many patients with myositis and antisynthetase antibodies or anti-SRP antibodies also appear to be relatively resistant to treatment.[10, 23] It is not clear whether this poor response correlates with the amount of interstitial pulmonary fibrosis encountered in these patients or relates to other factors. Nevertheless, therapeutic trials are warranted in each of these groups, and I begin as described earlier. If no improvement is observed at 6 weeks, I add a second agent as described. If no im-

provement is noted in the following 6 to 12 weeks, I discuss the option of adding a third agent versus discontinuing the medicines. It is bad enough to have treatment-resistant myositis; the additional problems of cost, inconvenience, and side effects that arise when potentially toxic medications are used should not compound the situation unless the patient is fully aware of the alternatives. This approach is similar to that recommended by other authors.[53]

When disease is refractory to treatment with corticosteroids, especially if there is no response whatsoever, the clinician should confirm the accuracy of the initial diagnosis. Patients with a wide variety of conditions that would not necessarily respond to corticosteroid therapy can satisfy some or all of the criteria for polymyositis (see Table 32–5). When the diagnosis is confirmed or when patients must discontinue the aforementioned treatments because of serious side effects, the potential risks and benefits of the more experimental therapies listed later must be weighed.

Pulmonary complications should be suspected when the patient complains of dyspnea or cough, when auscultation of the chest reveals crackles or "Velcro" rales, or when the chest radiograph is abnormal. These complications may include interstitial fibrosis, aspiration pneumonitis, or opportunistic infections. Each portends a poor prognosis, although some patients with interstitial fibrosis remain free of symptoms. Therapy often has little effect on interstitial fibrosis when it progresses. Aspiration usually occurs in severe disease with hypopharyngeal muscle involvement. Opportunistic infections are related to the degree of immunosuppression caused by corticosteroids or other agents.

No deviation from the described protocol for patients with interstitial lung disease is recommended unless the pulmonary status is deteriorating. Serial measurements of diffusing capacity are useful in assessing this decline. A gallium scan may also detect active inflammation in the lungs. Abnormal results in either of these parameters may be an indication for use of higher dosage corticosteroid therapy (up to 2 mg/kg/day) and addition of another immunosuppressant agent, if one is not already being used. Maximal immunosuppressive therapy should also be considered when there is evidence of aspiration. Although the risk of complications from such therapy are great, that risk is outweighed by the potential good, inasmuch as aspiration is almost always followed by death. If an opportunistic infection develops, the dosage of corticosteroids should be reduced to one that would cover for stress (the lowest dosage tolerated but no more than 40 mg of prednisone per day), and the dosages of other immunosuppressive agents should be lowered to a level that allows a leukocytosis to develop. (This lowering may necessitate discontinuing these agents.)

Finally, the pulmonary complications of methotrexate must be considered for patients who are taking that medication. Methotrexate should be discontinued immediately in the presence of cough, dyspnea, or an abnormal chest radiograph and not reinstituted until the cause of the pulmonary problem is defined and determined not to be methotrexate.

Clinically significant cardiac complications are unusual, although conduction abnormalities may be seen on electrocardiograms and congestive heart failure can result from hypoxia or cardiomyopathy. Most cardiac problems should be managed as they would be if they developed in a patient who did not have myositis. An exception would be the patient with cardiomyopathy, who might benefit from a trial of higher dosage corticosteroid therapy and other immunosuppressive agents.

## DRUG SIDE EFFECTS AND RECOMMENDED MONITORING SCHEDULES

The methods used to monitor for side effects of corticosteroids, azathioprine, or methotrexate are the same as when those agents are used to treat other rheumatic diseases. However, two potential side effects of corticosteroids—steroid myopathy and steroid-induced osteoporosis—warrant special consideration.

The possibility of steroid-induced myopathy poses a unique problem. The question of steroid myopathy is very difficult to deal with in patients with myositis, especially in those whose improvement has reached a plateau or those who have had a partial, if not gratifying, response to therapy and then become weaker. In those situations, it must be determined whether the decline in muscle strength is caused by a flare of the inflammatory process or by steroid-induced myopathy.[54, 55] Unfortunately, no specific test provides the answer; even a muscle biopsy is of little value. Active inflammatory changes can be observed even when steroid-induced myopathy is contributing to the weakness. Further complicating the situation, type 2 fiber atrophy, the typical histologic change of steroid-induced myopathy, is a nonspecific finding and may be seen with disuse atrophy or as a change induced by inflammation. A provocative challenge with higher dosage corticosteroids or a trial of rapid tapering of the dosage may be the only way to determine the cause of weakness in this situation.

The risk of corticosteroid-induced osteoporosis is significant for patients with myositis, especially if they are immobilized by weakness. Vertebral compression fractures are a significant long-term morbidity in these patients.[56] Thus, weight-bearing exercises, such as walking, should be emphasized when possible, and the use of supplemental calcium (1000 to 1500 mg/day) should be encouraged. Vitamin D and estrogen may also be appropriate. (See Chapter 40 for additional detailed information about management of osteoporosis.)

Azathioprine can be used safely in most patients with inflammatory muscle disease. The major concern with this agent is bone marrow suppression. Initiating treatment with lower doses and monitoring blood counts before increasing the dosage helps avoid problems. If anemia, leukopenia, or thrombocytopenia is encountered, azathioprine should be discontinued. It

may be reinstituted after blood counts have returned to normal, but at a lower dosage. Dosages as low as 25 mg every other day have been used safely and effectively in some patients who are very sensitive to azathioprine. Other rare side effects include hepatotoxicity and pancreatitis. A hypersensitivity reaction consisting of fever and hypotension may occur. The issue of whether azathioprine induces cancer is of concern to some authorities. Although azathioprine-related neoplasia has been reported among renal transplant recipients, this relationship has not been established for patients with rheumatic diseases. The issue is further complicated because of the relationship between myositis and cancer. I do not believe that the concern about cancer should be used as a reason to withhold azathioprine therapy from patients with myositis.

When methotrexate is selected, AST and ALT levels should be measured and pulmonary function should be considered before the start of treatment in order to minimize confusion between changes in these parameters caused by the basic disease and the potential hepatic and pulmonary toxic effects of the medication. The intramuscular route is usually avoided because of the resulting elevation in CK levels. However, if blood is sampled just before a dose (i.e., 6 or 7 days after the last injection), the elevation of CK as a result of the trauma of the injection is rarely a problem. This timing also avoids confusion caused by transient elevations in transaminases that may develop immediately after a dose of methotrexate, regardless of the route of administration.

## INVESTIGATIONAL DRUGS, ADDITIONAL APPROACHES, AND FUTURE DIRECTIONS

A number of therapies have been employed in an attempt to help the patient with refractory myositis. The approaches used include a variety of modalities and agents used singly or in combination. Each has been chosen in the hopes of improving muscle strength and of avoiding the side effects of corticosteroids. In refractory cases, I prefer to add a third agent: azathioprine if methotrexate is the second agent, methotrexate if azathioprine is the second. The use of combinations is attractive; theoretically, improved results may occur because the different agents act through different mechanisms and might work synergistically. The combination of methotrexate and azathioprine has been used successfully anecdotally[57] and in a controlled trial involving patients who had previously failed to respond to either agent alone.[33] Other combinations have been tried with some reported benefit, but numbers of patients treated to date are very small.[58] I believe that the available data suggest that the combination of azathioprine and methotrexate should be employed in refractory cases before choosing other potentially toxic regimens.

Two alkylating agents, chlorambucil and cyclophosphamide, have been reported to be effective for some patients with myositis. Chlorambucil was used in combination with prednisone and methotrexate in two patients with dermatomyositis[58, 59] and was successfully used in five others who had not responded to azathioprine and methotrexate.[60] The initial dosage of chlorambucil used is 2 to 4 mg/day with adjustments up to a maximum of 8 mg/day as necessary to obtain a response. Leukopenia was the only side effect encountered in these subjects, but more profound bone marrow suppression and seizures are potential complications of this treatment. The potential for development of cancer is higher with chlorambucil than with azathioprine or methotrexate. The risk of development of cancer with or after chlorambucil therapy increases with both duration of treatment and total dosage.[61]

Cyclophosphamide has been used orally on a daily schedule with anecdotal reports of success.[62, 63] Intravenous administration has received some attention. Advocates of intravenous administration believe that it should be as effective as oral administration, primarily on the basis of experience in treating lupus nephritis. Results have been mixed, however. Cyclophosphamide was ineffective in 10 of 11 patients with corticosteroid-refractory polymyositis and dermatomyositis at a monthly dose of 0.75 to 1.25 g/m². [64] The remaining patient experienced unsustained improvement. In another study, four of seven patients with refractory polymyositis given intravenous cyclophosphamide at a dose of 500 mg/week were reported "recovered."[65] Additional reports have demonstrated efficacy of monthly pulse cyclophosphamide in patients with myositis or lupus, Sjögren's syndrome, and interstitial lung disease.[66–68] The patients in these reports had longstanding refractory disease. Perhaps earlier treatment would produce better results, and smaller, more frequent doses would prove more effective.

Cyclosporine is an immunosuppressive agent that inhibits calcium-dependent T cell activation and blocks transcription of genes that code for some cytokines, including interleukin-2. Through these actions, cyclosporine prevents proliferation of T helper cells and development of cytotoxic lymphocytes. Experience with cyclosporine in the treatment of myositis is quite limited, but reports from the late 1980s to 1990s appear favorable.[69–78] Lower doses (2.5 to 5.0 mg/kg/day) may be as effective as higher doses (7.5 to 10 mg/kg/day) for treating myositis. It is presumed that lower doses would be less toxic.

Cyclosporin was effective in a patient with anti–Jo-1 antibodies and refractory polymyositis[77] and in combination with intravenous immune globulin in two patients with dermatomyositis.[78]

Monitoring blood levels of cyclosporine helps keep toxicity to a minimum. Strength generally begins to improve within the first month to 6 weeks of treatment in patients who respond to cyclosporine. More frequently encountered toxic effects include tremors, hypertrichosis, gingival hyperplasia, hypertension, renal insufficiency, anemia, and, very rarely, lymphoproliferative cancer. Cyclosporine can also cause a myopathy,[79] a side effect that may complicate its use in myositis. The reversibility of these side effects is in question, especially with regard to renal insufficiency.

Although the serum creatinine value may return to normal after the agent is discontinued, the creatinine clearance may not.

Tacrolimus (FK 506), another agent that inhibits calcium-associated CD4+ T cell activation is currently used to prevent allograft rejection in transplant recipients. This agent has been used with beneficial results in six patients with anti–Jo-1 antibody and two with anti-SRP antibody.[80] Each exhibited a drop in serum CK level, improvement in functional status, lessening of extramuscular manifestations (arthropathy, interstitial lung disease, and mechanic's hands), and a lowered corticosteroid requirement.

Perhaps because of its effectiveness in Kawasaki disease, intravenous immune globulin has been touted as a therapeutic agent for multiple disorders, including the inflammatory myopathies. This agent has proved variably effective in a number of uncontrolled trials.[80–93] The largest of these studies involved 20 patients with disease duration ranging from 6 months to 14 years.[82] In all but one patient, prior therapies had failed. Fifteen patients experienced moderate or better improvement, four patients experienced no improvement, and one patient's condition worsened. Improvement usually occurred within 2 months, and better responses were observed in patients with shorter duration of disease. Improvement was noted in only 3 of 11 patients with myositis who received intravenous immune globulin as first-line therapy.[83]

A small, uncontrolled trial suggested that intravenous immune globulin might be beneficial for patients with inclusion body myositis.[84] In one larger study, one third of 19 patients showed objective improvement in functional status and a significant improvement in swallowing.[85] In another study, of nine patients, two demonstrated subjective improvement, but all experienced a decrease in motor function.[86]

Intravenous immune globulin should perhaps receive strongest consideration for treatment of refractory dermatomyositis; this assertion is based on the findings of a controlled trial that showed it to be effective over the short term for patients with this disease.[32] There is reason to believe that intravenous immune globulin therapy would be effective in dermatomyositis. The pathologic change in that form of inflammatory myopathy appears to be initiated by antibodies bound to microvascular components. With activation of the classic complement pathway, C5b, C6, C7, C8, and C9 membranolytic attack complexes are deposited in capillaries bound to those antibodies.[87–89] Fiber damage is mediated by the membranolytic attack complex.[90] These processes eventuate in fiber necrosis and regeneration, inflammatory cell infiltration, perifascicular atrophy, capillary loss, and ischemia. A T cell–mediated and major histocompatibility complex-1 (MHC-1)–restricted cytotoxic process has also been implicated in dermatomyositis.[88] The mechanisms whereby immune globulin modulate the immune system are far from understood. Of the postulated mechanisms, immune globulins may block crystallizable Fragment (Fc) receptors on vessel walls.[91, 92] Immune globulin may also inhibit the effector functions of activated T cells[91-93] or decrease the expression of MHC-1 molecules.[94, 95] High levels of immunogobulin neutralize complement neoantigens[96] and inhibit formation of membrane attack complexes from activated C4b and C3b fragments.[97] Any of these actions would interfere with the pathogenesis of dermatomyositis. If those actions do contribute to the efficacy of immune globulin in dermatomyositis, that therapy is probably also effective in other forms of myositis in which the complement membrane attack complexes or MHC-1–restricted T cell cytotoxicity are involved in the pathogenesis.

It is truly difficult to assess the efficacy of intravenous immune globulin because of the lack of consistent measures of disease activity, the variation in regimens, and the heterogeneity of the patients studied. In addition, because immune globulin is prepared from pooled plasma, different batches may have different strengths and activities. The long-term efficacy of this treatment is not known, and tachyphylaxis has been observed.[98] Intravenous immune globulin is generally well tolerated; flushing, myalgias, headache and aseptic meningitis rarely occur.[99] However, it is very expensive. I am not convinced of its long-term efficacy and would reserve it for use in the patient with refractory disease as an interval therapy while waiting for other agents to take effect.

Apheresis, predominantly plasmapheresis, has been advocated as a very effective therapy in refractory polymyositis. Before 1992, all reports were uncontrolled, unblinded trials in which patients also received other therapies. Interestingly, many patients also received immune globulin or took cyclophosphamide as a routine component of the plasmapheresis protocol. A controlled trial showed that plasmapheresis was not effective.[31] Although that study does not prove total ineffectiveness of this expensive and time-consuming procedure, it does show that plasmapheresis is unlikely to help patients with circulating myositis-specific autoantibodies. However, two patients with refractory polymyositis were reported to have responded dramatically to the combination of plasma exchange and intravenous immune globulin.[100] The advantage of apheresis with intravenous immune globulin or cyclophosphamide over immune globulin or cyclophosphamide alone is yet to be demonstrated.

Total body or total nodal irradiation (TBI) has been used with varying results in patients with polymyositis.[101-103] The use of TBI has been reported in five patients. Two patients achieved remission; one patient responded, suffered relapse, and responded to repeat therapy; one patient did not respond; and one patient died of bone marrow suppression. The potential side effects of TBI are numerous and serious, causing lasting effects on the immune system. Death has occurred after this therapy.[101] Previous cytotoxic therapy may well potentiate the serious bone marrow–suppressive effects of TBI. This therapy can be effective in patients in whom disease has been refractory to multiple other treatments, but it should be reserved for the sickest of patients whose disease is refractory to other modalities.

## SELECTED CONSIDERATIONS

Today it is very difficult to determine the most appropriate treatment for inclusion body myositis because there is simply too little information available. Although inclusion body myositis may be responsible for perhaps 30% of the cases in some series of idiopathic inflammatory myopathy, many physicians still are unaware of its existence. Initially, patients with inclusion body myositis were thought to be totally resistant to therapy. Two studies added support to the position that treatment may be beneficial. Nevertheless, physicians' expectations should probably be different when they are treating patients with inclusion body myositis. The first report was a retrospective analysis of 32 patients.[50] Four patients received no therapy, and their condition deteriorated, as would be predicted. Thirteen received prednisone alone; of those, seven deteriorated, four seemed to stabilize, and two experienced temporary improvement. The remainder received prednisone in combination with methotrexate or azathioprine; six deteriorated, one stabilized, five experienced transient improvement, and three achieved remission. Methotrexate appeared to provide better results than did azathioprine. These results suggest that although remission is quite rare in inclusion body myositis, the patient's weakness may be stabilized or the rate of progression of the disease may be slowed with therapy. The possible long-term benefits must still be weighed against the long-term toxic effects and the expense of treating this condition. Therefore, it is essential that objective guides for determining efficacy are followed. The second study reported improvement in strength in three of four patients treated with two monthly infusions of high-dose intravenous immune globulin (2 g/kg/month).[84] Greatest improvement was seen in the proximal and less atrophic muscles. In that study, CK levels fell after each treatment but rose again after the second infusion, and no relationship was found between the fall in CK levels and improvement. Two subsequent studies were not encouraging.[85, 86]

The treatment of children with recalcitrant myositis is of concern because of the potential long-term effects that therapy might have on developing systems. Methotrexate currently seems to be the preferred choice for children whose disease is resistant to corticosteroids.[104] Support for this view is provided by a study of 16 children with dermatomyositis who had failed to respond to prednisone.[46] Patients received methotrexate orally at a dosage of 20 mg/m². Twelve children who took the medication for more than 8 months achieved normal muscle strength at a median of 5 weeks after beginning treatment, and 11 of the 12 were able to decrease the daily prednisone dosage to 5 mg or less. As encouraging as those data appear, 31% of the patients in the study were unable to take methotrexate because of side effects, poor compliance, or complications. Furthermore, myositis recurred, as evidenced first by elevated CK levels and then by weakness, in all five patients in whom this agent was discontinued after they achieved remission. Thus, methotrexate appears to be useful in refractory childhood dermatomyositis. However, the drug cannot be used in all cases and may have only suppressive effects for patients who can tolerate it.

Cyclosporine has been used in children with dermatomyositis at doses of 2.5 to 7.5 mg/kg/day with some beneficial results.[105–107] Strength improved in all patients. Similarly, CK levels fell, but not always to normal limits. Daily corticosteroid dosage was reduced in all patients and eventually discontinued in some. Side effects and toxic effects were similar to those in adults, with the added occasional report of flulike symptoms.

Intravenous immune globulin has been suggested as a safe therapy for childhood dermatomyositis. An uncontrolled trial from two centers involving 11 patients indicated that this approach may be useful in corticosteroid-resistant patients.[108] Strength improved or was maintained in all patients. CK levels fell, but not always to within normal limits. Prednisone dosage was decreased or discontinued in all patients. As with other forms of myopathy, additional information is necessary to determine the most appropriate role for this expensive therapy.

# REFERENCES

1. Bohan A, Peter JB: Polymyositis and dermatomyositis (first of two parts). N Engl J Med 1975; 292:344.
2. Walton JN, Adams RD: Polymyositis. Baltimore: Williams & Wilkins, 1958.
3. Research Group for Neuromuscular Diseases of the World Federation of Neurology: Classification of neuromuscular disorders. J Neurol Sci 1968; 6:165.
4. DeVere R, Bradley WG: Polymyositis: Its presentations, morbidity and mortality. Brain 1975; 98:637.
5. Engel AG, Hohfeld R, Banker BQ: The polymyositis and dermatomyositis syndromes. *In* Engel AG, Franzini-Armstrong C (eds): Myology, 2nd ed, vol 2. New York: McGraw-Hill, 1994:1335.
6. Tanimoto K, Nakano K, Kano S, et al: Classification criteria for polymyositis and dermatomyositis. J Rheumatol 1995; 22:668.
7. Targoff IN, Miller FW, Medsger TA, et al: Classification criteria for the idiopathic inflammatory myopathies. Curr Opin Rheum 1997; 9:527.
8. Wortmann RL: Inflammatory diseases of muscle and other myopathies. *In* Kelley WN, Harris ED Jr, Ruddy S, et al. (eds): Textbook of Rheumatology, 5th ed. Philadelphia: WB Saunders, 1997:1177.
9. Calabrese LH, Mitsumoto H, Chou SM: Inclusion body myositis presenting as treatment-resistant polymyositis. Arthritis Rheum 1987; 30:397.
10. Targoff IN: Autoantibodies. *In* Wortmann RL (ed): Clinical Disorders of Skeletal Muscle. Philadelphia: Lippincott, Williams & Wilkins, 2000:267.
11. Love LA, Leff RL, Fraser DD, et al: A new approach to the classification of idiopathic inflammatory myopathy: Myositis specific autoantibodies define useful homogeneous patient groups. Medicine 1991; 70:360.
12. Mastaglia FL, Phillips BA, Zilko P: Treatment of inflammatory myopathies. Muscle Nerve 1997; 20:651.
13. Miller FW: Inflammatory myopathies: Polymyositis, dermatomyositis, and related conditions. *In* Koopman WT (ed): Arthritis and Allied Conditions, 13th ed, vol 2. Baltimore: Williams & Wilkins, 1997:1407–1432.
14. Oddis, CV: Idiopathic inflammatory myopathy. *In* Wortmann RL (ed): Clinical Disorders of Skeletal Muscle. Philadelphia: Lippincott, Williams & Wilkins, 2000:45.
15. Tuffanelli DJ, Lavoie PE: Prognosis and therapy of polymyositis/dermatomyositis. Clin Dermatol 1988; 6:93.
16. Morand BF: Corticosteroids in the treatment of rheumatologic diseases. Curr Opin Rheumatol 1998; 10:179.
17. Medsger TA, Robinson H, Masi AT: Factors affecting survivorship in polymyositis: A life-table study of 124 patients. Arthritis Rheum 1986; 15:168.
18. Henriksson KG, Sandstedt P: Polymyositis—Treatment and prognosis: A study of 107 patients. Acta Neurol Scand 1982; 65:280.
19. Hochberg MC, Feldman D, Stevens MB: Adult onset polymyositis/dermatomyositis: An analysis of clinical and laboratory features and survival in 76 patients with a review of the literature. Semin Arthritis Rheum 1986; 15:168.
20. Oddis CV, Medsger TA Jr: Relationship between serum creatinine, kinase level and corticosteroid therapy in polymyositis-dermatomyositis. J Rheumatol 1988; 15:807.
21. Fafalak RG, Peterson MGE, Kagen LJ: Strength in polymyositis and dermatomyositis: Best outcome in patients treated early. J Rheumatol 1994; 21:643.
22. Lilley H, Dennett X, Byrne E: Biopsy proven polymyositis in Victoria 1982–1987: Analysis and prognostic factors. J R Soc Med 1994; 87:323.
23. Joffe MM, Love LA, Leff RL, et al: Drug therapy of the idiopathic inflammatory myopathies: Predictors of response to prednisone, azathioprine, and methotrexate and a comparison of their efficacy. Am J Med 1993; 94:379.
24. Hochberg MC, Lopez-Acuna D, Gittelsohn AM: Mortality from polymyositis and dermatomyositis in the United States, 1968–1978. Arthritis Rheum 1983; 26:1465.
25. Benbassat J, Gefel D, Larholt K, et al: Prognostic factors in polymyositis/dermatomyositis: A computer-assisted analysis of ninety-two cases. Arthritis Rheum 1985; 28:249.
26. McKendry RJR: Influence of age at onset on the duration of treatment in idiopathic adult polymyositis and dermatomyositis. Arch Intern Med 1987; 117:1989.
27. Arsura EL, Greenberg AS: Adverse impact of interstitial pulmonary fibrosis on prognosis in polymyositis and dermatomyositis. Semin Arthritis Rheum 1988; 18:29.
28. Clarke AE, Bloch DA, Medsger TA Jr, et al: A longitudinal study of functional disability in a national cohort of patients with polymyositis/dermatomyositis. Arthritis Rheum 1995; 38:1218.
29. Hoffman GS, Franck W, Raddatz DA, et al: Presentation, treatment and prognosis of idiopathic inflammatory muscle disease in a rural hospital. Am J Med 1983; 75:433.
30. Bunch TW: Prednisone and azathioprine for polymyositis: Long-term follow up. Arthritis Rheum 1981; 24:45.
31. Miller FW, Leitman SF, Cronin ME, et al: A randomized controlled trial of plasma exchange and leukapheresis in polymyositis and dermatomyositis. N Engl J Med 1992; 326:1380.
32. Dalakas MC, Illa I, Dambrosia JM, et al: A controlled trial of high-dose intravenous immune globulin infusions as treatment for dermatomyositis. N Engl J Med 1993; 329:1993.
33. Villalba L, Hicks JE, Adams EM, et al: Treatment of refractory myositis. Arthritis Rheum 1998; 41:392.
34. Mahowald ML, Dykstra DD: Rehabilitation of patients with muscle weakness. *In* Wortmann RL (ed): Clinical Disorders of Skeletal Muscle. Philadelphia: Lippincott, Williams & Wilkins, 2000:349.
35. Csuka ME, McCarty DJ: A rapid method for measurement of lower extremity muscle strength. Am J Med 1985; 78:77.
36. Hu W, Chan D, Min H: Study of 45 cases of nasopharyngeal carcinoma with dermatomyositis. Am J Clin Oncol 1996; 19:35.
37. Cox NH, Langtry JAA, Lawrence CM, et al: Dermatomyositis and malignancy: An audit of the value of extensive investigations. Br J Dermatol 1989; 121:47.
38. Callen JP: Relationships of cancer to inflammatory muscle diseases. Dermatomyositis, polymyositis, and inclusion body myositis. Rheum Dis Clin North Am 1994; 20:943.
39. Hicks JE: Comprehensive rehabilitative management of patients with polymyositis and dermatomyositis. *In* Dalakas MC (ed): Polymyositis and Dermatomyositis. Boston: Butterworths, 1988:293.
40. Hicks JE: Role of rehabilitation in the management of myopathies. Curr Opin Rheum 1998; 10:548.

41. Spector SA, Lemmer JT, Koffman BM, et al: Safety and efficacy of strength training in patients with sporadic inclusion body myositis. Muscle Nerve 1997; 20:1242.

42. Kagan LJ, Aram S: Creatine kinase activity inhibitor in sera from patients with muscle disease. Arthritis Rheum 1987; 30:213.

43. Oddis CV: Therapy for myositis. Curr Opin Rheumatol 1991; 3:919.

44. Dalakas MC: Polymyositis, dermatomyositis, and inclusion-body myositis. N Engl J Med 1991; 325:1486.

45. Yangisawa T, Sueshi M, Nawata Y, et al: Methylprednisolone pulse therapy in dermatomyositis. Dermatologica 1983; 167:47.

46. Miller LC, Sisson BA, Tucker LB, et al: Methotrexate treatment of recalcitrant childhood dermatomyositis. Arthritis Rheum 1992; 35:1143.

47. Newman ED, Scott DW: The use of low-dose methotrexate in the treatment of polymyositis and dermatomyositis. J Clin Rheumatol 1995; 1:99.

48. Wilke WE: Methotrexate use in miscellaneous inflammatory diseases. Rheum Dis Clin North Am 1997; 23:855.

49. Woo TY, Callen JP, Voorhees JJ, et al: Cutaneous lesions of dermatomyositis are improved by hydroxychloroquine. J Am Acad Dermatol 1984; 10:592.

50. Sayers ME, Chou SM, Calabrese LH: Inclusion body myositis: Analysis of 32 cases. J Rheumatol 1992; 19:1385.

51. Barohn RJ, Amato AA, Sabenk Z, et al: Inclusion body myositis: Explanation for poor response for immunosuppressive therapy. Neurology 1995; 45:1302.

52. Cohen MR, Sulaiman AR, Garancis JC, et al: Clinical heterogeneity and treatment response in inclusion body myositis. Arthritis Rheum 1989; 32:734.

53. Calabrese LH, Chou SM: Inclusion body myositis. Rheum Dis Clin North Am 1994; 20:955.

54. Afifi AK, Bergman RA, Harvey JC: Steroid myopathy: Clinical, histologic, and cytologic observations. Johns Hopkins Med J 1968; 123:158.

55. Askari A, Vignos PJ, Moskowitiz RW: Steroid myopathy in connective tissue disease. Am J Med 1976; 61:485.

56. Oddis CV, Hill P, Medsger TA Jr: Functional outcome in a national cohort of polymyositis-dermatomyositis (PM-DM) patients. Arthritis Rheum 1992; 35(suppl):S88.

57. Trotter D, McCarty DJ, Csuka ME: Treatment of dermatomyositis/polymyositis with combination chemotherapy in early disease. Arthritis Rheum 1991; 34(suppl):S149.

58. Wallace DJ, Metzger AL, White KK: Combination immunosuppressive treatment of steroid resistant dermatomyositis/polymyositis. Arthritis Rheum 1985; 28:590.

59. Cagnoli M, Marchesoni A, Tosi S: Combined steroid, methotrexate, and chlorambucil therapy for steroid-resistant dermatomyositis. Clin Exp Rheumatol 1991; 9:658.

60. Sinoway PA, Callen JP: Chlorambucil: An effective corticosteroid-sparing agent for patients with recalcitrant dermatomyositis. Arthritis Rheum 1993; 36:319.

61. Cameron S: Chlorambucil and leukemia. N Engl J Med 1977; 296:1065.

62. al-Janadi M, Smith CD, Karsh J: Cyclophosphamide treatment of interstitial pulmonary fibrosis in polymyositis/dermatomyositis. J Rheumatol 1989; 16:1592.

63. Bombardieri S, Hughes GH, Neri R, et al: Cyclophosphamide in severe polymyositis [Letter]. Lancet 1989; 1:1138.

64. Cronin ME, Miller FW, Hicks JE, et al: The failure of intravenous cyclophosphamide therapy in refractory idiopathic inflammatory myopathy. J Rheumatol 1989; 16:1225.

65. Haga H, D'Cruz D, Asherson R, et al: Short term effects of intravenous pulses of cyclophosphamide in the treatment of connective tissue disease crisis. Ann Rheum Dis 1992; 51:885.

66. Kono WH, Klashman DJ, Gilbert RC: Successful IV pulse cyclophosphamide in refractory polymyositis in 3 patients with systemic lupus erythematosus. J Rheumatol 1990; 17:982.

67. LeRoy JP, Drosos AA, Yiannapoulos DI, et al: Intravenous pulse cyclophosphamide therapy in myositis and Sjögren's syndrome. Arthritis Rheum 1990; 33:1579.

68. Boulware DW, Makkena R: Monthly cyclophosphamide in lupus pneumonitis and myositis. J Rheumatol 1991; 18:153.

69. Lueck CJ, Trend P, Swash M: Cyclosporine in the management of polymyositis and dermatomyositis. J Neurol Neurosurg Psychiatry 1991; 54:1007.

70. Correia O, Polonia J, Nunes JP, et al: Severe acute form of adult dermatomyositis treated with cyclosporine. Int J Dermatol 1992; 31:517.

71. Pugh MT, Collins NA, Rai A, et al: Case of adult dermatomyositis treated with cyclosporin A. Br J Rheumatol 1992; 31:855.

72. Mehregan DR, Su WPD: Cyclosporine treatment for dermatomyositis/polymyositis. Cutis 1993; 51:59.

73. Jongen PJ, Joosten EM, Berden JM, et al: Cyclosporine therapy in chronic slowly progressive polymyositis—Preliminary report of clinical results in three patients. Transplant Proc 1988; 20(suppl):335.

74. Casato M, Benomo I, Cuccavo C, et al: Clinical effects of cyclosporine in dermatomyositis. Clin Exp Dermatol 1990; 15:121.

75. Grau JM, Herrero C, Casademont J, et al: Cyclosporin A as first choice therapy for dermatomyositis. J Rheumatol 1994; 21:381.

76. Langford CA, Klippel JH, Barlow JE, et al: Use of cytotoxic agents and cyclosporine in the treatment of autoimmune diseases: Part I. Rheumatic and renal diseases. Ann Intern Med 1998; 128:121.

77. Tellus MM, Buchanan RRC: Effective treatment of anti-Jo-1 antibody-positive polymyositis with cyclosporine. Br J Rheumatol 1995; 34:1187.

78. Saddeh C, Bridges W, Burwick F: Dermatomyositis: Remission induced with combined oral cyclosporine and high-dose intravenous immune globulin. South Med J 1995; 88:866.

79. Noppen M, Velkeniers B, Dierckx R, et al: Cyclosporine and myopathy. Ann Intern Med 1987; 107:945.

80. Roifman CM, Schaffer FM, Wachsmuth SE, et al: Reversal of chronic polymyositis following intravenous immune serum globulin therapy. JAMA 1987; 258:513.

81. Lang BA, Laxer RM, Murphy G, et al: Treatment of dermatomyositis with intravenous gammaglobulin. Am J Med 1991; 91:169.

82. Cherin P, Herson S, Wechsler B, et al: Efficacy of intravenous immunoglobulin G therapy on chronic refractory polymyositis and dermatomyositis: An open study with 20 adult patients. Am J Med 1991; 91:162.

83. Cherin P, Piette JC, Wechsler B, et al: Intravenous gammaglobulin as first line therapy in polymyositis and dermatomyositis: An open study in 11 patients. J Rheumatol 1994; 21:1092.

84. Soiueidan SA, Dalakas MC: Treatment of inclusion body myositis with high-dose intravenous immunoglobulin. Neurology 1993; 43:876.

85. Dalakas MC, Dambrosia JM, Sekul EA, et al: The efficacy of high-dose intravenous immunoglobulin in patients with inclusion-body myositis. Neurology 1995; 45:S208.

86. Amato AA, Barohn RJ, Jackson CE, et al: Inclusion body myositis: Treatment with intravenous immunoglobulin. Neurology 1994; 44:1516.

87. Kissel JT, Mendell JR, Rammohan KW: Microvascular deposition of complement membrane attack complex in dermatomyositis. N Engl J Med 1986; 314:329.

88. Emslie-Smith AM, Engel AG: Microvascular changes in early and advanced dermatomyositis: A quantitative study. Ann Neurol 1990; 27:343.

89. Stein DP, Jordan SC, Toyoda M, et al: Antiendothelial cell antibodies (AECA) in dermatomyositis (DM). Neurology 1993; 43(suppl):356.

90. Engel AG, Biesecker G: Complement activation in muscle fiber necrosis: Demonstration of the membrane attack complex of complement in necrotic fibers. Ann Neurol 1982; 12:289.

91. Dwyer JM: Manipulating the immune system with immune globulin. N Engl J Med 1991; 326:107.

92. Ballow M: Mechanisms of action of intravenous immunoglobulin therapy and potential use in autoimmune connective tissue diseases. Cancer 1991; 68(suppl):1430.

93. Gelfand EW: Intervention in autoimmune disorders: Creation of a niche for intravenous gamma-globulin therapy. Clin Immunol Immunopathol 1989; 53:S1. [Erratum, Clin Immunol Immunopathol 1990; 53:492]

94. Blasczyk R, Westhoff U, Grosse-Wilde H: Soluble CD4, CD8, and HLA molecules in commercial immunoglobulin preparations. Lancet 1993; 341:789.

95. Dustin ML, Springer TA: Role of lymphocyte adhesion receptors in transient interactions and cell locomotion. Annu Rev Immunol 1991; 9:27.

96. Bacchi VF, Maillet F, Berlan L, et al: Neutralizing antibodies against C3NeF in intravenous immunoglobulin. Lancet 1992; 340:63.

97. Basta M, Kirshbom P, Frank MM, et al: Mechanism of therapeutic effect of high-dose intravenous immunoglobulin: Attenuation of acute, complement-dependent immune damage in a guinea pig model. J Clin Invest 1989; 84:1974.

98. Reimhold AAM, Weinblatt ME: Tachyphylaxis of intravenous immunoglobulin in refractory inflammatory myopathy. J Rheumatol 1994; 21:1144.

99. Sekal EA, Cupler EJ, Dalakas MC: Aseptic meningitis associated with high-dose intravenous immunoglobulin: Frequency and risk factors. Ann Intern Med 1994; 121:259.

100. Hersan S, Cherin P, Coutellier A: The association of plasma exchange synchronized with intravenous gamma globulin therapy in severe intractable polymyositis. J Rheumatol 1992; 19:828.

101. Morgan SH, Bernstein RM, Coppen J, et al: Total body irradiation and the course of polymyositis. Arthritis Rheum 1985; 28:831.

102. Kelly JJ, Mudoc-Jones H, Adelman LS, et al: Response to total nodal irradiation in dermatomyositis. Muscle Nerve 1988; 11:120.

103. Cherin P, Herson S, Coutellier A, et al: Failure of total body irradiation in polymyositis: Report of three cases. Br J Rheumatol 1992; 31:282.

104. Pachman LM: Inflammatory myopathy in children. *In* Wortmann RL (ed): Clinical Disorders of Skeletal Muscle. Philadelphia: Lippincott, Williams & Wilkins, 2000:87.

105. Heckmatt J, Hasson N, Saunders C, et al: Cyclosporine in juvenile dermatomyositis. Lancet 1988; 1:1063.

106. Pistola V, Buoncompagni A, Scribans R, et al: Cyclosporin A in the treatment of juvenile chronic arthritis and childhood polymyositis-dermatomyositis: Results of a preliminary study. Clin Exp Rheumatol 1993; 11:203.

107. Rawlings DJ, Herson S, Wechsler B, et al: Cyclosporine is safe and effective in refractory JRA and JDMS: Results of an open clinical trial. Arthritis Rheum 1992; 35:C130.

108. Barron KS, Sher MR, Silverman ED: Intravenous immunoglobulin therapy: Magic or black magic. J Rheumatol 1992; 19:94.

# 33 | Juvenile Rheumatoid Arthritis and the Pediatric Spondyloarthropathies

*Bernhard H. Singsen*

Juvenile rheumatoid arthritis (JRA) and the pediatric spondyloarthropathies are a heterogeneous group of clinically defined conditions. Onset subsets of JRA include systemic, polyarticular, and early- and late-onset pauciarticular. Ankylosing spondylitis, Reiter's syndrome, psoriatic arthritis, and the gut-associated arthropathies are all described in children. Among the spondyloarthropathies in children, the major differences from adults are the intermittence, absence, or late onset of clinical and radiologic abnormalities of the sacroiliac joints, a low frequency of spine and costochondral involvement, and the incomplete and/or late expression of diagnostic rashes. Children with an early-onset spondylarthritis often manifest only enthesitis; an asymmetric, predominantly lower-extremity arthritis; and a suggestive family history. Unexplained recurrent conjunctivitis, uveitis, minimal dysuria, and/or diarrhea may also be present. In such patients, testing for the human leukocyte antigen B27 (HLA-B27) allele can be a very helpful diagnostic adjunct.

During the past 20 years, pediatric rheumatologists have progressively treated JRA and the spondyloarthropathies of childhood earlier and more aggressively. Nonsteroidal anti-inflammatory drugs (NSAIDs) have largely replaced aspirin, and NSAID dosages per body weight have slowly increased. The trend toward more rapid addition of disease-modifying antirheumatic drugs (DMARDs) started with gold 20 years ago, now widely includes methotrexate (MTX), and is evolving with the introduction of etanercept. Combination therapy that adds either hydroxychloroquine (HCQ) or sulfasalazine (SSZ) to an NSAID and a DMARD is increasingly common for children with active arthritis of longer than 6 to 12 months' duration. Although it was once the norm to add a DMARD only after the onset of erosions (e.g., after 1 to 3 years), the goal now is to avoid both erosions and flexion contractures. Similarly, early intervention clearly promotes more normal growth and development for children with arthritis. Because it is difficult to evaluate the long-term efficacy of any pediatric medication regimen, and because unpredictable improvement often occurs in children, pharmacotherapy is focused on helping to "control" synovitis, minimize joint destruction and deformities, and maximize age-appropriate activities of daily living until disease quiescence or spontaneous remission occurs.

Until recently, there have been few prospective, multidimensional, long-term observations of disease outcomes related to drug therapy in children with arthritis—partly because of a paucity of health status assessment instruments available for children with chronic diseases[1] and partly because the pediatric rheumatology community has focused its major efforts on important short-term dose-finding, safety, and efficacy trials to increase the therapeutic alternatives available for children with arthritis. Several pediatric arthritis health assessment questionnaires are now available,[2] core sets of outcome variables for JRA have been developed and used to compare improvement among treatments,[3] and these models have been applied specifically to MTX.[4]

Data from retrospective, one-center studies reveal that prognosis in JRA is highly dependent on the type of disease onset.[5] One review of 147 JRA patients[6] showed the following remission rates: (1) 50% for systemic-onset JRA at 5 years and 57% at 10 years; (2) 0% for rheumatoid factor–positive, polyarticular-onset JRA at 10 years, but 60% for seronegative, polyarticular-onset JRA; (3) 70% for early-onset pauciarticular JRA at 10 years but 55% for late-onset pauciarticular JRA. The relative impact of specific drugs on outcome could not be established and in most studies is difficult to ascertain because of the absence of control groups and of standardized long-term treatment protocols. Overall, synovitis may be adequately controlled in only 50% of JRA patients receiving NSAIDs alone,[7] and this may be insufficient to prevent growth suppression and deformity.

## ASPIRIN

Aspirin is still the least expensive of the NSAIDs, but its use for children with arthritis is now largely unknown to a new generation of physicians. The analgesic action of the leaves, bark, and roots of the willow have been known since Hippocrates, its antipyretic action was confirmed in the 18th century, and the active ingredient (salicin) was identified in the 19th century. In 1876, Maclagan[8] used salicin to treat acute rheumatism.

Since 1980, the known association of aspirin with Reye's syndrome has led to a dramatic decline in use and a coincident reduction in the frequency of Reye's syndrome.[9] Rarely, aspirin remains a good choice for a child with arthritis who has already had definite chickenpox and is not currently exposed to influenza. Multiple enteric-coated, buffered, liquid, and nonacetylated preparations are available.

Anti-inflammatory dosages of aspirin in children are 75 to 90 mg/kg/day in pauciarticular and polyarticular JRA and occasionally up to 100 to 110 mg/kg/day in systemic disease with marked fever, polyserositis, or both. It should be administered in four or five divided daily doses and should be given at the *beginning* of a meal, to minimize gastritis. Aspirin is rapidly absorbed in the proximal gastrointestinal (GI) tract but is optimally effective only when stable serum levels of 150 to 250 $\mu$g/L are achieved after 3 to 5 days of treatment. The maximal anti-inflammatory action of aspirin is usually achieved within 2 to 4 weeks. Increasing of dosages beyond 100 mg/kg/day (or 3 g/day for adolescents and adults) should be done carefully, because small changes can lead to significant elevation in blood levels of aspirin. Metabolism is by hepatic microsomal enzymes; aspirin is conjugated to glycine to form salicyluric acid, which then undergoes renal excretion. If the urine is alkalinized, clearance is enhanced and serum aspirin levels will be reduced.

## Toxicity and Monitoring

If aspirin is used, parents and children should be regularly questioned about eating habits, abdominal pain or diarrhea, tinnitus or subtle hearing loss, behavioral changes, bruising, and epistaxis. In small children, anorexia may herald the presence of gastritis or mild hepatotoxicity. The prevalence and significance of stool blood loss due to aspirin in children with arthritis is not known. However, children with arthritis have multiple reasons to be anemic, and iron supplementation, if tolerated, often raises the serum hemoglobin level by about 1 g/dL.

Patients with newly diagnosed JRA often have mild hepatic inflammation; if aspirin is chosen, pretreatment transaminase values should be determined. Mild, reversible hepatic toxicity caused by salicylates occurs at some time in 60% to 70% of JRA cases; this often appears as anorexia or nausea and may be exacerbated by intercurrent infection or dehydration.[10] A brief (3- to 4-day) stoppage of aspirin, followed by reintroduction at a 15% to 20% lower dosage, usually permits continued treatment. Aspirin should be immediately discontinued after exposure to influenza and also after contact with varicella unless previous clinical chickenpox is certain. Increased bruising, related to altered platelet function, is common and benign with aspirin and many other NSAIDs. Recurrent epistaxis is reason to discontinue aspirin. If elective surgery is planned, aspirin should be stopped 7 to 10 days before surgery;

low-dose corticosteroids may be required in the perioperative period.

Aspirin-induced peptic ulcer disease is rare, but gastritis is common. GI distress can be managed by administration of antacids, cimetidine, ranitidine, famotidine, or omeprazole and by attention to possible colonization with *Helicobacter pylori*. Regarding antacids, children are particular about flavor and about tablets versus liquids; the purchase of several trial types is useful. Constipation and diarrhea are potential complications. Chewable antacids permit much greater social flexibility in patients older than 7 to 8 years of age.

Other rare side effects of aspirin include severe bleeding, disseminated intravascular coagulation (mainly in systemic JRA), interstitial nephritis, urticaria, bronchospasm, and hypersensitivity pneumonitis. Severe salicylism may manifest as hyperpyrexia, hyperpnea, metabolic acidosis, central nervous system (CNS) stimulation or depression, and cardiovascular shock. When there is a risk of dehydration, aspirin should be immediately discontinued. Salicylates are contraindicated in children with glucose-6-phosphate dehydrogenase or pyruvate kinase deficiency, hemophilia, or von Willebrand's disease and in those who are receiving anticoagulant therapy.

Among adults, aspirin compliance rates are 50%; the percentages among children may be similar and are probably worse among adolescents. Serum aspirin levels can be checked after 5 to 10 days of treatment, and pill counts may be helpful. However, many compliance studies suggest that simply asking patient and parent whether the medication is being taken is less expensive and usually quite reliable.

## NONSTEROIDAL ANTI-INFLAMMATORY DRUGS

NSAIDs are now frequently prescribed for JRA and the spondyloarthropathies. However, there is little consistency in their use because there are so few studies, controlled or otherwise. Although only tolmetin and naproxen have received regulatory approval with specific indications for children, ibuprofen and indomethacin are also widely used, and diclofenac and sulindac are occasionally used. Fenoprofen, ketoprofen, piroxicam, and sodium meclofenamate have also been studied by the Pediatric Rheumatology Collaborative Study Group (PRCSG) and others.

As a group, the NSAIDs have antipyretic, anti-inflammatory, analgesic, and platelet-inhibitory properties. Although they differ chemically, in both pharmacokinetics and pharmacodynamics, the clinical consequences of these differences appear limited.[11] Most NSAIDs are weakly acidic, which may cause preferential concentration in the synovium, but those that are lipid soluble also appear to cause more CNS side effects, which can be subtle but important in children. Mechanisms of actions include inhibition of cyclooxygenase and lipoxygenase enzymes with reduced production of prostaglandins, decreased leukocyte or synovial cell generation of leukotrienes, lowered

## TABLE 33–1
## Pediatric Dosages of Nonsteroidal Anti-inflammatory Drugs

| DRUG | SCHEDULE | DOSE (mg/kg/d) | COMMENTS |
| --- | --- | --- | --- |
| Naproxen | BID–TID | 15–20 | Good initial treatment. Suspension useful (25 mg/mL); OTC available. |
| Ibuprofen | TID–QID | 30–40 | Good initial therapy. Suspension (20 mg/mL); drops (50 mg/1.25 mL); OTC available. |
| Tolmetin | BID–TID | 20–35 | Expensive. Low GI toxicity, occasional headaches. |
| Diclofenac | QD–BID | 2–3 | For older children; extended-release tablets may be used. |
| Aspirin | QID | 75–100 | Inexpensive. GI and hepatotoxicity; rare Reye's syndrome; salicylism with dehydration. |
| Indomethacin | TID | 2–4 | GI toxicity common; upward taper helps reduce headaches. Good for spondyloarthropathies. |
| Indomethacin | HS | 0.5–1 | Relieves morning stiffness; useful in both JRA and the spondyloarthropathies. |
| Prednisone | QD–BID–QOD | 0.1–1 | Controls acute flare; anti-inflammatory bridge to await onset of new medication. Systemic complications. |

GI = gastrointestinal; JRA = juvenile rheumatoid arthritis; OTC = over-the-counter formulation.

proteoglycan synthesis, interference with cell membrane functions, and inhibition of some neutrophil actions, perhaps related to the uncoupling of protein-protein interactions within plasma membrane lipid bilayers.[12]

Generally, NSAIDs are well absorbed, highly albumin bound (more than 95%), and not rapidly metabolized. NSAIDs may be grouped into those with half-lives shorter than 6 hours and those with half-lives longer than 10 hours; however, relationships between dosage and serum levels and both efficacy and toxicity are often not linear. There is little to suggest that compliance with NSAIDs differs appreciably from that with aspirin. The NSAIDs are more expensive, and hopes for significantly lower toxicity profiles have not been borne out. It is not possible to predict which NSAID will be best for a given child with arthritis. Simultaneous use of two NSAIDs can lead to increased risk of toxicity. Evidence also suggests that oral and ophthalmic NSAIDs are helpful in controlling inflammatory eye disease in JRA. In addition, direct instillation into the eyes as NSAID drops can be used to replace corticosteroid ophthalmic preparations in patients with no, the same, or different NSAIDs.

The NSAIDs most commonly used by pediatric rheumatologists in the United States are tolmetin, naproxen, and ibuprofen. However, all NSAIDs studied in adults with rheumatoid arthritis (RA) and marketed in the United States or Europe are occasionally employed in children. Summaries of pediatric dosage, toxicity monitoring, side effects, and approach to associated peptic disease for several NSAIDs are provided in Tables 33–1, 33–2, 33–3, and 33–4, respectively.

TOLMETIN. This drug has been approved and widely used in children with JRA since 1979, although it remains costly. It is well absorbed from the GI tract. Although tolmetin causes less CNS and GI toxicity than indomethacin, similar fatigue, dizziness, and gastritis can occur. It is equal to aspirin in the treatment of JRA[13] and is more effective for the spondyloarthropathies. At a dosage of 20 to 30 mg/kg/day, it may be given three or four times a day. A false-positive result of a sulfosalicylic urine test for protein can be seen in patients taking the drug. The dye-impregnated reagent strips do not register falsely positive.

IBUPROFEN. This drug, in a dosage of 30 to 40 mg/kg/day, is moderately effective for JRA and is usually given four times daily because of its short half-life.[14]

## TABLE 33–2
## Laboratory Monitoring for Drug Toxicity in Children

| DRUG | BASELINE TESTS | FOLLOW-UP TESTS |
| --- | --- | --- |
| Nonsteroidal anti-inflammatory drugs | CBC, AST, ALT, urinalysis, creatinine | Not needed if asymptomatic |
| Methotrexate | CBC, platelet count, AST, urinalysis, creatinine (or BUN) | CBC, platelet count, AST, BUN 3 wk later; then 6 wk later, then every 3 mo |
| Intramuscular gold | CBC, platelet count, urinalysis, creatinine | CBC, platelet count, urinalysis weekly for 3–6 mo; then every 3–4 wk |
| Hydroxychloroquine | Detailed eye examination, CBC, platelet count | Same, every 6–12 mo |
| D-Penicillamine | Urinalysis, creatinine, ANA, immunoglobulins, CK, CBC, platelet count, AST, ALT | CBC, platelet count, urinalysis monthly |
| Sulfasalazine | CBC, AST, urinalysis | Same every 3 mo |

ALT = alanine aminotransferase; ANA = antinuclear antibody; AST = aspartate aminotransferase; BUN = blood urea nitrogen; CBC = complete blood count; CK = creative kinase.

**TABLE 33–3**
## Common Effects of Nonsteroidal Anti-inflammatory Drugs

| DRUG | GASTRITIS | CENTRAL NERVOUS SYSTEM | TRANSAMINASE ELEVATIONS |
|------|-----------|------------------------|-------------------------|
| Aspirin | + | + | + + |
| Tolmetin | + | + + | – |
| Naproxen | + | + | – |
| Ibuprofen | + | + | – |
| Indomethacin | + + + | + + + | + + |

– = none; + = mild; + + = moderate; + + + = marked; + + + + = severe.

It has little GI toxicity; the liquid form is well liked by children.[15] It has rarely been associated with white cell aplasia and hemolytic anemia. In school-aged children, giving doses at breakfast, after school with a snack, at dinner, and at bedtime avoids the stigma of taking medication at school. Its low cost and over-the-counter (OTC) availability can be an advantage, although some families believe that nonprescription drugs are "less potent" and resist their use.

NAPROXEN. The safety, efficacy, and toxicity of this drug have been described in 11 published reports, as well as in several unpublished studies, in a total of 530 children with "juvenile arthritis," more than half of whom received the suspension.[16–19] It was approved by the US Food and Drug Administration (FDA) for children in 1987. Absorption, metabolism, and side effects are similar to those observed in adults with RA. Naproxen is given in a dosage of 10 mg/kg/day; twice-daily administration, because of its longer half-life, may more effectively reduce morning stiffness and preclude the need for in-school administration. About 50% of children with JRA respond well to naproxen, but a 3-month trial may be required. Its tolerability, taste, and schedule make this drug a good choice for early-onset pauciarticular JRA. GI toxicity occurs in 5% to 10% of children; it is important to emphasize taking all NSAIDs at the beginning of a meal. Idiosyncratic reactions include an increasingly recognized photosensitive rash, which is more common in light-skinned patients.[20] Rarely, pseudoporphyria may occur.[21]

**TABLE 33–4**
## Management of Peptic Ulcer Disease Induced by Nonsteroidal Anti-inflammatory Drugs

| MEASURE | TREATMENT | PREVENTION |
|---------|-----------|------------|
| Dietary measures | + + | + + + |
| Antacids | + + + | – |
| Cimetidine | + + + | – |
| Sucralfate | + * | + + + |
| Omeprazole | + + + | + + + + |
| Famotidine | + + + | + + + + |

* For duodenal ulcers.
– = not effective; + = minimally effective; + + = mildly effective; + + + = moderately effective; + + + + = markedly effective.

INDOMETHACIN. This drug is a very potent NSAID, but headaches, dizziness, fatigue, and gastric distress can be limiting factors. It is particularly useful for the pediatric spondyloarthropathies, the fever and pericarditis of systemic-onset JRA, and as a single night-time dose to ameliorate morning stiffness. In one study of indomethacin, 50% of children had reduced symptoms of arthritis and 75% showed improved fever control, but the drug had to be discontinued in 40% of the cases because of adverse reactions.[22] It is somewhat more effective than ketoprofen.[23] The usual dosage of indomethacin is 2 to 3 mg/kg/day, or 0.5 to 1.0 mg/kg at bedtime; it should always be taken with food or an antacid. Initiation of therapy with 25% of the final calculated dose, followed by increases in 25% increments every 4 to 5 days, may avert the onset of headaches.

DICLOFENAC. This drug is widely used in Europe, and it is used as a second-line agent to treat JRA and the spondyloarthropathies in the US. An early open-label, 8-month study of diclofenac, 2 mg/kg/day, in 50 children with JRA, in which no other NSAIDs were taken and all slow-acting antirheumatic drugs (SAARDs) were left unchanged, revealed 68% to be improved or in remission.[24] Forty-five of these patients were still receiving diclofenac after 2 years, with almost no toxicity. One randomized, double-blind study compared aspirin (50 to 100 mg/kg/day), diclofenac (2 to 3 mg/kg/day), and placebo, with 15 children in each treatment group; however, therapy lasted only 2 weeks.[25] Diclofenac was judged as effective as aspirin but had fewer side effects. A 12-week, single-blind, crossover study of 28 children with juvenile chronic arthritis (JCA) compared diclofenac, naproxen, and tolmetin and found all to have mild side effects, with no significant differences in efficacy or tolerability.[26]

KETOPROFEN AND PIROXICAM. Preliminary data from a 4-week, open-label, noncontrolled study of JRA suggested that ketoprofen, 100 to 200 mg/m²/day, had safety and efficacy comparable to those of other NSAIDs.[26] There have been two studies of piroxicam in JRA. In one, 26 patients were randomly assigned to receive piroxicam or naproxen; piroxicam appeared to be slightly more efficacious and better tolerated.[27] In the other, an 8-week, double-blind, crossover comparison of piroxicam and naproxen in 47 children with JCA, no significant differences were found in clinical response or side effects.[28] One advantage of piroxicam may be its once-daily dosing.

## Adverse Reactions to NSAIDs in Children

The spectrum of adverse reactions to NSAIDs is broad, but full appreciation of toxicity in children may be delayed because of fewer and smaller studies, the often greater functional and reserve capabilities of young healthy organs involved in drug metabolism and elimination, the greater pain tolerance and limited communication skills of children, and less experience on the part of both child and parent with what is "abnormal" or unacceptable.

Because most NSAIDs cause some degree of GI irritation in children, they are preferably given with food (i.e., with a snack or at the beginning of a meal); many parents incorrectly give NSAIDs at the end of a meal, which may increase the likelihood of gastritis. Gastrotoxicity is partly caused by prostaglandin inhibition, which leads to increased gastric acid synthesis and decreased esophageal sphincter tone; direct epithelial damage by NSAIDs may also occur. Elevation of hepatic enzymes is less common than with aspirin, although hepatitis can occur during treatment with sulindac.[29] It is advisable to check serum liver enzyme levels every 6 months. Flato and coworkers found side effects in 21% of NSAID versus 31% of DMARD exposures in a pediatric rheumatology clinic population of 117 children, after a mean follow-up period of 8.6 years.[30] Rates of drug discontinuation due to toxicity were 17% with NSAIDs and 14% with DMARDs.

Among adults, NSAID-related renal toxicity has a reported prevalence of 1% to 2%, but renal complications appear rare in children.[31] In a 4-year prospective study, Szer and colleagues[31] evaluated 226 children with JRA who received one or several NSAIDs for a median of 1.3 years (range, 0.5 to 8 years). One child had persistent, unexplained proteinuria, whereas 21 of 22 children with abnormal urinalyses had resolution of abnormalities without discontinuation of the NSAID. The overall prevalence of hematuria/proteinuria was no different than in normal schoolchildren. Renal parenchymal disease rarely occurs in JRA, although hematuria may be associated with fever. Therefore all children should have a urinalysis before starting an NSAID. Although renal papillary necrosis is a rare complication, many NSAIDs have been implicated in its occurrence. It is important to emphasize sufficient fluid intake, especially in the summer or if the child is active in athletics. If cardiovascular complications or hypovolemia develops in a child, it is advisable to discontinue NSAIDs because of potential inhibition of prostaglandin-mediated renal function. The relationship of NSAID administration to the rare occurrence of renal tubular dysfunction in JRA is unclear.

Although the mechanisms are not known, experience has shown that CNS side effects are quite common in children receiving NSAIDs. Manifestations include dizziness or lightheadedness; mild headaches; tinnitus; behavioral changes such as confusion, euphoria, or depression; difficulty in concentrating; and declining school performance. Fatigue is also a common complaint and can be difficult to separate from underlying disease activity. Visual complaints may occur. CNS toxicity in children may become known only after prolonged NSAID administration (months to years). Because the NSAID has often greatly ameliorated the child's arthritis, the physician may be reluctant to stop the medication. Our practice is to regularly take a behavioral history and immediately discontinue NSAIDs if CNS abnormalities are suspected. If present, parents usually report a dramatic change within days. The number of children who rapidly improve, despite no evidence of other significant side effects, has been impressive. Most children tolerate another NSAID well, suggesting that at least some CNS side effects are idiosyncratic. There is no evidence of an association between NSAIDs and Reye's syndrome.

Other rare NSAID-related complications that occur in children with arthritis include anaphylaxis, hypoplasia or aplasia of bone marrow cell lines, decreased platelet adhesiveness, fluid and electrolyte imbalance, edema, bruising, and a variety of rashes.

## CORTICOSTEROIDS

### General Principles

Earlier diagnosis and referral of children with arthritis, a wide choice of NSAIDs, rapid addition and prolonged use of MTX or SAARDs or both, and increased use of combination therapy during the past decade have greatly diminished use of corticosteroids to treat JRA and the spondyloarthropathies. The potentially severe and lifelong negative effects of corticosteroids on growth and development are now well appreciated. Systemic and local steroids should be given in the lowest possible dosages, for minimal periods, and only to achieve specific objectives.[32] Indications include (1) a therapeutic "bridge" for early, disabling arthritis before achieving control with MTX or other DMARDs; (2) uveitis that does not respond to topical treatment or MTX; (3) uncontrolled fever or visceral manifestations of systemic-onset JRA; (4) intra-articular injection to restore functional use in one or a few joints.

### Dosage

Prednisone, prednisolone, and methylprednisolone are common oral preparations. If possible, alternate-day steroid therapy should be tried first. However, in new or severely flaring patients exhibiting loss of ambulation, intractable fever, or visceral manifestations, a brief (2- to 3-week) course of oral prednisone, 1 to 2 mg/kg/day in divided doses, may be required. Alternatively, intravenous methylprednisolone (Solu-Medrol) pulse therapy, 30 mg/m$^2$/day (1 g maximum) for 3 days can lead to rapid improvement. In either case, appropriate dosages of NSAIDs, DMARDs, and/or MTX should be started simultaneously. Plans for consolidation, provision of a tapering schedule, and education of the child and family about possible consequences should begin immediately. Intercurrent exacerbations of JRA or a spondyloarthropathy often respond to brief, low dosages (0.25 to 0.5 mg/kg/day) of oral prednisone given daily or every other day, or to a Medrol Dosepak, or equivalent. It is often difficult for families to accept that total control of JRA by steroids is accompanied by many unwanted side effects. A randomized, double-blind trial compared deflazacort with prednisone in JRA; deflazacort had a similar anti-inflammatory effect but better maintained spinal bone mineral content.[33]

When high divided doses of oral steroids are necessary, tapering begins with consolidation to a single daily dose; this can be associated with worsening of disease and may require a few days to implement (e.g., 10 mg three times daily, to 15 mg twice daily, to 30 mg every morning over a period of 10 to 15 days). Reductions of about 10% of the dosage every 5 to 7 days should then be attempted. When one fourth of the original dosage is reached, the rate of reduction should be slowed to 5% per week. After a total dosage of 5 mg/day is achieved, weekly reductions of only 0.25 to 0.50 mg/day (or every other day) are often necessary. At low dosages, for reasons that are not clear, children with JRA are exquisitely sensitive to small decremental changes. As much as 3 to 6 months may be needed to complete weaning, but this approach usually averts the cyclic need to treat recurrent disease exacerbations, and the total corticosteroid dosage, over the years, is much lower.

Single daily doses of corticosteroids should be given in the early morning to minimize pituitary inhibition. Methylprednisolone bypasses hepatic activation by methylation, which may be useful in the presence of liver disease. Dexamethasone and other long-acting fluorinated oral preparations are contraindicated in JRA because of the high incidence of associated steroid myopathy. Tablets can be crushed and mixed with food; liquid preparations are widely available. Restrictions of fat and caloric intake must be emphasized. Some parents report improved appetite control with high-bulk low-calorie snacks.

## Toxicity

Steroid side effects pose special problems for children and teenagers, often impairing school attendance and social development. These problems include (1) poor self-image because of acne, striae, cushingism, and hirsutism; (2) reduced growth velocity, in combination with inflammatory JRA, which also often limits ultimate height; (3) osteopenia leading to fractures; (4) increased likelihood of peptic ulceration and infections; (5) mood and behavioral disturbances; (6) posterior subcapsular cataracts; and (7) occasional myopathy. The development of toxicity is unpredictable, but there are clear relationships to total dose and length of therapy. Hypertension, aseptic necrosis, pseudotumor cerebri, and glaucoma are now infrequent with the newer steroid treatment regimens.

As little as 5 mg/m$^2$ of prednisone daily for 1 month may affect linear growth. The likely mechanism is peripheral resistance to somatomedin-C. With short treatment courses, recovery from growth delay can be seen by 4 to 6 weeks after steroids are stopped. The ability to exhibit "catch-up" growth is inversely related to age; alternate-day regimens are associated with less growth retardation.

## Intravenous Pulse Corticosteroids

Large intravenous dosages of methylprednisolone (30 mg/kg/day; 1 g maximum), given over 20 to 60 minutes, are often used for severe or life-threatening JRA, systemic lupus erythematosus (SLE), childhood dermatomyositis, vasculopathies, and other rheumatic conditions.[34] The goal is to achieve a rapid and profound anti-inflammatory effect, with minimum toxicity. Various daily or every-other-day protocols, up to three total doses, have been employed. Reports have documented the efficacy, mild and transient side effects, and occasional prolonged benefits of pulse therapy in children with arthritis,[35, 36] but individual patient responses remain highly variable, and most physician experience is anecdotal. Most centers perform pulse therapy on an outpatient basis.

Uncontrolled fever, disabling arthritis, myocarditis, pneumonitis, other systemic features, and disseminated intravascular coagulopathy are all potential indications for intravenous pulse corticosteroids. The anti-inflammatory and pain-reducing actions of methylprednisolone may last only a few days, or up to 4 to 8 weeks, allowing time for other interventions to become effective. Although intravenous pulse corticosteroids are less toxic than long-term oral steroids, several rare complications are possible, including acute osteonecrosis, sudden hypokalemia, electrolyte imbalance, seizures or psychosis, and increased infections.[37]

## Intra-articular Corticosteroids

If one or a few inflamed joints are unresponsive to NSAIDs and MTX or have caused severe disability in a patient with newly diagnosed JRA, intra-articular corticosteroids may be used. The rationale is to relieve pain, facilitate physical therapy or activity, improve joint range, and assist correction of joint deformity. Although this treatment is often rapidly effective, improvement may last only a few days, or it may be sustained for months. Common preparations are triamcinolone hexacetonide and prednisone tertiary butyl acetate, which have high potency and a prolonged half-life. The dosage is 0.5 mg/kg (10 to 20 mg) in small joints and 1.0 mg/kg (20 to 40 mg) in large joints, depending on age. Mixing the steroid solution with an equal volume of a nonpreservative containing local anesthetic may reduce discomfort. The correct frequency of injections has not been established; recommendations range from once only, to monthly, up to a total of three times. Children who respond well may be younger and have shorter disease durations; in one study 37% had joint relapse by 6 months after injection, and 50% by 1 year.[38] Several reports describe excellent short- and long-term results,[39–41] with 60% to 80% having articular remission for 6 months. One study described full joint remission in 81.6% of pauciarticular patients, with discontinuation of oral medications in 61% to 74% of cases.[40] Good outcome after multiple injections was reported in 51 joints among a total of 145 joints in 51 children.[38]

Rigorous aseptic technique, topical anesthesia with ethyl chloride, and both local and deep infiltration with lidocaine are important. Younger children and those requiring multiple or hip joint injections usually require general anesthesia, but the risks of this have not been independently assessed. Both ultrasound- and magnetic resonance imaging–guided injection have been recommended.

The incidence of side effects is extremely low, although subcutaneous atrophy, local depigmentation, infection, crystal-induced synovitis, avascular necrosis, and osteoporosis are known.[41–43] Changing to a new lidocaine-filled syringe after steroid instillation, and then continuously injecting lidocaine as the needle is withdrawn, appears to markedly reduce subcutaneous atrophy and depigmentation. Intra-articular or periarticular calcification occurs in 15% to 20% of cases, but the long-term implications of this are not yet known.[41–43]

## METHOTREXATE

### Background and Efficacy

The efficacy of aminopterin, a folic acid antagonist, in ameliorating RA was first described in 1951.[44] By 1985 several placebo-controlled clinical trials, involving more than 200 RA patients, had demonstrated the benefits of MTX in suppressing manifestations of disease activity such as swelling, morning stiffness, and erythrocyte sedimentation rate (ESR).[45, 46] One early controlled study in adult RA could not show a reduction in radiologic evidence of joint destruction[47]; however, another suggested that use of MTX alone or in combination with auranofin had a trend toward statistically significant slowing of erosions in RA.[48] Use of auranofin alone did not. In JRA, measurements of carpal bone length revealed limited radiologic evidence of progression among children who also had evidence of a positive clinical response.[49]

In 1986 MTX was first reported to be efficacious for JRA,[50] and other studies with similar findings quickly followed.[51–53] Subsequently, a double-blind, placebo-controlled, multicenter trial showed that MTX was effective for children with "resistant" JRA at a dosage schedule of either 5 or 10 mg/m²/week.[54]

### Mechanism of Action

MTX is a folic acid analog with potent inhibitory binding to the enzyme dihydrofolate reductase (DHFR). It appears to alter several folate-dependent pathways that affect immune response and the reactivity of inflammatory cells, but with relatively little cytotoxic effect. Although much of its toxicity seems to be related

to DHFR inhibition, whether such inhibition is responsible for the anti-inflammatory and/or the antiproliferative action of MTX is not clear. In vitro, MTX is capable of affecting several metabolic pathways, including the following:

1. De novo synthesis of purines. The inhibition of DHFR limits the conversion of dihydrofolic to tetrahydrofolic acid, which in turn is the universal donor of one-carbon units involved in de novo manufacture of purines. This effect is mainly mediated through inhibition of 5-aminoimidazole-4-carboxamide ribonucleotide transformylase (AICAR) and glycinamide ribonucleotide transformylase (GAR), both of which require one-carbon units in the purine synthesis pathway.
2. Formation of thymidylate synthase, which also uses one-carbon units and is crucial for manufacture of thymidine.
3. Serine formation from methionine, which requires tetrahydrofolate as a donor of a one-carbon unit.

Although there are few studies that relate specific in vitro MTX effects to defined alterations in clinical outcomes, it is known that the binding of MTX to DHFR is easily reversed by low concentrations of dihydrofolic acid, which permits "rescue" therapy when significant clinical toxicity occurs.[55]

MTX selectively inhibits both peripheral blood mononuclear cell (PBMC) proliferation in RA patients[56] and T- and B-cell proliferative and mitogen responses, which may amplify its anti-inflammatory activity.[57] Its suppression of rheumatoid factor production is striking.[58, 59] MTX also exhibits folate-dependent inhibition of the actions of interleukin-1 (IL-1), a potent mediator of local and systemic inflammation, and markedly inhibits IL-1–induced IL-2 synthesis and proliferation of T cells in vitro when added to PBMCs.[60] This mechanism is reversible by the addition of leucovorin.[61, 62]

Other observed MTX actions include (1) an effect on neutrophil leukotriene B₄ production in the lipoxygenase pathway[63]; (2) diminished expression of Ia antigens on the surface of peritoneal macrophages of rats with adjuvant arthritis; and (3) inhibition of the folate-dependent regeneration of methionine from homocysteine, which leads to (a) an antiproliferative action on lymphocytes because of interference with the manufacture of polyamines, which are essential for the synthesis of DNA, and (b) reduced production of proteins such as immunoglobulins, rheumatoid factor, and IL-2.[64]

### Kinetics

Data on the kinetics of MTX in children are limited. According to animal and adult human studies, oral MTX is effectively absorbed at a variable rate, with peak serum levels achieved 2 hours after ingestion. Its serum half-life is 6 hours, and its volume of distribution is 0.25 L/kg. Half of MTX is free in the serum, while the remaining 50% is protein bound and transported to the liver, where it is partially converted to 7-hydroxymethotrexate before being removed by active renal tubular secretion.[65] Biliary elimination of up to 30% of MTX occurs via the enterohepatic circulation[66]; this may act as a safety valve to reduce the risk of toxicity in patients with decreased renal function.

Bioavailability of MTX is similar after oral, subcutaneous, or intramuscular administration. However, uncontrolled observations in both adults and children suggest that selected patients receiving oral therapy who do not respond, who reach a plateau after variable degrees of improvement, or who experience an exacerbation after significant disease regression may benefit from switching to either the intramuscular or the subcutaneous route at a similar dosage.[67–71] It is not clear whether changes in response are caused by delayed MTX absorption, altered bioavailability, or coincidental changes in disease activity.

MTX is actively transported into cells and then polyglutamated, which increases its inhibitory action on DHFR and also prevents MTX from "escaping" from the cell. Polyglutamation may play an important role in conservation of MTX, because very low intracellular levels are required to be effective, and these are readily achieved with weekly oral pulses.[55, 65, 72]

In adults with RA, drugs known to interact with MTX include salicylates, indomethacin, naproxen, ketoprofen, and phenylbutazone.[73] Although an investigation by Dupuis and associates[73] of children with arthritis showed that MTX half-life was prolonged by tolmetin, indomethacin, aspirin, and naproxen, no interactions were found by Skeith and coworkers[74] for ibuprofen or flurbiprofen. Whether clinically significant interactions of MTX with other medications occur in JRA is uncertain at present.

## Toxicity

MTX is well tolerated by children with JRA. Giannini and colleagues[54] found that only 3% of patients had to discontinue the drug because of toxicity. Overall, as collated from five reports involving MTX treatment of 203 children with JRA, the most commonly observed side effects were upper GI upset (9%), diarrhea (4.5%), and abdominal pain (4%).[50–54] Such reactions are usually self-limited,[53] may be caused by folic acid depletion,[75] and often resolve if MTX is withheld for 1 week and then reinstituted at a 15% to 25% lower dosage. MTX toxicity in adults with RA may also rarely include alopecia, gynecomastia, transient azoospermia, impotence, and CNS disease, but these side effects have not been reported in children. MTX is potentially teratogenic and should be discontinued if pregnancy is being considered. Long-term studies of fertility in patients with JRA are not available.

Initial parental anxiety about MTX, commonly related to reproductive, teratogenic, or mutagenic issues, is often allayed by negotiating a 4- to 6-week trial of low-dosage oral treatment. This allows families to make an informed benefit-risk decision by contrasting actual clinical improvement in a disabled child with an incompletely studied group of possible future complications. In our experience, this approach has been highly successful in initiating therapy.

Bone marrow suppression due to MTX has been reported, but it is rare and idiosyncratic[65]; megaloblastic changes are more common and are caused by a relative folic acid depletion. In adults with RA, studies suggest that folic acid supplementation does not reduce MTX efficacy and does decrease GI toxicity.[57, 75] Children with JRA have not been studied in detail. We routinely begin oral folate in children 2 years of age or younger at 0.5 mg/day or 1 mg every other day; in older children the dosage is 1 mg/day. Folate is now commonly available in OTC preparations. It should be emphasized to families that the 400 $\mu$g of folate contained in OTC multivitamins is often not sufficient to eliminate toxicity. Some patients are unusually sensitive to folate depletion and do well when they are given 2 mg/day the day before, the day of, and the day after their MTX dose. The practice of skipping folate dosing on the day MTX is given does not appear to improve efficacy and may promote side effects.

Some clinicians commonly warn about MTX-induced alopecia in children. In our experience, this problem is rare. When we find alopecia in a child already receiving MTX, it is most frequently caused by the comorbidity of poor scalp hygiene, tinea capitis, or elaborate hairstyles leading to infrequent hair washing. Increased use of medicated shampoos usually alleviates this problem.

Among 117 children with JRA for whom data on liver enzymes were available, 9% demonstrated one or more episodes of enzyme elevations.[50–53] Persistent aspartate aminotransferase (AST) elevations usually precede development of liver fibrosis,[76, 77] but their absence does not preclude asymptomatic fibrosis. Most serial liver biopsy studies of adults with RA indicate that significant liver fibrosis is not associated with MTX intake,[78–80] although one report using electron microscopy suggested that an unspecified subset of RA patients receiving MTX may be prone to progressive liver fibrosis.[77] Graham and associates described liver biopsies in seven JRA patients after an average cumulative MTX dose of 1709 mg and found normal tissue in each child.[81] Clinical MTX-related liver fibrosis in JRA is rare.[82]

Although idiosyncratic interstitial pneumonitis is seen with antitumor dosages of MTX, it is only rarely reported in children with arthritis. Three retrospective clinical, radiographic, and pulmonary function studies, including two involving a total of 40 JRA patients[83, 84] and one involving adults,[85] found no evidence of interstitial pneumonitis. One prospective follow-up study of 200 cases of adult RA, over 41.5 months, revealed no MTX-related pulmonary toxicity.[57]

Methods of monitoring children receiving MTX for evidence of toxicity vary somewhat among practitioners. Early and frequent follow-up, including detailed oral and written education and assessment of understanding, is particularly important for young, anxious parents. Compliance tends to be excellent once the clinical benefits are perceived. We perform the following laboratory studies: complete blood cell count (CBC), mean corpuscular volume (MCV), liver enzyme determinations, renal function tests, and urinalysis at baseline. Repeat CBC, AST, and blood urea nitrogen determinations are recommended 2 to 3 weeks later, 4 to 6 weeks after that, and then every 3 months. We are not aware of any pediatric rheumatologists who are regularly performing liver biopsies, except via study protocol or in special circumstances. Wallace and co-workers[51] did not find plasma MTX levels in children with JRA to correlate with efficacy or likelihood of liver abnormalities, and side effects have been observed even within the range of "safety."

In children receiving MTX, in the complete absence of clinical complaints, it is common for serum liver enzyme levels to rise and then stabilize at two to three times baseline values. In about 40% of these cases, a further elevation of liver enzymes appears to develop after 6 to 9 months of therapy. In such cases MTX may be withheld for one or several weekly doses, depending on the degree and duration of rise in enzymes. Liver enzymes should then again be monitored weekly until they normalize. Normalization often occurs within 1 week, in which case the drug is often successfully restarted at the same dosage. If enzyme levels again rise after rechallenge at the same dosage, MTX is once more withheld and then restarted after several weeks at a dosage that is reduced by 15% to 25%. Mild GI upset or a few oral mucosal ulcerations, each of 24 hours' duration, and a single episode of elevated liver enzymes are the most commonly observed adverse reactions.

## Routes of Administration

Oral administration of MTX is the least expensive and most convenient method for most children and their families. Rarely, when socioeconomic disruption suggests a high likelihood of noncompliance with an oral MTX regimen in a significantly involved patient with JRA, we start directly with subcutaneous treatment. Injectable MTX is now also routinely used if children do not respond, reach a clinical plateau, do not comply, or develop GI reactions to oral MTX. In patients who have an initial good response but then develop plateau or flare, larger parenteral dosages (0.5 to 1 mg/kg/week) can be tried. We now routinely have a rheumatology nurse teach the patient, parent, friend, or family member how to administer subcutaneous MTX at home, much as with insulin. The "ultrafine" needle significantly reduces injection pain and is preferred. A local laboratory can communicate toxicity monitoring results directly to the consulting rheumatologist.

In our experience, about 60% of children with inflammatory arthropathies are eventually converted to injectable MTX, in order to minimize arthritis or side effects or both, and to maximize clinical and social function. Rapid GI transit times in younger children, binding by food, variations in absorption by the normal gut, partial metabolism by the liver before systemic distribution, compliance issues, or impaired absorption by the microscopically inflamed gut may all play roles in reducing MTX bioavailability.

## Clinical Use

Essentially all children with JRA of longer than 6 months' duration are candidates for MTX therapy. Historically, MTX was reserved for the child who had persistent or progressive polyarticular JRA despite adequate trials of NSAIDs and SAARDs. Increasing pediatric experience with MTX has led to its earlier use, including use in patients with pauciarticular JRA, especially if such a child has impaired ambulation, disturbed bone growth, or iridocyclitis unresponsive to topical therapy. We routinely initiate MTX at first confirmation of either pauciarticular or polyarticular JRA if it is clear that the diagnosis has been *missed* for long enough that deformity, growth failure, disabling fatigue or pain, loss of age-appropriate activities of daily living, or impaired schooling is present. Alternatively, some pediatric rheumatologists begin MTX only after a 6- to 12-month trial of NSAIDs. In severely compromised patients, to avoid hospitalization, allow ambulation, or restore lost age-appropriate physical activities and school attendance, a 3-day course of intravenous Solu-Medrol (30 mg/kg/day, up to a maximum of 1 g/day) may be an effective therapeutic "bridge" until MTX becomes effective.

Injectable, weekly MTX is also a useful alternative in children with ulcerative colitis or Crohn's disease who have a flare of arthritis while already receiving oral azathioprine, SSZ, or mesalamine. Often, oral MTX is not efficacious or well tolerated in the presence of gut inflammation, but significant improvement may occur with subcutaneous administration.

## INJECTABLE GOLD

### Background and Efficacy

Gold was the first drug ever tested in a controlled clinical trial in adult RA, and it long was an excellent option for treatment of progressive or severe polyarticular JRA. A total of 12 studies of intramuscular gold in 372 children with JRA were published between 1964 and 1988. Six were retrospective, four were open-label and compared gold with another SAARD, and three were randomized.[86] In only 56% was the type of JRA onset reported. Where noted, the usual dosage was 1 mg/kg/weekly to a maximum of 50 mg weekly, and mean treatment durations were 0.5 to 3.8 years, with a range of 3 months to 8 years. Rates of remission, variously defined, ranged from 0% to 57%, with a cumulative rate of 16% among the 372 patients, when adjusted for study size. Similarly, "improvement" was found in 18% to 78% of cases, with a combined rate of 48%. Among the 10 reports that detailed gold toxicity, the rates were 20% to 52% and the combined rate was 38%, whereas toxicity requiring drug termination occurred in 7% to 58% of patients (noted in 11 studies), with a combined rate of 23%.

In two other reports, Brewer and colleagues[87] showed that gold reduced the severity of disease in 63% and reduced joint counts in 49% of 51 patients with JRA, while Fink[32] suggested that a 50% rate of efficacy can be expected, particularly in polyarthritis. Gold is generally not effective for the systemic manifestations of JRA, and indeed it may be associated with neutropenia or intravascular coagulation.

## Mechanism of Action

The mechanism of action of gold remains poorly understood. In vitro, gold inhibits the growth of some viruses and bacteria, alters classical and alternate complement pathway functions, may block T-lymphocyte activation by impairing monocyte function, can suppress mitogen-induced immunoglobulin M (IgM) and IgM-RF (rheumatoid factor) synthesis, alters the chemotactic response of human peripheral monocytes and neutrophils, and may reduce overactive phagocytosis in patients with RA. Gold compounds may also decrease the activity of endothelial leukocyte adhesion molecule 1 and thereby reduce recruitment of leukocytes to sites of inflammation. In vitro inhibition of macrophage differentiation[88] and decreased HLA-DR expression after interferon-gamma stimulation[89] have also been described. In animals and human beings gold inhibits many enzymes, including cathepsin, $\beta$-glucuronidase, acid phosphatase, and malic dehydrogenase. Therefore gold may reduce inflammation by retarding the production or release of lysosomal enzymes.

## Administration

Gold aurothioglucose and sodium thiomalate are the common injectable forms. Gold salts are given by weekly intramuscular injection. In children an initial test dose of 0.25 to 0.33 mg/kg is administered and then increased weekly by 25% to 33% until a final weekly dosage of 1 mg/kg is reached (maximum, 50 mg/week). Beneficial effects usually occur after 6 to 12 weeks but may require 20 weeks, and optimal response may take 12 months. After 20 weeks, or a total cumulative dose of 500 to 1000 mg, the patient is reassessed, and if there is no improvement the drug is discontinued.

In children who respond well, gold should be continued indefinitely, or at least until growth and development are complete; dosage is adjusted as the patient gains weight. After 20 weeks it may be possible to gradually decrease the frequency of injections to once a month at 1 mg/kg; if the arthritis worsens, however, weekly injections must be resumed. Occasionally, concomitant NSAIDs can be discontinued. Some physicians treat patients with monthly gold injections for several years after remission is achieved. MTX has now largely displaced injectable gold because of the shorter time required to determine efficacy, fewer side effects, lower cost, less frequent monitoring, fewer office visits, and less discomfort. Nonetheless, for many children intramuscular gold remains an excellent first-line remittive agent.

## Toxicity and Monitoring

Major side effects caused by injectable gold involve the skin, kidneys, and bone marrow. Rashes are usually mildly red and maculopapular; they are pruritic in 15% of cases, they may be scaly, and they subside after drug discontinuation. Less common effects include alopecia; photosensitivity; urticarial, bullous, or severe exfoliative reactions; and skin pigmentation. Stomatitis occurs in 5% to 10% of cases. Hematuria, proteinuria, or both may indicate an immune complex–mediated membranous glomerulonephritis (10% to 20% of cases). If toxicity develops, in some cases injections can be restarted at a lower dosage after a 1-month interruption. Otherwise, termination of the drug is usually effective, although corticosteroids may be required. Some children with JRA have mild hematuria or proteinuria before any drug treatment, and NSAID administration can also be associated with renal abnormalities; these causes must be separated from those related to gold. Urine must be collected fresh and midstream and must not involve vigorous cleansing. If gold therapy is started in the presence of unexplained urinary abnormalities, future therapeutic decisions are rendered very difficult.

Hematologic toxicity is infrequent (1% to 2% of cases), except for eosinophilia. Thrombocytopenia, leukopenia, and aplastic anemia have been described. In adults, bone marrow, skin, and renal toxicity are all increased in patients who have HLA-DR3. Other less common toxic effects include fever, postinjection arthralgias, chest pain or tachycardia, pneumonitis, hepatitis, GI distress, hematochezia, the nitritoid reaction, headaches, and various behavioral disturbances. These essentially all disappear on drug cessation.

Toxicity is monitored with a weekly urinalysis, CBC, and platelet count; many practitioners reduce the frequency of testing to every 2 to 3 weeks if there is no evidence of side effects after 6 to 12 months. Regular evaluation must continue indefinitely. Although optimal compliance and monitoring may occur when treatment is performed by a rheumatologist, for family convenience it is common for laboratory tests and injections to be administered by a local physician. For reasons of cost and convenience, some families obtain local laboratory test results, fax them to their rheumatologist, and then give the injections themselves at home.

## ORAL GOLD (AURANOFIN)

Auranofin is 29% gold by weight; about 25% of that amount is absorbed, and serum levels stabilize after about 3 months of daily administration. The first trial of auranofin was reported in adult RA in 1979; several thousand patients have now been evaluated in open-label, placebo-controlled, comparative studies with most SAARDs.[90] Although auranofin is superior to placebo, dropouts because of lack of efficacy are higher when auranofin is compared with intramuscular gold. Auranofin may be more effective in patients with early disease; however, it has not been successful in sustaining remission in those who have switched to it after a good response to intramuscular gold. Auranofin also produces a later response, and more side effects, than does MTX.

Six open-label, noncontrolled studies of auranofin for children with JRA were published between 1983 and 1988.[91] At dosages of 0.1 to 0.2 mg/kg/day, most patients demonstrated some improvement by 6 months. However, in a 6-month double-blind, randomized, placebo-controlled investigation in which the PRCSG evaluated safety in 231 JRA patients and efficacy in 191, auranofin, 0.15 mg/kg/day, resulted in only a modest, nonsignificant improvement over placebo among the primary study variables (66% vs. 56%).[7] As a result, auranofin is now very rarely used in the treatment of pediatric arthritis.

Common adverse reactions with auranofin include diarrhea, dermatitis, stomatitis, and a metallic taste; renal complications are rare. Intolerance causes only one fourth as many withdrawals as injectable gold (5% vs. 20%). Monitoring includes an initial CBC, urinalysis, and chemistry profile, followed by repeat CBC and urinalysis in 2 weeks and then monthly. A careful history and examination are mandatory. Diarrhea often subsides with dosage reduction or if the dosage is skipped 1 or 2 days per week. Auranofin is not recommended for pregnant or nursing mothers.

## SULFASALAZINE

SSZ was developed in Sweden in the 1940s to treat RA, which was then thought to be caused by infection. Sulfapyridine (a sulfonamide) was linked to 5-aminosalicylic acid (an anti-inflammatory agent) by an azo bond in order to effect delivery to the colon, where SSZ undergoes bacterial cleavage. About one third of the 5-aminosalicylic acid is absorbed, but it does not achieve effective anti-inflammatory levels. Almost 90% of the sulfapyridine is absorbed from the colon, but its mechanism of action is not understood. In controlled trials in adult RA, SSZ was found to be superior to placebo and similar to gold and to D-penicillamine (D-PEN).[92] It is also effective in ankylosing spondylitis,[93] the reactive arthropathies,[94] and inflammatory bowel disease.

In 1986, Ozdogan and associates[95] reported significant improvement in 12 of 18 patients in an open-label study of JRA treated with SSZ, although toxicity was a limiting factor. Joos and coworkers[96] employed enteric-coated SSZ (30 to 50 mg/kg/day; median dosage, 1 g/day) for 41 patients 16 years of age or younger who had been unsuccessfully treated for at least 3 months with NSAIDs. Remission occurred in 21 patients and substantial improvement in 12; 4 were unchanged, and 3 worsened. A significant decrease in the number of swollen joints was observed after 3 months and then maintained; the ESR was significantly reduced after 6 months of therapy. Toxicity was observed in five children, of whom four stopped taking SSZ (one each because of GI intolerance, leukopenia, rash, and agitation), but all side effects were reversible on withdrawal of the drug.

Grondin and colleagues[86] retrospectively studied SAARD treatment in 43 children with JCA; 12 received SSZ. Improvement occurred in six, remission in one, no change in four, and worsening in one. Their literature review noted toxicity in 37% of patients, with 10% requiring discontinuation. Five trials of SSZ in children for whom NSAIDs alone had failed used SSZ alone or in combination with another SAARD in 270 patients with JRA or a spondyloarthropathy.[97–101] SSZ dosages were 30 to 50 mg/day, usually administered twice daily. Treatment durations were 3 to 12 months, and efficacy measures varied, but overall 161 children (60%) were deemed to have significant clinical improvement. SSZ was discontinued because of adverse reactions in 45 cases (16.6%). One report of four patients treated for a mean of 3.3 years suggested a role for SSZ in the treatment of chronic uveitis in JRA or juvenile ankylosing spondylitis.[102]

## Monitoring, Toxicity and Clinical Use

The most common toxicity is an allergic skin reaction, including urticarial, maculopapular, and multiforme rashes.[103] GI toxicity may include nausea, vomiting, anorexia, or abdominal pain in up to 30% of children, and hematologic complications such as anemia, granulocytopenia, or hemolysis develop in up to 23% of cases. Headaches, agitation, and depression are occasionally described, but renal toxicity is almost never seen. There may be idiosyncratic reactions, including serum sickness.[99] SSZ-related side effects almost always cease after drug discontinuation. Hepatotoxicity and fulminant hepatic failure may rarely occur.[104] Monthly monitoring includes history, examination, AST determination, and CBC.

Clinical response to SSZ may occur as rapidly as several weeks, more often develops by 3 months, and in severe cases may require 12 months. It appears to be more useful in the spondyloarthropathies[100] and in HLA-B27—positive "pauciarthritis."[97] The usual starting dosage is 40 to 60 mg/kg/day, beginning with one fourth of the calculated dosage and then increasing weekly by another one fourth, up to a maximum of 1 to 2 g/day. The most frequent problem at higher dosages is GI upset. Administration with food can be helpful, and enteric-coated preparations are often better tolerated.

SSZ is usually a third-line medication, added when NSAIDs and MTX have not been sufficient to adequately control the disease process. One may add SSZ to a combination of an NSAID, HCQ, and MTX in severe cases of JRA or spondyloarthropathy. SSZ may be useful as second-line therapy for children with mild juvenile ankylosing spondylitis, nonspecific arthritis with enthesitis, psoriatic arthritis, or Reiter's syndrome.

## HYDROXYCHLOROQUINE

### Background and Efficacy

Antimalarial compounds have long been employed by pediatric rheumatologists as adjunctive therapy for

JRA, but their use varies widely among centers and may reflect success with HCQ in other conditions such as childhood SLE and dermatomyositis. Early studies of HCQ in JRA suggested that it was effective and less toxic than D-PEN or gold.[105, 106] Five later trials (three retrospective, one open-label, and one prospective) evaluated antimalarials (mostly HCQ) in 245 patients with JRA (76 with polyarticular disease, 77 with oligoarticular JRA, and 35 with systemic onset). Overall, 41% (range, 16% to 75%) showed improvement, and 28% (range, 0% to 45%) achieved remission. Rates of toxicity ranged from 8% to 61%, but the drug was stopped in only 6.5% of the cases. One randomized, open-label, controlled comparison of HCQ, injectable gold, and D-PEN showed similar efficacy for all three but fewer side effects with HCQ.[107] A double-blind, multicenter, placebo-controlled study of *severe* JRA suggested that HCQ alone is little better than placebo in this situation.[108]

Oral chloroquine and HCQ are rapidly absorbed and have a half-life of 3 to 12 days; the serum level plateaus at 2 to 5 weeks. Tissue concentrations are much higher than plasma levels, particularly in fat, bone, cornea, and pigmented organs such as the iris and choroid. Proposed mechanisms of action for HCQ include direct intracellular enzyme inhibition; stabilization of lysosomal membranes; reduced immune complex formation; decreased function of lymphocytes, macrophages, and polymorphonuclear leukocytes; inhibition of DNA and RNA synthesis; and interference with prostaglandin manufacture.[109]

The starting dosage of HCQ is 5 to 6.5 mg/kg/day, with a maximum of 200 mg in children weighing less than 40 kg and of 400 mg in teenagers. HCQ has a delayed onset of action (3 to 6 months); 88% of the patients who respond do so by 6 months. Otherwise, the drug usually should be discontinued. Therapy with HCQ generally should not exceed 2 to 3 years, although in some cases treatment can be extended for longer periods.

### Toxicity and Monitoring

The frequency of side effects with antimalarials is usually dose related and is generally lower than with other SAARDs; only 8.5% of adult patients, and 4% to 6% of children, drop out because of toxicity.[86,103] The most common toxic reactions are lichenoid, urticarial, morbilliform, or maculopapular rashes. Pruritus and photosensitivity can also occur. GI toxicity may mimic that of concomitant NSAIDs but is generally milder. Neurologic side effects are usually minimal and easily reversible, but headaches, insomnia, agitation, and reduced concentration may impair school performance. Questions about psychoneurologic performance should be asked at each visit. The skin should also be monitored for depigmentation. Antimalarials have not been shown to be safe during pregnancy, and they also must be safely stored; death from respiratory failure occurred after a child ingested as few as four tablets (1 g) of chloroquine.

There are three types of ophthalmologic side effects, although their frequency is very low: (1) neurally mediated defects in convergence or accommodation, with blurred vision; (2) corneal deposits (keratopathy), which are reversible, appear to be dose related, and suggest a safe upper HCQ dosage of 5 to 6.5 mg/kg/day;[105] and (3) retinopathy, including pigmentary stippling, mottling, clumping, central scotomata, or reduced peripheral fields. So-called "premaculopathy" is manifested by changes in red-green color vision or early pigmentary abnormalities and is usually reversible. More serious retinopathy, which often occurs in those who receive higher than recommended daily doses, may cause irreversible visual loss and can progress after HCQ is withdrawn.

At baseline and then every 6 months, a pediatric ophthalmologist should question children and parents about visual changes, determine acuity, assess red-green color vision, and evaluate the retina for pigmentary changes.

## PENICILLAMINE

### Background and Efficacy

Early studies of D-PEN in adult RA suggested that it was as effective as gold, had similar therapeutic indications, and was little more toxic, leading to much initial enthusiasm. There have been nine trials of D-PEN in children (three retrospective, four open/randomized and compared with gold, and two double-blind and placebo-controlled).[86] Among a total of 505 patients, most received dosages ranging from 10 to 30 mg/kg/day; disease subtype at onset often was not specified. Overall, although operational definitions of levels of disease activity either were not given or varied widely, 14 (2.8%) achieved remission and 308 (61%) were "improved." The total rate of toxicity was 20% (92/415), whereas the rate of toxicity necessitating drug termination was 13.7% (68/495).[86]

A 1986 prospective, placebo-controlled, double-blind, randomized study of HCQ and D-PEN in 162 children with active, poorly controlled JRA who had not responded adequately to NSAIDs did not show significant differences from placebo for either drug, using 30% clinical change as its arbitrary level for significance.[108] These findings coincided with recognition of the efficacy of oral MTX for JRA, and the use of D-PEN rapidly declined thereafter. It may retain a limited role in combination therapy and in severe cases where multiple other therapies have failed.

### Dosage and Toxicity

Oral D-PEN is absorbed well on an empty stomach and achieves peak blood levels at 1 hour; a single dose is completely eliminated by 48 hours. Treatment is 10 to 20 mg/kg/day in one or two doses, which should be taken on an empty stomach. Dosage is increased slowly by 62.5 mg/week in children weighing less than 40 kg and by 125 mg/week in larger patients, to minimize GI intolerance. Maximum dosages rarely exceed 750 mg/day. To combat vitamin $B_6$ deficiency, 25 mg/day of pyridoxine may be given simultaneously. Efficacy appears slowly, but D-PEN should be discontinued if there is no clear benefit in 9 to 12 months.

Adverse reactions include thrombocytopenia, agranulocytosis, aplastic anemia, membranous nephropathy, rashes, and cholestatic hepatitis. Autoimmune toxicity includes an SLE-like syndrome, thyroiditis, polymyositis, myasthenia, and Goodpasture's syndrome. Nausea, vomiting, diarrhea, alterations in taste, headache, and dizziness have also been described in children.[86] Urinalysis, CBC, platelet count, and liver enzyme studies should be performed initially and then monthly; antinuclear antibodies (ANA) and immunoglobulin levels may be obtained annually. Idiosyncratic allergic reactions are fairly common and occur more often in patients with certain HLA types, such as Dw3, DR2, and the C4 null allele. Some patients who experience toxic reactions to gold may also manifest allergies to D-PEN.

# IMMUNOSUPPRESSIVE AGENTS

Immunosuppressive and cytotoxic agents should be used only for severe or life-threatening disease that has not responded to NSAIDs and SAARDs. Severe uveitis and amyloidosis may be specific indications.[110, 111] Major concerns include high rates of infection, bone marrow suppression, sterility, and late mutagenic and oncogenic potential.

AZATHIOPRINE. This drug has been used in 12 controlled trials in adult RA,[112] is similar in efficacy to SAARDs, but is not remittive. Anecdotally, azathioprine has been widely used for small numbers of severely ill children, but most pediatricians are not enthusiastic. At 1 to 2 mg/kg/day orally, it may be effective in up to 50% of cases, in comparison with placebo, for controlling arthritis.[113] In a prospective study of 129 consecutive patients with treatment-"refractory" JCA between 1980 and 1989, 38% of those receiving azathioprine demonstrated significant clinical and laboratory evidence of improvement.[114] The drug had notable steroid-sparing effects but was not effective for iridocyclitis. Azathioprine is associated with frequent infections, particularly herpes zoster. Leukopenia, biochemical hepatitis, rash, and GI intolerance are other complications.

CHLORAMBUCIL. This is an effective but toxic alkylating agent whose side effects may be cumulative and delayed; it carries significant risks of thrombocytopenia, leukopenia, infections in 10%, herpes zoster in 15%, acute monoblastic leukemia in children with JRA,[111] and other late malignant diseases. The dosage is 0.1 to 0.3 mg/kg/day orally. Because it does not cause hair loss or bladder complications, it may be more acceptable than cyclophosphamide for some families and teenagers, particularly for uncontrollable amyloidosis, uveitis, aortitis, vasculitis, or other complications of far-advanced JRA.[110]

CYCLOPHOSPHAMIDE. Because of severe alopecia and bladder complications, oral cyclophosphamide is now rarely used to treat JRA, although intravenous pulses (0.4 to 1.0 g/m$^2$) are occasionally given every 4 weeks for profound, destructive, often systemic JRA.[115, 116] There have been nine clinical trials of cyclophosphamide in adult RA which indicate that it may decrease the rate of formation of new articular erosions. Its major role may be in the treatment of severe, unresponsive vasculitis.

CYCLOSPORINE. This drug has been used to treat many autoimmune disorders; several studies have shown efficacy in adult RA. Its postulated mechanism of action is an inhibition of IL-2 transcription; the absence of generalized bone marrow suppression is notable.[117] However, GI intolerance, hirsutism, hypertension, and renal toxicity are major complications. Cyclosporine, at a dosage of 4 to 15 mg/kg/day, was first reported in 14 children with severe JRA in 1988; there were 11 withdrawals, 4 for lack of efficacy and 7 because of side effects.[118] Cyclosporine may be useful along with MTX for treatment-resistant JRA or dermatomyositis[119] and in cases of JRA with the macrophage activation syndrome.[120]

# BIOLOGIC AGENTS

INTRAVENOUS IMMUNE GLOBULIN. There have been several studies of intravenous immune globulin (IVIG) to treat systemic-onset JRA. In one report of 27 children who received monthly IVIG for 3 to 54 months, the main benefit was a significant improvement in systemic features and fever, but the efficacy for arthritis was limited.[121] The PRCSG evaluated IVIG in a multicenter trial of polyarticular JRA, using 1.5 to 2 g/kg infusion (100 g maximum) bimonthly for 2 months and monthly for 6 months in 25 patients.[122] Substantial clinical improvement was found in three fourths of cases during open-label administration, but the duration of benefit was short after discontinuation of IVIG. Overall, IVIG therapy is extremely expensive, there is always the risk of transmission of previously unknown infectious agents (most recently, hepatitis C), and it is often in short supply. It is still anecdotally used in very severe cases of JRA, where all other therapies have been inadequate, but efficacy is difficult to establish.

STEM CELL TRANSPLANTATION. This is a highly experimental approach that has been used in five children with refractory JRA,[123, 124] with a preparative regimen of antithymocyte globulin and cyclosporine. However, follow-up has been only 1 to 18 months, and life-threatening infectious complications may occur.

GROWTH HORMONE. The possible adjunctive use of growth hormone to ameliorate short stature in children with arthritis, particularly those also treated with corticosteroids, has been discussed for many years. However, expense and difficulties in study design have been limiting factors. Some reports have described low levels of 24-hour growth hormone secretion in JRA,[125] whereas others have noted low-normal to normal levels of growth hormone and of insulin-like growth factor I (IGF-1).[126–128] Approximately 40 children have been treated, usually for 1 year, some with human and others with recombinant growth hormone. Most patients demonstrated increased growth velocity, but follow-up durations were only 1 to 2 years, and a number of these children entered puberty during the investigations. At this point the risk-benefit ratio of using growth hormones in children is totally unknown, and reducing corticosteroid dosages and durations in children with arthritis seems a more effective way to minimize growth suppression.

ETANERCEPT. Etanercept was studied in 69 patients, aged 4 to 17 years, with polyarticular-course JRA refractory to or intolerant of MTX. A twice-weekly injectable dose of 0.4 mg/kg/dose, up to a maximum of 25 mg/dose,[129] was employed. In part I of the study, which lasted 3 months, all patients received etanercept; 74% demonstrated a positive clinical response (30% or better improvement in three or more of six core set variables). In part II, the positive responders were randomly assigned to receive etanercept or placebo for 4 more months; 24% of the etanercept patients withdrew due to disease flare, compared with 77% of those receiving placebo ($P$ = .007). Etanercept was well tolerated; the most common side effects were mild injection site reactions and mild to moderate upper respiratory tract infections that did not require treatment interruption.

Etanercept was approved by the FDA in June, 1999, for use in patients with moderate to severely active polyarticular-course JRA who have had an inadequate response to one or more DMARDs. Most pediatric centers now have small numbers of severely impaired patients receiving etanercept, often in combination with MTX, and in many cases the degree of improvement has been dramatic. However, treatment durations are still very short, rates of long-term complications are unknown, and examples of diminishing efficacy are beginning to be described.

MEASURES TO IMPROVE BONE MINERAL DENSITY. Abnormalities of bone mineral density in children with arthritis have been evident on radiographs for decades, but information about corticosteroid, nutritional, and physical activity influences; abnormalities in bone metabolism; responses to treatment; fracture rates; and long-term outcomes have all been limited. A 1998 study of 111 children with JRA, using factor analysis of 13 explanatory variables, followed by multiple linear regression analyses, showed that physical activity, calcium intake, and body size were significant positive determinants in bone mineral density in JRA,[130] whereas disease activity and glucocorticoids were significant negative determinants. It is highly likely that failure to achieve adequate bone mass in children and adolescents with arthritis will lead to clinically important osteopenia in later life, regardless of subsequent disease activity.[37] Therefore, we routinely advise calcium and vitamin D supplementation and maximal physical activity, to tolerance, in all children with arthritis.

## PRACTICAL MANAGEMENT STRATEGIES

The four cases that follow illustrate our approach to common patient care problems in children with arthritis.

## Case 1

An 18-month-old girl had 3 months of right knee swelling, a 5-degree flexion contracture, and morning toe-walking (i.e., morning stiffness); review of systems and family history were noncontributory. The following laboratory studies were obtained: CBC, urinalysis, ESR, liver enzyme studies, and ANA. The ESR was 28 mm/hour (more than 15 mm/hour is abnormal), and the ANA titer was 1:320. The most likely diagnosis is pauciarticular JRA, and regular ophthalmologic evaluation is mandatory. At present, she has no evidence of uveitis on slit-lamp examination, but in view of the positive ANA, she should have evaluations every 3 to 4 months for at least 5 years, because iridocyclitis in children is usually asymptomatic and young patients rarely complain of changes in visual acuity. The ANA determination should be repeated every 1 to 2 years.

Physical therapy evaluation revealed muscle wasting, with a 1-cm decrease in both thigh and gastrocnemius circumference. The child was given a home physical therapy program; a night splint will be added if the knee is not straight within 3 weeks (the normal 18-month-old knee can hyperextend to −15 degrees). The parents were encouraged to allow full play and athletic activities to tolerance. Detailed, written education pamphlets about JRA were provided.

Radiographs of involved joints were obtained (and studies of newly affected ones should be obtained in the future). This child demonstrated mild epiphyseal overgrowth at the femur, suggesting more chronic inflammation and the potential need for aggressive management if initial therapy is not optimally beneficial. Follow-up radiographs should be performed annually.

PHARMACOLOGIC MANAGEMENT. Liquid or crushed-tablet NSAIDs are good initial choices. We prescribe naproxen at 10 to 15 mg/kg/day, which for a 15-kg child is 3 to 4 mL of naproxen (25 mg/mL suspension) twice daily, given at the *beginning* of meals. Ibuprofen may be given at 30 to 35 mg/kg/day—for example, 5 to 7 mL (1 to 1.25 teaspoons) of the 20-mg/mL suspension three times daily is a good starting dosage. Tolmetin sodium is an alternative, although it is expensive. Renal and liver function should be checked at baseline only. Further laboratory testing should depend on symptoms. If after 3 months and one NSAID switch the inflammation continues, intra-articular injection of triamcinolone hexacetonide (up to twice per year) or the addition of MTX may be considered. This patient can be expected to need uninterrupted medical therapy for at least 2 years. Children complain little of, and rapidly adapt to, joint pain and also may have only subtle persistent synovitis. Nonetheless, the potential for major growth abnormalities is high, and parents should be initially prepared for a 2-year course of treatment. If deformity progresses or if growth and development are impaired, then MTX becomes mandatory. Ophthalmologic follow-up should continue for 5 years after articular remission is achieved. Evidence of gastritis may include declining appetite or epigastric discomfort. Mood changes may reflect medication toxicity or advancing arthritis.

## Case 2

Over a period of 2 months, a 6-year-old Hispanic girl developed progressive synovitis that included both knees, one ankle, one midfoot, the left first metatarsophalangeal joint, and a proximal interphalangeal finger joint. She had severe morning stiffness and could not attend school; there was a history of "eczema," and three fingernail pits were present. An aunt has psoriasis, and a grandmother has classic RA. A diagnosis of extended pauciarticular JRA is possible, although an early presentation of psoriatic arthritis should also be considered. The ESR was 35 mm/hour, the hemoglobin level was 11.9 g/dL, rheumatoid factor was absent, and the ANA titer was 1:160.

The principles of radiologic investigation, physical therapy evaluation, emphasis on remaining athletically active, ophthalmologic assessment and follow-up, patient indifference to pain, and family education are the same as in case 1. The prognosis for the ultimate number of joints involved is guarded, and this should be clearly communicated to the family.

MANAGEMENT. Initial pharmacologic management is the same as in case 1, but early preparation of the parents about the potential need for DMARDs should be added. If there is little or no visible improvement in the child's joints after 2 months of therapy, one may try Azulfidine while remembering that this drug is safe but may have limited efficacy. We prescribe 40 to 50 mg/kg/day in two divided doses, with a stepwise upward increase to achieve the full dosage in 2 to 4 weeks, and obtain a CBC with platelet count after 2 weeks of therapy. For example, if the weight is 20 kg, the initial dosage would be one-half tablet (250 mg) per day; if this is tolerated, the dosage is increased every 5 days in 250-mg increments, to one tablet twice daily. Experience with the taste of the suspensions has been disappointing. Tablets of most medications are "crushable," although enteric-coated preparations should be avoided if there is need for tablet crushing.

Some experienced physicians add HCQ at this point, but improvement may then require another 6 to 12 months of observation. We prefer to start oral MTX if there has been no improvement after 8 weeks. In this case, the child's body surface area is approximately 0.8 m². We start MTX at 10 mg/m²/week, so an appropriate starting dosage in this case would be 7.5 mg one time each week. Folic acid, 1 mg/day, should also be given. After a 12-week trial, MTX can be increased approximately every 8 weeks, up to 15 to 20 mg/m², and ultimately changed to injection, if required. Morning baths can be highly effective for morning stiffness, but they often disrupt busy family routines. We advise the use of an electric blanket set on medium-high and plugged into an electric timer that is set to activate 1 hour before the child arises.

## Case 3

A 14-year-old girl had a 6-month history of prominent swelling in 17 joints, including one elbow, both wrists, shoulders, knees, and ankles, 3 metacarpophalangeal joints, and 4 proximal interphalangeal joints; she also had limitation and discomfort at the neck. Her mother noted 45 minutes of morning stiffness and progressive withdrawal from physical activities, both of which the teenager denied. There had been no height or weight gain for 9 months; school performance was deteriorating. There was no family history of SLE and no evidence of butterfly rash, mucosal ulcerations, or alopecia. Laboratory data revealed an ESR of 45 mm/hour, a hemoglobin level of 10 g/dL, and a leukocyte count of 6300 cells/μL with normal differential; urinalysis was normal. The patient most likely has polyarticular JRA, but a gut-associated arthropathy or psoriatic arthritis is possible.

MANAGEMENT. In this setting of progressive, disabling JRA we immediately start both an NSAID and oral MTX, 10 mg/m²/week, with an expected response time of 4 to 6 weeks. If, at the time of initial presentation, the patient cannot attend school, is experiencing severe fatigue, or cannot adequately ambulate, a 3-day course of intravenous pulse prednisolone or methylprednisolone, 30 mg/kg/day (up to a maximum of 1 g) for three consecutive or alternate days is also indicated. After the usual 7- to 21-day poststeroid "honeymoon period," the patient may slowly worsen. The dosage of MTX may then be increased by 2.5 mg/week every 4 to 6 weeks. Often, these patients inexorably develop more joint involvement, and the *addition* of Azulfidine or HCQ or both may then become necessary. Such children commonly also have interval disease flares that respond only to brief courses of oral steroids. It is highly preferable to start with alternate-day prednisone, and the patient and parents should clearly be given a firm stopping date, in order to avoid the long-term consequences of steroid dependence, such as irreversible growth failure. Many practitioners would increase either oral or parenteral MTX to 15 mg/m²/week before adding any corticosteroids. A single bedtime dose of indomethacin, 25 to 50 mg (one or two 25-mg capsules), can help alleviate morning stiffness.

## Case 4

A 5-year-old boy developed arthralgias, hectic fever, inanition, and lymphadenopathy. After 1 week of unsuccessful treatment with antibiotics, a faint salmon-colored rash and splenomegaly were detected. Viral titers were negative, the leukocyte count was 14,600 cells/mm³ but with normal differential, the ESR was 96 mm/hour, and the hemoglobin level had progressively fallen to 7.6 g/dL; the platelet count was 900,000 cells/mm³. There was no family history of rheumatic disease, and there had been no unusual infectious disease exposure. Both rheumatoid factor and ANA were absent. Although the patient does not yet have synovitis, the most likely diagnosis is systemic-onset JRA.

This child will not presently benefit from a radiologic arthritis survey or physical therapy evaluation, but both should be done with the advent of synovitis. A chest radiograph, electrocardiogram, and echocardiogram should be obtained if there is any suspicion of pericarditis or myocarditis. Ophthalmologic assessment may be done annually.

MANAGEMENT. Although most NSAIDs are beneficial in patients with arthralgias, aspirin and indomethacin are the most effective antipyretics. Indomethacin is also an excellent choice for the pain and inflammation of pericarditis. A "therapeutic bridge" of oral prednisone, 1 to 2 mg/kg/day divided into two or three doses per day, is often needed for several days or weeks to ameliorate systemic symptoms, and occasionally a severely compromised child requires intravenous pulse steroids as outlined earlier. The use of steroids should be tailored to the severity of illness and the organs involved, particularly if vasculitis is present. It is essential to outline the therapeutic approach in detail to the parents, including alternative "What if?" strategies, intermediate- or long-term timelines, and events that might lead to changes. MTX should be introduced early if articular involvement occurs. Although they are investigational, immunosuppressive agents and/ or IVIG may be needed for uncontrollable systemic features.

Essentially, pediatric ankylosing spondylitis, Reiter's syndrome, psoriatic arthritis, and the limited enthesopathic syndromes can be managed like polyarticular JRA, although many practitioners favor tolmetin sodium or indomethacin among the NSAIDs. We have found that the early addition of oral MTX is also very useful in this group of illnesses. Psoriatic arthritis can be treated early with Azulfidine, whereas the protean weight loss and fever of some children with Reiter's syndrome responds to management similar to that for systemic-onset JRA. The principles of physical therapy and radiographic and laboratory evaluation are essentially the same. We have found HLA-B27 testing useful for family counseling when a parent has long-neglected back or articular difficulties or a sibling develops enthesitis-like symptoms and the family desires early intervention.

## General Considerations

Throughout the management of childhood arthritis it is important to be positive and optimistic about prognosis and to emphasize physical activity, independence, and athletic participation to *the child's* perception of tolerance. In this manner, the patient learns about self-efficacy and appropriate setting of limits. The parents, and progressively the child, should be encouraged to undertake a primary role in making decisions regarding school, family, social, vocational, and other aspects of life that relate to the illness.

## THERAPEUTIC HINTS

## Pain, Morning Stiffness, Medications, and Education

The presence of joint pain, morning stiffness, and limp should be reviewed at each visit. Older children often

deny discomfort, and it is well known that children acclimate to "pain" and have fewer complaints. This may occur to avoid a perceived risk of physician- or parent-mandated limitation of activities (in school, sports, family, or play). In younger patients irritability, frequent crying, and reduction or change in play routines may be nonverbal indicators of inflammation or inadequate response to therapy.

Physical measures to reduce morning stiffness, such as the use of a sleeping bag, can be helpful. However, evening baths are not useful and morning baths often conflict with hectic family routines. We recommend connecting an electric blanket, preset at medium to high, to a plug-in timer that is set to activate 1 hour before the child arises. Thus, the child will not be too hot while sleeping but, after 1 hour of concentrated warmth, will be easier to arouse and will require less assistance from the busy parent. Setting an alarm to sound 1 hour before arising and supervising the child to awake briefly and take the first morning dose of medication from the bedside table can also be helpful.

Most patients and families misinterpret giving NSAIDs "with meals" to mean *at the end*. Rather, NSAIDs should be given with the first bite of food, in order to optimize mixing and buffering. NSAIDs taken at the end of meals amplify GI distress at the time of maximal postprandial gastric acid production. Similarly, it is important to use sufficient, preferably chewable, antacids, 2 hours after meals, to minimize any residual GI distress.

Better quality and greater breadth of *written* patient-family education materials about arthritis in children have contributed to improved acceptance, compliance, and outcomes. High-quality, comprehensive take-home brochures concerning diagnosis and treatment of many pediatric rheumatic disorders are now available from most centers. Important functions of brochures include the following:

1. Validation of disease presence and type.
2. Clarification of disease severity, despite the child's often appearing "active and well."
3. Ease of brochure reproduction to achieve uniform knowledge among relatives, absent parents, school personnel, and so on.
4. Stated rationales for laboratory testing and information about alternative treatments.
5. Discussion of prognosis.

It is important that education handouts be given to all newly diagnosed children with rheumatic disease and their families. The Arthritis Foundation, the American Juvenile Arthritis Organization, and the Arthritis Information Clearinghouse are other resources for materials.

Patients with JRA usually wish to be physically active; they tolerate exercise and sports surprisingly well, and their parents welcome loosening of restrictions in this area, particularly because enforcement is difficult and often leads to family conflict. Although children with JRA often exhibit prolonged exercise recovery and are deconditioned relative to age- and sex-matched healthy children, fitness levels in JRA do not correlate with disease activity.[131] Often, poor fitness in JRA is related to activity restrictions by concerned physicians, teachers, and parents that lead to unfamiliarity with many physical skill activities. It has been shown that aerobic conditioning programs are safe, effective, and enjoyed by patients with JRA, as well as those with many other chronic childhood illnesses (e.g., cystic fibrosis, Down's syndrome, asthma, spina bifida).[132] Conditioning or sports activities for patients with JRA can be accomplished in community settings, monitored with validated and age-normed tests, and administered by persons who are not health professionals; such activities may have a beneficial impact on social activities, school attendance, and self-efficacy. Similarly, summer camps for patients with JRA are widely enjoyed and promote social and physical growth and development.

## When to Stop Treatment

Most pediatric rheumatologists continue treatment of all patients with any evidence of persistent disease activity, particularly if epiphyses are open and there is still growth potential. About 20% of children with JRA exhibit synovial swelling even with a normal ESR and therefore a normal ESR alone should not lead to discontinuation of treatment. Although parents can be very perceptive about when their children are "normal," patients with JRA subtly but constantly alter their physical behaviors to accommodate joint involvement. Parents dislike the presence of arthritis and the costs and risks of medications; therefore, the physician may need to urge continued treatment to maximize outcome, despite variable levels of family resistance.

Conversely, some rheumatologists elect not to treat some patients with low disease activity and no current "morbidity." These patients are often those children who deny pain and whose range of motion and growth are nearly normal but who have persistent pauciarticular or polyarticular joint bogginess (mild) without erosions. The decision to stop, or not start, treatment despite mild ongoing inflammation may appear to be justified, particularly if the patient and family have strong feelings against taking medications or if they perceive no discernible benefit. However, the potential for long-term impairment of normal growth and development must be clearly explained.

For the patient who achieves complete laboratory and clinical remission, many physicians suggest that the child be sustained on medication for another 6 to 12 months. Treatment is then slowly tapered over several weeks to months.

## Compliance

Cost, denial of illness, drug side effects, poor understanding of treatment goals, unrealistic expectations, guilt about causality, desire to avoid drug "addiction," equation of absence of pain with wellness, and familial pressures to try alternative remedies are just a few of the reasons for noncompliance that we regularly encounter. Numerous studies of adult RA estimate compliance with NSAIDs at about 50%. In general pediatrics, compliance rates of 50% to 54% have been reported,[133] whereas two retrospective studies of aspirin in JRA both yielded values of 55% in teenagers as well as younger children.[134] Children both overmedicate and undermedicate themselves; they exhibit negative reactions to medications in 43% of cases, to exercise regimens in 60%, and to splints in 43%.[135] Direct refusal of treatment by a child is a frequent problem, and yet it often is not directly addressed by physicians. One investigation showed that up to 70% of JRA patients use unconventional remedies. Often, when physicians acknowledge their own forgetfulness in medication use, they empower patients and parents to ingest missed doses. Altering schedules to fit social situations, and being positive despite suboptimal compliance, will actually improve future behaviors.

## Patients with Arthritis in the Operating Room

All children with rheumatic disease who undergo surgery should have a CBC, platelet count, and determinations of prothrombin time, partial thromboplastin time, and template bleeding time to assess in vivo platelet function. NSAIDs should be stopped 3 to 4 days before surgery if the operation is expected to be associated with significant bleeding. Bleeding times may need to be checked more than once, and this should not be delayed until the day of hospitalization. If NSAIDs are discontinued, a short course of steroids may be necessary to control disease activity. Patients undergoing long-term corticosteroid therapy (>15 mg/day for 1 week, or >5 to 15 mg for 1 month) should receive 30 mg/m² of intramuscular hydrocortisone every 6 hours during the 12 to 24 hours preceding surgery (depending on dosage and duration of prior oral treatment). Some surgeons administer intravenous hydrocortisone to all patients during surgery, whereas others use it only if complications develop. Another intramuscular dose of hydrocortisone should be given 1 hour later in the recovery room. While receiving nothing by mouth, children should be given the parenteral equivalent of any regularly prescribed preoperative steroid. In our experience, MTX has been continued without difficulty. The potential to develop or exacerbate bone marrow depression induced by immunosuppressive agents should be closely monitored in the postoperative period.

## CONCLUSION

Therapeutic interventions for JRA and the pediatric spondyloarthropathies have continuously become more aggressive during the past 20 years. This development may be attributed to the following:

1. Earlier and more accurate diagnoses.
2. Availability of well-studied, relatively safe, and effective NSAIDs.

3. Recognition of the potential for arrested growth and development and severe late disability if remittive therapy is delayed.

4. Earlier use of SAARDs, often in combinations.

5. The advent of MTX as a major treatment modality.

6. The recent introduction of etanercept.

Other important advances include the following:

1. Improved education of patients, parents, schools, and referring physicians.

2. Emphasis on patient and family self-efficacy.

3. Use of both individual and group support techniques.

4. Less external setting of limits by parents, physicians, and schools.

5. Greater patient participation in exercise and athletics.

Such changes may contribute to better compliance, more age-appropriate social behaviors, and better scholastic performance in children with arthritis. Parents and patients have become more active participants in decision making, and the global impact on functional outcomes appears to be positive.

Exciting research in pediatric rheumatology continues and is leading to:

1. Better understanding of the relationship between genetics and treatment responses.

2. New protocols for combination therapy.

3. Safer corticosteroids.

4. Immunotherapy and other biologic treatments.

5. Permissible limits of exercise and physical conditioning for the child with arthritis.

# REFERENCES

1. Singsen BH: Health status (arthritis impact) in children with chronic rheumatic diseases. Arthritis Care Res 1991; 4:87.
2. Duffy CM, Duffy KN: Health assessment in the rheumatic diseases of childhood. Curr Opin Rheumatol 1997; 9:440.
3. Moroldo MB, Giannini EH: Estimates of the discriminant ability of definitions of improvement for juvenile rheumatoid arthritis. J Rheumatol 1998; 25:986.
4. Ruperto N, Ravelli A, Falcini F, et al: Performance of the preliminary definition of improvement in juvenile chronic arthritis patients treated with methotrexate. Ann Rheum Dis 1998; 57:38.
5. Schaller JG: Juvenile rheumatoid arthritis: Series I. Arthritis Rheum 1977; 20(suppl 2):165.
6. Ansell BM: Juvenile chronic arthritis. Scand J Rheumatol 1987; 66(suppl):47.
7. Giannini EH, Brewer EJ, Kuzmina N, et al: Auranofin in the treatment of juvenile rheumatoid arthritis. Arthritis Rheum 1990; 33:466.
8. Maclagan TJ: The treatment of acute rheumatism with salicin. Lancet 1876; 1:342.
9. Belay ED, Bresee JS, Holman RC, et al: Reye's syndrome in the United States from 1981 through 1997. N Engl J Med 1999; 340:1377.
10. Athreya BH, Moser G, Cecil HS, et al: Aspirin-induced hepatotoxicity in juvenile rheumatoid arthritis: A prospective study. Arthritis Rheum 1975; 18:347.
11. Brooks PM, Day RO: Nonsteroidal antiinflammatory drugs: Differences and similarities. N Engl J Med 1991; 324:1716.
12. Abramson SB, Weissman G: The mechanism of action of nonsteroidal anti-inflammatory drugs. Arthritis Rheum 1989; 32:1.
13. Levinson JE, Baum J, Brewer E, et al: Comparison of tolmetin sodium and aspirin in the treatment of juvenile rheumatoid arthritis. J Pediatr 1977; 91:799.
14. Price T, Venning H, Ansell BM: Ibuprofen in juvenile chronic arthritis. Clin Exp Rheumatol 1985; 3:59.
15. Giannini EH, Brewer EJ, Miller ML, et al: Ibuprofen suspension in the treatment of juvenile rheumatoid arthritis. J Pediatr 1990; 117:645.
16. Ansell BM, Hanna B, Moran H, et al: Naproxen in juvenile chronic polyarthritis. Eur J Rheumatol Inflamm 1979; 2:79.
17. Makela AL: Naproxen in the treatment of juvenile rheumatoid arthritis. Scand J Rheumatol 1977; 6:193.
18. Kvien TK: Naproxen and acetylsalicylic acid in the treatment of pauciarticular and polyarticular juvenile rheumatoid arthritis. Scand J Rheumatol 1984; 13:342.
19. Laxer RM, Silverman ED, St.-Cyr C, et al: A six-month open safety assessment of a naproxen suspension formulation in the therapy of juvenile rheumatoid arthritis. Clin Ther 1988; 10:381.
20. Suarez SM, Cohen PR, DeLeo V: Bullous photosensitivity to naproxen: "Pseudoporphyria." Arthritis Rheum 1990; 33:903.
21. Lang BA, Finlayson LA: Naproxen-induced pseudoporphyria in patients with juvenile rheumatoid arthritis. J Pediatr 1994; 124:639.
22. Brewer EJ: A comparative evaluation of indomethacin, acetaminophen and placebo as antipyretic agents in children. Arthritis Rheum 1968; 11:645.
23. Bhettay E, Thompson AJ: Double-blind study of ketoprofen and indomethacin in juvenile chronic arthritis. S Afr Med J 1978; 54:276.
24. Sanger L: Long-term treatment of juvenile chronic arthritis (juvenile rheumatoid arthritis) and systemic juvenile chronic arthritis (Still's syndrome) with diclofenac. Aktuelle Rheum 1978; 3:5.
25. Haapasaari J, Wuolijoki E, Ylijoki H: Treatment of juvenile rheumatoid arthritis with diclofenac sodium. Scand J Rheumatol 1983; 12:325.
26. Leak AM, Richter MR, Clemens LE, et al: A crossover study of naproxen, diclofenac and tolmetin in seronegative juvenile chronic arthritis. Clin Exp Rheumatol 1988; 6:157.
27. Garcia-Morteo O, Maldonado-Cocco JA, Cuttica R, et al: Piroxicam in juvenile rheumatoid arthritis. Eur J Rheumatol Inflamm 1987; 8:49.
28. Williams PL, Ansell BM, Bell A, et al: Multicentre study of piroxicam versus naproxen in juvenile chronic arthritis, with special reference to problem areas in clinical trials of nonsteroidal anti-inflammatory drugs in childhood. Br J Rheumatol 1986; 25:67.
29. Kaul A, Reddy JC, Fagman E, et al: Hepatitis associated with use of sulindac in a child. J Pediatr 1981; 99:650.
30. Flato B, Vinje O, Forre O: Toxicity of antirheumatic and anti-inflammatory drugs in children. Clin Rheumatol 1998; 17:505.
31. Szer IS, Goldenstein-Schainberg C, Kurtin P: Paucity of renal complications associated with nonsteroidal antiinflammatory drugs in children with chronic arthritis. J Pediatr 1991; 119:815.
32. Fink CW: Medical treatment of juvenile arthritis. Clin Orthop 1990; 259:60.
33. Loftus J, Allen R, Hesp R, et al: Randomized, double-blind trial of deflazacort versus prednisone in juvenile chronic arthritis: A relatively bone-sparing effect of deflazacort. Pediatrics 1991; 88:428.
34. Miller JJ: Prolonged use of large intravenous steroid pulses in the rheumatic diseases of children. Pediatrics 1980; 65:989.
35. Job-Deslandre C, Menkes CJ: Administration of methylprednisolone pulse in chronic arthritis in children. Clin Exp Rheumatol 1991; 9(suppl 6):15.
36. Adebajo AO, Hall MA: The use of intravenous pulsed methylprednisolone in the treatment of systemic onset juvenile chronic arthritis. Br J Rheumatol 1998; 37:1240.
37. Cassidy JT, Petty RE: Basic concepts of drug therapy. In Textbook of Pediatric Rheumatology, 3rd ed. Philadelphia: WB Saunders, 1995:85.
38. Allen RC, Gross KR, Laxer RM, et al: Intraarticular triamcinolone hexacetonide in the management of chronic arthritis in children. Arthritis Rheum 1986; 29:997.

39. Hertzberger-ten Cate R, de Vries-van der Vlugt BC, van Suijlekom-Smit LW, et al: Intra-articular steroids in pauciarticular juvenile chronic arthritis, type 1. Eur J Pediatr 1991; 150:170.

40. Padeh S, Passwell JH: Intraarticular corticosteroid injection in the management of children with chronic arthritis. Arthritis Rheum 1998; 41:1210.

41. Sparling M, Malleson P, Wood B, et al: Radiographic followup of joints injected with triamcinolone hexacetonide for the management of childhood arthritis. Arthritis Rheum 1990; 33:821.

42. Gilsanz V, Bernstein BH: Joint calcification following intra-articular corticosteroid therapy. Radiology 1984; 151:647.

43. Job-Deslandre C, Menkes CJ: Complications of intra-articular injections of triamcinolone hexacetonide in chronic arthritis in children. Clin Exp Rheumatol 1990; 8:413.

44. Gubner R, August S, Ginsberg V: Therapeutic suppression of tissue reactivity: Effects of aminopterin in rheumatoid arthritis and psoriasis. Am J Med Sci 1951; 221:176.

45. Weinblatt ME, Coblyn JS, Fox DA, et al: Efficacy of low-dose methotrexate in rheumatoid arthritis. N Engl J Med 1985; 312:818.

46. Williams HJ, Wikens RF, Samuelson CO, et al: Comparison of low-dose oral pulse methotrexate and placebo in the treatment of rheumatoid arthritis. Arthritis Rheum 1985; 28:721.

47. Nordstrom DM, West SG, Andersen PA, et al: Pulse methotrexate therapy in rheumatoid arthritis: A controlled prospective roentgenographic study. Ann Intern Med 1987; 107:797.

48. Lopez-Mendez A, Daniel WW, Reading JC, et al: Radiographic assessment of disease progression in rheumatoid arthritis patients enrolled in the cooperative systematic studies of the rheumatic diseases program randomized clinical trial of methotrexate, auranofin, or a combination of the two. Arthritis Rheum 1993; 36:1364.

49. Harel L, Wagner-Weiner L, Poznanski AK, et al: Effects of methotrexate on radiologic progression in juvenile rheumatoid arthritis. Arthritis Rheum 1993; 36:1370.

50. Truckenbrodt H, Hafner R: Methotrexate therapy in juvenile rheumatoid arthritis. Arthritis Rheum 1986; 29:801.

51. Wallace CA, Bleyer WA, Sherry DD, et al: Toxicity and serum levels of methotrexate in children with juvenile rheumatoid arthritis. Arthritis Rheum 1989; 32:677.

52. Danao T, Steinbrunner J, Medendorp S, et al: Methotrexate in juvenile rheumatoid arthritis. Arthritis Rheum 1989; 32:S28.

53. Rose CD, Singsen BH, Eichenfield, et al: Safety and efficacy of methotrexate therapy in juvenile rheumatoid arthritis. J Pediatr 1990; 117:653.

54. Giannini EH, Brewer EJ, Kuzmina N, et al: Methotrexate in resistant juvenile rheumatoid arthritis. N Engl J Med 1992; 346:1043.

55. White C: Reversal of methotrexate binding to dihydrofolate reductase by dihydrofolate. J Biol Chem 1979; 254:10889.

56. Olsen NJ, Murray LM: Antiproliferative effects of methotrexate on peripheral blood mononuclear cells. Arthritis Rheum 1989; 32:378.

57. Stewart KA, Mackenzie AH, Clough JD, et al: Folate supplementation in methotrexate-treated rheumatoid arthritis patients. Semin Arthritis Rheum 1991; 20:1.

58. Olsen NJ, Callahan LF, Pincus T: Immunologic studies of rheumatoid arthritis patients treated with methotrexate. Arthritis Rheum 1987; 30:481.

59. Alarcon G, Schrohenlocher RE, Bartolucci AA, et al: Suppression of rheumatoid factor production by methotrexate in patients with rheumatoid arthritis. Arthritis Rheum 1990; 33:1156.

60. Segal R, Mozes E, Yaron M, et al: The effects of methotrexate on the production and activity of interleukin-1. Arthritis Rheum 1989; 32:370.

61. Segal R, Yaron M, Tartakovsky B: Rescue of interleukin-1 activity by leucovorin following inhibition by methotrexate in a murine in vitro system. Arthritis Rheum 1990; 33:1745.

62. Hine RJ, Everson MP, Hardin JM, et al: Methotrexate therapy in rheumatoid arthritis patients diminishes lectin-induced mononuclear cell proliferation. Rheumatol Int 1990; 10:165.

63. Sperling RI, Coblyn JS, Larkin JK, et al: Inhibition of leukotriene B4 synthesis in neutrophils from patients with rheumatoid arthritis by a single oral dose of methotrexate. Arthritis Rheum 1990; 33:1149.

64. Nesher G, Moore T: The in vitro effects of methotrexate on peripheral blood mononuclear cells. Arthritis Rheum 1990; 33:954.

65. Furst DE, Kremer JM: Methotrexate in rheumatoid arthritis. Arthritis Rheum 1988; 31:305.

66. Nuernberg B, Koehnke R, Solsky M, et al: Biliary elimination of low-dose methotrexate in humans. Arthritis Rheum 1990; 33:898.

67. Gabriel S, Creagan EC, O'Fallon WM, et al: Treatment of rheumatoid arthritis with higher dose intravenous methotrexate. Rheumatol 1990; 17:460.

68. Shiroky JB, Neville C, Skelton JD: High dose intravenous methotrexate for refractory rheumatoid arthritis. J Rheumatol 1992; 19:247.

69. Wallace CA, Sherry DD: Preliminary report of higher dose methotrexate treatment in juvenile rheumatoid arthritis. J Rheumatol 1992; 19:1604.

70. Singsen BH, Rose CD: Parenteral methotrexate for juvenile rheumatoid arthritis. Arthritis Rheum 1993; 36:S137.

71. Onel KB, Lehman TJA: High dose intramuscular methotrexate for juvenile rheumatoid arthritis. Arthritis Rheum 1993; 36:S122.

72. Goldman D, Matherly LH: The cellular pharmacology of methotrexate. Pharmacol Ther 1985; 28:77.

73. Dupuis LL, Koren G, Shore A, et al: Methotrexate-nonsteroidal antiinflammatory drug interaction in children with arthritis. J Rheumatol 1990; 17:1469.

74. Skeith KJ, Russell AS, Fakkreddin J, et al: Lack of significant interaction between low dose methotrexate and ibuprofen or flurbiprofen in patients with arthritis. J Rheumatol 1990; 17:1008.

75. Morgan SL, Baggot JE, Vaughn WH, et al: The effect of folic acid supplementation on the toxicity of low-dose methotrexate in patients with rheumatoid arthritis. Arthritis Rheum 1990; 33:98.

76. Walker AM, Funch D, Dreyer NA: Determinants of serious liver disease among patients receiving low-dose methotrexate for rheumatoid arthritis. Arthritis Rheum 1993; 36:329.

77. Bjorkman DJ, Boschert M, Tolman KG, et al: The effect of long-term methotrexate therapy on hepatic fibrosis in rheumatoid arthritis. Arthritis Rheum 1993; 36:1697.

78. Aponte J, Petrelli M: Histopathologic findings in the liver of rheumatoid arthritis patients treated with long-term bolus methotrexate. Arthritis Rheum 1988; 31:1457.

79. Kremer JM, Lee RG, Tolman KG: Liver histology in rheumatoid arthritis patients receiving long-term methotrexate therapy. Arthritis Rheum 1989; 32:121.

80. Rau R, Karger T, Herborn G, et al: Liver biopsy findings in patients with rheumatoid arthritis undergoing long-term treatment with methotrexate. J Rheumatol 1989; 16:489.

81. Graham LD, Rivas-Chacon RF, Myones BL: Lack of hepatotoxicity with chronic administration of methotrexate in juvenile rheumatoid arthritis. Arthritis Rheum 1990; 33:S144.

82. Keim D, Ragsdale C, Heilderberger K, et al: Hepatic fibrosis with the use of methotrexate for juvenile rheumatoid arthritis. J Rheumatol 1990; 17:846.

83. Rose CD, Padman R, Wesdock KA, et al: Methotrexate safety in juvenile rheumatoid arthritis (JRA). Arthritis Rheum 1990; 33:S95.

84. Graham LD, Myones BL, Rivas-Chacon RF, et al: Morbidity associated with long-term methotrexate therapy in juvenile rheumatoid arthritis. J Pediatr 1992; 120:468.

85. Croock AD, Furst DE, Helmers RA, et al: Methotrexate dose does not alter pulmonary function in patients with rheumatoid arthritis. Arthritis Rheum 1989; 32:S60.

86. Grondin C, Malleson P, Petty RE: Slow acting anti-rheumatic drugs in chronic arthritis of childhood. Semin Arthritis Rheum 1988; 18:38.

87. Brewer EJ, Giannini EH, Barkley E: Gold therapy in the management of juvenile rheumatoid arthritis. Arthritis Rheum 1980; 23:404.

88. Littman BH, Carlson PL, Loose LD, et al: Effects of gold sodium thiomalate and tenidap sodium (CP-66,2482-2) on a model of macrophage differentiation using HL-60 cells. Arthritis Rheum 1990; 33:29.

89. Kawakami A, Eguchi K, Migita K, et al: Inhibitory effects of gold sodium thiomalate on proliferation and interferon-γ induced HLA-DR expression in human endothelial cells. J Rheumatol 1990; 17:430.

90. Abruzzo JL: Auranofin: A new drug for rheumatoid arthritis. Ann Intern Med 1986; 105:274.

91. Marcolongo R, Mathieu A, Pala R, et al: The efficacy and safety of auranofin in the treatment of juvenile rheumatoid arthritis. Arthritis Rheum 1988; 31:979.

92. Pinals RS: Sulfasalazine in the rheumatic diseases. Semin Arthritis Rheum 1988; 17:246.

93. Nissila M, Lehtinen K, Leirisalo-Repo M, et al: Sulfasalazine in the treatment of ankylosing spondylitis. Arthritis Rheum 1988; 31:1111.

94. Nordstrom DM, West SG, Freeman S, et al: HLA-B27 positive enterogenic reactive arthritis: Response of arthritis and microscopic colitis to sulfasalazine. Arthritis Rheum 1987; 30:S24.

95. Ozdogan H, Turunc M, Deringol B, et al: Sulphasalazine in the treatment of juvenile rheumatoid arthritis: A preliminary open trial. J Rheumatol 1986; 13:124.

96. Joos R, Veys EM, Mielants H, et al: Sulfasalazine treatment in juvenile chronic arthritis. J Rheumatol 1991; 18:880.

97. Ansell BM, Hall MA, Loftus JK, et al: A multcentre pilot study of sulfa-salazine in juvenile chronic arthritis. Clin Exp Rheumatol 1991; 9:201.

98. Gedalia A, Barash J, Press J, et al: Sulphasalazine in the treatment of pauciarticular-onset juvenile chronic arthritis. Clin Rheumatol 1993; 12:511.

99. Imundo LF, Jacobs JC: Sulfasalazine therapy for juvenile rheumatoid arthritis. J Rheumatol 1996; 23:360.

100. Huang JL, Chen LC: Sulphasalazine in the treatment of children with chronic arthritis. Clin Rheumatol 1998; 17:359.

101. van Rossum MA, Fiselier TJ, Franssen MJ, et al: Sulfasalazine in the treatment of juvenile chronic arthritis: A randomized, double-blind, placebo-controlled, multicenter study. Arthritis Rheum 1998; 41:808.

102. Huang JL, Hung IJ, Hsieh KH: Sulphasalazine therapy in chronic uveitis of children with chronic arthritis. Asian Pac J Allerg Immunol 1997; 15:71.

103. Furst DE: Toxicity of antirheumatic medications in children with juvenile arthritis. J Rheumatol 1992; 19(suppl 33):11.

104. Huang JL, Hung IJ, Chen LC, et al: Successfully treated sulphasalazine induced fulminant hepatic failure, thrombocytopenia and erythroid hypoplasia with intravenous gammaglobulin. Clin Rheumatol 1998; 17:349.

105. Laaksonen A, Koskiahde V, Juka K: Dosage of antimalarial drugs for children with juvenile rheumatoid arthritis and systemic lupus erythematosus: A clinical study with determination of serum concentration of chloroquine and hydroxychloroquine. Scand J Rheumatol 1974; 3:103.

106. Stillman S: Antimalarials. In: Moore TD, ed. Arthritis in Childhood: Report of the 80th Ross Conference on Pediatric Research. Columbus, Ohio: Ross Laboratories, 1981:125.

107. Kvien TK, Hoyeraal HM, Sandstad B: Slow acting antirheumatic drugs in patients with juvenile rheumatoid arthritis— Evaluated in a randomized, parallel 50-week clinical trial. J Rheumatol 1985; 12:533.

108. Brewer EJ, Giannini EH, Kuzmina N, et al: Penicillamine and hydroxychloroquine in the treatment of severe juvenile rheumatoid arthritis. N Engl J Med 1986; 314:1269.

109. van Kerckhove C, Giannini EH, Lovell DJ: Temporal patterns of response to D-penicillamine, hydroxychloroquine and placebo in juvenile rheumatoid arthritis. Arthritis Rheum 1988; 31:1252.

110. Deschenes G, Prieur AM, Hayem F, et al: Renal amyloidosis in juvenile chronic arthritis: Evolution after chlorambucil treatment. Pediatr Nephrol 1990; 4:463.

111. Savolainen HA: Chlorambucil in severe juvenile chronic arthritis: Longterm followup with special reference to amyloidosis. J Rheumatol 1999; 26:898.

112. Arnold M, Schrieber L, Brooks PM: Immunosuppressive drugs and corticosteroids in the treatment or rheumatoid arthritis. Drugs 1988; 36:340.

113. Kvien TK, Hoyeraal HM, Standstad B: Azathioprine versus placebo in patients with juvenile rheumatoid arthritis. J Rheumatol 1986; 13:118.

114. Savolainen HA, Kautiainen H, Isomaki H, et al: Azathioprine in patients with juvenile chronic arthritis: A longterm followup study. J Rheumatol 1997; 24:2444.

115. Shaikov AV, Maximov AA, Speransky AI, et al: Repetitive use of pulse therapy with methylprednisolone and cyclophosphamide in addition to oral methotrexate in children with systemic juvenile rheumatoid arthritis: Preliminary results of a longterm study. J Rheumatol 1992; 19:612.

116. Wallace CA, Sherry DD: Trial of intravenous pulse cyclophosphamide and methylprednisolone in the treatment of severe systemic-onset juvenile rheumatoid arthritis. Arthritis Rheum 1997; 40:1852.

117. Kahan BD: Cyclosporin. N Engl J Med 1989; 321:1725.

118. Ostensen M, Hoyeraal HM, Kass E: Tolerance of cyclosporin A in children with refractory juvenile rheumatoid arthritis. J Rheumatol 1988; 15:1536.

119. Reiff A, Rawlings DJ, Shaham B, et al: Preliminary evidence for cyclosporin A as an alternative in the treatment of recalcitrant juvenile rheumatoid arthritis and juvenile dermatomyositis. J Rheumatol 1997; 24:2436.

120. Mouy R, Stephan JL, Pillet P, et al: Efficacy of cyclosporine A in the treatment of macrophage activation syndrome in juvenile arthritis: Report of five cases. J Pediatr 1996; 129:750.

121. Uziel Y, Laxer RM, Schneider R, et al: Intravenous immunoglobulin therapy in systemic onset juvenile rheumatoid arthritis: A followup study. J Rheumatol 1996; 23:910.

122. Giannini EH, Lovell DJ, Silverman ED, et al: Intravenous immunoglobulin in the treatment of polyarticular juvenile rheumatoid arthritis: A phase I/II study. Pediatric Collaborative Study Group. J Rheumatol 1996; 23:919.

123. Wulffraat N, van Royen A Bierings M, et al: Autologous haemopoietic stem-cell transplantation in four patients with refractory juvenile chronic arthritis. Lancet 1999; 353:550.

124. Quartier P, Prieur AM, Fischer A: Haemopoietic stem-cell transplantation for juvenile chronic arthritis. Lancet 1999; 353:1885.

125. Hopp RJ, Degan J, Corley K, et al: Evaluation of growth hormone secretion in children with juvenile rheumatoid arthritis and short stature. Nebr Med J 1995; 80:52.

126. Allen RC, Jimenez M, Cowell CT: Insulin-like growth factor and growth hormone secretion in juvenile chronic arthritis. Ann Rheum Dis 1991; 50:602.

127. Davies UM, Rooney M, Preece MA, et al: Treatment of growth retardation in juvenile chronic arthritis with recombinant human growth hormone. J Rheumatol 1994; 21:153.

128. Simon D, Touati G, Prieur AM, et al: Growth hormone treatment of short stature and metabolic dysfunction in juvenile chronic arthritis. Acta Pediatr 1999(suppl); 88:100.

129. Lovell DJ, Giannini EH, Whitmore JB, et al: Safety and efficacy of tumor necrosis factor receptor P75 fusion protein (TNF:FC; Enbrel™) in polyarticular course juvenile rheumatoid arthritis. Arthritis Rheum 1998; 41(suppl):S130.

130. Kotaniemi A, Savolainen A, Kroger H, et al: Weight bearing physical activity, calcium intake, systemic glucocorticoids, chronic inflammation, and body constitution as determinants of lumbar and femoral bone mineral in juvenile chronic arthritis. Scand J Rheumatol 1999; 28:19.

131. Klepper SE, Darbee J, Effgen SK, et al: Physical fitness levels in children with polyarticular juvenile rheumatoid arthritis. Arthritis Care Res 1992; 5:93.

132. Singsen BH: Physical fitness in children with juvenile rheumatoid arthritis and other chronic pediatric illnesses. Pediatr Clin North Am 1995; 42:1035.

133. Jay S, Litt IF, Durant RH: Compliance with therapeutic regimens. J Adolesc Health Care 1984; 5:124.

134. Litt IR, Cuskey WR, Rosenberg BA: Role of self-esteem and autonomy in determining medication compliance among adolescents with juvenile rheumatoid arthritis. Pediatrics 1982; 69:15.

135. Rapoff MA: Compliance with treatment regimens for pediatric rheumatic diseases. Arthritis Care Res 1989; 2:S40.

# 34 | The Rheumatic Diseases of Childhood

*Bracha Shaham and Bram H. Bernstein*

Rheumatic diseases in childhood pose special challenges to the treating physician: in addition to control of active symptoms, prevention of irreversible damage, and surveillance and early detection of disease flares, improved outcomes require that normal physical and emotional development be fostered in the face of serious and long-term illness. In addition to the pediatric rheumatologist, a team including nurse, social worker, physical therapist, and occupational therapist is essential to provide support to the child and family. With the prime goal of achieving normal function and growth while increasing survival, a long-term focus is necessary.

Treatment of both inflammatory and noninflammatory rheumatic diseases of childhood is discussed. The inflammatory diseases include systemic lupus erythematosus (SLE), neonatal lupus (NLE), juvenile dermatomyositis (JDMS), Henoch-Schönlein purpura (HSP), Kawasaki syndrome (KS), polyarteritis nodosa (PAN), Wegener's granulomatosis (WG), and limited scleroderma. Noninflammatory conditions include reflex neurovascular dystrophy (RND) and fibromyalgia syndrome (FMS).

## SYSTEMIC LUPUS ERYTHEMATOSUS

SLE is an autoimmune, multisystem disease characterized by inflammation of blood vessels and connective tissue with variable clinical manifestations and unpredictable course. Rare in childhood, the disease incidence is estimated at 0.4 per 100,000 population.[1] Although childhood lupus can start at any age up to 16 years, most children are 10 years or older at presentation, and onset under 4 years of age is very rare. As is the case in adults, childhood SLE is predominantly a female disease. However, more males are affected in childhood than in adult onset because of the increased incidence in prepubertal children (3:1 female-to-male ratio, in comparison with 7:1 in postpubertal onset and 8:1 in adults).[2] The disease is more prevalent and more severe in blacks, Hispanics, and Asians.[1] Multiple etiologic factors involved are immunologic, environmental, hormonal, ethnic, and genetic. Cutting-edge research into the genetic factors involved in disease expression is paramount to the development of innovative therapies for SLE. Studies currently in progress in adults and in murine models confirm the importance of gene polymorphism at several loci, including the major histocompatibility complex (MHC), complement proteins, immunoglobulin receptors, cytokines, and yet unidentified sites.[3] Similar studies to define the genetics of the disease in childhood are ongoing.

Clinical manifestations of SLE in children are similar to those in adults, and the same guidelines are used for diagnosis. However, very few children have mild disease manifesting primarily in the skin, whereas renal involvement occurs in two thirds and neuropsychiatric disease in 20% to 40%.[4, 5] If unresponsive to treatment or untreated, the disease can be fulminant, resulting in death within months from infection or organ failure. Poor survival is associated with male sex, nephritis, seizures, and thrombocytopenia.[6] Advances in supportive therapies, such as antibiotics and antihypertensive drugs, critical care and dialysis, and better means of identifying children at high risk of organ involvement or life-threatening complications, have improved the prognosis. Current survival rates of children with lupus are 93% at 5 years, 85% at 10 years, and 79% at 15 years[4]; therefore, the course of the disease and its ultimate prognosis may no longer be worse in children than in adults.[7] However, the prognosis for children with end-stage renal disease who are receiving dialysis has been shown to be worse.[8, 9] Similarly, the experience in some pediatric rheumatology centers, including ours, is that children have more severe organ system involvement than do adults,[4, 5] and few children with SLE achieve adequate disease control without the use of steroids. The episodic nature of the disease, with spontaneous exacerbations not always predictable before organ damage, and the effects of chronic illness and potentially toxic medications on emotional as well as physical growth and development make the treatment of lupus particularly challenging in children.

The goals of treatment are to control active inflammation, to prevent or resolve organ damage, to protect normal growth, and to improve quality of life and survival. Milder symptoms may be treated with nonsteroidal anti-inflammatory drugs (NSAIDs) and antimalarials. When disease manifestations are potentially damaging to organs, disabling, or life-threatening, corticosteroid and immunosuppressive therapies are used. Specialized therapies, such as anticoagulation, intravenous immune globulin (IVIG), or psychotropic drugs, may be required to treat such features as thromboses, uncontrolled thrombocytopenia, and psychosis.

It is essential to help the child and the family establish support systems and effective coping mechanisms. A team approach, in which a designated physician (pediatric rheumatologist) and specialized allied health personnel monitor the child and family, is important in enhancing trust and communication. In our unit, patients and families are encouraged to participate in a support group. The team nurse or social worker provides school liaison. Education about the disease process and its therapy is begun at the first visit and continues throughout follow-up.

## General Therapeutic Measures

Supportive measures include management of nutritional status, blood pressure, fluid and electrolyte balance, and superimposed infections. Easy fatigability, a common feature of active disease, may require adjustment of the child's schedule to provide rest periods and adequate sleep at night. Although the school schedule and physical education program may need to be altered initially, return to normal school activities as soon as possible is encouraged. Practice of sun protection techniques is emphasized. Children are taught to use sunscreen and to avoid direct sun exposure. Daily application of sunscreen with a sun protection factor (SPF) of 15 or higher is recommended. Waterproof preparations are preferred for younger children. Local reactions such as erythema or stinging can occur, so patients must establish a personal choice of product by trial and error. Sun-protective clothing items are also available. For adolescents, makeup can be applied over sunscreen or makeup that contains a sunblock may be used.

Lupus dermatitis, which occurs in more than two thirds of children at presentation, responds well to hydroxychloroquine (Plaquenil) or systemic steroids, which may be indicated for other disease manifestations. Topical steroids for treatment of persistent rashes should be used cautiously, because prolonged use, particularly of the high-potency fluorinated products, can cause local skin atrophy or depigmentation. For facial lesions, we start with 1% hydrocortisone cream, increasing the strength to 2.5% or changing to 0.1% betamethasone (Valisone) as necessary. Nonfacial lesions may be treated with high-potency preparations such as 0.05% betamethasone dipropionate (Diprolene) or 0.05% fluocinonide (Lidex). Mucosal ulcers are common with active disease. If they are symptomatic, sucralfate suspension applied topically or local application of 0.1% triamcinolone acetonide (Kenalog in Orabase) every 2 to 3 hours may be helpful. Severe mucositis is treated with systemic steroids.[10]

## Salicylates and Nonsteroidal Anti-inflammatory Drugs

### Indications

Indications for the use of salicylates and NSAIDs include arthralgia, myalgia, and mild arthritis. When disease symptoms are mild, children can be treated with NSAIDs, often in combination with an antimalarial agent (see later discussion). Because the use of aspirin (ASA) in children is associated with increased risk of liver toxicity[11] as well as other adverse effects, we favor use of NSAIDs over salicylates. When NSAID therapy is indicated, our preference is to use ibuprofen (40 to 45 mg/kg/day divided into three doses), or naproxen (Naprosyn; 15 to 20 mg/kg/day divided into two doses). NSAIDs inhibit the enzyme cyclooxygenase (COX), of which two distinct forms have been described: COX-1, which functions as a housekeeping enzyme in multiple tissues including gastric mucosa, kidney, and brain, and COX-2, which is active at sites of inflammation. The anti-inflammatory action of NSAIDs is attributed to inhibition of COX-2; however, all NSAIDs inhibit COX-1 as well, thereby creating the potential for toxic effects. By their inhibitory effect on both enzymes, NSAIDs may cause multiple adverse effects. For similar reasons, COX-2 inhibitors may not provide protection from renal or other NSAID-associated side effects in pediatric SLE.[12, 13] COX-2 inhibitors have not yet been approved for pediatric use.

### Side Effects

GASTRITIS, PEPTIC ULCER, GASTROINTESTINAL BLEEDING. Concomitant use of steroids increases this risk. Barrier agents such as sucralfate, antacids or histamine$_2$ (H$_2$)–blockers may be used.[14]

HEPATIC. Mild elevation of transaminases is usually transient and may resolve with dosage adjustment or withdrawal of medication. NSAIDs are highly protein bound; low levels of serum albumin (a common feature in lupus) may expose patients to high levels of potentially toxic unbound drug.

RENAL. Decreased renal blood flow and decreased glomerular filtration rate (GFR) are of concern especially in the presence of glomerulonephritis, congestive heart failure, or ascites. Idiosyncratic interstitial nephritis, manifested by proteinuria without cellular casts, can complicate the clinical picture, because differentiation from active lupus nephritis is necessary.[15]

CENTRAL NERVOUS SYSTEM. Episodes of aseptic meningitis and nonspecific febrile reactions have been described with many NSAIDs, particularly ibuprofen, tolmetin, and sulindac.[16, 17]

OTHER. Reversible skin rashes and ocular dryness may confuse the clinical picture. Pseudoporphyria can occur in children receiving naproxen.[18] Cytopenia may be aggravated by drug effect on the bone marrow. NSAIDs potentiate the anticoagulation effect of coumarin and should not be used concomitantly.

# Antimalarial Drugs

## Indications

Indications for the use of antimalarial drugs include cutaneous manifestations, arthritis, and steroid-sparing effect. Antimalarials have been used in the treatment of SLE for the past 100 years, and studies continue to demonstrate their effectiveness.[19] Current research into their mechanism of action demonstrates that both hydroxychloroquine (Plaquenil) and chloroquine (Atabrine) inhibit production of tumor necrosis factor-$\alpha$ (TNF-$\alpha$), interferon-$\gamma$, and interleukin-6 (IL-6) by peripheral blood mononuclear cells and induce apoptosis in T lymphocytes.[20, 21]

Hydroxychloroquine is the most commonly used antimalarial for childhood lupus. Major indications are to treat skin involvement and to provide a steroid-sparing effect. Studies have shown additional benefits in prevention of disease and of treatment-induced complications, including hyperlipidemia, hyperglycemia, liver enzyme elevation, and thrombosis.[22] Hydrochloroquine (5 to 6.5 mg/kg/day) has a slow onset of action (2 to 4 months) with peak effect at 6 to 12 months.[10]

Chloroquine is rarely used in children because of its potential toxicity (see later discussion). However, it can be more effective than hydroxychloroquine.[19] Onset of action is shorter (3 to 4 weeks), and maximal beneficial effect is usually evident by 6 to 8 weeks. There is no retinal toxicity, and it has a stronger effect in alleviating fatigue.[10] Chloroquine is indicated in selected cases of severe cutaneous manifestations, especially in children with subacute cutaneous lupus who are not responsive to combined therapy with hydroxychloroquine and low- to moderate-dose steroids. The dosage is 1 to 2 mg/kg/day, to a maximum of 100 mg/day.

## Hydroxychloroquine Side Effects

RETINAL TOXICITY. Possible visual impairment resulting from hydroxychloroquine has been studied extensively. Review of those studies suggests that the incidence of sight-threatening retinopathy is minimal at dosages less than 6.5 mg/kg/day and a cumulative dose of less than 200 g.[23–25] Retinopathy is usually but not always reversible. There is no agreement as to the best method or ideal interval for ophthalmology screening.[25] We recommend that pediatric patients have a baseline ophthalmologic evaluation within 1 month after starting hydroxychloroquine therapy and then at 6-month intervals, depending on dosage and length of therapy.

GASTROINTESTINAL. Nausea, abdominal bloating, cramps, and diarrhea occur infrequently.

CUTANEOUS. A variety of reversible rashes, including urticaria, may occur.

CENTRAL NERVOUS SYSTEM. A stimulatory effect, which may be beneficial, can rarely produce nervousness, insomnia, confusion, migraine headaches, tinnitus, nerve deafness, and vestibular dysfunction.[10]

## Chloroquine Side Effects

The side effects of chloroquine include the following.[10]

CUTANEOUS. Chloroquine binds to melanin, causing yellowish skin discoloration in one third of patients. Dark pigmentation of nails and pretibial skin, resembling ecchymoses, is also reported.

HEMATOLOGIC. Bone marrow suppression with leukopenia or agranulocytosis is a major concern. A lichenoid skin rash is noted in most cases before the development of cytopenia; therefore, the drug must be discontinued immediately if a rash occurs. A complete blood count (CBC) should be obtained at least every 6 weeks.

## Other Considerations

Although bone marrow suppression can occur with either antimalarial, it is far more common with chloroquine. In addition, because antimalarials have oxidant properties, they are contraindicated in patients who are deficient in glucose-6-phosphate dehydrogenase.

In the absence of side effects, tapering of either antimalarial should be gradual and slow, because disease flare has been associated with discontinuation.[26]

# Steroids

## Indications

Indications for the use of steroids include significant constitutional symptoms, progressive rash or mucositis, major organ involvement, life-threatening crises, anemia and cytopenia, and serologic evidence of increasing disease activity. When corticosteroids are necessary, the lowest possible dosages or appropriate steroid-sparing measures should be used, so as to minimize side effects and protect normal growth. Severe changes in appearance from steroids are a major concern and can lead to serious depressive reactions. Noncompliance is a major issue in the teenagers, and sudden withdrawal has resulted in death from the disease in some cases.[27, 28]

The mechanisms of action of glucocorticoids are currently being investigated, including selective inhibition of proinflammatory responses and immunomodulatory effects.[29] Short-acting preparations such as prednisone, prednisolone, and methylprednisolone are most frequently used. Because steroids are metabolic, deactivated mainly in the liver, concurrent use of other drugs such as phenobarbital or the presence of associated conditions (e.g., hyperthyroidism) that stimulate hepatic microsomal enzyme activity may hasten steroid deactivation.[16]

## Low-Dose, High-Dose, and Intravenous Pulse Steroid Therapy

Even with relatively mild symptoms and without major organ involvement, many children do not respond adequately to NSAIDs and antimalarials alone but do improve when given low-dose prednisone. Such a regimen may also be used in selected patients in whom a drop in the levels of complement C3 and C4 and a rise in anti–double-stranded DNA antibodies signify possible disease exacerbation.[30] A dosage of 0.25 to 0.5 mg/kg/day, divided into two to four daily doses to increase the therapeutic effect, is prescribed. With good clinical and laboratory response, the drug is gradually consolidated to a single daily dose and then tapered off completely, or to the minimum effective dose. Another option, when the disease is well controlled with a single daily dose, is to switch to alternate-day therapy with slightly more than twice the previous daily dose. Alternatively, the amount taken every other day may be slowly reduced until alternate-day dosing is reached. The exact extent and rate of steroid reduction are individualized as determined by the patient's condition, the quality of clinical and serologic response, and the severity of side effects. In lupus the general rule is to *taper slowly!*

Steroid therapy for renal disease varies according to the particular histology of the renal lesion. An unusual lesion in children is pure membranous glomerulonephritis without a proliferative component. This lesion may not show much response to steroids or cytotoxic drugs.[31] However, progression to chronic renal failure is uncommon. Treatment is with intermediate dosages of steroids: 1 mg/kg/day for 6 to 12 weeks, followed by gradual tapering.

With more serious renal or other internal organ disease, or when anemia, thrombocytopenia, or pancytopenia is significant, oral prednisone or intravenous methylprednisolone is administered (1 to 2 mg/kg/day in divided doses). Initial intravenous treatment for 3 to 5 days or longer may be needed for the acutely ill child. With improvement, parenteral therapy can be converted to oral therapy.

Pulse intravenous methylprednisolone therapy has been used in patients with severe progressive or life-threatening manifestations.[32, 33] This strategy can be particularly useful for lupus cerebritis.[34] Although there are reports of beneficial results from this treatment in patients with acute lupus nephritis,[35] experience in our center with several patients who developed worsening renal failure and anasarca after pulse methylprednisolone suggests that caution should be exercised in this situation. A dosage of 30 mg/kg/day, up to 1 g per dose, is infused over 1 to 2 hours on 3 consecutive days and may be repeated at 3- to 4-week intervals. After pulse treatment, daily administration of steroids at a dosage determined by the patient's condition (0.5 to 2 mg/kg/day) is usually continued. When marked response to the pulse and stability of the patient's condition are observed, pulses may be repeated every 3 to 4 weeks without interim steroid therapy. Pulse methylprednisolone has been associated with potentially serious side effects, such as arrhythmia, sudden death, seizures, and anaphylaxis[36]; therefore, the patient's vital signs and general condition must be closely monitored. Opportunistic infections, avascular necrosis of bone, and glucose intolerance are also potential risks.[37] Children who respond

well benefit by avoiding the side effects of prolonged daily use of steroids.

## Side Effects

Major concerns *in children* are as follows.

STUNTED LINEAR GROWTH. Most children with SLE have not reached normal adult height at onset. If the child reaches puberty before steroid dosages are lowered enough to allow "catch-up" growth, growth retardation becomes permanent, sometimes leading to serious difficulty with social and psychological development and adjustment.[38] In general, linear growth is delayed with prednisone dosages of more than 5 mg/day. Strategies to reduce steroid dosages include using the use of antimalarial or cytotoxic drugs.

CHANGES IN APPEARANCE. Steroid side effects include cushingoid features, obesity, hirsutism, striae, acne, bruising, and thin fragile skin. Body image and appearance are of extreme importance to adolescents, and alteration in these traits can lead to noncompliance, depression, and even suicide.[39] Dietary education and support by the treatment team are essential to limit weight gain and to help the teenager cope with unavoidable changes. Hirsutism can be treated cosmetically, and acne may respond to topical therapy.

OSTEOPOROSIS, AVASCULAR NECROSIS, AND PATHOLOGIC FRACTURES. These side effects are also of concern.[40, 41] Minimizing steroid dosage, ensuring adequate intake of calcium and vitamin D, and encouraging load-bearing activities serve to reduce osteoporosis.[42] Severe avascular necrosis may eventually necessitate joint replacement.

EMOTIONAL LABILITY. Psychological turmoil associated with diagnosis or flare-up can be further aggravated by steroid-induced mood changes. Reduction in steroid dosage, together with providing emotional support to the child and family, is the main strategy used to minimize this effect.

HYPERTENSION. Antihypertensive therapy may be necessary, especially in children with renal disease.

GASTROINTESTINAL. Peptic ulcer disease and pancreatitis caused by steroid therapy can confuse the clinical picture.[2] The incidence of gastritis increases with concomitant use of steroids and NSAIDs. Barrier agents such as sucralfate, $H_2$-blockers, or antacids can be given. Monitoring of abnormal abdominal symptoms, unexplained drop in hemoglobin, and presence of blood in the stool is essential to early detection and intervention.

## Cytotoxic Drugs

Cytotoxic agents are indicated for severe organ involvement or life-threatening disease, for steroid-resistant disease, and for steroid sparing when unacceptable side effects occur. Cyclophosphamide (Cytoxan) and azathioprine (AZA, Imuran) are most commonly used. Methotrexate (MTX) has limited use in selected cases. Nitrogen mustard therapy is reserved for exceptional life-threatening circumstances. New investigative therapies include mycophenolate mofetil

(MMF, CellCept)[43] and immunoablation with high-dose chemotherapy followed by stem-cell transplantation (HDC/SCT)[44] for progressive, severe disease.

## Cyclophosphamide

Cyclophosphamide is indicated for control of progressive or life-threatening disease, including proliferative nephritis, uncontrolled vasculitis, neuropsychiatric or pulmonary involvement, uncontrolled thrombocytopenia, pancytopenia, and hemolytic anemia.[45–48]

Cyclophosphamide is an alkylating agent that acts throughout the cell cycle and inhibits DNA replication. It is toxic to rapidly proliferating lymphoid tissues, causing a prolonged decrease in T cells and a transient decrease in B cells. T-cell function and antibody production are inhibited, and immunologic tolerance is induced. The drug has a short serum half-life (2 to 10 hours). It is mainly metabolized in the liver into compounds that are themselves alkylating agents.[49]

CYCLOPHOSPHAMIDE THERAPY IN LUPUS NEPHRITIS. Two thirds of children with SLE eventually have renal involvement, usually diffuse proliferative glomerulonephritis (DPGN), which, without aggressive treatment, leads to end-stage renal disease and renal dialysis. Especially in children, end-stage renal disease and dialysis are associated with poor quality of life and reduced survival.[8, 50] For this reason, aggressive treatment is indicated to prevent or delay progression of lupus nephritis.

Controlled studies from the National Institutes of Health (NIH) concluded that parenteral cyclophosphamide was superior to steroids alone and to AZA in preventing irreversible renal damage and end-stage renal disease in adults.[48] Therefore, protocols for its use in childhood lupus nephritis have been adapted by pediatric rheumatology centers. Although questions remain as to the lowest possible effective dosage[51] and controversial opinions have been expressed regarding the possible use of AZA as first-line agent in pediatric lupus DPGN,[52] cumulative experience strongly supports cyclophosphamide as the gold standard therapy for childhood lupus nephritis.[53]

In our center, renal biopsy is not always obtained before the initiation of cyclophosphamide therapy for pediatric lupus nephritis. Because in the majority of affected children the kidney histopathology is that of DPGN, treatment of children with typical presentation is initiated as soon as possible. In these patients, biopsy is obtained if poor response is observed after the first three to six monthly cyclophosphamide treatments. When the diagnosis is in question or the presentation of renal disease is atypical, renal biopsy is recommended before initiation of treatment.

Patients receiving intravenous pulse cyclophosphamide therapy (IVCY) are evaluated before each treatment, by physical examination and laboratory studies, to assess for potential side effects and contraindications to treatment (e.g., neutropenia, acute infection) and to evaluate disease activity and response. To provide adequate monitoring, hydration, and control of nausea, patients are hospitalized overnight for the first three to four treatments, until dosage stability is achieved and good tolerance of treatment is established. From then on, treatments may be administered at a daytime infusion clinic with a slightly shorter intravenous hydration period, compensated by increased oral fluid intake for 24 hours.

IVCY treatments are begun with a dosage of 500 mg/m², increased to 750 mg/m² the following month and to a maintenance dosage of 1000 mg/m² by the third month, leukocyte count permitting. If the leukocyte count is less than 3000 cells/mm³ at the nadir or less than 4000 cells/mm³ at month's end, the dosage is adjusted downward. Treatment is continued at monthly intervals for the first 6 months after the initial dose. With satisfactory response to seven monthly infusions, cyclophosphamide is continued at 3-month intervals for an additional 2 years. At the completion of this regimen, many patients show no evidence of active renal disease and the drug can be discontinued.

Improvement with cyclophosphamide is usually apparent within 3 to 6 months after treatment initiation. If there has been no improvement by 6 months, reevaluation of renal disease by kidney biopsy is strongly suggested. Biopsy evidence of severe scarring and high chronicity at this point would suggest that no further cytotoxic treatment be given,[54] whereas evidence of uncontrolled active disease would lead to other therapy options, such as oral cyclophosphamide, MMF, AZA, or cyclosporine.

Children who show an initial response but suffer relapse while receiving cyclophosphamide at 3-month intervals may benefit from monthly cyclophosphamide for three doses followed by a gradual increase of the interval between treatments. A few patients experience relapse after completion of the full treatment course[55] and should be considered for resumption of therapy. Children who respond well to monthly cyclophosphamide but experience relapse whenever the interval increases pose a difficult management problem. Currently, most continue treatment at intervals of 1 to 2 months as tolerated, and these patients may be considered for MMF or oral cyclophosphamide therapy.

Selected children with rapidly progressive lupus nephrotic syndrome have responded well to one or more injections of nitrogen mustard during the course of cyclophosphamide therapy (unpublished observations). In this case, resumption of cyclophosphamide administration is postponed so as to avoid additive bone marrow depression.

CYCLOPHOSPHAMIDE THERAPY IN OTHER DISEASE MANIFESTATIONS. Cyclophosphamide therapy is indicated in generalized vasculitis, central nervous system (CNS) lupus, transverse myelitis, peripheral neuritis, pneumonitis or pulmonary hemorrhage, uncontrolled hemolytic anemia, and leukopenia or thrombocytopenia.

INTRAVENOUS THERAPY. In our experience, intravenous cyclophosphamide at 10 mg/kg every 2 weeks has been life-saving in some children in whom high-dose steroid therapy alone had failed. Precautions and monitoring are similar to those of the renal protocol, and response may be apparent within 2 weeks. Length of treatment is determined by individual response.

After control of acute disease has been achieved, the cyclophosphamide dosage may be reduced or the treatment interval prolonged.

ORAL THERAPY. Daily oral cyclophosphamide carries a higher risk of hemorrhagic cystitis, other adverse effects and, possibly, eventual malignant disease.[56, 57] Nevertheless, some children whose response to IVCY has been inadequate benefit from daily oral therapy (1 to 2 mg/kg/day). It can also be considered for children whose quality of life with IVCY is poor because of frequent hospitalizations or side effects. With good response, conversion to intermittent treatment (3 to 5 days per week) may be acceptable as a means of reducing toxicity. Patients are instructed to take cyclophosphamide in the morning, to increase fluid intake and urinate frequently, and to report promptly any sign of infection. CBC, urinalysis, and clinical assessment are performed at 2- to 4-week intervals.

SIDE EFFECTS. The side effects of cyclophosphamide therapy include the following.[58, 59]

NAUSEA AND VOMITING. These may occur within a few hours after treatment and are dosage related. Patients are premedicated intravenously with ondansetron hydrochloride (Zofran),[60] 0.15 mg/kg (maximum, 12 mg), 30 minutes before cyclophosphamide administration and at 4 and 8 hours after infusion. Oral ondansetron at similar dosage and interval is used for delayed nausea. Nausea and vomiting refractory to ondansetron are effectively treated with granisetron (Kytril),[61] 10 to 20 μg/kg. It is usually sufficient to administer granisetron intravenously or orally once, just before cyclophosphamide therapy; however, the dose may be repeated at 12 hours (maximum, 40 μg/kg/day divided every 12 hours).

HAIR LOSS. Significant alopecia may occur during treatment, but hair growth usually recovers when cyclophosphamide frequency is reduced. Although benefit has not been proved, the use of an ice cap during treatment may be considered. The team provides support to the child and the family. Wigs and head coverings are used creatively.

BONE MARROW SUPPRESSION. This effect is usually transient, because stem cells are spared. Maximal leukopenia is expected 7 to 14 days after cyclophosphamide administration (nadir point) and resolves by 21 to 25 days. Anemia can accompany the leukopenia, but severe thrombocytopenia is rare. A CBC should be obtained before cyclophosphamide administration and 7 to 14 days after each treatment. In the event that leukocyte, hemoglobin, or thrombocyte levels drop significantly, the next cyclophosphamide dose should be adjusted down accordingly.

HEMORRHAGIC CYSTITIS. The metabolite acrolein is toxic to bladder transitional cell epithelium and may cause severe hemorrhagic cystitis that is not completely preventable with vigorous hydration.[56] Mesna (sodium 2-mercaptoethane sulfonate), a chelating agent, binds acrolein to form a nontoxic compound without interfering with the desired cyclophosphamide effect.[62] Our practice is to administer mesna to all patients receiving IVCY. Mesna at 20% of the cyclophosphamide dosage is infused over 15 to 30 minutes just before cyclophosphamide administration; this dose is repeated twice at 6- to 8-hour intervals.

INFECTION. Immunosuppression may lead to opportunistic bacterial or fungal infections. These are difficult to differentiate from active lupus and can be life-threatening. Maintaining the absolute neutrophil count higher than 2000 cells/mm[3] minimizes this risk. Immunoglobulin levels should be monitored, and prophylactic immune globulin should be considered if hypogammaglobulinemia develops.[63] Patients are taught to promptly report symptoms of infections or exposure to varicella. Children exposed to varicella who do not have prior immunity receive varicella-zoster immunoglobulin within 96 hours. Children with lupus benefit from pneumococcal as well as meningococcal vaccines. Live attenuated vaccines, such as the measles, mumps, and rubella (MMR) or the oral polio vaccine, are contraindicated in pediatric patients receiving immunosuppressive therapy.[48]

STERILITY. Ovarian failure has been reported in female adults with SLE treated with cyclophosphamide. Risk of sterility increases with age at onset of cyclophosphamide therapy (less than 30 years, 14%; more than 40 years, 50%) and with cumulative dose (less than 10 g, 4%; more than 30 g, 70%).[57] Studies to determine risk of gonadal failure are not available in the pediatric lupus population; however, significant risk probably exists, especially for postpubertal patients. Because the cumulative dose is usually higher with oral therapy, we consider those patients to be at higher risk as well. For older boys, consideration should be given to sperm banking before cyclophosphamide therapy is initiated.

TERATOGENICITY. A teratogenic effect may occur during the first trimester of pregnancy.[64] Although pregnancy outcome in patients with SLE who received cytotoxic treatment during pregnancy was found to be similar to that in patients not treated with such drugs,[65] counseling to avoid pregnancy during cyclophosphamide treatment should be provided. Sexually active girls should have a negative pregnancy test result before treatment is given.

LATE MALIGNANT DISEASE. This has been reported in adults treated with cyclophosphamide.[66] Although not reported in children, this complication remains a concern.

SUMMARY. Patients undergoing cyclophosphamide treatment require careful clinical and laboratory monitoring. Vigorous hydration and intravenous Mesna are used to prevent hemorrhagic cystitis. The new antiemetics, ondansetron and granisetron control nausea and vomiting in most patients. Blood counts at the nadir point and at frequent intervals are used to assess treatment effect and marrow suppression. The treatment team and the family maintain vigilance in monitoring for infection and other side effects. Although some controversy still exists regarding the use of this drug as first-line therapy in childhood lupus nephritis because of the possibility of long-term side effects, we believe its potential organ and lifesaving effects outweigh its risks in appropriate patients.

## Azathioprine

AZA is a purine analog of hypoxanthine that suppresses the antibody response and reduces B-cell numbers.[67] Indications include active generalized disease, steroid sparing,[68] significant cutaneous involvement,[69] and selected cases of nephritis requiring prolonged use of high-dose steroids.[52]

Side effects include leukopenia and possible bone marrow suppression, elevation of liver transaminases, nausea, diarrhea, headaches, mild hair loss, and possible abnormalities of menstrual cycle.[70] Development of malignancy (leukemia) was reported in adults as well as in young adults who received this drug for connective tissue disease, but not in children.[71] Increased incidence of infections, especially herpes zoster, is of concern.[72]

AZA is given in a dosage of 1.5 to 2.5 mg/kg/day, with benefit usually apparent by 6 to 8 weeks. If no effect has been observed after 12 weeks, the drug should be discontinued. When maximal beneficial effect has been achieved, the dosage may be gradually reduced to the lowest effective maintenance dosage.

Monitoring includes frequent clinical and laboratory evaluations. A CBC and liver panel are obtained at initiation of therapy, after 1 to 2 weeks, and then at monthly intervals.

## Methotrexate

MTX, administered as a low-dose weekly therapy, is used successfully in childhood arthritis and other rheumatic conditions as a potent anti-inflammatory drug. The anti-inflammatory and immune-modulating effects of MTX are not mediated by inhibition of cellular proliferation but via promotion of adenosine release and subsequent increase in extracellular adenosine levels.[73] Studies show benefit of MTX in carefully selected patients with lupus arthritis or other nonvisceral involvement who do not have renal disease.[74] A steroid-sparing effect has not been consistently demonstrated.[75–77]

MTX is administered orally once a week on an empty stomach, at a dosage of 0.3 to 0.5 mg/kg. Folinic acid (leucovorin) was shown to lower the risk of adverse effects; it is given as a weekly oral dose of 5 to 10 mg, 12 to 24 hours after MTX.[78]

Side effects include nausea, vomiting, abdominal discomfort, sun sensitivity, transient elevation of liver enzymes, increased susceptibility to infections, reversible leukopenia, and oral mucosal lesions. Severe bone marrow suppression is rare, as are severe stomatitis, confusion, seizures, and idiosyncratic pneumonitis.[79] Of concern is a case report of Hodgkin's lymphoma in a 6-year-old child after low-dose MTX therapy for systemic juvenile rheumatoid arthritis.[80] Similarly, a small number of older patients developed lymphoma during MTX therapy for rheumatoid arthritis and dermatomyositis, in association with Epstein-Barr virus.[81]

Monitoring includes determination of CBC and transaminase concentrations at monthly intervals. Careful evaluation of renal status is essential, because MTX is primarily cleared by the kidney and a creatinine clearance of less than 60 mL/minute may be associated with increased risk of toxicity.

## Nitrogen Mustard

Nitrogen mustard is an alkylating agent that is toxic to rapidly proliferating cells. Clinical studies have documented its efficacy and a steroid-sparing effect in rapidly progressive nephrotic syndrome in adults with SLE.[82] In our center, the drug is used cautiously in selected children with life-threatening renal, pulmonary, or CNS disease that is unresponsive to steroids and cyclophosphamide. Although treatment can be repeated, our experience with acquired irreversible agammaglobulinemia in one patient has led us to exercise extreme caution in repetitive usage. A dose of 0.4 mg/kg is given in the hospital as a single infusion or split into two daily doses. Nitrogen mustard is a powerful vesicant and causes vein irritation or, with extravasation, local necrosis. Contact with skin or mucosal membranes must be avoided. Therefore, a secure intravenous line should be used. Methylprednisolone is flushed through that line at a concentration of 1 mg/mL during the nitrogen mustard infusion to prevent phlebitis. Because the drug is unstable in solution, its crystals should be dissolved immediately before administration and slowly infused as an intravenous "push" by a physician who wears protective gloves and mask.

Side effects of nitrogen mustard include the following:

- Local irritation or necrosis.
- Nausea and vomiting expected within 1 to 3 hours after the infusion and lasting up to 24 hours. Antiemetics are given as with cyclophosphamide.
- Predictable granulocytopenia (and occasional thrombocytopenia) within 6 to 8 days. It usually resolves in 10 to 21 days. It is uncommon for bone marrow depression to be prolonged; in rare cases, it progresses to aplasia.
- Infection related to granulocytopenia.
- Risk of infertility and of malignancy.

In summary, cytotoxic drugs offer the possibility of improved survival and quality of life for selected children with lupus who might otherwise die or have to endure dialysis or disabling steroid side effects. Careful monitoring of clinical and laboratory parameters is indispensable to their use.

## Investigational Treatments

MYCOPHENOLATE MOFETIL. This new immunosuppressive agent inhibits proliferation of B and T lymphocytes through noncompetitive, reversible inhibition of a key enzyme: inosine monophosphate dehydrogenase in the de novo synthetic pathway of guanine nucleotides.[83] MMF has been used effectively in the treatment of refractory organ transplant rejection in children and adults, in combination with steroids and with cyclosporine.[84, 85] Investigational studies and experience in adults show that MMF is also effective and safe in the treatment of refractory inflammatory glomerulonephritis, including lupus renal disease,[43] vasculitis,[86] rheumatoid arthritis, psoriasis, and hemolytic anemia.[87] In our center, selected children with refractory lupus nephritis are treated with MMF. Young children receive 600 mg/m² twice daily. For adolescent and older children, the starting dosage is 250 mg orally twice daily; pending good tolerance and efficacy, the dosage is gradually increased to a maximum of 1000 mg twice a day.

Adverse effects include abdominal cramping, diarrhea and nausea that improve over time in most patients, leukopenia, anemia and thrombocytopenia, and risk of infection, as well as a few case reports of lymphoproliferative disease in adult patients (not reported in children).[86] Absorption is decreased with aluminum and magnesium hydroxide antacids. MMF is diesterified in vivo into its active compound, mycophenolic acid, which is strongly albumin bound; therefore, high dosages of salicylates or furosemide that may displace it from albumin and increase toxicity are to be avoided. It has no adverse interactions with steroids or cyclosporine.[86] Patients are assessed frequently for infections as well as other adverse effects. A CBC is obtained within 1 week after onset of treatment and is repeated weekly until stable dosage is achieved. Thereafter, blood tests are done every 2 to 4 weeks.

PLASMAPHERESIS. Plasma is selectively removed and replaced with albumin, saline solution, or fresh-frozen plasma, whereas all other blood components are returned to the patient. Plasmapheresis removes circulating immune complexes, reduces serum immunoglobulin G (IgG) and autoantibody levels, and restores normal phagocytic activity of reticuloendothelial cells.[88] Repeated plasmapheresis followed by IVCY is used to prevent reactivation of B cells after IgG removal. However, in lupus nephritis no benefit over IVCY alone was found in two controlled trials.[89, 90] Case reports describe benefit in adult lupus patients with thrombotic thrombocytopenic purpura and in CNS disease.[91, 92] We use plasmapheresis in children with life-threatening fulminant vasculitis who have not responded to steroids and cyclophosphamide. This includes children with severe generalized disease, pulmonary hemorrhage, and CNS involvement. The frequency and duration of treatment are individualized. Treatment is administered daily for the first 5 days and changed to alternate-day therapy (three times weekly) as improvement is seen, with subsequent tapering as tolerated. The usual course of plasmapheresis lasts 1 to 3 months.

Plasmapheresis is an invasive procedure that usually requires surgical insertion of a venous catheter. Removal of some red blood cells, platelets, and leukocytes occurs, resulting in varying degrees of anemia, thrombocytopenia, and leukopenia, as well as hypogammaglobulinemia. Because of manipulation of the intravascular volume, hypotension and hemodynamic instability are possible. The procedure is performed in the dialysis or critical care unit. Patients are closely monitored for stability of vital signs, fluid balance, change in serum mineral and electrolyte levels, and any evidence of bleeding, cytopenia, anemia, or infection.

INTRAVENOUS IMMUNOGLOBULIN. Although IVIG is effective in the treatment of some inflammatory diseases, controlled studies showing efficacy in SLE are lacking, and its use in this disease remains controversial.[93] Case reports suggest benefit in neurologic manifestations as well as in thrombocytopenia, antiphospholipid syndrome, and refractory pneumonitis.[94] Multiple mechanisms of action in SLE are identified, with current research emphasizing anti-idiotype activity.[95] The IVIG dose for each treatment is 2 g/kg, which may be slowly infused over 10 to 12 hours or divided over 2 to 5 days; the rate of infusion is individualized according to tolerance, and therapy may be repeated at intervals of 3 to 4 weeks. Patients are premedicated with diphenhydramine (Benadryl) and acetaminophen (Tylenol).

Significant adverse effects include chills, fever, abdominal pain, nausea, vomiting, thromboembolic events, increased serum viscosity, headaches, aseptic meningitis, exacerbation of renal disease, and possible transfer of viral disease.[96, 97]

CYCLOSPORINE. Cyclosporine is an immune modulator that inhibits T-cell activation and expression of inflammatory cytokines, as well as release of TNF-$\alpha$ by macrophages.[98, 99] Prospective uncontrolled clinical trials and case reports suggest that low-dose oral cyclosporine can be moderately effective in patients with steroid- or cytotoxic-resistant SLE renal disease, as well as in thrombocytopenia, and can have a steroid-sparing effect.[100, 101] An open, randomized study of 40 children with lupus nephritis in whom steroid therapy had failed or had led to unacceptable side effects showed a significant decrease in proteinuria and a steroid-sparing effect with cyclosporine.[102] The dosage is 2 to 5 mg/kg/day, and it should be kept as low as possible because of the potential side effects. Those can be significant, especially increased serum creatinine and hypertension. The dosage is reduced by 0.5 mg/kg if the serum creatinine concentration rises more than 30% from baseline. A 1-year pilot study of cyclosporine in adult patients with renal lupus found no pathologic evidence of cyclosporine toxicity on renal biopsies.[103] Other side effects include gingival hyperplasia and hirsutism. Major concerns regarding the use of cyclosporine in lupus are its long-term safety in renal disease and possible disease reactivation after discontinuation of the drug.[104] We view this drug as a possible treatment in selected children with heavy and recalcitrant proteinuria or thrombocytopenia.

IMMUNOABLATION WITH HIGH-DOSE CHEMOTHERAPY AND AUTOLOGOUS OR ALLOGENEIC STEM CELL TRANSPLANTATION. Experiments in animal models of SLE and other autoimmune diseases showed improved survival after ablation of the bone marrow followed by transplantation of healthy marrow progenitors (CD34 cells) or stem cells.[105] Case reports of patients in whom HDC/SCT was indicated for malignancies or blood disorders who also had lupus or other autoimmune disease showed improvement of SLE and autoimmune conditions after this therapy.[44] This led to sporadic reports of use of HDC/SCT as specific therapy for severe and refractory SLE.[106] The rationale suggested by those reports is that the newly developing T cells might be tolerant to self-antigens.[107] Multicenter studies of HDC/SCT in adult and pediatric lupus to define possible indications for this intervention and effective and safe ablation protocols are currently in early organizational stages.

## Antiphospholipid Syndrome

Antiphospholipid syndrome (lupus anticoagulant syndrome) is defined by the presence of circulating antibodies to phospholipids (aPLs) in association with clinical hypercoagulability (venous or arterial thrombosis, stroke, fetal loss, myocardial infarction, atherosclerosis), cognitive function deficits or other CNS manifestations, thrombocytopenia, hemolytic anemia, and livedo reticularis.[108, 109] Although most patients with this phenomenon have SLE, some have no other manifestations of lupus and their condition is referred to as

"the antiphospholipid syndrome." The epidemiology, pathogenesis, and treatment of this disorder have been the focus of many clinical and laboratory studies.[109] The protein targets of aPLs were identified as a variety of plasma proteins (e.g., $\beta_2$-glycoprotein-I) that are sometimes bound to phospholipids.[110] This explains the variability in the results of aPL assays and the difficulty in detecting such antibodies in some patients who clearly have the clinical syndrome. Patients may demonstrate false-positive tests for syphilis (Venereal Disease Research Laboratory [VDRL] or rapid plasma reagin [RPR]), prolonged activated partial thromboplastin time (aPTT) or direct Russell viper venom time (DRVVT) not corrected by adding plasma (lupus anticoagulant), anticardiolipin antibodies (aCL), anti–$\beta_2$-glycoprotein antibodies, antibodies to prothrombin, and others. Binding of aPLs to endothelial or trophoblast cells was shown in in vitro studies to provoke the tissue to develop a prothrombotic surface and accelerate coagulation.[111, 112] Pathogenic aPLs can also develop as a result of exogenous estrogen, drugs (pro-

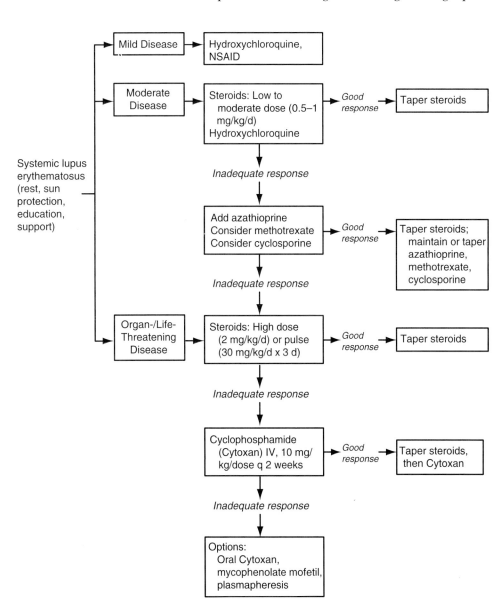

**FIGURE 34–1**
Treatment of childhood lupus (excluding renal disease). AZA, azathioprine; CSA, cyclosporine; MMF, mycophenolate mofetil; MTX, methotrexate; NSAID, nonsteroidal anti-inflammatory drug.

cainamide), and viral infections (human immuno-deficiency virus and parvovirus B19).[109] Patients with antiphospholipid syndrome are clearly at risk for thromboembolic complications and may benefit from antithrombotic therapy.[113] Children with a documented thrombotic event caused by antiphospholipid syndrome are given anticoagulation by heparin, followed by conversion to oral warfarin.[114] In our center, patients with circulating aPLs but without thrombotic manifestations are given daily low-dose aspirin for platelet antagonist effect. Studies are needed to determine which patients are at significant risk for thrombosis, the efficacy of prophylactic therapy in asymptomatic patients, and the length of anticoagulation therapy in those who have had a thrombotic event.

## Management of Childhood Lupus

Algorithms outlining the treatment of childhood lupus are presented in Figures 34–1 and 34–2. The terms used are defined as follows:

- *Mild disease:* mild constitutional symptoms, alopecia, aphthous lesions, arthralgia or arthritis not limiting

of function, nonulcerating rash, asymptomatic small pleural effusion, slight abnormality of serologic studies.
- *Moderate disease:* significantly limiting constitutional symptoms, progressive rash or mucosal lesions, functionally limiting arthritis or myositis, pleural or pericardial effusion, myocarditis, abdominal symptoms, moderate anemia or leukopenia, significant decrease of complement C3 or increase of anti–double-stranded DNA antibody titer or both.
- *Organ or life-threatening disease:* lupus crisis with diffuse multisystem disease, necrotizing vasculitis, CNS involvement, pulmonary disease, progressive serositis or myocarditis, renal disease, progressive GI or pancreatic disease, significant cytopenia or hemolysis.

## NEONATAL LUPUS

This rare syndrome in newborn babies is characterized by at least one of the following clinical manifestations: discoid skin lesions, thrombocytopenia, hemolytic ane-

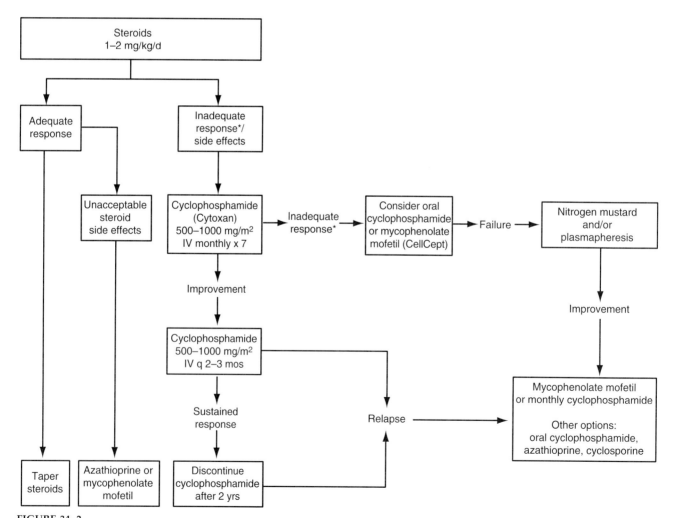

**FIGURE 34–2**
Treatment of lupus nephritis in childhood. AZA, azathioprine; CSA, cyclosporine; MMF, mycophenolate mofetil. *Consider renal biopsy.

mia, hepatic inflammation, and congenital heart block, in association with maternal-fetal transmission of autoreactive antibodies to intracellular cytoplasmic ribonucleoproteins SSA/Ro and SSB/La.[115] Most mothers (40% to 60%) are not identified as having an autoimmune illness at the time of birth of an affected infant, and many of them remain healthy; only a few have or eventually develop mild SLE, Sjögren's syndrome, or an undifferentiated connective tissue disease.[116]

Noncardiac manifestations usually resolve spontaneously and completely. Hematologic and hepatic manifestations resolve within weeks to months, and discoid skin lesions within 1 year.[117] Thrombocytopenia or anemia may necessitate platelet or red blood cell transfusions. Steroids have been used successfully in infants with serious or persistent hematologic or hepatic manifestations.[118] Case reports of NLE with CNS vasculitis or with unusual skin atrophy or pancytopenia have also been published.[119, 120] The most serious manifestation of NLE is congenital complete heart block, which occurs in approximately one half of affected babies and is associated with significant morbidity and mortality.[121] The majority of affected infants require placement of a pacemaker within the first 3 months of life.[122] Cardiomyopathy can also develop in utero or later in life.[123] Mortality approaches 30% within the first 3 months to 3 years of life; the greatest risk of death occurs in affected infants born before 34 weeks of gestation.[116, 124] Irreversible damage to the fetal heart is caused by anti–SS-A or anti–SS-B antibodies that are transferred from the mother to the fetus via the placenta. Although not pathogenic in the mothers, studies have shown that they cross-react with fetal cardiac laminin[125] and interfere with L-type calcium channels,[126] leading to destruction of the conduction system and other areas of the developing heart. Aggressive intervention to reduce the antibody load in the pregnant mother (high-dose steroids and plasmapheresis) have so far not succeeded in preventing complete heart block or associated hydrops fetalis.[127] However, successful outcome with intensive management of hydrops fetalis and heart failure in two infants with NLE has been reported.[128]

The risk that a pregnant woman with anti–SS-A or anti–SS-B antibodies will bear an infant with complete heart block is 6%. This risk significantly increases with subsequent pregnancies to 16%; the risk for any NLE manifestation is 26%.[2, 116]

Early detection of fetal cardiac involvement might permit earlier intervention. Pregnant women who are at risk (women known to have anti–SS-A or anti–SS-B antibodies or a history of previous babies with NLE) should be monitored with serial fetal echocardiography, especially between 18 and 24 weeks of gestation, to detect fetal bradyarrhythmias or myocarditis.[2] There have been a few reports of connective tissue disease occurring in patients who had NLE at birth.[129] Therefore, we recommend long-term rheumatology follow-up of these babies as well. A national registry of NLE, through the National Institute of Arthritis and Musculoskeletal Diseases, has been created to collect and study clinical data, which are essential to the development of better understanding and management strategies for this disorder.[2]

## JUVENILE DERMATOMYOSITIS

JDMS is an autoimmune multisystem inflammatory illness that primarily affects proximal skeletal muscle and skin, with typical heliotrope rash and Gottron's papules. Smooth muscle of the GI tract and myocardium can also be involved. Small-vessel vasculitis is a prominent feature of the disease in childhood and can involve the CNS, peripheral nerves, and other internal organs. Calcinosis of cutaneous and subcutaneous tissues, muscles, tendons, and ligaments is a late manifestation unique to the childhood disease that can develop while inflammation is still active or even years after resolution of active disease.

Although spontaneous recovery sometimes occurs, without treatment the disease is fatal in more than one third of affected children and results in serious morbidity in another third. Treatment with corticosteroids and other drugs has greatly improved both survival and outcome in JDMS. Most children recover completely, with residual disability in fewer than one third. Nevertheless, early respiratory failure and complications of severe vasculitis continue to be leading causes of death in 5% to 10% of patients.[130]

### Mild to Moderate Disease

A few children have minimal skin and muscle disease and no systemic involvement. They usually recover fully without treatment.

Corticosteroids are the mainstay of therapy in most patients.[131, 132] Dosages of 1 to 2 mg/kg/day are given during the acute phase. Maximal therapeutic effect is achieved by administration of steroids in divided doses at 6- to 8-hour intervals. With clinical improvement and decreasing muscle enzyme levels, usually by 3 to 6 weeks, gradual tapering of steroids is instituted while the divided daily dose schedule is maintained. Once muscle enzymes have returned to normal and strength has shown consistent improvement, steroids can be consolidated to a single daily dose and slowly tapered. Total duration of steroid therapy is usually months to years.

Studies of muscle biopsy specimens show that early in the course of inflammation complement C5b-9 membranohemolytic attack complex is deposited in intramuscular capillaries resulting in capillary necrosis, ischemia, and destruction of muscle fibers.[133] For this reason, we recommend that patients take low-dose aspirin (one 81-mg tablet daily) early in the course of the disease. Hydroxychloroquine, 5 to 6.5 mg/kg/day, may be effective therapy in those with persistent JDMS skin manifestations and may provide a steroid-sparing effect.[134] However, worsening of rash with this drug has also been described.[135] In most cases, MTX in dosages of 0.3 to 0.5 mg/kg once weekly by mouth is added to improve disease control and provide a steroid-sparing effect.[79] As in other uses of MTX for rheumatic disorders, leucovorin (folinic acid) is given within 12 to 24 hours after the MTX dose, to minimize potential toxicities.[78] With clinical and laboratory evidence of improvement, steroids are gradually tapered, followed by slow reduction of MTX dosage over months to years.

## Severe Disease

A variety of treatments have been used for children with progressive disease whose response to corticosteroids has been inadequate or in whom steroid side effects have been unacceptable.

METHOTREXATE. Oral dosages of 0.6 to 1 mg/kg once a week (up to 20 mg/m$^2$), or parenteral administration of 1 to 10 mg/kg with folinic acid rescue every 3 weeks has resulted in improved muscle strength and serum muscle enzyme levels within a few weeks from the start of therapy, together with steroid sparing.[136–139] MTX dosage reduction can result in a disease flare.

CYCLOSPORINE. Retrospective studies found that cyclosporine is an effective and safe treatment for JDMS when the disease is refractory to steroids, MTX, or cytotoxic agents.[140, 141] Significant steroid-sparing effect was reported as well. Added to steroids alone or in combination with MTX, the cyclosporine dosage is 2 to 5 mg/kg/day. Onset of action may take a few weeks. Careful monitoring of renal function is essential, and effort should be made to keep the dosage at the lowest effective range to minimize renal toxicity. Clearance of this drug is increased in young children, who may require a higher dosage. Presence of GI inflammation may reduce absorption. For this reason we use Neoral, a microemulsion formulation of cyclosporine that was shown to have a more predictable absorption, independent from food intake.[142] The development of *Pneumocystis carinii* pneumonia in one girl who received combined prednisone, MTX, and cyclosporine treatment for extremely severe disease has led us to carefully monitor such patients for complicating opportunistic infections. Relapse of disease after discontinuation of cyclosporine is of concern[53]; we recommend that patients keep receiving therapeutic dosages of cyclosporine for about 2 years after clinical remission is achieved and then undergo a very slow tapering.

AZATHIOPRINE. This purine analog was reported to be effective for control of childhood disease in a small number of cases.[130] In adult disease, when tested in a blinded and controlled study versus steroids alone, azathioprine was effective in severe and prolonged disease and in providing a steroid-sparing effect, although improvement was evident only after 3 years of therapy.[143] A more recent study found that the combination of azathioprine with oral low-dose MTX was effective in very recalcitrant cases.[138] The azathioprine dosage is 1 to 2.5 mg/kg/day. Onset of action is slow, at least 3 months, and the risk of a secondary malignancy is higher than with MTX; therefore we reserve azathioprine therapy for children for whom MTX, cyclosporine, IVIG, or combined therapies have failed.

INTRAVENOUS IMMUNE GLOBULIN. Open studies of IVIG in JDMS found significant improvement of muscle strength and skin rash in about one third of the patients.[144, 145] A placebo-controlled, double-blind study in adult subjects confirmed marked improvement in a significant number of patients clinically and by muscle enzyme levels and muscle histology. Improvement was evident early in the course of therapy and peaked after the second monthly infusion of 2 g/kg. This efficacy was of short duration: patients suffered relapse 4 to 8 weeks after discontinuation of therapy.[133] As a first-line therapy in JDMS, without steroids, IVIG produced mixed results.[130] The mechanism of action of IVIG in dermatomyositis is prevention of membrane attack complex deposition on the endomysial capillaries[133] and possibly also provision of neutralizing antibodies against occult viral agents that may trigger disease in a subset of patients.[131] We conclude that IVIG combined with steroids may be an effective short-term therapy in refractory and progressive JDMS. In addition to the adverse effects described earlier, patients who are deficient in IgA should receive IgA-depleted preparation to prevent anaphylaxis. Children should not receive immunization against measles during IVIG therapy because of the presence of neutralizing antibodies in the preparation.[96]

CHLORAMBUCIL. Case reports and a prospective study demonstrated this alkylating drug to be an effective steroid-sparing agent in adult patients with recalcitrant dermatomyositis for whom other immunosuppressive or cytotoxic therapies had failed.[146, 147] Beneficial effect was evident at 4 to 6 weeks with dosages of 0.1 to 0.2 mg/kg/day administered orally. Frequent monitoring for reversible leukopenia and bone marrow suppression is required. Other potential side effects include azoospermia, teratogenicity, development of malignant disease, GI irritation, elevation of transaminases, CNS irritability, and interstitial pneumonia.[148]

SUMMARY. As disease control is achieved, steroids are slowly tapered. The duration of therapy with these agents after complete disease control and discontinuation of steroids is still unknown. Our practice is to individualize length of therapy according to prior disease severity, response to treatment, and tolerance of the drugs. In all cases, tapering should be carried out slowly while patients are monitored for clinical and laboratory evidence of JDMS activity.

## Life-threatening Disease

Severe vasculitis of the GI tract, heart, lungs, or CNS may lead to potentially fatal complications such as GI perforation, arrhythmias, pulmonary alveolitis, pneumothorax, and neurologic disease. Cyclophosphamide may be effective in these situations when administered intravenously in a dosage of 10 mg/kg every 2 weeks.[149] With consistent control of vasculitis, the interval between doses may be gradually increased. Other approaches include the use of intravenous-pulse steroids (30 mg/kg of methylprednisolone, up to 1 g/day for 3 days),[130] AZA,[150] chlorambucil, or IVIG.[133] Patients who fail to respond adequately to such treatment are at great risk and may benefit from plasmapheresis in combination with steroids and cyclophosphamide.[151, 152, 130] Although we have seen several instances of desperately ill children who recovered with this treatment, a controlled trial in adults with dermatomyositis or polymyositis failed to show efficacy with either leukapheresis or plasmapheresis.[153]

SUPPORTIVE MEASURES. Patients with progressive or severe disease are at risk for aspiration, respiratory failure, dehydration, malnutrition, skin sores, and limb contractures caused by weakness and debilitation. Supportive measures include elevation of the head, suction, cardiorespiratory monitoring, soft foods or parenteral feeding, stool softeners, skin care, and positioning. Psychological support to the child and family and education about the disease and its treatment are provided by the rheumatology team.

CALCINOSIS. Calcium deposits in the skin, subcutaneous tissue, fat, and fascia occur in 23% to 39% of JDMS patients and are a unique and potentially debilitating complication of the childhood disease.[130, 132, 136] Risk factors for development of calcinosis include delay to initiation of treatment, polycyclic or recalcitrant course, local trauma, and therapy with lower steroid dosages.[131] Superficial masses of calcium may extrude spontaneously. Calcium "tumors" can liquefy and produce abscesses, which frequently require surgical drainage. Deep, chronic ulceration of skin with bacterial superinfection may occur. These are treated much like full-thickness burns, with whirlpool, débridement, antibiotics, possible skin grafting, pain control, fluids, and nutritional support. Sheets of calcium may limit mobility of joints or even chest expansion, leading to serious functional disability.[154] No effective treatment for calcinosis is known. Various past therapeutic approaches have failed, including warfarin, calcitonin, diphosphonates, and chelating agents.[130, 155, 156] Diltiazem in dosages of 3 to 6 mg/kg/day was reported to improve calcinosis in long-term therapy, especially when combined with the biphosphonate drug pamidronate.[157, 158] Lithotripsy has been used to treat calcific tendinitis,[159] but it may also cause increased inflammation.[131] Colchicine has been used successfully for reduction of local inflammation associated with development of new calcium deposits.[160] Calcinosis spontaneously undergoes complete or partial remission in up to 50% of patients after 5 or more years.[131, 136] Because improvement of calcinosis is associated with increased mobility, physical and occupational therapy should be strongly emphasized to prevent or correct contractures and maintain strength and range of motion.

REHABILITATION. Children with JDMS are at risk for long-term morbidity, with limited mobility and loss of independence in activities of daily living (ADL), even in the face of a good response to drug therapy. Prolonged muscle weakness with eventual scarring and development of calcinosis may lead to restricted joint motion and loss of function. Physical and occupational therapy should be included early in the treatment plan. In the initial phase of acute muscle inflammation, proper positioning of the extremities is essential to avoid development of contractures. This may involve the use of resting splints as well as gentle passive stretching. When inflammation subsides, methods to stretch tight muscles and tendons and active exercises are introduced gradually to facilitate strengthening and to increase range of motion, function, and endurance. The overall aim of the rehabilitative effort is to enable these children to achieve optimal functioning.

# CHILDHOOD VASCULITIC SYNDROMES

Idiopathic inflammation of blood vessels characterizes a spectrum of vasculitic disorders in childhood. Classification of these syndromes is complicated and takes into account histopathologic as well as clinical features such as the affected vessel size, pathologic characteristics of lesions, major organs involved, and clinical progression.[161] Understanding of the role of antineutrophil cytoplasmic antibodies (ANCA) in causing disease and their utility in clinical diagnosis and follow-up of vasculitic disorders is an evolving process and the subject of numerous studies.[162] Initial reports of high sensitivity and specificity of this test in certain syndromes (e.g., WG) are currently questioned.[162] Although the presence of ANCA is helpful in the diagnosis of systemic vasculitic syndromes, it cannot be used in lieu of biopsy,[163] and lack of ANCA does not rule out a systemic vasculitic disorder.[164] The presence of ANCA in children with vasculitis and glomerulonephritis is associated with high morbidity and progression to end-stage renal disease in as many as 60%. Therefore, detection of ANCA in pediatric patients with vasculitis and glomerulonephritis is an indication for prompt and aggressive treatment.[165]

HSP and KS are the most common idiopathic vasculitides occurring before the age of 20 years and are mostly unique to this age group. Management of these disorders and of the more rare forms of vasculitis in childhood is discussed here.

## Henoch-Schönlein Purpura

A wide spectrum of clinical manifestations, including nonthrombocytopenic purpura, GI pain and bleeding, and large-joint arthritis, may occur in HSP because of IgA-mediated necrotizing inflammation of small vessels.[166] This vasculitis can also involve the CNS, scrotum, testes, and lungs.[167, 168] The severity and extent of vasculitis determine the severity of the acute-phase manifestations as well as the long-term outcome.[169] About half of the patients experience occult or frank GI bleeding, which in 1.3% to 13.6% leads to intussusception.[170] Acute hematuria develops in half of the children but progresses to end-stage renal disease in fewer than 1%.[171] Death occurs in 2% of cases during the acute phase, usually as a result of rapidly progressive glomerulonephritis or bowel obstruction.[172] Long-term morbidity and mortality are determined by the extent and progression of renal involvement.[169] Despite the potential for serious manifestations and complications, HSP usually follows a self-limited course, with good prognosis and complete resolution in 6 to 12 weeks. This fact and the lack of controlled studies contribute to the controversy regarding efficacy of the various treatment modalities that are currently used.

MILD DISEASE. Patients with mild manifestations, such as rash, arthritis, abdominal pain, and malaise, are treated with supportive measures (hydration, pain control, nutritional support) and reassurance while being monitored for evidence of GI, renal, or other major organ involvement. Although NSAIDs may be effective for the joint manifestations, these drugs should be used with caution because they can confuse and aggravate the clinical picture if GI bleeding or glomerulonephritis develops.[167] Discomfort may result from the purpuric rash and its underlying edema. Steroid therapy is effective but should be reserved for exceptionally severe symptoms.[173] Monitoring for evidence of renal disease with urinalyses and periodic blood pressure checks should continue for 1 year after resolution of illness. Because the persistence of hematuria is a poor prognostic sign, such patients require more prolonged monitoring of renal function.

## Moderate to Severe Disease

GASTROINTESTINAL BLEEDING OR SEVERE PAIN. Although most patients respond rapidly to steroids at (1 to 2 mg/kg/day in divided doses),[174] controversy still exists about their use, with some studies reporting no advantage over supportive measures alone.[167] Complicating intussusception may be successfully reduced by barium enema, but persistent intussusception or perforation requires surgical intervention.[170]

RENAL INVOLVEMENT. The debate regarding whether steroids administered early in the course of HSP glomerulonephritis prevent development or progression of kidney disease is unresolved. One prospective study found prophylactic treatment with steroids to be effective in preventing renal disease,[174] but others found no such benefit.[175] Patients at increased risk for glomerulonephritis (onset after 9 years of age, persistent rash, bloody stools) and those at risk of progression to end-stage renal disease (proteinuria or nephrotic syndrome)[167] should probably receive a trial of steroid therapy at 1 to 2 mg/kg/day in divided doses, with slow tapering on improvement. Treatment regimens for HSP glomerulonephritis can be difficult to evaluate because of the high rate of spontaneous resolution and the lack of randomized controlled trials. Observations and case reports indicate that steroids alone or in combination with cyclophosphamide, AZA,[176, 177] or cyclosporine[178] can be effective in cases of severe renal involvement. Therefore, prolonged immunosuppressive therapy may be beneficial in progressive HSP kidney disease.[179] Patients who develop renal failure may require kidney transplantation.

CENTRAL NERVOUS SYSTEM VASCULITIS OR VASCULITIS IN OTHER ORGANS. Steroids given in moderate to high dosages of 1 to 2 mg/kg/day or via an intravenous pulse regimen are the mainstay of therapy.[167] Cyclophosphamide, plasmapheresis, and other cytotoxic agents may be used for progressive disease but are rarely required.

## Kawasaki Syndrome

KS is an acute vasculitis of small and medium-sized arteries in multiple organs that affects primarily infants and young children. The disease occurs worldwide in all racial groups, but it is most prevalent in Japan and in children of Japanese ancestry living outside of Japan. Infantile PAN, a serious and often fatal arteritis initially thought to be an early-age form of PAN, is now recognized as identical to KS.[180] Immune activation of T cells and monocyte-macrophages by bacterial-toxin superantigens is recognized as a major factor in the pathogenesis of disease.[181]

Most of the acute inflammatory manifestations of this disease follow a self-limited course and resolve without sequelae, even if untreated.[182] The most serious manifestation, coronary artery involvement, determines the long-term outlook. Without treatment, coronary aneurysms develop in 20% to 25% of patients.[182, 183] Giant aneurysms, larger than 8 mm in diameter, are especially dangerous because they do not undergo spontaneous regression and may result in stenosis and thrombosis, with resulting cardiac ischemia.[183, 184] ASA, one of the first drugs used for KS, was shown in a few retrospective studies to reduce the length of the febrile phase as well as the rate of coronary aneurysm formation.[185] The use of systemic steroids in KS remains controversial; several studies reported that treatment with steroids alone or in combination with ASA was associated with higher frequency of coronary aneurysms and complications.[186] However, an uncontrolled study of four patients who failed repeated IVIG courses suggested a beneficial response to intravenous pulse methylprednisolone therapy (30 mg/kg/day for 1 to 3 days).[187] For this reason, steroids are avoided in KS except for certain IVIG-resistant life-threatening manifestations, such as nonischemic myocarditis or massive lymphadenopathy causing complications such as airway obstruction.[188, 189]

High-dose IVIG, administered within the first 10 to 12 days of illness in conjunction with anti-inflammatory dosages of ASA, are the cornerstone of KS management. Several studies demonstrated the efficacy and safety of this regimen in reducing the prevalence of coronary abnormalities from 20% to 4%.[183] IVIG with ASA therapy was also shown to prevent the formation of giant aneurysms,[190] improve left ventricular function,[191] and reduce the length of the febrile and acute inflammatory phase.[185] Controlled study showed that a single dose of 2 g/kg of IVIG, in comparison with multiple-dose regimens of equivalent total dose, significantly reduced the incidence of coronary artery aneurysms and hastened resolution of acute manifestations, without greater risk of adverse effects.[192] The importance of treating early to prevent significant coronary disease is emphasized in all studies.[193] Research demonstrating that antibodies in IVIG block superantigen-mediated T-cell activation suggest this as a possible mechanism of IVIG action in KS.[194]

We recommend the following for treatment of KS:

1. Admission of the patients to the hospital for monitoring of acute inflammatory symptoms, possible complications, and response to therapy.

2. A single high-dose IVIG treatment (2 g/kg over 10 to 12 hours), in conjunction with anti-inflammatory ASA therapy (80 to 100 mg/kg/day in four divided doses). Patients are treated with IVIG provided that the diagnosis has been made within 10 days after the onset of fever or that symptoms and laboratory signs of inflammation persist. This may be repeated once if fever recurs 48 hours or longer after the initial dose.

3. Continuation of anti-inflammatory ASA therapy until resolution of fever and acute inflammatory symptoms (usually 10 to 14 days).

4. Reduction of the ASA dosage to 3 to 5 mg/kg/day for an antithrombotic effect after resolution of fever. If coronary abnormalities are not detected, ASA is discontinued after the platelet count and sedimentation rate have returned to normal (usually 7 to 8 weeks). Patients in whom coronary disease develops continue low-dose ASA therapy.

5. Cardiac follow-up. A second echocardiogram is performed 5 to 9 days after IVIG administration. Normal coronary appearance within 14 days after treatment is associated with virtually no risk of future aneurysms.[195] These patients are allowed to return gradually to normal levels of physical activity and are monitored clinically. An echocardiogram is repeated 1 year after onset, to verify normal cardiac structure and function. Further echocardiograms are not indicated unless symptoms are present. Children with coronary artery disease require close cardiology follow-up. The majority of coronary aneurysms show angiographic regression within 6 months to 2 years after onset; however, giant aneurysms are much less likely to regress and have the worst prognosis.[196]

6. Treatment of persistent arthralgia or arthritis with NSAIDs.

7. Recurrence of acute KS after complete resolution of the initial episode is reported in 2% of patients.[197] Treatment is identical.

## Polyarteritis Nodosa

PAN is a rare disease in childhood in which necrotizing vasculitis of unknown origin involves small and medium-sized muscular arteries with formation of nodular aneurysms along their walls in multiple sites, especially in the mesenteric, hepatic, renal, coronary, cutaneous, and central and peripheral nervous systems. Diversity of clinical manifestations is characteristic. These include fever, myalgia, arthralgia, rashes, abdominal pain, hypertension, glomerulonephritis, central or peripheral neurologic abnormalities, lung and cardiac findings, and laboratory evidence of acute phase reactants.[198] Group A streptococcal infection is sometimes associated with onset or exacerbation of childhood PAN.[199] The spectrum of disease severity in childhood ranges from a limited cutaneous form to progressive organ involvement.[200] Although attempts have been made to define clinical diagnostic criteria for childhood PAN,[201] definite diagnosis still requires

typical findings on biopsy or angiography. ANCA determination may contribute to the diagnostic process and provide a measure of prediction of outcome, inasmuch as P-ANCA (directed against myeloperoxidase) or atypical ANCA are detected in more than 47% of adult patients with severe systemic involvement.[202, 162]

The extent and reversibility of organ involvement determines the outcome of PAN. Early diagnosis and prompt institution of therapy are essential. Renal impairment and CNS or severe GI involvement are indications of poor prognosis.[200] Before steroids came into use, most children succumbed to these complications within the first year of disease. Survival increased markedly with the introduction of corticosteroids in the 1960s.[203] Prospective randomized trials in adults showed that combined steroid and cyclophosphamide therapy improved the clinical response and reduced the number of disease episodes, although overall survival remained similar to that achieved with steroids alone (i.e., 75% at 10 years).[204–207]

**APPROACH TO TREATMENT.** A few children have very limited cutaneous disease and may respond to NSAIDs. In general, however, steroids are the keystone of therapy.

**POLYARTERITIS NODOSA WITHOUT ORGAN OR LIFE-THREATENING INVOLVEMENT.** Steroids are administered intravenously or orally at 1 to 2 mg/kg/day in divided doses. With adequate response, usually in a few weeks, steroids are tapered. Patients are continued on low daily or alternate-day therapy until there is no evidence of active disease. Patients are closely monitored thereafter.

**ORGAN OR LIFE-THREATENING DISEASE.** Methylprednisolone pulse therapy (30 mg/kg up to 1 g per dose daily for 3 days) may be beneficial for CNS vasculitis.[208] Central or peripheral nervous system disease that does not respond to pulse steroids, as well as other severe disease manifestations such as significant GI vasculitis, progressive glomerulonephritis, and pulmonary hemorrhage, are treated with a combination of steroids (1 to 2 mg/kg/day in divided doses) and cyclophosphamide (10 mg/kg intravenously every 2 weeks). With adequate response, the interval between cyclophosphamide doses may be increased gradually. If necessary, efficacy may be enhanced by oral administration of cyclophosphamide (daily doses of 1 to 2 mg/kg); however, the risk of infections and other adverse reactions increases. To minimize these risks, the frequency of cyclophosphamide administration may be reduced to 3 to 4 days per week once improvement is evident. Although efficacy of plasmapheresis in PAN and other vasculitic disorders is not proven, patients with pulmonary bleeding, rapidly progressive glomerulonephritis, or other life-threatening complications who respond inadequately to steroids and cyclophosphamide may benefit from the addition of plasmapheresis.[204, 209] General supportive measures in all patients include control of hypertension, maintenance of normal hemodynamic status, and treatment of infection.

## Wegener's Granulomatosis

WG is a rare form of necrotizing granulomatous vasculitis that primarily involves the upper and lower respiratory systems and the kidneys. Clinical manifestations range from limited disease affecting nasal, sinus, ear, or upper airways to the more generalized form involving multiple systems, especially lungs and kidneys.[210, 211] Fever, arthralgia, and myalgia are common. Untreated, the disease progresses rapidly and is often fatal. Daily steroid and cyclophosphamide therapy has greatly improved the course and survival of this illness. Outcome still depends on early diagnosis and prompt institution of therapy, before the development of irreversible organ damage.[212] Antibodies to proteinase-3 (C-ANCA), which are highly sensitive and specific to this condition, are used to hasten diagnosis and onset of therapy.[213] ANCA titers can also be monitored to assess response and guide therapy.[214] However, a negative test result does not rule out this diagnosis or flare of disease.[162] Standard treatment of WG combines daily oral cyclophosphamide at 2 mg/kg with daily steroids at 1 mg/kg.[215, 216] As the initial symptoms resolve, usually in 3 to 12 months, steroids are gradually tapered. Cyclophosphamide is usually maintained for at least 1 year after complete remission and then gradually tapered while the patient is monitored for evidence of clinical or laboratory reactivation. This treatment regimen was shown to result in complete remission in 75% of patients and marked improvement in 91% after a median of 12 months. Remissions lasted longer than 5 years in a significant number of patients. However, more than half experienced one or more relapses within 3 months to 16 years after remission. A 13% mortality rate, from complications of disease as well as of therapy, was found.[217] Studies of IVCY versus oral cyclophosphamide treatment in WG are the subject of controversy. A large prospective, controlled study concluded that pulse cyclophosphamide therapy and oral therapy were equally effective in achieving initial remission,[218] but others dispute this form of treatment because of a higher rate of mortality and serious infectious complications.[219] Although a favorable response to trimethoprim-sulfamethoxazole was reported in selected patients,[220] this finding was not confirmed in a prospective NIH trial.[216, 217] More recent prospective trials in adults and in children reported improvement with weekly low-dose oral MTX.[221, 212] MTX currently appears to be an acceptable initial therapy in patients without immediately life-threatening disease.[222] Novel therapies in adults include MMF (reported in two patients) and a clinical trial of leflunomide, each used with steroids as a maintenance treatment after standard induction therapy.[173]

## LIMITED SCLERODERMA

Localized scleroderma is the most common form of scleroderma in childhood. The disease may be limited to one or a few patches of sclerotic skin, also termed *morphea*, or it may occur as a linear sclerotic band (linear scleroderma).[223] When linear lesions affect the face or scalp, they may resemble a saber scar, termed *en coup de sabre*. Although the disease is not life-threatening, linear bands may result in atrophy of

the face or extremities, joint contractures, and failure of limbs to grow and develop. In addition, there may be localized involvement of adjacent internal organs, including brain, subcutaneous structures, muscle, bone, synovium, and blood vessels.[224–226] Unlike localized morphea lesions, linear lesions seldom regress spontaneously.[227] The functional and cosmetic effects can lead to serious emotional difficulties.

Because the clinical condition changes very slowly in many cases, it is often difficult to determine which patients need treatment. Serum levels of soluble IL-2 receptor were shown to correlate with disease activity in limited scleroderma and may be used as a marker of disease activity and a guide to therapy.[228]

In very early stages of the disease, clinical signs of inflammation, including erythema and swelling, are sometimes seen. In such patients a short course of steroids may be prescribed. For children with more chronic, slowly progressive disease, steroids are not effective and should not be used.

D-Penicillamine was the major agent used to treat this condition in the past[229]; however, because of its slow action and significant profile of adverse effects,[230] it is seldom used today. MTX is the current mainstay of therapy. A controlled trial found that MTX given in a low-dose weekly oral regimen improved the skin score and other disease manifestations in adults with systemic sclerosis.[231] We recommend MTX for children whose disease appears to be progressive and likely to produce severe disfigurement or limb shortening. Our experience with this drug is that it is effective and well tolerated by patients with linear scleroderma. Surgical release of scar tissue and skin grafting may improve range of motion, even though the grafted area may become involved in the disease process. When limb shortening is severe, a surgical approach to limit growth of the uninvolved extremity (e.g., epiphysiodesis) may be considered. Timing is critical, because this procedure is beneficial only while the normal limb is still growing. In rare cases, amputation of a severely deformed distal extremity that is interfering with function may be necessary. Physical and occupational therapy as well as support by the team nurse and social worker are essential to enable these children to function with minimal physical and emotional disability.

## REFLEX NEUROVASCULAR DYSTROPHY

RND is also known as reflex sympathetic dystrophy, complex regional pain syndrome, causalgia, and Sudek's syndrome. It is a noninflammatory musculoskeletal pain syndrome characterized by severe extremity pain that typically is accompanied by diffuse local swelling, significant tenderness to light touch, and color and temperature changes of vasomotor instability (cold and mottled, painful area although well perfused). Under-recognized in children, it is most commonly seen in adolescent girls but can occur in younger children and in either sex. Although the outlook is better in children than in adults, RND can produce long-term disability and trophic changes, with eventual permanent damage to the affected extremity.[232, 233] The cause of RND is not known. Psychological factors may be important in predisposing to this disease, because certain trends are observed in most patients and their families.[234, 235] Characteristically, children with RND tend to be overachievers. They seem to be "perfect children from perfect families." Secondary gain (a respite from responsibilities?) is often operative. Enmeshment with one parent (usually the mother) is almost universal, whereas the other parent is seen as powerful but remote. Marital discord, subtle or overt, is frequently present. Families are perceived as solid but often are psychologically chaotic.

The goal of treatment is to improve function rather than to relieve pain. In RND pain is generally not amenable to direct therapeutic intervention. Furthermore, our experience has demonstrated that pain tends to resolve as function improves. Accordingly, pain complaints are acknowledged but not dwelt on. The basic therapeutic approach is to treat with a combination of physical and occupational therapy to regain full use of the involved extremity and psychological counseling to help the child deal with underlying feelings and conflicts in more appropriate ways. We make it clear to patients that the more they use the involved extremity, the quicker it will improve, whereas disuse will worsen the condition. Although there are reports of benefit from corticosteroids and sympathetic blocking agents in adult patients, experience in our unit has been that these modes of treatment generally produce short-lived or no benefit and may be associated with toxic effects. Furthermore, they may divert the patient from dealing with the underlying psychological issues. Except for the rare patient in whom emotional factors do not seem to be operative, our tendency has been to avoid these forms of therapy.

Treatment begins with a clear, straightforward discussion of the diagnosis and its implications with the child and parents. As soon as the diagnosis is established, the child and parents should be so informed in definite terms. The important role that emotional factors can play in causing the disease should be explained. The fact that, with treatment, the prognosis is good can be emphasized. This is the time to set the stage for ongoing psychotherapy. In our experience, it is crucial for the family to accept the emotional aspect of the disease in order to achieve a good outcome. Although the prognosis for short-term improvement with physical therapy alone is good, without psychological intervention there is likely to be an eventual relapse of RND or development of another somatization disorder.

In mild cases, outpatient management may suffice. If symptoms are more severe and longstanding, however, admission to a rehabilitation center is indicated.

## Management in the Rehabilitation Center

The initial approach is crucial, because the diagnosis and management plan, both physical and psychological, must be understood and accepted by the patient and the family. At this time a functional discharge goal, entailing full use of the affected extremity, is set up. A typical goal for a child with lower-extremity involvement might be ambulation for a reasonable distance, wearing shoes and socks, and no more than a minimal limp. Assistive devices such as wheelchairs, crutches, and braces are quickly withdrawn. Patients are permitted mild analgesics, such as acetaminophen, but they are advised that drugs are not likely to provide major pain relief. The multidisciplinary treatment team meets shortly after the initial evaluation and weekly thereafter to set a series of interim treatment objectives (short-term goals) and review progress. These objectives, usually exercises involving progressively more functional use of the affected extremity, must be quantifiable and sufficiently challenging that the patient will have to work hard to accomplish them within 1 week. At the same time, they must be realistic and attainable. Patients who meet their weekly treatment objectives by the weekend are awarded a pass; however, if objectives are not fully met by the end of the week, the child continues to work toward that goal until new interim objectives are set.

### Roles of Therapeutic Team Members

PHYSICIAN (PEDIATRIC RHEUMATOLOGIST). The physician sets the overall direction of the patient's management, determines the discharge goal, conducts team meetings, communicates with parents, and regularly evaluates the patient. The physician's approach to the patient must be compassionate but firm, emphasizing full compliance with the therapy program despite pain.

NURSE. The rheumatology team nurse serves as a liaison between the patient, the family, and the other team members. Most important is the nurse's role in establishing a relationship of trust with the patient and providing encouragement to express feelings.

PHYSICAL THERAPIST. The physical therapist provides weight-bearing exercises for the involved extremity. Desensitization techniques, such as vigorous toweling, use of lotion, or immersion in contrast baths, are applied. Atrophied muscles and endurance are improved. Those are instrumental to reverse physical symptoms of this disorder and regain full functional use of the involved extremity. Throughout this process, choices are permitted within limits, so that the child remains focused on the therapy objectives and is encouraged to assume a more proactive role in the treatment regimen. For example, the patient may be given the choice of vigorously toweling the involved extremity himself for a longer period or having the therapist do it for a shorter period. The therapist uses a firm but nonpunitive approach.

OCCUPATIONAL THERAPIST. Characteristically, children with RND are overachievers. The occupational therapist evaluates the patient's capabilities and the psychological costs involved in attempting to reach the patient's own or the family's high expectations. The team may work with the child or family to modify such expectations. The occupational therapist's role also extends to facilitation of age-appropriate activities and interactions. Opportunities are provided for the child to make choices and exercise independence. In childhood RND, the upper extremities are involved less commonly than the lower extremities. When upper-extremity involvement is present, the occupational therapist provides tasks that require hand and arm use in much the same way the physical therapist does for the lower extremity.

PARENTS. The parents form a vital component of the therapeutic team. Without their active participation, recovery tends to be slower and relapses more common. Their support of the child and of all aspects of the treatment plan, including the challenging physical exercise program, withdrawal of assistive devices, and participation in individual and family psychological therapy, is vital to good outcome.

SOCIAL WORKER/PSYCHOLOGIST. The role of this team member is crucial for the long-term outlook. Initially, patient and family psychosocial dynamics are evaluated. Although the patient presents with the symptoms, RND is frequently a family system disorder, and family therapy may be highly desirable. The social worker, often using a psychiatrist as a consultant, provides both family and individual therapy during the inpatient phase of treatment, as well as referral for outpatient counseling after discharge.

### Summary

The treatment program outlined here has evolved in our institution over many years. It has proved to be effective in returning the majority of patients to normal life, with a very low rate of disease recurrence.

## FIBROMYALGIA

Childhood FMS, a diffuse, noninflammatory pain syndrome previously under-recognized in children, currently represents about 7% of all new diagnoses in pediatric rheumatology centers in the United States.[236] FMS is characterized by chronic musculoskeletal pain, fatigue, and the presence of characteristic tender points.[237] Other symptoms frequently present in children with FMS include sleep disturbance, subjective stiffness or swelling, headaches, paresthesias, and irritable bowel syndrome.[238] In comparison with adults with FMS, children have fewer muscle tender points but more complaints of difficulty sleeping.[239] In addition, joint hypermobility is commonly identified in these children.[240] In contrast to RND, objective physical changes are not seen. Emotional factors, especially those related to family dysfunction, may play a role in some childhood cases. However, a controlled study of psychological adjustment, coping, family functioning, and disability in children with FMS and their families did not support the notion that FS is a psychogenic condition.[241] Further studies suggested that family environment and parental pain history may be related to how a child copes with FMS.[242]

With a few exceptions, treatment is carried out in the outpatient setting. The treatment program ad-

dresses the emotional as well as the somatic aspects of this condition by combining the efforts of physician, nurse, physical therapist, occupational therapist, and social worker. First, the child and the family are reassured that this is not a destructive chronic disease and that the long-term outlook is good.[235]

The social worker, physical therapist, occupational therapist, and rheumatology nurse evaluate the patient. Education of patient and family regarding FMS is coordinated by the team nurse. A social worker evaluation of the child and the family is essential to identify coping methods and possible psychological stress factors and to provide guidance and support. Often, relaxation techniques are taught. Community mental health referral is arranged if indicated. All team members emphasize the importance of participation in normal activities and advise the parents on how to avoid situations in which secondary gain may result from the child's complaints of pain.[243]

Children with FMS are frequently poorly conditioned because of physical inactivity and pain. The physical therapist develops a graduated program of reconditioning as well as strengthening and flexibility exercises to be followed daily at home or in regular outpatient therapy sessions. The exercise program also emphasizes postural awareness, energy conservation techniques, and activities to improve endurance.

The occupational therapist assesses the impact of FMS on the child's daily life. The child's use of body mechanics during typical activities is evaluated and modified if necessary. Relaxation techniques are practiced. Myofascial release as well as massage, pressure, and heating methods are used to relieve trigger points. Those are also taught to the patients and family members so that they may take an active role in treatment and reduce dependence on the medical team. With these various modalities, muscle stress and pain can be decreased and overall function and sense of well-being improved. Most important, the child begins to develop a sense of having some control over the disease.

Low-dose tricyclic antidepressants such as amitriptyline (Elavil) may be useful when sleep disturbance is significant and not amenable to exercise and relaxation.[244] We prescribe 10 to 25 mg at bedtime. The drug has an atropine-like effect and therefore may cause dryness of the mouth and other mucous membranes. We have not seen urinary retention or increased intraocular pressure in any of our patients. The drug should not be used in combination with cimetidine, which delays its elimination and may enhance toxicity. It should be used with caution in patients who are taking antihypertensive agents. Uncommon adverse effects include arrhythmia and nonspecific changes in the electrocardiogram, various CNS effects, and anticholinergic effects, including paralytic ileus. In addition, this drug is known to be teratogenic and to be excreted in breast milk. Amitriptyline has not been approved by the US Food and Drug Administration for use in children younger than 12 years of age. In our experience, however, the small dosages prescribed (much lower than those used to treat depression) are well tolerated.

# REFERENCES

1. Gare BA: Epidemiology of rheumatic disease in children. Curr Opin Rheumatol 1996; 8:449.
2. Sandborg CI: Childhood systemic lupus erythematosus and neonatal lupus syndrome. Curr Opin Rheumatol 1998; 10:481.
3. Tan FK, Arnett FC: The genetics of SLE. Curr Opin Rheumatol 1998; 10:399.
4. Tucker LB, Menon S, Schaller JG, et al: Adult and childhood onset systemic lupus erythematosus: A comparison of onset, clinical features, serology, and outcome. Br J Rheumatol 1995; 34:866.
5. Donadio JV, Hart GM, Bergstrahl EJ, et al: Prognostic determinations in lupus nephritis: A long-term clinicopathologic study. Lupus 1995; 4:109.
6. Ward MM, Pyun E, Studenski S: Mortality risks associated with specific clinical manifestations of systemic lupus erythematosus. Arch Intern Med 1996; 156:1337.
7. Graham TB, Lovell DJ: Outcome in pediatric rheumatic disease. Curr Opin Rheumatol 1997; 9:434.
8. Baqi N, Mozami S, Singh A, et al: Lupus nephritis in children: A longitudinal study of prognostic factors and therapy. J Am Soc Nephrol 1996; 7:924.
9. McCurdy DK, Lehman TJA, Bernstein B, et al: Lupus nephritis: Prognostic factors in children. Pediatrics 1992; 89:240.
10. Wallace DJ: Antimalarial agents and lupus. Rheum Dis Clin North Am 1994; 20:243.
11. Bernstein BH, Singsen BH, King KK, et al: Aspirin induced hepatotoxicity and its effects on juvenile rheumatoid arthritis. Am J Dis Child 1977; 131:659.
12. Simon LS: Biology and toxic effects of nonsteroidal anti-inflammatory drugs. Curr Opin Rheumatol 1998; 10:153.
13. Komonoff M, Grone HJ, Klein T, et al: Localization of cyclooxygenase-1 and -2 in adult and fetal human kidney: Implication for renal function. Am J Physiol 1997; 272:460.
14. Hermaszewski R, Hyllar J, Woo P: Gastro-duodenal damage due to non-steroidal anti-inflammatory drugs in children. Br J Rheumatol 1996; 32:69.
15. Blackshear JL, Napier JS, Davidman M, et al: Renal complications of nonsteroidal anti-inflammatory drugs: Identification and monitoring of those at risk. Semin Arthritis Rheum 1985; 14:163.
16. Kimberly RP: Corticosteroid and anti-inflammatory drugs. Rheum Dis Clin North Am 1988; 14:203
17. Samuelson CO, William HJ: Ibuprofen associated aseptic meningitis in systemic lupus erythematosus. West J Med 1979; 131:57.
18. Levy ML, Barron KS, Eichenfield A, et al: Naproxen induced pseudoporphyria: A distinctive photodermatitis. J Pediatr 1990; 117:660.
19. Avina-Zubieta JA, Galindo-Rodriguez G, Newman S, et al: Long-term effectiveness of anti-malarial drugs in rheumatic disease. Ann Rheum Dis 1998; 57:582.
20. Van den Bourne BEEM, Dijkmans BAC, De Rooij HH, et al: Chloroquine and hydroxychloroquine equally affect tumor necrosis factor-α, interleukin-6, interferon-gamma by peripheral blood mononuclear cells. J Rheumatol 1997; 24:55.
21. Meng XW, Feller JM, Ziegler JB, et al: Induction of apoptosis in peripheral blood lymphocytes following treatment in vitro with hydroxychloroquine. Arthritis Rheum 1997; 40:927.
22. Petri M: Hydroxychloroquine use in the Baltimore Lupus Cohort: Effects on lipids, glucose and thrombosis. Lupus 1996; 5(suppl 1):S16.
23. Grierson DJ: Hydroxychloroquine and visual screening in a rheumatology outpatient clinic. Ann Rheum Dis 1997; 56:188.
24. Levy GD, Munz SJ, Paschal J, et al: Incidence of hydroxychloroquine retinopathy in 1207 patients in a large multi-centre outpatient practice. Arthritis Rheum 1997; 40:1482.
25. Silman A, Shipley M: Ophthalmological monitoring for hydroxychloroquine toxicity: A scientific review of available data. Br J Rheumatol 1997; 36:599.
26. The Canadian Hydroxychloroquine Study Group: A randomized study of the effect of withdrawing hydroxychloroquine sulfate in systemic lupus erythematosus. N Engl J Med 1991; 324:150.
27. Platt JL, Burke BA, Fish AJ, et al: Systemic lupus erythematosus in the first two decades of life. Am J Kidney Dis 1982; 2(suppl 1):212.
28. White PH: Pediatric systemic lupus erythematosus and neonatal lupus. Rheum Dis Clin North Am 1994; 20:119.
29. Wilckens T, de Rijk R: Glucocorticoid and immune function: Unknown dimensions and new frontiers. Immunology Today 1997; 18:418.
30. Szer IS: The diagnosis and management of systemic lupus erythematosus in childhood. Pediatr Ann 1986; 15:596.
31. Sloan RP, Schwartz MM, Kobert SM, et al: Long-term outcome in systemic lupus erythematosus membranous glomerulonephritis. Lupus Nephritis Collaborative Study Group. J Am Soc Nephrol 1996; 7:299.
32. Evanson S, Passo MH, Aldo-Benson MA, et al: Methyl prednisolone pulse therapy for non-renal lupus erythematosus. Ann Rheum Dis 1980; 39:377.
33. Ballou SP, Kahn MA, Kushner I: Intravenous pulse methylprednisolone in lupus erythematosus: A prospective evaluation. J Rheumatol 1985; 12:944.
34. Hanmer O, Saltissi D: Response of acute cerebral lupus in childhood to pulse methylprednisolone in reduced dosage. Ann Rheum Dis 1986; 45:606.
35. Barron KS, Person DA, Brewer EJ, et al: Pulse methylprednisolone therapy in diffuse proliferative lupus nephritis. J Pediatr 1982; 101:137.
36. McDougal BA, Whittier FC, Cross DE: Sudden death after bolus steroid therapy for acute rejection. Transplant Proc 1976; 8:493.
37. Kimberly RP: Pulse methylprednisolone in SLE. Clin Rheum Dis 1982; 8:261.
38. Melo-Gomes JA: Problems related to systemic glucocorticoid therapy in children. J Rheumatol 1993; 20(suppl 37):35.
39. Urowitz MB, Gladman DD: Late mortality in SLE. "The price we pay for control." J Rheumatol 1980; 7:412.
40. Trapani S, Civinini R, Ermini M, et al: Osteoporosis in juvenile systemic lupus erythematosus: A longitudinal study on the effect of steroids on bone mineral density. Rheumatol Int 1998; 18:45.
41. Mok CC, Lau CS, Wong RW: Risk factors for avascular bone necrosis in systemic lupus erythematosus. Br J Rheumatol 1998; 37:895.
42. Adachi JD, Bensen WG, Bianchi F, et al: Vitamin D and calcium in the prevention of corticosteroid induced osteoporosis. J Rheumatol 1996; 23:995.
43. Briggs WA, Choi MJ, Scheel PJ: Successful mycophenolate mofetil treatment of glomerular disease. Am J Kidney Dis 1998; 31:213.
44. Musso M, Porretto F, Crescimanno A, et al: Autologous peripheral blood stem and progenitor (CD34+) cell transplantation for systemic lupus erythematosus complicated by Evans syndrome. Lupus 1998; 7:492.
45. Klipple JH, Austin HA, Balow JE, et al: Studies of immunosuppressive drugs in the treatment of lupus nephritis. Rheum Dis Clin North Am 1987; 13:47.
46. Grimbacher B, Huber M, Von Kempius J, et al: Successful treatment of gastrointestinal vasculitis due to systemic lupus erythematosus with intravenous pulse cyclophosphamide: A clinical case report and review of the literature. Br J Rheumatol 1998; 37:1023.
47. Mok CC, Lau CS, Chan EY, et al: Acute transverse myelopathy in systemic lupus erythematosus: Clinical presentation, treatment, and outcome. J Rheumatol 1998; 25:467.
48. McCune J, Singer NG: Immunosuppressive drug treatment. Curr Opin Rheumatol 1997; 9:191.
49. Yule SM, Buddy AV, Cole M, et al: Cyclophosphamide metabolism in children. Cancer Res 1995; 55:803.
50. McCurdy DK, Lehman TJA, Bernstein BH, et al: Lupus nephritis: Controlled trial of prednisone and cytotoxic drugs. Pediatrics 1992; 89:240.

51. Godfrey T, Kamashta MA, Hughes GRV: Therapeutic advances in systemic lupus erythematosus. Curr Opin Rheumatol 1998; 10:435.

52. Silverman E: What's new in the treatment of pediatric SLE. J Rheumatol 1996; 23:1657.

53. Szer IS: Clinical development in the management of lupus in the neonate, child, and adolescent. Curr Opin Rheumatol 1998; 10:431.

54. Lehman TJA: Current concepts in immunosuppressive drug therapy of systemic lupus erythematosus. J Rheumatol 1992; 33(suppl 2):20.

55. Wagner-Weiner L, Magilavy DB, Emery HM: Flare of childhood lupus after discontinuing treatment with intravenous pulse cyclophosphamide (IVCY). Arthritis Rheum 1988; 31(suppl):s117.

56. Plotz PH, Klipple JH, Decker JL, et al: Bladder complications in patients receiving cyclophosphamide for systemic lupus erythematosus or rheumatoid arthritis. Ann Intern Med 1979; 91:221.

57. Mok CC, Lau CS, Wong RWS: Risk factors for ovarian failure in patients with systemic lupus erythematosus receiving cyclophosphamide therapy. Arthritis Rheum 1998; 41:831.

58. Fox DA, McCune WJ: Immunosuppressive drug therapy of systemic lupus erythematosus. Rheum Dis Clin North Am 1994; 20:265.

59. Martin F, Lauwerys B, Lefebvre C, et al: Side effects of intravenous cyclophosphamide pulse therapy. Lupus 1997; 6:254.

60. Carden PA, Mitchell SL, Waters KD, et al: Prevention of cyclophosphamide/cytarabine-induced emesis with ondansetron in children with leukemia. J Clin Oncol 1990; 8:1531.

61. Hahlen K, Quintana E, Pinkerton CR, et al: A randomized comparison of intravenously administered granisetron versus chlorpromazine plus dexamethasone in the prevention of ifosfamide-induced emesis in children. J Pediatr 1995; 126:309.

62. Hows JM, Mehta A, Ward L, et al: Comparison of mesna with forced diuresis to prevent cyclophosphamide-induced haemorrhagic cystitis in marrow transplantation: A prospective randomized study. Br J Cancer 1984; 50:753.

63. Stiehm ER: Human intravenous immunoglobulin in primary and secondary antibody deficiencies. Pediatr Infect Dis J 1997; 16:696.

64. Kirshon B, Wasserstrum N, Willis, et al: Teratogenic effects of first trimester cyclophosphamide therapy. Obstet Gynecol 1988; 72:462.

65. Ramsey-Goldman R, Mientus JM, Kutzer JE, et al: Pregnancy outcome in women with systemic lupus erythematosus treated with immunosuppressive drugs. J Rheumatol 1993; 20:1152.

66. Rosenthal NS, Farhi DC: Myelodysplastic syndromes and acute myeloid leukemia in connective tissue disease after single-agent chemotherapy. Am J Clin Pathol 1996; 106:676.

67. Fox DA, McCune WJ: Immunosuppressive drug therapy for systemic lupus erythematosus. Rheum Dis North Am 1994; 20:265.

68. Sztenbok M, Stewart A, Diamond H, et al: Azathioprine in the treatment of systemic lupus erythematosus: A controlled study. Arthritis Rheum 1971; 14:639.

69. Tsokos GC, Caughman SW, Klipple JH: Successful treatment of generalized discoid skin lesions with azathioprine: Its use in patients with systemic lupus erythematosus. Arch Dermatol 1985; 121:1323.

70. Slack S, Furst DE: Disease modifying antirheumatic drugs. Drugs of Today 1996; 32:463.

71. Alexon E, Brandt KD: Acute leukemia after azathioprine treatment of connective tissue disease. Am J Med Sci 1977; 273:335.

72. Balow JE: Lupus as a renal disease. Hosp Pract 1988; 23:129.

73. Kornstein BN: Molecular therapeutics: Methotrexate and its mechanism of action. Arthritis Rheum 1996; 39:1951.

74. Ravelli A, Ballardini G, Viola S, et al: Methotrexate therapy in refractory pediatric onset systemic lupus erythematosus. J Rheumatol 1998; 25:572.

75. Rahman P, Humphrey-Murto S, Gladman D, et al: Efficacy and tolerability of methotrexate in antimalarial resistant lupus arthritis. J Rheumatol 1998; 25:243.

76. Cameiro JR, Sato EL: Prospective double blind randomized clinical trial comparing methotrexate and placebo in SLE. Arthritis Rheum 1997; 40(suppl):S324.

77. Kipen Y, Littlejohn G, Morand E: Methotrexate use in SLE. Lupus 1997; 6:385.

78. Shiroky JB, Neville C, Esdaile JM, et al: Low dose methotrexate with leucovorin (folinic acid) in the management of rheumatoid arthritis: Results of a multicenter randomized, double blind, placebo controlled trial. Arthritis Rheum 1993; 36:795.

79. Singsen BH, Goldbach-Mansky R: Methotrexate in the treatment of juvenile rheumatoid arthritis and other pediatric rheumatoid and non-rheumatic disorders. Rheum Dis Clin North Am 1997; 23:811.

80. Padeh S, Sharon N, Schiby G, et al: Hodgkin's lymphoma in systemic onset juvenile rheumatoid arthritis after treatment with low dose methotrexate. J Rheumatol 1997; 24:2035.

81. Kamel OW, Van De Rijn M, Weiss LM, et al: Brief report: Reversible lymphomas associated with Epstein-Barr virus occurring during methotrexate therapy for rheumatoid arthritis and dermatomyositis. N Engl J Med 1993; 328:1317.

82. Wallace DJ, Podell TE, Weiner JM, et al: Lupus nephritis: Experience with 230 patients in a private practice from 1950 to 1980. Am J Med 1982; 72:209.

83. Lipsky JJ: Mycophenolate mofetil (drug profile). Lancet 1996; 348:1357.

84. Sievers TM, Rossi SJ, Ghobrial RM, et al: Mycophenolate mofetil. Pharmacotherapy 1997;17:1178.

85. Birkeland SA, Larsen KE, Rhor N: Pediatric renal transplant without steroids. Pediatr Nephrol 1998; 12:87.

86. Nowack R, Birck R, van der Woude FJ: Mycophenolate mofetil for systemic vasculitis and IgA nephropathy. Lancet 1997; 349:774.

87. Zimmer-Molsberger B, Knauf W, Thiel E: Mycophenolate mofetil for severe autoimmune hemolytic anemia. Lancet 1997; 350:1003.

88. Lupus Plasmapheresis Study Group: Plasmapheresis and subsequent pulse cyclophosphamide versus pulse cyclophosphamide alone in severe lupus: Design of the LPSG trial. J Clin Apheresis 1991; 6:40.

89. Wallace D, Goldfinger D, Pepkowitz SH, et al: A prospective controlled trial of pulse synchronization cyclophosphamide/apheresis for proliferative lupus nephritis. Arthritis Rheum 1997; 40(suppl):S58.

90. Schroeder J, Schwab U, Zuener R, et al: Plasmapheresis and subsequent pulse cyclophosphamide in severe SLE: Preliminary results of the LPSG trial. Arthritis Rheum 1997; 40(suppl):S325.

91. Hess DC, Kapil S, Awad E: Thrombotic thrombocytopenic purpura in systemic lupus erythematosus and antiphospholipid antibodies: Effective treatment with plasma exchange and immunosuppression. J Rheumatol 1992; 19:1474.

92. Smith GM, Leyland MJ: Plasma exchange for cerebral lupus erythematosus [Letter]. Lancet 1987; 1:103.

93. Heyneman CA, Gudger CA, Beckwith JV: Intravenous immune globulin for inducing remissions in systemic lupus erythematosus. Ann Pharmacother 1997; 31:242.

94. Dalakas MC: Mechanism of action of intravenous immunoglobulin and therapeutic considerations in the treatment of autoimmune neurologic disease. Neurology 1998; 51:s2.

95. DeKeyser F, DeKeyser H, Kazatchkine MD, et al: Pooled human immunoglobulins contain anti-idiotypes with reactivity against the SLE-associated 4B4 cross-reactive idiotype. Clin Exp Rheumatol 1996; 14:587.

96. Barron KS, Sher MR, Silverman ED: Intravenous immunoglobulin therapy: Magic or black magic. J Rheumatol 1992; 19(suppl 33):94.

97. Hashkes PJ, Lovell DJ: Vasculitis in systemic lupus erythematosus following intravenous immunoglobulin therapy. Clin Exp Rheumatol 1996; 14:673.

98. Salmon SE, Dalton WS: Relevance of multidrug resistance to rheumatoid arthritis: Development of a new therapeutic hypothesis. J Rheumatol 1996; 44:97.

99. Schreiber SL, Crabtree GR: The mechanism of action of cyclosporin A and FK506. Immunology Today 1992; 13:136.

100. Caccavo D, Lagana B, Mitterhofer A, et al: Long term treatment of systemic lupus erythematosus with cyclosporin A. Arthritis Rheum 1997; 40:27.

101. Sugiyama M, Ogasawara H, Kaneko H, et al: Effect of extremely low dose cyclosporine treatment on the thrombocytopenia in systemic lupus erythematosus. Lupus 1998; 7:53.

102. Fu LW, Yang LY, Chen WP, et al: Clinical efficacy of cyclosporin A Neoral in the treatment of pediatric lupus nephritis with heavy proteinuria. Br J Rheumatol 1998; 37:217.

103. Dostal C, Tesar V, Rychlik I, et al: Effect of 1 year cyclosporin A treatment on the activity of renal involvement of systemic lupus erythematosus: A pilot study. Lupus 1998; 7:29.

104. Singer NG, McCune WJ: Update on immunosuppressive therapy. Curr Opin Rheumatol 1998; 10:169.

105. Hahn BH: The potential role of autologous stem cell transplantation in patients with systemic lupus erythematosus. J Rheumatol 1997; 48:89.

106. Burt RK, Traynor AE, Pope R, et al: Treatment of autoimmune disease by intense immunosuppressive conditioning and autologous hematopoietic stem cell transplantation. Blood 1998; 92:3505.

107. Marmont AM: Stem cell transplantation for severe autoimmune diseases: Progress and problems. Haematologica 1998; 83:733.

108. Von Scheven E, Athreya BH, Rose CD, et al: Clinical characteristics of antiphospholipid antibody syndrome in children. J Pediatr 1996; 129:339.

109. Petri M: 1998 Update on antiphospholipid antibodies. Curr Opin Rheumatol 1998; 10:426.

110. McIntyre JA, Wagenknecht DR, Suji T: Phospholipid binding plasma proteins required for antiphospholipid antibody detection: An overview. Am J Reprod Immunol 1997; 37:101.

111. Cockwell P, Tse WY, Savage CO: Activation of endothelial cells in thrombosis and vasculitis. Scand J Rheumatol 1997; 26:145.

112. Rand JH, Wu XX, Andree HAM, et al: Pregnancy loss in the antiphospholipid-antibody syndrome: A possible thrombogenic mechanism. N Engl J Med 1997; 337:154.

113. Wahl DG, Guillemin F, de Maistre E, et al: Risk for venous thrombosis related to antiphospholipid antibodies in systemic lupus erythematosus: A meta-analysis. Lupus 1997; 6:467.

114. Ravelli A, Martini A: Antiphospholipid antibody syndrome in pediatric patients. Rheum Dis Clin North Am 1997; 23:657.

115. Silverman ED, Laxer RM: Neonatal lupus erythematosus. Rheum Dis Clin North Am 1997; 23:599.

116. Brucato A, Franceschini F, Buyon JP: Neonatal lupus: Long-term outcomes of mothers and children and recurrence rate. Clin Exp Rheumatol 1997; 15:467.

117. Olsen NY, Lindsley CB: Neonatal lupus syndrome. Am J Dis Child 1987; 141:908.

118. Rider LG, Buyon JP, Rutledge J, et al: Treatment of neonatal lupus: Case report and review of the literature. J Rheumatol 1993; 20:1208.

119. Cabanas F, Pellicer A, Valverde E, et al: Central nervous system vasculopathy in neonatal luppus erythematosus. Pediatr Neurol 1996; 15:124.

120. Crowley E, Frieden IJ: Neonatal lupus erythematosus: An unusual congenital presentation with cutaneous atrophy, erosions, alopecia and pancytopenia. Pediatr Dermatol 1998; 15:38.

121. Buyon JP: Autoantibodies reactive with Ro(SSA) and anti-La(SSB)and pregnancy. J Rheumatol 1997; 24(suppl 50):12.

122. Finkelstein Y, Adler Y, Harel L, et al: Anti-Ro(SSA) and anti-La(SSB) antibodies and complete congenital heart block. Ann Med Interne (Paris) 1997; 148:205.

123. Taylor-Albert E, Reichlin M, Toews WT, et al: Delayed dilated cardiomyopathy as a manifestation of neonatal lupus: Case reports, autoantibody analysis, and management. Pediatrics 1997; 99:733.

124. Buyon JP, Hiebert R, Copel J, et al: Autoimmune-associated congenital heart block: Demographics, mortality, morbidity and recurrence rates obtained from a national neonatal lupus registry. J Am Coll Cardiol 1998; 31:1658.

125. Horsfall AC, Li JM, Maini RN: Placental and fetal cardiac laminin are targets for cross-reacting autoantibodies from mothers of children with congenital heart block. J Autoimmunity 1996; 4:561.

126. Boutjdir M, Chen L, Zhang ZH, et al: Arrhythmogenicity of IgG and anti-52-Kd SSA/Ro affinity-purified antibodies from mothers of children with congenital heart block. Circ Res 1997; 80:354.

127. Silverman ED: Congenital heart block and neonatal lupus erythematosus: Prevention is the goal [Editorial]. J Rheumatol 1993; 20:1101.

128. Deloof E, Devlieger H, Van Hoestendberghe R, et al: Management with a staged approach of the premature hydropic fetus due to complete congenital heart block. Eur J Pediatr 1997; 156:521.

129. Hubscher O, Carillo D, Reichlin M: Congenital heart block and subsequent connective tissue disorder in adolescence. Lupus 1997; 6:283.

130. Rider LG, Miller FW: Classification and treatment of the juvenile idiopathic inflammatory myopathies. Rheum Dis Clin North Am 1997; 23:619.

131. Ansell BM: Juvenile dermatomyositis. Rheum Dis Clin North Am 1991; 17:931.

132. Pachman LM, Hayford JR, Chung A, et al: Juvenile dermatomyositis at diagnosis: Clinical characteristics of 79 children. J Rheumatol 1998; 25:1198.

133. Dalakas MC: Controlled studies with high-dose intravenous immunoglobulin in the treatment of dermatomyositis, inclusion body myositis and polymyositis. Neurology 1998; 51(suppl 5):s37.

134. Olson NY, Lindsley CB: Adjunctive use of hydroxychloroquine in childhood dermatomyositis. J Rheumatol 1989; 16:1545.

135. Bloom BJ, Tucker LB, Klein-Gitelman M, et al: Worsening of the rash of juvenile dermatomyositis with hydroxychloroquine therapy. J Rheumatol 1994; 21:2171.

136. Spencer CH, Hanson V, Singsen BH, et al: Course of treated juvenile dermatomyositis. J Pediatr 1984; 105:399.

137. Miller LC, Sisson BA, Tucker LB, et al: Methotrexate treatment of recalcitrant childhood dermatomyositis. Arthritis Rheum 1992; 35:1143.

138. Zieglschmid-Adams ME, Pandya AG, Cohen SB, et al: Treatment of dermatomyositis with methotrexate. J Am Acad Dermatol 1995; 32:754.

139. Villalba L, Hicks JE, Adams EM, et al: Treatment of refractory myositis. Arthritis Rheum 1998; 41:392.

140. Reiff A, Rawlings DJ, Shaham B, et al: Preliminary evidence of cyclosporin A as an alternative in the treatment of recalcitrant juvenile rheumatoid arthritis and juvenile dermatomyositis. J Rheumatol 1997; 24:2436.

141. Zeller V, Cohen P, Prieur AM, et al: Cyclosporin A therapy in refractory juvenile dermatomyositis: Experience and long term followup of 6 cases. J Rheumatol 1996; 23:1424.

142. Ettenger RE, Smith HT, Kaiser B, et al: Use of Neoral in pediatric renal transplantation. Transplant Proc 1996; 28:2257.

143. Bunch TW: Prednisone and azathioprine for polymyositis: Long term follow up. Arthritis Rheum 1981; 24:45.

144. Vedanarayan V, Subramony SH, Ray LI, et al: Treatment of childhood dermatomyositis with high dose intravenous immunoglobulin. Pediatr Neurol 1995; 13:336.

145. Sansome A, Dubowitz V: Intravenous immunoglobulin in juvenile dermatomyositis: Four year review of nine cases. Arch Dis Child 1995; 72:25.

146. Sinoway PA, Callen JP: Chlorambucil: An effective corticosteroid-sparing agent for patients with recalcitrant dermatomyositis. Arthritis Rheum 1993; 36:319.

147. Mastaglia FL, Phillips BA, Zilko P: Treatment of inflammatory myopathies. Muscle Nerve 1997; 20:651.

148. Callen JP: Immunosuppressive and cytotoxic drugs: Uses in the dermatology patient. Adv Dermatol 1990; 5:3.

149. De Vita S, Fossaluzza V: Treatment of idiopathic inflammatory myopathies with cyclophosphamide pulses: Clinical experience and review of the literature. Acta Neurol Belg 1992; 92:215.

150. Ng YT, Ouvrier RA, Wu T: Drug therapy in juvenile dermatomyositis: Follow up study. J Child Neurol 1998; 13:109.

151. Brewer EJ Jr, Giannini EH, Rossen RD, et al: Plasma exchange therapy of childhood onset dermatomyositis patient. Arthritis Rheum 1980; 23:509.

152. Dau PC, Bennington JL: Plasmapheresis in childhood dermatomyositis. J Pediatr 1981; 98:237.

153. Miller FW, Leitman SF, Cronin ME, et al: Controlled trial of plasma exchange and leukapheresis in polymyositis and dermatomyositis. N Engl J Med 1992; 326:1380.

154. Maugars YM, Berthelot JM, Abbas AA, et al: Long-term prognosis of 69 patients with dermatomyositis or polymyositis. Clin Exp Rheumatol 1996; 14:263.

155. Metzger AL, Singer FR, Bluestone R, et al: Failure of disodium etindronate in calcinosis due to dermatomyositis and scleroderma. N Engl J Med 1974; 291:1294.

156. Lassoued K, Saiag P, Anglade MC, et al: Failure of warfarin in treatment of calcinosis universalis. Am J Med 1988; 84:795.

157. Palmieri GM, Sebes JI, Aelion JA, et al: Treatment of calcinosis with diltiazem. Arthritis Rheum 1995; 38:1646.

158. Olivieri MG, Palermo R, Mautalen C, et al: Regression of calcinosis during diltiazem treatment in juvenile dermatomyositis. J Rheumatol 1996; 23:2152.

159. Spindler A, Berman A, Braier M, et al: Lithotripsy: A novel therapeutic approach for calcific tendinitis refractory to conventional therapy. Arthritis Rheum 1996; 39(suppl):134.

160. Fuchs D, Fruchter L, Fishel B, et al: Colchicine suppression of local inflammation due to calcinosis in dermatomyositis and progressive systemic sclerosis. Clin Rheumatol 1986; 5:527.

161. Michel BA: Classification of vasculitis. Curr Opin Rheumatol 1992; 4:3.

162. Bajema IM, Christian-Hagen E: Evolving concepts about the role of antineutrophil cytoplasm antibodies in systemic vasculitides. Curr Opin Rheumatol 1999; 11:34.

163. Langford CA: The diagnostic utility of c-ANCA in Wegener's granulomatosis. Cleve Clin J Med 1998; 65:135.

164. Lesavre P, Kyndt X, Vanhille P, et al: Serial ANCA testing has limited value during the follow-up of disease activity in patients with ANCA associated vasculitis. Sarcoidosis Vasc Diffuse Lung Dis 1996; 13:246.

165. Valentini RP, Smoyer WE, Sedman AB, et al: Outcome of antineutrophil cytoplasmic autoantibodies-positive glomerulonephritis and vasculitis in children: A single-center experience. J Peds 1998; 132:325.

166. Coppo R, Cirina P, Amore A, et al: Properties of circulating IgA molecules in Henoch-Schönlein purpura nephritis with focus on neutrophil cytoplasmic antigen IgA binding (IgA-ANCA): New insight into a debated issue. Nephrol Dial Transplant 1997; 12:2269.

167. Szer IS: Henoch-Schönlein purpura. Curr Opin Rheumatol 1994; 6:25.

168. Mintzer CO, Nussinovitch M, Danziger Y, et al: Scrotal involvement in Henoch-Schönlein purpura in children. Scand J Urol Nephrol 1998; 32:138.

169. Coppo R, Mazzucco G, Cagnoli L, et al: Long term prognosis of Henoch-Schönlein nephritis in adults and children. Nephrol Dial Transplant 1997; 12:2277.

170. Choong CK, Kimble RM, Pease P, et al: Colo-colic intussusception in Henoch-Schönlein purpura. Pediatr Surg Int 1998; 14:173.

171. Lanzkowsky S, Lanzkowsky L, Lanzkowsky P: Henoch-Schönlein purpura. Pediatr Rev 1992; 13:130.

172. Emery H, Carter W, Schaler SG: Henoch-Schönlein vasculitis. Arthritis Rheum 1977; 20:385.

173. Gross WL: New concepts in treatment protocols for severe systemic vasculitis. Curr Opin Rheumatol 1999; 11:41.

174. Mollica F, Li Volti S, Garozzo R, et al: Effectiveness of early prednisone treatment in preventing the development of nephropathy in anaphylactoid purpura. Eur J Pediatr 1992; 151:140.

175. Salisbury FT: Corticosteroid therapy does not prevent nephritis in Henoch-Schönlein purpura. Pediatr Nephrol 1993; 7:69.

176. Mat C, Yurdakul S, Tuzuner N, et al: Small vessel vasculitis and vasculitis confined to skin. Baillieres Clin Rheumatol 1997; 11:237.

177. Bergstein J, Leiser J, Andreoli SP: Response of crescentic Henoch-Schönlein purpura nephritis to corticosteroid and azathioprine therapy. Clin Nephrol 1998; 49:9.

178. Schmaldeinst S, Winkler S, Breiteneder S, et al: Severe nephrotic syndrome in a patient with Schönlein-Henoch purpura: A complete remission after cyclosporin A. Nephrol Dial Transplant 1997; 12:790.

179. Allmaras E, Nowack R, Andrassy K, et al: Rapidly progressive IgA nephropathy with anti-myeloperoxidase antibodies benefit from immunosuppression. Clin Nephrol 1997; 48:269.

180. Landing BH, Larson EJ: Are infantile periarteritis nodosa with coronary involvement and fatal mucocutaneous lymph node syndrome the same? Comparison of 20 patients from North

181. Leung DYM, Schlievert PM, Meissner HC: The immunopathogenesis and management of Kawasaki syndrome. Arthritis Rheum 1998; 41:1538.

182. Rowley AH, Shulman ST: Kawasaki syndrome. Clin Microbiol Rev 1998; 11:405.

183. Kato H, Ichinose E, Yoshioka F, et al: Fate of coronary aneurysms in Kawasaki disease: Serial coronary angiography and long-term follow-up study. Am J Cardiol 1982; 49:1758.

184. Akagi T, Rose V, Benson LN, et al: Outcome of coronary artery aneurysms in patients after Kawasaki disease. J Pediatr 1992; 121:689.

185. Daniels SR, Specker B, Capannari TE, et al: Correlates of coronary artery aneurysm formation and prevention in patients with Kawasaki disease. Pediatr Res 1986; 20:169A.

186. Kato H, Koike S, Yokoyama T: Kawasaki disease: Effect of treatment on coronary artery involvement. Pediatrics 1979; 63:175.

187. Wright DA, Newburger JW, Baker A, et al: Treatment of immune globulin-resistant Kawasaki disease with pulse dose of corticosteroids. J Pediatr 1996; 128:146.

188. Barron KS: Kawasaki disease: Epidemiology, late prognosis, and therapy. Rheum Dis Clin North Am 1991; 17:907.

189. Shetty AK, Homsi O, Ward K, et al: Massive lymphadenopathy and airway obstruction in a child with Kawasaki disease: Success with pulse steroid therapy. J Rheumatol 1998; 25:1215.

190. Rowley AH, Duffy CE, Shulman ST: Prevention of giant coronary aneurysms in Kawasaki disease by intravenous gamma globulin therapy. J Pediatr 1989; 114:1065.

191. Newburger JW, Sanders SP, Burns JC, et al: Left ventricular contractility and function in Kawasaki syndrome: Effect of intravenous gamma globulin. Circulation 1989; 79:1237.

192. Newburger JW, Takahashi M, Beiser AS, et al: A single intravenous infusion of gamma globulin as compared with four infusions in the treatment of acute Kawasaki syndrome. N Engl J Med 1991; 324:1633.

193. Durongpisitkul K, Gururaj VJ, Part JM, et al: The prevention of coronary artery aneurysm in Kawasaki disease: A meta-analysis on the efficacy of aspirin and immunoglobulin treatment. Pediatrics 1995; 96:1057.

194. Takei S, Arora YK, Walker SM: Intravenous immunoglobulin contains specific antibodies inhibitory to activation of T cells by staphylococcal toxin superantigens. J Clin Invest 1993; 91:602.

195. Gernsoy WM: Long-term issues in Kawasaki disease [Editorial]. J Pediatr 1992; 12:121:731.

196. Kato H, Sugimura T, Akagi T, et al: Long-term consequences of Kawasaki disease: a 10–21 year follow-up study of 594 patients. Circulation 1996; 94:1379.

197. Dajani AS, Taubert KA, Gerber MA, et al: Diagnosis and therapy of Kawasaki disease in children. Circulation 1993; 87:1776.

198. Dillon MJ: Childhood vasculitis [Review]. Lupus 1998; 7:259.

199. Till SH, Amos RS: Long-term follow-up of juvenile-onset cutaneous polyarteritis nodosa associated with streptococcal infection. Br J Rheumatol 1997; 36:909.

200. Mocan H, Mocan MC, Peru H, et al: Cutaneous polyarteritis nodosa in a child and review of the literature. Acta Pediatr 1998; 87:3.

201. Ozen S, Besbas N, Saatci U, et al: Diagnostic criteria for polyarteritis nodosa in childhood. J Pediatr 1992; 120:206.

202. Hagen EC, Daha MR, Hermans J, et al: The diagnostic value of standardized assays for anti-neutrophil cytoplasmic antibodies (ANCA) in idiopathic systemic vasculitis: Results of an international collaborative study. Kidney Int 1998; 53:743.

203. Reynold EW, Weinberg AG, Fink CW, et al: Polyarteritis in children. Am J Dis Child 1976; 130:534.

204. Guillevin L, Jarrousse B, Lok C, et al: Long-term follow-up after treatment of polyarteritis nodosa and Churg-Strauss angiitis with comparison of steroids, plasma exchange and cyclophosphamide to steroids and plasma exchange: A prospective randomized trial of 71 patients. J Rheumatol 1991; 18:567.

205. Guillevin L, Fain O, Lhote F, et al: Lack of superiority of steroids plus plasma exchange to steroids alone in the treatment of polyarteritis nodosa and Churg-Strauss syndrome: A prospec-

tive, randomized trial in 78 patients. Arthritis Rheum 1992; 35:208.

206. Savage COS, Harper L, Adu D: Primary systemic vasculitis. Lancet 1997; 349:553.

207. Jennette JC, Falk RJ: Small-vessel vasculitis. N Engl J Med 1997; 337:1512.

208. Blau EB, Morris RF, Yunis EJ: Polyarteritis nodosa in older children. Pediatrics 1977; 60:227.

209. Gianviti A, Trompeter RS, Barrat TM, et al: Retrospective study of plasma exchange in patients with idiopathic rapidly progressive glomerulonephritis and vasculitis. Arch Dis Child 1996; 75:186.

210. Rottem M, Fauci AS, Hallahan CW, et al: Wegener's granulomatosis in children and adolescents: Clinical presentation and outcome. J Pediatr 1993; 122:26.

211. Cassan SM, Coles DT, Harrison EG Jr: The concept of limited forms of Wegener's granulomatosis. Am J Med 1970; 49:366.

212. Gottleib BS, Miller LC, Ilowite NT, et al: Methotrexate treatment of Wegener's granulomatosis in children: Clinical and laboratory observations. J Pediatr 1996; 129:604.

213. Van der Woude FJ, Rassmussen N, Lobato S, et al: Antibodies against neutrophils and monocytes: Tool for diagnosis and marker for disease activity in Wegener's granulomatosis. Lancet 1985; 1:425.

214. Cohen Tervaert JW, Huitema MG, Hene RJ, et al: Prevention of relapses in Wegener's granulomatosis by treatment based on antineutrophil cytoplasmic antibody titer. Lancet 1990; 336:709.

215. Moorthy AV, Chesney RW, Segar WE, et al: Wegener's granulomatosis in childhood: Prolonged survival following cytotoxic therapy. J Pediatr 1977; 91:616.

216. Fauci AS, Haynes BF, Katz P, et al: Wegener's granulomatosis: Prospective clinical and therapeutic experience with 85 patients for 21 years. Ann Intern Med 1983; 98:76.

217. Hoffman GS, Kerr GS, Leavitt RY, et al: Wegener's granulomatosis: An analysis of 158 patients. Ann Intern Med 1992; 116:488.

218. Guillevin L, Cordier JF, Lhote F, et al: A prospective, multicenter, randomized trial comparing steroids and pulse cyclophosphamide in the treatment of generalized Wegener's granulomatosis. Arthritis Rheum 1997; 40:2187.

219. Hoffman GS. Treatment of Wegener's granulomatosis: Time to change the standard of care? Arthritis Rheum 1997; 40:2099.

220. Yuasa K, Tokitsu M, Goto H, et al: Wegener's granulomatosis: Diagnosis by transbronchial lung biopsy, evaluation by gallium scintigraphy and treatment with sulfamethoxazole/trimetoprim. Am J Med 1988; 84:371.

221. Hoffman GS, Leavitt RY, Kerr GS, et al: The treatment of Wegener's granulomatosis with glucocorticoids and methotrexate. Arthritis Rheum 1992; 35:1322.

222. Langford CA: Use of cytotoxic agents and cyclosporine in the treatment of autoimmune diseases. Ann Intern Med 1998; 129:49.

223. Lehman TJ: Systemic and localized scleroderma in children [Review]. Curr Opin Rheumatol 1996; 8:576.

224. Menni S, Marzano AV, Passoni E: Neurological abnormalities in two patients with facial hemiatrophy and sclerosis coexisting with morphea. Pedtiatr Dermatol 1997; 14:113.

225. Moreno Alvarez MJ, Lazaro MA, Espada G, et al: Linear scleroderma and melorheostosis: Case presentation and literature review [Review]. Clin Rheumatol 1996; 15:389.

226. Tuffanelli DL: Localized scleroderma. Semin Cutan Med Surg 1998; 17:27.

227. Foldvari I: Progressive linear scleroderma and morphea in a child [Insights]. J Pediatr 1998; 133:308.

228. Uziel Y, Krafchik BR, Feldman B, et al: Serum soluble interleukin-2 receptor (S-IL2R) levels in localized scleroderma. Arthritis Rheum 1993; 36(suppl):S54.

229. Falanga V, Medsger TA Jr: d-Penicillamine in the treatment of localized scleroderma. Arch Dermatol 1990; 126:609.

230. Kunkle RW, Restronk A, Drachman DB, et al: The pathophysiology of penicillamine-induced myasthenia gravis. Ann Neurol 1986; 20:740.

231. Van den Hoogen FH, Boerbooms AM, Swaak AJ, et al: Comparison of methotrexate with placebo in the treatment of systemic sclerosis: A 24 week randomized double-blind trial, followed by a 24 week observational trial. Br J Rheumatol 1996; 35:364.

232. Bernstein BH, Singsen BH, Kent JT, et al: Reflex neurovascular dystrophy in childhood. J Pediatr 1978; 93:211.

233. Szer IS: Musculoskeletal pain syndromes that affect adolescents. Arch Pediatr Adolesc Med 1996; 150:740.

234. Sherry DD, McGuire T, Mellins E, et al: Psychosomatic musculoskeletal pain in childhood: Clinical and psychological analysis of 100 children. Pediatrics 1991; 88:1093.

235. Sherry DD, Weisman R: Psychologic aspects of childhood reflex sympathetic dystrophy. Pediatrics 1988; 81:572.

236. Siegel DM, Janeway D, Baum J: Fibromyalgia syndrome in children and adolescents: Clinical features at presentation and status at follow-up. Pediatrics 1998; 101:377.

237. Wolfe F, Smythe HA, Yunus MB, et al: The American College of Rheumatology 1990 criteria for the classification of fibromyalgia. Arthritis Rheum 1990; 33:160.

238. Yunus MB, Masi AT: Juvenile primary fibromyalgia syndrome: A clinical study of 33 patients and matched normal controls. Arthritis Rheum 1985; 28:138

239. Buskila D: Fibromyalgia, chronic fatigue syndrome, and myofascial pain syndrome. Curr Opin Rheumatol 1999; 11:119.

240. Gedalia A, Press J, Klein M, et al: Joint hypermobility and fibromyalgia in school children. Ann Rheum Dis 1993; 52:494.

241. Reid GJ, Lang BA, McGrath PJ: Primary juvenile fibromyalgia: Psychological adjustment, family functioning, coping and functional disability. Arthritis Rheum 1997; 40:752.

242. Schanberg LE, Keefe FJ, Lefebvre JC, et al: Social content of pain in children with juvenile fibromyalgia syndrome: Parental pain history and family environment. Clin J Pain 1998; 14:107.

243. Walco GA, Ilowite NT: Cognitive-behavioral intervention for juvenile primary fibromyalgia syndrome. J Rheumatol 1992; 19:1617.

244. Godfrey RG: A guide to the understanding and use of tricyclic antidepressants in the overall management of fibromyalgia and other chronic pain syndromes. Arch Intern Med 1996; 156:1047.

Since McCarty and Hollander first used polarized microscopy to identify monosodium urate (MSU) crystals in synovial fluids of patients with acute gout in 1961,[1] other crystals have been found to induce a similar inflammatory synovial reaction, particularly calcium pyrophosphate dihydrate (CPPD) and basic calcium phosphate (BCP) (Table 35–1). The pathophysiology of the synovitis induced by these crystals is not completely understood, and crystalline deposits may be asymptomatic. Self-limited acute attacks of monarthritis or polyarthritis are the most common presentation of gout and pseudogout in particular. However, in many patients, a chronic and destructive arthritis results after years of crystal deposition and inflammation. For a comprehensive review of the pathophysiology and diagnosis of these conditions, the reader is referred to Kelley and colleagues.[2, 3] This chapter reviews a practical approach to the management of patients with crystal-associated arthritis, with particular attention to patients who require individualized management strategies because of important underlying comorbid conditions.

## GOUT

Gout is a syndrome that results from tissue deposition of MSU crystals. Chronic hyperuricemia is considered necessary for the development of the clinical syndrome. In some persons, chronic hyperuricemia results in MSU crystal deposition in and around the joints. These deposits may remain unnoticed and asymptomatic, or they may be associated with recurrent attacks of self-limited arthritis. The clinical spectrum of gout or MSU deposition includes the following: (1) chronic hyperuricemia, (2) asymptomatic urate deposition, (3) acute gouty arthritis, (4) intercritical gout, (5) tophaceous gout and chronic arthritis, and (6) urolithiasis and urate nephropathy.

Uric acid is the final product of purine metabolism in human beings. Most other animals produce uricase, which breaks down uric acid into allantoin and carbon dioxide, resulting in much lower uric acid values. Humans do not produce uricase in significant amounts. In vitro studies have shown that uric acid behaves as a powerful antioxidant, and the higher levels found in humans may be protective against degenerative diseases and other disorders. At 37° C, the saturation value of urate in plasma is approximately 7.0 mg/100 mL. Hyperuricemia is defined as a serum urate level higher than 7.0 mg/100 mL by the uricase method, or 7.5 to 8.0 mg/100 mL by automated analysis. The incidence and prevalence of gout are parallel to those of hyperuricemia in the general population. Serum urate levels increase by 1 to 2 mg/dL in males at the time of puberty, but females exhibit little change in urate levels until after menopause, when concentrations approach those seen in men.[2] Most patients with increased serum uric acid levels do not have gout, and asymptomatic hyperuricemia should not be treated. However, hyperuricemia is clearly associated with an increased risk of developing gout.[4] For example, persons with serum urate levels greater than 10 mg/dL have an annual incidence of gout of 70 per thousand and a 5-year prevalence of 30%, whereas those with levels lower than 7 mg/dL have an annual incidence of only 0.9 per thousand and a prevalence of 0.6%. Additional factors that correlate strongly with serum urate levels and the prevalence of gout in the general population include serum creatinine concentration, body weight, height, blood pressure, and alcohol intake.

Gout may be associated with factors that increase production or decrease renal excretion of uric acid (Fig. 35–1). These include obesity, myeloproliferative disorders, psoriasis, heavy alcohol intake, and renal disease. In addition, a large number of drugs can interfere with renal excretion of uric acid, including diuretics, cyclosporine, low-dose salicylates, ethambutol, pyrazinamide, niacin, and didanosine. In most patients with gout, no single underlying cause can be identified, but most patients may have a relative defect in renal excretion of uric acid, despite apparently normal renal function.[2, 5]

In classical gout, the typical initial attack occurs in a middle-aged man after years of sustained hyperuricemia and deposition of MSU in the synovial tissue. The initial attack of gout is monoarticular in 85% to 90% of patients.[2] Patients experience a sudden, exquisite, and severe pain associated with redness and swelling. Lower-extremity joints are usually affected, with approximately 60% of first attacks involving the first metatarsophalangeal joints. Attacks last from a few days to 2 to 3 weeks, with a gradual resolution of all

**TABLE 35–1**
**Potentially Phlogistic Crystals Found in or Around Joints and Associated Diseases**

| CRYSTAL | ASSOCIATED DISEASES |
|---|---|
| Monosodium urate (MSU) | MSU deposition disease: <br> Gout <br> Asymptomatic tophaceous deposits <br> Symptomatic—acute arthritis, chronic arthritis <br> Urate nephropathy |
| Calcium pyrophosphate dihydrate (CPPD) | CPPD deposition disease or pseudogout: <br> Asymptomatic chondrocalcinosis <br> Acute arthritis and chronic arthritis |
| Basic calcium phosphate (BCP) <br> (hydroxyapatite, octacalcium <br> phosphate, tricalcium phosphate) | Subcutaneous calcifications <br> Calcific periarthritis <br> Acute arthritis <br> Chronic arthritis |
| Calcium oxalate | Arthritis (patients with chronic renal failure, <br> oxalosis) <br> Acute and chronic arthritis |
| Lipid liquid | Acute and chronic arthritis |
| Long-acting microcrystalline <br> corticosteroids | Postinjection (iatrogenic synovitis) |

inflammatory signs and a return to apparent normalcy. An "intercritical" period lasting weeks to months may elapse before a new attack occurs in the same or another joint. A few patients have no further attacks. As the disease progresses untreated, attacks occur more frequently; they may be polyarticular and associated with fever and with constitutional symptoms.[6,7] Tophaceous deposits become apparent over the elbows, fingers, or other areas over the years, and a chronic polyarticular arthritis may develop, sometimes resembling rheumatoid arthritis or degenerative joint disease.

In elderly patients, the presentation of gout is more likely polyarticular, with a higher frequency of women affected. The small joints of the fingers are more commonly involved, and tophaceous deposits may occur earlier in the course of the illness, sometimes becoming apparent even before any history of acute arthritis.[8]

Synovial fluid analysis, including a careful search for crystals, is a required step in the evaluation of patients with acute arthritis. The demonstration of intracellular, strongly negative, birefringent crystals with polarized light microscopy establishes the diagnosis. Concomitant infection should be ruled out in patients with fever, comorbid conditions, purulent effusions, or attacks refractory to therapy. Normal serum urate levels may be seen in 20% to 30% of patients during acute attacks.

## Untreated Gout

Without treatment, acute gout is considered to be a self-limited process, with mild attacks lasting only several hours. Most patients begin to note improvement in 2 to 5 days. By 7 days, resolution of redness, heat, and swelling occurs in almost all patients, but only about one third of patients have total resolution of pain.[9] A minority of patients never have another attack of gout after the initial event. In one large series, 62% of pa-

tients had a recurrence within 1 year, and 78% within 2 years, while only 7% never had another attack.[10] In general, the frequency of attacks tends to increase over time; attacks become less explosive, last longer, and are more likely to be polyarticular. Visible tophaceous deposits eventually occur in 72% of patients, at an average of 11.6 years after the first attack of gout, although this interval is highly variable.[11] The rate of formation of tophi depends on both the duration and the degree of hyperuricemia.[12] Renal stones are common in patients with gout, with between 10% and 40% of patients having an attack of renal colic before the first attack of gout.[2]

## Management of Gout

The goals of therapy in gout include termination of the acute attack, prevention of further attacks in the subsequent several weeks, assessment for associated and contributing factors, and consideration of long-term hypouricemic therapy. Each aspect of therapy should be considered separately, and there should be no confusion between efforts to suppress inflammation in the acute setting and those designed to lower serum urate levels and decrease the frequency of attacks in the future.

## Management of Acute Gouty Arthritis

### General Considerations

The management of acute gout in patients with no other aggravating or comorbid condition (e.g., renal failure, liver disease, peptic ulcer disease, postoperative state) is usually straightforward and should pose no dilemma for the treating physician. For best results, the diagnosis should be established as soon as possible and treatment initiated as early into the

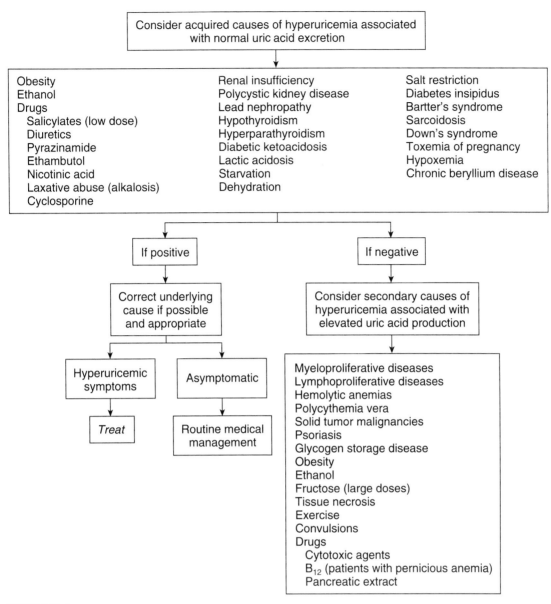

**FIGURE 35–1**

Evaluation of the patient with hyperuricemia. (Modified from Kelley WN, Wortmann RL: Gout and hyperuricemia. *In* Kelley WN, Harris ED, Ruddy S, et al [eds]: Textbook of Rheumatology, 5th ed. Philadelphia: WB Saunders, 1997:1341.)

attack as possible. Agents available for terminating the acute attack include nonsteroidal anti-inflammatory drugs (NSAIDs), colchicine, corticotropin (ACTH), and corticosteroids (Table 35–2). Each agent has a toxicity profile that offers advantages and disadvantages in individual circumstances. The choice among agents is usually based on the patient's overall medical condition, with underlying renal and gastrointestinal (GI) disease being the most important considerations in most patients.

### Nonsteroidal Anti-inflammatory Drugs

The term *nonsteroidal anti-inflammatory drug* was first applied to phenylbutazone in 1949. Since then, many other NSAIDs have been introduced, all having in com-

mon the suppression of cyclooxygenase-mediated prostaglandin synthesis. This suppression explains in part some of their anti-inflammatory potential and side effects. NSAIDs have also been shown to interfere with neutrophil activation and the release of cytotoxic substances, including free radicals, lysosomal enzymes, and lipoxygenase products.[13] Although the many currently available NSAIDs differ by chemical class, plasma half-life, and dosage, they have similar anti-inflammatory properties and potential for toxicity.

In the absence of comorbid conditions or risk factors (Table 35–3), NSAIDs are effective with an acceptable risk profile in the treatment of acute gout. Indomethacin in dosages of 100 to 200 mg during the first 2 or 3 days of the acute attack usually begins to provide relief within a few hours after the initial oral dosage. As the

**TABLE 35–2**
**Therapeutic Options in Acute Gout**

| THERAPY | CONSIDERATIONS |
| --- | --- |
| Nonsteroidal anti-inflammatory drugs (e.g., indomethacin) | Ideal for healthy patients without gastrointestinal or renal disease<br>Use with caution for limited periods and in lower doses with comorbid conditions and in the elderly |
| Corticosteroids or corticotropin (ACTH) (intra-articular, oral, parenteral) | Preferable in patients with comorbid conditions, elderly patients<br>Use with caution in diabetes |
| Colchicine (oral) | Useful at BID-TID dose for milder attacks<br>Higher doses usually not tolerated<br>Use with caution in elderly or with renal or hepatic disease<br>Intravenous preparation rarely used; concerns about toxicity |

inflammatory process subsides, the dosage is reduced to 75 mg/day. Unfortunately, many patients—particularly the elderly—are unable to tolerate the high doses required because of toxic effects such as headache, problems with mentation, fluid retention, GI intolerance, or even acute reversible renal problems (Table 35–4). Other available NSAIDs that are useful in acute gout include naproxen (500 mg two to three times daily), ibuprofen (800 mg three to four times daily), sulindac (200 mg twice daily), and diclofenac (75 mg twice daily). As an attack is controlled, maintenance doses of the NSAID can be used for prophylaxis if necessary. If one NSAID is not tolerated, another NSAID or colchicine may be used. GI, renal, and central nervous systemic toxicity, all of which are more common in elderly patients, play a significant role in limiting the usefulness of NSAIDs in managing acute gout.[14, 15]

## Corticosteroids

Corticosteroids have become increasingly popular in recent years for the treatment of acute gout.[16] In cases in which one or two large joints are involved, an intra-

**TABLE 35–3**
**Potential Risk Factors for NSAID-Induced Toxicity**

Decreased renal function
Liver disease
Peptic ulcer disease
Congestive heart failure
Elderly patient
Allergic, hypersensitive: asthma, rhinitis, nasal polyps
Drug interactions
  Anticoagulants (avoid combination)
  Lithium (monitor carefully)
  Oral hypoglycemics (monitor)
  Potassium-sparing diuretics (avoid combination)
  Digoxin (avoid if possible in renal insufficiency)
  Cyclosporine (avoid combination)
  Probenecid (increases NSAID levels)

articular injection with microcrystalline corticosteroid (e.g., 40 to 80 mg of methylprednisolone acetate or triamcinolone acetonide) is usually very effective, with control of the pain and inflammatory signs achieved within a few hours. In the absence of infection, and under strict aseptic technique, the joint is aspirated, the diagnosis is confirmed, and the joint is injected. Smaller joints may be injected with one third to one half of the dose needed for larger joints. Intra-articular injections are well tolerated in almost all cases. Rare complications seen after local corticosteroid injection include transient increase in pain, skin atrophy, local hypopigmentation, tendon rupture, and even iatrogenic joint infection. For this reason, patients should be advised to call or return if any adverse event that occurs after an injection lasts more than 48 hours.

Single intramuscular (IM) injections of triamcinolone acetonide, 60 mg, have been found effective and comparable to indomethacin. A few patients may require a second injection.[17] However, significant tissue atrophy may occur. We have used 40 to 80 mg of IM methylprednisolone acetate with similar good results. Oral or parenteral courses of corticosteroids have been used in selected cases, primarily in patients with polyarticular gout and in those with contraindications for NSAIDs or colchicine. Initial dosages of 20 to 50 mg of oral prednisone were used, and therapy was required for 10 to 15 days because of slow resolution of symptoms. No significant side effects were noted, except for mild hyperglycemia in 1 of 12 patients so treated.[18] Wolfson and coworkers[19] first reported the use of ACTH in acute gout in 1949. More recently, Axelrod and Preston compared IM injection of ACTH with oral indomethacin in 76 patients.[20] In the 36 patients who received ACTH, pain relief was noted within a few hours and there were no apparent side effects; in contrast, of 40 patients who received indomethacin, 12 had problems with mentation and pain relief was delayed. Siegel and associates compared single doses of IM ACTH (40 units) and triamcinolone acetonide (60 mg) in acute gout.[21] Repeat injection was required in 9 of 15 patients receiving ACTH but in only 5 of 16 receiving triamcinolone, and many ACTH

**TABLE 35–4**
**Adverse Reactions to NSAIDs**

| SYSTEM | REACTIONS |
|---|---|
| Gastrointestinal | Dyspepsia, erosive gastritis, peptic ulcer disease, diarrhea, small bowel ulceration, colitis, liver dysfunction |
| Renal | Decreased renal function, acute renal failure, interstitial nephritis, papillary necrosis, hyperkalemia, chronic renal failure(?) |
| Neurologic | Headache, dizziness, aseptic meningitis (ibuprofen, sulindac, tolmetin), decreased mentation, psychosis |
| Skin | Fixed drug reaction, erythema multiforme, urticaria, pseudoporphyria (naproxen) |
| Other | Pneumonitis, aplastic anemia, bone marrow suppression |

patients required a third injection to treat rebound attacks. Therefore, triamcinolone acetonide may be more effective than ACTH in the treatment of acute gouty arthritis.

Patients treated with oral or systemic corticosteroid therapy for acute gout should be started on low-dose colchicine (0.6 mg once to twice daily) if no contraindications to colchicine therapy exist. This serves to prevent "rebound" after the steroid effect wears off, and also provides prophylaxis for recurrent attacks.

### Colchicine

Colchicine is a derivative of the meadow saffron (*Colchicum autumnale*).[22] Extracts of this plant, as a cathartic, were introduced for the treatment of gout in 600 A.D. The alkaloid colchicine was isolated in 1820 by Pelletier and Caventon.[5, 23] Because of its selective anti-inflammatory properties and effectiveness in the management of acute gout, colchicine was the drug of choice in these patients for many years, with reported complete resolution in about 80% of patients within 48 hours.[10] The striking improvement noted with its use also served diagnostic purposes. Because of its poor therapeutic benefit/toxicity ratio and because many other effective drugs have become available, the use of colchicine in this setting has decreased. However, it continues to be useful and is quite safe if used according to established guidelines.[24]

In the absence of comorbid conditions or risk factors (Table 35–5), colchicine can be given orally, one 0.5- to 0.6-mg tablet every hour or two tablets every 2 hours, until improvement occurs or toxic effects are noted (usually diarrhea or vomiting, which may be severe),

**TABLE 35–5**
**Risk Factors for Colchicine Toxicity**

Sepsis
Bone marrow depression
Decreased renal function
Hepatic disease or biliary obstruction
Prior maintenance colchicine
Older patient
Medications—cimetidine, tolbutamide, cyclosporine

or until a total dose of about 6 mg has been given. Unfortunately, more than half of patients treated with such a regimen experience toxic effects coincident with improvement or before improvement is noted. In a controlled study of 45 patients with acute gout, all of the 22 subjects given oral colchicine developed diarrhea or vomiting at a median time of 24 hours, or after a mean dose of 6.6 mg.[25]

To avoid or minimize GI toxicity, intravenous (IV) colchicine has been used to treat acute gout, particularly in the past. However, the increasing recognition of the potential for bone marrow suppression and other systemic toxicities from IV colchicine has resulted in guidelines for restricting dosage and even a lack of availability in some countries.[24] A dosage of 1 to 2 mg, diluted in 20 mL of normal saline, can be administered slowly (over several minutes), preferably through an established IV access line to avoid extravasation, because colchicine can be very irritating and tissue damage may occur. A smaller dose (0.5 to 1.0 mg) may be repeated every 6 hours without giving more than 4 mg as a total IV dose for acute attacks, but no more colchicine by any route should be given for 1 week. Absolute contraindications to IV colchicine therapy include a creatinine clearance rate of less than 10 mL/min, combined renal and hepatic disease, and extrahepatic biliary obstruction. Because many other therapeutic options exist, we believe it is best to avoid colchicine in high doses for the management of acute gout.

In recent years, the most common use of colchicine in gout has been to prevent an early recurrence after treatment of an acute attack or to provide long-term prophylaxis. In patients treated with corticosteroids acutely, we begin a low dose of colchicine, 0.5 to 1.2 mg/day, unless the drug is contraindicated. Higher doses are usually not well tolerated because of GI toxicity. Patients treated with NSAIDs may begin colchicine prophylaxis immediately or wait until their attack is under good control. This strategy prevents acute attacks of gout in about 85% of patients, but it does not prevent the further deposition of urate and development of tophi.[26]

METABOLISM. Colchicine is rapidly absorbed after oral administration, with a bioavailability of 25% to 50% and peak concentrations of 0.3 μg/mL after 30 to

120 minutes; it concentrates in leukocytes, and about 50% is bound to plasma proteins. The drug is deacetylated in the liver and is excreted in the bile, feces, and urine. The frequency of intestinal toxicity is partly explained by the presence of large concentrations of the drug in the bile and intestinal secretions. Colchicine affects rapidly dividing cells, most notably those of the bone marrow and intestinal mucosa. It is still detectable in white blood cells and in the urine 10 days after a single dose.[27] In studies done in patients with familial Mediterranean fever, the plasma half-life of colchicine increased from 4.4 hours in patients with normal renal function to 18.8 hours in patients with renal failure, and it has been reported to be as long as 50 hours in patients with end-stage renal disease and hepatic cirrhosis.[28] Therefore, colchicine should be given with extreme caution in patients with renal disease, and it should be avoided in patients receiving chronic dialysis therapy (because it is not dialyzed) and in patients with combined renal and hepatic disease.

Colchicine interferes with steps of the inflammatory reaction mediated by neutrophils. Its interference with microtubular systems may lead to decreased neutrophil motility, chemotaxis, formation of digestive vacuoles, degranulation, and suppression of a chemotactic factor released by neutrophils during phagocytosis of urate.[13, 22]

TOXICITY. The frequency and severity of side effects associated with colchicine administration depend on multiple factors, including dose, route of administration, presence of comorbid conditions (e.g., renal and liver disease), previous maintenance doses, age, and drug interactions. The most common and best recognized side effects are GI effects, with most patients experiencing diarrhea, vomiting, or both at the doses used to treat the acute attacks. The main circumstances in which severe toxicity occurs are suicide attempts and inappropriate therapeutic overdoses. The correlation between amount ingested, severity of toxicity, and prognosis is not straightforward, inasmuch as fatalities have been reported after oral doses of 7 mg over 3 days and after single doses of 7.5 to 11 mg, and survival has been reported after ingestion of more than 300 mg.[23]

Many manifestations have been associated with colchicine toxicity (Table 35–6). Hematologic manifestations include disseminated intravascular coagulation and bone marrow depression. In some patients, severe diarrhea and leukopenia may lead to hypotension, sepsis, and death. A colchicine-induced myoneuropathy mimicking polymyositis has been described in several reports. In one series, all 12 patients affected had decreased renal function and were receiving long-term low-dose prophylaxis (1.2 mg/day).[29] Muscle weakness, distal areflexia, and elevation of creatine kinase were noted. Electromyography showed myopathic changes, and muscle biopsy revealed a distinctive vacuolar myopathy with no apparent inflammatory changes. Prompt recovery followed discontinuation or use of a reduced dosage of colchicine.

The treatment of severe colchicine toxicity is supportive. The drug's short half-life and its ability to bind to tissues make hemodialysis and exchange transfusions useless.[23, 30] It may be useful to administer gastric lavage, emetics, activated charcoal, or cathartics in the absence of diarrhea. Using an approach similar to one used in digoxin overdose, Baud and colleagues reported the successful treatment of a colchicine overdose with colchicine-specific antibody (Fab) fragments.[31] In a patient who had taken a 60-mg intentional overdose, the infusion of Fab fragments resulted in a dramatic reversal of hypotension and improvement in cardiac output, with an eventual full recovery after transient marrow suppression, hair loss, and polyneuropathy.

## Management of Intercritical Gout

Patients remain at increased risk of another attack for several weeks after resolution of an acute attack of

---

TABLE 35–6
**Manifestations of Colchicine Toxicity**

| SYSTEM | MANIFESTATIONS |
| --- | --- |
| Gastrointestinal | Abdominal pain, nausea/vomiting, ileus, hepatocellular damage, pancreatitis |
| Respiratory | Respiratory distress, acute respiratory distress syndrome |
| Hematologic | Leukocytosis (early), bone marrow hypoplasia, coagulopathy, hemolytic anemia |
| Skin | Rash, alopecia |
| Cardiovascular | Hypovolemia, hypotension, depressed myocardial function, peripheral vasodilatation, arrhythmias, myocarditis |
| Renal | Proteinuria, hematuria, acute renal failure |
| Metabolic | Metabolic acidosis, hyponatremia, hypocalcemia, hypophosphatemia, hypomagnesemia |
| Neuromuscular | Mental status changes, coma, ascending paralysis, seizures, peripheral neuropathy, rhabdomyolysis |
| Fertility | Azoospermia, sterility |
| Miscellaneous | Fever, hypothermia |

From Putterman C, Ben-Chetrit E, Caraco Y, et al: Colchicine intoxication: Clinical pharmacology, risk factors, features, and management. Semin Arthritis Rheum 1991; 21:143, and Ben-Chetrit E, Scherrmann J-M, Zylber-Katz E, et al: Colchicine deposition in patients with familial Mediterranean fever with renal impairment. J Rheumatol 1994; 21:710.

**TABLE 35–7**
**Initial Prophylaxis and Follow-up of Gout After First Attack in Uncomplicated Cases**

| TYPE OF THERAPY | SPECIFIC TREATMENT |
|---|---|
| Short-term prophylaxis | Low-dose NSAID or colchicine |
| Lifestyle modifications | Medications, diuretics, diet, obesity, alcohol consumption |
| Metabolic evaluation | Consider 24-hr urine analysis for uric acid excretion<br><700 mg/d—underexcretor<br>>700 mg/d—overproducer |
| Clinical observation | For recurrent attacks, renal function, renal stones, tophi |

NSAID, nonsteroidal anti-inflammatory drug.

gout. For this reason, prophylaxis with small doses of colchicine or NSAIDs should be used in most cases (Table 35–7). Colchicine in a dosage of 0.6 mg once or twice daily prevents attacks in more than 80% of patients. Prophylaxis should be continued for 1 to 2 months after an acute attack or for several months in patients with a history of frequent attacks, as well as when urate-lowering drugs are initiated.[26, 32] The dose of colchicine should be reduced or its duration limited in patients with reduced renal function, because bone marrow suppression and myoneuropathy have been reported in patients receiving chronic low-dose colchicine therapy who had a creatinine clearance of less than 50 mL/min.[33] In patients without renal disease and with no visible tophaceous deposits, colchicine may be given as prophylaxis for several months to years, depending on the individual case and whether urate-lowering drugs are used. In patients with tophaceous gout, several years of colchicine prophylaxis may be required.

During the period of follow-up after an acute attack, a patient can be monitored for recurrent attacks and assessed for possible causes of hyperuricemia. A 24-hour urine collection for determination of urate excretion helps classify the patient as an "overproducer" or "underexcretor" of urate, so that the optimal drugs for lowering of serum urate levels can be selected, if these are indicated.[5] Daily excretion of more than 700 mg of urate indicates that allopurinol is most appropriate for lowering urate levels by decreasing production, whereas lower levels suggest that a uricosuric drug might be useful.

Correctable environmental factors that play a role in hyperuricemia should be sought. Patients with renal disease may be hyperuricemic due to decreased renal excretion, whereas patients with obesity or a myeloproliferative disorder have an increased production of urate. Alcohol consumption contributes to hyperuricemia by increasing production and reducing renal excretion of urate. A review of the patient's diet occasionally reveals heavy consumption of purine-rich foods, such as organ meats, seafood, and various legumes or other vegetables. However, the purine content of the diet contributes only about 1.0 mg/dL to the serum urate concentration.[34] A number of medica-

tions can interfere with renal urate excretion, most notably thiazide diuretics.[35]

Some patients have only a single attack of gout, or several months or years may elapse before a second attack. In patients with a single or a few gouty attacks, normal renal function, no history of renal stones, and no apparent tophaceous deposits, gout may be managed conservatively with education, lifestyle modifications including weight control and reduction in alcohol consumption, avoidance of diuretics, and possibly maintenance colchicine. A 1995 analysis of the cost effectiveness of urate-lowering drugs suggested that for patients who have two or more attacks of gout annually the cost of treatment with urate-lowering drugs is lower than the cost of treatment of acute attacks only.[36]

## Control of Hyperuricemia

### General Considerations and Indications

Drugs that lower serum uric acid levels are indicated in patients who continue to have frequent attacks of gout and in patients with tophaceous deposits, renal disease, chronic deforming or erosive arthritis, or kidney stones (Table 35–8). In general, it is best to start antihyperuricemic therapy after an attack is well con-

**TABLE 35–8**
**Hypouricemic Drug Therapy in Gout**

Indications
  Tophaceous gout
  Urate renal stones
  Chronic erosive gouty arthritis
  Recurrent acute gout (probably more than 2 attacks per year)
Choice of agents
  Allopurinol
    24-hr urate excretion at any level
    History of renal stones
    Renal insufficiency
  Uricosuric drugs
    24-hr urate excretion <700 mg
    Normal renal function
    No history of renal stones

trolled and the patient is free of symptoms, usually at about 2 weeks after the attack. Urate-lowering medication begun during attacks may have some potential to delay response or lead to rebound exacerbations. However, urate-lowering drugs should not be stopped in patients who develop acute gout while taking them. The initiation of urate-lowering drugs may increase the risk of gouty attacks for the first month or two, although this has never been substantiated in controlled trials.[37, 38] For this reason, low-dose colchicine or NSAIDs should be used in most patients when therapy is initiated with urate-lowering drugs. The length of this prophylactic therapy must be individualized; in some patients, a few months to a year may be sufficient, whereas those with tophaceous gout may require years of such therapy. A 1993 study of patients receiving allopurinol for tophaceous gout demonstrated that recurrent attacks occur in 81% of patients and tophi recur in 43% of patients within 3 years after stopping therapy.[39] Therefore, most patients with severe tophaceous gout are probably better off remaining on hypouricemic therapy indefinitely, even after tophi have resolved and attacks have subsided completely.

## Allopurinol

Allopurinol was first developed as a chemotherapeutic agent, but it had little or no effect on experimental tumors. As an inhibitor of xanthine oxidase, allopurinol was first given to human patients in 1963 to achieve reduced values of both serum and urinary uric acid.[5, 40] Uric acid is the final product of purine metabolism in human beings. In the final steps, hypoxanthine is oxidized to xanthine and xanthine to uric acid; these reactions are catalyzed by xanthine oxidase. Both allopurinol and oxypurinol inhibit xanthine oxidase, thereby decreasing uric acid production and resulting in increased xanthine and hypoxanthine concentrations. Allopurinol also inhibits de novo purine synthesis, decreasing total urinary purine excretion.[41]

Allopurinol is well absorbed after oral administration, reaching peak levels within 30 to 60 minutes and having a plasma half-life of 2 to 3 hours. Some is excreted in the feces and urine; however, most is converted to oxypurinol, which has a much longer half-life, up to 20 hours in patients with normal renal function. Most of the oxypurinol is excreted by the kidney. Therefore, a decrease in renal function may markedly increase its half-life. A similar increase may occur with a low-protein diet in malnourished persons, increasing the risk of toxicity. The long half-life of oxypurinol may be responsible for most of the urate-lowering effect and toxicity of allopurinol. Although allopurinol increases the half-life of probenecid and uricosurics increase the clearance of oxypurinol, these interactions have minimal practical consequences and both medications have been used together without altering their usual doses.[41]

The administration of allopurinol is followed by a decrease in serum and urinary uric acid values within 24 to 48 hours. Maximal reductions are reached within 2 weeks and then values remain relatively constant for prolonged periods.[5] Optimally, serum urate levels should be lowered below the saturation point, 6 mg/100 mL or less if possible. In patients with normal renal function, 200 to 300 mg/day in one dose should be given in combination with prophylactic doses of colchicine or low-dose NSAIDs. The allopurinol dose may be gradually increased if necessary. Occasionally a patient may require 600 to 800 mg/day. Patients should be informed that, during the initial months of treatment, they may experience an increase in the frequency of attacks. This is thought to result from increased mobilization of urates from tophaceous deposits and shedding of crystals into joints. Good control of the hyperuricemia should lead to gradual resolution of tophaceous deposits, control of arthritis, and preservation of joint and renal function. In patients with decreased renal function in whom allopurinol therapy is definitely indicated, the medication should be started at a much lower dose based on renal function. Hande and coworkers have suggested the protocol in Table 35–9 for maintenance allopurinol dosage based on creatinine clearance.[42]

In patients with mild renal insufficiency (creatinine clearance, 60 to 80 mL/min), we prefer initial therapy at low doses beginning with only 100 mg/day. If the medication is tolerated and there are no side effects, the dose is gradually increased.

TOXICITY. After 35 years of clinical use, allopurinol continues to be a standard therapy for most patients with chronic tophaceous gout, urate nephropathy, and nephrolithiasis and in cases of gout and renal insufficiency. Although uricosurics may be of value in controlling hyperuricemia in patients with mild renal insufficiency (unless contraindicated by urate nephropathy, nephrolithiasis, or overproduction), allopurinol is mainly indicated in cases of significant renal insufficiency (glomerular filtration rate, less than 60 mL/min) and severe gout. However, the medication should be used very cautiously in these patients, with initial low doses of 50 to 100 mg only (see Table 35–9) and a gradual increase if necessary to avoid toxicity. Renal and liver function should be carefully monitored. Although most patients tolerate allopurinol without toxic reactions, some experience significant

**TABLE 35–9**

**Allopurinol Dose Adjustment Based on Renal Function**

| CREATININE CLEARANCE (mL/min) | ALLOPURINOL DOSE |
|---|---|
| 0 | 100 mg every 3 days |
| 10 | 100 mg every 2 days |
| 20 | 100 mg daily |
| 40 | 150 mg daily |
| 60 | 200 mg daily |
| 80 | 250 mg daily |
| 100 | 300 mg daily |

From Hande KR, Noone RM, Stone WJ: Severe allopurinol toxicity: Description and guidelines for prevention in patients with renal insufficiency. Am J Med 1984; 76:47.

side effects. There is ample evidence that allopurinol is given inappropriately to many patients. Hande and associates[42] and Singer and Wallace[43] have described a life-threatening allopurinol hypersensitivity syndrome in 158 patients. High fever, severe dermatitis in more than 90% of patients (erythema multiforme, toxic epidermal necrolysis, or exfoliative rash), hepatitis, eosinophilia, and worsening of renal function were noted, and 38 (24%) of the 158 patients died. In one of these series, 33 of 59 patients had been given allopurinol for asymptomatic hyperuricemia.[43] Risk factors for this syndrome are the presence of renal insufficiency, concomitant diuretic therapy, and perhaps the use of full loading doses of allopurinol (300 mg). Because allopurinol metabolizes to oxypurinol and the half-life of the latter substance is very prolonged in the presence of renal insufficiency, accumulation of oxypurinol occurs.[42] Oxypurinol has been implicated in allopurinol-induced toxicity.

Allopurinol may induce milder rashes that do not require discontinuation of the medication; however, these patients must be very carefully monitored, and the dose of medication should be reduced. The presence of fever, worsening dermatitis, decreased renal function, abnormal liver enzymes, or eosinophilia should prompt discontinuation of the drug. Bone marrow suppression, aplastic anemia, agranulocytosis, granulomatous hepatitis, and jaundice have been described.

Allopurinol has important interactions with several frequently used medications. Some of these interactions include a higher incidence of rashes (in combination with ampicillin) and bone marrow suppression (with cyclophosphamide). The dose of azathioprine or mercaptopurine should be reduced to about one third of the usual dose if given with allopurinol, because these drugs are inactivated by xanthine oxidase. Allopurinol prolongs the half-life of warfarin and theophylline.[41] Rarely, in patients with uric acid overproduction and excretion, such as those with enzyme deficiencies and those undergoing cytolytic therapy, allopurinol induces xanthinuria or xanthine stone formation.

## Uricosuric Agents

Uric acid is almost completely freely filtered at the glomerulus. More than 90% undergoes tubular reabsorption and then tubular secretion, reabsorption, and excretion; this explains the final product in the urine. Uricosurics compete with urate for the tubular brush border transporter, thus inhibiting urate reabsorption. The net result is increased uric acid excretion and decreased serum urate levels. The uricosurics available in the United States are probenecid, sulfinpyrazone, and salicylates.

PROBENECID. This drug was initially developed to sustain high levels of penicillin and para-aminosalicylic acid by interfering with their renal excretion. Probenecid is well absorbed from the GI tract, with a half-life ranging from 6 to 12 hours. It is highly bound to plasma proteins and is excreted in the urine.[41] Gutman and Yu[44] and Talbott and colleagues[45] noted increased urinary uric acid excretion and normalization of serum urate in patients treated with doses of probenecid ranging from 0.5 to 2 g/day. A precipitous drop in serum urate levels was noted in a few days. As with allopurinol, an increase in acute gouty attacks was seen, and 2 of 18 patients receiving 2 g/day of probenecid in the Gutman and Yu study experienced a recurrence of renal colic. Because uricosurics increase urine uric acid excretion, they may precipitate uric crystals (primarily in uric acid overproducers) or lead to uric acid stones when given initially at high doses. It is advisable to begin therapy at low doses to prevent crystallization. Precipitation is unusual in the normal producer of uric acid. Initial doses of 0.5 to 1 g/day are given and may be increased to 1.5 to 2 g/day in divided doses. Higher doses may be needed. Uricosurics are highly effective for most gouty patients. However, they should not be used in patients with uric acid overproduction and overexcretion or in those with urate nephropathy or nephrolithiasis because of the propensity for crystal precipitation and stone formation. To minimize the risk of crystalluria and stone formation, fluid intake should be increased, particularly at the beginning of therapy, when larger quantities of uric acid are excreted. Urine alkalinization increases uric acid solubility, thereby decreasing the chance of crystallization. It has been suggested that patients be given 2 to 6 g of sodium bicarbonate during the first days of therapy, but this is impractical in clinical practice. Acetazolamide, 200 mg taken at night during the first 7 to 10 days, helps to alkalinize the urine throughout the night. Uricosurics are ineffective in patients with impaired renal function (glomerular filtration rate, less than 30 to 40 mL/min).

In long-term studies, 20% of probenecid-treated patients developed side effects, including GI intolerance, fever, hypersensitivity reactions, and rashes. Probenecid decreases the renal excretion of salicylates, acetazolamide, dapsone, indomethacin, ampicillin, penicillin, cephradine, and methotrexate. It delays heparin metabolism, which may lead to increased anticoagulation.[41]

SULFINPYRAZONE. This drug is a derivative of a phenylbutazone metabolite. It lacks anti-inflammatory properties but is a strong uricosuric. It is rapidly absorbed from the GI tract. It is highly bound to plasma proteins and has a half-life of 1 to 3 hours.[5] Most of the drug is excreted in the urine. An added advantage is its antiplatelet effect. This medication is administered in divided doses of 200 to 800 mg/day. GI intolerance of sulfinpyrazone is similar to that of probenecid. Occasional bone marrow toxicity has been observed. Because of its strong uricosuric effect, sulfinpyrazone should not be given to patients with overproduction of uric acid, urate nephropathy, or a history of uric acid stones.

SALICYLATES. Aspirin or salicylates in a dose of 4 to 6 g/day are effective uricosurics. Most patients are unable to tolerate such high doses, however, and there are other options. Low doses (<2.4 g/day) of aspirin or salicylates appear to inhibit the renal tubular secretion of uric acid, leading to hyperuricemia. At any dose, they inhibit the uricosuric effect of probenecid or sulfinpyrazone and should not be used with these drugs.

## Management of Complicated Gout

In most cases, gout is a very treatable disease and good control can be achieved. However, some patients with severe disease have comorbid conditions that make therapeutic decisions difficult. As previously discussed, colchicine and NSAIDs are often contraindicated for acute attacks. Uricosurics often cannot be used for long-term control, and patients may not tolerate allopurinol. In such patients, more careful attention to education, lifestyle changes, and medication adjustment may be enough to allow better long-term control of hyperuricemia. In addition, an individualized approach to management based on the severity of the patient's gout and specific comorbid conditions is usually successful.

### Patients with Renal Disease and/or Edematous States

In patients with renal disease or edematous states, NSAIDs should be used with caution in treating acute attacks, owing to the effect of these drugs on renal function and renal handling of sodium and water. In such patients, the best choices appear to be intra-articular steroid preparations for patients with one or a few joints involved. In patients with polyarticular attacks, a regimen of systemic corticosteroids (oral prednisone or IM triamcinolone or ACTH) should be effective in controlling acute attacks. Low-dose colchicine can still be used for long-term prophylaxis with caution. Maintenance doses of colchicine in patients with chronic renal insufficiency may lead to neuromyopathy or bone marrow suppression; careful monitoring of blood counts, peripheral nerve function, and muscle enzymes is essential. Doses of 0.6 mg daily or every other day may be sufficient to prevent attacks in such patients without toxicity. In addition, earlier discontinuation of chronic prophylactic colchicine should be considered in patients with renal disease. For long-term control of hyperuricemia, uricosuric agents are ineffective in patients with renal insufficiency and should be avoided. Allopurinol should be effective in most patients, but the dose should be reduced as discussed previously.

### Patients at Risk for NSAID Gastropathy

In patients with a history of peptic ulcer disease or GI bleeding, and in elderly patients, NSAIDs should be used with extreme caution for treatment of acute attacks or for long-term prophylaxis. NSAIDs should be avoided altogether in patients with active or recently active peptic ulcer disease. In patients with past GI intolerance to NSAIDs, concomitant misoprostol, high-dose histamine-2 antagonists (e.g., famotidine), or proton pump inhibitors (e.g., omeprazole) should theo-

retically reduce the risk of complications of short- or long-term NSAID therapy. However, one of the various corticosteroid regimens or colchicine represents a more practical and less expensive option for the treatment of acute gout in patients at risk for GI complications from NSAID therapy.

### Transplantation Patients Receiving Cyclosporine Therapy

The management of gout in transplantation patients taking cyclosporine poses another dilemma for the clinician. For patients with acute gout, NSAIDs and colchicine should be avoided in most cases because of reduced renal function. Because most of these patients are receiving long-term corticosteroids and may have some adrenal suppression, ACTH may be less effective. Therefore, intra-articular or systemic steroids are the best option for treating acute gout in this setting. If required, analgesics may be added. For prophylaxis between attacks, NSAIDs and colchicine should be avoided because of tenuous renal function in most patients taking cyclosporine. In addition, a 1994 report describes a possible additive risk for toxicity in patients taking colchicine and cyclosporine together.[46] In many patients, it is probably safest to use no such prophylactic regimen, but to rely on the prompt use of corticosteroids for acute attacks along with an aggressive urate-lowering regimen. Uricosurics should be avoided because of the renal dysfunction that usually is present. Small doses of allopurinol (i.e., 50 mg/day) may be given with close observation for possible toxicity; if tolerated, the dose may be increased after 1 or 2 months. Patients receiving concurrent azathioprine should have the dose of this drug reduced to about one third of the usual amount, because allopurinol inhibits xanthine oxidase, which is required in azathioprine degradation.

### Refractory Gout

Refractory gout is uncommon. In patients with acute gout that is unresponsive to NSAIDs, colchicine, or corticosteroids, alternative diagnoses and concurrent problems should be investigated.[47] In particular, coexistent bacterial infectious arthritis in patients with gout is well described, and synovial fluid cultures should be obtained from those patients with acute gout accompanied by fever or an attack that is not responding to therapy. Occasionally, other conditions, such as pseudogout, cellulitis, calcific periarthritis, Reiter's syndrome, or even atypical rheumatoid arthritis, can manifest with acute attacks. In patients who have never had a diagnosis of gout confirmed by crystal analysis and in those with known gout and refractory attacks, careful analysis of synovial fluid for the presence of crystals is essential. Once a diagnosis of acute gout is confirmed or reconfirmed and other conditions are appropriately excluded, repeat doses of intra-articular or systemic corticosteroids are most likely to bring a refractory attack of gout under control.

Some gout patients do not respond to allopurinol with the expected reduction in uric acid levels or frequency of acute gouty attacks. In such patients, concomitant medications that might affect urate metabolism, diet, alcohol consumption, and the patient's understanding of the importance of compliance with the regimen of daily allopurinol should all be reviewed again. Although poor compliance usually explains a poor response, incomplete absorption of allopurinol may be responsible in some cases.[48] In patients who are compliant with allopurinol dosage regimens but do not have an adequate lowering of their serum uric acid concentration, doses can be raised as high as 600 to 800 mg/day, and some patients may respond to a combination of allopurinol and uricosuric drug.[49]

### Allopurinol Hypersensitivity

Oxypurinol (not available in the United States) has been tried as an alternative in allopurinol-sensitive patients. Although toxic events similar to previous allopurinol allergy occurred in 40% of the patients, slow incremental doses were tolerated by 60% of patients with complicated hyperuricemia.[50] Patients who are sensitive to allopurinol and require the same medication as those with severe tophaceous gout may need a desensitization trial. Oral and IV desensitization methods have been successful in a few patients.[51–54] Close monitoring is necessary, because serious toxicity has occurred. Patients should be fully informed about the potential for severe reactions even at low doses. Oral desensitization should be tried first, because it may be safer. Gradually increasing doses of an oral solution, beginning at 0.008 mg and increasing by 0.008 mg each day for 10 days, reaching 20 mg/day at day 20 and 300 mg at 1 month, have been successful in a few cases.[52] An alternative regimen for slow oral desensitization was published by Fam and coworkers, who used a starting dose of 0.5 mg/day, with increases every 3 to 7 days.[53, 54] With this regimen, 26 of 30 patients were able to reach a therapeutic effect at a mean of 44 days, although 12 of these patients experienced transient rashes during the period of desensitization. Walz-LeBlanc and associates used IV desensitization after failure of the oral route.[51] After a negative result of a skin test with 0.1 $\mu$g, they arbitrarily gave IV doses of 1, 10, 50, 100, and 500 $\mu$g at 15-minute intervals, followed by 1, 2, 5, 10, 20, and 50 mg at 30-minute intervals; 100 mg was given 1 hour later with no apparent problem (200 mg of allopurinol was diluted in 500 mL of 5% dextrose in water).

Uricosuric agents should be used in patients with normal renal function, low uric acid excretion, and no history of renal stones. In addition, uricosuric drugs could be considered in some patients with moderate renal insufficiency, high urate excretion, or a history of renal stones, although the efficacy may be decreased. In such patients, every effort should be made to decrease the risk of renal stones through high fluid intake and alkalinization of the urine.

## CALCIUM PYROPHOSPHATE DEPOSITION DISEASE

CPPD deposition disease, or pseudogout, was first described in 1962.[55] The term *pseudogout* was used to characterize an acute arthropathy similar to gout, with calcifications in cartilage (chondrocalcinosis) and CPPD crystals in the synovial fluid. Other clinical presentations have been described. The acute variety may be monoarticular or polyarticular and is sometimes associated with fever. Tophaceous deposits in tendons and periarticular tissues have been described, but they are not as common or as characteristic as in gout. As with gout, the disease may be chronic, destructive, and incapacitating. CPPD deposition disease may follow patterns other than the typical one of intermittent acute attacks, including a symmetric "pseudorheumatoid" disease, "pseudo-osteoarthritis," a "pseudoneuropathic" pattern, or even asymptomatic (lanthanic) patterns. Joints commonly involved include the knees, wrists, shoulders, hips, and ankles. The disease has been associated with hyperparathyroidism, hemochromatosis, hypophosphatasia, and hypomagnesemia, and it is more common in the elderly. The diagnosis is established by the clinical presentation, radiographic features, and demonstration of intracellular, weakly birefringent crystals by polarized microscopy. The pathophysiologic mechanisms by which CPPD deposition disease develops are uncertain, and the events leading to the inflammatory reaction are probably similar to those seen with MSU crystals in gout.[3]

No treatment is known to halt the progression of crystal deposition in CPPD disease. In addition, even correction of underlying associated metabolic abnormalities, such as hyperparathyroidism and hemochromatosis, has not been shown to lead to improvement of radiographic cartilage calcification. Therefore, the treatment of CPPD deposition disease is symptomatic, with the object of therapy being to control pain and inflammation as quickly as possible. In acute attacks, drainage of the joint by arthrocentesis may be sufficient in some patients. Other options include intra-articular injection of corticosteroids or NSAIDs. Colchicine is effective in acute pseudogout. However, we prefer to avoid colchicine because of the risk of toxicity in elderly patients at the doses required to control the acute attack (see earlier discussion). At lower doses of 0.6 mg once or twice daily, colchicine can be helpful in preventing further attacks.[56] Corticosteroids seem to have efficacy in acute pseudogout similar to that seen in gout. Two uncontrolled studies have reported an excellent response to parenteral steroid regimens, one with 60 mg of IM triamcinolone and the other with a combination of IM and IV steroids.[57, 58] For patients with chronic pain and inflammation, physiotherapy, analgesics, colchicine, and NSAIDs are alternatives for management. For patients with chronic "pseudorheumatoid" CPPD disease, hydroxychloroquine in doses of 200 to 400 mg daily was shown to be superior to placebo in one small, controlled study.[59] Magnesium carbonate (30 mEq/day) was also shown to decrease the severity of symptoms in one small series of patients with chronic CPPD disease.[60]

## BASIC CALCIUM PHOSPHATE CRYSTAL DEPOSITION

A number of articular syndromes may be associated with the deposition of BCP crystals in and around the joints. In most cases periarticular calcifications are radiographically evident, and in some cases such calcifications partially or completely disappear in the weeks after an acute attack. Deposits may be asymptomatic or associated with acute periarthritis. Acute calcific periarthritis is common in patients undergoing chronic hemodialysis. An acute arthritis involving the first metatarsophalangeal joint in young women, mimicking acute gout, has been described.[61] In the older patient, a very destructive intra-articular process of the shoulder and knee (Milwaukee shoulder-knee syndrome) has been described.[62, 63] The management of this crystal-induced process is symptomatic. Locally injected corticosteroids or oral NSAIDs are the treatments of choice, but NSAIDs should be avoided in those patients with renal failure. For acute attacks, marked improvement within 5 days has been noted with NSAIDs, with the mean duration of attacks being 10 days and no recurrence in follow-up periods ranging from 9 months to 14 years.[61] For those with chronic disease, NSAIDs and analgesics may be used with appropriate attention to physiotherapy and exercise, as in the management of osteoarthritis.

## INVESTIGATIONAL DRUGS AND FUTURE DIRECTIONS

### Cyclooxygenase-2–Specific Inhibitors

In the early 1990s, several investigators discovered that cyclooxygenase (COX) had at least two isoforms, called COX-1 and COX-2, both of which were inhibited to some degree by the NSAIDs available at that time.[13] These two isoforms appear to have distinct patterns of expression, with COX-2 being a more "inducible" enzyme that is more important in the inflammatory process, while COX-1 is a more "constitutive" enzyme that is responsible in particular for protection of the gastric mucosa and platelet function. Two NSAIDs with a high specificity for COX-2 are currently available for the treatment of rheumatoid arthritis and osteoarthritis (celecoxib and rofecoxib). These agents should be much less toxic in general, and they appear to have very low potential for GI toxicity and inhibition of platelet function in clinical studies.[64] These COX-2–specific NSAIDs should be useful in the treatment of acute gout, and possibly in long-term prophylaxis, in patients at risk for GI toxicity from other NSAIDs.

## Urate Oxidase

The availability of uricase (urate oxidase) as a therapeutic agent would allow direct degradation of uric acid to allantoins, which are more highly soluble than the hypoxanthines and xanthines that are the products of urate metabolism in humans. The successful use of an injectable polyethylene glycol–modified uricase in humans has been reported in patients with lymphoma and leukemia undergoing chemotherapy,[65, 66] and this drug has been available in Europe for years. A recombinant urate oxidase was reported to result in a rapid decrease in uric acid levels within hours after a single injection.[67] The availability of uricase would be important mostly for patients with hematologic malignancies who are undergoing chemotherapy, in whom a rapid lowering of uric acid levels would help prevent acute intrarenal precipitation and renal failure. Such an agent might be useful in the rare patient with gout who is unable to take allopurinol or uricosuric drugs, but it would be impractical in most patients with gout because it is available only in parenteral forms.

## Benzbromarone

Benzbromarone is a uricosuric agent that has been available in Europe for more than 20 years. Doses of 50 to 150 mg daily reduce uric acid levels by 50% to 60% in patients with low uric acid secretion. Benzbromarone has been shown to be useful in some organ transplantation patients who are receiving cyclosporine and have reduced renal function.[68] More recently, it has been shown to be at least as effective as allopurinol in lowering plasma uric acid concentrations in underexcretors.[69] Availability of this agent in the United States might allow for more effective uricosuric therapy in patients with refractory gout, in organ transplantation patients, and in patients with allopurinol hypersensitivity.

## REFERENCES

1. McCarty DJ, Hollander JL: Identification of urate crystals in gouty synovial fluids. Ann Intern Med 1961; 54:452.
2. Kelley WN, Wortmann RL: Gout and hyperuricemia. *In* Kelley WN, Harris ED, Ruddy S, et al (eds): Textbook of Rheumatology, 5th ed. Philadelphia: WB Saunders, 1997:1313.
3. Reginato AL, Reginato AM: Diseases associated with deposition of calcium pyrophosphate or hydroxyapatite. *In* Kelley WN, Harris ED, Ruddy S, et al (eds): Textbook of Rheumatology, 5th ed. Philadelphia: WB Saunders, 1997:1352.
4. Campion ES, Glynn RJ, DeLabry LO: Asymptomatic hyperuricemia: Risks and consequences in the Normative Aging Study. Am J Med 1987; 82:421.
5. Wyngaarden JB, Kelly WN: Gout and hyperuricemia. New York: Grune & Stratton, 1976.
6. Hadler NM, Franck WA, Bress NM, et al: Acute polyarticular gout. Am J Med 1974; 56:715.
7. Lawry GV, Fan PG, Bluestone R: Polyarticular versus monoarticular gout: A prospective, comparative analysis of clinical features. Medicine (Baltimore) 1988; 67:335.
8. Agudelo CA, Wise CM: Crystal-associated arthritis. Clin Geriatr Med 1998; 14:495.
9. Bellamy N, Wilson Downie W, Buchanan WW: Observations on spontaneous improvement in patients with podagra: Implica-

tions for therapeutic trials of non-steroidal anti-inflammatory drugs. Br J Clin Pharmacol 1987; 24:33.

10. Gutman AB: Gout. *In* Beeson PB, McDermott W (eds): Textbook of Medicine, 12th ed. Philadelphia: WB Saunders, 1958:595.

11. Hench PS: The diagnosis of gout and gouty arthritis. J Lab Clin Med 1936; 220:48.

12. Gutman AG: The past four decades of progress in the knowledge of gout, with an assessment of the present status. Arthritis Rheum 1973; 16:431.

13. Clements PJ, Paulus HE: Nonsteroidal antirheumatic drugs. *In* Kelley WN, Harris ED, Ruddy S, et al (eds): Textbook of Rheumatology, 5th ed. Philadelphia: WB Saunders, 1997:707.

14. Allison MC, Howatson AG, Torrance CJ, et al: Gastrointestinal damage associated with the use of nonsteroidal antiinflammatory drugs. N Engl J Med 1992; 327:749.

15. Altman RD, Honig S, Levin JM, et al: Ketoprofen versus indomethacin in patients with acute gouty arthritis: A multicenter double-blind comparative study. J Rheumatol 1988; 15:1422.

16. Fam AG: Current therapy of acute microcrystalline arthritis and the role of corticosteroids. J Clin Rheumatol 1997; 3:35.

17. Alloway JA, Moriarty MJ, Hoogland YT, et al: Comparison of triamcinolone acetonide with indomethacin in the treatment of acute gouty arthritis. J Rheumatol 1993; 20:111.

18. Groff GD, Franck WA, Raddatz DA: Systemic steroid therapy for acute gout: A clinical trial and review of the literature. Semin Arthritis Rheum 1990; 34:1766.

19. Wolfson WQ, Cohn C, Levine R: Rapid treatment of acute gouty arthritis by concurrent administration of pituitary adrenocorticotropic hormone (ACTH) and colchicine. J Lab Clin Med 1949; 34:1766.

20. Axelrod D, Preston S: Comparison of parenteral adrenocorticotropic hormone with oral indomethacin in the treatment of acute gout. Arthritis Rheum 1988; 31:803.

21. Siegel LB, Alloway JA, Nashel DJ: Comparison of adrenocorticotropic hormone and triamcinolone acetonide in the treatment of acute gouty arthritis. J Rheumatol 1994; 21:1325.

22. Ben-Chetrit E, Levy M: Colchicine: 1998 update. Semin Arthritis Rheum 1998; 28:48.

23. Putterman C, Ben-Chetrit E, Caraco Y, et al: Colchicine intoxication: Clinical pharmacology, risk factors, features, and management. Semin Arthritis Rheum 1991; 21:143.

24. Wallace SL, Singer JZ: Systemic toxicity associated with the intravenous administration of colchicine: Guidelines for use. J Rheumatol 1988; 15:495.

25. Ahern MJ, Reid C, Grodon TP, et al: Does colchicine work? The results of the first controlled study in acute gout. Aust N Z J Med 1987; 17:301.

26. Yu TF, Gutman AB: Efficacy of colchicine prophylaxis: Prevention of recurrent gouty arthritis over a mean of five years in 208 gout subjects. Ann Intern Med 1961; 55:179.

27. Wyngarden JB, Kelley WN: Pharmacology of colchicine, indomethacin, and phenylbutazone. *In* Wyngarden JB, Kelley WN (eds): Gout and Hyperuricemia. New York: Grune and Stratton, 1976:421.

28. Ben-Chetrit E, Scherrmann J-M, Zylber-Katz E, et al: Colchicine disposition in patients with familial Mediterranean fever with renal impairment. J Rheumatol 1994; 21:710.

29. Kuncl RW, Duncan G, Watson D, et al: Colchicine myopathy and neuropathy. N Engl J Med 1987; 316:1562.

30. Elwood MG, Robb JH: Self-poisoning with colchicine. Postgrad Med 1971; 47:129.

31. Baud FJ, Sabouraud A, Vicaut E, et al: Brief report: Treatment of severe colchicine overdose with colchicine-specific Fab fragments. N Engl J Med 1995; 332:642.

32. Yu T-F: The efficacy of colchicine prophylaxis in articular gout: A reappraisal after 20 years. Semin Arthritis Rheum 1982; 12:256.

33. Wallace SL, Singer JZ, Duncan GJ, et al: Renal function predicts colchicine toxicity: Guidelines for the prophylactic use of colchicine in gout. J Rheumatol 1992; 18:264.

34. Emmerson BT: The management of gout. N Engl J Med 1996; 334:445.

35. Scott JT, Higgins CS: Diuretic induced gout: A multifactorial condition. Ann Rheum Dis 1992; 51:259.

36. Ferraz MB, O'Brien B: A cost effectiveness analysis of urate lowering drugs in nontophaceous recurrent gouty arthritis. J Rheumatol 1995; 22:908.

37. Ferraz MB: An evidence based appraisal of the management of nontophaceous interval gout [Editorial]. J Rheumatol 1995; 22:1618.

38. Fam AG: Should patients with interval gout be treated with urate lowering drugs? [Editorial]. J Rheumatol 1995; 22:1621.

39. van Lieshout-Zuidema MF, Breedveld FC: Withdrawal of long-term antihyperuricemic therapy in tophaceous gout. J Rheumatol 1993; 20:1383.

40. Rundles RW, Wyngarden JB, Hitchings GH, et al: Effects of a xanthine oxidase inhibitor on thiopurine metabolism, hyperuricemia, and gout. Trans Assoc Am Physicians 1963; 76:126.

41. Schumacher HR, Fox IR: Antihyperuricemic drugs. *In* Kelley WN, Harris ED, Ruddy S, et al (eds): Textbook of Rheumatology, 5th ed. Philadelphia: WB Saunders, 1997:829.

42. Hande KR, Noone RM, Stone WJ: Severe allopurinol toxicity: Description and guidelines for prevention in patients with renal insufficiency. Am J Med 1984; 76:47.

43. Singer JZ, Wallace SL: The allopurinol hypersensitivity syndrome: Unnecessary morbidity and mortality. Arthritis Rheum 1986; 29:82.

44. Gutman AB, Yu TF: Benemid (p-di-n-propylsulfamyl-benzoic acid) as a uricosuric agent in chronic gouty arthritis. Trans Assoc Am Physicians 1951; 64:372.

45. Talbott JM, Bishop C, Norcross BM, et al: The clinical and metabolic effects of Benemid in patients with gout. Trans Assoc Am Physicians 1951; 64:430.

46. Yussim A, Bar-Nathan N, Lustig S, et al: Gastrointestinal, hepatorenal, and neuromuscular toxicity caused by cyclosporine-colchicine interaction in renal transplantation. Transplant Proc 1994; 26:2825.

47. Rosenthal AK, Ryan LM: Treatment of refractory crystal-associated arthritis. Rheum Dis Clin North Am 1995; 21:151.

48. Simmonds HA, Gibson T, Huston GJ, et al: Gout resistant to allopurinol: Poor compliance or non-response. Adv Exp Med Biol 1984; 165:171.

49. Kersely GD: Allopurinol in primary gout with and after the administration of uricosuric agents. Ann Rheum Dis 1966; 25:643.

50. O'Duffy JD: Oxipurinol therapy in allopurinol-sensitive patients. Arthritis Rheum 1993; 36:S159.

51. Walz-LeBlanc B, Reynolds WJ, MacFadden DK: Allopurinol sensitivity in a patient with chronic tophaceous gout: Success of intravenous desensitization after failure of oral desensitization. Arthritis Rheum 1991; 34:1329.

52. Webster E, Panush RS: Allopurinol hypersensitivity in a patient with severe chronic tophaceous gout. Arthritis Rheum 1985; 78:707.

53. Fam AG, Lewtas J, Stein J, et al: Desensitization to allopurinol in patients with gout and cutaneous reactions. Am J Med 1992; 93:299.

54. Dunne SM, Fam AG, Iazzetta J, et al: Efficacy and safety of desensitization to allopurinol following cutaneous reactions. Arthritis Rheum 1998; 41:S151.

55. McCarty DJ, Kohn NN, Faires JS: The significance of calcium phosphate crystals in the synovial fluid of arthritis patients: The "pseudogout syndrome": I. Clinical aspects. Ann Intern Med 1962; 56:711.

56. Alvarellos A, Spilberg I: Colchicine prophylaxis in pseudogout. J Rheumatol 1986; 13:804.

57. Roane DW, Harris MD, Carpenter MT, et al: Prospective use of intramuscular triamcinolone acetonide in pseudogout. J Rheumatol 1997; 24:1168.

58. Werlin D, Gabay C, Vischer TL: Corticosteroid therapy for the treatment of acute attacks of crystal-induced arthritis: An effective alternative to nonsteroidal antiinflammatory drugs. Rev Rheum Engl Ed 1996; 63:248.

59. Rothschild B, Yakabov LE: Prospective 6 month double blind trial of hydroxychloroquine treatment of CPPD. Compr Ther 1997; 23:327.

60. Doherty M, Dieppe PA: Double blind placebo controlled trial of magnesium carbonate in chronic pyrophosphate arthropathy. Ann Rheum Dis 1983; 42(suppl):106.

61. Fam AG, Rubenstein J: Hydroxyapatite pseudopodagra: A syndrome of young women. Arthritis Rheum 1989; 32:741.

62. McCarty DJ, Halverson PB, Carrera GF, et al: "Milwaukee shoulder": Association of microspheroids containing hydroxyapatite

crystals, active collagenase, and neutral protease with rotator cuff defects: I. Clinical aspects. Arthritis Rheum 1981; 24:464.

63. Halverson PB, Carrera GF, McCarty DJ: Milwaukee shoulder syndrome: Fifteen additional cases and a description of contributing factors. Arch Intern Med 1990; 150:677.

64. Simon LS, Lanza FL, Lipsky PE, et al: Preliminary study of the safety and efficacy of SC-58635, a novel cyclooxygenase-2 inhibitor: Efficacy and safety in two placebo-controlled trials in osteoarthritis and rheumatoid arthritis, and studies of gastrointestinal and platelet effects. Arthritis Rheum 1998; 41:1591.

65. Chua CC, Greenberg ML, Viau AT: Use of polyethylene glycol-modified uricase (PEG-URICASE) to treat hyperuricemia in a patient with non-Hodgkin lymphoma. Ann Intern Med 1988; 109:114.

66. Pui CH, Relling MV, Lascombes F, et al: Urate oxidase in prevention and treatment of hyperuricemia associated with lymphoid malignancies. Leukemia 1997; 11:1813.

67. Mahmoud HH, Leverger G, Patte C, et al: Advances in the management of malignancy-associated hyperuricemia. Br J Cancer 1998; 77(suppl 4):18.

68. Zurcher RM, Bock HA, Thiel G: Excellent uricosuric efficacy of benzbromarone in cyclosporine-A-treated renal transplant patients: A prospective study. Nephrol Dial Transplant 1994; 9:548.

69. Perez-Ruiz F, Alonso-Ruiz A, Calabozo M, et al: Efficacy of allopurinol and benzbromarone for the control of hyperuricemia: A pathogenic approach to the treatment of primary chronic gout. Ann Rheum Dis 1998; 57:545.

# 36 | Osteoarthritis

*Boris Ratiner, Deirdre A. Gramas, and Nancy E. Lane*

Osteoarthritis (OA) is a slowly evolving disease of articular cartilage degeneration characterized by the gradual development of joint pain, stiffness, and limitation of motion. OA is considered common if the radiographic definition of the disease—that more than 75% of persons over 70 years of age show some radiographic evidence of the OA—is accepted.[1] It affects the joints of the hands, including the distal interphalangeal joints, the proximal interphalangeal joints, and the carpometacarpal joint of the thumb. Other joints involved include the cervical spine, the lumbosacral spine, the hip, the knee, and the first metatarsophalangeal joint. The ankle, wrist, elbow, and shoulder are much less frequently involved. There are known inconsistencies between findings on radiographs and clinical symptoms; only 50% to 60% of patients in whom OA is diagnosed by radiograph are clinically symptomatic.[2]

A number of factors have been implicated in the pathogenesis of OA: the genetic predisposition of the individual, previous trauma, previous occupation, inflammation, exercise, and biochemical and metabolic abnormalities.[2,3] The disease process of OA probably begins in the articular cartilage, but it eventually involves the surrounding bone, the synovium, and other surrounding soft tissues. When cartilage is absent from the articular surface, the underlying bone is subjected to greater local stress. Wolff's law of bone remodeling predicts new bone formation in these areas, resulting in bony sclerosis that is often seen on radiographs.[4] Subarticular bone cysts are also commonly seen on radiographs and generally exist only in the absence of overlying cartilage. Bone cysts are the result of the transmission of intra-articular pressure on the marrow spaces of the subchondral bone. Cysts increase in size until the pressure in the cyst is equal to the intra-articular pressure. If the joint becomes covered with reparative cartilage, the cysts regress.[5] Finally, the breakdown of both cartilage and bone produces a chronic inflammatory response in the synovium of the joint.[2,3,6]

Because OA results from a degeneration of articular cartilage, an understanding of the biochemical events of OA is important. We begin with a description of pathophysiologic changes in articular cartilage.

## PATHOPHYSIOLOGY OF OSTEOARTHRITIS

Although there may be different precipitating factors in OA, there are similar biochemical changes. These changes affect the joints in OA in two major matrix components: proteoglycan and type II collagen. There is a progressive depletion of cartilage proteoglycan that parallels the severity of the disease.[7] At a certain stage, the chondrocytes appear unable to fully compensate for the proteoglycan depletion; this results in a net loss of matrix. The structural changes of the proteoglycan macromolecules include a decrease in hyaluronic acid content, a diminution in the size of the proteoglycan aggregates to monomers, and a decrease in the size and aggregation of monomers.[7-9] The latter changes are probably related to the enzymatic cleavage of the proteoglycan monomer core protein in several areas, including the hyaluronic acid–binding region.[10]

Although the content of type II collagen remains unchanged in OA, increased cartilage hydration and ultrastructural changes of the collagen fibers represent important alterations in the collagen fiber network.[11] The increase in minor collagen types such as type I collagen, particularly in the pericellular area, suggests a change in chondrocyte metabolism. Together with the damaged collagen structure, changes in the proteoglycan content of the matrix lead to a functional deterioration of the cartilage. This makes the cartilage less resistant to compression or mechanical stress and leads to the appearance of cartilage loss.

Cartilage loss in OA occurs by enzymatic and mechanical degradation.[12] The enzymatic process appears to be a cascade of events. Whereas the synovium is the most important source of degradative enzymes in rheumatoid arthritis, the chondrocytes appear to be the most significant source of enzyme responsible for cartilage matrix catabolism in OA.[13,14] The matrix metalloproteinase enzymes (MMPs) are implicated in cartilage matrix degradation in OA.[15,16] Collagenase (MMP-1) appears to be responsible for the breakdown of the collagen network in OA cartilage, inasmuch as increased collagenase level has been detected both in experimental OA and in human OA cartilage.[11,16] The collagenase level has also been found to correlate with the severity of OA cartilage lesions. Likewise, stromelysin (MMP-2) and gelatinase (MMP-7 and MMP-9) have been identified in human articular cartilage, and their levels correlate with the severity of the OA lesions.[17,18]

The biologic activity of metalloproteinases is controlled by both physiologic inhibitors and activators. At least two tissue inhibitors of metalloproteinases

(TIMP-1 and TIMP-2) are known to exist in humans. In OA cartilage, there is an imbalance between synthesis of TIMP and metalloproteinases. A relative deficiency in the amount of the inhibitor[19, 20] favors an increased level of active metalloproteinases and, secondarily, matrix degradation.

The early changes in the course of OA—cartilage swelling and increased hydration—can be attributed to a breakdown of the collagenous framework that allows further hydration of the matrix.[3, 7] Synthesis of proteoglycans (especially those richer in chondroitin sulfate) increases early in OA, presumably as attempted repair mechanisms are overwhelmed and then overall proteoglycan degradation of the aggregate to monomers ensues. With further breakdown of the collagen framework and depletion of matrix proteins, structural changes, such as blistering, fibrillation, and fissuring, appear. There are concomitant changes in the subchondral bone, and the articular surface is eventually denuded.[3, 7]

After the initial stages of cartilage degeneration, which may have resulted from an injury, there may be a delay of many years before the affected person feels any joint pain or before a radiograph shows evidence of cartilage degeneration (joint space narrowing or osteophyte formation). This delay in the appearance of symptoms is attributable in part to the lack of innervation of the cartilage. There is a rich nerve supply to the surrounding structures, including the periosteum, subchondral bone, and the joint capsule.[3] Therefore, significant and irreversible cartilage damage has occurred before inflammation and attendant joint pain appear.

No therapy has yet been shown to arrest the progression of OA. The challenge for the clinician is to find a way to best preserve joint function, treat joint pain, and treat concurrent inflammation. The remainder of this chapter covers the current therapeutic approaches for OA.

## THERAPY FOR OSTEOARTHRITIS

The key to the effective management of OA rests in an accurate and appropriate diagnosis. As noted earlier, OA has a long asymptomatic period, and there is

## TABLE 36–1
### Classification Criteria for Hand Osteoarthritis

Hand pain, aching, or stiffness *and* at least three of the following:
  Hard tissue enlargement of 2 or more of 10 selected joints*
  Hard tissue enlargement of 2 or more DIP joints
  Deformity of at least 1 of 10 selected joints
  Fewer than 3 swollen MCP joints

CMC = carpometacarpal; DIP = distal interphalangeal; MCP = metacarpophalangeal; PIP = proximal interphalangeal.
  * These include the second and third DIP, the second and third PIP, and the first CMC joint on each hand.
  Sensitivity, 94%; specificity, 87%.
  From Deal CL, Schnitzer TJ, Lipstein E, et al: Treatment of arthritis with topical capsaicin: A double blind trial. Clin Ther 1991; 13(3):383–395.

## TABLE 36–2
### Classification Criteria for Hip Osteoarthritis

Hip pain *and* at least two of the following:
  Erythrocyte sedimentation rate < 20 mm/hour
  Radiographic femoral or acetabular osteophytes
  Radiographic joint space narrowing

Sensitivity, 89%; specificity, 91%
From Altman R, Avea A, Holmburg CE, et al: Capsaicin cream 0.025% as monotherapy for osteoarthritis: A double blind study. Semin Arthritis Rheum 1994; 23(suppl 3):25–33.

little justification for its treatment during this stage. Joint space narrowing, subchondral sclerosis, and osteophytosis may be radiographic incidental findings in someone with musculoskeletal pain from another cause. A careful history and physical examination, radiographs, and well-directed laboratory tests are required if there is a clinical indication. The American College of Rheumatology has published guidelines to guide the clinician in establishing a diagnosis of hand (Table 36–1), hip (Table 36–2), and knee (Table 36–3) OA. When the diagnosis of OA is secure, therapeutic decisions are made on the basis of the patient's pain, discomfort, and level of disability; the joint involved; and, to some extent, the degree of radiographic damage.

## NONPHARMACOLOGIC THERAPIES

### General Principles and Weight Loss

Simple, nonpharmacologic measures should be used initially in the treatment of OA. If the problem suggests a "mechanical" component, such as worsening of pain by the end of the day or after strenuous activity, therapy should be directed toward reduction of the stress or load on that joint and emphasis on periarticular muscle strengthening, so as to promote optimal biomechanical alignment of that joint. If the appropriate physical therapy has not ameliorated pain or disability, other modalities should be considered. These include oral and/or topical analgesics, intra-articular glucocorticoids, intra-articular hyaluronic acid, and nonsteroidal anti-inflammatory drugs (NSAIDs). After pharmacologic treatment, other nonpharmacologic treatment methods will avoid further mechanical damage; they include the use of assistive devices, muscle-

## TABLE 36–3
### Classification Criteria for Knee Osteoartheritis

Knee pain *and* osteophytes *and* at least one of the following:
  Age > 50 years
  Crepitus on motion
  Stiffness < 30 minutes

Sensitivity, 91%; specificity, 86%
From McCarthy GM, McCarty DJ: Effect of topical capsaicin in the therapy of painful osteoarthritis of the hands. J Rheumatol 1992; 19(4):604–607.

strengthening techniques, and avoidance of previously destructive habits. Strategies used to prevent excessive use and to reduce mechanical strain on the hands, knees, and hips are simple and straightforward:

1. Use light-weight utensils.
2. Wrap utensils with foam rubber for grip.
3. Use a ring or loop on a zipper to pull up and down.
4. Use electric appliances whenever possible.
5. Use Velcro fasteners and zippers instead of buttons.
6. Use a single-lever faucet.
7. Avoid lifting heavy objects; get help.
8. If you must lift heavy items, use both hands and forearms, and place them under the object.
9. Avoid standing for prolonged periods.

Poor body mechanics and improper posture may be a leading factor in the causation and exacerbation of pain in OA. Numerous epidemiologic studies have shown that obesity is commonly associated with OA and causes abnormal stresses on the articular cartilage in weight-bearing joints. Therefore, weight loss may provide additional symptomatic relief of pain as well as reduce mechanical joint damage.[21] To best maintain independent and active living, collaboration and close contact with the family, physical therapist, and occupational therapist are important.

An occupational or physical therapist can also help with avoidance of repetitive-motion injury during recreation or at work. They can provide a number of ergonomic and assistive devices that can both decrease joint load and repetitive motion. Examples of assistive devices include a cane for hip and knee problems, a knee brace for exercise, a tool to improve handgrip, and an elevated toilet seat. OA patients who walk for occupation or recreation may need special shoes with good shock absorption and extra depth, extra width, or metatarsal bars to improve toe alignment and relieve pain.

Physicians should initiate patient education, in the form of pamphlets and referral to a community arthritis support group (both of which are available through the Arthritis Foundation) and possibly a referral to a physical or occupational therapist. The support groups and the therapists can be very helpful, both as educators and as motivators, to patients with OA. There is strong evidence that health education for self-management of chronic arthritis can decrease pain, number of visits to physicians' offices, and the patient's overall disability.[22–27]

## Rehabilitation and Exercise

Rehabilitation is essential for the prevention of joint destruction, restoration of joint function after damage has occurred, and maintenance of joint function. Rehabilitation assists the patient in reaching his or her maximal potential. An individualized program is developed to meet the needs of every patient. This program includes occupational therapy, physical therapy, vocational counseling, and social work services. Rehabilitation is limited by the extent of arthritis, motor and neurologic skills, and the patient's own motivation.

The first goal for a patient with symptomatic OA of a joint is to reduce, control, and prevent pain. The second goal is to preserve the patient's functional level and prevent further pain, weakness, and disability. Muscles are key to maintaining joint stability and flexibility, and aerobic conditioning and muscle-strengthening exercises have been shown to be helpful in improving overall function and decreasing pain in patients with knee OA.[28, 29] This can include a low-impact aerobic regimen, such as walking or aquatics for 30 minutes, three times per week, and local muscle strengthening, such as quadriceps exercises for knee OA.[30] Energy conservation, in the form of maximizing function and decreasing muscle fatigue, is also necessary for success. Adaptive equipment or substitutive devices are employed as needed to compensate for lost function. Education and guidance must be available to patients, because they are needed to develop the coping strategies necessary for an effective rehabilitative program.

Other modalities that can be helpful include application of local heat or cold packs, isometric exercise programs, ultrasonography, and splinting of affected joints. These modalities can decrease joint pain, local muscle spasm, stiffness, and swelling, and they help protect the joint.[31–33] Improving body mechanics and posture training, often with the help of physical therapists, can also help control pain and prevent further injury. These methods can be used separately or in combination.

More controversial therapies include the use of transcutaneous electrical nerve stimulation (TENS) devices, acupuncture, auricular stimulation, and laser therapy.[34, 35] Although these methods are not used routinely and have not been studied in a scientific manner, many patients attest to satisfactory results. Patients with OA who cannot tolerate medical therapy for OA may have significant relief from the pain of OA with any or all of these modalities. More detailed descriptions of these modalities for the treatment of OA are available in several reviews.[36, 37]

## PRINCIPLES OF PHARMACEUTICAL THERAPY IN OSTEOARTHRITIS

OA is a chronic disease with intermittent exacerbations and disease flares that often resolve without intervention. The natural history of OA with its intermittent exacerbations of pain can make it difficult to demonstrate a difference between the effects of an investigational drug and those of placebo in clinical trials. In addition, investigators are just beginning to validate and standardize radiographic and histologic parameters that can be used in clinical studies for the measurement of progression of disease. Traditionally, the lack of standardized disease definitions and study designs has made it difficult to compare efficacy in different treatments of OA.[23]

Nevertheless, many studies have focused on drug efficacy in OA.[23] These studies use outcome measures such as pain relief, joint mobility, walking time, quality of life, time lost from work, and global assessment by patient and physician. Other studies use radiographic or histologic end points, determined by serial radiographs, arthroscopic scores, and cartilage or synovial specimens. Reviews of common outcome measurements for OA have been recommended and appear in other publications.[38-41]

In the next sections of this chapter, we discuss the most common medications used to treat the pain and inflammation of OA, recommend guidelines for prescribing them, and discuss clinically important side effects.

## Pure Analgesics

On the basis of the degree of pain, amount of functional disability, and lack of improvement with nonpharmaceutical therapies, medications for relief of pain should be considered (Table 36–4). For a single joint, therapy can be directed locally. When multiple joints are involved, systemic therapy should be considered. Treatment for OA is often multifactorial and consists of a combination of analgesics and anti-inflammatory agents.[23, 42]

Topical analgesics can be tried as sole therapy for mild to moderate OA of the hand, elbow, shoulder, and knee; however, most trials have focused on such agents as adjuncts in the treatment of OA. Local application of capsaicin or salicylate cream over the affected joint has been shown, in randomized controlled trials, to be more effective than placebo in reducing joint pain and improving joint function.[43-45] In one study, 70 patients with knee OA were randomly assigned to receive capsaicin, which works by locally depleting substance P, or placebo for 4 weeks. The capsaicin was applied four times per day, and patients were allowed to continue their previous arthritis medications. Patients treated with the capsaicin had significant reductions in pain scores after both 2 and 4 weeks.[43, 45] Pain relief is only local, however, and the cream must be applied multiple times per day to have maximal effect.

Local skin irritation is the most commonly cited side effect but is tolerable for most patients; with continued use, the burning sensation seems to fade, whereas the analgesic effect persists. These medications can be particularly helpful in patients who do not want oral treatments, cannot tolerate NSAIDs, or have intermittent painful OA joint flares in a single joint.

Non-narcotic mild oral analgesics, such as acetaminophen, may be the initial and sole therapy for some patients with OA. Acetaminophen is generally safe in dosages of less than 4000 mg/day (eight 500-mg tablets/day or twelve 325-mg tablets/day). This is not true, however, for patients with preexisting liver disease or known ongoing alcohol use.[46] In such patients, acetaminophen should be prescribed with caution, usually in dosages of less than 2 g/day, and liver function test results should be monitored closely.

Multiple studies have reinforced the benefit of acetaminophen in OA. Whether it is equivalent to NSAIDs, especially over months or years, remains controversial. In 1981, Doyle and associates compared ketoprofen with propoxyphene/acetaminophen in the treatment of OA.[47] In this double-blind, crossover trial of 44 patients with OA, there were no observed differences in the relief of pain. However, the articular index score and "patient preference" scale favored ketoprofen as the drug of choice. In a second randomized, double-blind study of 864 patients with OA of the hip, knee, wrist, or ankle, there was a significant decrease in pain with slow-release diclofenac in comparison with propoxyphene/acetaminophen.[48] Finally, in a small, double-blind, crossover study comparing flurbiprofen with nefopam (an analgesic) for the treatment of pain in 30 patients with OA of the knee, no differences were found between the study agents.[49]

Bradley and coworkers compared two dosages of ibuprofen with high-dosage acetaminophen in the treatment of a flare of mild to moderate OA of the knee.[50] In this study, 195 subjects were randomly assigned to three treatment groups: low or analgesic dosage of ibuprofen (1200 mg/day), high or anti-inflammatory levels of ibuprofen (2400 mg/day), and acetaminophen (4000 mg/day). Baseline characteristics for these individuals with OA of the knee were

## TABLE 36–4
## Commonly Used Analgesics

| DRUG NAME | USUAL TOTAL DAILY DOSAGE FOR PATIENTS WITH OSTEOARTHRITIS | SHORT (S) OR LONG (L) ACTING | MOST COMMON SIDE EFFECTS |
|---|---|---|---|
| Acetaminophen | 650–3000 mg | S | Liver Toxicity |
| Codeine (alone or in combination with acetaminophen or aspirin) | 30–180 mg | S | Lightheadedness, dizziness, sedation Shortness of breath, nausea, respiratory distress |
| Tramadol | 100–400 mg | S | Dizziness/vertigo, nausea, constipation, headache, somnnolence, pruritis, central nervous system stimulation, and rarely seizures |

From Harris ED Jr, Genovese M (eds): *Primary Care Rheumatology*. Philadelphia: WB Saunders, 2000.

similar. After 4 weeks of therapy, changes in pain and disability score,[51] walking pain score, walking distance, 50-foot walk time, and physician assessment were comparable between groups. However, there was a statistically significant improvement in rest pain in both groups of ibuprofen-treated patients in comparison with the acetaminophen-treated patients ($P = .05$). The results of this study suggest that high daily doses of acetaminophen may be equivalent to high- and low-dosage ibuprofen for a flare of knee OA. However, in this study there was no placebo group with which to assess the degree of spontaneous improvement in comparison to drug effect. Also, OA is a disease that occurs over years, not 30 days; therefore, the long-term effects of acetaminophen on reducing joint pain in knee OA are not clear.

To compare the long-term efficacy and safety of analgesics (acetaminophen) and NSAIDs (naproxen), a 2-year, double-blind, multicenter parallel trial was performed.[52] One hundred seventy-eight patients with OA of the knee were monitored for up to 2 years. The primary end points of the study were radiographic progression of OA and withdrawal of the drug because of lack of efficacy. Only 62 (35%) of the original 178 patients completed the 2-year study. The only significant difference between the two groups was slightly higher efficacy for naproxen, but in view of the high drop-out rate from both study groups, it could be concluded that neither drug was efficacious in the long-term treatment of knee OA. The reasons for the high dropout rate among the patients receiving acetaminophen (Tylenol) were more likely lack of response and noncompliance, whereas for the naproxen recipients, the reasons were more likely gastrointestinal side effects, lack of efficacy, and noncompliance (in that order).

Tramadol, a new type of analgesic, has been approved by the US Food and Drug Administration for the treatment of acute and chronic pain. Its analgesic effect is likely derived from a combination blockade of opioid receptors and inhibition of norepinephrine and serotonin reuptake. This helps explain why its effect can be only partially blocked by naloxone, a pure opioid antagonist. Preliminary studies show that it is effective for breakthrough pain in patients with OA who are currently taking an NSAID.[53, 54] In a randomized 3-week study of 40 patients with knee OA pain not relieved by NSAIDs, tramadol, 50 mg TID, was superior in relieving rest pain over propoxyphene, 65 mg TID.[54] In a similar study of 14 days' duration, tramadol was significantly more effective than placebo in relieving breakthrough rest pain of the knee.[53] Long-term studies of efficacy and toxicity for tramadol in OA patients are not currently available, but because it does have some opioid-like effects, its use is not recommended in patients with a history of physical dependence to opioids.

More potent analgesics, consisting of opiates, either alone or in combination with acetaminophen or aspirin, have also been shown to be most helpful for acute, painful flares of OA. Traditionally, these agents have been best used in occasional short (2- to 4-week) courses during times of severe pain that does not respond to other medications.[55] However, it has been shown that in several rheumatic diseases, including OA, opiates can be safe and effective even as longer term (>3 months) therapy.[56] Although abuse and dependence should remain a concern in all patients taking narcotic medications, the above study concluded that when used for well-defined rheumatic diseases, including OA, tolerance and dependence were not a significant problem.[56] Only 4 of 32 patients in this cohort exhibited abuse behaviors. Side effects included nausea, constipation, headache, dizziness, and sedation. These can be of special concern in elderly patients because of increased risk of falls. There is also the theoretical risk of masking symptoms of joint infection or ligamental damage, an issue that was not addressed in this study.

## Nonsteroidal Anti-inflammatory Drugs (Table 36–5)

### General Principles

NSAIDs are widely used in the treatment of OA. In low dosages, NSAIDs are effective analgesics; in higher dosages, they have anti-inflammatory activity. Low dosages provide an analgesic effect by inhibiting prostaglandin sensitization of peripheral pain receptors.[57] In higher dosages, they exert their anti-inflammatory actions through a number of biologic systems:

- Prostaglandin production
- Leukotriene function
- Lymphocyte function
- Neutrophil aggregation and granule release
- Rheumatoid factor production
- Alteration of membrane viscosity
- Superoxide generation
- Lysosomal enzyme release
- Cell membrane function
- Inhibition of diacylglycerol production

First, NSAIDs inhibit the production of the enzyme cyclooxygenase (COX), especially the isoenzyme COX-1, which catalyzes the formation of prostaglandins from arachidonic acid (Fig. 36–1). Prostaglandins mediate the process of inflammation by causing erythema, vasodilatation, and pain. Aspirin (acetylsalicylic acid) irreversibly acetylates COX, thereby permanently interfering with prostaglandin production for the life of the platelet or cell. All other NSAIDs reversibly interfere with the active site of COX and antagonize its activity. After COX inhibition, arachidonic acid may build up and be directed to leukotriene synthesis regulated by lipoxygenase. Some in vitro lipoxygenase inhibition by sodium meclofenamate,[58] diclofenac,[59] and ketoprofen[60] has been reported. The clinical significance of this is currently unknown.

In the early 1990s, the existence of multiple several forms of the COX enzyme was reported. The first isoenzyme, COX-1, also known as the *constitutive* form, and the second isoenzyme, COX-2, also known as *inducible*. The constitutive form is present in most tissues and is responsible for "housekeeping" issues in the body by synthesizing prostaglandins that regulate normal cellular activities.[61] These prostaglandins play a role in

## TABLE 36–5
## Nonsteroidal Anti-Inflammatory Drugs

| CLASS | CATEGORY | DRUG NAME | USUAL TOTAL DAILY DOSAGE FOR OA PATIENTS | SHORT (S) OR LONG (L) ACTING | GI BLEED RISK | NAUSEA OR DYSPEPSIA | RISK OF DYSURIA, RENAL INSUFFICIENCY, OR PAPILLARY NECROSIS | RASH OR PRURITIS | DIZZINESS, HEADACHE, OR TINITUS | OTHER |
|---|---|---|---|---|---|---|---|---|---|---|
| Nonselective COX inhibitors | Arylcarboxylic acids | Acetylsalicylic acid (aspirin) | 650–3000 mg | S | ++ | +++ | + | +++ | ++++ | Enteric-coated and available |
| | | Salsalate (Salflex Disalcid) | 750–3000 mg | L | + | +++ | + | + | ++++ | |
| | Arylalkanoic acids | Diflunisal (Dolobid) | 500–1000 mg | L | + | +++ | + | +++ | +++ | Enteric-coated and long-acting (XL) available |
| | | Diclofenac (Voltaren) | 100–150 mg | S | ++ | +++ | + | ++ | ++ | |
| | | Ibuprofen (Motrin, Advil) | 1200–2400 mg | S | + | +++ | + | +++ | +++ | Edema |
| | | Naproxen (Naprosyn, Aleve) | 500–1000 mg | L | + | +++ | + | +++ | +++ | Edema |
| | | Oxaprozin (Daypro) | 600–1200 mg | L | + | +++ | ++ | +++ | ++ | |
| | | Tolmetin (Tolectin) | 600–1800 mg | S | +– | ++++ | ++ | ++ | ++ | Edema |
| | | Ketorolac tromethamine (Toradol) | 30 mg IV/IM (max 5 days) or 10–60 mg PO | S | | | | | | |
| | | Indomethacin (Indocin) | 75–2000 mg | S | + | +++ | + | + | ++++ | Long-acting (SR) available |
| | | Sulindac (Clinoril) | 300–400 mg | L | + | ++++ | + | +++ | +++ | Edema |
| | | Etodolac (Lodine) | 600–1200 mg | S | + | ++++ | ++ | ++ | ++ | Edema |
| | | Flurbiprofen (Ansaid) | 100–300 mg | S | + | +++ | +++ | ++ | ++ | Edema |
| | | Ketoprofen (Orudis, Actron) | 75–300 mg | S | + | ++++ | +++ | ++ | +++ | |
| | Enolic acid | Piroxicam (Feldene) | 10–20 mg | L | +– | ++++ | ++ | ++ | ++ | Edema |
| | Nonacidic agent | Nabumetone (Relafen) | 1000–2000 mg | L | +– | ++++ | + | +++ | +++ | Edema |
| Selective COX-2 Inhibitors | | Celecoxib (Celebrex) | 200–400 mg | L | + | ++ | + | ++ | ++++ | No detected effect on platelet function |
| | | Rofecoxib (Vioxx) | 12.5–25 mg | L | | | | | | |

COX = cyclooxygenase; GI = gastrointestinal; IM = intramuscularly; IV = intravenously; OA = osteoarthritis; PO = per os (orally).
Adapted from Harris ED Jr, Genovese M (eds): Primary Care Rheumatology. Philadelphia: WB Saunders, 2000.

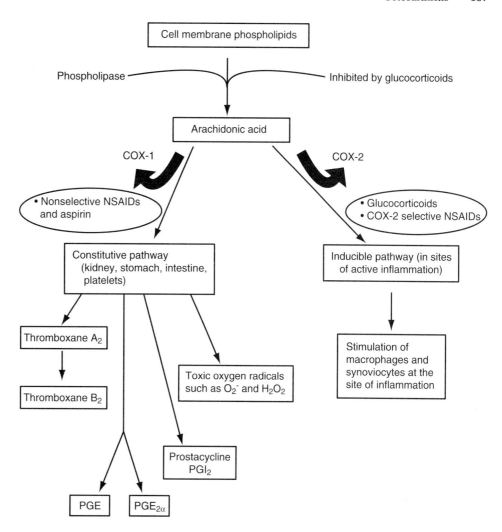

**FIGURE 36–1**
Cyclooxygenase pathway for arachidonic acid metabolism. COX-1 = cyclooxygenase-1; COX-2 = cyclooxygenase-2; NSAIDs = nonsteroidal anti-inflammatory drugs; PGE = prostaglandin E.

normal physiologic functions such as gastrointestinal cytoprotection, vascular homeostasis, and renal function. COX-2, on the other hand, is almost undetectable in most tissues until active inflammation begins to take place, and it is likely that the inhibition of this form of the enzyme is responsible for most of the anti-inflammatory effect seen with traditional NSAIDs.[61] Other anti-inflammatory agents, specifically glucocorticoids that down-regulate COX-2 expression, can also prevent the induction of COX-2 activity by other proinflammatory cytokines,[61] through similar mechanisms.

The anti-inflammatory activity of NSAIDs, however, extends beyond their ability to inhibit COX and lipoxygenase. Cell membrane–linked processes such as superoxide generation,[62] phospholipase C activity,[63] and oxidative phosphorylation[64] may be inhibited by the ability of NSAIDs to disrupt lipid membranes.[65] Inhibition of diacylglycerol production and alteration of membrane viscosity may also occur.[66]

The concept that NSAIDs might alter the course of OA was first described in vitro by Annefeld in 1983.[67] NSAIDs may influence cartilage degradation by either stimulation or inhibition of the extracellular matrix production. Using a semiquantitative method, Annefeld measured the ultrastructural changes in lap-

ine chondrocytes induced by steroids and classified the changes as either stimulatory or inhibitory on the basis of semiqualitative changes in the endoplasmic reticulum, nucleus, and mitochondria of the cell.[68] As Annefeld proceeded to evaluate NSAIDs in this in vitro system, these agents were referred to as chondroprotective because some NSAIDs stimulated ultrastructural changes in the chrondrocyte. We prefer not to use that term because the protection of cartilage degradation by NSAIDs has not been determined or established. To our knowledge, no clinical study documents the ability of NSAIDs to protect articular cartilage or slow the progression of OA. To determine whether NSAIDs alter the degradation of articular cartilage in OA, a 10- to 15-year longitudinal study of patients with early OA would be needed.

Not surprisingly, NSAIDs have had both a positive and a negative effect on cartilage metabolism in several different experimental systems. For example, tiaprofenic acid (an NSAID not available in the United States) was found to increase proteoglycan production in cartilage explants of patients with OA, as well as increase proteoglycan aggregate size and decrease aggregate fragments.[69] Alternatively, aspirin, fenoprofen, and ibuprofen inhibit proteoglycan synthesis in normal canine articular cartilage slices, whereas indomethacin and sulindac do not.[70–74] Although these data are intriguing, their clinical significance is yet to be determined. Caution must be exercised in interpreting the effects of medications of cartilage explant cultures. In vitro studies do not account for the mechanical stimulus of an active joint or the chondrocyte's interaction with the extracellular matrix compartment. Furthermore, investigators have shown that there is marked variability in chondrocyte metabolism.[75, 76]

Choosing a nonsteroidal agent in the treatment of OA is not simple task. Patient response is influenced by factors other than pain relief and is not predictable.[77] In choosing an NSAID, it is prudent to recommend the drug with the least severe side effects. If the patient has current other illnesses or is elderly, a trial of an NSAID with a *short* half-life (4 to 6 hours) is warranted, with close follow-up. The elderly are at increased risk for the development of toxicity because of a reduction in hepatic mass, blood flow, glomerular filtration rate, and lean mass and because of an increase in body fat.[78] These factors change the distribution, protein binding, metabolism, and excretion of the medication. Although no conclusive studies to this effect have been performed it is hoped that the selective COX-2 inhibitors are the least toxic to this group of patients.

NSAIDs interact with commonly used drugs that need to be evaluated per patient and condition. The most common and potentially serious interaction is between nonselective NSAIDs and warfarin. NSAIDs may effect the metabolism of s-warfarin, cause an increase in the prothrombin time and potentiate a bleeding diathesis.[79] NSAIDs displace warfarin from binding to serum proteins and result in an increase in free warfarin, leading to an increased tendency to bleed. Of more importance, nonselective NSAIDs themselves cause asymptomatic damage and bleeding in the gastrointestinal mucosa. This intestinal damage, coupled with an inhibition of thromboxane and decreased platelet aggregation ("plugging"), increases the risk significantly for gastrointestinal hemorrhage. On the basis of risk/benefit analysis, there has been no indication for the use of nonselective NSAIDs in OA for the patient who is taking anticoagulants. An open question is whether the selective (inducible) COX-2 inhibitors have the same interaction with warfarin as do their nonselective predecessors (see discussion of inducible COX-2 inhibitors, in the later section on hematologic complications). Until further studies can be done, we suggest prescribing alternative medications such as analgesics and/or corticosteroid injections before prescribing NSAIDs to patients taking warfarin.

In considering analgesia and arthritis, it is important to consider pain a physiologic response. If an analgesic is effective, overuse of the joint may occur. The goals for the clinician and the patient are to decrease pain and improve well-being but to avoid overuse and accelerated joint degeneration. In 1989 Rashad and colleagues randomly assigned 105 subjects with hip OA to treatment with either indomethacin or azapropazone (a weak prostaglandin inhibitor) and monitored the progression of OA to determine need for surgical

arthroplasty.[80] They reported that the azapropazone-treated subjects took 5 months longer than the indomethacin recipients to reach the arthroplasty end point (15.6 vs. 10.4 months) and had less radiographic progression of OA than did the indomethacin recipients. This suggests that potent inhibitors of prostaglandin synthesis, such as indomethacin, may actually accelerate OA of the hip. Although the mechanism responsible for this effect was not determined, indomethacin may have created an "analgesic arthropathy" by effective pain relief and worsened the course of OA of the humoral head. These results suggest that analgesic compounds may have a role in the treatment of OA in patients who have pain out of proportion to the degree of inflammation or have contraindications to the use of NSAIDs.

In the rest of this section, these agents are discussed separately as nonselective COX inhibitors (primarily constitutive, or COX-1, agents) and selective COX inhibitors (primarily inducible, or COX-2, agents). Although the second category currently consists of only a few agents, it has a different side effect profile and has been used in only a small number of patients, in comparison with the first category, which have been studied for many decades and for which there is a large volume of data.

## Nonselective Cyclooxygenase Inhibitors

The NSAIDs in this category are primarily COX-1 inhibitors. They are categorized according to their molecular structure, as seen in Table 36–5, and are categorized as either salicylates or nonsalicylate NSAIDs. The salicylates may be either acetylated or nonacetylated. The acetyl group is responsible for increased potency and toxicity of aspirin (acetylsalicylic acid) in comparison with the nonacetylated salicylates and nonsalicylate NSAIDs. The propionic acid derivatives, indole/indene acetic acid derivatives, heteroaryl acetic acid derivatives, arylacetic acid derivatives, and fenamic acid derivatives are nonsalicylate NSAIDs. Enolic acid, pyranocarboxylic acid, and naphthalkone are also nonsalicylates; only one agent in each group (piroxicam, etodolac, and nabumetone) is currently used in the United States.

Differences in the half-lives of the NSAIDs do not correlate with their molecular structures and are important to recognize. The NSAIDs with long half-lives include naproxen, phenylbutazone, sulindac, diflunisal, piroxicam, and nabumetone. The longer half-life, which ranges from 12 to 38 hours, allows the agent more time to equilibrate between the plasma and synovial fluid. The average half-life of piroxicam is 38 hours, but it has been reported to last for up to 158 hours.[81] The short-acting NSAIDs include indomethacin, ibuprofen, fenoprofen, ketoprofen, tolmetin, meclofenamate, diclofenac, etodolac, flurbiprofen, and ketorolac. The half-lives of these agents range between 1 and 8 hours. When there is concern about the toxicity of NSAIDs in elderly patients or in those with preexisting conditions, the short-acting agents are recommended.

All NSAIDs are metabolized in the liver by hydroxylation, carboxylation, or glucuronidation and are excreted in the urine. In some patients with renal insufficiency, the inactive metabolites may be resynthesized or converted back into their active compounds. Indomethacin and sulindac, both of which are indole acetic acid derivatives, undergo enterohepatic circulation and should be used with caution in patients with liver and cholestatic disease. There is more than 95% protein binding of NSAIDs to serum albumin, so that drugs or medical conditions that decrease the protein binding increase the percentage of free drug, and this may increase toxicity. The pro-drugs sulindac and nabumetone are converted to the active compounds after absorption. This pro-drug effect may spare some (but not all) of the gastrointestinal tract toxicity and may be useful for patients who are prone to gastrointestinal side effects.

## Gastrointestinal Toxicity

The inhibition of prostaglandins locally, in the gastric mucosa, and systemically can result in nausea, gastritis, esophagitis, intestinal perforation, and gastroduodenal bleeding.

Gastrointestinal toxicity is the most clinically significant side effect of NSAIDs. The mechanism by which NSAIDs damage the mucosa is complex. NSAIDs reduce mucosal defenses by the depletion of endogenous prostaglandins, decrease the magnitude of the mucus-bicarbonate barrier, disrupt the epithelial layer, reduce the surface hydrophobicity of epithelial cells, and diminish mucosal blood flow.[82] Clinical NSAID-induced gastrointestinal toxic effects include gastritis, esophagitis, mucosal erosions, peptic ulcers, gastrointestinal perforation, gastrointestinal hemorrhage, gut dysmotility, and dyspermeability. Toxicity may occur throughout the alimentary tract, but lesions are most commonly found near the prepyloric region and antrum of the stomach.[82] Esophagitis and duodenitis may develop and cause strictures.

The gastrointestinal lesions caused by NSAIDs are often asymptomatic; therefore, determination of the true incidence and relative risk is impossible. It has been estimated that NSAIDs are responsible for 100,000 to 200,000 complicated ulcers in the United States each year. Gastrointestinal toxicity caused by NSAIDs account for more than 70,000 hospitalizations and 10,000 to 20,000 deaths annually in the United States alone.[83] However, not all patients taking NSAIDs are at the same risk for the development of life-threatening events. Longitudinal data from Arthritis, Rheumatism, and Aging Medical Information System (ARAMIS) permit the identification of several risk factors.[84] The relative risk of hospitalization for patients with rheumatoid arthritis taking NSAIDs is 5.2, in comparison with such patients who are not taking NSAIDs.[83] Major risk factors identified for gastrointestinal toxicity include age, level of disability, previous history of NSAID-induced peptic ulcer disease, history of taking antiulcer medications, NSAID dosage, and concomitant glucocorticoid use.[83] Gastrointestinal hemorrhage

with NSAID use is a cause of increased morbidity and mortality in rheumatoid arthritis patients and has been called "the second most deadly rheumatic disease."[83]

The evaluation of antiulcer agents for patients at increased risk of NSAID-related gastrointestinal hemorrhage is ongoing. In patients on NSAIDs, no study has shown that a decrease in endoscopically recognized ulcers is related to a decrease in gastrointestinal hemorrhage, perforation, or death.[85] Currently, the available antiulcer strategies include (1) the prevention of gastric acid secretion, (2) the neutralization of gastric acid, and (3) mucosal cytoprotection. Histamine ($H_2$) receptor antagonists (cimetidine, ranitidine, famotidine) and adenosine triphosphatase inhibitors (omeprazole and lansoprazole) prevent the secretion of gastric acid. Inorganic antacids, such as Maalox and Mylanta, neutralize gastric acids. Sucralfate (Carafate) and the prostaglandin analog misoprostol are cytoprotective agents.

Misoprostol (Cytotec) is a prostaglandin $E_1$ analog that supplies prostaglandin locally to the gastrointestinal tract for protection. A large, multicenter, randomized, double-blind, placebo-controlled trial evaluated the protective effect of misoprostol on NSAID-related gastrointestinal ulcer formation.[86] The investigators described 638 arthritis patients on a variety of NSAIDs and monitored them endoscopically at baseline and after 4, 8, and 12 weeks on misoprostol or placebo. A duodenal or gastric ulcer was defined as a circumscribed mucosal defect 0.5 cm in diameter or larger, with perceptible depth. By 12 weeks, duodenal ulcers had developed in 2 (0.6%) of 320 patients taking 200 $\mu$g of misoprostol four times daily, in comparison with 15 (4.6%) of 323 patients taking placebo. Gastric ulceration developed in 6 (1.9%) of 320 patients taking misoprostol, in comparison with 25 (7.7%) of 323 patients taking placebo. The authors concluded that misoprostol lowered the frequency of duodenal and gastric ulcers. These results must be interpreted with caution, because the rate of compliance with NSAID and prednisone regimens, the NSAID dosage, and the prednisone dosage are not known. Furthermore, we do not know the clinical significance of these asymptomatic, endoscopically determined ulcerations. Misoprostol did cause diarrhea in 32.3% of patients and 17.9% of controls. If gastrointestinal symptoms from misoprostol cause patients to skip their nonsteroidal medication, the beneficial effect observed may be from erratic NSAID use or noncompliance, rather than from misoprostol cytoprotection, as the authors concluded.

Two previous studies had evaluated misoprostol with placebo[87] and misoprostol with sucralfate[88] in the prevention of NSAID-induced ulcers. Using endoscopic evaluation, both studies concluded that misoprostol was superior in the protection of gastric ulcers for patients on NSAIDs. In the first study of 420 patients, after 3 months, new gastric ulcers developed in 12.3% of patients receiving placebo, in 4.2% of patients receiving 100 $\mu$g of misoprostol four times a day, and 0.7% of those receiving 200 $\mu$g of misoprostol four times a day.[87] Of 253 patients available for analysis in the second study, an NSAID-induced ulcer developed in 1.6% of patients receiving misoprostol, in comparison with 16% of patients receiving sucralfate.[88] The only inclusion criteria for these two studies were abdominal pain and NSAID use. Although these results are intriguing, NSAID-induced ulcers associated with morbidity are often asymptomatic, and so the clinical significance of these results is not determined.

In two published controlled trials, ranitidine has been shown to be effective in decreasing duodenal ulcer formation associated with NSAIDs but relatively ineffective against gastric ulceration.[89, 90] Therefore, on the basis of these studies, misoprostol appears more effective than an H₂ blocker in preventing NSAID-induced gastrointestinal toxicity. However, the side effects and costs associated with misoprostol may limit its use.

More recent trials have focused on the use of proton pump inhibitor agents (and lansoprazole) for both prevention and treatment of gastroduodenal erosions and ulcerations. The Scandinavian Collaborative Ulcer Recurrence (SCUR) study found that patients taking omeprazole had a peptic ulcer rate of 4.7%, as opposed to 16.7% among those taking placebo, and a dyspepsia rate of 8.2%, as opposed to 20.0% among those taking placebo. In the same study, 16.5% of patients taking placebo developed one or more peptic ulcers, in comparison with 3.6% of patients taking omeprazole.[91] The Omeprazole Versus Misoprostol for NSAID-Induced Ulcer Management (OMNIUM) study consisted of a healing phase and a prophylactic phase. In the 8-week healing phase, 20 mg/day of omeprazole, 40 mg/day of omeprazole, and 200 g QID of misoprostol were highly effective in treatment of gastroduodenal ulcers and erosions (75%, 75%, and 71%, respectively; no placebo). Patients who successfully completed the healing phase were randomly reassigned to receive 20 mg/day of omeprazole, 200 g QID of misoprostol, or placebo for up to 6 months. In patients receiving omeprazole, 36.5% experienced treatment failure, in comparison with 48.6% of those taking misoprostol and 67.7% of those taking placebo.[92]

THE ACID-SUPPRESSION TRIAL. The Ranitidine Versus Omeprazole for NSAID-Associated Ulcer Treatment (ASTRONAUT) study also consisted of a healing phase and a prophylactic phase. In the healing phase, patients were assigned to one of three treatments: 20 mg/day of omeprazole, 40 mg/day of omeprazole, or 150 mg BID of ranitidine. The results after 8 weeks of treatment showed that 80% of the patients in the group given 20 mg/day of omeprazole, 79% of those given 40 mg/day of omeprazole, and 63% of those given ranitidine experienced significant improvement in their NSAID-induced gastroduodenal ulcers and erosions. However, the rates of healing of all types of lesions were higher with omeprazole than with ranitidine. Patients who successfully completed the healing phase were then randomly reassigned to receive either omeprazole or ranitidine for up to 6 months. In patients receiving omeprazole, 26.2% experienced treatment failure, in comparison with 37.7% of those on ranitidine. Peptic ulcer relapse occurred in 5.7% of patients

taking omeprazole and 19.5% of those taking ranitidine.[93]

From these clinical studies,[92–95] we conclude that omeprazole, 20 mg/day, is effective both in preventing the significant gastrointestinal consequences of NSAIDs and in healing those that do occur. This dosage is also more effective than placebo, H₂ blockers, and misoprostol in the clinical setting of NSAID-induced gastrointestinal toxicity.

Finally, it is important to mention that the organism Helicobacter pylori, a gastric pathogen, may also play a role in NSAID-induced gastrointestinal toxicity. The bacteria are strongly associated with peptic ulcers, and Chan and associates showed that its eradication before NSAID treatment reduced the occurrence of NSAID-induced ulcers (26% with infection vs. 7% without).[96]

### Renal Toxicity

Prostacyclin and prostaglandins contribute to the maintenance of renal hemodynamics under normal and adverse conditions. Nonsteroidal medications, by inhibiting prostaglandin production, may decrease glomerular filtration and cause renal insufficiency. Patients at higher risk of renal toxicity have had previous impairment of renal function, diabetes, hypertension, atherosclerosis, and congestive heart failure and are hypovolemic or hypoalbuminemic.[97] In a study by Heerdink and colleagues,[98] there was a twofold increased risk of hospitalization for congestive heart failure in elderly patients taking diuretics who started taking NSAIDs. Most of the increase in hospitalization risk occurred in the first 20 days after initiation of NSAID therapy, and by 40 days the incidence density was back to the same level as before concomitant use. This effect is likely caused by decreases in renin release, renal blood flow, and tubular transport reported with NSAIDs.

Interstitial nephritis and proteinuria are also not uncommon in NSAID usage and are likely the result of local T lymphocyte activation and infiltration. It is often reversible with discontinuation of the offending NSAID.[99] Fenoprofen, indomethacin, naproxen, and tolmetin are the agents more commonly associated with interstitial nephritis.[100] Papillary necrosis is unusual and most likely related to marked renal medullary ischemia from inhibition of prostaglandins.[101]

Some investigators have suggested that sulindac may spare renal function. In a study comparing renal prostaglandin synthesis in normal women taking sulindac, indomethacin, or placebo, the investigators found decreased renal excretion of prostaglandin E₂, prostaglandin F₂ₐ, and 6-keto prostaglandin F₁ₐ in patients taking indomethacin, in comparison with those taking sulindac or placebo.[102] It is suggested that sulindac and its metabolite sulindac sulfone are renally inactive and similar to placebo, and do not inhibit renal prostaglandin H synthetase (COX). The active metabolite of sulindac, sulindac sulfide, is converted to sulindac sulfone within the kidneys before excretion. Therefore, sulindac may spare the renal vasculature from prostaglandin inhibition and may subsequently decrease nephrotoxicity. Although decreased renal toxicity was shown in this study, other investigators have not reproduced these findings.[103, 104] Many authors have concluded that sulindac does not decrease the risk of renal toxicity.

### Hepatic Side Effects

Abnormal liver function may occur with NSAID use and is usually manifested as a mild to moderate chemical hepatitis that is reversible with removal of the offending agent. In rare cases, hepatic dysfunction progresses to hyperbilirubinemia and hepatic necrosis.[105] A meta-analysis found elevations in serum glutamic oxaloacetic transaminase (SGOT) to be related to baseline SGOT levels, diclofenac use by patients with OA, aspirin use by patients with rheumatoid arthritis, duration of treatment, and daily dose of medication.[106] Factors such as other medications, disease duration, and gender did not contribute to SGOT elevations. The majority of SGOT elevations for the patients were minimal and not related to clinical hepatitis. There is additional evidence that advanced age, polypharmaceuticals, high dosages of NSAIDs, decreased renal function, and prolonged treatment are risk factors for NSAID-related hepatotoxicity.[105] Phenylbutazone has been causal in a number of fatalities from hepatocellular injury and cannot be recommended for routine use.[107]

### Cutaneous and Hypersensitivity Side Effects

NSAIDs may cause a morbilliform rash, urticaria, photosensitivity, vesiculobullous changes, vasculitis, serum sickness, exfoliative dermatitis, erythema multiforme/Stevens-Johnson syndrome, and toxic epidermal necrolysis.[108] The American Academy of Dermatology reported increased skin reactions with piroxicam, sulindac, and meclofenamate.[109] Severe reactions have occurred with phenylbutazone and oxyphenylbutazone. If an allergic skin reaction occurs, the medication should be discontinued. If the patient requires the use of an NSAID and the adverse reaction was limited to the skin, another agent may be used, but it should be from a different class. NSAIDs from one class react similarly to agents from the same class and should not be given to patients with a history of a previous reaction.

Hypersensitivity reactions characterized by urticaria, laryngospasm, bronchospasm, angioedema, and anaphylaxis may occur in patients with nasal polyps, asthma, and vasomotor rhinitis.[110] With the inhibition of COX, prostaglandin precursors are shunted away from the bronchodilating regulatory prostaglandins and toward leukotriene formation. An excess of a leukotriene product such as leukotriene B4 (LTB4, the slow-reacting substance of anaphylaxis) is responsible for the bronchospasm and anaphylaxis of this syndrome. Under these circumstances, patients with this syndrome should avoid aspirin and all NSAIDs.

### Other, Less Common Side Effects

In rare cases, blood dyscrasias occur with the use of NSAIDs. Aplastic anemia, hemolytic anemia, neutropenia, agranulocytosis, and thrombocytopenia have been reported. Phenylbutazone and oxyphenbutazone are most strongly associated with these adverse effects, and these two agents should not be used for OA.[111]

Neutropenia is associated with the use of NSAIDs. A population-based, case-control study was performed with Medicaid claims from six states.[112] Cases were noted as hospitalized patients with neutropenia. For each case, four controls were randomly chosen and matched for age, sex, state, and year. The frequency of exposure to NSAIDs within 30 days of hospitalization was compared with the frequency in the control cases. The odds ratio for the development of neutropenia was 4.2. No single class of medication was associated with increased risk because of the low incidence of neutropenia and the inability to evaluate individual drugs. A previous study found that for patients taking NSAIDs, an incidence rate of neutropenia was 45 cases per million per year, and for agranulocytosis, 7.2 cases per million per year.[113] The low incidence rate and relative risk of 4.2 suggests that 145 cases of neutropenia and 23 cases of agranulocytosis would occur for every one million people taking NSAIDs for a year.[112]

Both aspirin and NSAIDs result in a bleeding tendency by blocking the synthesis of thromboxane $A_2$ in platelets. Nonaspirin NSAIDs reversibly bind to and inhibit COX for the life of the platelet. The antithrombotic effect is reversed when the NSAID is metabolized or excreted. On the other hand, aspirin permanently inactivates COX. For approximately 1 week after aspirin is taken, inhibition of thromboxane exists. Therefore, the bleeding abnormality persists after the discontinuation of aspirin.

Because of this effect and the tendency of NSAIDs to decrease metabolism of warfarin, the use of NSAIDs (including aspirin) in patients receiving warfarin remains controversial. The combined use of the two medications makes finding a stable dosage of warfarin difficult and is associated with increased risk of gastrointestinal and intracerebral hemorrhage.[114-117] There is some evidence that this interaction is predominately a COX-1 phenomenon and that the more COX-2–specific agents do not produce this interaction.[118-120]

### Central Nervous System Side Effects

NSAIDs are associated with central nervous system side effects because they are lipophilic and diffuse easily across the blood-brain barrier. Aspirin may cause reversible tinnitus and hearing loss, which may limit therapy in some patients.[121] Other side effects include altered moods, confusion, insomnia, depression, paranoia, headaches, lightheadedness, and drowsiness. These central effects are most prominent with indomethacin but are noticed with all NSAIDs. Aseptic meningitis has been reported with ibuprofen, indomethacin, sulindac, and tolmetin, but it is uncommon.[122] Salicylate overdose with serum levels of

250 mg/L or greater can cause confusion, hallucinations, agitation, seizures, and coma and may be fatal if not diagnosed and treated appropriately.

## Pregnancy

NSAIDs are not recommended for use during pregnancy, because their safety has not been established. They are designated category B, meaning that reproduction studies performed in rats, rabbits, and mice with dosages up to six times the human dosage have revealed no evidence of impaired fertility or harm to the fetus caused by the drug.[123] Unfortunately, animal reproduction studies are not always predictive of human response. Therefore, these drugs should not be used during pregnancy for any condition unless clearly needed. Because OA and the pregnant patient do not often occur together, the chance that this issue will become a clinical problem is extremely remote. In addition, the patency of the fetus's ductus arteriosus is dependent on prostaglandins, and so NSAID use may cause premature closure of the ductus. Use of NSAIDs during late pregnancy should be avoided. In animal models and lactating humans, some NSAIDs have been found excreted in milk.[123]

## Selective Inhibitors of Inducible Cyclooxygenase

Selective COX-2 inhibitors (SCIs) are a new group of promising medications that potentially have equivalent anti-inflammatory and analgesic properties of traditional (nonselective) NSAIDs but produce far fewer gastrointestinal and hematologic side effects. There are currently two such medications, celecoxib and rofecoxib, and the published literature on either is scarce at this point. In a short-term study of patients with dental pain, however, celecoxib appeared to have an analgesic effect similar to that of aspirin.[120] More recently, a randomized placebo phase II trial by Simon and coworkers[119] tested the efficacy and safety of celecoxib at 2- and 4-week intervals in patients with OA and those with rheumatoid arthritis. The study found that patients treated with celecoxib had a significant dose-dependent improvement in their Visual Analogue Scale and Global Assessment scores in comparison with those receiving placebo. The side effect arm of the trial compared celecoxib, 100 mg twice daily; naproxen, 500 mg twice daily; and placebo. Gastric ulcers were found in none of the placebo and celecoxib recipients but in six patients (19%) taking naproxen ($P \leq .011$). Gastric erosions developed in 9% to 13% of the placebo and celecoxib recipients, as opposed to 72% of the naproxen recipients ($P \leq .011$). Duodenal erosions were present in 0% to 6% of the placebo and celecoxib recipients, as opposed to 19% of the naproxen recipients ($P \leq .047$).

Rofecoxib also seems to be effective and well tolerated in knee and hip OA. In a double-blind, randomized, multicenter study by Cannon and associates, a total of 784 patients with clinical and radiographic hip or knee OA were randomly assigned to receive rofecoxib, 12.5 mg/day or 25 mg/day, or diclofenac, 50 mg TID. They were then assessed at 2, 4, 8, 12, and 26 weeks according to multiple clinical parameters. Rofecoxib was generally well tolerated, and its efficacy was comparable to that of diclofenac; however, significantly more patients discontinued the diclofenac than rofecoxib ($P < .05$).[124] In a very similar study by Saag and coworkers, rofecoxib, 12.5 mg/day and 25 mg/day, had similar efficacy to ibuprofen, 800 mg TID.[125]

Another benefit of these agents seems to be their lack of platelet inhibition. A small cohort of six healthy patients received celecoxib, 400 mg twice per day, and subsequently a single dose of aspirin, 650 mg. The pretreatment and post-treatment levels of collagen-induced platelet aggregation were measured. The results showed that up to 12 hours after dosing with celecoxib, there was no change in the platelet aggregation in comparison with pretreatment levels (86.5% [pretreatment] vs. 87.2% [2 hours], 90% [4 hours], and 81.5% [12 hours]). For aspirin, however, there were major changes: the pretreatment aggregation value was 84.3%, and after treatment the values were 20.7% and 35% at 2 and 4 hours, respectively.[119]

The lack of effect on platelet aggregation makes this drug safer to use with warfarin (Coumadin). Karim and colleagues studied the effect of adding celecoxib, 200 mg BID, as opposed to placebo to 24 healthy patients on a stable dosage of warfarin and with a prothrombin time (PT) of 1.2 to 1.7 times their baseline level. After 7 days of cotreatment, the authors found that celecoxib had no effect on the pharmacokinetics of warfarin and that there was no significant difference between the PT of the celecoxib group and placebo group.[126]

The renal and hepatic effects of selective COX inhibitors are not clear at this time. Initial studies indicate that these drugs may have a better renal safety profile than traditional NSAIDS.[125, 127–129] Because the inhibition of physiologic prostaglandin synthesis is primarily a COX-1–mediated process, these agents would presumably cause little effect on renal blood flow. In a study of patients with mild renal failure (creatinine clearance, 25 to 60 mL/min), meloxicam, 15 mg/day given for 28 days, had no effect on the creatinine clearance, the serum $N$-acetyl-$\beta$-glucosaminidase/creatinine ratio (a marker for renal tubular damage), the serum urea level, or the serum potassium level.[129]

## Intra-articular Glucocorticoids

In 1951, hydrocortisone became available for intra-articular injection and was employed for the treatment of OA. The rationale for its use as an anti-inflammatory agent in OA can be considered similar to that for NSAID use (discussed earlier). Systemic glucocorticoid treatment is not recommended, because the beneficial effects are minimal or negligible and the side effects of prolonged use are significant. It is thought that glucocorticoids decrease joint inflammation by decreasing the production of the enzyme phospholipase $A_2$, which results in decreased production of prostaglandin and leukotriene.

Glucocorticoids have many biologic effects in the human body. They affect leukocyte movement and leukocyte function and alter humoral factors.[130] They have been noted to have a greater effect on leukocyte movement and on cell-mediated inflammation than on leukocyte function and humoral processes. Saxne and colleagues compared the use of intra-articular glucocorticoids with placebo and found a reduction of interleukin-1 and some protease enzymes involved in cartilage degradation.[131] In addition, corticosteroids may reduce synovial vascular permeability and inhibit angiogenesis.[132, 133] These factors help suppress intra-articular inflammation.

A possible protective effect of intra-articular corticosteroids has been noted in experimentally induced OA. In 1985, Williams and Brandt found a dose-dependent protective effect of triamcinolone hexacetonide in chemically (iodoacetate-) induced articular damage in the guinea pig model of OA.[134] Also, in the anterior cruciate ligament resection model of OA in Pond-Nuki dogs, intra-articular triamcinolone hexacetonide and/or oral prednisone at 0.25 mg/kg/day decreased femoral cartilage erosions and significantly reduced osteophyte size, in comparison to untreated or placebo-treated controls.[135]

A theoretical protective effect of intra-articular corticosteroids is to relieve joint pain and swelling, even temporarily, thereby causing the joint to become more usable. The increase in piezoelectric forces across the joint and periarticular muscle strength may help stabilize the joint and decrease pain. This can lead to overall symptomatic improvement for the patient and delay the need for joint replacement. Most clinicians describe favorable results with intra-articular corticosteroids in OA, although little scientific data from randomized, double-blind, placebo-controlled clinical trials exist.

Intra-articular corticosteroid use should be considered palliative and temporary (short-lived). It is used in single or multiple joints that are not responsive to other therapies or by patients who cannot tolerate NSAIDs. It has been used to facilitate rehabilitation, to aid patients undergoing physical therapy, to decrease effusions, and to prevent stretching and laxity in the capsule and ligaments. The size of the joint, volume of effusion, type and dosage of corticosteroid preparation, injection technique, and severity of synovitis are factors that influence the efficacy of intra-articular injections (Table 36–6). Contraindications to glucocorticoid articular injection include the presence or suspicion of a skin or joint infection, bacteremia, and recent trauma to neighboring structures.

Side effects of glucocorticoid injection include skin, articular, and systemic infection; postinjection flare; crystal-induced synovitis; cutaneous atrophy; and fat necrosis. Repeated corticosteroid use may induce "analgesic arthropathy," whereby a decrease or absence of pain may allow overuse of the joint and a more rapid deterioration.[136] In rare cases, there may be some systemic absorption of corticosteroids from the joint that may result in fluid retention, hyperglycemia, and hypertension. We recommend no more than two to three injections per joint per year in routine cases. Each intra-articular injection for weight-bearing joints should be followed by a short period of rest (recommended time period, 1 to 7 days). An occasional patient may need up to three or four injections in a single joint during 1 year; this situation is exceedingly unusual and should force the clinician to rethink the treatment plan for that patient. For example, is there another reason for the patient's symptoms or another cause of the problem? Finally, repeated injections into the same joint seem to lose efficacy over time; reasons for this well-documented clinical phenomenon are not known.

## Intra-articular Viscosupplementation

Hyaluronic acid, or hyaluronan, is the major nonsulfated glycosaminoglycan component of synovial fluid and cartilage. It has been extracted from rooster combs for veterinary/medical use. Intra-articular injection of hyaluronan has been used in race horses with OA since the 1970s in an attempt to limit glucocorticoid injections. The material is viscous, but it does not act as an intra-articular lubricant, inasmuch as its half-life is less than 48 hours. It may provide a local anti-inflammatory effect or may stimulate cartilage and synovial metabolism.

The mechanism of hyaluronan in pain relief is not well understood. High-molecular-weight hyaluronan ($1.9 \times 10^6$ d) is able to inhibit leukocyte chemotaxis while having no effect on the production of free radicals in vitro.[137, 138] Some investigators have postulated that hyaluronate may localize in the extracellular matrix around the synoviocytes and stimulate biosynthetic activity.[137, 138] This might improve the viscosity and elasticity of the cartilage. Hyaluronan may physically bind to and entrap noxious substances from synovial fluid to protect the intra-articular cells from their

**TABLE 36–6**
## Steroidal Joint Injection Recommendations

| JOINT SIZE (EXAMPLE) | RECOMMENDED TRIAMCINOLONE ACETONIDE DOSE PER INJECTION | NEEDLE SIZE |
|---|---|---|
| Small (PIP, DIP, CMC) | 5–10 mg | 27–30 Gauge |
| Medium (wrist, elbow, ankle) | 10–20 mg | 22–25 Gauge |
| Large (knee, hip, shoulder) | 30–40 mg (alternative for hip and knee is triamcinolone hexacetonide, 20–40 mg | 19–22 Gauge |

CMC = carpometacarpal; DIP = distal interphalangeal; PIP = proximal interphalangeal.
Adapted from Harris ED Jr, Genovese M (eds): Primary Care Rheumatology. Philadelphia: WB Saunders, 2000.

effect.[137] When injected into animals and humans, hyaluronan has a half-life of less than 48 hours. In postulating a mechanism of action of hyaluronan, investigators must account for the benefit of the material with a short intra-articular half-life.

Early reports on the efficacy and safety of intra-articular hyaluronic acid (hylan G-F 20 [Synvisc]) were reported Moreland and associates[139] and Adams and colleagues[140] in 1993. Both studies were randomized, double-blind, multicenter trials with hylan G-F 20 that involved patients with OA of the knee. Moreland and associates evaluated three weekly intra-articular injections of hylan G-F 20 in 104 patients after a 4-week period of washout from NSAIDs and glucocorticoids. All patients who received one treatment (three weekly injections) showed statistically significant improvement in several clinical parameters in comparison with controls (sham injection). In those who had two treatments (two courses of three weekly injections), there was also significant improvement in pain parameters from baseline. Furthermore, two treatment courses of hylan G-F 20 were found to be superior to one treatment course after 26 weeks ($P <.05$). In the second study, Adams and colleagues studied the safety and efficacy of three weekly injections of hylan G-F 20 alone and in combination with continuous NSAID treatment. The groups were divided as follows: (1) NSAID continuation and three weekly injections of hylan G-F 20, (2) NSAID continuation and three weekly "sham" injections, and (3) NSAID discontinuation at baseline and three weekly injections of hylan G-F 20. At 12 and 26 weeks after injection, the three groups studied showed significant improvement in most of the measured pain parameters from baseline. However, NSAIDs alone was found to be ineffective for reduction in rest pain and lateral tenderness. The patients who received the hylan G-F 20 injections with or without NSAID therapy had statistically significantly better results than did the patients who received continuous NSAID therapy alone ($P <.05$). Local, transient pain and swelling rarely occurred at the injection sites in both studies. Also, no systemic adverse effects were observed. In these two preliminary studies, three weekly intra-articular injections of hylan G-F 20 were safe and effective.

Two more recent clinical trials with hyaluronan were conducted by Dahlberg and associates[141] and Lohmander and colleagues.[142] Dahlberg and associates compared the effect of intra-articular hyaluronan injections with those of placebo in patients with exertional knee pain and with joint cartilage abnormalities. Fifty-two patients with knee pain and arthroscopically verified deep cartilage fissures were randomly assigned to receive weekly intra-articular injections of 2.5 mL of either hyaluronan or placebo, for a total of 5 weeks. The treatment effects were assessed at 2, 4, 13, 26, and 52 weeks. At the follow-up visits, both groups had some improvement in joint pain and function from baseline; however, there was no significant difference between the treatment and placebo groups in any of the outcome variables at any time point.

Lohmander and colleagues randomly assigned 240 patients with symptomatic, radiologically confirmed knee OA to either treatment with five weekly injections of 25 mg of hyaluronan or placebo. Results were evaluated at weeks 1, 2, 3, 4, 5, 13, and 20 by visual analogue scales (pain, function, motion, activity), algofunctional index (a validated scale of knee OA severity on which 0 represented no pain and full function and 24 represented maximal pain and disability), and global evaluation by patient and investigator. No serious side effects were reported. At 20 weeks, both groups improved in comparison to baseline; there were no difference between patients treated with placebo and those treated with hyaluronan. An additional analysis that compared the treatment groups after stratification by age and baseline algofunctional index revealed a statistically significant difference in favor of hyaluronan over placebo for patients older than 60 years and with a baseline algofunctional index greater than 10. There was no clinically relevant difference between the two treatments for the other three stratified subgroups.

In summary, there are currently two preparations of hyaluronan (Hyalgan and Synvisc) approved for use in knee OA. Both of these require three to five joint injections to be administered over a period ranging from 3 to 5 weeks and can be given only every 6 months. Although results of initial trials in animal models were promising, prospective controlled studies in humans have shown only modest efficacy, the overall difference in pain between the group and placebo being very small ($<10\%$).[141] However, patients older than 60 years with significant symptoms and functional disability had slightly more amelioration in pain and improvement in function after hyaluronate injections than other groups of patients.[142]

## JOINT LAVAGE

Individuals with OA who do not respond to analgesics, NSAIDs, or intra-articular corticosteroid injections may be candidates for joint lavage. The technique was developed when investigators observed improvement of knee pain in OA when the joint was treated with only lavage and arthroscopic surgery was not performed. Saline lavage of the arthritic knee may be performed in an office setting with arthroscopic visualization and guidance or with a large-bore (14-gauge) needle and syringe. A total of about 1 L of normal saline is then infused and removed from the joint. Some investigators have suggested that this improvement results from a washout effect of inflammatory mediators in the joint, and others believe that mechanically stretching the joint capsule is responsible for the relief of pain.

Two investigational groups, Chang and colleagues[143] and Ike and associates,[144] have shown that closed joint lavage may be beneficial in a subgroup of patients with OA. In the study by Chang and colleagues, 32 individuals with OA of the knee were randomly assigned to arthroscopic surgery or to closed-needle joint lavage. The patients were compared at baseline, 3 months, and 12 months by standard clinical outcome measures. After 1 year, 58% of all subjects who underwent joint lavage reported clinical improvement, in comparison to 44% of all subjects who underwent arthroscopy. For the patients who underwent arthroscopic surgery, predictors for successful outcome included meniscal tears of the anterior two thirds of the medial meniscus and any lateral meniscal tear. In this study, no clinical signs or symptoms (i.e., McMurray's sign, locking or giving way of the knee) predicted the presence or absence of meniscal pathology. Unfortunately, predictors for success of the lavage remains unknown, because intra-articular features of patients randomly assigned to receive lavage were unknown. Of interest is that the cost of arthroscopy was significantly higher than that of closed needle lavage, but other postprocedure costs were not significantly different between the two groups.

Ike and associates evaluated tidal irrigation in the treatment of patients with refractory OA of the knee.[144] They randomly assigned 77 patients from seven centers to receive physical therapy with or without tidal knee irrigation. They found statistically significant differences after 4 weeks of follow-up. The lavage group had decreased stiffness, decreased recall stiffness, and decreased knee tenderness in comparison with controls treated with physical therapy. The interpretation of their short-term results is limited because there was no placebo or sham irrigation group in the study. However, the results do suggest that lavage of the joint may provide short-term improvement in flares of pain and inflammation in knee OA.

## ARTHROSCOPY

OA of the knee is characterized by the breakdown, softening, fragmentation, and erosion of the articular cartilage of partial or full thickness. Arthroscopy aids in the inspection of the supporting structures of the joint. Through arthroscopy, underlying subchondral bone and varying degrees of synovitis along the capsule may be visualized. Along the articular surfaces, osteophytes often develop and may be seen. Partial or complete tears of the anterior cruciate ligament and posterior cruciate ligament can also be seen, as can tears of the meniscal cartilage. Arthroscopy often provides an earlier method of establishing the diagnosis of OA in the absence of radiographic findings and may identify other factors contributing to the patient's symptom complex. Arthroscopy may be helpful in the therapy of OA in the interim before joint replacement is required, although longitudinal studies must be done to confirm this possibility.

With the aid of specialized instruments, arthroscopy allows physicians to remove or repair meniscal tears, to remove loose bodies, and to shave the articular cartilage and synovium. These procedures may relieve symptoms, improve range of motion, and prolong the use of the osteoarthritic joint. Although pain is decreased and range of motion is improved with the removal of loose bodies and meniscal tears, the long-term outcomes of arthroscopic débridement of the articular damage in the presence of OA are not yet known.

Arthroscopic surgery may be performed as a temporizing measure to avoid partial or total knee replacement. Several studies have reported some improvement in pain after a tear in the anterior two thirds of the medial meniscus and a tear in the lateral meniscus is repaired.[143] However, the long-term consequence of meniscal débridement and the progression of joint degeneration is just beginning to be studied. For example, Chang and colleagues reported that 1 year after closed knee lavage or arthroscopic débridement, more patients had improvement in pain with saline lavage than with arthroscopy.[143] These results suggest patient selection for arthroscopic surgery is critical and the procedure may not be justified for every patient with non–end-stage OA of the knee. Success rates for arthroscopic débridement have varied between 50% and 67%, depending on the age of the patient, degree of arthritis, activity level of the patient, anatomic abnormality, and length of patient follow-up.[145, 146]

Arthroscopy for OA of the hip, ankle, shoulder, wrist, and elbow is currently being performed for both diagnostic and therapeutic procedures. Arthroscopy is available for both rheumatologists and orthopedists to perform in their offices because newer fiberoptics has permitted the development of arthroscopes of 1.6 mm in diameter. Office arthroscopy of the knee allows for both diagnosis and guided articular saline lavage. More experienced arthroscopists can perform more complex procedures. The patient remains awake (local and intra-articular anesthetic is used), and the diagnoses are known immediately. At this time it is viewed as a diagnostic tool for both orthopedists and rheumatologists to diagnose early OA and internal derangements. Some investigators have postulated that it can also be used as a "bridge" to joint surgery or replacement, but the population that would benefit most from such a procedure has yet to be established from randomized and controlled studies.[144, 147]

## ARTHROPLASTY

In general, when patients with OA develop joint pain and swelling, damage to the articular cartilage is irreversible. Many patients have a period of time when analgesic and anti-inflammatory medications control the pain long enough for patients to perform most of their activities of daily living. Eventually, medical therapy is less effective, and patients with OA may require surgical intervention. A large number of open surgical procedures can benefit OA patients; these include ligament repairs and total joint replacements.

Pain and disability are the key factors involved in the timing of arthroplasty. When the level of pain and disability is almost or completely unacceptable, the operation is indicated. Other factors that can influence the timing of surgery include deformity that interferes with joint function, the number of procedures that the surgeon has performed, and the patient's cooperation with the prescribed rehabilitation regimen.[148] Good medical health and psychological health, in addition to cooperation with postoperative care, are mandatory for surgical success. Active infection, poor medical health, morbid obesity, neurologic abnormalities, and muscular abnormalities are relative contraindications for joint replacement surgery.

Timing for surgery and joint replacement is crucial because most prosthetic joints wear out with time. The patient's general medical condition and age are also important considerations. In a patient who is less than 50 years old and is likely to outlive the artificial joint, a second procedure may be required in the future. In this case, it may be better to postpone replacement, by maximizing the medical regimen and physical therapy, for as long as possible. On the other hand, the longer that patients are inactive, the more obese and deconditioned they become and the more likely it is that they will have a worse outcome during surgery and immediately postoperatively.

The hip and knee are the most commonly replaced joints, as involvement of these joints has a great impact on patients' daily activities. Unfortunately, artificial joints have a limited lifetime: prostheses last from 12 to 16 years for both the hip and the knee, depending on the type of joint used.[149] Because of the limited lifetime of the artificial joint, some physicians delay arthroplasty in order to avoid repeated joint replacements. A significant amount of research is devoted to developing prostheses with longer lifetimes. Predictors of failure of prostheses include an imperfect surgical fit, a high level of activity, and obesity.[150]

Osteotomy, which literally means "a cut in the bone," is a procedure less common than joint replacement. The technique is best used for younger and more motivated patients with knee deformities, such as genu valgum, and with hip diseases such as congenital hip dysplasia, nonunion after femoral neck fracture, slipped femoral epiphysis, Legg-Calvé-Perthes disease, and osteonecrosis.[151] It can be quite effective for pain relief, can improve bony alignment, can improve stability, and can delay the need for knee replacement for up to 10 years.[152]

Total joint replacement is reserved for patients who have bicompartmental or tricompartmental joint disease and may not benefit from osteotomy. An in-depth discussion of the types of orthopedic procedures, materials, and options is beyond the scope of this section but they are discussed in other reviews.[150]

## COMPLEMENTARY AND INVESTIGATIONAL AGENTS

### Proteoglycans and Glycosaminoglycans

The oral supplements glucosamine and chondroitin sulfate, which are available in drug and health food stores, are under investigation for the treatment of knee OA. Both glucosamine and chondroitin are components of articular cartilage and are crucial to its stability. Proponents theorize that taking these supplements orally may replenish the articular cartilage in affected joints. To date, the published trials on these supplements are few in number, have involved relatively small numbers of patients, and have very short follow-up times. However, they show that glucosamine is superior to placebo and similar to ibuprofen in improving pain and function in patients with OA.[153, 154] There appear to be few side effects from these agents, and so, other than the cost of the supplements, there is little risk to the patients who choose to try these supplements. Clinical studies are currently in progress and should provide a better understanding as to the efficacy of these supplements in the treatment of knee OA.

### Doxycycline

Doxycycline has been shown to reduce breakdown of articular cartilage in human and animal models.[155] Laboratory studies suggest this may result from its ability to block the metalloproteinase enzymes that are responsible for some of the cartilage breakdown process.[156] Clinical studies are currently under way to determine the ability of doxycycline to decrease the incidence and progression of knee OA.

### Vitamin D

It has been recognized that pathophysiologic changes in periarticular bone have a role in progression of OA. This has led to the idea that the nature of bone response in OA may influence the rate of degeneration of the articular cartilage in the OA joint. Normal bone remodeling and cartilage matrix turnover are contingent on the presence of vitamin D. Therefore, it has been theorized that low concentrations of vitamin D impair the bone remodeling cycle and cartilage matrix turnover, which may accelerate the development and progression of OA.[157, 158]

In a longitudinal study of the knee, McAlindon and coworkers evaluated 556 patients over a 10-year period for knee OA and found that low serum levels and low dietary intake of vitamin D were associated with a threefold increase in the risk for knee OA progression in comparison with serum levels and higher dietary intake of vitamin D. Low serum levels of vitamin D were also predictive of loss of joint space on radiograph (odds ratio, 2.3; 95% confidence interval [CI], 0.9 to 5.5) and osteophyte growth (odds ratio 3.1; CI, 1.3 to 7.5).[159]

Lane and associates studied the association of serum vitamin D levels and the development of incident hip OA in elderly women. These investigators reported that subjects with low serum levels of vitamin D had a threefold increased risk of incident hip OA.[94] Therefore, dietary intake of vitamin D that maintains a normal serum vitamin D level can decrease the incidence of hip OA development and decrease the rate of progression of knee OA.

### Vitamin C and E

In laboratory studies, chondrocytes have been found to be potent producers of free radicals known as reactive oxygen species (ROS). ROS have been shown to adversely affect collagen integrity and depolymerize synovial fluid hyaluronate.[158] Vitamins C and E and beta-carotene (a vitamin A precursor) can act as antioxidants, neutralizing these free radicals and preventing their damage.

In the Framingham Knee OA Cohort Study published by McAlindon and coworkers,[160] the authors specifically examined whether higher intake of vitamin C, vitamin E, and beta-carotene reduced the incidence and progression of knee OA in comparison to a non-antioxidant "control" vitamin group. They found that patients who took the highest dosages of vitamin C (119 to 1599 mg/day) did have a reduced risk (adjusted odds ratio, 0.3; 95% CI, 0.1 to 0.8) of developing incident knee OA during the study period. Also, they found a one-third reduction of knee OA progression in the two groups with the highest vitamin C intake (119 mg to 1599 mg/day). The results for low-dosage vitamin E group (6.2 to 18 mg/day) were less impressive (adjusted OR, 0.7; 95% CI, 0.3 to 1.6) and observed only in men. No significant effects were observed for beta-carotene. Again, these data suggest that moderate to high dosages of vitamin C may slow the development of incident knee OA and decrease the rate of progression of knee OA.

Vitamin C may affect the development and progression of OA through other mechanisms. Vitamin C is a cofactor for lysylhydroxylase, which is an enzyme essential for the stabilization of mature collagen fibrils. It also assists in the incorporation of sulfate groups in glycosaminoglycan synthesis and affects cartilage growth factors in ways that are not clear at this time. In an animal model of OA in guinea pigs, the animals treated with higher dosages of vitamin C (human equivalent dosage of >500 mg/day) showed less joint damage than animals treated with lower dosages.[158]

## Plaquenil and Sulfasalazine

Plaquenil and sulfasalazine, which are often used in rheumatoid arthritis and systemic lupus erythematosus, may also have a role in the treatment of inflammatory OA; however, these agents are only now being studied in OA. They have relatively few side effects and can be good adjunct medications in specific cases. However, until the results from the ongoing studies are completed, we cannot recommend widespread use of these agents in OA.

Other novel therapies such as intra-articular NSAIDS and electromagnetic radiation show some promising results in initial trials in OA but have yet to be used on large numbers of patients.[161, 162]

## RECOMMENDATIONS FOR MANAGEMENT OF OSTEOARTHRITIS

Effective management of OA rests on an accurate diagnosis (Figs. 36–2 to 36–4). The clinician must rule out other conditions that can mimic OA, including chronic infection, systemic disease, osteonecrosis, and malignancy. We recommend physical and occupational therapy for all of our patients to strengthen the supporting muscles and for protection of the joint. For patients who are functionally disabled, we recommend the early use of appropriate assistive devices. For obese patients, weight reduction is strongly advised.

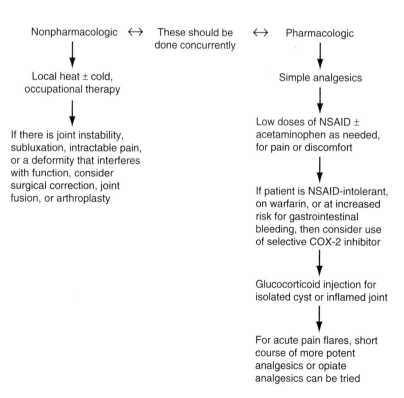

**FIGURE 36–2**
Suggested protocol for confirmed hand osteoarthritis. COX-2 = cyclooxygenase-2; NSAID = nonsteroidal anti-inflammatory drug.

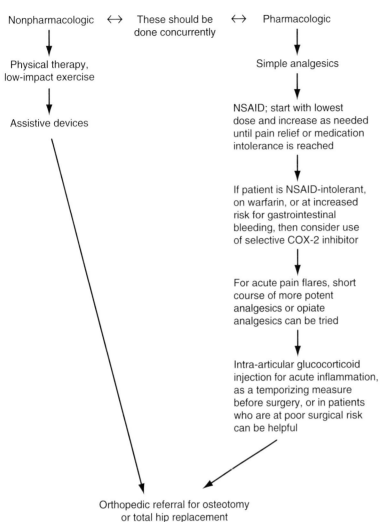

FIGURE 36–3
Suggested protocol for confirmed hip osteoarthritis. COX-2 = cyclooxygenase-2; NSAID = nonsteroidal anti-inflammatory drug.

We encourage a symptomatic and regional approach to therapy in patients with OA (see Figs. 36–2 to 36–4). On initial evaluation, we focus on the patient's quality of life, specifically on inflammatory and noninflammatory (or mechanical) signs and symptoms. Morning stiffness, joint swelling, erythema, warmth, and joint stiffness after sitting or resting for a period of time (known as the "gel phenomenon") are attributed to inflammation of the joint or synovitis. This is because the capillary network that supplies blood to the synovium is responsible for the production of synovial fluid. Inflammation increases the blood supply to the joint, which results in increased synovial fluid production. In inflammatory arthritis, the increase in the volume of fluid within each joint produces swelling, stiffness, and "gelling." These patients often experience improvement in their symptoms after activity as the mechanical pumping action of the joints and muscles reverses this process and decreases the volume of fluid within the joint. Mechanical joint pain often occurs during and after the patient makes use of the joint. For example, mechanical pain in the hip and knee occurs when the patient is climbing up and down stairs or after an extended walk. It occurs at the end of the

day rather than upon waking. However, structural and mechanical joint abnormalities often lead to inflammation within the joint, so the distinction between inflammatory and noninflammatory joint pain is, in reality, less defined.

In the patient with OA, if inflammatory findings predominate, we concentrate on anti-inflammatory medications such as NSAIDs, selective COX-2 inhibitors, and glucocorticoid injections. For the patient with primarily mechanical symptoms, we recommend rest, analgesia, assistive devices, occupational therapy, and physical therapy.

## The Hand

Primary OA of the hand involves the first carpometacarpal (CMC) joint, the proximal interphalangeal (PIP) joint, and the distal interphalangeal (DIP) joint. Osteophytes may cause a decrease in the range of motion of the fingers and may be painful. For single, isolated mechanical DIP, PIP, and CMC joint involvement, acetaminophen or low-dosage NSAIDs and occupational therapy are recommended. For involvement of a single joint of the hand with signs of inflammation, we use

**FIGURE 36–4**
Suggested protocol for confirmed knee osteoarthritis. COX-2 = cyclooxygenase-2; NSAID = nonsteroidal anti-inflammatory drug.

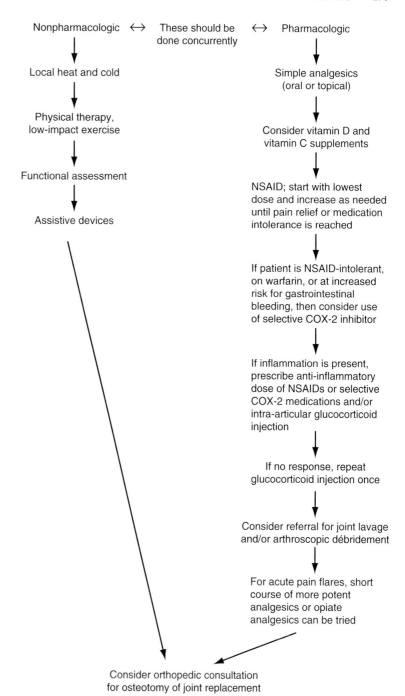

Nonpharmacologic ↔ These should be done concurrently ↔ Pharmacologic

Local heat and cold

Physical therapy, low-impact exercise

Functional assessment

Assistive devices

Simple analgesics (oral or topical)

Consider vitamin D and vitamin C supplements

NSAID; start with lowest dose and increase as needed until pain relief or medication intolerance is reached

If patient is NSAID-intolerant, on warfarin, or at increased risk for gastrointestinal bleeding, then consider use of selective COX-2 inhibitor

If inflammation is present, prescribe anti-inflammatory dose of NSAIDs or selective COX-2 medications and/or intra-articular glucocorticoid injection

If no response, repeat glucocorticoid injection once

Consider referral for joint lavage and/or arthroscopic débridement

For acute pain flares, short course of more potent analgesics or opiate analgesics can be tried

Consider orthopedic consultation for osteotomy of joint replacement

a 27- to 30-gauge needle to inject a small volume of glucocorticoid into the joint (see Table 36–3). Intra-articular cysts may occur and cause local symptoms. If an intra-articular cyst has formed and is symptomatic, we carefully isolate it, aspirate the joint fluid, and similarly inject triamcinolone acetonide into it. If more than three joints are involved and the patient has mechanical, noninflammatory symptoms, we recommend analgesics and occupational therapy (Fig. 36–5). If more than three joints are involved with inflammatory symptoms, we consider the use of daily anti-inflammatory doses of NSAIDs after assessing the patient's risk for NSAID-associated toxic effects. If the patient is taking warfarin, is predisposed to gastrointestinal bleeding, or is elderly and frail, we recommend considering the use of selective COX-2 inhibitors rather than traditional NSAIDs. For very unstable and painful joints (the first CMC or interphalangeal joints with OA), we consider joint fusion or replacement. This is considered only if the patient has suffered irreversible loss of function in the hand or has considerable pain that is not relieved by glucocorticoid injections, oral medications, physical therapy, and assistive devices. Surgery for cosmetic purposes is not recommended.

Disease in the first CMC joint of the thumb is always a major therapeutic challenge because of the marked

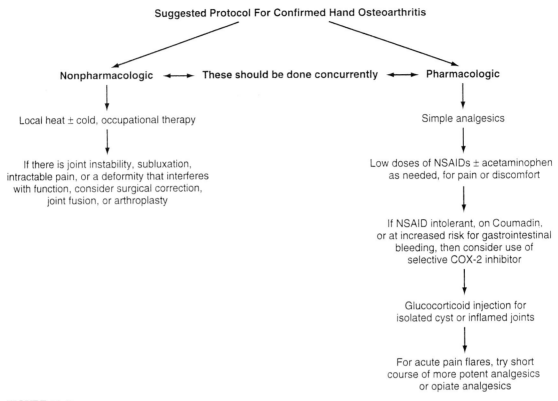

**FIGURE 36–5**
Suggested protocol for confirmed hand osteoarthritis. (From Ratiner B, Lane NE: Osteoarthritis of the extremities. *In* Harris ED Jr, Genovese MC [eds]: Primary Care Rheumatology. Philadelphia: WB Saunders, 2000, p 340.)

functional impairment produced by loss of pinch and grasp. Consultation with a occupational therapy hand specialist in the early stages is useful. Careful consideration should be given to an integrated program consisting of judicious use of specialized splints, intra-articular injections, joint protection methods, assistive devices, and reorganization of the work and recreational environments.

## The Hip

OA of the hip is problematic for the patient because it is a weight-bearing joint. Disease in weight-bearing joints creates a disproportionate amount of pain and disability in those joints. In patients with isolated OA of the hip, we assess symptoms (mechanical or inflammatory) and functional status. As in the approach used for OA of the hand, we recommend NSAIDs at anti-inflammatory dosages for inflammatory symptoms and rest, physical therapy, and analgesia for non-inflammatory symptoms (Fig. 36–6). If the patient is being treated with warfarin, is predisposed to gastrointestinal bleeding, or is elderly and frail, we recommend considering the use of selective COX-2 inhibitors rather than traditional NSAIDs. For patients who weigh more than 20% of their ideal body weight, we recommend weight loss and refer them to a dietitian. To avoid abnormal stress on the knees and contralateral hip, we take precautions to ensure the proper use of appro-

priate assistive devices when needed. If a patient's symptoms do not improve or worsen and if the range of motion greatly limits the function of the patient, we consider a referral to the orthopedist for joint replacement. We do not routinely inject glucocorticoids into the hip unless those drugs are used diagnostically to differentiate hip pain from knee and back pain when the pain is poorly defined and when knee and back disease are also present. If injection of the hip is considered necessary, we recommend fluoroscopic or computerized tomographic guidance.

## The Knee

OA of the knee is a common rheumatologic problem that is associated with pain and functional disability. As with hand and hip OA, we treat inflammatory symptoms with anti-inflammatory therapies and treat mechanical symptoms with analgesics, rest, assistive devices, and physical therapy (Fig. 36–7). We focus our initial examination on the presence or absence of inflammation and on the specific compartment involved. The knee is composed of three compartments: the patellofemoral compartment, the medial tibiofemoral compartment, and the lateral tibiofemoral compartment. For isolated patellofemoral compartment involvement, we use analgesics and recommend physical therapy and joint protection. If inflammation is present, we add NSAIDs in anti-inflammatory dosages

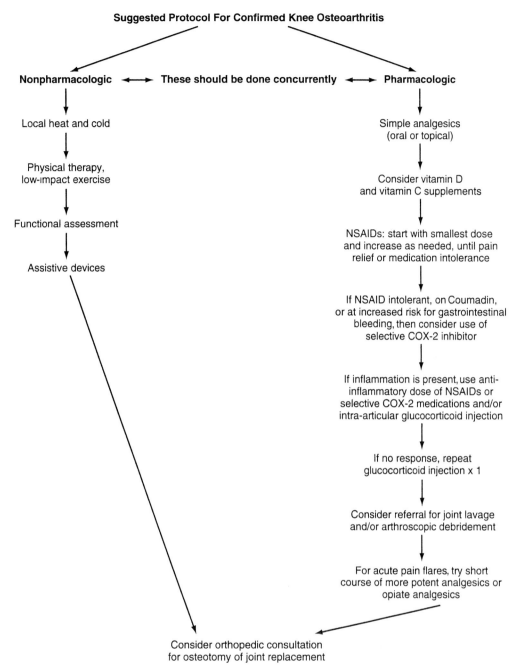

**Suggested Protocol For Confirmed Knee Osteoarthritis**

**FIGURE 36–6**
Suggested protocol for confirmed hip osteoarthritis. (From Ratiner B, Lane NE: Osteoarthritis of the extremities. *In* Harris ED Jr, Genovese MC [eds]: Primary Care Rheumatology. Philadelphia: WB Saunders, 2000, p 341.)

or inject a glucocorticoid into the knee (see Table 36–3). For patients with medial and/or lateral compartment mechanical pain, we recommend conservative management with rest, physical therapy, assistive devices, and analgesics. We initially prescribe NSAIDs for treatment of inflammatory symptoms of the medial and lateral compartment of the knee. If the patient is taking warfarin, is predisposed to gastrointestinal bleeding, or is elderly and frail, we recommend considering the use of selective COX-2 inhibitors instead of traditional

NSAIDs. This is followed by a trial of intra-articular glucocorticoids and may be repeated. An occasional patient may develop a symptomatic synovial effusion and/or popliteal (Baker's) cyst. This may necessitate aspiration to decrease the intra-articular pressure. The direct communication between the popliteal cyst and the patellofemoral joint provides safe and easy access to the joint space and the posterior fossa for aspiration and injection. If the patient's knee symptoms persist or become worse and if clicking, locking, and falling

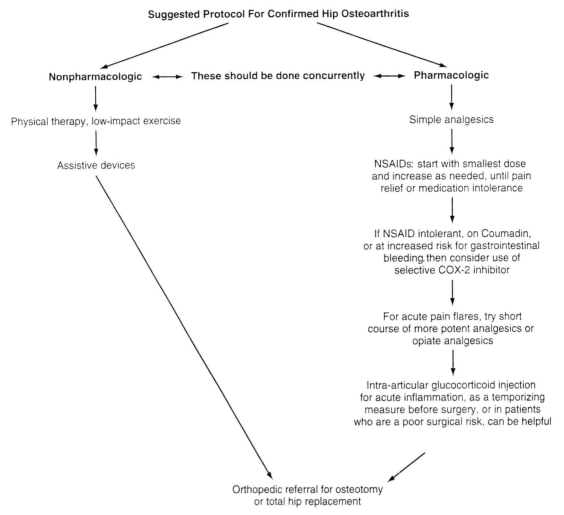

**Suggested Protocol For Confirmed Hip Osteoarthritis**

Nonpharmacologic ←→ These should be done concurrently ←→ Pharmacologic

Physical therapy, low-impact exercise

Assistive devices

Simple analgesics

NSAIDs: start with smallest dose and increase as needed, until pain relief or medication intolerance

If NSAID intolerant, on Coumadin, or at increased risk for gastrointestinal bleeding, then consider use of selective COX-2 inhibitor

For acute pain flares, try short course of more potent analgesics or opiate analgesics

Intra-articular glucocorticoid injection for acute inflammation, as a temporizing measure before surgery, or in patients who are a poor surgical risk, can be helpful

Orthopedic referral for osteotomy or total hip replacement

**FIGURE 36–7**
Suggested protocol for confirmed knee osteoarthritis. (From Ratiner B, Lane NE: Osteoarthritis of the extremities. *In* Harris ED Jr, Genovese MC [eds]: Primary Care Rheumatology. Philadelphia: WB Saunders, 2000, p 342.)

occur, further diagnostic testing is required. Magnetic resonance scanning or diagnostic arthroscopy may be used to determine whether the new symptoms are associated with an internal derangement such as a meniscal tear or a lose body in the knee joint.

Some patients with knee OA suffer a significant loss of function. We refer patients for surgical consultation when they have intractable pain, have a history and physical examination findings consistent with instability of the knee, or have a significant loss of knee function. Figures 36–1 to 36–7 are provided to guide the internist in the work-up and management of OA.

## FOR THE FUTURE

Our goal is to detect the onset of OA at a point when the disease is reversible. Earlier diagnoses will be obtained with the advent of needle arthroscopy, higher resolution magnetic resonance imaging, and the identification of serologic markers of the disease. Patients from our rheumatology clinic are currently involved in

many ongoing studies involving both diagnostic and therapeutic interventions for OA. Novel therapeutic modalities now under study in the treatment of OA include compounds that inhibit enzymatic breakdown of cartilage at an early, possibly reversible, stage of OA; cartilage transplantation; growth factors to stimulate cartilage matrix production; and orthopedic devices with improved longevity.

As the population ages and the proportion of elderly people grows, so does the prevalence of OA. Physicians need to have a better understanding of the pathogenesis of early OA in order to develop preventive measures and better therapeutic options for patients with this disease. The therapeutic options that we have discussed provide an exciting and more optimistic future for persons with OA.

## REFERENCES

1. National Center for Health Statistics: Prevalence of osteoarthritis in adults by age, sex, race, and geographic area: United

States 1960–1962. Vital and Health Statistics, No. 15, Series 11. Washington, DC: US Government Printing Office, 1966.

2. Howell D, Treadwell DV, Tripple SB: The Pathogenesis of Osteoarthritis. Kalamazoo, MI: Upjohn, 1983.

3. Howell DS: Etiopathogenesis of osteoarthritis. In Moskowitz RW, Howell DS, Goldberg VM (eds): Osteoarthritis: Diagnosis and Medical/Surgical Management, 2nd ed. Philadelphia: WB Saunders, 1992:233.

4. Wolff J: The Law of Bone Remodeling [Maquet P, Transl]. Springer-Verlag, 1986. [Originally published 1892]

5. Telhas H, Lindberg L: A method of inducing osteoarthritic changes in rabbit's knees. Clin Orthop 1972; 86:66.

6. Buckwalter JA, Rosenberg LC, Hunzker EB: Articular cartilage: Composition, structure, response to injury and methods of facilitating repair. In Ewing JW (ed): Articular Cartilage and Knee Joint Function: Basic Science of Arthroscopy. New York: Raven, 1990:19.

7. Mankin H: The reaction of articular cartilage to injury and osteoarthritis. N Engl J Med 1990; 291:1285.

8. Martel-Pelletier J, Pelletier J, Malemud C: Activation of neutral metalloproteinase in human osteoarthritic knee cartilage: Evidence for degradation in the core protein of sulphated proteoglycan. Ann Rheum Dis 1988; 47:801.

9. Tyler J: Chondrocyte-mediated depletion of articular cartilage proteoglycans in vitro. Biochem J 1985; 225:493.

10. Sandy J, Nearne PJ, Boynton RE, et al: Catabolism of aggrecan in cartilage explants. Identification of a major cleavage site within the interglobular domain. J Biol Chem 1981; 266:8683.

11. Pelletier J, Martel-Pelletier J, Altman RD, et al: Collagenolytic activity and collagen matrix breakdown of the articular cartilage in the Pond-Nuki dog model of osteoarthritis. Arthritis Rheum 1983; 26:866.

12. Proceedings of the Symposium on Osteoarthritis: Proteases: Their involvement in osteoarthritis. J Rheumatol 1987; 106(Suppl):1.

13. Dean D: Proteinase-mediated cartilage degradation in osteoarthritis. Semin Arthritis Rheum 1991; 20(suppl):2.

14. Pelletier J, Rougley P, DiBattista JA, et al: Are cytokines involved in osteoarthritic pathophysiology? Semin Arthritis Rheum 1991; 20(suppl):63.

15. Sapolsky A, Malemud CJ, Norby DP, et al: Neutral proteinases from articular chondrocytes in culture: 2. Metal-dependent latent neutral proteoglycanase and inhibitory activity. Biochem Biophys Acta 1981; 658:138.

16. Pelletier J, Martel-Pelletier J, Howell DS, et al: Collagenase and collagenolytic activity in human osteoarthritic cartilage. Arthritis Rheum 1983; 26:63.

17. Martel-Pelletier J, Pelletier JP, Cloutier JM, et al: Neutral protease capable of proteoglycan digesting activity in osteoarthritic and normal human articular cartilage. Arthritis and Rheum 1984; 27:305.

18. Pelletier J, Martel-Pelletier J, Cloutier JM, et al: Proteoglycan-degrading acid metalloprotease activity in human osteoarthritic cartilage, and the effect of intraarticular steroid injections. 1987; 19:541.

19. Dean D, Martel-Pelletier J, Pelletier JP, et al: Evidence for metalloproteinase and metalloprotease inhibitor (TIMP) imbalance in human osteoarthritic cartilage. J Clin Investigation 1989; 84:678.

20. Dean D, Woessner J Jr: Extracts of human articular cartilage contain an inhibitor of tissue metalloproteinases. Biochem J 1984; 218:277.

21. Felson D, Zhang Y, Anthony JM, et al: Weight loss reduces the risk for symptomatic knee osteoarthritis in women. Ann Intern Med 1992; 116:535.

22. Lorig KR, Mazonson PD, Holman HR: Evidence suggesting that health education for self-management in patients with chronic arthritis has sustained health benefits while reducing health care costs. Arthritis Rheum 1993; 36(4):439–446.

23. Batchlor E, Paulus H: Principles of drug therapy. In Moskowitz RW, Goldberg VN, Mankin HJ (eds): Osteoarthritis: Diagnosis and Management. Philadelphia: WB Saunders, 1992:465.

24. Creamer P, Hochberg MC: The relationship between psychosocial variables and pain reporting in osteoarthritis of the knee. Arthritis Care Res 1998; 11(1):60–65.

25. Cronan TA, Hay M, Groess IE, et al: The effects of social support and education on health care costs after three years [In process citation]. Arthritis Care Res 1998; 11(5):326–334.

26. Balint G, Szebenyi B: Non-pharmacological therapies in osteoarthritis. Baillière's Clin Rheumatol 1997; 11(4):795–815.

27. Mazzuca SA, Brandt KD, Katz BP, et al: Effects of self-care education on the health status of inner-city patients with osteoarthritis of the knee [see comments]. Arthritis Rheum 1997; 40(8):1466–1474.

28. Fisher NM, Gresham GE, Abrams M, et al: Quantitative effects of physical therapy on muscular and functional performance in subjects with osteoarthritis of the knees. Arch Phys Med Rehabil 1993; 74(8):840–847.

29. O'Reilly S, Jones A, Doherty M: Muscle weakness in osteoarthritis. Curr Opin Rheumatol 1997; 9(3):259–262.

30. Puett DW, Griffin MR: Published trials of nonmedicinal and noninvasive therapies for hip and knee osteoarthritis [see comments]. Ann Intern Med 1994; 121(2):133–140.

31. Hashish I, Harvey W, Harris M: Anti-inflammatory effects of ultrasound therapy: Evidence for a major placebo effect. Br J Rheumatol 1986; 25(1):77–81.

32. Feibel A, Fast A: Deep heating of joints: A reconsideration. Arch Phys Med Rehabil 1976; 57(11):513–514.

33. O'Sullivan S, Schmitz T: Physical Rehabilitation: Assessment and Treatment. Philadelphia: FA Davis, 1994:438–440.

34. Magura G, Aladjemoff L, Tennebaum J, et al: Treatment of pain by transcutaneous electrical stimulation. Acta Anaesthesiol Scand 1978; 22(6):589–592.

35. Gaw AC, Chang LW, Shaw LC: Efficacy of acupuncture on osteoarthritic pain. A controlled, double-blind study. N Engl J Med 1975; 293(8):375–378.

36. Nicholas J: Rehabilitation of patients with rheumatic disease. In Kelley WN, Harris ED Jr, Ruddy S, et al (eds): Textbook of Rheumatology, 5th ed. Philadelphia: WB Saunders, 1993:1728.

37. Cosgrove JL, Nicholass JJ, Barwak J, et al: Team treatment. Does a specialized unit improve team performance? Am J Phys Med Rehabil 1988; 67(6):253–260.

38. Fife R, Brandt K: Experimental modes of therapy in osteoarthritis. In Moskowitz RW, Goldberg VN, Mankin HJ (eds): Osteoarthritis: Diagnosis and Management. Philadelphia: WB Saunders, 1992:511.

39. Thonar EJ, Shinmei M, Lohmander LS: Body fluid markers of cartilage changes in osteoarthritis. Rheum Dis Clin North Am 1993; 19(3):635–657.

40. Bellamy N, Kaloni S, Pope J, et al: Quantitative rheumatology: A survey of outcome measurement procedures in routine rheumatology outpatient practice in Canada. J Rheumatol 1998; 25(5):852–858.

41. Ellrodt AG, Cho M, Cush JJ, et al: An evidence-based medicine approach to the diagnosis and management of musculoskeletal complaints. Am J Med 1997; 103(6A):3S–6S.

42. Lane NE, Thompson JM: Management of osteoarthritis in the primary-care setting: An evidence-based approach to treatment. Am J Med 1997; 103(6A):25S–30S.

43. Deal CL, Schnitzer TJ, Lipstein E, et al: Treatment of arthritis with topical capsaicin: A double-blind trial. Clin Ther 1991; 13(3):383–395.

44. Altman R, Avea A, Holmburg CE, et al: Capsaicin cream 0.025% as monotherapy for osteoarthritis: A double blind study. Semin Arthritis Rheum 1994; 23(suppl 3):25–33.

45. McCarthy GM, McCarty DJ: Effect of topical capsaicin in the therapy of painful osteoarthritis of the hands. J Rheumatol 1992; 19(4):604–607.

46. Koch-Weser J: Drug therapy: Acetaminophen. N Engl J Med 1979; 295:1297.

47. Doyle D, Dieppe PA, Scott J, et al: An articular index for the assessment of osteoarthritis. Ann Rheum Dis 1981; 40:75.

48. Parr G, Darekar B, Fletcher A, et al: Joint pain and quality of life; Results of a randomised trial. Br J Clin Pharmac 1989; 27:235.

49. Stamp J, Rhind V, Haslock I: A comparison of nefopam and flurbiprofen in the treatment of osteoarthrosis. Br J Clin Pract 1989; 1(43):24.

50. Bradley JD, Brandt KD, Katz BP, et al: Comparison of an anti-inflammatory dose of ibuprofen, an analgesic dose of ibuprofen, and acetaminophen in the treatment of patients with osteoar-

484    *Boris Ratiner, Deirdre A. Gramas, and Nancy E. Lane*

thritis of the knee [see comments]. N Engl J Med 1991; 325(2):87–91.

51. Fries JF, Spitz PW, Young DY: The dimensions of health outcomes: The health assessment questionnaire, disability and pain scales. J Rheumatol 1982; 9(5):789–793.

52. Williams HJ, Ward JR, Egger MJ, et al: Comparison of naproxen and acetaminophen in a two-year study of treatment of osteoarthritis of the knee [see comments]. Arthritis Rheum 1993; 36(9):1196–1206.

53. Roth SH: Efficacy and safety of tramadol HCl in breakthrough musculoskeletal pain attributed to osteoarthritis. J Rheumatol 1998; 25(7):1358–1363.

54. Rousi T, Pohjoli R, Matio J: Tramadol in the treatment of osteoarthritic pain; A double blind crossover study versus dextropropoxyphene. Budapest: Meeting Report, 12th European Congress in Rheumatology, 1991.

55. Quiding H, Grimstad J, Rusten K, et al: Ibuprofen plus codeine, ibuprofen, and placebo in a single- and multidose cross-over comparison for coxarthrosis pain. Pain 1992; 50(3):303–307.

56. Ytterberg SR, Mahowald ML, Woods SR: Codeine and oxycodone use in patients with chronic rheumatic disease pain. Arthritis Rheum 1998; 41(9):1603–1612.

57. Lim R, Guzman F, Rodger DW, et al: Site of action on narcotic and non-narcotic analgesics determined by blocking bradykinin-evoked visceral pain. Arch Int Pharmacodyn Ther 1964; 152:25.

58. Boctor AM, Eickholt M, Pugsley TA: Meclofenamate sodium is an inhibitor of both the 5-lipoxygenase and cyclooxygenase pathways of the arachidonic acid cascade in vitro. Prostaglandins Leukot Med 1986; 23(2–3):229–38.

59. Ku E, Lee W, Koathari HV, et al: The Effects of Diclofenac on Arachidonic Acid Metabolism. Semin in Arthritis Rheum 1985; 15:36.

60. Abramson S, Edelson H, Kaplan H, et al: The neutrophil in rheumatoid arthritis: Its role and the inhibition of its activation by non-steroidal antiinflammatory drugs. Semin Arthritis Rheum 1983; 13(suppl 1):148.

61. Needleman P, Isakson PC: The discovery and function of COX-2. J Rheumatol 1997; 24(suppl 49):6–8.

62. Biemond P, Swaak AJ, Peners JM, et al: Superoxide production by polymorphonuclear leucocytes in rheumatoid arthritis and osteoarthritis: In vivo inhibition by the antirheumatic drug piroxicam due to interference with the activation of the NADPH-oxidase. Ann Rheum Dis 1986; 45(3):249–255.

63. Bomalaski JS, Hirata F, Clark MA: Aspirin inhibits phospholipase C. Biochem Biophys Res Commun 1986; 139(1):115–121.

64. Minta JO, Williams MD: Some nonsteroidal antiinflammatory drugs inhibit the generation of superoxide anions by activated polymorphs by blocking ligand-receptor interactions. J Rheumatol 1985; 12(4):751–757.

65. Abramson S, Weismann G: The mechanism of action of nonsteroidal antiinflammatory drugs. Arthritis Rheum 1989; 32:1.

66. Hochberg M: NSAIDs: Mechanism and pathways of action. Hosp Pract 1989; 24:185.

67. Annefeld M: The chondrocyte—The living element of articular cartilage. *In* Annefeld M (ed): Articular Cartilage and Osteoarthrosis. Bern: Hans Huber, 1983:30.

68. Annefeld M: A new test method for the standardized evaluation of changes in the ultrastructure of chondrocytes. Int J Tissue React 1985; 7(4):273–289.

69. Muir H, Carney SL, Hall LG: Effects of tiaprofenic acid and other NSAIDs on proteoglycan metabolism in articular cartilage explants. Drugs 1988; 35(suppl 1):15–23.

70. Palmoski M, Brandt K: In vivo effect of aspirin on canine osteoarthritic cartilage. Arthritis Rheum 1989; 48:619.

71. Doherty M: "Chondroprotection" by non-steroidal antiinflammatory drugs [see comments]. Ann Rheum Dis 1989; 48(8):619–621.

72. Ghosh P: Anti-rheumatic drugs and cartilage. Baillière's Clin Rheumatol 1988; 2(2):309–338.

73. Herman JH, Appel AM, Hess EV: Modulation of cartilage destruction by select nonsteroidal antiinflammatory drugs. In vitro effect on the synthesis and activity of catabolism-inducing cytokines produced by osteoarthritic and rheumatoid synovial tissue. Arthritis Rheum 1987; 30(3):257–265.

74. McKenzie LS, Horsburgh BA, Ghosh P, et al: Effect of anti-inflammatory drugs on sulphated glycosaminoglycan synthesis in aged human articular cartilage. Ann Rheum Dis 1976; 35(6):487–497.

75. Verbruggen G, Malfait AM, Veys EM, et al: Proteoglycan metabolism in isolated chondrocytes from human cartilage and in short-term tissue-cultured human articular cartilage. Clin Exp Rheumatol 1989; 7(1):13–17.

76. Morales TI, Hascall VC: Factors involved in the regulation of proteoglycan metabolism in articular cartilage. Arthritis Rheum 1989; 32(10):1197–1201.

77. Joyce C: Patient cooperation and the sensitivity of clinical trials. J Chron Dis 1962; 15:1025.

78. Ouslander JG: Drug therapy in the elderly. Ann Intern Med 1981; 95(6):711–722.

79. Vebeeck R: Pharmacologic drug interactions with NSAIDs. Clin Pharmacokinet 1990; 19:44.

80. Rashad S, Hemingway A, Rainsford K, et al: Effect of nonsteroidal antiinflammatory drugs on the course of osteoarthritis [see comments]. Lancet 1989; 2(8662):519–522.

81. Hobbs DC, Twomey TM: Piroxicam pharmacokinetics in man: Aspirin and antacid interaction studies. J Clin Pharmacol 1979; 19(5–6):270–281.

82. Shorrack C, Rees W: Mechanism of gastric damage by nonsteroidal antiinflammatory drugs. Scand J Rheumatol 1989; 78(suppl):5.

83. Fries JF: NSAID gastropathy: The second most deadly rheumatic disease? Epidemiology and risk appraisal. J Rheumatol Suppl 1991; 28:6–10.

84. Fries JF, McShane DJ: ARAMIS (the American Rheumatism Association Medical Information System). A prototypical national chronic-disease data bank. West J Med 1986; 145(6):798–804.

85. Bjorkman DJ, Kimmey MB: Nonsteroidal anti-inflammatory drugs and gastrointestinal disease: Pathophysiology, treatment and prevention. Dig Dis 1995; 13(2):119–129.

86. Graham, DY, White RH, Moreland LW, et al: Duodenal and gastric ulcer prevention with misoprostol in arthritis patients taking NSAIDs. Misoprostol Study Group [see comments]. Ann Intern Med 1993; 119(4):257–262.

87. Roth S: Misoprostol in the prevention of NSAID-induced gastric ulcers: A multi-center, double blind, placebo controlled trial. J Rheumatol 1990; 17(suppl 20):20.

88. Agrawal NM, Roth SH, Graham DY, et al: Misoprostol compared with sucralfate in the prevention of nonsteroidal anti-inflammatory drug-induced gastric ulcer. A randomized, controlled trial [see comments]. Ann Intern Med 1991; 115(3): 195–200.

89. Robinson MG, Griffin JW, Bowers J, et al: Effect of ranitidine on gastroduodenal mucosal damage induced by nonsteroidal antiinflammatory drugs. Dig Dis Sci 1989; 34(3):424–428.

90. Ehsanullah RS, Page MC, Tidesley C, et al: Prevention of gastroduodenal damage induced by non-steroidal anti-inflammatory drugs: Controlled trial of ranitidine. BMJ 1988; 297(6655):1017–1021.

91. Ekstrom P, Carling L, Wetterhus S, et al: Prevention of peptic ulcer and dyspeptic symptoms with omeprazole in patients receiving continuous non-steroidal anti-inflammatory drug therapy. A Nordic multicentre study [see comments]. Scand J Gastroenterol 1996; 31(8):753–758.

92. Hawkey CJ, Karrasch JA, Szczepanski L, et al: Omeprazole compared with misoprostol for ulcers associated with nonsteroidal antiinflammatory drugs. Omeprazole versus Misoprostol for NSAID-induced Ulcer Management (OMNIUM) Study Group [see comments]. N Engl J Med 1998; 338(11):727–734.

93. Yeomans ND, Tulassay Z, Juhasz L, et al: A comparison of omeprazole with ranitidine for ulcers associated with nonsteroidal antiinflammatory drugs. Acid Suppression Trial: Ranitidine versus Omeprazole for NSAID-associated Ulcer Treatment (ASTRONAUT) Study Group [see comments]. N Engl J Med 1998; 338(11):719–726.

94. Lane NE, Gore LR, Cumming SR, et al: Serum vitamin D levels and incident changes of radiographic hip osteoarthritis: A longitudinal study. Arthritis Rheum 1999; 42:854–860.

95. Hawkey CJ: Progress in prophylaxis against nonsteroidal antiinflammatory drug-associated ulcers and erosions. Omeprazole NSAID Steering Committee. Am J Med 1998; 104(3A):67S–74S [discussion 79S–80S].

96. Chan FK, Sung JJ, Chung SC, et al: Randomised trial of eradication of Helicobacter pylori before non-steroidal antiinflammatory drug therapy to prevent peptic ulcers [see comments]. Lancet 1997; 350(9083):975–979.

97. Clements P, Paulus H: Non-steroidal antiinflammatory drugs. *In* Kelley WN, Harris ED Jr, Ruddy S, et al (eds): Textbook of Rheumatology, 5th ed. Philadelphia: WB Saunders, 1993:707.

98. Heerdink ER, Leufkens HG, Herings RM, et al: NSAIDs associated with increased risk of congestive heart failure in elderly patients taking diuretics. Arch Intern Med 1998; 158(10):1108–1112.

99. Blackshear JL, Napier JS, Davidman M, et al: Renal complications of nonsteroidal antiinflammatory drugs: Identification and monitoring of those at risk. Semin Arthritis Rheum 1985; 14(3):163–175.

100. Abraham PA, Keane WF: Glomerular and interstitial disease induced by nonsteroidal anti-inflammatory drugs. Am J Nephrol 1984; 4(1):1–6.

101. DiBona GF: Prostaglandins and nonsteroidal anti-inflammatory drugs. Effects on renal hemodynamics. Am J Med 1986; 80(1A):12–21.

102. Sedor JR, Williams SL: Effects of sulindac and indomethacin on renal prostaglandin synthesis. Clin Pharmacol Ther 1984; 36(1):85–91.

103. Whelton A, Stout RL, Spilman PS, et al: Renal effects of ibuprofen, piroxicam, and sulindac in patients with asymptomatic renal failure. A prospective, randomized, crossover comparison [see comments]. Ann Intern Med 1990; 112(8):568–576.

104. Berg KJ, Talseth T: Acute renal effects of sulindac and indomethacin in chronic renal failure. Clin Pharmacol Ther 1985; 37(4):447–452.

105. Katz L, Love P: Hepatic dysfunction in association with nonsteroidal antiinflammatory drugs. *In* Famey J, Paulus H (eds): Non-steroidal Anti-inflammatory Drugs: Subpopulation Therapy and Drug Delivery Systems. New York: Marcel Dekker, 1991.

106. Furst DE, Anderson W: Differential effects of diclofenac and aspirin on serum glutamic oxaloacetic transaminase elevations in patients with rheumatoid arthritis and osteoarthritis. Arthritis Rheum 1993; 36(6):804–810.

107. Benjamin SB, Isha KG, Zimmerman HJ, et al: Phenylbutazone liver injury: A clinical-pathologic survey of 23 cases and review of the literature. Hepatology 1981; 1(3):255–263.

108. O'Brien WM, Bagby GF: Rare adverse reactions to nonsteroidal antiinflammatory drugs: Part 4. J Rheumatol 1985; 12(4):785–90.

109. Stern RS, Bigby M: An expanded profile of cutaneous reactions to nonsteroidal anti-inflammatory drugs. Reports to a specialty-based system for spontaneous reporting of adverse reactions to drugs. JAMA 1984; 252(11):1433–1437.

110. Szczeklik A: Antipyretic analgesics and the allergic patient. Am J Med 1983; 75(5A):82–84.

111. Inman WH: Study of fatal bone marrow depression with special reference to phenylbutazone and oxyphenbutazone. BMJ 1977; 1(6075):1500–1505.

112. Strom BL, Carson JL, Schinnar R, et al: Nonsteroidal antiinflammatory drugs and neutropenia. Arch Intern Med 1993; 153(18):2119–2124.

113. Strom BL, Carson JL, Schinnar R, et al: Descriptive epidemiology of agranulocytosis. Arch Intern Med 1992; 152(7):1475–1480.

114. Younossi ZM, Strum WB, Schatz RA, et al: Effect of combined anticoagulation and low-dose aspirin treatment on upper gastrointestinal bleeding. Dig Dis Sci 1997; 42(1):79–82.

115. Buckley NA, Dawson AH: Drug interactions with warfarin [see comments]. Med J Aust 1992; 157(7):479–483.

116. Chan TY, Lui SF, Chung SY, et al: Adverse interaction between warfarin and indomethacin [see comments]. Drug Saf 1994; 10(3):267–269.

117. Chan TY: Prolongation of prothrombin time with the use of indomethacin and warfarin. Br J Clin Pract 1997; 51(3):177–178.

118. Turck D, Su CA, Heinzel G, et al: Lack of interaction between meloxicam and warfarin in healthy volunteers. Eur J Clin Pharmacol 1997; 51(5):421–425.

119. Simon LS, Lanza FL, Lipsky PE, et al: Preliminary study of the safety and efficacy of SC-58635, a novel cyclooxygenase 2 inhibitor: Efficacy and safety in two placebo-controlled trials in osteoarthritis and rheumatoid arthritis, and studies of gastrointestinal and platelet effects. Arthritis Rheum 1998; 41(9):1591–1602.

120. Lane NE: Pain management in osteoarthritis: The role of COX-2 inhibitors. J Rheumatol 1997; 24(suppl 49):20–24.

121. Day RO, Graham GG, Bieri D, et al: Concentration-response relationships for salicylate-induced ototoxicity in normal volunteers. Br J Clin Pharmacol 1989; 28(6):695–702.

122. Sylvia LM, Forlenza SW, Brocavich JM: Aseptic meningitis associated with naproxen. Drug Intell Clin Pharm 1988; 22(5):399–401.

123. Physicians Desk Reference (PDR), 47th ed. Montvale, NJ: Medical Economics Co., 1993:1485.

124. Cannon G, Caldwell J, Holt P, et al: A specific COX-2 inhibitor, has clinical efficacy comparable to diclofenac in the treatment of knee and hip osteoarthritis in a 26-week controlled clinical trial. Arthritis Rheum 1998; 41(9, suppl):S196.

125. Saag K, Fisher C, McKay J, et al: A specific COX-2 inhibitor, has clinical efficacy comparable to ibuprofen in the treatment of knee and hip osteoarthritis in a 6-week controlled clinical trial. Arthritis Rheum 1998; 41(9, suppl):S196.

126. Karim A, Tolbert D, Piergies A, et al: Celecoxib, a specific COX-2 inhibitor, lacks significant drug-drug interactions with methotrexate or warfarin. Arthritis Rheum 1998; 41(9, suppl): S315.

127. Furst DE: Meloxicam: Selective COX-2 inhibition in clinical practice. Semin Arthritis Rheum 1997; 26(6, suppl 1):21–27.

128. Bernareggi A: Clinical pharmacokinetics of nimesulide [in process citation]. Clin Pharmacokinet 1998; 35(4):247–274.

129. Bevis PJ, Bird HA, Lapham R: An open study to assess the safety and tolerability of meloxicam 15 mg in subjects with rheumatic disease and mild renal impairment. Br J Rheumatol 1996; 35(suppl 1):56–60.

130. Parrillo JE, Fauci AS: Mechanisms of glucocorticoid action on immune processes. Annu Rev Pharmacol Toxicol 1979; 19:179–201.

131. Saxne T, Heinegard D, Wollheim FA: Therapeutic effects on cartilage metabolism in arthritis as measured by release of proteoglycan structures into the synovial fluid. Ann Rheum Dis 1986; 45(6):491–497.

132. Ebert R, Barclay W: Changes in connective tissue reaction induced by cortisone. Ann Intern Med 1952; 37:506.

133. Folkman J, Ingber D: Angiostatic steroids. *In* Schleimer R, Claman H, Oronsky A (eds): Anti-inflammatory Steroid Action: Basic and Clinical Aspects. San Diego, CA: Academic Press, 1989.

134. Williams JM, Brandt KD: Triamcinolone hexacetonide protects against fibrillation and osteophyte formation following chemically induced articular cartilage damage. Arthritis Rheum 1985; 28(11):1267–1274.

135. Pelletier JP, Martel-Pelletier J: Protective effects of corticosteroids on cartilage lesions and osteophyte formation in the Pond-Nuki dog model of osteoarthritis. Arthritis Rheum 1989; 32(2):181–193.

136. Miller W, Restifo R: Steroid arthropathy. Radiology 1966; 86:652.

137. Adams ME: An analysis of clinical studies of the use of cross-linked hyaluronan, hylan, in the treatment of osteoarthritis. J Rheumatol Suppl 1993; 39:16–18.

138. Balazs EA, Denlinger JL: Viscosupplementation: A new concept in the treatment of osteoarthritis. J Rheumatol Suppl 1993; 39:3–9.

139. Moreland L, Arnold WJ, Saway A, et al: Efficacy and safety of intra-articular hylan G-F (Synvisc), a viscoelastic derivative of hyaluronan, in patients with osteoarthritis of the knee. Arthritis Rheum 1993; 37:S165.

140. Adams M, Atkinson M, Lussler AJ, et al: Comparison of intra-articular hylan G-F (Synvisc), a viscoelastic derivative of hyalur-

onan, and continuous NSAID therapy in patients with osteoarthritis of the knee. Arthritis Rheum 1993; 37:S165.

141. Dahlberg L, Lohmander LS, Ryd L: Intraarticular injections of hyaluronan in patients with cartilage abnormalities and knee pain. A one-year double-blind, placebo-controlled study. Arthritis Rheum 1994; 37(4):521–528.

142. Lohmander LS, Dalen N, Englund G, et al: Intra-articular hyaluronan injections in the treatment of osteoarthritis of the knee: A randomised, double blind, placebo controlled multicentre trial. Hyaluronan Multicentre Trial Group [see comments]. Ann Rheum Dis 1996; 55(7):424–431.

143. Chang RW, Falconer J: A randomized, controlled trial of arthroscopic surgery versus closed-needle joint lavage for patients with osteoarthritis of the knee. Arthritis Rheum 1993; 36(3): 289–296.

144. Ike RW, Arnold WJ: Tidal irrigation versus conservative medical management in patients with osteoarthritis of the knee: A prospective randomized study. Tidal Irrigation Cooperating Group. J Rheumatol 1992; 19(5):772–779.

145. Timoney JM, Kneisl JS, Barrack RL, et al: Arthroscopy update #6: Arthroscopy in the osteoarthritic knee. Long-term follow-up. Orthop Rev 1990; 19(4):371–373, 376–379.

146. Richards R, Lonergan R: Arthroscopic surgery for the relief of pain in the osteoarthritic knee. Orthopedics 1984; 7:1705.

147. Gramas D, Lane N, Antounian F: Needle arthroscopy: Our preliminary experience. Arthritis Rheum 1993; 37(suppl):164.

148. Peterson MG, Hollenberg P, Szatrowski TP, et al: Geographic variations in the rates of elective total hip and knee arthroplasties among Medicare beneficiaries in the United States [see comments]. J Bone Joint Surg Am 1992; 74(10):1530–1539.

149. Emery DF, Clarke HJ, Grover ML: Stanmore total hip replacement in younger patients: Review of a group of patients under 50 years of age at operation. J Bone Joint Surg Br 1997; 79(2):240–246.

150. Sledge C, Poss R: Orthopedic surgery and degenerative arthritis. Rheum Dis Clin North Am 1988; 14:xi.

151. Santore RF, Dabezies EJ Jr: Femoral osteotomy for secondary arthritis of the hip in young adults. Can J Surg 1995; 38(suppl 1):S33–S38.

152. Paley D, Maar DC, Herzenberg JE: New concepts in high tibial osteotomy for medial compartment osteoarthritis. Orthop Clin North Am 1994; 25(3):483–498.

153. Lopes Vaz A: Double-blind clinical evaluation of the relative efficacy of ibuprofen and glucosamine sulphate in the management of osteoarthrosis of the knee in out-patients. Curr Med Res Opin 1982; 8(3):145–149.

154. McAlindon TE, LaValley MP, Gulin JP: Glucosamine and chondroitin for treatment of osteoarthritis. A systematic quality assessment and meta-analysis. JAMA 2000; 283(11):1469–1474.

155. Cole AA, Chubinskaya S, Luchene LJ, et al: Doxycycline disrupts chondrocyte differentiation and inhibits cartilage matrix degradation. Arthritis Rheum 1994; 37(12):1727–1734.

156. Kuettner K, Goldberg V: Osteoarthritic disorders. Osteoarthritis Workshop. Monterey, CA: February 1994.

157. Dieppe P, Cushnaghan J, Young P, et al: Prediction of the progression of joint space narrowing in osteoarthritis of the knee by bone scintigraphy. Ann Rheum Dis 1993; 52(8):557–563.

158. McAlindon T, Felson DT: Nutrition: Risk factors for osteoarthritis. Ann Rheum Dis 1997; 56(7):397–400.

159. McAlindon TE, Felson DT, Zhang Y, et al: Relation of dietary intake and serum levels of vitamin D to progression of osteoarthritis of the knee among participants in the Framingham study. Ann Intern Med 1996; 125(5):353–359.

160. McAlindon TE, Jacques P, Zhang Y, et al: Do antioxidant micronutrients protect against the development and progression of knee osteoarthritis? Arthritis Rheum 1996; 39(4):648–656.

161. Trock DH, Bollet AJ, Markoll R, et al: A double-blind trial of the clinical effects of pulsed electromagnetic fields in osteoarthritis [see comments]. J Rheumatol 1993; 20(3):456–460.

162. Pelletier JP, McCollum R, DiBattista J, et al: Regulation of human normal and osteoarthritic chondrocyte interleukin 1 receptor by antirheumatic drugs. Arthritis Rheum 1993; 36(11):1517–1527.

# 37 | Uncommon Rheumatic Diseases

*Sterling G. West and Gene V. Ball*

The rheumatic syndromes discussed in this chapter are uncommon disorders with poorly understood etiology and pathogenesis. Clinical manifestations are often variable, making it difficult to find adequate numbers of similar patients for controlled therapeutic trials. Consequently, treatment is often empiric and not always satisfactory. This chapter reviews treatment for the systemic as well as rheumatic aspects of sarcoidosis, Behçet's disease (BD), amyloidosis, familial Mediterranean fever (FMF), relapsing polychondritis (RP), hereditary hemochromatosis (HH), and Paget's disease. For many of these disorders, drug therapies have not been shown to alter their natural history.

## SARCOIDOSIS

Sarcoidosis is a systemic inflammatory disorder defined histologically by the presence of noncaseating granulomas. In the United States, African Americans have a 2.4% and Caucasians a 0.85% lifetime risk for development of sarcoidosis. The clinical spectrum is protean, ranging from an abnormal chest radiograph in an asymptomatic individual to severe multiorgan involvement.[1] The most common sites of clinical involvement are the lungs (95%), lymph nodes, (80%), skin (25%), and eyes (25%). Other areas that may be involved are the heart (10%), central nervous system (5%), bones (5%), joints, muscles, liver, and upper respiratory tract.[2] Because of overproduction of 1,25-dihydroxyvitamin D by activated macrophages, up to 10% of sarcoid patients have hypercalcemia and 40% have hypercalciuria. Sarcoidosis has also been reported to coexist with various other connective tissue diseases, including rheumatoid arthritis, systemic lupus erythematosus, Sjögren's syndrome, scleroderma, and vasculitis.[3]

Joint manifestations, including arthritis, periarthritis, and arthralgias, occur in 2% to 38% of patients with sarcoidosis. Rheumatic involvement is generally divided into acute and chronic types. The first consists of articular involvement during the acute presentation of the illness. The triad of arthritis, erythema nodosum, and hilar adenopathy comprise Löfgren's syndrome, which may be accompanied by fever. Arthritis arises most often in knees and ankles, and periarticular pain can be severe. Symptoms tend to remit spontaneously

over a period of several weeks. The less common type of joint involvement consists of synovitis that accompanies the slower-onset, more chronic, and systemic form of the disease. The arthritis may be mild and transient, recurrent, or protracted. It is usually a nondestructive polyarthritis, oligoarthritis, or monoarthritis involving the shoulders, wrists, knees, ankles, and/or small joints of the hands and feet. Dactylitis resulting from sarcoid bone and soft tissue involvement can occur. In contrast to the acute type, chronic sarcoid arthropathy is characterized by inflammatory joint fluid and histologic granulomas within the synovium and frequently coexists with chronic cutaneous sarcoidosis.

The natural history of untreated sarcoidosis is difficult to predict in an individual patient. Most patients (66%) undergo spontaneous remission, but the course is chronic in 10% to 30%. Of those having a chronic course, half will have progressive pulmonary disease and half will display involvement of critical extrapulmonary organs such as the eye, brain, and heart. The probability of a spontaneous remission can be predicted by the patient's clinical and radiologic presentation. Up to 80% of patients presenting with hilar adenopathy alone (radiographic stage I disease) have a spontaneous resolution. Patients with Löfgren's syndrome have the best overall prognosis for remission. Fifty percent to 60% of patients with radiographic stage II signs (hilar adenopathy with pulmonary infiltrates) experience remission, in contrast to fewer than 30% of those with stage III disease (infiltrates without adenopathy).[4] The mortality rate of patients with pulmonary fibrosis (radiographic stage IV, vital capacity less than 1.5 L) is 25% to 40%. Although the overall prognosis for sarcoidosis is good, at least 50% of patients have some degree of permanent organ dysfunction. In addition, there is a 5% mortality rate, with progressive pulmonary disease accounting for half and cardiac/neurologic disease causing the other half of all deaths from sarcoidosis. In general, the more severe the involvement and the more organ systems (greater than three) involved at the time of diagnosis, the worse the prognosis. Cutaneous sarcoidosis is a poor prognostic sign, as is black race, onset of disease after 40 years of age, and symptoms lasting longer than 6 months.[1, 5]

Because the cause of sarcoidosis is unknown, therapy is empiric (Tables 37–1 and 37–2). If possible, patients with good prognostic signs should be observed

## TABLE 37–1
## Immunosuppressive Therapy Used in Selected Patients with Severe Rheumatic Disease

| DRUG | TRADE NAME | DOSE/TABLET (mg) | DOSAGE | SIDE EFFECTS | COMMENTS |
|------|-----------|------------------|--------|--------------|----------|
| Methotrexate | Rheumatrex | 2.5 | 10–25 mg once a week, oral or SC | Hematologic Nausea, mouth sores Hepatic Lung Lymphoma (rare) | Use with folate 1 mg/d Avoid use with Septra/ Bactrim Avoid use in renal insufficiency |
| Azathioprine | Imuran | 50 | 2 mg/kg/d | Hematologic Nausea, mouth sores Hepatic Infection/herpes zoster Carcinogenicity | Avoid use with allopurinol Avoid use with Septra/ Bactrim |
| Cyclophosphamide | Cytoxan | 25, 50 | 2 mg/kg/d orally or 0.75–1 g/m$^2$ every 4 wk IV | Hematologic Nausea Bladder Carcinogenicity | Use mesna for bladder prophylaxis* Force fluids |
| Chlorambucil | Leukeran | 2 | 0.1 mg/kg/d | Hematologic Carcinogenicity | Do not use longer than 12 mo |
| Cyclosporine | Neoral | 25, 100 | 5–10 mg/kg/d | Nausea Hypertension Renal Tremors | Many drug interactions |
|  | Sandimmune | 25, 50, 100 |  |  |  |
| Tacrolimus (FK-506) | Prograf | 1, 5 | 0.1–0.15 mg/kg/d | Nausea Renal Tremors Hyperglycemia | Keep whole blood trough level lower than 20 ng/ mL |

\* Give four doses of mesna (one dose every 3 hr intravenously) on the day of cyclophosphamide administration. Each dose of mesna (in milligrams) is 20% of the total cyclophosphamide dose.

## TABLE 37–2
## Immunomodulatory Therapy Used in Selected Patients with Rheumatic Disease

| DRUG | TRADE NAME | DOSE/TABLET (mg) | DOSAGE | SIDE EFFECTS | COMMENTS |
|------|-----------|------------------|--------|--------------|----------|
| Hydroxychloroquine | Plaquenil | 200 | 200–400 mg/d | Nausea Retinal | Eye examination every 6–12 mo |
| Pentoxifylline | Trental | 400 | 400 mg three times per day | Nausea |  |
| Colchicine | Colchicine | 0.5, 0.6 | 1.0–2.4 mg/d | Nausea Diarrhea Neuromyopathy | Decrease dose if renal or liver disease |
| Sulfasalazine | Azulfidine | 500 | 2–4 g/d | Hematologic Nausea Rash | Avoid if sulfa allergy |
| Interferon alfa | Roferon-A Intron-A | Injection* SC | 9 × 10$^6$ units SC three times per week for 3 mo, followed by 3 × 10$^6$ units three times per wk for maintenance | Flu-like symptoms Leukopenia Alopecia | Dosage listed is for Behçet's disease; may be different for other diseases |
| Dapsone | Dapsone | 25, 100 | 50–200 mg/d | Hematologic Nausea | Avoid in patients with glucose-6-phosphate dehydrogenase deficiency |
| Thalidomide | Thalomid | 50 | 50–300 mg/d | Neuropathy (irreversible) | Use lowest dose possible to avoid neuropathy |

\* Roferon-A is supplied in 1-mL vials containing 3, 6, or 9 million IU. Intron-A is supplied in 1-mL vials containing 3, 5, or 10 million IU.

for the first 6 months without therapy because of the potential of spontaneous resolution. In patients with progressive disease, the recommended doses of corticosteroids and adjunctive therapies vary depending on the organ system involved. There have been no controlled, randomized trials to establish the appropriate dose and duration of any therapy for sarcoidosis. Despite a lack of well-controlled clinical trials proving that corticosteroids improve long-term outcome, oral corticosteroids are used as first-line treatment for symptomatic and progressive (a decrease in forced vital capacity of 10% or more, or 20% or greater lung diffusion of carbon monoxide), stage II and III pulmonary disease, malignant hypercalcemia, and severe ocular, neurologic, cardiac, skin, and musculoskeletal involvement.[6]

## Pulmonary

Two prospective, nonrandomized studies showed short-term benefits of corticosteroid therapy for patients with deteriorating lung function or serious extrapulmonary disease.[7, 8] For the 15% of patients who develop progressive lung involvement, current guidelines suggest the use of 30 to 60 mg (1 mg/kg/day) of prednisone daily for 8 to 12 weeks, with a gradual tapering of the dose to 30 mg every other day by 6 months, 20 mg every other day by 9 months, and 10 mg every other day by 12 months. More than 70% of patients respond favorably, but relapses occur in 25% to 50% of patients after tapering or discontinuation of corticosteroids. Some patients need 10 to 20 mg every other day indefinitely to prevent relapses.[1] Inhaled corticosteroids have been found to be more efficacious than low-dose corticosteroids as maintenance therapy in stage II and III pulmonary disease.[9]

A variety of other medications have been tried to reduce oral corticosteroid dependence and in patients who do not respond or have intolerable side effects (see Tables 37–1 and 37–2). Two double-blind, randomized studies failed to demonstrate that inhaled budesonide was more efficacious than placebo for preventing pulmonary deterioration.[10, 11] Although inhaled corticosteroids may have a role in patients with mild endobronchial sarcoidosis, they have none in patients with severe pulmonary parenchymal involvement. Experience with immunosuppressive medications including azathioprine, cyclophosphamide, chlorambucil, cyclosporine, and methotrexate has been limited to small, uncontrolled trials and anecdotal case reports.[12] Of these, azathioprine and methotrexate are used most often. In one report, 70% of 50 patients with chronic sarcoidosis treated with methotrexate were able to reduce their prednisone use after 6 months. However, relapses were frequent after methotrexate was discontinued.[13] The therapeutic effectiveness of cyclosporine in pulmonary sarcoidosis has generally been disappointing, in contrast to methotrexate.[14] In patients for whom corticosteroids and immunosuppressive drugs have failed, mechanical dilatation of bronchial stenosis can be effective but often needs to be repeated.[1, 15] In patients with end-stage pulmonary fibrotic disease,

lung transplantation offers a potential cure, although higher-than-normal rates of rejection and recurrence of sarcoidosis in the allograft have been observed.[16]

## Arthritis

Acute sarcoidosis with arthritis/periarthritis (Löfgren's syndrome) requires no specific therapy other than analgesics or nonsteroidal anti-inflammatory drugs (NSAIDs) such as indomethacin, since spontaneous resolution is the most likely outcome. Colchicine appears to shorten attacks in some patients.[17] For chronic synovitis, low-dose corticosteroids may be helpful if NSAIDs or analgesics fail. Hydroxychloroquine, azathioprine, and methotrexate have been used successfully in patients with severe musculoskeletal manifestations refractory to corticosteroids.[18]

## Dermatologic

Topical corticosteroids and monthly intralesional injections of triamcinolone are often effective therapy for small sarcoid papules or plaques. Large or disfiguring skin lesions require systemic corticosteroid therapy (30 mg every day to every other day).[19] Several small studies have found chloroquine and hydroxychloroquine to be useful, with an overall 35% response rate.[20, 21] Mucosal lesions of the upper respiratory tract have also been reported to respond to antimalarial therapy.[22] Methotrexate has been reported to be an effective steroid-sparing agent for severe cutaneous sarcoid.[23] Thalidomide, allopurinol, and tranilast have been anecdotally successful in a few patients with refractory sarcoid skin lesions.[24, 25]

## Ophthalmic

Eye manifestations are treated with topical, injectable, and systemic corticosteroids. Topical steroids and cycloplegics are usually sufficient for anterior uveitis, although granulomatous involvement of ocular structures and posterior segment inflammation require oral corticosteroid or periocular steroid injections. Azathioprine and methotrexate have been effective for steroid-refractory, chronic uveitis[13] (see Chapter 16).

## Renal

Hypercalciuria usually responds rapidly to 10 to 20 mg/day of prednisone. Chloroquine and ketoconazole act more slowly but produce more sustained lowering of calcium after cessation of treatment.[26] A low-calcium diet, avoidance of vitamin D supplements, and limited exposure to sunlight are helpful adjunctive measures.

## Cardiovascular

Cardiac and neurologic sarcoid are uncommon, but they are leading causes of mortality. Large doses of prednisone (60 mg/day or greater) should be initiated in patients with ventricular arrhythmias or cardiomyopathy.[27] Antiarrhythmic agents and medications for heart failure should be used as adjunctive therapies. Magnetic resonance imaging of the heart and myocardial scintigraphy may be useful in monitoring the response to therapy.[28] In patients with severe or refractory disease, high-dose pulse methylprednisolone, azathioprine, methotrexate, chlorambucil, and cyclophosphamide have been used with some success.[29, 30] Implantable pacemakers and heart transplantation have been used for patients in whom medical management failed.[31] Sarcoid vasculitis is uncommon and may require treatment with immunosuppressive drugs.

## Neurologic

Neurologic sarcoidosis is treated with oral prednisone, 40 to 80 mg/day.[32, 33] Antiseizure medications are used as adjunctive therapy in patients with seizures. Patients with severe and refractory disease have been treated with immunosuppressive therapy, as for cardiac sarcoidosis. However, uncontrolled reports have also suggested that antimalarials, cyclosporine, and cranial radiation may be effective.[34–36] Surgical intervention is necessary for hydrocephalus and mass lesions that are expanding or causing increased intracranial pressure.

New therapies for sarcoidosis will depend on a better understanding of its cause and immunopathogenesis.[37, 38] An infectious or environmental trigger has long been suspected. Tumor necrosis factor-$\alpha$ (TNF-$\alpha$), interleukin-12 (IL-12), and other cytokines involved in T helper 1 (Th1) response have been shown to be increased in active sarcoidosis. Pentoxifylline (400 mg three times daily) inhibits the synthesis of TNF-$\alpha$ and reversed the loss of pulmonary function in 11 of 18 patients.[39] Other TNF-$\alpha$ inhibitors, including monoclonal antibodies and TNF-$\alpha$ receptors currently used to treat rheumatoid arthritis and inflammatory bowel disease, may be useful in sarcoidosis. Furthermore, IL-4 and IL-10, which are potent suppressors of Th1 activity and granuloma formation, and transforming growth factor-$\beta$, which inhibits IL-2 production by T cells, may be useful as future therapies.

## BEHÇET'S DISEASE

BD is an episodic, inflammatory disease first described in 1937 by the Turkish dermatologist, Hulushi Behçet.[40] Because the cause of this multisystem disorder is unknown, the diagnosis is based on fulfillment of various clinical criteria. The International Study Group criteria, proposed in 1990, have had the best discriminatory performance.[41] Diagnosis requires at least three episodes of oral ulcerations over a 12-month period, plus at least two of four other manifestations: recurrent genital ulcerations (occurring in 80% of patients), eye inflammation including uveitis or retinal vasculitis (60% to 70%), inflammatory skin lesions (60% to 80%), and pathergy (erythematous papule occurring at entry site of needle stick). These clinical features can evolve in a single patient over time. Other possible features are gastrointestinal lesions (50%), thrombophlebitis and

arteritis with aneurysms (25%), and involvement of the central and peripheral nervous systems (5%). Arthritis, which occurs in 40% of patients, is characteristically inflammatory, nondeforming, monoarticular or oligoarticular, and most commonly involves the knee, ankle, or wrist. Episodes last 2 to 8 weeks. BD uncommonly is associated with relapsing polychondritis, the combination being designated *MAGIC syndrome* (*m*outh *a*nd *g*enital ulcerations with *i*nflamed *c*artilage).[42]

BD occurs mainly in young adults (average age at onset, 25 years). It is most common in Japan, eastern Asia, and the eastern Mediterranean. Its prevalence in the United States is less than 7 per 100,000 population. The course of BD is variable. Its onset may be acute or insidious, and its natural history tends to be one of recurrent attacks that last several weeks or longer. Overall the prognosis is generally good, with a 10-year survival rate of 95%. Younger age at onset, male sex, neurologic involvement, vascular thromboses, arterial aneurysms, and certain ethnic backgrounds predict a poor prognosis. Clearly, mortality is increased and sequelae are severe if vital organs are involved. Life-threatening complications such as meningoencephalitis and major venous and arterial thromboses are rare. However, these manifestations, as well as uveitis with its attendant risk of visual loss, constitute the most compelling basis for the use of immunosuppressive drug therapy.[13]

Treatment of BD is aimed at control of inflammation and thromboses (see Tables 37–1 and 37–2).[44] There are few prospective, controlled, or large trials that have demonstrated a substantial or sustained benefit of any anti-inflammatory or immunosuppressive medication. However, there have been numerous case reports and small clinical trials supporting the use of several medications for specific disease manifestations. Topical agents are initially used to treat oral and genital ulcers.[45] Triamcinolone paste or other corticosteroid gels help palliate the symptoms. A topical tetracycline solution made by dissolving the contents of a 250-mg capsule in 5 mL of water and holding the mixture on the lesion for 2 minutes has also been reported to be helpful.[43] If needed, intralesional corticosteroids and topical interferon-$\alpha$2c (INF-$\alpha$2c) can be tried.[46] Fever and arthritis should be treated first with antipyretics and NSAIDs. Because many episodes of BD are mild and self-limited, symptomatic therapy is warranted for minor symptoms. However, for severe and recurrent symptoms, additional therapies are also necessary.

Colchicine is a potent inhibitor of neutrophil chemotaxis, which has been observed to be accelerated in BD. In doses of 1 to 2 mg/day, colchicine can ameliorate mucocutaneous symptoms including orogenital ulcers and erythema nodosum.[47] For severe mucocutaneous lesions, low-dose prednisone (20 mg/day or less), dapsone, levamisole, methotrexate, or azathioprine can be helpful. Masuda et al. reported in a randomized, double-blind trial that high-dose cyclosporine (10 mg/kg/day) was more effective than colchicine in controlling mucocutaneous and genital ulceration in BD.[48] A randomized, controlled trial of 96 male BD patients who had primarily mucocutaneous lesions showed thalidomide (100–300 mg/day) to be superior to placebo in suppressing oral and genital ulcers and follicular skin lesions. However, complete response occurred in fewer than 20% of patients, and peripheral neuropathy and an increase in erythema nodosum lesions were seen in patients receiving thalidomide.[49]

Joint involvement is initially treated with NSAIDs, although a double-blind, controlled trial failed to show significant effect after the first week of therapy.[50] Colchicine also has not been found to be effective. A double-blind, controlled trial showed improvement in arthralgias but no measurable change in arthritis in patients receiving colchicine.[51] However, in a randomized trial, prophylactic benzathine penicillin (1.2 million U) every 3 weeks with colchicine 1.5 mg/day resulted in a decreased number of episodes of BD compared to colchicine alone.[52] This has been interpreted as evidence that *Streptococcus* may be an environmental trigger in some patients with BD. For patients with severe arthritic involvement, low-dose prednisone (20 mg/day or less), sulfasalazine, methotrexate, azathioprine, levamisole, and INF-α2b have been reported to be effective in open trials. Patients with arthritis and/or gastrointestinal ulcers may respond particularly well to sulfasalazine and prednisone. For persistent monoarthritis, intra-articular corticosteroids are recommended.

Corticosteroids are widely used for the minor manifestations of BD, but there is little evidence that they have a substantial impact on any of the major clinical manifestations when used alone. Consequently, other immunosuppressive agents have been given in conjunction with high-dose corticosteroids to small numbers of patients with chorioretinitis, uveitis, vasculitis, and/or central nervous system disease. Anterior uveitis is initially treated with topical corticosteroid drops and mydriatics. Severe or unresponsive cases are treated with systemic corticosteroids. Posterior uveitis and retinal vasculitis are treated with corticosteroid injections and systemic corticosteroids (1 mg/kg/day) in conjunction with other immunosuppressive agents.[53] In a 2-year randomized, controlled trial of 70 BD patients, azathioprine was found to be superior to placebo in controlling serious eye disease in addition to orogenital ulcerations and arthritis.[54] In addition, a long-term, controlled trial showed that BD patients treated early on with azathioprine had a better prognosis overall than those who received placebo over a mean of 8 years.[55] Methotrexate, sulfasalazine, and chlorambucil have also been used in a few patients with ocular disease (see Chapter 16).

Cyclosporine has been used by several groups for the treatment of uveitis and retinal vasculitis. Cyclosporine inhibits the function of CD4-positive lymphocytes by decreasing the production of IL-2 and other cytokines. Cyclosporine is reported to be comparable to cytotoxic agents and better than colchicine in controlling acute ocular attacks.[48, 56–58] It also appears to be more effective early on than monthly bolus cyclophosphamide but not after 2 years of therapy.[59] Cyclosporine in combination with azathioprine may

improve eye manifestations in patients for whom either medication alone has failed. Tacrolimus (FK 506) in doses of 0.1 to 0.15 mg/kg/day reduces calcineurin activity of T cells and may also be useful in ocular disease that is unresponsive to cyclosporine alone.[60, 61]

Central nervous system disease, arteritis, and major vein thromboses are usually treated with a combination of high-dose prednisone and alkylating agents. Patients with severe presenting manifestations can be treated with a bolus of methylprednisolone (1 g/day) for 3 days. In addition, daily oral or monthly intravenous boluses of cyclophosphamide are used.[62, 63] Chlorambucil has also been recommended as therapy for severe central nervous system and ocular disease. O'Duffy et al. describe 21 patients with meningoencephalitis or uveitis treated with various drug regimens.[64] Eight of nine patients studied retrospectively improved after receiving chlorambucil at doses of 0.1 mg/kg/day for at least 3 months. After a remission of at least 1 year, alkylating agents should be stopped to lessen the chance of developing a malignancy. Relapses may occur. For recurrent thromboses, aspirin and anticoagulants can be used with caution, but immunosuppressive medications are also required to control the underlying vasculitis.[65] Anticoagulants should be avoided in patients with pulmonary arterial aneurysms because of the risk of fatal hemoptysis. Surgery in patients with active vasculitis is associated with a risk of recurrence of aneurysm or thrombosis after vascular surgery and bowel perforations after bowel resection.[66, 67] Consequently, the underlying vasculitis should be controlled with medical therapy before surgery if at all possible.

Better therapies for BD in the future will depend on an improved understanding of its etiopathogenesis.[68] The success of intramuscular benzathine penicillin in decreasing flares of BD is of interest. A report that pentoxifylline (600 mg/day for 2 weeks tapered to 300 mg/day) improved mild orogenital ulceration and uveitis in three patients with BD suggests that oxpentifylline in its current 400 mg dosage may be a useful adjunctive agent in mild disease.[69] Systemic administration of tolerizing agents such as retinal protein S may represent a future therapy for uveitis. For more severe or recurrent disease, systemic INF-α has shown some success. A review of 144 BD patients reported in the literature who had received INF-α in various regimens showed partial or complete response within 1 to 4 months in 74% of those with mucocutaneous lesions, 95% of those with uveitis, and 93% of those with arthritis.[70] After analysis, the recommended regimen was a 3-month high-dose induction followed by a low maintenance dose. However, this does not represent a cure, and clinical manifestations will recur after therapy is stopped. Any reports of successful new therapies need to be interpreted cautiously, because BD can exhibit spontaneous exacerbations and remissions.

## AMYLOIDOSIS

Amyloidosis is a heterogeneous group of diseases characterized by the extracellular deposition of insoluble fibrillar proteins in various organs and tissues.[71] There are at least 17 different amyloid proteins described, and each shares a common structural conformation (β-pleated sheet) that is responsible for amyloid's unique staining properties with Congo red. Amyloid can be acquired or familial, and the deposits can be systemic or localized. The most common systemic amyloidoses are primary or myeloma-associated AL amyloidosis, AA amyloidosis secondary to chronic inflammation, β₂-microglobulin amyloidosis associated with chronic hemodialysis, and familial amyloidosis associated with abnormal transthyretin. Each has a unique clinical onset, natural history, and treatment strategy. Treatment strategies focus on treating any underlying disease, preventing the synthesis and deposition of amyloid components, and removing amyloid deposits[72] (Table 37–3). In general, corticosteroids alone have little role in the treatment of amyloidosis.

## AL Amyloidosis

AL amyloidosis is a plasma cell dyscrasia with an excess of clonal plasma cells in the bone marrow. The amyloid deposits are primarily the variable regions of light chains. The incidence is approximately 4.5 per 100,000 population, and the disease usually affects persons over 40 years of age. Patients typically (85% to 90%) have an abnormal serum or urine protein electrophoresis showing a monoclonal immunoglobulin protein. Extensive multisystem involvement is common, with heart, kidney, liver, nerves, skin, tongue, and musculoskeletal system most commonly affected. Overall, survival without treatment is less than 2 years depending on the extent of organ system involvement. Patients with cardiac deposition resulting in a restrictive cardiomyopathy or conduction disturbances have a median survival time of 4 to 6 months, whereas those with primarily kidney involvement have a median survival time of 18 to 21 months.[71]

Because of the poor overall prognosis, treatment should be started as soon as the diagnosis is confirmed. In a large clinical trial, colchicine was found to improve the median survival time to 17 months, compared with 6 months for untreated controls.[73] Although colchicine

may slow progression, patients eventually die. Consequently, therapies to eliminate clonal plasma cells have been used. Cyclic chemotherapy with oral melphalan and prednisone is the mainstay of therapy. Kyle and Gertz have published several reports on the benefits of melphalan and prednisone in AL amyloidosis.[74] In the most recent of these, 220 patients with biopsy-proven primary amyloidosis were randomly assigned to receive (1) colchicine, (2) melphalan and prednisone, or (3) melphalan, prednisone, and colchicine. Median duration of survival in the three groups was 8.5, 18, and 17 months, respectively. The authors concluded that melphalan plus prednisone was superior to colchicine alone. However, in a previous trial, 10 patients died of acute leukemia or myelodysplastic syndromes attributed to melphalan therapy.[75]

Skinner et al. conducted a randomized trial of 100 patients with AL amyloidosis treated with melphalan, prednisone, and colchicine compared with patients treated only with colchicine.[76] Although the difference was not statistically significant, median survival time was 12.2 months from study entry for the melphalan treatment group and 6.7 months for those treated only with colchicine. Patients with neuropathy and hepatomegaly fared better than those with cardiomyopathy. Survival was most likely to improve in patients who received chemotherapy for at least 4 months. Consequently, patients with cardiomyopathy, who have a particularly poor prognosis and frequently do not survive 4 months, should be considered for heart transplantation. Heart transplantation has been successful in a few selected patients, although amyloidosis can recur in the transplanted heart.[77]

Future therapy in selected patients with AL amyloidosis may be dose-intensive chemotherapy with vincristine, doxorubicin, and dexamethasone[78] or high-dose melphalan with autologous stem cell transplantation.[79, 80] Another potential therapy is with an iodinated analog of doxorubicin (IDOX), which has been shown to cause resorption of amyloid deposits through unknown mechanisms.[81] In patients with organ failure, the use of both dose-intensive chemotherapy with stem cell support and IDOX may improve survival in the future.

## TABLE 37–3
## Treatment Recommendations for Systemic Amyloidosis

| | |
|---|---|
| AL (primary) | Oral melphalan, 0.15–0.25 mg/kg/d for 4 d; prednisone, 1.5–2.0 mg/kg/d for 4 d. Repeat every 6 wk for 1 y. Colchicine, 0.6 mg BID can be given with cyclic melphalan/prednisone but should not be taken during the 4 d of chemotherapy.<br>OR<br>Intravenous melphalan, 100–200 mg/m² over 2 d, with autologous stem cell rescue (experimental) |
| AA (secondary) | Aggressive treatment of underlying inflammatory or infectious disease. Surgical excision of infectious focus when possible. Trial of colchicine, 0.6 mg BID. |
| ATTR (familial) | Orthotopic liver transplantation. |

Adapted from Skinner M: Amyloidosis. *In* Kelley WN, Harris ED, Ruddy S, et al (eds): Textbook of Rheumatology. Philadelphia: WB Saunders, 1997:1415.

## Secondary Amyloidosis

AA amyloidosis occurs as a complication of chronic inflammation or infection. It is seen uncommonly in patients with tuberculosis, leprosy, rheumatoid arthritis, juvenile rheumatoid arthritis, ankylosing spondylitis, BD, or other conditions. In the United States, fewer than 1% of rheumatoid arthritis patients develop amyloidosis, whereas 5% of such patients in Europe and Scandinavia develop this complication. The amyloid fibrils are composed of the terminal portion of an acute-phase reactant, serum amyloid A (SAA). The most common presentation is renal insufficiency and proteinuria. Hepatomegaly and autonomic neuropathy frequently appear as the disease progresses. Cardiomyopathy and musculoskeletal involvement are rare. Disease progression is slow, and survival is often greater than 10 years with supportive treatment including dialysis.[82]

Treatment of the underlying inflammatory or infectious disease is the primary goal in all patients with secondary amyloidosis. Although successful anti-inflammatory therapy, including cytotoxic drugs, may arrest or retard deposition, there are no controlled trials that demonstrate regression of amyloid or reduction in mortality with standard anti-inflammatory or immunosuppressive therapy.[83–85] Measurement of serum SAA levels and possibly serum amyloid P scintigraphy can be used to monitor effectiveness of therapy.[86] There are case reports of regression of proteinuria in patients with ankylosing spondylitis and juvenile rheumatoid arthritis treated with colchicine.[87] Certainly, patients with amyloidosis secondary to FMF should be treated with colchicine 1.2 to 2.0 mg/day.[88] Future therapy may involve use of specifically-designed ribozymes to suppress SAA gene expression.[89]

## Hemodialysis-Associated Amyloidosis

Hemodialysis-associated amyloidosis arises only after 7 years of chronic hemodialysis treatment for end-stage renal disease.[90] Between 50% to 100% of patients undergoing dialysis for longer than 12 to 15 years develop this complication. It is thought that inefficient clearance of $\beta_2$-microglobulin by dialyzers over many years leads to the accumulation and subsequent deposition of amyloid. Clinical manifestations are primarily musculoskeletal and include carpal tunnel syndrome, persistent noninflammatory joint effusions of large joints (shoulders, knees, wrists, hips), spondyloarthropathy with destructive changes of intervertebral discs, cystic bone lesions filled with $\beta_2$-microglobulin amyloid deposits which can result in pathologic fractures, and soft tissue tumors. Deposition in other organs is rare.

Treatment is difficult because the $\beta_2$-microglobulin is too large to pass through a dialysis membrane. One prospective, controlled study showed that over 6 years none of the patients dialyzed with a high-flux polysulfone membrane developed amyloidosis, whereas 8 of 10 patients dialyzed with the standard low-flux cuprophane dialysis membrane developed amyloidosis.[91] Therefore, new membranes of the high-flux type appear to be more efficient at removing $\beta_2$-microglobulin than older membranes. In addition, renal transplantation has been observed to arrest the progression and even cause regression of hemodialysis-associated amyloidosis.[92, 93] Surgical removal of amyloid deposits from the carpal tunnel, spine, and bony cystic lesions is often indicated to relieve neural compression and treat or prevent pathologic fractures. Therapies such as plasma filtration and use of immunoadsorption columns to remove $\beta_2$-microglobulin from the circulation may be used in the future.[94]

## Familial Transthyretin Amyloidosis

The heredofamilial amyloidoses are a rare and diverse group. The most common is familial amyloid polyneuropathy, which is an autosomal dominant disease.[82] The amyloid deposits are an abnormal form of transthyretin caused by a mutated gene. Patients present in midlife with a peripheral sensory motor and autonomic neuropathy. Pathognomonic vitreous opacities occur in 25%. Cardiac and renal involvement is less common, and macroglossia does not occur. Survival time after disease onset is 7 to 15 years. Patients with onset before 30 years of age have a more rapid progression of their disease. There is no effective medical therapy for transthyretin amyloidoses. However, because most of the transthyretin protein is produced in the liver, liver transplantation with a liver from a normal donor corrects the underlying metabolic abnormality. Patients who undergo liver transplantation before irreversible organ failure experience improvement in their symptoms, function, quality, and extent of life.[95] Gene therapy is an attractive but untested option for future treatment.

## FAMILIAL MEDITERRANEAN FEVER

FMF is an autosomal recessive disease that primarily affects Sephardic Jews, Arabs, Turks, and Armenians in areas surrounding the Mediterranean basin.[96, 97] It is characterized by relapsing episodes of fever (100% of patients) with peritonitis (89% to 96%), pleuritis (25% to 80%), arthritis (21% to 76%), and an erysipelas-like skin rash (12% to 41%). Episodes typically last from several hours to 4 days. Less common manifestations can also occur. In 1997 a new set of diagnostic criteria was proposed.[98] Disease manifestations have their onset during childhood or adolescence in 80% to 90% of patients.

The underlying genetic defect that leads to expression of the disease has been discovered.[99, 100] The responsible gene, *MEFV* (Mediterranean fever), is located on the short arm of chromosome 16. The gene is 10 kb long, consists of 10 exons, and encodes a 781-amino-acid basic protein named marenostrin/pyrin. This novel protein shows significant homology with a family of nuclear effector molecules and transcription factors. It is expressed exclusively in polymorphonuclear leukocytes and eosinophils. Four missense mutations have been identified in the distal part of exon 10 in about 75% of FMF patients. Other mutations or genes are expected to be discovered.[101] It is hypothesized that the presence of a mutation in this protein leads to uncontrolled neutrophil activation and migration to serosal tissues, although the responsible mechanism is not completely understood. Assays are being developed to detect the gene as a diagnostic test for FMF.[102]

The most significant complication of FMF is amyloidosis of the AA type. It usually affects the kidneys, resulting in renal insufficiency progressing to end-stage renal disease. Other organs, including the gastrointestinal tract, liver, spleen, and heart, may also be involved. The prevalence of amyloidosis increases progressively with age; up to 30% of patients acquire it by age 40 years if they do not receive colchicine therapy. The occurrence of amyloidosis is not related to frequency or severity of attacks. However, the risk of developing amyloidosis with FMF is related to ethnic background, with Sephardic Jews, Turks, and Armenians having a higher prevalence than Arabs or other ethnic groups. Rarely, a patient manifests amyloidosis before experiencing any attacks of FMF (phenotype II).[103] Amyloidosis is the only fatal complication of FMF. Additional morbidity from untreated FMF results from a chronic, destructive arthritis (2% to 5%) most commonly affecting the hips and knees. Infertility, vasculitis, constrictive pericarditis, and ascites resulting from sclerosing peritonitis also occur.

Colchicine was first used in 1972 to treat acute manifestations of FMF.[104] Since then large, randomized, placebo-controlled trials have shown that continuous daily colchicine use prevents the attacks of FMF and the subsequent development of amyloidosis.[105–108] The established effective dose is 1 to 2 mg/day. Up to 95% of treated patients note marked improvement in their disease, and 45% to 65% have complete arrest of attacks. Only 2% of 906 patients compliant with therapy developed proteinuria after 11 years of disease, whereas 49% of 54 noncompliant patients developed proteinuria after 9 years of disease. Colchicine is also beneficial for FMF patients who have already developed proteinuria. Improvement or stabilization of renal function and proteinuria is best achieved if serum creatinine is less than 1.5 mg/dL and high doses of colchicine (>1.5 mg/day) are used.[88]

Although a minority of patients treated with colchicine continue to have attacks, the clear benefits seen in most patients have led to its accepted use in all FMF patients who tolerate the drug. Dosing of colchicine should begin at 0.5 to 1.0 mg/day regardless of the patient's weight or age. The dose is titrated upward to 2 mg/day or until episodes stop. There is no evidence that higher doses are any more effective for those patients who do not respond completely to 2 mg/day. Compliance with daily administration is the key to successful treatment: missing even one dose can result in an attack. Colchicine concentrates mainly in neutrophils, possibly because of the absence of a P-glycoprotein efflux pump on the membranes of these cells. Once in the neutrophils, colchicine inhibits the increased chemotactic activity during FMF attacks by acting on microtubules and possibly by up-regulating

*MEFV* gene expression.[96] The most common side effects are diarrhea (10% to 20%) and nausea.[109] These can be minimized by initiating therapy with gradually increasing doses, by dividing higher doses for twice-daily administration, and by using antidiarrheal agents and a lactose-free diet. Rash, angioedema, reversible leukopenia, reversible myopathy with elevated creatine kinase concentrations, azoospermia, and a peripheral neuropathy are relatively uncommon. These side effects are more common in patients with hepatic disease or renal insufficiency and in patients who are also receiving cimetidine, tolbutamide, or cyclosporine. Some patients who experience leukopenia or allergic reactions may be desensitized to colchicine.

Despite the effectiveness of colchicine, concerns have been raised concerning long-term treatment, especially of young children. To date, in both boys and girls treated with colchicine for FMF, there have been no adverse effects on growth and development. In addition, observed problems with female and male reproductive functions are unusual. Rates of conception and sperm production and function do not appear to be affected by colchicine therapy.[110, 111] Small series have not shown that colchicine used during pregnancy is associated with an adverse fetal outcome, but conclusive evidence for its complete safety is lacking. There have been two case reports of trisomy 21 in fetuses of FMF patients treated with colchicine. For this reason, amniocentesis has been recommended for all pregnancies in which one or both parents are being treated with colchicine. Finally, the incidence of malignant neoplasm does not appear to be increased in those patients treated over a long term, although experience is relatively limited.

Colchicine is not thought to be abortive for acute attacks, although patients who experience a prodrome such as transient abdominal or articular symptoms may be able to prevent the attack by taking an additional dose of colchicine. As many as 5% of FMF patients do not respond to colchicine. Nonresponders have been shown to have low serum colchicine concentrations, suggesting poor drug absorption or abnormal metabolism.[112] In selected patients, intravenous administration of colchicine (1 mg/week) in addition to daily oral colchicine may reduce the number of attacks. The risk of serious colchicine toxicity is, however, increased with intravenous administration and needs to be closely monitored. INF-$\alpha$ (3 to 10 million IU subcutaneously) was shown in an open-label study to abrogate 18 of 21 attacks in patients with FMF resistant to colchicine.[113] In the future, therapies may be directed at correcting the lack of regulation caused by a defective marenostrin/pyrin protein.

Patients who develop an attack of FMF are treated symptomatically with analgesics, antipyretics, and NSAIDs. Chronic use of narcotics should be avoided. Prednisone and intra-articular corticosteroid administration are usually ineffective for the arthritis, although prednisone may be useful in patients with protracted febrile myalgias. Prednisone and cyclophosphamide may be required for treatment of FMF in patients who develop polyarteritis nodosa or rapidly progressive glomerulonephritis. Although controversial, elective appendectomy is usually not recommended because of risk of causing peritoneal adhesions and obstructive ileus.[97] In rare patients who develop chronic synovitis, synovectomy may be beneficial.[114] Total hip replacement is associated with a higher risk of loosening, and some orthopedists recommend the use of cementless hip prostheses. Patients who develop renal failure are treated in the standard fashion. FMF patients frequently have increased abdominal febrile attacks with continuous peritoneal dialysis, so this is usually avoided. They may also have an increased tendency for arteriovenous shunt closure. Patients with FMF and renal failure can undergo kidney transplantation; higher doses of daily colchicine (1.5 mg/day or greater) are necessary to prevent recurrence of amyloidosis in the kidney graft.[115] In patients receiving cyclosporine to prevent graft rejection, the dose must be reduced by half to prevent colchicine intoxication.

## RELAPSING POLYCHONDRITIS

RP is an uncommon multisystem disorder characterized by recurrent episodes of inflammation of cartilaginous tissues.[116] RP typically affects young adults (average age, 47 years) but it is well described in both children and the elderly. Patients typically first present with sudden onset of pain and erythema involving the cartilage of the external ear (but sparing the soft lobule) (26% to 91%), the larynx/trachea (14% to 38%), or the nose (13% to 33%). A nonerosive, seronegative polyarthritis or oligoarthritis affecting small, large, or costochondral joints (23% to 47%), ocular inflammation including episcleritis/scleritis (14% to 24%), and audiovestibular disturbances (4% to 9%) may also be presenting symptoms. RP is presumably an autoimmune disease, supported by its association with the human leukocyte antigen HLA-DR4 allele and the demonstration of antibodies to type II collagen and cell-mediated immune responses to various cartilage components.[117] It is diagnosed clinically since there are no confirmatory laboratory tests. McAdams and colleagues suggested that RP could be diagnosed in patients with three of the above six cardinal features and histologic confirmation of chondritis.[118] Diagnosis is delayed more than 1 year in at least two thirds of patients. Inflammatory episodes of chondritis may last from days to weeks, resulting in chronic degeneration and deformity of cartilaginous structures. Many patients have persistent symptoms between flares, and most develop some degree of disability. The most common late complications are loss of hearing and olfaction, reduced vision (8%), and neurologic dysfunction. Potentially life-threatening complications include airway compromise from tracheal narrowing or collapse (14%), aortic or mitral valvular incompetence or rupture (8%), heart block, aortic involvement, and arterial or venous thromboses.[116] In the past, overall survival rates were 74% or less at 5 years and 55% at 10 years,[119] perhaps reflecting referral bias and less advanced medical and surgical management of complications. More recent studies showed an improved survival rate of 94% in 66 patients with average disease duration of 8 years.[116] Pneumonia is the most common cause of death, followed by respiratory failure from airway collapse and complications of valvular heart disease and vasculitis. Patients frequently have associated diseases, including systemic vasculitis, various connective tissue diseases, neoplastic disease (particularly myelodysplastic syndromes), thyroid disease, and others, that may affect prognosis and therapy.[117, 120]

The low prevalence of RP prevents controlled clinical trials of drug therapies. Consequently there is no standard medical therapy, although systemic corticosteroids are used most often. NSAIDs or low-dose colchicine can sometimes control mild episodes of inflammation. However, in most cases, prednisone in doses of 0.5 to 1.0 mg per kilogram of body weight per day are needed to suppress inflammation. The dose is then tapered to the lowest amount that prevents relapse. Episodes of acute airway obstruction have been treated successfully with pulses of intravenous methylprednisolone (1000 mg/day for 3 days) and nebulized racemic ephedrine.[121, 122] Whether corticosteroid therapy should be continued during clinically quiescent periods is not clear. There are several reports of aortic valve disease progressing despite control of other symptoms, and there is little convincing evidence that corticosteroids alter aortic valve dilatation.[123] However, despite concerns for side effects of long-term steroid use, most RP patients require long-term corticosteroids.

Several immunosuppressive drugs have been used empirically in patients who developed resistance to corticosteroids and in those who would benefit from corticosteroid-sparing regimens (see Tables 37–1 and 37–2). Azathioprine, cyclophosphamide, cyclosporine, and plasmapheresis have all been used as adjunctive therapies.[118, 124–126] Dapsone (50 to 200 mg/day) has been advocated as effective therapy for patients without cardiopulmonary involvement, but results have been mixed.[116, 127, 128] Most patients experience side effects including nausea, headache, rashes, fever, and anemia, which is severe in patients with glucose-6-phosphate dehydrogenase deficiency. Methotrexate has been an efficacious and well-tolerated steroid-sparing medication.[116, 129] Trentham and colleagues reported that 23 of 31 patients receiving methotrexate at an average weekly dose of 17.5 mg responded to therapy and were able to taper their prednisone dose from 19 mg/day to 5 mg/day. Patients who develop cardiorespiratory complications despite medical therapy may require surgery. Tracheostomy or stenting may be required to alleviate localized or extensive tracheobronchial disease.[130] In addition, more than 33% of patients with valvular regurgitation need valve replacement.[131, 132] Frequent postoperative complications include perivalvular leak and dehiscence resulting from valvular ring dilatation and friable tissue from the chronic inflammation. The 2-year mortality rate of patients undergoing cardiac valve surgery was approximately 50% in one review of 20 patients.[133]

The management of RP is confounded by its intermittent nature, multiorgan involvement, and association with other diseases. Patients with "minor" manifestations of nasal or auricular chondritis, polyarthritis, eye inflammation, and skin involvement should first receive moderate doses of prednisone for control. NSAIDs, colchicine, dapsone, and methotrexate may be used successfully alone or in combination as steroid-sparing therapies. Patients receiving dapsone or methotrexate should also be given daily folate (1 to 2 mg/day) to limit side effects. Patients with "major" manifestations of respiratory tract inflammation, cardiovascular involvement, systemic vasculitis (particularly with renal or central nervous system involvement), cochlear or vestibular damage, or severe ocular inflammation, may need aggressive treatment with pulse or high-dose corticosteroids. Initially, daily cyclophosphamide may be the best medication to bring steroid-resistant disease under control. After RP is quiescent, the patient may be switched to methotrexate to maintain remission and allow further tapering of corticosteroids. Other immunosuppressive agents may also be used, but experience is anecdotal. In the future, treatment with biologic agents may prove effective.[134, 135]

## HEREDITARY HEMOCHROMATOSIS

HH is the most common type of primary iron-overload disease. It is caused by an inherited defect in iron regulation that results in continuous over-absorption of iron from the gastrointestinal tract.[136] The mode of inheritance is autosomal recessive, with the responsible gene being tightly linked to the HLA-A locus on a short arm of chromosome 6. A candidate gene for HLA-linked hemochromatosis (*HFE*), has been cloned, and a single G-to-A mutation resulting in a cysteine to tyrosine substitution (Cys 282 Tyr) has been identified in 60% to 100% of patients.[137] Other mutations (His 63 Asp) have been identified in a few patients. The exact mechanism by which these genetic mutations result in iron overabsorption is not completely understood. People who are homozygous for the gene are at risk for development of severe iron overload and damage to a number of organs, including liver, pancreas, heart, joints, and endocrine glands.

The HLA-linked iron-loading gene, *HFE* is present in approximately 10% of subjects of European descent, most of whom are unaffected heterozygotes (97%). In contrast, 1 to 5 of every 1000 people (1 in 400 births) are homozygous and at risk of developing overt clinical manifestations of hemochromatosis. However, only 50% of men and 25% of women who are homozygous for the *HFE* gene are likely to develop severe and potentially life-threatening complications of iron overload.[138]

The first expression of hemochromatosis is an elevation in serum transferrin saturation. As iron accumulates in tissue, the serum ferritin concentration increases relative to total body iron stores. Patients usually begin to manifest symptoms between 30 and 50 years of age, although symptoms can occur earlier in some patients. Early symptoms include severe fatigue, impotence, arthralgias, and elevated liver enzymes. Later, patients may experience arthritis, skin pigmentation, cardiomyopathy, and endocrine disorders including diabetes mellitus and hypogonadism. Once hepatic iron concentration exceeds 400 $\mu$mol per gram of dry weight, cirrhosis and the risk of hepatocellular carcinoma are increased.[139]

Detectable joint involvement occurs in 40% to 75% of patients with HH.[140] The metacarpophalangeal joints, wrists, knees, and hips are most often involved.[141] The arthropathy resembles degenerative joint disease, but with involvement of atypical joints such as the metacarpophalangeal joints and wrists it may be indistinguishable from calcium pyrophosphate deposition disease (CPDD). Chondrocalcinosis, which is present in 20% to 50% of patients, is typically asymptomatic but in some patients can cause attacks of acute inflammatory synovitis (pseudogout).[142] The prevalence of overt arthritis increases with age and may be only minimally symptomatic when the disease is discovered in other organs. It is not uncommon, however, for articular pain to be the initial presenting complaint. For this reason, all patients with premature osteoarthritis occurring in atypical joints, especially the metacarpophalangeal joints, should be screened for HH.

Diagnosis of HH is made by the demonstration of pathologic iron deposition in tissue in the absence of other conditions known to cause transferrin overload.[143] Diagnostic evaluation should begin with the determination of fasting serum transferrin saturation and serum ferritin levels. If neither value is substantially elevated, HH can be excluded. If serum iron saturation is repeatedly 55% or greater, an elevated serum ferritin value (more than 200 $\mu$g/L in premenopausal women, more than 300 $\mu$g/L in men and postmenopausal women) indicates iron overload and warrants further evaluation. Definitive diagnosis is made with liver biopsy showing hepatic iron concentration greater than 80 $\mu$mol/g of dry weight and/or a hepatic iron index score of 1.9 or higher. Newer technologies in magnetic resonance imaging may prove useful as noninvasive methods of demonstrating increased hepatic iron stores. The use of genetic testing to detect the *HFE* gene as a diagnostic or family screening test is currently being evaluated.[144]

The prognosis of untreated HH is poor. In an early retrospective analysis, the 5-year survival rate after the clinical diagnosis was 18% and the 10-year rate was 6%.[145] Patients died from cardiomyopathy, complications of diabetes mellitus, and cirrhosis. Of patients with cirrhosis, 8% to 30% died from hepatoma.[146, 147] Removal of iron through therapeutic venesection improves prognosis dramatically. Removal of excess iron before it is deposited in target tissues prevents clinical manifestations of disease. If therapy is started after the patient is symptomatic, life expectancy is normal provided cirrhosis is not present when phlebotomies are initiated. In those patients with cirrhosis, the 10-year survival rate after removal of the iron is 50% to 80%, which is better than in other causes of cirrhosis.[146] Therapeutic phlebotomy also improves clinical features of HH. Removal of the excess iron leads to a decrease in skin hyperpigmentation, and 50% of patients get a reduction in insulin resistance. The cardiomyopathy usually improves with therapy, and cardiac function may return to normal. Hepatic fibrosis may decrease, but cirrhosis and the increased risk of hepatoma are irreversible. Phlebotomy therapy has little or no effect on the arthropathy or the hypogonadism.[141, 148]

HH is treated with repeated therapeutic phlebotomy at any stage when excess iron stores are detected.[149] Five hundred milliliters of blood is removed weekly until mild anemia (hemoglobin greater than 10 g/dL) develops and the ferritin concentration is 50 g/dL. Maintenance phlebotomy at 2- to 4-month intervals is continued indefinitely with monitoring of the ferritin level. Dietary therapy of hemochromatosis includes avoidance of medicinal iron, mineral supplements, excess vitamin C, and uncooked seafood due to increased risk of *Vibrio* infection. Patients with liver disease, diabetes mellitus, or cardiac abnormalities often require additional specific management. The treatment of established arthropathy is similar to the treatment of osteoarthritis and CPDD. Hypogonadism should be treated to prevent osteoporosis. Family members including siblings and children should be screened with transferrin saturation, ferritin level, and genotyping to determine whether they have HH or are at risk of developing HH.

## PAGET'S DISEASE OF BONE

Paget's disease of bone (osteitis deformans) is a focal disorder of bone remodeling in which excessive osteoclastic resorption followed by increased osteoblastic activity leads to structurally disorganized bone (woven bone) which is mechanically weaker.[150] In the United States, it is estimated to affect 2% to 3% of the population older than 50 years of age. Familial aggregation occurs in up to 14% of patients, with a first-degree relative being seven times more likely to develop Paget's disease than an individual who does not have an affected relative.

Approximately 70% to 90% of patients with Paget's disease are asymptomatic. The condition may be monostotic (17%) but is more frequently multifocal, with predilection for the axial skeleton (spine, pelvis, femur, sacrum, and skull in descending order or frequency), although any bone may be affected.[151] After onset, the disease does not spread from bone to bone but may become progressively worse at preexisting sites. In symptomatic patients, local bone pain is the most common symptom. Pain is described as a dull ache that is usually not severe but is present at rest and often is exacerbated by weight bearing. Frequently there is local skin warmth as a result of increased bone microvasculature. Skeletal complications include deformity, secondary osteoarthritis, fractures of weight-bearing limb bones (6% to 7%), deafness (13%), dental malocclusion and sarcomatous change (fewer than 1%). Neurologic complications include cranial nerve

compression, noncommunicating hydrocephalus, spinal stenosis, and vascular steal syndromes affecting spinal cord and cerebral blood supply. In patients with extensive Paget's disease, the increased bone vascularity may rarely cause high-output cardiac failure, and immobilization may precipitate hypercalcemia.[152]

The cause of Paget's disease is unknown, and development of a cure has not been possible. However, the following indications for treatment of patients with Paget's disease have been proposed based on clinical experience and theoretic consideration: (1) the presence of symptoms likely to respond to therapy, including bone or articular pain, bone deformity, bone warmth, and, in some patients, neural compression; (2) prevention of local progressive and future complications even in an asymptomatic patient (spine, weight-bearing long bones, skull); and (3) preoperative treatment of patients scheduled for elective orthopedic surgery involving highly vascular pagetic bone to decrease bleeding complications.[150, 152] Because effective and safe antipagetic drugs are now available, treatment should be withheld only in an asymptomatic patient in whom the disease is associated with little or no risk of complications (i.e., iliac crest, sacrum, scapula, upper limbs, ribs) and possibly in the patient with advanced age and poor general health.

A number of drugs are available that are potent inhibitors of osteoclastic-mediated bone resorption (Table 37–4). These can alleviate pain and limit complications by allowing bone formation to proceed at a more normal pace, with development of relatively normal new bone. Synthetic salmon calcitonin is available for parenteral and intranasal use. Treatment of Paget's disease is not an approved indication for nasal calcitonin, although it has been used in this disease (200 to 400 U/day).[153, 154] After a 10- to 25-U test dose, the usual starting dose for subcutaneous calcitonin is 50 U three times a week, increasing to 100 U/day. Some patients (20% to 30%) experience problems with flushing, nausea, and other gastrointestinal symptoms. These adverse reactions can be avoided by starting with a low dose and gradually increasing the dosage and by administering calcitonin after dinner or at bedtime. Calcitonin therapy can induce a 30% to 55% lowering of biochemical markers of bone turnover in approximately 50% to 66% of patients within 3 to 6 months of therapy.[155–157] Patients with severe disease are less likely to respond initially. After response has been achieved, the dosage can be reduced to 50 to 100 U three times a week with maintenance of response. The duration of therapy depends on clinical response and disease activity. Patients with moderate or severe disease may require continuous treatment. Disadvantages of calcitonin are the rapid loss of therapeutic effect after treatment is stopped and the approximately 20% of patients who become resistant to ongoing therapy after a variable period as a result of the development of neutralizing antibodies or down-regulation of calcitonin receptors.[158] Calcitonin has been superseded by the new bisphosphonates as the treatment of first choice.

## TABLE 37–4
## Medications Used in the Treatment of Paget's Disease of Bone

| DRUG | TRADE NAME | DOSE/TABLET (mg) | DOSAGE | SIDE EFFECTS |
|---|---|---|---|---|
| Calcitonin | Calcimar Miacalcin | Injection[†] SC | Gradual increase to 100 U/d SC | Flushing, hypotension, gastrointestinal symptoms |
| Bisphosphonates (oral) | | | | |
| Etidronate | Didronel | 200 | 5 mg/kg/d (400 mg) for 6 mo | Mineralization defect |
| Tiludronate | Skelid | 200 | 400 mg/d for 3 mo | Gastrointestinal (GI) symptoms |
| Alendronate | Fosamax | 40 | 40 mg/d for 6 mo | Upper GI symptoms |
| Risedronate | Actonel | 30 | 30 mg/d for 2 mo | Upper GI symptoms |
| Clodronate* | Ostac, Bonefos | | 400–1600 mg/d for 3–6 mo | Mild GI symptoms |
| Bisphosphonates (intravenous) | | | | |
| Pamidronate | Aredia | Vials of 30, 60, 90 mg | 30 mg weekly for 6 wk 60 mg every 2 wk for 3 doses 90 mg/wk for 2 wk Other regimens reported | Transient, acute, influenza-like reaction |
| Clodronate* | Ostac, Bonefos | | 300 mg/d for 5 d | |

* Not available in the United States.
† Calcimar and miacalcin injection supplied as a 2-mL vial containing 400 IU.

Bisphosphonates, analogs of pyrophosphate, are poorly absorbed from the gastrointestinal tract (1%); they are rapidly taken up by bone, and about 50% of an oral dose is cleared by the kidney.[159] Bisphosphonates bind to bone through the phosphorous-carbon-phosphorous structure and localize to resorbing surfaces. Osteoclasts are exposed to a high concentration of bisphosphonates as they resorb bone. The main action of bisphosphonates is to induce marked and prolonged inhibition of bone resorption by decreasing osteoclast numbers and activity. The potency of bisphosphonates is influenced by the structure of the particular compound side chain, ranging from 1 for etidronate to 10,000 for ibandronate.

Etidronate was the first bisphosphonate used in Paget's disease and is well tolerated. A good symptomatic response with 50% suppression of total alkaline phosphatase (TAP) occurs in 30% of patients within 6 months. Etidronate, 5 mg/kg, is taken with a 2-hour fast before and after ingestion.[160–162] In 33% of severely affected patients, the efficacy wanes, and up to 25% of all Paget's disease patients become resistant to repeated courses of etidronate.[162] The side effects of etidronate include abdominal cramps and diarrhea, increased bone pain, and defective mineralization of newly-formed bone matrix (osteomalacia) if it is used in high doses (10 to 20 mg/kg/day) or is used continuously for longer than 6 months at a time. Etidronate is contraindicated in patients with renal failure, those with a history of osteomalacia, those who have lytic lesions in weight-bearing bones or healing fractures, and those who are planning to undergo orthopedic surgery.[152] With the availability of more potent bisphosphonates that do not impair mineralization at clinically effective doses, etidronate is used less often today.

The new oral bisphosphonates available in the United States include tiludronate, alendronate, and risedronate. Clodronate is available only in Europe. In comparison trials, all have been shown to be more effective than etidronate.[163–166] In controlled clinical trials, tiludronate normalized biochemical markers in 35% of patients and decreased TAP by 50% in 50% to 60% of patients treated with 400 mg/day (with a 1-hour fast before and after ingestion) for 3 months.[163, 167, 168] Alendronate normalized biochemical markers in 48% of patients and decreased TAP by 73% and N-telopeptide excretion by 86% in patients treated with 40 mg/day for 6 months. At 12 months after discontinuation of alendronate, 91% of patients (29/32) remained in biochemical remission.[164, 169, 170] In open-label, single-center and multicenter trials, risedronate eliminated bone pain and decreased TAP by at least 77% in all patients treated with one or two courses of 30 mg/day for 2 months.[165, 171–173] In a double-blind, active control study, risedronate normalized TAP in 77% of 56 Paget's patients compared with 11% of 57 patients treated with etidronate. At 16 months after discontinuation of risedronate, 53% of patients (17/32) remained in biochemical remission.[174] Clodronate normalized TAP in 71% of patients with mild Paget's disease treated with 1600 mg/day for 6 months.[166] The most common side effects in patients treated with bisphosphonates were gastrointestinal disturbances such as abdominal pain, esophagitis, diarrhea, nausea, and vomiting. To facilitate absorption, patients should take the medication in the morning after arising and 30 to 60 minutes before the first food, beverage, or medication of the day. To minimize gastrointestinal side effects, bisphosphonates should be taken with 8 ounces of plain water, and the patient should remain upright for at least 30 minutes after it is ingested.

Intravenous pamidronate has been reported to be effective in a variety of therapeutic regimens.[175, 176] Response seems to correlate with the total dose of medication. In patients with mild disease, a single 60- to

90-mg infusion (in 500 to 1000 mL normal saline) administered over 4 to 6 hours (15 mg/h) completely suppresses disease activity. Patients with more severe polyostotic disease frequently require higher doses administered over several weeks to months. Intravenous pamidronate can normalize TAP values in up to 90% of patients, with subsequent biochemical remission lasting 2 years in 50%.[177] Adverse effects are usually mild and include a transient febrile, flu-like reaction, which is seen in 10% to 30% of patients. Symptoms begin 1 to 48 hours after the infusion (usually after the first but not subsequent infusions) and are probably caused by cytokine (IL-6) release. Transient hypocalcemia, hypophosphatemia, lymphopenia, exacerbation of bone pain, and venous irritation can also occur. Clodronate can also be administered intravenously.[178]

The newer oral bisphosphonates (alendronate, risedronate) should be the first choice of therapy. In countries where they are not available, etidronate is appropriate for many patients. Intravenous pamidronate is indicated for patients who cannot tolerate oral therapy, have severe disease, or have a neurologic complication. Daily supplementation with 1 g of elemental calcium and 800 IU of vitamin D is indicated in all patients treated with bisphosphonate to prevent secondary hyperparathyroidism. Attention should also be paid to simple analgesia using NSAIDs for symptomatic relief. Physiotherapy and simple aids are useful adjuncts, and patients with marked secondary osteoarthritis, deformity, and neurologic complications may benefit from surgery. In patients with joint involvement, bone pain from Paget's usually responds to bisphosphonate therapy (especially intravenous pamidronate) but secondary osteoarthritis does not.

The appropriate follow-up for a treated patient varies with the severity of disease. Symptomatic patients should be monitored every 3 to 6 months for changes in pain and neurologic status. Disease activity can be effectively monitored by measurement of serum or bone alkaline phosphatase and urinary hydroxyproline, pyridinoline cross-links, or N-telopeptide. The degree of suppression of biochemical markers of bone turnover is predictive of the long-term risk for development of complications. Failure to normalize these markers results in development of new complications of Paget's disease in more than 60% to 70% of patients despite a favorable effect on pain.[179] Therefore, therapy should be aimed at normalizing these biochemical markers, which usually occurs several months after the end of therapy. Recurrence of biochemical markers 20% to 30% above the upper limit of normal justifies retreatment.[150, 180]

Other medications are being investigated for future therapy. Intravenous zoledronate and ibandronate are new bisphosphonates that are effective in microgram doses. Plicamycin (previously mithramycin) is an antibiotic shown to be effective for severe Paget's when administered as a 4- to 8-hour infusion in doses of 15 to 25 $\mu$g/kg/day.[181] Doses can be repeated every 2 to 3 days if necessary. Because of bone marrow, liver, and kidney toxicity, its use is limited to patients with severe refractory disease. Gallium nitrate adsorbs to hydroxyapatite and reversibly inhibits the adenosine triphosphate–dependent proton pump of osteoclasts. A multicenter trial showed that 0.5 mg/kg/day given by subcutaneous injection in two 14-day cycles separated by 4 weeks was safe and effective for patients with severe Paget's disease.[182] Although gallium nitrate holds promise, experience and follow-up are limited, and its role in the treatment of patients with Paget's disease is yet to be determined.

# REFERENCES

1. Newman LS, Rose CS, Maier LA: Sarcoidosis. N Engl J Med 1997; 336:1224.
2. Ishak KG: Sarcoidosis of the liver and bile ducts. Mayo Clin Proc 1998; 73:467.
3. Enzenauer R, West S: Sarcoidosis in autoimmune disease. Semin Arthritis Rheum 1992; 22:1.
4. Consensus conference: Activity of sarcoidosis. Eur Respir J 1994; 7:624.
5. Mana J, Salazar A, Manresa F: Clinical factors predicting persistence of activity in sarcoidosis: A multi-variate analysis of 193 cases. Respiration 1994; 61:219.
6. Winterbauer RH: Sarcoidosis. In Lichtenstein LM, Fauci AS (eds): Current Therapy in Allergy Immunology and Rheumatology. St. Louis: Mosby–Year Book, 1996:272.
7. Gibson GJ, Prescott RJ, Muers MF, et al: British Thoracic Society Sarcoidosis Study: Effects of long-term corticosteroid treatment. Thorax 1996; 51:238.
8. Hunninghake GW, Gilbert S, Pueringer R, et al: Outcome of the treatment of sarcoidosis. Am J Respir Crit Care Med 1994; 149:893.
9. Zych D, Pawlicka L, Zielinski J: Inhaled budesonide vs. prednisone in the maintenance treatment of pulmonary sarcoidosis. Sarcoidosis 1993; 10:56.
10. Milman N, Graudal N, Grode G, et al: No effect of high-dose inhaled steroids in pulmonary sarcoidosis: A double blind, placebo-controlled study. J Intern Med 1994; 236:285.
11. Alberts C, van der Mark TW, Jansen HM: Dutch Study Group on Pulmonary Sarcoidosis. Inhaled budesonide in pulmonary sarcoidosis: A double blind, placebo-controlled study. Eur Respir J 1995; 8:682.
12. Baughman RP, Lower EE: Steroid-sparing alternative treatments for sarcoidosis. Clin Chest Med 1997; 18:853.
13. Lower EE, Baughman RP: Prolonged use of methotrexate for sarcoidosis. Arch Intern Med 1995; 155:846.
14. Rebuck A, Sander B, MacFadden D, et al: Cyclosporin in pulmonary sarcoidosis. Lancet 1987; i:1486.
15. Fouty BW, Pomeranz M, Thigpen TP, et al: Dilatation of bronchial stenoses due to sarcoidosis using a flexible fiberoptic bronchoscope. Chest 1994; 106:677.
16. Judson MA: Lung transplantation for pulmonary sarcoidosis. Eur Respir J 1998; 11:738.
17. Kaplan H: Sarcoid arthritis with a response to colchicine. N Engl J Med 1960; 268:778.
18. Kaye O, Palazzo E, Grossin M, et al: Low-dose methotrexate: An effective corticosteroid-sparing agent in the musculoskeletal manifestations of sarcoidosis. Br J Rheumatol 1995; 34:642.
19. Russo G, Millikan LE: Cutaneous sarcoidosis: Diagnosis and treatment. Compr Ther 1994; 20:418.
20. Jones E, Callen JP: Hydroxychloroquine is effective therapy for control of cutaneous sarcoidal granulomas. J Am Acad Dermatol 1990; 23:487.
21. Zic JA, Horowitz DH, Arzubiaga C, et al: Treatment of cutaneous sarcoidosis with chloroquine. Arch Dermatol 1991; 127:1035.
22. Hassid S, Choufani G, Saussez S, et al: Sarcoidosis of the paranasal sinuses treated with hydroxychloroquine. Postgrad Med J 1998; 74:172.
23. Webster GF, Razsi LK, Sanchez M, et al: Weekly low-dose methotrexate therapy for cutaneous sarcoidosis. J Am Acad Dermatol 1991; 24:451.

24. Rousseau L, Beylot-Barry M, Doutre M-S, et al: Cutaneous sarcoidosis successfully treated with low doses of thalidomide. Arch Dermatol 1998; 134:1045.

25. Yamada H, Ide A, Sugiura M, et al: Treatment of cutaneous sarcoidosis with tranilast. J Dermatol 1995; 22:149.

26. Sharma OP: Vitamin D, calcium, and sarcoidosis. Chest 1996; 109:535.

27. Veinot JP, Johnson B: Cardiac sarcoidosis: An occult cause of death. A case report and literature review. J Forensic Sci 1998; 43:715.

28. Doherty MJ, Kumar SK, Nicholson AA, et al: Cardiac sarcoidosis: The value of magnetic resonance imaging in diagnosis and assessment of response to treatment. Respir Med 1998; 92:697.

29. Sharma OP: Cardiac and neurologic dysfunction in sarcoidosis. Clin Chest Med 1997; 18:813.

30. Demeter SL: Myocardial sarcoidosis unresponsive to steroids: Treatment with cyclophosphamide. Chest 1988; 94:202.

31. Barbers RG: Role of transplantation in sarcoidosis. Clin Chest Med 1997; 18:865.

32. Sharma OP, Sharma AM: Sarcoidosis of the nervous system: A clinical approach. Arch Intern Med 1991; 151:1317.

33. Lower EE, Broderick JP, Brott TG, et al: Diagnosis and management of neurological sarcoidosis. Arch Intern Med 1997; 157:1864.

34. Sharma OP: Effectiveness of chloroquine and hydroxychloroquine in treating selected patients with sarcoidosis with neurological involvement. Arch Neurol 1998; 55:1248.

35. Stern BJ, Schonfeld SA, Sewell C, et al: The treatment of neurosarcoidosis with cyclosporine. Arch Neurol 1992; 49:1065.

36. Rubinstein I, Gray TA, Moldofsky H, et al: Neurosarcoidosis associated with hypersomnolence treated with corticosteroids and brain irradiation. Chest 1988; 94:205.

37. Rizzato G, Montemurro L, Colombo P: The late follow-up of chronic sarcoid patients previously treated with corticosteroids. Sarcoidosis Vasc Diffuse Lung Dis 1998; 15:52.

38. Moller DR: Etiology of sarcoidosis. Clin Chest Med 1997; 18:695.

39. Zabel P, Entzian P, Dalhoff K, et al: Pentoxifylline in treatment of sarcoidosis. Am J Respir Crit Care Med 1997; 155:1665.

40. Behçet's H: Uber rezidivierende, aphthose, durch ein Virus verursachte Gershwure am Mund, Auge und an den Genitalien. Derm Wschr 1937; 105:1152.

41. International Study Group for Behçet's Disease: Criteria for diagnosis of Behçet's disease. Lancet 1990; 335:1078.

42. Imai H, Motegi M, Mizuki N, et al: Mouth and genital ulcers with inflamed cartilage (MAGIC syndrome): A case report and literature review. Am J Med Sci 1997; 314:330.

43. Kaklamani V, Vaiopoulos G, Kaklamanis PG: Behçet's disease. Semin Arthritis Rheum 1998; 27:197.

44. Bang D: Treatment of Behçet's disease. Yonsei Med J 1997; 38:401.

45. Lehner T: Progress report: Oral ulceration and Behçet's syndrome. Gut 1977; 18:491.

46. Hamuryudan V, Yurdakul S, Serdaroglu S, et al: Topical alpha interferon in the treatment of oral ulcers in Behçet's syndrome: A preliminary report. Clin Exp Rheumatol 1990; 8:51.

47. Miyachi Y, Taniguchi S, Ozaki M, et al: Colchicine in the treatment of the cutaneous manifestations of Behçet's disease. Br J Dermatol 1981; 104:67.

48. Masuda K, Urayama A, Kogure M, et al: Double-masked trial of cyclosporin versus colchicine and long-term open study of cyclosporin in Behçet's disease. Lancet 1989; 1:1093.

49. Hamuryudan V, Mat C, Saip S, et al: Thalidomide in the treatment of the mucocutaneous lesions of the Behçet's syndrome. Ann Intern Med 1998; 128:443.

50. Moral F, Hamuryudan V, Yurdakul S, et al: Inefficacy of azapropazone in the acute arthritis of Behçet's syndrome: A randomized, double-blind, placebo controlled study. Clin Exp Rheumatol 1995; 13:494.

51. Yurdakul S, Yazici H, Tuzun Y, et al: The arthritis of Behçet's disease: A prospective study. Ann Rheum Dis 1983; 42:505.

52. Calguneri M, Kiraz S, Ertenli I, et al: The effect of prophylactic penicillin treatment on the course of arthritis episodes in patients with Behçet's disease: A randomized clinical trial. Arthritis Rheum 1996; 39:2062.

53. Nussenblatt RB: Uveitis in Behçet's disease. Int Rev Immunol 1997; 14:67.

54. Yazici H, Pazarli H, Barnes C, et al: A controlled trial of azathioprine in Behçet's syndrome. N Engl J Med 1990; 322:281.

55. Hamuryudan V, Ozyazgam Y, Hizli N, et al: Azathioprine in Behçet's syndrome: Effects on long-term prognosis. Arthritis Rheum 1997; 40:769.

56. Ben Ezra D, Cohen E, Chajek T, et al: Evaluation of conventional therapy versus cyclosporine A in Behçet's syndrome. Transplant Proc 1988; 20(suppl 4):136.

57. Nussenblatt RB, Palestine AG, Chan C-C, et al: Effectiveness of cyclosporin therapy for Behçet's disease. Arthritis Rheum 1985; 28:671.

58. Shahram E, Davatchi F, Chams H, et al: Cyclosporine for severe ocular lesions of Behçet's disease. *In* Eighth International Conference on Behçet's Disease. Abstract K05. Rev Rhum Engl Ed 1996; 63:559.

59. Ozyazgan Y, Yurdakul S, Yazici H, et al: Low-dose cyclosporin A versus pulsed cyclophosphamide in Behçet's syndrome: A single masked trial. Br J Ophthalmol 1992; 76:241.

60. Mochizuki M, Masuda K, Sakane T, et al: A multicenter clinical open trial of FK 506 in refractory uveitis, including Behçet's disease. Transplant Proc 1991; 23:3343.

61. Ishioka M, Ohno S, Nakamura S, et al: FK506 treatment of noninfectious uveitis. Am J Ophthalmol 1994; 118:723.

62. Hamuryudan V, Ozdogan H, Yazici H: Other forms of vasculitis and pseudovasculitis. *In* Vasculitis. Baillieres Clin Rheumatol 1997; 11:335.

63. Erkan F, Cavdar T: Pulmonary vasculitis in Behçet's disease. Am Rev Respir Dis 1992; 146:232.

64. O'Duffy JD, Robertson D, Goldstein N: Chlorambucil in the treatment of uveitis and meningoencephalitis of Behçet's disease. Am J Med 1984; 76:75.

65. O'Duffy JD: Vasculitis in Behçet's disease. Rheum Dis Clin North Am 1990; 16:423.

66. Tuzun H, Besirli K, Sayin A, et al: Management of aneurysms in Behçet's syndrome: An analysis of 24 patients. Surgery 1997; 121:150.

67. Lee KS, Kim SJ, Lee BC, et al: Surgical treatment of intestinal Behçet's disease. Yonsei Med J 1997; 38:455.

68. Sakane T, Suzuki N, Nagafuchi H: Etiopathology of Behçet's disease: Immunological aspects. Yonsei Med J 1997; 38:350.

69. Yasui K, Ohta K, Kobayashi M, et al: Successful treatment of Behçet disease with pentoxifylline. Ann Intern Med 1996; 124:891.

70. Zouboulis CC, Orfanos CE: Treatment of Adamantiades-Behçet disease with systemic interferon alfa. Arch Dermatol 1998; 134:1010.

71. Falk RH, Comenzo RL, Skinner M: The systemic amyloidoses. N Engl J Med 1997; 337:898.

72. Husby G: Treatment of amyloidosis and the rheumatologist. Scand J Rheumatol 1998; 27:161.

73. Cohen AS, Rubinow A, Anderson JJ, et al: Survival of patients with primary (AL) amyloidosis and the effect of colchicine treatment. Am J Med 1987; 82:1182.

74. Kyle RA, Gertz MA, Greipp PR, et al: A trial of three regimens for primary amyloidosis: Colchicine alone, melphalan and prednisone, and melphalan, prednisone and colchicine. N Engl J Med 1997; 336:1202.

75. Gertz MA, Kyle RA, Greipp PR: Response rates and survival in primary systemic amyloidosis. Blood 1991; 24:257.

76. Skinner M, Anderson J, Simms R, et al: Treatment of 100 patients with primary amyloidosis: A randomized trial of melphalan, prednisone, and colchicine versus colchicine alone. Am J Med 1996; 100:290.

77. Pelosi F, Capehart J, Roberts WC: Effectiveness of cardiac transplantation for primary (AL) cardiac amyloidosis. Am J Cardiol 1997; 79:532.

78. Persey MR, Lovat LB, Apperley JF, et al: Intensive chemotherapy for AL amyloidosis. Br J Rheumatol 1996; 35(suppl 1):12.

79. Comenzo RL, Vosburgh E, Falk RH, et al: Dose-intensive melphalan with blood stem-cell support for the treatment of AL (amyloid light-chain) amyloidosis: Survival and responses in 25 patients. Blood 1998; 91:3662.

80. Moreau P, Leblond V, Bourquelot P, et al: Prognostic factors for survival and response after high-dose therapy and autologous stem cell transplantation in systemic AL amyloidosis: A report on 21 patients. Br J Haematol 1998; 101:766.

81. Gianni L, Bellotti V, Gianni AM, et al: New drug therapy of amyloidoses: Resorption of AL-type deposits with 4′-iodo-4′ deoxydoxorubicin. Blood 1995; 86:855.

82. Skinner M: Amyloidosis. In Kelley WN, Harris ED, Ruddy S, et al (eds): Textbook of Rheumatology. Philadelphia: WB Saunders, 1997:1409–1417.

83. Berglund K, Keller C, Thysell H: Alkylating cytostatic treatment in renal amyloidosis secondary to rheumatic disease. Ann Rheum Dis 1987; 46:757.

84. Maezawa A, Hiromura K, Matsuhashi H, et al: Combined treatment with cyclophosphamide and prednisolone can induce remission of nephrotic syndrome in patients with renal amyloidosis associated with rheumatoid arthritis. Clin Nephrol 1994; 42:30.

85. Ahlmen M, Ahlemn J, Svalander C, et al: Cytotoxic drug treatment of reactive amyloidosis in rheumatoid arthritis with special reference to renal insufficiency. Clin Rheumatol 1987; 6:27.

86. Hawkins PN, Lavender JP, Pepys MB: Evaluation of systemic amyloidosis by scintigraphy with $^{123}$I-labeled serum amyloid P component. N Engl J Med 1990; 323:508.

87. Escalante A, Ehresmann GR, Quismorio FP Jr: Brief report: Regression of reactive systemic amyloidosis due to ankylosing spondylitis following the administration of colchicine. Arthritis Rheum 1991; 34:920.

88. Livneh A, Zemer D, Langevitz P, et al: Colchicine treatment of AA amyloidosis of familial Mediterranean fever. Arthritis Rheum 1994; 37:1804.

89. Gaughan DJ, Steel DM, Whitehead AS: Ribozyme mediated cleavage of acute phase serum amyloid A (A-SAA) mRNA in vitro. FEBS Lett 1995; 374:241.

90. Drüeke TB: Dialysis-related amyloidosis. Nephrol Dial Transplant 1998; 13(suppl 1):58.

91. Küchle C, Friche H, Held E, et al: High flux hemodialysis postpones clinical manifestation of dialysis-related amyloidosis. Am J Nephrol 1996; 16:4484.

92. Jadoul M, Drüeke T, Zingraff J, et al: Does dialysis-related amyloidosis regress after transplantation. Nephrol Dial Transplant 1997; 12:655.

93. Tan SY, Irish A, Winearls CG, et al: Long-term effect of renal transplantation on dialysis-related amyloid deposits and symptomatology. Kidney Int 1996; 50:282.

94. Gejyo F, Teramura T, Ei I, et al: Long-term clinical evaluation of an adsorbent column (BM-01) of direct hemoperfusion type for B2-microglobulin on the treatment of dialysis-related amyloidosis. Artif Organs 1995; 19:1222.

95. Suhr OB, Holmgren G, Steen L, et al: Liver transplantation in familial amyloidotic polyneuropathy. Transplantation 1995; 60:933.

96. Ben-Chetrit E, Levy M: Familial Mediterranean fever. Lancet 1998; 351:659.

97. Livneh A, Langevitz P, Zemer D, et al: The changing face of familial Mediterranean fever. Semin Arthritis Rheum 1996; 26:612.

98. Livneh A, Langevitz P, Zemer D, et al: Criteria for the diagnosis of familial Mediterranean fever. Arthritis Rheum 1997; 40:1879.

99. The International FMF Consortium: Ancient missense mutations in a new member of the RoRet gene family are likely to cause familial Mediterranean fever. Cell 1997; 90:797.

100. The French FMF Consortium: A candidate gene for familial Mediterranean fever. Nat Genet 1997; 17:25.

101. Samuels J, Aksentijevich I, Torosyan Y, et al: Familial Mediterranean fever at the millennium. Medicine (Baltimore) 1998; 77:268.

102. Eisenberg S, Aksentijevich I, Deng Z, et al: Diagnosis of familial Mediterranean fever by a molecular genetics method. Ann Intern Med 1998; 129:539.

103. Heller H, Sohar E, Gafni J, et al: Amyloidosis in familial Mediterranean fever: An independent genetically determined character. Arch Intern Med 1961; 107:539.

104. Goldfinger SE: Colchicine for familial Mediterranean fever. N Engl J Med 1972; 287:1302.

105. Zemer D, Revach M, Pras M, et al: A controlled trial of colchicine in preventing attacks of familial Mediterranean fever. N Engl J Med 1974; 291:932.

106. Dinarello CA, Wolff SM, Goldfinger SE, et al: Colchicine therapy for familial Mediterranean fever: A double-blind trial. N Engl J Med 1974; 291:934.

107. Goldstein RC, Schwabe AD: Prophylactic colchicine therapy for familial Mediterranean fever: A controlled, double-blind study. Ann Intern Med 1974; 81:792.

108. Ben-Chetrit E, Levy M: Colchicine prophylaxis in familial Mediterranean fever: Reappraisal after 15 years. Semin Arthritis Rheum 1994; 20:241.

109. Putterman C, Ben-Chetrit E, Caraco Y, et al: Colchicine intoxication: Clinical pharmacology, risk factors, features, and management. Semin Arthritis Rheum 1991; 21:143.

110. Haimov-Kochman R, Ben-Chetrit E: The effect of colchicine treatment on sperm production and function: A review. Hum Reprod 1998; 13:360.

111. Rabinovitch O, Zemer D, Kukia E, et al: Colchicine treatment in conception and pregnancy: Two hundred thirty-one pregnancies in patients with familial Mediterranean fever. Am J Reprod Immunol 1992; 28:245.

112. Zylber E, Ehrenfeld M, Levy M, et al: Plasma colchicine concentration in patients with recurrent polyserositis (familial Mediterranean fever) on long-term prophylaxis. Arthritis Rheum 1982; 25:227.

113. Tunca M, Tankurt E, Akpinar HA, et al: The efficacy of interferon alpha on colchicine-resistant familial Mediterranean fever attacks: A pilot study. Br J Rheumatol 1997; 36:1005.

114. Garcia-Gonzalez A, Weisman MH: The arthritis of familial Mediterranean fever. Semin Arthritis Rheum 1992; 22:139.

115. Livneh A, Zemer D, Siegal B, et al: Colchicine prevents kidney transplant amyloidosis in familial Mediterranean fever. Nephron 1992; 60:418.

116. Trentham DE, Le CH: Relapsing polychondritis. Ann Intern Med 1998; 129:114.

117. Hochberg MC: Relapsing polychondritis. In Kelley WN, Harris ED, Ruddy S, et al (eds): Textbook of Rheumatology. Philadelphia: WB Saunders, 1997:1404–1408.

118. McAdam LP, O'Hanlan MA, Bluestone R, et al: Relapsing polychondritis: Prospective study of 23 patients and a review of the literature [Review]. Medicine (Baltimore) 1976; 55:193.

119. Michet CJ, McKenna CH, Luthra HS, et al: Relapsing polychondritis: Survival and predictive role of early disease manifestations. Ann Intern Med 1986; 104:74.

120. Hebbar M, Brouillard M, Wattel E, et al: Association of myelodysplastic syndrome and relapsing polychondritis: Further evidence. Leukemia 1995; 9:731.

121. Lipnick RN, Fink CW: Acute airway obstruction in relapsing polychondritis: Treatment with pulse methylprednisolone. J Rheumatol 1991; 18:98.

122. Gaffney RJ, Harrison M, Blayney AW: Nebulized racemic ephedrine in the treatment of acute exacerbation of laryngeal relapsing polychondritis. J Laryngol Otol 1992; 106:63.

123. Buckley LM, Ades PA: Progressive aortic valve inflammation occurring despite apparent remission of relapsing polychondritis. Arthritis Rheum 1992; 35:812.

124. Ruhlen JL, Huston KA, Wood WG: Relapsing polychondritis with glomerulonephritis: Improvement with prednisone and cyclophosphamide. JAMA 1981; 245:847.

125. Stewart KA, Mazanec DJ: Pulse intravenous cyclophosphamide for kidney disease in relapsing polychondritis [Letter]. J Rheumatol 1992; 19:498.

126. Svenson KLG, Homdahl R, Klareskog L, et al: Cyclosporine A treatment in a case of relapsing polychondritis. Scand J Rheumatol 1984; 13:329.

127. Barranco VP, Minor DB, Soloman H: Treatment of relapsing polychondritis with dapsone. Arch Dermatol 1976; 112:1286.

128. Martin J, Roenigk HH, Lynch W, et al: Relapsing polychondritis treated with dapsone. Arch Dermatol 1976; 112:1272.

129. Park J, Gowin KM, Schumacher HR: Steroid sparing effect of methotrexate in relapsing polychondritis. J Rheumatol 1996; 23:937.

130. Dunne JA, Sabanathan S: Use of metallic stents in relapsing polychondritis. Chest 1994; 105:864.

131. Del Rosso A, Petix NR, Pratesi M, et al: Cardiovascular involvement in relapsing polychondritis. Semin Arthritis Rheum 1997; 26:840.
132. Van Decker W, Panidis IP: Relapsing polychondritis and cardiac valvular involvement. Ann Intern Med 1988; 109:340.
133. Lang-Lazdunski L, Hvass U, Paillole C, et al: Cardiac valve replacement in relapsing polychondritis: A review. J Heart Valve Dis 1995; 4:227.
134. Choy EH, Chikanza IC, Kingsley GH, et al: Chimeric anti-CD4 monoclonal antibody for relapsing polychondritis [Letter]. Lancet 1991; 338:450.
135. Van der Lubbe PA, Miltenburg AM, Breedveld FC: Anti-CD4 monoclonal antibody for relapsing polychondritis [Letter]. Lancet 1991; 337:1349.
136. Bothwell TH, MacPhail AP: Hereditary hemochromatosis: Etiologic, pathologic, and clinical aspects. Semin Hematol 1998; 35:55.
137. Feder JN, Gnirke A, Thomas W, et al: A novel MHC class I-like gene is mutated in patients with hereditary hemochromatosis. Nat Genet 1996; 134:399.
138. Adams PC, Gregor JC, Kertesz AE, et al: Screening blood donors for hereditary hemochromatosis: Decision analysis model based on a thirty-year database. Gastroenterology 1995; 109:177.
139. Bassett ML, Halliday JW, Powell LW: Value of hepatic iron measurements in early hemochromatosis and determination of the critical iron levels associated with fibrosis. Hepatology 1986; 6:24.
140. Niederau C, Fischer R, Sonnenberg A, et al: Survival and causes of death in cirrhotic and noncirrhotic patients with primary hemochromatosis. N Engl J Med 1985; 313:1256.
141. Schumacher HR, Straka PC, Krikker MA, et al: The arthropathy of hemochromatosis: Recent studies. Ann N Y Acad Sci 1988; 526:224.
142. Huaux JP, Geubel A, Koch MC, et al: The arthritis of hemochromatosis: A review of 25 cases with special reference to chondrocalcinosis, and a comparison with patients with primary hyperparathyroidism and controls. Clin Rheumatol 1986; 5:317.
143. Powell LW, George K, McDonnell SM, et al: Diagnosis of hemochromatosis. Ann Intern Med 1998; 129:925.
144. Edwards CQ, Griffen LM, Ajioka RS, et al: Screening for hemochromatosis: Phenotype versus genotype. Semin Hematol 1998; 35:72.
145. Williams R, Smith PM, Spicer EFJ, et al: Venesection therapy in idiopathic hemochromatosis. Q J Med 1969; 38:1.
146. Niederau C, Fischer R, Pursehel A, et al: Long-term survival in patients with hereditary hemochromatosis. Gastroenterology 1996; 110:1107.
147. Adams PC, Valberg LS: Evolving expression of hereditary hemochromatosis. Semin Liver Dis 1996; 16:47.
148. Stremmel W, Niederau C, Berger M, et al: Abnormalities in estrogen, androgen, and insulin metabolism in idiopathic hemochromatosis. Ann N Y Acad Sci 1988; 526:209.
149. Barton JC, McDonnell SM, Adams PC, et al: Management of hemachromatosis. Ann Intern Med 1998; 129:932.
150. Delmas PD, Meunier PJ: The management of Paget's disease of bone. N Engl J Med 1997; 336:558.
151. Ooi CG, Fraser WD: Paget's disease of bone. Postgrad Med J 1997; 73:69.
152. Tiegs RD: Paget's disease of bone: Indications for treatment and goals of therapy. Clin Ther 1997; 19:1309.
153. Luboshitzky R, Bar Shalom R: Calcitonin nasal spray for Paget's disease of the bone. Harefuah 1995; 128:358.
154. Gonzales D, Vega E, Ghiringhelli G, et al: Comparison of the acute effect of the intranasal and intramuscular administration of salmon calcitonin in Paget's disease. Calcif Tissue Int 1987; 41:313.
155. Singer FR, Keutman HT, Neer RM, et al: Pharmacologic effects of salmon calcitonin in man. *In* Talmage RV, Munson PL (eds). Calcium, Parathyroid Hormone and the Calcitonins. Amsterdam: Excerpta Medica, 1972:89–96.
156. DeRose J, Singer F, Avramides A, et al: Response of Paget's disease to porcine and salmon calcitonin: Effects of long-term treatment. Am J Med 1974; 47:9.
157. Singer FR, Fredericks RS, Minkin C: Salmon calcitonin therapy for Paget's disease of bone: The problem of acquired clinical resistance. Arthritis Rheum 1980; 23:1148.
158. Haddad JG Jr, Caldwell JG: Calcitonin resistance: Clinical and immunologic studies in subjects with Paget's disease of bone treated with porcine and salmon calcitonin. J Clin Invest 1972; 51:3133.
159. Rodan GA: Mechanism of action of bisphosphonates. Annu Rev Pharmacol Toxicol 1998; 38:375.
160. Altman R, Johnston CC, Khairi MRA, et al: Influence of disodium etidronate on clinical and laboratory manifestations of Paget's disease of bone (osteitis deformans). N Engl J Med 1973; 289:1379.
161. Khairi MRA, Altman RD, DeRosa GP, et al: Sodium etidronate in the treatment of Paget's disease of bone. Ann Intern Med 1977; 87:656.
162. Siris E, Canfield RE, Jacobs TP, et al: Clinical and biochemical effects of EHDP treatment of Paget's disease of bone: Patterns of response to initial treatment and to long term therapy. Metab Bone Dis Rel Res 1981; 3:301.
163. Roux C, Gennari C, Farrerons JP, et al: Comparative prospective, double-blind, multicenter study of the efficacy of tiludronate and etidronate in the treatment of Paget's disease of bone. Arthritis Rheum 1995; 38:851.
164. Siris ES, Weinstein RS, Altman R, et al: Comparative study of alendronate versus etidronate for the treatment of Paget's disease of bone. J Clin Endocrinol Metab 1996; 81:961.
165. Singer FR, Clemens TL, Eusebio RA, et al: Risedronate, a highly effective oral agent in the treatment of patients with severe Paget's disease. J Clin Endocrinol Metab 1998; 83:1906.
166. Khan SA, McCloskey EV, Nakatsuka K, et al: Duration of response with oral clodronate in Paget's disease of bone. Bone 1996; 18:185.
167. Fraser WD, Stump TC, Creek RA, et al: A double-blind, multicentre, placebo-controlled study of tiludronate in Paget's disease of bone. Postgraduate Med J 1997; 73:496.
168. McClung MR, Tou CK, Goldstein NH, et al: Tiludronate therapy for Paget's disease of bone. Bone 1995; 17(5 suppl):493S.
169. Reid IR, Nicholson GC, Weinstein RS, et al: Biochemical and radiologic improvement in Paget's disease of bone treated with alendronate: A randomized, placebo-controlled trial. Am J Med 1996; 101:341.
170. Khan SA, Vasikaran S, McCloskey EV, et al: Alendronate in the treatment of Paget's disease of bone. Bone 1997; 20:263.
171. Hosking DJ, Eusebio RA, Chines AA: Paget's disease of bone: Reduction of disease activity with oral risedronate. Bone 1998; 22:51.
172. Siris ES, Chines AA, Altman RD, et al: Risedronate in the treatment of Paget's disease of bone: An open label, multicenter study. J Bone Miner Res 1998; 13:1032.
173. Brown JP, Hosking DJ, Ste-Marie LG, et al: Risedronate, a highly effective, short-term oral treatment for Paget's disease: A dose-response study. Calcif Tissue Int 1999; 64:93.
174. Miller PD, Brown JP, Siris EM, et al: A randomized, double-blind comparison of risedronate and etidronate in the treatment of Paget's disease of bone. Am J Med 1999; 106:513.
175. Fitton A, McTavish D: Pamidronate: A review of its pharmacological properties and therapeutic efficacy in resorptive bone disease. Drugs 1991; 41:289.
176. Siris ES: Perspectives: A practical guide to the use of pamidronate in the treatment of Paget's disease. J Bone Miner Res 1994; 9:303.
177. Harinck HIJ, Bijovet OLM, Blanksma HJ, et al: Efficacious management with aminobisphosphonate (APD) in Paget's disease of bone. Clin Orthop 1987; 217:79.
178. Khan SA, McCloskey EV, Eyres KS, et al: Comparison of three intravenous regimens of clodronate in Paget's disease of bone. J Bone Miner Res 1996; 11:178.
179. Meunier PJ, Vignot E: Therapeutic strategy in Paget's disease of bone. Bone 1995; 17(suppl):489S.
180. Patel S, Coupland CAC, Stone MD, et al: Comparison of methods of assessing response of Paget's disease to bisphosphonate therapy. Bone 1995; 16:193.
181. Ryan WG, Schwartz TB, Perlia CP: Effects of mithramycin on Paget's disease of bone. Ann Intern Med 1969; 70:549.
182. Bockman RS, Wilhelm F, Siris ES, et al: A multicenter trial of low dose gallium nitrate in patients with advanced Paget's disease of bone. J Clin Endocrinol Metab 1995; 80:595.

# 38 | Infectious Agent Arthritis

*James S. Louie and Milton H. Louie*

The effective treatment of an infectious arthritis begins with a prompt and specific diagnosis, followed by therapies that destroy the offending microorganism and remove the detritus that damages the host tissues. Of equal importance are the processes that monitor the effectiveness of these therapies. A knowledge of the hosts and their defenses, the microorganisms, and the factors that mediate these interactions may change the observation that "despite better antimicrobial agents and improved hospital care, the case fatality for bacterial arthritis has not changed substantially in the past 25 years."[1] Accordingly, we review here the traditional and newer methods of specific diagnosis, discuss the choices of antibiotics for empirical and specific therapy, and outline the procedures that are useful in the sequential evaluation of outcome.

## EARLY AND SPECIFIC DIAGNOSIS

A monoarthritis, or any arthritis with fever, positions infectious arthritis at the top of the differential diagnosis. Less typical presentations occur when the hosts are at the extremes of the age spectrum, have significant comorbid disease, relate prior joint surgeries (including placement of prosthetic joints), or take drugs that alter the inflammatory and immune responses. Risk factors that alert the clinician include skin infections, hip or knee prosthesis, recent joint surgery, rheumatoid arthritis, diabetes mellitus, and age greater than 80 years.[2, 3] Prompt diagnosis demands the recovery of synovial fluid or tissue for specific identification of the infective microorganisms by appropriate culture. When preexisting arthritis or problematic joints with unique anatomic relationships are affected, immediate collaboration with a radiologist to outline the affected structures and with an orthopedist to facilitate aspiration or biopsy is warranted. Because virtually all cases of infectious agent arthritis are disseminated via the blood stream, blood cultures are a necessary part of the diagnostic work-up in all patients. It is axiomatic that a diligent search for the source of the septicemia should be undertaken immediately.

A *tentative* identification is derived from the Gram stain of any bacteria within the cells recovered from the synovial fluid. Although the technique is not commonly used, Gram stain preparations are more easily viewed when the cells are concentrated and dispersed by means of a cytocentrifuge. Organisms should be visible in 60% of cases of nongonococcal bacterial arthritis.

The *specific* identification of the offending microorganisms traditionally depends on their culture and growth on supportive media. Many bacteria require special attention to maximize growth in media. For example, if gonococcal arthritis is suspected, synovial fluid should be cultured on chocolate agar and transported quickly to the laboratory for incubation in 5% to 7% carbon dioxide. If Lyme disease is suspected, the fluid should be cultured in Barbour-Stoenner-Kelley (BSK) medium (Sigma B3528) and incubated at 33° C to recover *Borrelia burgdorferi*. Even with typical infections, inoculation of larger volumes of synovial fluid into blood culture bottles may enhance the 90% recovery rate reported for nongonococcal bacterial infections.

Although it is not yet available in most clinical laboratories, a new molecular technique to identify pathogens that are difficult to culture uses the polymerase chain reaction (PCR) to amplify small quantities of specific bacterial DNA. Two different primers of oligonucleotides are selected to encompass a DNA sequence that codes for a characteristic bacterial protein. When the specific primers, nucleotides, and a polymerase are added to synovial fluid samples with bacterial DNA and placed within a thermocycler, a process occurs that sequentially changes the temperature to dissociate the double strands of the bacterial DNA (approximately 96° F), anneals the primers by base alignment to the single strands of bacterial DNA (56° F), and fills in the intervening nucleotides between the primers (72° F). This process constructs sufficient copies of the specific DNA fragment for identification by Southern blot. With this technique, *Neisseria gonorrhoeae*, *Staphylococcus aureus*, *B. burgdorferi*, *Chlamydia trachomatis*, and other bacteria have been identified in synovial fluid, and *Mycobacterium tuberculosis* and *Tropherema whippelii*, the gram-positive actinomycete that produces Whipple's disease, have been identified in synovial fluid biopsies of synovial tissue.[4-10] Sets of oligonucleotide primers for various bacteria are offered or under development for clinical laboratory use, and in the near future it is proposed that universal primers based either on the ribosomal nucleic acid (rRNA) gene or on some other conserved region of the microorganism genome and more efficient DNA identification procedures will enable documentation of infection in a clinical specimen within hours.[11, 12] In addition, PCR can identify several genes that code for antibiotic resistance in some bacteria, including the *mecA* gene, which encodes for synthesis of a penicillin-binding protein.[12] The marked sensitivity of PCR and other molecular methods of identification requires great care in collection and assay procedures to prevent contamination and false-positive identifications and to remove inhibitor substances in the collection media that would lead to false-negative results.[13, 14]

## SELECTION OF ANTIBIOTICS

Because rapid destruction of cartilage and joint may ensue in acute bacterial joint infections, antibiotics should be instituted by an intravenous route immediately after synovial fluid and other clinical fluids and tissue have been recovered and processed for culture or PCR. An increasing array of antibiotics of different classes are available (Table 38–1). The clinical setting, the age of the host, local patterns of bacterial resistance, and a careful review of the Gram stain of the synovial fluid cells all influence the empirical choice of antibiotics (Table 38–2). Of course, unique clinical settings raise suspicions for specific infections, as when an intravenous drug user presents with *Pseudomonas aeruginosa* in the sternoclavicular joint or when a patient with rheumatoid arthritis is infected with *S. aureus* in a pannus-laden joint. The age of the host confers a spectrum of different infections that may disseminate to joint tissue. Neonates and young children are prone to upper respiratory infections of *Haemophilus influenzae,* although the rates are decreasing as a result of improved immunization practices. Young adults demonstrate *S. aureus, Streptococcus pneumoniae,* or *N. gonorrhoeae* associated with skin, lung, or venereal infections, and the elderly are susceptible to gram-negative bacilli attendant to genitourinary and gastrointestinal infections. In addition, because patterns of bacterial resistance differ in each locality, the experience of the local hospital microbiology laboratory may influence the initial choices of antibiotics.

Gram's stains of bacteria within synovial fluid cells modulate this empirical decision for antibiotics. The presence of gram-positive cocci suggests *Staphylococcus* or *Streptococcus* species. Because most *S. aureus* organisms produce a β-lactamase, empirical coverage calls for a β-lactamase–resistant penicillin. Nafcillin or oxacillin is given four times a day; cefazolin is given three times a day and is less expensive, and ceftriaxone is given only once a day, offering a greater convenience. The antibacterial activity of the β-lactam antibiotics, the penicillins, and the cephalosporins is dependent on their ability to penetrate the bacterial cell wall through protein-lined channels called *porins,* resist inactivation by bacterial enzymes (β-lactamases), and bind and inactivate the penicillin-binding proteins. The β-lactamase–resistant penicillins such as nafcillin

have a bulky acyl side chain at the R position that prevents hydrolysis by steric hindrance. Another strategy that avoids hydrolysis uses a β-lactamase inhibitor, such as clavulanate or sulbactam, which acts as a suicide inhibitor to form the acyl intermediate with a β-lactamase–susceptible penicillin or cephalosporin. The treatment of gram-positive cocci in a setting where *S. aureus* is resistant to methicillin (MRSA) and to other β-lactamase–resistant penicillins requires the use of vancomycin. These bacteria have developed chromosomal mutations that have decreased the affinities of the penicillin-binding proteins for the antibiotics. Vancomycin succeeds by binding to a different cellular constituent to inhibit bacterial cell wall synthesis. Vancomycin also changes the bacterial wall permeability and impairs RNA synthesis. These multiple mechanisms may be responsible for the low frequency of resistance.

When gram-negative bacilli are observed in cells of the synovial fluid in a clinical situation suggestive of Enterobacteriaceae, a third-generation cephalosporin (e.g., ceftriaxone) or a quinolone (e.g., ciprofloxacin) should be given. The third-generation cephalosporins have complex additions at two positions which confer a broad spectrum of activity against gram-positive and gram-negative bacteria, with particular resistance to the β-lactamases located in the periplasmic space between the inner and outer membranes of the gram-negative bacteria. In addition, the side chain may extend the half-life and allow less frequent and more convenient dosing. Gram-negative bacilli in an immunocompromised host should receive antibiotic coverage for *P. aeruginosa.* Again, a third-generation cephalosporin with antipseudomonal activity (e.g., ceftazidime), a quinolone such as ciprofloxacin, or an antipseudomonal extended-spectrum penicillin such as piperacillin and an aminoglycoside may be selected.

Gram-negative cocci suggest neisserial infections. Because more than 5% of gonococci are resistant to penicillin, all infected patients should be given a third-generation cephalosporin, such as ceftriaxone, or a quinolone. Similarly, when *no bacteria* are identified on Gram's stain from a young adult or an elderly person, a third-generation cephalosporin provides coverage against the most likely offending organisms, *N. gonorrhoeae* and Enterobacteriaceae, respectively. Because *S. aureus* remains a major pathogen in all age groups, antistaphylococcal coverage should be initiated in this situation until synovial fluid culture results are available to modify this empirical regimen. A patient who has previously been given antibiotics poses special difficulties because the antibiotics inhibit the culture results. PCR identification is useful in these instances because bacterial DNA can persist for 10 weeks after antibiotic therapies.[4] When culture results are not available to guide therapy, some or all components of the empirical treatment may need to be continued for weeks.

After the culture and susceptibility results become available, the antibiotic regimen should be modified to a more specific spectrum on the basis of the antibiotic susceptibility profile of the offending organism and

## TABLE 38–1
## Antibiotic Classification

| GENERIC NAME | TRADE NAME | ADMINISTRATION ROUTES |
|---|---|---|
| Penicillins | | |
| β-lactamase–susceptible, nonantipseudomonal | | |
| Penicillin G | | IV, IM, PO |
| Benzathine penicillin G | Bicillin | IM |
| Penicillin V (phenoxymethyl) | Pen Vee K | PO |
| Ampicillin | Amcill, Polycillin | IV, PO |
| Amoxicillin | Amoxil | PO |
| β-lactamase–susceptible, antipseudomonal | | |
| Azlocillin | Azlin | IV |
| Mezlocillin | Mezlin | IV, IM |
| Piperacillin | Pipracil | IV |
| Ticarcillin | Ticar | IV, IM |
| Combination β-lactamase inhibitors and β-lactamase agents | | |
| Amoxicillin plus clavulanate | Augmentin | PO |
| Ticarcillin plus clavulanate | Timentin | IV |
| Ampicillin plus sulbactam | Unasyn | IV, IM |
| Piperacillin plus tazobactam | Zosyn | IV |
| β-lactamase–resistant | | |
| Cloxacillin | Tegopen | PO |
| Dicloxacillin | Dynapen, Pathocil | PO |
| Nafcillin | Unipen, Nafcil | IV |
| Oxacillin | Prostaphlin, Bactocill | IV, IM |
| Methicillin | Staphcillin, Celbenin | IV |
| Cephalosporins | | |
| First-generation | | |
| Cefazolin | Ancef, Kefzol | IV, IM |
| Cephalothin | Keflin | IV, IM |
| Cephapirin | Cefadyl | IV, IM |
| Cephradine | Velosef, Anspor | IV, IM, PO |
| Cephalexin | Keflex | PO |
| Cefadroxil | Duricef, Ultracef | PO |
| Second-generation | | |
| Cefonicid | Monocid | IV, IM |
| Cefotetan | Cefotan | IV, IM |
| Cefoxitin | Mefoxin | IV, IM |
| Cefuroxime | Zinacef, Kefurox | IV, IM |
| Cefuroxime axetil | Ceftin | PO |
| Cefaclor | Ceclor | PO |
| Cefprozil | Cefzil | PO |
| Loracarbef | Lorabid | PO |
| Third-generation | | |
| Cefotaxime | Claforan | IV |
| Ceftizoxime | Cefizox | IV, IM |
| Ceftriaxone | Rocephin | IV, IM |
| Cefixime | Suprax | PO |
| Cefpodoxime proxetil | Vantin | PO |
| Good antipseudomonal activity | | |
| Cefoperazone | Cefobid | IV |
| Ceftazidime | Fortaz, Tazicef, Tazidime | IV, IM |
| Aminoglycosides | | |
| Amikacin | Amikin | IV, IM |
| Gentamicin | Garamycin | IV, IM |
| Netilmicin | Netromycin | IV, IM |
| Spectinomycin | Trobicin | IV, IM |
| Streptomycin | | IM |
| Tobramycin | Nebcin | IV, IM |
| Macrolides and lincomycins | | |
| Clindamycin | Cleocin | IV, IM, PO |
| Erythromycin | | |
| Base, stearate, estolate, ethyl succinate, | E-mycin, Erythrocin, Ilosone, E.E.S. | PO |
| lactobionate, gluceptate | | IV |
| Clarithromycin | Biaxin | PO |
| Azithromycin | Zithromax | PO |
| Tetracyclines | | |
| Tetracycline, oxytetracycline | Terramycin | IV, PO |
| Doxycycline | Vibramycin, Doryx, Vibra-tabs | IV, PO |
| Minocycline | Minocin | PO |

*Table continued on following page*

**TABLE 38–1**
**Antibiotic Classification Continued**

| GENERIC NAME | TRADE NAME | ADMINISTRATION ROUTES |
|---|---|---|
| Fluoroquinolones | | |
| Ciprofloxacin | Cipro | IV, PO |
| Levofloxacin | Levaquin | IV, PO |
| Trovafloxacin | Trovan | IV, PO |
| Carbapenems | | |
| Imipenem plus cilastatin | Primaxin | IV, IM |
| Meropenem | Merrem | IV |
| Monobactams | | |
| Aztreonam | Azactam | IV |
| Chloramphenicol | Chloromycetin | IV, PO |
| Vancomycin | Vancocin, Vancoled | IV, PO |
| Trimethoprim-sulfamethoxazole | Bactrim, Septra | IV, PO |
| Metronidazole | Flagyl, Metric 21, Prostat | IV, PO |

the clinical response (Table 38–3). Clinical laboratories use a variety of methods that correlate with standards promoted by the National Committee for Clinical Laboratory Standards (NCCLS). The minimal inhibitory concentration (MIC) is the lowest concentration of an antimicrobial agent that does not permit visible growth of the retrieved microorganism. The results of broth dilution methods in test tubes are read by eye, while those of automated microdilution techniques are read by optical scanner. The minimum bactericidal concentration (MBC) is defined as the concentration that kills 99.9% of the initial inoculum of viable organisms after incubation for a fixed length of time under a given set of conditions read by serial dilutions in a pour plate.

Time-kill curves can be generated with both methods. The disc diffusion method records the diameters of zones of inhibition around antibiotic-impregnated paper discs. The diameters of inhibited growth are reported to correlate inversely with MICs derived from broth microdilutions and are read as sensitive, intermediately sensitive, or resistant to the antibiotic tested.[15] The serum bactericidal test (SBT) is performed by diluting serum from a patient receiving antimicrobial therapy that is bactericidal to the infective microorganism. SBT values of 1:8 or higher ensure measurable bactericidal activity in the serum for at least three half-lives of the antibiotic being tested.[15] Practically, bactericidal tests are used only to monitor endocarditis, although

**TABLE 38–2**
**Antibiotic Therapy of Bacterial Arthritis Prior to Culture and Susceptibility Results**

| SYNOVIAL FLUID GRAM'S STAIN | PROBABLE PATHOGEN | THERAPEUTIC REGIMEN |
|---|---|---|
| Gram-positive cocci | *Staphylococcus aureus,* "methicillin"-susceptible *Staphylococcus epidermidis* *Streptococcus pneumoniae* *Streptococcus pyogenes* *Streptococcus agalactiae* | Nafcillin, 2 g q6h IV; or cefazolin, 1–2 g q8h IV |
| | *Staphylococcus aureus,* "methicillin"-resistant | Vancomycin, 1 g q12h IV |
| Gram-negative cocci | *Neisseria gonorrhoeae* | Ceftriaxone,* 1 g IV in a single dose |
| Gram-negative bacilli | Enterobacteriaceae | Levofloxacin, 500 mg IV or PO q24h or aminoglycoside |
| | *Pseudomonas aeruginosa* | Ceftazidime, 2 g q8h IV; or piperacillin,† 4–5 g q6h IV, plus an aminoglycoside‡ |
| Indeterminate | | |
| Young adult | *N. gonorrhoeae* | As above |
| Older adult | Enterobacteriaceae | As above |

\* Ceftizoxime or cefotaxime may also be used.
† Azlocillin or mezlocillin may be substituted if they are equally active and less expensive.
‡ Tobramycin, netilmicin, or amikacin should not be used unless the isolate is resistant to gentamicin but susceptible to an alternative (the dose of amikacin is three times higher than that for the other drugs); the doses of these aminoglycosides should be regulated according to assays of peak-trough concentrations in the blood.
Adapted from Parker RH: Septic arthritis. *In* Hoeprich P (ed): Infectious Diseases, 4th ed. Philadelphia: JB Lippincott, 1989:1380.

## TABLE 38–3
## Antimicrobial Treatment of Septic Arthritis After Culture Results

| PRIMARY ANTIMICROBIAL AGENTS | ALTERNATIVE AGENTS | ORAL DRUG FOR COMPLETION |
|---|---|---|
| *Staphylococcus aureus,* "methicillin"-susceptible | | |
| Nafcillin | Cefazolin | Dicloxacillin |
| Oxacillin | Vancomycin | Cephalexin |
| *S. aureus,* "methicillin"-resistant | | |
| Vancomycin | Teichoplanin (not available) | Clindamycin or trimethoprim sulfamethoxazole if susceptible |
| *Streptococcus pyogenes* or *S. pneumoniae* | | |
| Penicillin G | Cefazolin | Penicillin V Cephalexin (cephradine or cefadroxil) |
| *Neisseria gonorrhoeae,* β-lactamase (−) | | |
| Penicillin G | Cefazolin Ampicillin | Amoxicillin Tetracycline or doxycycline |
| *N. gonorrhoeae,* β-lactamase (+) | | |
| Ceftriaxone | Cefotaxime Ceftizoxime Levofloxacin | Levofloxacin Cefuroxime axetil Amoxicillin-clavulanic acid |
| Enterobacteriaceae | Levofloxacin | Levofloxacin |
| Specific agent chosen according to in vitro susceptibility of isolate | | |
| *Pseudomonas aeruginosa* | | |
| Either piperacillin, azlocillin, mezlocillin, or ticarcillin plus an aminoglycoside | Ceftazidime ± aminoglycoside | Ciprofloxacin |
| *Bacteroides fragilis* | | |
| Metronidazole | Clindamycin | Metronidazole Clindamycin |
| *Peptococcus* species and other gram-positive anaerobes | | |
| Penicillin G/ampicillin | Clindamycin | Penicillin VK, amoxicillin, clindamycin |

Adapted from Parker RH: Septic arthritis. In Hoeprich P (ed): Infectious Diseases, 4th ed. Philadelphia: JB Lippincott, 1989:1381.

some have recommended the SBT to verify the effectiveness of antibiotics in the treatment of children with septic arthritis or osteomyelitis.

One should remain aware that these in vitro susceptibility tests show good but not absolute correlation with the in vivo activity of an antimicrobial. The predictive value of susceptibility tests that identify bacterial resistance to an antibiotic is about 95% in most laboratories. Both chromosomal mutations and acquisitions of new DNA from plasmids can result in the development of a wide variety of resistance mechanisms, including the elaboration of β-lactamases, which inactivate the β-lactam antibiotics; alteration of the antibiotic target by decreasing the efficiency of the penicillin-binding protein; restriction of the permeability of the bacteria to antibiotic; or bypass of the metabolic inhibition accorded by the antibiotic. The predictive value of bacterial sensitivity to an antibiotic is only 80% to 85%, with most discrepancies related to β-lactam therapies for *Pseudomonas* and enterococci. Most laboratories know and adjust for the poor reliability of sensitivities of *Pseudomonas* by rapid-identification microtiter techniques, and of *Salmonella* by disc

diffusion methods. In addition, antibiotics that deter growth of *Pseudomonas* in vitro may not be effective in vivo because of the high bacteria inoculum, low pH, and poor antibiotic penetration in the closed spaces of infected joints. Careful monitoring is essential for adjusting therapy in these clinical situations.

There are no controlled studies on the optimal duration and route of antibiotic therapy for infectious arthritis. Accordingly, general experience recommends that prolonged treatment with intravenous antibiotics continue for at least 2 weeks, followed by a course of oral antibiotics for another 1 to 4 weeks for nongonococcal infections of the joint. Because parenterally administered antibiotics achieve high concentrations in infected synovial fluid, intra-articular antibiotics are rarely necessary. Indeed, the concentration of some antibiotics given intra-articularly may injure tissue. All antibiotics, except erythromycin, attain synovial fluid concentrations that are much higher than the average MIC or MBC for most microorganisms.[16-18] Efforts to administer intravenous antibiotics at home and to change early to oral antibiotics at two to three times the usual dosage have been successful in children and in adults, with less cost and better patient satisfaction.[19-23]

Relative contraindications for the use of some antibiotics occur in specific clinical situations. Patients with a history of penicillin allergy can be treated with cephalosporins, vancomycin, or clindamycin with caution. In patients who are pregnant, penicillins, cephalosporins, and erythromycin base can safely be used, but tetracyclines, chloramphenicol, erythromycin estolate, aminoglycosides, quinolones, and sulfonamides should be avoided. Mothers who are breast-feeding should not take chloramphenicol or sulfonamides.

## DOCUMENTING CLINICAL RESPONSE

All the clinical data that prompt and validate the diagnosis and constitute the therapy should be recorded and displayed in a sequential fashion to document the effectiveness of the treatment regimen (Table 38-4). Clinically, in acute infectious arthritis, fever and malaise as well as local tenderness and erythema should improve within 24 to 48 hours. Within 3 to 5 days, the synovial fluid volume and the white cell count should decrease by 30% to 50% and the synovial fluid glucose should have increased to within 75% of normal. When the diagnosis of infectious arthritis is secure, lack of clinical improvement should prompt procedures to identify a sequestered infection that requires surgical drainage. If the diagnosis of septic arthritis is not secure, concomitant nonsteroidal anti-inflammatory drugs (NSAIDs) should be avoided for 5 to 7 days so that any clinical improvement may be correctly attributed to the empirical antibiotic therapy. Concomitant use of NSAIDs with antibiotics cleared by the kidney, such as the aminoglycosides or vancomycin, requires monitoring of renal function and antibiotic drug levels.

Joints that are clinically difficult to evaluate or that have a complex anatomic structure, such as the hip or shoulder, may require imaging by radionuclide scanning, computed tomography (CT), or magnetic resonance imaging (MRI). Radionuclide scanning procedures are sensitive but not very specific because all radiolabeled agents localize to infections and to inflammatory foci of any cause, including the acute joints of rheumatoid, psoriatic, and other inflammatory arthritides. Technetium phosphate bone scans become abnormal within days after the onset of a bone infection, within minutes describing a "hot" area of increased vascular flow that persists for hours. Occasionally, a "cold" photodeficient area is noted initially. Gallium binds to transferrin, lactoferrin, and related receptors of metabolically active cells such as leukocytes within inflammatory foci. Therefore, because of restricted blood flow from increased intramedullary pressure, gallium scans may identify infected bone when the bone scans are negative. Finally, reinfusion of indium-labeled peripheral blood white cells can also outline foci of inflammation in bones, joints, and soft tissue.

CT scanning identifies bony lesions early, particularly at a time when conventional radiographs may be difficult to interpret. MRI affords early detection of fluid, loculations, and soft tissue abnormalities.[24, 25] Most prefer the T2-weighted images, in which the bone is dark and the fluid is white, and the use of gadolinium, which localizes within inflamed tissue. Standard radiographs taken at the time of initial diagnosis can provide information to rule out other possible diagnoses (e.g., fractures), but they are not sensitive enough for monitoring cartilage space loss or the development of osteomyelitis.

## TABLE 38-4
## Clinical Response*

| PARAMETER | DAY 0 (DIAGNOSIS) | DAY 1-4 | DAY 5-7 (REVIEW DIAGNOSIS) | WEEK 1-2 |
|---|---|---|---|---|
| Clinical | | | | |
| Fever | Present | GC: Afebrile | NGC: Afebrile | |
| Joint | Inflamed | GC: Improved | NGC: Improved | Clinical cure |
| Laboratory | | | | |
| SF volume | +++ | 1 | ± Postinfectious effusion | ± Postinfectious effusion |
| SF WBC | NGC: 20,000–100,000 cells/mm³ GC: 10,000–50,000 cells/mm³ | GC: 30%–50% ↓ | NGC: 30%–50% ↓ | |
| SF culture [PCR] | +++ | — [+] | — [±] | — [±] |
| Radiology | | | | |
| [MRI, CT scan] | [Difficult arthrocentesis] | | [Sequestered infection] | |
| Antibiotics | Empirical IV | GC: Adjust to susceptibilities; day 3: change to oral | | NGC: Change to oral |

\* If course is atypical, consider items in brackets.
   CT = computed tomography; GC = gonococcal arthritis; MRI = magnetic resonance imaging; NGC = nongonococcal arthritis; PCR = polymerase chain reaction; SF = synovial fluid; WBC = leukocyte count.

## REMOVAL OF DETRITUS

Closed-needle aspiration should be the initial method of drainage in all cases of infectious arthritis in accessible joints. Aspiration with a large-bore needle is attempted daily for 5 days in joints such as the knee, wrist, ankle, and smaller joints when an effusion is clinically detectable.[26, 27] Because closed-needle drainage may not remove all the detritus, it is prudent to request an orthopedic consultation for consideration of drainage procedures early in the clinical course. Open surgical drainage of the hips and shoulders is generally preferred because complete drainage is difficult, particularly in children, whose anatomy predisposes to avascular necrosis.[1, 27, 28] Although they are not difficult to aspirate, the redundant spaces within the shoulder allow for sequestered infection, especially if there is a delay in diagnosis. The multiple articulations of the wrist, including the intercarpal and radiocarpal joints, and of the sacroiliac and sternoclavicular joints are difficult to aspirate. In general, more complex anatomy, the presence of preexisting joint damage, and delay in the institution of therapy point toward an earlier use of open surgical drainage.

Arthroscopic surgery is the procedure of choice in accessible joints such as the knee. Diagnostically, arthroscopy allows biopsy of the infected synovium to be performed under direct vision. Therapeutically, arthroscopy enables more effective removal of inflammatory debris through irrigation of all of the joint spaces, including the posterior compartment of the knee. The frequency of introduction of bacteria into the joint during arthroscopy is less than 1%, particularly when small-needle arthroscopes are used.[29] In comparison with arthrotomy, arthroscopy also carries the advantage of decreased morbidity of the procedure (no need for general anesthesia), improved joint mobility, and shorter hospital stay.[28, 29]

If pain, fever, effusion, and synovial leukocytosis persist after needle aspiration or arthroscopy, an open drainage procedure to explore and to débride loculations, adhesions, and bony sequestrum should be undertaken promptly. Open surgical drainage procedures are usually followed by a decreased range of motion in the affected joint, and this may be permanent.

## INFECTIONS OF PROSTHETIC JOINTS

Prosthetic joint infections represent a special kind of bacterial arthritis.[30] Early infections after joint replacement are usually caused by *Staphylococcus epidermidis*, *S. aureus*, or gram-negative bacilli. To decrease the risk of infection, attention must be given to improved surgical technique, laminar flow environments, and the prophylactic use of antibiotics given 30 to 60 minutes before and continued for 1 to 2 days after surgery.[31, 32] Cefazolin, 1 to 2 g every 8 hours given intravenously, is the recommended antistaphylococcal antibiotic. Intravenous vancomycin, 1 g every 8 hours, is used in hospitals with a high frequency of MRSA and for patients who are allergic to penicillins or cephalosporins.[33] When patients with prosthetic joints undergo other surgical procedures in which bacteremia is likely to occur, antistaphylococcal antibiotics are recommended.

If an infection develops within the prosthetic site and continues despite antibiotic therapies, the usual recommendation is to remove the prosthesis, perform a wide surgical débridement, and administer antibiotics intravenously for 2 months and orally for a few months before attempting a second prosthetic joint placement.[34, 35] Serial joint aspirations to record the culture, volume, cell count, and glucose level are more helpful than an erythrocyte sedimentation rate, Gram's stain, radiographs, and scans. In an English multicenter study of 41 prosthetic joint infections, the most effective microbiologic diagnosis of infection at elective revision arthroplasty required culture and histologic studies of seven or more surgical samples. Gram's stains of the tissues were unrevealing.[36] After cultures from the prosthetic site become sterile, a custom-made implant is often necessary to compensate for the deficient bone and soft tissues. The implant and cement are soaked in antibiotics, and intravenous antibiotics are continued for another 4 to 6 weeks. This two-stage reimplantation protocol eradicated infection in 95% of cases with 65% good-to-excellent clinical results at an average of 4 years' follow-up in one series.[34] Others have reported a poorer outcome, with only 31% retention of the infected prosthesis, especially in the hip and elbow.[35]

Therefore, if an infection of the prosthesis is discovered within the first weeks, antibiotics may suffice, particularly if the organism is gram-positive and sensitive to the antibiotics. In most late infections, the prolonged immobilization required for the reimplantation may be hazardous for a patient of advanced age or one with comorbid disease such as rheumatoid arthritis.[35] In some instances, it may be necessary to retain the infected prosthesis and suppress the infection with continual administration of antibiotics. In rare instances, amputation may be necessary. In an attempt to shorten the prolonged hospitalization and rehabilitation period, various antibiotics configured to a slow-release solid bead have been placed in the prosthetic site, but the efficacy of these procedures has not been rigorously assessed. Future studies using PCR will most likely change this paradigm.[10]

## JOINT REHABILITATION

The acute phase of infection mandates the use of protected rest with the joint in a functional anatomic position. Splints are often necessary. Passive range of motion and exercises are initiated as soon as the acute stage of infection has subsided. Studies in animals suggest that continuous passive motion facilitates rehabilitation.[37]

To prevent muscle atrophy, isotonic or muscle-tightening exercises are initiated in the acute phase of the infection. For example, quadriceps-setting exercises are recommended for infections in the knee. As the joint pain resolves, the patient is instructed in a program of stretching, active range of motion exercises, and muscle strengthening at least twice each day. Some patients develop a postinfectious arthritis that manifests as a sterile, recurrent, inflammatory effusion when function is resumed.[38] This is attributed to sequestered bacterial products such as antigenic bacterial cell-wall components, exotoxins, or endotoxins. Differentiation from an incompletely treated infection or a superinfection may require repeated culture. NSAIDs can be helpful in these patients once infection is ruled out.

## CHRONIC INFECTIOUS AGENT ARTHRITIS

Many pathogenic microorganisms are capable of circumventing host defenses by residing within the cells. Infectious arthritis induced by these agents, such as *Chlamydia,* manifests less typically than acute infections, particularly when it has progressed to more chronic phases. Because diagnosis is delayed by the slow growth in culture, PCR may find greater applicability. Antibiotics that attain effective intracellular concentrations are preferred, but susceptibility testing of these slower-growing organisms and the duration of therapy are not standardized. Furthermore, the clinical response is more prolonged, making recommendations for removal of infected material and rehabilitation less precise. Continuing experience is necessary.

## MYCOBACTERIAL INFECTIONS

The increase of pulmonary tuberculosis in the United States as a result of new immigration and immunocompromised disease states is expected to spawn greater recognition of bone and joint involvement, which occurs in 1% to 5% of patients infected with *M. tuberculosis.*[39, 40] The two most common rheumatic manifestations are spinal tuberculosis, also known as Pott's disease, and peripheral tuberculous arthritis. Pott's disease is treated with the standard chemotherapy for pulmonary tuberculosis, consisting of 9 months of isoniazid (INH), 5 mg/kg/day orally up to a maximum of 300 mg/day, and rifampin, 10 mg/kg/day orally to a maximum of 600 mg/day. Pyrazinamide (PZA), 25 mg/kg/day orally to a maximum of 2 g/day, is added for the first 2 months of the 9-month regimen.[41] If the spine is not stable and if neurologic involvement is anticipated, spinal fusion prevents vertebral collapse and neurologic sequelae in more than 93% of cases.[42] Paravertebral cold abscesses respond to the chemotherapeutic regimen and usually do not require surgical drainage. Others recommend surgical excision of all tuberculous granulation tissue and disc material to facilitate greater access of chemotherapeutic agents to the area of infection.[43] Similarly, early peripheral arthritis responds to the chemotherapy regimen, but late lesions with sequestrum require surgical débridement.

Because multidrug-resistant tuberculosis is becoming more common, susceptibility testing is required on all isolates. For patients at increased risk, particularly those who have received incomplete courses of therapy, empirical treatment requires the use of four antituberculosis drugs, usually INH, ethambutol, rifampin, and PZA.

In most urban centers, any patients with tuberculosis that has disseminated to the joint or to other extrapulmonary sites should be tested for human immunodeficiency virus (HIV) infection. HIV-positive patients coinfected with tuberculosis should receive the same regimens as HIV-negative patients, even though bacteremia and extrapulmonary involvement occur in most of these patients. If INH and rifampin are used without PZA, duration of treatment is extended from 9 to at least 12 months. Most therapeutic regimens are continued for 12 months after the culture becomes negative.[44]

Other mycobacterial infections that induce arthritis in immunocompromised hosts include *Mycobacterium kansasii,* which responds to the same regimen outlined for *M. tuberculosis; Mycobacterium marinum,* which is treated with rifampin and ethambutol; and *Mycobacterium gastri,* which responds to streptomycin for 2 months combined with rifampin and ethambutol for 9 months.[45] *Mycobacterium avium-intracellulare* is treated with ethambutol and various regimens that include clarithromycin, rifampin, amikacin, and ciprofloxacin.[46–48]

*Mycobacterium leprae* infections reflect the importance of the immune status of the host in the expression of disease. Those patients with the tuberculoid form demonstrate a good cell-mediated response and a positive lepromin skin test. Those in the lepromatous state demonstrate an anergy of the cell-mediated immunity and a proliferation of *M. leprae* in the skin, nerves, and joints. The lepra bacillus is identified in synovial fluid cells by acid-fast stains in one third of cases and in synovial tissue in one half.[49, 50] Lepromatous leprosy is treated with rifampin, 600 mg at least once a month or even daily; dapsone, 100 mg/day; and clofazimine, 300 mg once a month and 50 mg daily, for a period of 2 years.[51] The erythema nodosum leprosum reaction that occurs with specific chemotherapy necessitates prednisone, 60 mg in divided doses, or thalidomide, 200 mg twice daily, tapering to 50 to 100 mg at night.[51] With the chronic sequelae attendant to untreated disease, consultations with specialists in neurology, orthopedics, and physical medicine are required for the evaluation of nerve, bone, and functional impairment. Chronic arthritis affects the peripheral small joints and the sacroiliac joints.[52]

## FUNGAL ARTHRITIS

Traditionally, most fungal arthritis is treated with the polyene amphotericin B (AMB), which binds to ergosterol and damages the fungal cell wall. AMB is given intravenously at a maximum dosage of 1 mg/kg (up to 70 mg) in 500 mL of dextrose and water over 2 to 4 hours daily or three times a week for a total of 2 to

2.5 g. Initially, 1 mg is administered to test for acute toxicity, followed by 10 or 20 mg/day to maximal tolerated dosage. To forestall fever and severe chills, patients are premedicated with aspirin or acetaminophen, and hydrocortisone (25 mg) is administered within the infusion. Occasionally, narcotics such as meperidine, 25 mg, are required during the infusion to prevent rigors. Toxicity in the kidneys requires monitoring of serum creatinine; if it approaches 2.5 mg/dL, the dosage and frequency of AMB are attenuated. Adequate hydration is essential, and saline loading is helpful.[53] These toxicities and a variable efficacy have prompted the search for different formulations. AMB administered in lipid complexes or liposomes showed increased efficacy and decreased toxicity in experimentally produced fungal infections.[54] AMB is rarely given intra-articularly because of the induction of a chemical synovitis.

The azoles are broad-spectrum antifungal agents that inhibit fungal cytochrome P450–dependent enzymes and the synthesis of membrane ergosterol. They are less toxic than AMB and can be given orally. As a group, the imidazoles, miconazole and ketoconazole, are more toxic and less effective than the triazoles, fluconazole and itraconazole.[55, 56] Combinations of azoles with AMB may confer improved efficacy with decreased toxicities, but further studies are needed. Inasmuch as the orally administered azoles require gastric acid for absorption, they should not be used in patients who are achlorhydric or who are taking antacids or histamine-2 (H$_2$) blockers. However, oral absorption of fluconazole is decreased in patients with the acquired immunodeficiency syndrome (AIDS) who are taking H$_2$-blocking agents. Flucytosine, a competitive antimetabolite of uracil in the synthesis of yeast RNA, is used adjunctively with AMB because of early resistance. It is never used alone, because rapid resistance develops. Other azoles, polypeptides, echinocandins, and nikkomycins represent new drugs that may also broaden antifungal therapeutic options. Current treatment recommendations for selected fungal arthritides appear in Table 38–5.

Treatment of coccidioidomycosis involves medical and surgical interventions. AMB produces cure rates of 50% to 70%, and relapses are frequent. Azoles may become the drug of choice. Itraconazole, 200 mg twice daily by mouth, and fluconazole, 400 to 800 mg once a day by mouth, provide response rates similar to AMB against coccidioidomycosis arthritis. Ketoconazole provides limited efficacy and relapses of infection are frequent. Intra-articular AMB has been used successfully despite the local toxicity. Synovectomy to débride the joint and reduce the fungal burden alone does not effect a cure.[57-60] Improved outcome is obtained by combining synovectomy and débridement with intravenous AMB, and this is the recommended treatment.[59]

The role for antifungal susceptibility testing remains to be standardized. Inconsistencies have been noted in monitoring the treatment of coccidioidomycosis, as well as candidiasis.[52] Coccidioidomycosis complement fixation titers of serum and/or synovial fluid may be prognostic and should be obtained every other month. Complement fixation titers of 1:16 or more at the completion of therapy are likely to result in clinical relapse, but titers of less than 1:4 may persist for years. Skeletal radiographs are not reliable markers for progress because abnormalities may persist for months after clinical and microbiologic cure.

Isolated *Candida* arthritis responds to AMB or fluconazole, although the duration of therapy is not clear. Open drainage is rarely necessary except where there is hip involvement. If antifungal drugs are ineffective, synovectomy is an alternative.[61]

Histoplasmosis arthritis is uncommon. If the disease is severe, itraconazole, 400 mg/day orally for 6 months,

## TABLE 38–5
### Treatment of Fungal Arthritis

| ORGANISM | PRIMARY ANTIFUNGAL AGENTS | ALTERNATIVE AGENTS |
|---|---|---|
| *Coccidioides immitis* | Amphotericin B | Fluconazole<br>Itraconazole<br>Amphotericin B, intra-articular |
| *Candida* species | | |
| Localized | Fluconazole | Itraconazole |
| Disseminated | Amphotericin B | Amphotericin B plus flucytosine |
| *Histoplasma capsulatum* | | |
| Mild | Itraconazole | Fluconazole |
| Moderate | Itraconazole or amphotericin | |
| Blastomycosis | | |
| Non-AIDS patients | Itraconazole | Amphotericin B |
| AIDS patients | Amphotericin B | |
| *Cryptococcus neoformans* | Amphotericin B plus flucytosine | Fluconazole |
| *Sporothrix schenckii* | Amphotericin B | Amphotericin B, intra-articular |

*Dosing:* Amphotericin B: 0.6 mg/kg/d IV × 7 d, then 0.8 mg/kg qod IV; start test dose 1 mg on day 1, 10 mg day 2, 20 mg day 3, up to 50 mg/d; adjust dose by renal function; total dose = 2.5 g. Fluconazole, itraconazole, and ketoconazole: 400 mg PO qd. Flucytosine: 150 mg/kg/d in four divided doses.

represents the drug of choice in patients who do not have AIDS. Alternatively, a short course of AMB, up to 500 mg total, can be used. If severe systemic infection is present, a total dose of 2 g is needed.[62, 63] NSAIDs and, less often, corticosteroids can be used against the arthritis associated with erythema nodosum.

Disseminated blastomycosis leads to death in 30% to 80% of cases. Treatment includes AMB or itraconazole. Because loculations are common, open drainage is often necessary.[64]

Cryptococcal arthritis occurs in patients with impaired cell-mediated immunity, such as those with AIDS or lymphoreticular cancers and those receiving corticosteroids. Treatment includes high-dose AMB with flucytosine for a period sufficient to yield conversion of cultures with minimal or no toxicity.[65] Surgical drainage and excision are often required for an adjacent osteomyelitis.

*Sporothrix schenckii* is the most reported fungal arthritis. AMB for 12 weeks, combined with surgery, is the treatment of choice. Intra-articular AMB has been successfully used in a patient whose infection was refractory to a full course of intravenous AMB.[66, 67]

# SUMMARY

Clinical awareness, prompt identification of the infectious agent and initiation of therapy, a considered choice of antibiotics, and continuing attention to host factors, particularly the removal of pus, remain the primary determinants for successful treatment of infectious arthritis. In the future, DNA hybridization techniques such as PCR should increase the capabilities for specific diagnosis of infections by organisms that are difficult to identify. Furthermore, the ability to identify an infective organism within hours, particularly when prior antibiotic administration obviates reliable cultural identification, will enable less discriminate and more effective use of broad-spectrum antibiotics while culture results are awaited. As increasing patterns of antibiotic resistance are reported, it is hoped that newer methods to facilitate host defenses for bacterial killing may be forthcoming.[68] For the present, effective care for this most treatable group of patients demands continued vigilance.[69]

# REFERENCES

1. Goldenberg DL: Septic arthritis. Lancet 1998; 351:197.
2. Kaandorp CJE, Van Schaardenburg D, Krijnen P, et al: Risk factors for septic arthritis in patients with joint disease. Arthritis Rheum 1995; 38:1819.
3. Gardner GC, Weisman MH: Pyarthroses in patients with rheumatoid arthritis: A report of 13 cases and a review of the literature from the past 40 years. Am J Med 1990; 88:503.
4. Liebling MR, Nishio MJ, Rodriguez A, et al: The polymerase chain reaction for the detection of *Borrelia burgdorferi* in human body fluids. Arthritis Rheum 1993; 36:665–675.
5. Canvin JMG, Goutcher SC, Hagig M, et al: Persistence of *Staphylococcus aureus* as detected by polymerase chain reaction in the synovial fluid of a patient with septic arthritis. Br J Rheumatol 1997; 36:203.
6. Liebling MR, Arkfeld DG, Michelini GA, et al: Identification of *Neisseria gonorrhoeae* in synovial fluid using the polymerase chain reaction. Arthritis Rheum 1994; 37:702.
7. Kuipers JG, Nietfeld L, Dreses-Werringloer U, et al: Optimised sample preparation of synovial fluid for detection of *Chlamydia trachomatis* DNA by polymerase chain reaction. Ann Rheum Dis 1999; 38:103.
8. Relman DA, Schmidt TM, Mac Dermott RP, et al: Identification of the uncultured bacillus of Whipple's disease. N Engl J Med 1992; 327:293.
9. O'Duffy JD, Griffing WL, Li CY, et al: Whipple's arthritis: Direct detection of *Tropheryma whippelii* in synovial fluid and tissue. Arthritis Rheum 1999; 42:812.
10. Mariani BD, Martin DS, Levine MJ, et al: The Coventry Award: Polymerase chain reaction detection of bacterial infection in total knee arthroplasty. Clin Orthop 1966; 331:11–22.
11. Bergeron MG, Oullette M: Preventing antibiotic resistance through rapid genotypic identification of bacteria and of their antibiotic resistance genes in the clinical microbiology laboratory. J Clin Microbiol 1998; 36:2169.
12. Wallet F, Roussel-Delvallez M, Courcol RJ: Choice of a routine method for detecting methicillin resistance in staphylococci. J Antimicrob Chemother 1996; 37:901.
13. Fredericks DN, Relman DA: Improved amplification of microbial DNA from blood cultures by removal of the PCR inhibitor sodium polyanetholesulfonate. J Clin Microbiol 1998; 36:2810.
14. Gibb AP, Wong S: Inhibition of PCR by agar from bacteriological transport media. J Clin Microbiol 1998; 36:275.
15. Stratton CW: In vitro testing: Correlations between bacterial susceptibility, body fluid levels and effectiveness of antibacterial therapy. *In* Lorian V (ed): Antibiotics in Laboratory Medicine, 3rd ed. Baltimore: Williams & Wilkins, 1991:849.
16. Parker RH, Schmid FR: Antibacterial activity of synovial fluid during treatment of septic arthritis. Arthritis Rheum 1971; 14:96.
17. Nelson JD: Antibiotic concentrations in septic joint effusions. N Engl J Med 1971; 284:349.
18. Baciocco EA, Lies RL: Ampicillin and kanamycin concentrations in joint fluid. Clin Pharmacol Ther 1971; 12:858.
19. Tetzlaff TR, McCracken GH, Nelson JD: Oral antibiotic therapy for skeletal infections of children: II. Therapy of osteomyelitis and suppurative arthritis. J Pediatr 1978; 92:485.
20. Prober CG, Yeager AS: Use of the serum bactericidal titer to assess the adequacy of oral antibiotic therapy in the treatment of acute hematogenous osteomyelitis. J Pediatr 1979; 95:131.
21. Bryson YJ, Conner JD, LeClerc M, et al: Brief clinical and laboratory observation: High-dose oral dicloxacillin treatment of acute staphylococcal osteomyelitis in children. J Pediatr 1979; 94:673.
22. Kolyvas E, Ahronheim G, Marks MI, et al: Oral antibiotic therapy of skeletal infections in children. Pediatrics 1980; 65:867.
23. Black J, Hunt TL, Godley PJ, et al: Oral antimicrobial therapy for adults with osteomyelitis or septic arthritis. J Infect Dis 1987; 155:968.
24. Resnick CS, Ammann AM, Walsh JW: Chronic septic arthritis of the adult hip: Computed tomographic features. Skeletal Radiol 1987; 16:513.
25. Rosenberg D, Baskies AM, Deckers PJ: Pyogenic sacroiliitis: An absolute indication for computerized scanning. Clin Orthop 1984; 184:128.
26. Goldenberg DL, Reed JI: Bacterial arthritis. N Engl J Med 1985; 312:764.
27. Broy SB, Schmid FR: A comparison of medical drainage (needle aspiration) and surgical drainage (arthrotomy or arthroscopy) in the initial treatment of infected joints. Clin Rheum Dis 1986; 12:501.
28. Bulmer JH: Septic arthritis of the hip in adults. J Bone Joint Surg Br 1966; 48:289.
29. Broy S, Stulberg SD, Schmid FR: The role of arthroscopy in the diagnosis and management of the septic joint. Clin Rheum Dis 1986; 12:489.
30. Saccente M: Periprosthetic joint infections: A review for clinicians. Infect Dis Clin Pract 1998; 7:431–441.
31. Lidwell OM, Elson RA, Lowbury EJ, et al: Ultra clean air and antibiotics for prevention of post operative infection: A multi center study of 8052 joint replacement operations. Acta Orthop Scand 1987; 58:4.

32. Antimicrobial prophylaxis in surgery. Med Lett Drugs Ther 35:91, 1993.
33. Maki D, Bohn MJ, Stolz SM, et al: Comparative study of cefazolin, cefamandole, and vancomycin for surgical prophylaxis in cardiac and vascular operations. J Thorac Cardiovasc Surg 1992; 104:1423.
34. Wilson MG, Kelley K, Thornhill TS: Infection as a complication of total knee replacement in arthroplasty: Risk factors and treatment in sixty seven cases. J Bone Joint Surg Am 1990; 72:878.
35. Tsukayama DT, Estrada R, Gustilo RB: Infection after total hip arthroplasty: A study of the treatment of one hundred and six infections. J Bone Joint Surg Am 1996; 78:512–523.
36. Atkins BL, Athanasou N, Deeks JJ, et al: Prospective evaluation of criteria for microbiological diagnosis of prosthetic-joint infection at revision arthroplasty: The OSIRIS Collaborative Study Group. J Clin Microbiol 1998; 36:2932–2939.
37. Salter RB, Bell RS, Keeley FW: The protective effect of continuous passive motion on living articular cartilage in acute septic arthritis: An experimental investigation in the rabbit. Clin Orthop 1981; 159:223.
38. Goldenberg DL: ''Post infectious'' arthritis: New look at an old concept with particular attention to disseminated gonococcal infection. Am J Med 1983; 74:925.
39. Evanchick CC, Davis DE, Harrington TM: Tuberculosis of peripheral joints: An often missed diagnosis. J Rheumatol 1986; 13:187.
40. Berney S, Goldstein M, Bishko F: Clinical and diagnostic features of tuberculous arthritis. Am J Med 1972; 53:36.
41. Gilbert DN, Moellering RC, Sande MA: The Sanford Guide to Antimicrobial Therapy—1998. Hyde Park, VT: Antimicrobial Therapy, Inc, 1998:80.
42. Chakirgil GS: Evaluation of anterior spinal fusion for treatment of vertebral tuberculosis. Orthopedics 1991; 14:601.
43. Alarcon GS: Arthritis due to tuberculosis, fungal infections, and parasites. Curr Opin Rheumatol 1992; 4:516.
44. Small PM, Schecter GF, Goodman PC, et al: Treatment of tuberculosis in patients with advanced human immunodeficiency virus infection. N Engl J Med 1991; 324:289.
45. Perandones CE, Roncoroni AJ, Frega NS, et al: *Mycobacterium gastri* arthritis: A case report—Septic arthritis due *to Mycobacterium gastri* in a patient with a renal transplant. J Rheumatol 1991; 18:777.
46. Ahn CH, Ahn SS, Anderson RA, et al: A four-drug regimen for initial treatment of cavitary disease caused by *Mycobacterium avium* complex. Am Rev Respir Dis 1986; 134:438.
47. Chiu J, Nussbaum J, Bozzette S, et al: Treatment of disseminated *Mycobacterium avium* complex infection in AIDS with amikacin, ethambutol, rifampin, and ciprofloxacin. Ann Intern Med 1990; 113:358.
48. Jones AR, Bartlett J, McCormack JG: *Mycobacterium avium* complex (MAC) osteomyelitis and septic arthritis in an immunocompetent host. J Infect 1995; 30:59–62.
49. Pernambuco JCA, Opromolla DUA, Tolentin MM, et al: Arthritis in lepromatous Hansen's disease [Abstract]. Int J Leprosy 1979; 47:353–354.
50. Louie JS, Koransky JR, Cohen AH: Lepra cells in synovial fluid of a patient with erythema nodosum leprosum. N Engl J Med 1973; 289:1410–1411.
51. WHO Study Group: Chemotherapy of Leprosy for Control Programmes. WHO Technical Report 675. Geneva: World Health Organization, 1982.
52. Cossermelli-Messina W, Cossermelli W: Possible mechanisms of chronic leprosy-related arthritis. Rev Paul Med 1997; 115:1406–1409.
53. Graybill JR: Future directions of antifungal chemotherapy. Clin Infect Dis 1992; 14(suppl 1):170.
54. Lopez-Berestein G, Bodey GP, Fainstein V: Treatment of systemic fungal infections with liposomal amphotericin B. Arch Intern Med 1989; 149:2533.
55. Perez-Gomez A, Prieto A, Torresano M, et al: Role of the new azoles in the treatment of fungal osteoarticular infections. Semin Arthritis Rheum 1998; 27:226–244.
56. Terrell CL: Antifungal agents: Part II. The azoles. Mayo Clin Proc 1999; 74:78.
57. Bayer AS, Guze LB: Fungal arthritis: II. Coccidioidal synovitis: Clinical, diagnostic, therapeutic, and prognostic considerations. Semin Arthritis Rheum 1979; 8:200.
58. Gillespie R: Treatment of cranial osteomyelitis from disseminated coccidioidomycosis. West J Med 1986; 145:694.
59. Bried JM, Galgiani JN: *Coccidioides immitis* infections in bones and joints. Clin Orthop 1986; 211:235.
60. Galgiani JN: Coccidioidomycosis: A regional disease of national importance. Ann Intern Med 1999; 130:293.
61. Hansen BL, Anderson K: Fungal arthritis: A review. Scand J Rheumatol 1995; 24:248.
62. Goodwin RA, Loyd JE, Des Prez RM: Histoplasmosis in normal hosts. Medicine (Baltimore) 1989; 60:231.
63. Fowler VG Jr, Nacinovich FM, Alspaugh JA, et al: Prosthetic joint infection due to *Histoplasma capsulatum*. Clin Infect Dis 1998; 26:1017.
64. Abril A, Campbell MD, Cotten VR Jr, et al: Polyarticular blastomycotic arthritis. J Rheumatol 1998; 25:1019–1021.
65. Ricciardi DD, Sepkowitz DV, Berkowitz LB, et al: Cryptococcal arthritis in a patient with AIDS: Case report and review of the literature. J Rheumatol 1986; 13:455.
66. Downs NJ, Hinthorn DR, Mhatre VR, et al: Intra-articular amphotericin B treatment of *Sporothrix schenckii* arthritis. Arch Intern Med 1989; 149:954.
67. Zacharias J, Crosby LA: Sporotrichal arthritis of the knee. Am J Knee Surg 1997; 10:171.
68. Davies J: Inactivation of antibiotics and the dissemination of resistance genes. Science 1994; 264:375.
69. Kaandorp CJE, Krijnen P, Moens HJB, et al: The outcome of bacterial arthritis. Arthritis Rheum 1997; 40:884.

# 39 | Lyme Disease

*Nancy A. Shadick*

Lyme disease is a tick-borne illness caused by the spirochete *Borrelia burgdorferi*, which causes disease of the skin, nervous system, heart, and joints.[1] Although the clinical manifestations, may vary, the disease usually begins with erythema migrans accompanied by flu- or meningitis-like symptoms. Weeks later, meningitis, facial palsy, atrioventricular nodal block, or migratory musculoskeletal pain may develop, followed months to years later by episodes of oligoarticular arthritis, encephalopathy, polyneuropathy, or acrodermatitis.[2, 3]

## EPIDEMIOLOGY

Lyme disease is the most common vector-borne illness in the United States. Over 80,000 cases from 49 states have been reported to the Centers for Disease Control and Prevention since 1992.[4] The highest density of cases is found in three endemic areas: the Northeast (extending from Maryland to northern Massachusetts), the upper Midwest (including Wisconsin and Minnesota), and the Far West (including Northern California and Oregon).[5, 6] Two members of the Ixodidae family, *Ixodes scapularis* (found in the Northeast and Midwest) and *Ixodes pacificus* (found in the Far West), are the most common vectors of Lyme disease in the United States.[7]

Endemic areas of Lyme disease are located worldwide and include Europe, China, Russia, and Japan.[8, 9] Transmission is by ixodid ticks in these areas as well. The *Ixodes ricinus* tick has been known since 1950 to cause erythema migrans in Europe.[10]

Erythema migrans was first described in Europe[11] in 1909. The first cases in the United States were identified in Wisconsin in 1969[12] and in Lyme, Connecticut,[13] in 1975, but polymerase chain-reaction technology has identified *B. burgdorferi* in tick specimens as far back as 1940.[14] The more recent increase in Lyme disease is thought to have resulted partially from the increase in the density and population of deer, the most common host of the adult *I. scapularis* tick. Deforestation of much of the Northeast eliminated the conditions favorable for deer and deer ticks, but certain areas, such as Long Island, New York, and some islands off Cape Cod, maintained their deer and tick populations. As farming decreased and suburban metropolitan areas proliferated, deciduous forests returned along with the deer, creating ecologic conditions suitable for endemicity.

Competent reservoir hosts and tick vectors are necessary for maintaining endemicity. A reservoir host must be frequently infected and capable of sustaining borrelial infection. A competent vector must, in turn, be able to receive and transmit infection from a competent reservoir host. In the Northeast, the white-footed mouse (*Peromyscus leucopus*) is the most important reservoir for the larval and nymphal tick and appears to be the means through which high rates of infectivity are maintained in endemic areas.[15] The *I. scapularis* tick has a 2-year, three-stage life cycle (larva, nymph, and adult).[16] Both larval and nymph forms feed on the white-footed mouse and other small mammals. The nymphal tick, which feeds during the late spring and summer, commonly transmits the disease to humans. The adult form also transmits *B. burgdorferi* to humans during the late fall or winter when it feeds on larger mammals, such as deer, horses, cows, or dogs.

Infection with *B. burgdorferi* occurs by horizontal transmission.[17] Infected nymphal ticks transmit *B. burgdorferi* to the white-footed mouse, which then passes it on to larval ticks. Larvae then molt into nymphs and transmit infection to either other mice or humans. Between 20% and 80% of ticks may harbor the spirochete in endemic areas, but infection rates vary considerably within these endemic areas.[18] Dormant, infected ticks can sustain infection until the next season and, as adults, can transmit the spirochete while feeding on deer and/or humans.

In the Far West, the wood rat serves as reservoir host for Lyme disease, and the non–human-biting tick *Ixodes neotomae* is the rodent- and rabbit-feeding vector responsible for maintaining infection. *I. pacificus*, which feeds mostly on lizards, is responsible for the transmission to humans. When no lizards are available, *I. pacificus* feeds on small mammals and, at a relatively low rate (1%), transmits *B. burgdorferi* to humans.[19] Other vectors, *I. scapularis* and *Amblyomma americanum*, are likely vectors in the southeast United States and Texas, respectively.

## BIOLOGY OF *BORRELIA BURGDORFERI*

The causative agent of Lyme disease was first isolated from *I. scapularis* ticks captured on Shelter Island, New

York.[1] The organism is a member of the phylum spirochete, which has a spiral-shaped body with 7 to 11 flagella arranged along an axial filament that lies between the outer and inner membranes of the cell.[20] Linear and circular plasmids encode for the organism's outer surface lipoproteins (Osp) (i.e., the 31-kd OspA and the 34-kd OspB).[21] The expression of these proteins varies between isolates and sometimes loses pathogenicity through multiple passages in culture.[22] Other immunologically important peptides include the 41-kd flagellar protein, which bears resemblance to other spirochetes; the 60-kd, 66-kd, and 83-kd heat shock proteins; and the low-molecular-weight proteins between 18 and 25 kd.

The organism grows very slowly, dividing every 12 to 24 hours in vitro and more slowly in vivo. It is grown in Barbour-Stoenner-Kelly medium at 33° F and has been cultured from blood, skin, spinal fluid, and joint fluid.[23] Spirochetes are extracellular organisms, although studies have demonstrated that *B. burgdorferi* can live inside phagocytes.[24] (For more detail on pathogenesis, the reader is referred to the chapter on Lyme disease in Kelley et al.[24a])

## DIAGNOSIS

The diagnosis of Lyme disease is made clinically with supportive serologic and epidemiologic data. A history of a tick bite in an area with known Lyme disease and erythema migrans is the most important information in diagnosing Lyme disease. The risk of developing Lyme disease after a tick bite in an endemic area is low (approximately 5% in one study).[25] Because culture or direct visualization of *B. burgdorferi* in tissue is difficult, infection can rarely be proved. In early Lyme disease, 53% of patients have an elevated erythrocyte sedimentation rate (ESR), 19% have liver function abnormalities, and 12% have a hematocrit value less than 37%, but these findings are nonspecific.[26] Erythema migrans, a red patch at the site of the tick bite that clears centrally and expands over a period of days to weeks to form a large, round lesion, usually more than 5 cm in diameter, is pathognomonic for Lyme disease. The lesions can be pleomorphic, however. Not all of these lesions necessarily have central clearing; some may be vesiculated, and "satellite" lesions can be observed. Moreover, nearly one third of the patients with Lyme disease do not have erythema migrans.[27] In such cases, a flu-like syndrome with fever, headache, shaking chills, arthralgias, or lymphadenopathy after a tick bite may provide a clue to the diagnosis. A small percentage of patients may have asymptomatic infection with *B. burgdorferi*. In the United States, the frequency of asymptomatic infection in endemic areas ranges between 3% and 5%, but with active surveillance, it can be up to 25%.[28] The Centers for Disease Control and Prevention national surveillance case definition is weighted heavily toward serologic confirmation, and late manifestations cannot be the sole basis for clinical diagnosis.[29]

## Antibody Tests

Early in the course of infection, T lymphocytes proliferate preferentially to *B. burgdorferi* antigens.[30] Approximately 3 to 6 weeks after infection, a specific immunoglobulin M (IgM) response becomes detectable.[31] A specific immunoglobulin G (IgG) response appears anytime from 6 to 8 weeks after infection but may not peak until months later and can remain elevated indefinitely. The IgG response expands over time to novel *B. burgdorferi* antigens, which supports the theory that live spirochetes persist throughout the course of Lyme disease.[32]

The two most commonly used methods for detecting antibodies to *B. burgdorferi* are the enzyme-linked immunosorbent assay (ELISA) and the indirect immunofluorescent assay (IFA), both of which use sonicated homogenates of the whole organism.[31] Because of its greater sensitivity and specificity, the ELISA is preferred over the IFA. Serologic testing remains unstandardized, and results vary between laboratories. False-positive serologic results are seen with a number of other diseases, including syphilis, relapsing fever, Rocky Mountain spotted fever, infectious mononucleosis, autoimmune disease, and neurologic illnesses such as amyotrophic lateral sclerosis.[31, 33] Even a borderline positive level of rheumatoid factor or antinuclear antibody can result in a false-positive Lyme ELISA titer. The prevalence of false-positive results ranges from 5% to 10% in the United States.[34]

False-negative serologic findings occur, particularly in early infection and in cases in which antibiotic treatment early in the disease may attenuate the specific antibody response.[31] Serum samples during the acute illness are negative in most patients by standard ELISA. By antibody capture immunoassay (ELISA capture) to IgM, 90% of patients have a detectable IgM response.[35] IgG, IgM, and immunoglobulin A (IgA) capture enzyme immunoassay decreases nonspecific binding to cross-reactive epitopes by adsorption of the test serum with *Escherichia coli* and thus is able to detect small increases in *B. burgdorferi*–specific antibody in comparison with total antibody. Both indirect ELISA and ELISA capture assays can be used to measure intrathecal antibody production in response to *B. burgdorferi*, the most specific diagnostic test for neurologic Lyme disease.[36] Increased cerebrospinal fluid (CSF) serum ratios of specific IgG and IgA provide evidence for active central nervous system (CNS) infection in early and late neuroborreliosis. The antibody capture immunoassay is currently available from only a few specialty laboratories.[35]

## Western Blot Analysis

Expansion of the immunoglobulin G response to novel *B. burgdorferi* polypeptides occurs over time[32] and includes immune reactivity to a 31-kd OspA, a 34-kd OspB, and a 23-kd OspC outer surface protein. The 41-kd flagellar protein shares homology with other spirochetes, and the 58-, 66-, and 74-kd heat shock proteins share homology with other heat shock proteins in the *E. coli* family, making these polypeptides less specific for Lyme disease.[37] The 31-kd (OspA) and 34-kd (OspB) reactivity is found in persons with prolonged episodes of arthritis.[37a] The functions of the 21-, 28-, and 93-kd proteins, which are more specific for Lyme disease, are not known. The requirement of 5 of 10 IgG bands (bands 18, 21, 28, 30, 39, 41, 45, 58, 66, and 93) after the first weeks of infection had a sensitivity of 83% and a specificity of 95% in one prospective analysis.[38] The Western blot's utility is primarily in confirming exposure in the presence of a borderline or positive ELISA titer or a presumed false-positive result or in monitoring the specific immune response over time. The Centers for Disease Control and Prevention recommends that all borderline or positive antibody tests be followed up with a Western Blot analysis.

## Polymerase Chain Reaction

Polymerase chain reaction (PCR) is a highly sensitive technique that amplifies *B. burgdorferi* DNA. It has been used to identify *B. burgdorferi* DNA in patients' CSF, blood, urine, and skin and to test ticks for infectivity.[14] PCR is a difficult test to perform and has a high rate of contamination. There also have been few studies demonstrating its clinical utility. One report, however, demonstrated that PCR testing can detect *B. burgdorferi* DNA in synovial fluid and that the test may be helpful in elucidating whether prolonged arthritis after antibiotic therapy is caused by active infection or by an autoimmune reaction that persists after eradication of the spirochete.[39]

Physicians should test for Lyme disease initially with ELISA or ELISA capture assay for IgM or IgG, followed by a Western blot analysis. Work-up of neurologic Lyme disease should include analysis of the CSF for IgG, IgA, or IgM antibody.

## CLINICAL MANIFESTATIONS AND TREATMENT RECOMMENDATIONS
(Table 39–1)

### In Vitro and In Vivo Studies

Results of in vitro antimicrobial studies of 18 agents demonstrate that *B. burgdorferi* is susceptible to the action of tetracyclines, semisynthetic penicillins, macrolides, and second- and third-generation cephalosporins. *B. burgdorferi* was noted to be moderately sensitive to penicillin G and resistant to chloramphenicol, aminoglycosides, trimethoprim-sulfamethoxasole, quinolones, and rifampin.[40, 41] Cefuroxime demonstrated a higher in vitro minimum bactericidal concentration (MBC) (1.0 $\mu$g/mL) than did ceftriaxone (0.08 $\mu$g/mL) or erythromycin (0.32 $\mu$g/mL), but the MBC was similar to that of amoxicillin (0.8 $\mu$g/mL) and doxycycline (1.6 $\mu$g/mL). *B. burgdorferi* was less susceptible to tetracycline (MBC, 3.2 $\mu$g/mL) and penicillin G (MBC, 6.4 $\mu$g/mL). Penicillin G, which demonstrated a high in vitro MBC, had weak protective activity in a Syrian hamster model; it binds to *B. burg-*

*dorferi* immediately but remains sensitive to $\beta$-lactamase for only 4 to 7 days.[40]

With the exception of erythromycin, the findings of in vivo studies in the Syrian hamster models paralleled those of the in vitro studies. Three antibiotics with similar in vitro MBCs—cefuroxime, doxycycline, and amoxicillin—demonstrated comparable activities in preventing borreliosis in the hamster model. The in vivo activity of cetotoxime improved when the treatment schedule was modified from once a day to three times a day for 5 days. Penicillin G, when given at a high dosage of 150 mg/kg, showed a similar improvement when given more frequently.[40]

The in vivo and in vitro susceptibilities of *B. burgdorferi* to azithromycin, clarithromycin, and vancomycin have also been investigated. In one study, *B. burgdorferi* was more susceptible to azithromycin (MBC, 0.04 $\mu$g/L) than to erythromycin (MBC, 0.16 mg/L) or to tetracycline (MBC, 1.6 mg/L).[42] Azithromycin was more effective than both tetracycline and erythromycin in vivo in eliminating infection from the hamster model. Tissue concentrations exceeding the MBC were present for 24 hours after the last dose. Clarithromycin was effective in vivo against *B. burgdorferi*–induced arthritis in the hamster, being more than 1 log stronger than tetracycline.[42] *B. burgdorferi* has in vivo and in vitro susceptibility to vancomycin. Vancomycin, a glycopeptide antibiotic not previously known to be active against spirochetes, demonstrates synergy with penicillin at one fourth the minimum inhibitory concentration (MIC) of each drug.[43a] *B. burgdorferi* was shown to be susceptible in vitro to roxithromycin, a new semisynthetic macrolide, but treatment with this drug failed in five of nine animals in a gerbil model. Roxithromycin is therefore not recommended for treatment of Lyme disease.

### Early Lyme Disease

Acute, localized disease consisting of erythema migrans, with or without flu-like symptoms, can be treated with oral antibiotics, although untreated erythema migrans resolves on its own (median duration of eruption, 28 days). Steere and colleagues[45] reported that either penicillin or tetracycline was associated with a more rapid resolution of erythema migrans than was no therapy. In another study, tetracycline was compared with phenoxymethylpenicillin and erythromycin at doses of 250 mg four times daily for 10 days and was found to be more effective in preventing major late manifestations, such as meningoencephalitis, myocarditis, and recurrent attacks of arthritis.[46] However, with all three antibiotic agents, half the patients experienced symptoms of headache, musculoskeletal pain, fatigue, and lethargy at 1 year of follow-up.

Treatment failures with penicillin and tetracycline have been reported[47] and have led to longer durations of therapy and to the use of other tetracyclines and $\beta$-lactam drugs. In a 21-day trial comparing amoxicillin/probenecid, 500 mg three times daily, with doxycycline, 100 mg twice a day, there was a 100% response rate for both regimens and protection against major

## TABLE 39–1
## Treatment Recommendations

| SYSTEM | REGIMEN |
|---|---|
| Early infection* (local or disseminated) | |
| Adults | Doxycycline 100 mg orally BID for 20–30 d† |
| | Amoxicillin 500 mg orally TID for 20–30 d† |
| | Cefuroxime axetil 500 mg orally BID for 20–30 d† |
| Children (age 8 or less) | Amoxicillin 250 mg orally TID or 20 mg/kg/d in divided doses for 20–30 d† |
| | Alternative in case of allergy to penicillin: |
| | Erythromycin‡ 250 mg orally TID or 30 mg/kg/d in divided doses for 20–30 d† |
| Arthritis* (intermittent or chronic) | Doxycycline 100 mg orally BID for 30–60 d |
| | Amoxicillin and probenecid, 500 mg of each TID orally for 30–60 d |
| | Cefriaxone 2 g IV once a day for 14–30 d |
| | Penicillin G 20 million IU in 4 divided doses for 30 d |
| Neurologic abnormalities* | |
| Early or late | Ceftriaxone 2 g IV once daily for 14–30 d§ |
| | Penicillin G 20 million IU in 4 divided doses daily for 14–30 d§ |
| | Alternatives in case of allergy to penicillin or cephalosporin |
| | Doxycycline 100 mg orally TID for 30 d |
| Facial palsy alone | Oral regimens may be adequate |
| Cardiac abnormalities | |
| First-degree AV block (PR interval >0.3 s) | Oral regimens, as for early infection |
| High-degree AV block | Parenteral regimens, as for neurologic abnormalities |
| Acrodermatitis | Oral regimens for 1 month are usually adequate |
| Pregnancy | |
| Localized, early disease | Amoxicillin 500 mg TID for 21 d |
| All other manifestations | Ceftriaxone 2 g IV once a day for 14–30 d |
| | Penicillin G 20 million IU IV in 6 divided doses for 14–30 d |

AV = atrioventricular.

* Treatment failures have occurred with any of the regimens given. Re-treatment may be necessary.
† The duration of therapy is based on clinical response.
‡ These antibiotics have not yet been tested systematically for this indication in Lyme disease.
§ For early neurologic abnormalities, 2 weeks of therapy is generally adequate. The appropriate duration of therapy is not yet clear for patients with late neurologic abnormalities, and 4 weeks of therapy may be preferable.
Modified from Steere AC: ACR State of the Art Lecture: Update on Lyme disease. Presented at the Annual Scientific Meeting of the American College of Rheumatology, Boston, 1999.

sequelae; 15% of the patients, however, had fatigue and arthralgias for 3 months after taking the antibiotics, but these symptoms resolved in 6 months.[48] In a study of 198 patients with erythema migrans,[49] 2 g/day of oral penicillin V or tetracycline for 10 days produced a response. In another study of higher doses of oral penicillin V (1 million U three times a day) for 12 days in comparison with ceftriaxone (1 g intramuscularly per day for only 5 days), ceftriaxone was superior in preventing minor symptoms in 19 patients who had had two or more symptoms before therapy.[50]

Doxycycline, 100 mg twice daily, has replaced tetracycline as a recommended agent for early localized Lyme disease because of its better gastrointestinal absorption, longer half-life, and superior CNS penetration. Amoxicillin is recommended over penicillin because of its better in vitro activity against *B. burgdorferi*. Although there are no studies addressing the optimal duration of therapy, the recommended duration of therapy is 10 to 30 days. Doxycycline is also effective against human granulocytic ehrlichiosis, which can coexist with *Ixodes scapularis* infection.

Penicillin allergy, which occurs in 1% to 10% of the general population, can produce significant morbidity.[51] Tetracyclines are contraindicated during pregnancy and lactation and are associated with photosensitivity reactions during the summer months, a time when early[52] Lyme disease is commonly detected. Erythromycin is the usual alternative agent prescribed, although it is less effective in treating erythema migrans and in preventing late manifestations. The need for alternative therapies for early Lyme disease has led to clinical studies of newer and related antibiotics.

Azithromycin, an analog of erythromycin, is an azalide antibiotic with greater in vivo activity against *B. burgdorferi* in the hamster model.[42] In addition, azithromycin has a longer half-life and better tissue penetration, and there is less gastrointestinal intolerance. In a randomized, controlled trial of 246 patients, azithromycin, 500 mg PO QD for 7 days, was compared with amoxicillin/probenecid, 500 mg three times a day for 10 days. Amoxicillin was superior in lessening the likelihood of relapse and increasing the likelihood of complete remission.[52a] In a study of 201 children with early Lyme disease who received either amoxicillin or doxycycline, 94% experienced a rapid recovery and none had residual symptoms 2 years after infection.[53]

Clarithromycin also shows promise as an agent in treating early Lyme disease. In an open study of 500 mg BID for 21 days, the therapeutic response was rapid, all patients recovering within 6 months.[54]

Cefuroxime, a second-generation cephalosporin, has good in vitro and in vivo activity against *B. burgdorferi* in a Syrian hamster model.[40] In a prospective, blinded, multicenter clinical trial comparing cefuroxime axetil (an oral form of cefuroxime), 500 mg twice a day, with doxycycline, 100 mg three times a day, for 20 days, the two regimens appeared equally effective in treating Lyme disease and preventing late Lyme disease at 1 year of follow-up. Doxycycline was associated with more photosensitivity reactions (15% vs. 0%) and cefuroxime with more diarrhea (21% vs. 7%).[55] In another study in which 20 days of cefuroxime axetil was compared with 20 days of doxycycline (100 mg BID of either drug) among 232 patients, the efficacy rates were equally high (95% vs. 100%, respectively). Doxycycline caused more photosensitivity reactions, and cefuroxime caused more diarrhea.[56]

The author's current recommendation for the treatment of early Lyme disease is oral doxycycline (100 mg twice daily) or amoxicillin (500 mg three times daily). The optimal duration of therapy is unknown, and the treatment duration is based on clinical response. The author recommends 3 or 4 weeks of therapy, depending on clinical response.

## Early Disseminated Lyme disease

### Multiple Erythema Migrans

In a randomized controlled study comparing doxycycline with ceftriaxone for disseminated Lyme disease with multiple erythema migrans and arthralgias, but without meningitis, the rates of response were similar for the two drugs. In each group of patients, there was one failure. Arthralgias were the only persistent symptoms, occurring with similar frequency in both groups (14% vs. 27%, nonsignificant). Doxycycline is therefore recommended for the treatment of early disseminated Lyme disease without meningitis.[57]

### Meningitis or Meningoencephalitis

The most common acute neurologic manifestation of disseminated Lyme disease is meningitis.[26] The meningitis is self-limited, but antibiotic treatment shortens its duration.[46] There is both clinical and experimental evidence of early invasion of the CNS by *B. burgdorferi*. Headache and meningismus are found in 64% of patients with symptoms of early Lyme disease.[26] Garcia-Monco and associates,[58] in a study of Lyme disease in Lewis rats, demonstrated changes in blood-brain barrier permeability within 12 hours of inoculation. Concomitantly with these changes, white blood cells and spirochetes were found in the CSF within 24 hours of inoculation. Using frozen CSF serum samples from patients with erythema migrans and early neurologic symptoms (but no antibody of *B. burgdorferi* in the serum or CSF), the investigators found spirochetal antigens by Immunoblot in three of five samples.[58] The findings suggest that *B. burgdorferi* may be found in the CNS early in the course of acute, disseminated disease.

Persons with suspected neurologic Lyme disease should undergo a spinal tap to confirm meningeal inflammation with lymphocytic pleocytosis and an elevated level of CSF protein. Selective concentration of CSF antibody should be confirmed by obtaining simultaneous serum and CSF samples. Most patients with meningitis have evidence of locally synthesized IgG, IgM, and/or IgA antibody to *B. burgdorferi* in the CSF, but among American patients with late neurologic abnormalities, selective concentration of specific antibody is less common and typically consists of only the IgG or IgA isotype.[36]

A third-generation cephalosporin is the agent of choice for the treatment of meningitis or meningoencephalitis. Cephalosporins have an overall safe and efficacious profile for a variety of infections.[59] They may be used as therapy for patients with penicillin allergy, although they share certain structural similarities with penicillin, and up to 15% of the patients may have both penicillin and cephalosporin allergy. Ceftriaxone and cefotaxime can be given once or twice daily; they have an excellent in vitro activity against *B. burgdorferi* and good CSF penetration. Ceftriaxone[59a] and cefotaxime[60, 61] appear superior to benzylpenicillin for neurologic Lyme disease. In one small randomized study, 2 g per day of parenteral ceftriaxone for 14 days had a better response rate than 20 million U of penicillin for 10 days in the treatment of late neurologic findings.[59a] The duration of effective therapy ranges from 2 to 4 weeks.

In one Swedish study, oral doxycycline appeared effective in the treatment of meningitis compared with penicillin.[62] A single case report noted the efficacy of chloramphenicol, 1 g intravenously every 6 hours for 10 days, in the treatment of neurologic Lyme disease,[63] and one report noted success with tetracycline for Lyme meningitis.[64]

Lyme disease can produce a subtle encephalopathy with deficits in verbal memory and concentration.[65] A positive serum serologic finding and intrathecal production of IgG can assist in diagnosing the disease. Both parenteral ceftriaxone and penicillin have been reported to be effective therapy for encephalopathy, although the optimal dosage and duration of therapy have not been established.

The author's current recommendation for the treatment of neurologic manifestations of Lyme disease is a 30-day course of 2 g of parenteral ceftriaxone. Effective alternative parenteral medications are cefotaxime and penicillin. In the case of a penicillin allergy, doxycycline, 100 mg twice daily for 30 to 60 days, may be prescribed. In the case of a treatment failure, retreatment may be necessary.

## Bell's Palsy

Bell's palsy (facial nerve paralysis) is the most common cranial nerve abnormality in Lyme disease; it is found in up to 5% of untreated cases.[26] With or without antibiotics, it usually resolves within 2 months, so the primary reason for treating Bell's palsy is to shorten its course and prevent late manifestations. The author recommends that an isolated seventh nerve palsy without concurrent CSF inflammatory changes be treated with doxycycline (100 mg twice daily) for 21 to 30 days. With concurrent meningitis or radiculoneuritis, parenteral therapy with ceftriaxone (2 g/day) is recommended.

## Peripheral Neuropathy

Peripheral neuropathy in Lyme disease occurs in acute and chronic forms. In the acute form, an early, severe, but spontaneously resolving axonal radiculoneuropathy is often associated with meningitis or cranial neuritis. The chronic form appears later in the course of disease, sometimes along with acrodermatitis, and is clinically and electrophysiologically milder.[66] This form resolves slowly with antibiotic therapy. Lyme disease–related radiculoneuritis or polyneuropathy manifests with numbness, paresthesias, or burning pain in an extremity, often followed by sensory loss, hyporeflexia, or weakness.[65] Nerve conduction studies reveal mild to moderate reduction in motor and sensory conduction velocities. To date, no intraneural *B. burgdorferi* have been demonstrated in biopsy specimens.

Lyme disease–related neuropathy is responsive to antibiotics; improvement is demonstrable both clinically and electrophysiologically. In a series of 25 patients with chronic peripheral neuropathy resulting from Lyme disease, neuropathic symptoms began a median of 8 months after the onset of erythema migrans. Approximately half the patients had symmetric nonpainful paresthesias; the others had asymmetric radicular pain. Both groups had denervation of paraspinal and limb muscles, but 6 months after treatment with intravenous ceftriaxone, 76% showed improvement. In general, the clinical response is not as dramatic as in meningitis, reflecting slow recovery from axonal injury.[66] The intravenous antibiotic regimens used for the treatment of meningitis are recommended for the treatment of Lyme disease–related peripheral neuropathy.

The author's current recommendation for the treatment of Lyme disease–related neuropathy is parenteral ceftriaxone, 2 g/day for 30 days. Parenteral penicillin G, 20 million U in divided doses is an effective alternative. Oral doxycycline, 100 mg twice daily for 30 days, can also be used as an alternative, although experience with this drug is limited.

## Lyme Disease–Induced Carditis

Carditis, present in approximately 8% of untreated persons with Lyme disease,[67] typically consists of varying degrees of atrioventricular block, but myopericarditis, mild congestive heart failure, and bradyarrhythmias have been reported. Common presenting symptoms consist of fatigue or lightheadedness, palpitations, syncope, and exertional dyspnea. Spirochete-like structures have been demonstrated in cardiac tissue,[68, 69] and *B. burgdorferi* was cultured from the myocardium in a patient with dilated cardiomyopathy.[70] One fatality from cardiac complications associated with Lyme disease occurred in a patient with concurrent babesiosis who had pancarditis and spirochetes in myocardial tissue.[69]

Although Lyme disease–related carditis has been treated successfully with oral antibiotics,[71] intravenous antibiotics are currently recommended in all cases except the most benign form (PR interval of <0.30 second). Antimicrobial therapy has been reported to be successful in improving the ejection fraction of patients with dilated cardiomyopathy from Lyme disease.[72, 73] There is a relationship between duration of infection and improvement in left ventricular function: Improvement is unlikely after more than 6 months of symptoms. Both intravenous benzylpenicillin[71] and ceftriaxone[74] for 2 weeks resolve carditis. Corticosteroids are used only in severe carditis that does not respond to antibiotics within the first few days. Although the optimal duration of therapy has not been established, 2 to 3 weeks of intravenous penicillin or ceftriaxone appears sufficient. Lyme disease–related carditis frequently necessitates hospitalization with cardiac monitoring and placement of a temporary pacemaker for bradyarrhythmias. Although Lyme disease–related carditis is usually self-limited, there have been case reports of complete heart block[68, 75] and persistent first-degree block after infection with *B. burgdorferi*. However, in one long-term follow-up study, there was no increased frequency of electrocardiographic abnormalities among patients with and without a history of Lyme disease a mean of 6 years after infection.[76]

The author currently recommends 2 g intravenous ceftriaxone for 30 days for the treatment of Lyme carditis. Oral antibiotic therapies with doxycycline, 100 mg twice daily, or amoxicillin, 500 mg three times daily, can be given for 30 days if the PR interval is less than 0.30 second.

## Arthritis

Sixty percent of patients with untreated Lyme disease develop arthritis. Common manifestations include migratory musculoskeletal pain in the early stages of disease, sometimes followed by intermittent oligoarticular asymmetric arthritis, particularly of the knee. Without treatment, persons with Lyme disease–related arthritis improve at a rate of 10% per year.[77] Eleven percent of persons in one study who had untreated arthritis developed chronic synovitis.[77] Erosive synovitis, cartilage loss, cysts, and enthesopathy have been reported.[78] A subgroup of persons with chronic arthritis were found to have HLA-DR2 and HLA-DR4 phenotypes more frequently than other phenotypes.[79] The presence of the DR4 phenotype was associated with a lack of response to antibiotic therapy, which suggests that *B. burgdorferi* may trigger an autoimmune response that is independent of the organism's viability. Patients with DR4 (DRB0401) specificity developed strong IgG responses to OspA near the beginning of prolonged episodes of arthritis, from 5 months to 7 years after disease onset in one report.[37a]

During acute arthritis, laboratory abnormalities include a mild peripheral leukocytosis and an elevated ESR. Synovial fluid characteristics include leukocytosis, with measurements ranging from 500 cells/mm$^3$ to 110,000 cells/mm$^3$, mostly polymorphonuclear leukocytes, an elevated protein level, but a normal glucose value.[67,77] In one study, 10 days of intravenous benzylpenicillin treatment cured 55% of cases with Lyme arthritis, whereas intramuscular benzathine penicillin each week for 3 weeks cured only 35% of the cases.[80] In a randomized study, intravenous ceftriaxone was compared with intravenous penicillin for the treatment of persistent and remitting arthritis. At 3 months of follow-up, two of seven penicillin-treated patients showed improvement, in comparison with 17 of 18 ceftriaxone-treated patients.[59a] Oral treatment with amoxicillin/probenecid or doxycycline is successful in curing most cases of Lyme disease–related arthritis, although these regimens may not have CNS penetration adequate for treating concomitant neuroborreliosis.[81]

It may take up to 3 months for a response to antibiotics to appear. Intra-articular corticosteroid injections should be avoided, because they may prolong synovitis. Refractory chronic Lyme disease–related arthritis with early joint damage may be treated with hydroxychloroquine or synovectomy.[80]

The author's current recommendation for the treatment of Lyme disease–related arthritis is 2 g of parenteral ceftriaxone for 4 weeks, although oral doxycycline, 100 mg twice daily, for 30 to 60 days can be used. Treatment failure occurs with any regimen, and retreatment may be necessary.

## TREATING THE PREGNANT PATIENT

Transplacental transmission of *B. burgdorferi* has been documented with Dieterle's silver stain in three infants, both from mothers with untreated or inadequately treated Lyme disease contracted in the first trimester. Two infants died shortly after birth, one of a congenital cardiac malformation[82] and the other of encephalitis[83]; the third infant was stillborn.[84] In a retrospective review of 19 women with Lyme disease contracted in all three trimesters, five adverse outcomes were reported, including syndactyly, cortical blindness, intrauterine fetal death, prematurity, and hyperbilirubinemia and rash.[85] Thirteen of these patients had received appropriate antibiotic therapy. In another study, 10 pregnancies complicated by localized Lyme disease that was treated had no adverse outcomes, and in six samples no IgM antibody existed to suggest intrauterine infection.[86]

The author recommends the treatment of all manifestations other than early, localized Lyme disease with parenteral therapy: either ceftriaxone, 2 g/day, or penicillin G, 20 million U/day in divided doses, for 14 to 30 days. Doxycycline is contraindicated during pregnancy because of its potential toxic effects on the fetus; therefore, erythema migrans should be treated with oral amoxicillin, 500 mg three times daily for 21 days.

## THE POST-LYME SYNDROME

A 4-week course of intravenous therapy for disseminated Lyme disease is usually curative, although in some cases resolution of symptoms may be delayed for 6 to 8 months. Whether a "post–Lyme disease syndrome" exists is controversial. Dinerman and Steere[87] described fibromyalgia after Lyme disease in 8% of their cohort (15 patients) that was not responsive to antibiotics. Fatigue, arthralgias, and memory complaints may persist after treatment; in one series, up to 30% of the patients reported persistent complaints such as myalgias, arthralgias, persistent fatigue, and attention and concentration difficulties, despite a lack of objective abnormalities to suggest active infection.[88] In some cases, residual morbidity from disseminated infection is present; in others, fibromyalgia or the chronic fatigue syndrome has occurred.

## MONITORING THE SIDE EFFECTS OF TREATMENT

Parenteral intravenous therapy is well tolerated for 4 weeks with the use of a peripherally inserted central catheter. Phlebitis can occur; axillary vein thrombosis is a rare but potential side effect of the catheter placement.

No studies have documented a benefit from prolonged antibiotic treatment. Indeed, long-term antibiotic therapy can be associated with significant morbidity. $\beta$-Lactam antibiotics can be associated with leukopenia, and liver function measurements may be elevated. Cephalosporins can be associated with biliary complications ("sludge") and, like amoxicillin and doxycycline (photosensitivity), with diarrhea and/or a drug rash. In one series, 25 patients who had received intravenous ceftriaxone for close to 6 months developed biliary disease; 14 of them required cholecystectomy.[89] Twenty-two patients developed a total of 29 blood stream infections. In an extreme case, one patient with suspected seronegative Lyme disease was treated with 3 weeks of intravenous ceftriaxone and developed granulocytopenia, fever, hepatitis, and *Clostridium difficile*–induced diarrhea.[89]

Diagnostic serologic testing for Lyme disease remains imperfect and unstandardized, and false-positive findings occur.[34] Several investigators have re-

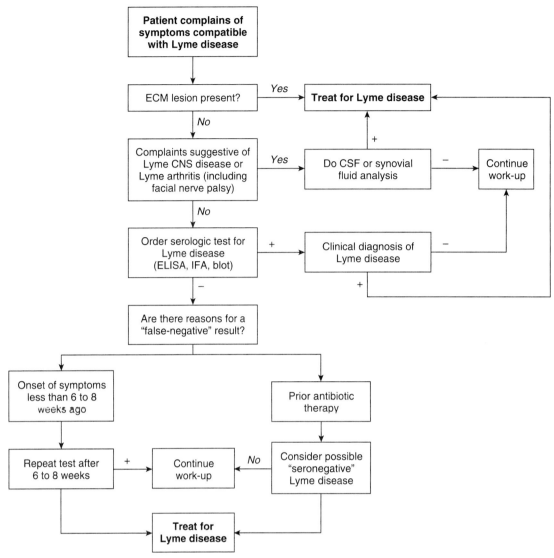

**FIGURE 39–1**
Diagnostic work-up for Lyme disease. (From Sigal LH: Current recommendations for the treatment of Lyme disease. Drugs 1992; 43:683–699.)

ported a high rate of misdiagnosis among patients with Lyme seropositivity and complaints of fatigue, arthralgias, and memory difficulties who were evaluated at a Lyme disease referral center.[90, 91] Every effort should be made to document objective abnormalities before embarking on a course of treatment for presumed Lyme disease (Fig. 39–1). A cost-effectiveness analysis examined the consequences of treating patients with parenteral antibiotic therapy who had chronic fatigue, myalgia, and a positive serologic test result for Lyme disease but lacked classic manifestations.[92] According to the model, it would cost $86,221 for each true positive case treated, and 29 cases of drug toxicity would occur. Only when patients would be willing to pay $3485 out of pocket to eliminate anxiety about not treating possible true Lyme disease would the model's strategy break even. For most patients with a positive

Lyme titer and only nonspecific symptoms, the risks and costs of empirical parenteral antibiotic therapy exceed the benefits.

The author recommends monitoring home parenteral therapy with weekly complete blood cell count and liver function tests. The parenteral central catheter should be closely inspected daily to detect phlebitis or venous thrombosis.

## PREVENTION

Tick bite control is an important initiative to prevent Lyme disease and other tick-borne illnesses. Evidence from the occupational literature suggests that preventive measures such as avoiding tick-infested areas, wearing long pants tucked into socks and long-sleeved shirts, and light-colored clothing and applying insect repellent are effective in reducing the risk of Lyme disease.[93-95] Repellent containing diethyltoluamide (DEET) can by sprayed on clothing and exposed skin other than the face. A safe concentration in adults is between 30% and 35% and in children, excluding infants, 10% to 15%. The application of outdoor insecticides (such as Dursban, Tempo, or Sevin) is the only available method of reducing tick density in residential neighborhoods. When applied in late spring, the number of nymphal deer ticks decreases throughout the summer.

Performing daily tick checks is an important and effective precaution against Lyme disease.[94] Ixodes ticks require a minimum of 24 hours to transmit the B. burgdorferi organism.[96] Persons should be instructed on how to perform a tick check, including inspection of the whole body that consists of looking and feeling for ticks. If one is found, it should be grabbed closest to the person's skin at the tick's mouthparts and pulled straight out with a strong tug. Alcohol, petroleum jelly, and matches should not be used, because they will harm the tick and increase the chance of regurgitation of the B. burgdorferi into the host.

Although knowledge of Lyme disease among residents of endemic areas is adequate, precautions are generally underperformed.[97, 98] In one study, people traveling to an endemic area had very good knowledge of Lyme disease, but only between 40% and 60% regularly practiced precautions. In another study of high school students living in Connecticut, 90% believed that taking tick bite precautions prevented Lyme disease; however, fewer than half reported practicing preventive behaviors.[97] More accurate predictors of precautionary behaviors related to attitudinal and health belief variables, particularly self-efficacy related to performing successful tick checks and recognizing Lyme disease symptoms. Believing that the avoidance behavior is effective in reducing Lyme disease and that the precaution's benefit outweighed its inconvenience was also predictive of performance. Because general knowledge about Lyme disease symptoms and transmission was not associated with taking precautions, public health departments and health educators are currently targeting persons at risk by employing these methods of modeling and social learning theory.[99]

## Tick Bite Prophylaxis

Treating patients for Lyme disease after an Ixodes dammini tick bite remains a controversial subject despite studies on the risks and benefits of empirical therapy.[25] Ixodes ticks must feed for a minimum of 24 hours to transmit B. burgdorferi, at which time their risk of transmission is only 5%. After a tick has fed for 2 days, the risk of transmission increases to 50%, and almost all infected ticks transmit the spirochete to their host after more than 4 days of attachment.[100] Nymphal Ixodes ticks measure approximately 1.5 mm in length and transmit pathogens to human hosts more frequently than do larval or adult forms.[100] Larvae are rarely infected, and adults, which are 5 mm in length, are gener-

ally large enough to be removed before B. burgdorferi can be transmitted. Because adults feed mostly in the winter and nymphs mostly in the spring, nymphal bites are most likely to result in Lyme disease.

Some investigators have proposed the use of the scutal index (measuring the chest/scutum:abdomen ratio) to approximate the amount of engorgement, and therefore feeding time, which can estimate the risk of B. burgdorferi transmission[101] or propose that replete nymphal Ixodes ticks can be detected when the branches of the tick's gut cannot be readily distinguished by means of a hand lens. To the untrained eye this may be difficult and therefore an unreliable measure.

The question of whether to provide prophylaxis against Lyme disease after a tick bite was systematically studied in a cost-effectiveness analysis by Magid and coworkers.[102] The model incorporated the outcomes' cost and the cost effectiveness of three alternatives to treating patients bitten by Ixodes ticks in areas of endemic Lyme disease: (1) empirically treating all patients with 2 weeks of doxycycline; (2) treating only patients in whom erythema migrans developed; or (3) treating only patients with erythema migrans or a positive serologic test result for Lyme disease 1 month after exposure. Empirical treatment of patients with tick bites was indicated when the probability of B. burgdorferi infection after a tick bite was 0.036 or higher. The authors stated that treatment may be preferred when the probability of infection ranges from 0.01 to 0.035 but is not recommended for a probability of infection lower than 0.01. Two studies reported that B. burgdorferi transfer occurred in approximately 10% of persons bitten by infected ticks.[26, 102] Those authors suggested that empirical therapy is therefore not warranted in areas where the prevalence of tick infection is less than 10%, because the product prevalence would be equal to 0.001.

This decision model was confirmed by a controlled trial of antimicrobial prophylaxis for Lyme disease after deer tick bites in an endemic area of Connecticut.[103] The study compared treatment consisting of amoxicillin, 250 mg three times a day for 10 days, with placebo for the development of symptoms of Lyme disease. The area's proportion of infected nymphal ticks was 12%, which resulted in a 1.2% infection rate. Although there were two cases of erythema migrans in the placebo recipients, there were no cases of late Lyme disease. The authors concluded that routine prophylactic therapy for tick bites in such an endemic area of Lyme disease was not indicated, inasmuch as the risk of Lyme disease among persons with a recognized deer tick bite was low. The 1.2% infection rate falls at the lower end of the discretionary range of treatment, according to the cost-effectiveness model of Magid and coworkers,[102] and confirms their findings.

Although discouraged, antibiotic prophylaxis for tick bites is administered. In one study of 232 consecutive patients seen for an evaluation for possible Lyme disease in Maryland, 142 presented with tick bites; 55% were given antibiotic therapy. No patients with a tick bite developed clinical Lyme disease; however, $15,230 was attributable to the care, treatment, and testing of those who presented to the physician with an *Ixodes* tick bite.[104]

The decision to treat a tick bite should be made on an individualized basis, because the anxiety associated with watching and waiting for symptoms often drives the physician and patient toward prophylactic therapy. This is especially true for pregnant patients, in whom risking possible dissemination of the spirochete to the fetus can be an unacceptable alternative. Empirical treatment can also be justified in a patient in whom disseminated disease would be of dire consequence. Currently, the most effective means of preventing Lyme disease is to practice tick bite control measures, such as wearing protective clothing, avoiding tick-infested areas, and checking for ticks after potential exposure if living in or traveling to endemic areas (Table 39–2).

No data on the optimal dose or duration of prophylactic therapy exist. If empirical therapy is chosen, the author recommends oral doxycycline, 100 mg twice daily, or amoxicillin, 250 mg three times daily, for 10 days.

## Vaccination

A vaccine consisting of a purified OspA of *B. burgdorferi* is currently available for the prevention of Lyme disease (L-OspA). The OspA, OspB, and OspC lipoproteins are B cell and T cell immunogens in human infection and are protective against Lyme disease in rabbits, mice, and hamsters.[105] Immunization with recombinant flagellar protein, however, provides no protection against *B. burgdorferi*. Mice immunized with recombinant OspA were protected against *B. burgdorferi* by means of syringe and tick inoculation.

The OspA vaccine has a dual mode of action[106] in that *B. burgdorferi* is cleared from the infected tick after ingesting blood from the vaccinated host. *B. burgdorferi* organisms express primarily OspA in the tick's midgut but switch to expressing predominantly OspC when entering the host. Because transmission takes at least 36 hours, this allows the serum antibodies to OspA to neutralize the organism in the tick's midgut before it enters the host. Persons with natural *B. burgdorferi* infection do not have a prominent OspA antibody response.

Two pivotal efficacy studies[107, 108] demonstrated that three shots of OspA given at 0, 1, and 12 months pre-

vented between 76% and 90% of Lyme disease cases. After only two shots the efficacy was only between 49% and 68%. The vaccine was safe; up to 24% of the subjects experienced soreness at the infection site and 2% experienced fever, which resolved in a median of 3 days. Alternate vaccination schedules (0, 1, and 2 months and 0, 1, and 6 months) produce protective levels of antibody against *B. burgdorferi* infection.[109, 110] The vaccine is not currently approved for children less than 15 years of age or in adults older than 70 years, although efficacy studies with children are under way.

Of some concern is that in natural infection, antibody responses to OspA correlate with prolonged-treatment–resistant Lyme disease–induced arthritis in patients with human leukocyte antigen (HLA)–DR4.[37a] One study detailed the molecular mimicry between the predominant T cell epitope of OspA and the HLA-1 as a possible mechanism of autoimmunity in Lyme disease–induced arthritis.[110]

Whom to vaccinate has been addressed by the Centers for Disease Control and Prevention; this institution proposed that vaccination be considered in persons at high risk for Lyme disease, who both ''reside or otherwise spend time in high or moderate risk areas'' and ''engage in activities (recreation, property management, occupational or leisure) that result in frequent or prolonged exposure to tick-infested habitats.'' For persons at moderate risk, vaccination is considered optional; for persons at low risk, meaning from a nonendemic state and who do not reside in or otherwise spend time in moderate- or high-risk areas, vaccination is considered unnecessary.

Lyme disease vaccination alters the laboratory diagnosis of subsequent infection. Individuals with erythema migrans can be treated empirically, but serologic analysis should include a Western blot with examination of other bands exclusive of the 31-kd band. Several laboratories have started testing with an OspA-free strain to aid in diagnosing the disease in vaccinated patients.

Lyme disease remains a public health problem. Persons at risk need to be educated about prevention and about the signs and symptoms of Lyme disease. Early recognition and treatment of erythema migrans and neurologic symptoms can prevent later morbidity.

## TABLE 39–2
## Guidelines for Tick Prevention

When living in or traveling to a known endemic area:
1. Wear long-sleeved shirts.
2. Tuck long pants into socks or boots.
3. Wear light-colored clothing so that ticks can be easily spotted.
4. Stay on hiking paths; avoid brush.
5. Search exposed skin every 4 hours when outside.
6. Once inside, check your skin, particularly skin folds.

## REFERENCES

1. Burgdorfer W, Barbour AG, Hayes SF, et al: Lyme disease—A tick-borne spirochetosis? Science 1982; 216:1317–1319.
2. Steere AC, Malawista SE, Hardin JA, et al: Erythema chronicum migrans and Lyme arthritis. The enlarging clinical spectrum. Ann Intern Med 1977; 86:685–698.
3. Steere AC: Lyme disease. N Engl J Med 1989; 321:586–596.
4. Orloski K, Haye E, Campbell G, et al: Surveillance for Lyme disease. United States 1992–1998. MMWR CDC Surveill Summ 2000; 49(5503):1–11.
5. Tsai TF, Bailey RE, Moore PM: National surveillance of Lyme disease, 1987–1988. Conn Med 1992; 53:324.
6. Ciesielski CA, Markowitz LE, Horsley R, et al: The geographic distribution of Lyme disease in the United States. Ann N Y Acad Sci 1988; 539:283–288.
7. Anderson JF: Epizootiology of *Borrelia* in *Ixodes* tick vectors and reservoir hosts. Rev Infect Dis 1989; 2(suppl):1451.

8. Stanek G, Pletschette M, Flamm H, et al: European Lyme borreliosis. Ann N Y Acad Sci 1988; 539:274–282.

9. Dekonenko EJ, Steere AC, Berardi VP, et al: Lyme borreliosis in the Soviet Union: A cooperative US-USSR report. J Infect Dis 1988; 158:748–753.

10. Hellerstrom S: Erythema chronicum migrans afzelius with meningitis. Acta Der Venereol 1951; 31:227.

11. Afzelius A: Erythema chronicum migrans. Acta Derm Venereol 1921; 2:120.

12. Scrimenti RJ: Erythema chronicum migrans. Arch Dermatol Syphil 1970; 102:104–105.

13. Steere AC, Malawista SE, Snydman DR, et al: Lyme arthritis: An epidemic of oligoarticular arthritis in children and adults in three Connecticut communities. Arthritis Rheum 1977; 20:7–17.

14. Persing DH, Telford SR, Spielman A, et al: Detection of Borrelia burgdorferi infection in Ixodes dammini ticks with the polymerase chain reaction. J Clin Microbiol 1990; 28:566.

15. Levine JF, Wilson ML, Spielman A: Mice as reservoirs of the Lyme disease spirochete. Am J Trop Med Hyg 1985; 34:355–360.

16. Spielman A, Wilson ML, Levine JF: Ecology of Ixodes dammini–borne babesiosis and Lyme disease. Annu Rev Entomol 1985; 30:439.

17. Burgdorfer W: Vector/host relationships of the Lyme disease spirochete, Borrelia burgdorferi. Rheum Dis Clin North Am 1989; 15:775–787.

18. Burgdorfer W, Hayes SF, Benach JL: Development of Borrelia burgdorferi in ixodid tick vectors. Ann N Y Acad Sci 1988; 539:172–179.

19. Brown RN, Lane RS: Lyme disease in California: A novel enzootic transmission cycle of Borrelia burgdorferi. Science 1992; 256:1439.

20. Barbour AG, Hayes SF: Biology of Borrelia species. Microbiol Rev 1986; 50:381–400.

21. Howe TR, Mayer LW, Barbour AG: A single recombinant plasmid expressing two major outer surface proteins of the Lyme disease spirochete. Science 1985; 227:645–646.

22. Barbour AG, Heiland RA, Howe TR: Heterogeneity of major proteins in Lyme disease borreliae: A molecular analysis of North American and European isolates. J Infect Dis 1985; 152:478–484.

23. Barbour AG: Isolation and cultivation of Lyme disease spirochetes. Yale J Biol Med 1984; 57:521–525.

24. Georgilis K, Steere AC, Klempner MS: Infectivity of Borrelia burgdorferi correlates with resistance to elimination by phagocytic cells. J Infect Dis 1991; 163:150–155.

24a. Kelley WN, Harris ED Jr, Ruddy S, et al (eds): Textbook of Rheumatology, 6th ed. Philadelphia: WB Saunders, 2000.

25. Costello CM, Steere AC, Pinkerton RE, et al: A prospective study of tick bites in an endemic area for Lyme disease. J Infect Dis 1989; 159:136–139.

26. Steere AC, Bartenhagen NH, Craft JE, et al: The early clinical manifestations of Lyme disease. Ann Intern Med 1983; 99:76–82.

27. Malane MS, Grant-Kels JM, Feder HM, et al: Diagnosis of Lyme disease based on dermatologic manifestations. Ann Intern Med 1991; 114:490.

28. Steere AC, Taylor E, Wilson ML, et al: Longitudinal assessment of the clinical and epidemiological features of Lyme disease in a defined population. J Infect Dis 1986; 154:295–300.

29. Case definition for public health surveillance. MMWR Morb Mortal Wkly Rep 1990; 39:19–21.

30. Dattwyler RJ, Volkman DJ, Luft BJ, et al: Seronegative Lyme disease. Dissociation of specific T- and B-lymphocyte responses to Borrelia burgdorferi. N Engl J Med 1988; 319:1441–1446.

31. Craft JE, Grodzicki RL, Steere AC: Antibody response in Lyme disease: Evaluation of diagnostic tests. J Infect Dis 1984; 149:789–795.

32. Craft JE, Fischer DK, Shimamoto GT, et al: Antigens of Borrelia burgdorferi recognized during Lyme disease. Appearance of a new immunoglobulin M response and expansion of the immunoglobulin G response late in the illness. J Clin Invest 1986; 78:934–939.

33. Magnarelli LA, Miller JN, Anderson JF, et al: Cross-reactivity of nonspecific treponemal antibody in serologic tests for Lyme disease. J Clin Microbiol 1990; 28:1276.

34. Schwartz BS, Goldstein MD, Ribeiro JMC, et al: Antibody testing in Lyme disease: A comparison of results in four laboratories. JAMA 1989; 262:3431.

35. Berardi VP, Weeks KE, Steere AC: Serodiagnosis of early Lyme disease: Analysis of IgM and IgG antibody responses by using an antibody-capture enzyme immunoassay. J Infect Dis 1988; 158:754–760.

36. Steere AC, Berardi VP, Weeks KE, et al: Evaluation of the intrathecal antibody response to Borrelia burgdorferi as a diagnostic test for Lyme neuroborreliosis. J Infect Dis 1990; 161:1203–1209.

37. Hansen K, Bangsborg JM, Fjordvang H: Immunochemical characterization of an isolation of the gene for a Borrelia burgdorferi immunodominant 60 kD antigen common to a wide range of bacteria. Infect Immun 1988; 56:2047.

37a. Kalish RA, Leong JM, Steere AC: Association of treatment resistant chronic Lyme arthritis with HLA-DR4 and antibody reactivity to OspA and OspB of Borrelia burgdorferi. Infect Immun 1993; 61:2774–2779.

38. Dressler F, Whalen JA, Reinhardt BN, et al: Western blotting in the serodiagnosis of Lyme disease. J Infect Dis 1993; 167:392–400.

39. Nocten JJ, Dresler F, Rutledge BJ, et al: Detection of B. burgdorferi by polymerase chain reaction in synovial fluid from patients with Lyme disease. N Engl J Med 1994; 330:229–234.

40. Johnson RC, Kodner C, Jurkovich PJ, et al: Comparative in vitro and in vivo susceptibilities of the Lyme disease spirochete Borrelia burgdorferi to cefuroxime and other antimicrobial agents. Antimicrob Agents Chemother 1990; 34(11):2133.

41. Johnson SE, Klein GC, Schmid GP, Feeley JC: Susceptibility of the Lyme disease spirochete to seven antimicrobial agents. Yale J Biol Med 1984; 57:549–553.

42. Johnson RC, Kadner C, Russell M, Girard D: In-vitro and in-vivo susceptibility of Borrelia burgdorferi to azithromycin. J Antimicrob Chemother 1990; Suppl A:33–38.

43. Alder J, Mitten M, Jarvis K: Efficacy of clarithromycin for treatment of experimental Lyme disease in vivo. Antimicrob Agents Chemother 1993; 37(6):1329.

43a. Dever LL, Jorgensen JH, Barbour AG: In vitro activity of vancomycin against the spirochete Borrelia burgdorferi. Antimicrob Agents Chemother 1993; 37(5):1115.

44. Hansen K, Hovmark A, Lebech AM: Roxithromycin in Lyme borreliosis: Discrepant results of an in vitro and in vivo animal susceptibility study and a clinical trial in patients with erythema migrans. Acta Derm Venereol 1992; 72(4):297.

45. Steere AC, Malawista SE, Newman JH, et al: Antibiotic therapy in Lyme disease. Ann Intern Med 1980; 93:1–8.

46. Steere AC, Hutchinson GJ, Rahn DW, et al: Treatment of the early manifestations of Lyme disease. Ann Intern Med 1983; 99:22–26.

47. Dattwyler RJ, Halperin JJ: Failure of tetracycline therapy in early Lyme disease. Arthritis Rheum 1987; 30:448–450.

48. Dattwyler RJ, Volkman DJ, Conaty SM, et al: Amoxicillin plus probenecid versus doxycycline for treatment of erythema migrans borreliosis. Lancet 1990; 336:1404–1406.

49. Asbrink E, Hovmark A: Early and late cutaneous manifestations in Ixodes-borne borreliosis (erythema migrans borreliosis, Lyme borreliosis). Ann N Y Acad Sci 1988; 539:4–15.

50. Weber K, Preac-Mursic V, Wilske B, et al.: A randomized trial of ceftriaxone versus oral penicillin for the treatment of early European Lyme borreliosis. Infection 1990; 18:91–96.

51. Green CR, Rosenblum A: Report of the penicillin study group—American Academy of Allergy. J Allergy Clin Immunol 1971; 48:331.

52. Standiford HC: Tetracyclines and chloramphenicol. In Mandell GL, Douglas RG, Bennett JE (eds): Principals and Practice of Infectious Diseases, 3rd ed. New York: Churchill Livingstone, 1990:284.

52a. Massarotti EM, Luger SW, Rahn DW, et al: Treatment of early Lyme disease. Am J Med 1992; 92(4):396–403.

53. Gerber MA, Shapiro ED, Burke GS, et al: Lyme disease in children in southeastern Connecticut. N Engl J Med 1996; 335:1270.

54. Dattwyler RJ, Grunwaldt E, Luft BJ: Clarithromycin in treatment of early Lyme disease: A pilot study. Antimicrob Agents Chemother 1996; 40:468–469.

55. Nadelman RB, Luger SW, Frank E: Comparison of cefuroxime axetil and doxycycline in the treatment of early Lyme disease. Ann Intern Med 1992; 117:273.

56. Luger SW, Paparone P, Wormser GP, et al: Comparison of cefuroxime axetil and doxycycline in treatment of patients with early lyme disease associated with erythema migrans. Antimicrob Agents Chemother 1995; 39:661–667.

57. Dattwyler RJ, Luft BJ, Kunkel MJ, et al: Ceftriaxone compared with doxycycline for the treatment of acute disseminated Lyme disease. N Engl J Med 1997; 337:289.

58. Garcia-Monco JC, Villar BF, Alen JC, et al: Borrelia burgdorferi in the central nervous system: Experimental and clinical evidence for early invasion. J Infect Dis 1990; 161:1187–1193.

59. Donowitz GR, Mandell GL: Cephalosporins. In Mandell GL, Douglas RG, Bennett JE (eds): Principals and Practice of Infectious Diseases, 3rd ed. New York: Churchill Livingstone, 1990:246.

59a. Dattwyler RJ, Halperin JJ, Volkman DJ, et al: Treatment of late Lyme borreliosis—Randomised comparison of ceftriaxone and penicillin. Lancet 1988; 1:1191–1194.

60. Bojar M, Hercogova J, Valesova M, et al: Cefotaxime in the Treatment of Lyme Borreliosis. Presented at the Fourth European Congress of Clinical Microbiology, Nice, France, 1989.

61. Pfister HW, Preac-Mursic V, Wilske B, et al: Randomized comparison of ceftriaxone and cefotaxime in Lyme neuroborreliosis. J Infect Dis 1991; 163:311–318.

62. Karlsson M, Hammers-Berggren S, Lindquist L, et al: Comparison of intravenous penicillin G and oral doxycycline for treatment of Lyme disease: Recognition and management. Neurology 1994; 44:1203.

63. Diringer MN, Halperin JJ, Dattwyler RJ: Lyme meningoencephalitis: Report of a severe, penicillin-resistant case. Arthritis Rheum 1987; 30:705–708.

64. Dotevall L, Alestig K, Hanner P: The use of doxycycline in nervous system Borrelia burgdorferi infection. Scand J Infect Dis 1988; 53(suppl):74.

65. Logigian EL, Kaplan RF, Steere AC: Chronic neurologic manifestations of Lyme disease. N Engl J Med 1990; 323:1438–1444.

66. Logigian EL, Steere AC: Clinical and electrophysiologic findings in chronic neuropathy of Lyme disease. Neurology 1992; 42:303–311.

67. Steere AC, Broderick TF, Malawista SE: Erythema chronicum migrans and Lyme arthritis: Epidemiologic evidence for a tick vector. Am J Epidemiol 1978; 108:312–321.

68. de Koning J, Hoogkaamp-Korstanje JAA, van der Line MR: Demonstration of spirochete in cardiac biopsies of patients with Lyme disease. J Infect Dis 1989; 160:150.

69. Marcus LC, Steere AC, Duray PH, et al: Fatal pancarditis in a patient with coexistent Lyme disease and babesiosis. Demonstration of spirochetes in the myocardium. Ann Intern Med 1985; 103:374–376.

70. Stanek F, Klein J, Bittner R, et al: Isolation of Borrelia burgdorferi from the myocardium of a patient with longstanding cardiomyopathy. N Engl J Med 1990; 322:249.

71. McAlister HF, Klementowicz PT, Andrews C, et al: Lyme carditis: An important cause of reversible heart block. Ann Intern Med 1989; 110:339–345.

72. Gasser R, Dusleag J, Fruhwald F: Early antimicrobial treatment of dilated cardiomyopathy associated with Borrelia burgdorferi. Lancet 1992; 340:982.

73. Vegsundvag J, Nordeide J, Reikvam A, et al: Late cardiac manifestation of infection with Borrelia burgdorferi (Lyme disease). BMJ 1993; 307:173.

74. Blaauw AA, van der Linden SJ, Kuiper J: Lyme carditis in the Netherlands. Ann Intern Med 1989; 111:261.

75. Artigao R, Torres G, Guerrero A: Irreversible complete heart block in Lyme disease. Am J Med 1991; 90:531.

76. Sangha O, Phillips CB, Fleischmann KE, et al: Lack of cardiac manifestations among patients with previously treated Lyme disease. Ann Intern Med 1998; 128:346–353.

77. Steere AC, Schoen RT, Taylor E: The clinical evolution of Lyme arthritis. Ann Intern Med 1987; 107:725–731.

78. Lawson JP, Steere AC: Lyme arthritis: Radiologic findings. Radiology 1985; 154:37–43.

79. Steere AC, Dwyer E, Winchester R: Association of chronic Lyme arthritis with HLA-DR4 and HLA-DR2 alleles. N Engl J Med 1990; 323:219–223. [Published erratum appears in N Engl J Med 1991; 324(2):129]

80. Steere AC, Malawista SE, Craft JE, et al: International symposium on Lyme disease. Yale J Biol Med 1984; 57:445.

81. Steere AC, Levin RE, Molloy PJ, et al.: Treatment of Lyme arthritis. Arthritis Rheum 1994; 37:878–888.

82. Schlesinger PA, Duray PH, Burke BA, et al: Maternal-fetal transmission of the Lyme disease spirochete, Borrelia burgdorferi. Ann Intern Med 1985; 103:67–68.

83. Weber K, Bratzke HJ, Neubert U: Borrelia burgdorferi in a newborn despite oral penicillin for Lyme borreliosis during pregnancy. Pediatr Infect Dis J 1988; 7:286–289.

84. MacDonald AB, Benach JL, Burgdorfer W: Stillbirth following maternal Lyme disease. N Y State J Med 1987; 87:615.

85. Markowitz LE, Steere AC, Benach JL, et al: Lyme disease during pregnancy. JAMA 1986; 255:3394–3396.

86. Sigal LH: Therapy for Lyme disease. Drugs 1992; 43:683.

87. Dinerman H, Steere AC: Lyme disease associated with fibromyalgia. Ann Intern Med 1992; 117:281–285.

88. Shadick NA, Phillips CB, Sangha DS, et al: Musculoskeletal and neurological outcomes in patients with previously treated Lyme disease. Ann Intern Med 1999; 131:919–926.

89. Nadelman RB, Arlin Z, Wormser GP: Life-threatening complication of empiric ceftriaxone therapy for "seronegative Lyme disease." South Med J 1991; 84(10):1263.

90. Sigal LH: Summary of the first 100 patients seen at a Lyme disease referral center. Am J Med 1990; 117:281.

91. Steere AC, Taylor E, McHugh GL, et al: The overdiagnosis of Lyme disease. JAMA 1993; 269:1812.

92. Lightfoot RW Jr, Luft BJ, Rahn DW, et al: Empiric parenteral antibiotic treatment of patients with fibromyalgia and fatigue and a positive serologic result for Lyme disease. A cost-effectiveness analysis. Ann Intern Med 1993; 119:503–509.

93. Schwartz BS, Goldstein MD, Childs JE: Longitudinal study of Borrelia burgdorferi infection in New Jersey outdoor workers, 1988–1991. Am J Epidemiol 1994; 139:504–512.

94. Schwartz BS, Goldstein MD: Lyme disease in outdoor workers: Risk factors, preventive measures, and tick removal methods. Am J Epidemiol 1990; 131:877–885.

95. Spielman A: Prospects for suppressing transmission of Lyme disease. Ann N Y Acad Sci 1988; 539:212–220.

96. Piesman J, Mather IN, Sinsky RJ, Spielman A: Duration of tick attachment and Borrelia burgdorferi transmission. J Clin Microbiol 1987; 25:557–558.

97. Cartter ML, Farley TA, Ardito HA, et al: Lyme disease prevention—Knowledge, beliefs, and behaviors among high school students in an endemic area. Conn Med 1989; 53:354–356.

98. Herrington JEJ, Campbell GL, Bailey RE, et al: Predisposing factors for individuals' Lyme disease prevention practices: Connecticut, Maine, and Montana. Am J Public Health 1997; 87:2035–2038.

99. Shadick NA, Daltroy LH, Phillips CB, et al: Determinants of tick avoidance behaviors in an endemic area for Lyme disease. Am J Prev Med 1997; 13:264–270.

100. Matuschka FR, Fischer P, Heiler M: Stage-associated risk of transmission of the Lyme disease spirochete by European Ixodes ticks. Parsitol Res 1992; 78:695.

101. Matuschka FR, Spielman A: Risk of infection from and treatment of Lyme disease. Lancet 1993; 342:529.

102. Magid D, Schwartz B, Craft J, et al: Prevention of Lyme disease after tick bites. A cost-effectiveness analysis. N Engl J Med 1992; 327:534–41.

103. Shapiro ED, Gerber MA, Holabird NB: A controlled trial of antimicrobial prophylaxis for Lyme disease after deer tick bites. N Engl J Med 1992; 327:1769.

104. Fix AD, Strickland GT, Grant J: Tick bites and Lyme disease in an endemic setting: Problematic use of serologic testing and prophylactic antibiotic therapy. JAMA 1998; 279:206–210.

105. Fikrig E, Bathold SW, Kantor FS, et al: Protection of mice against the Lyme disease agent by immunizing with recombinant Osp A. Science 1990; 250:553.

106. Shih CM, Spielman A, Telford SR. Short report: Mode of action of protective immunity to Lyme disease spirochetes. Am J Trop Med Hyg 1995; 52:72–74.

107. Steere AC, Sikand V, Meurice F, et al: Vaccination against Lyme disease with recombinant *Borrelia burgdorferi* outer-surface lipoprotein A with adjuvant. N Engl J Med 1998; 339:209–215.

108. Sigal LH, Zahradnik JM, Lavin P, et al: A vaccine consisting of recombinant *Borrelia burgdorferi* outer-surface protein A to prevent Lyme disease. N Engl J Med 1998; 339:216–222.

109. Van Hoecke C, Lebacq E, Beran J, et al: Alternative vaccination schedules (0, 1, and 6 months and 0, 1, and 12 months) for a recombinant OspA Lyme disease vaccine. Clin Infect Disease 1999; 28:1260–1264.

110. Parent D, Schoen R, Sikand V, et al: Evaluation of reactogenicity and immunogenicity of Lymerix, recombinant 2-OspA vaccine against Lyme disease administered on two different schedules [Abstract]. Denver: Meeting of the Infectious Disease Society of America, 1998:705.

111. Gross DM, Forsthuber T, Tary-Lehmann M, et al: Identification of LFA-1 as a candidate autoantigen in treatment-resistant Lyme arthritis. Science 1998; 281:703–706.

# 40 | Osteoporosis and Rheumatic Disorders

*Miriam F. Delaney, John Wade, and Meryl S. LeBoff*

Osteoporosis is a disease characterized by generalized loss of bone mass, which leads to increased risk of fracture. Twenty-eight million Americans have osteoporosis or are at risk for osteoporosis. Of the population over 51 years of age, 40% of women and 13% of men suffer one or more osteoporotic fractures during their lifetime, at a cost to the health care system in excess of $13.8 billion per year. The number of elderly people in the population is increasing rapidly, and because fractures are associated with increasing age, it is estimated that the number of fractures and associated costs could triple by the year 2040.[1] Strategies to prevent bone loss in patients at risk of osteoporosis may have a substantial impact on reducing the anticipated number of fractures, morbidity, and health care costs.

The skeleton is composed of 20% of trabecular bone, which is more metabolically active and is located in the spine, epiphyses, and pelvis, and 80% of cortical bone, which is concentrated in the appendicular skeleton. Bone mass is normally maintained by the tight coupling of bone resorption by osteoclasts and bone formation by osteoblasts. Peak bone mass is achieved after puberty until the third decade; thereafter, there are age-related decreases in bone mass in both sexes. In women, there is a phase of accelerated bone loss during early menopause; this loss slows after 5 to 8 years. During the course of a lifetime, women lose approximately 50% of the bone in the spine and proximal femur and 30% of the bone in the appendicular skeleton; men lose approximately 33% and 20%, respectively.[1] Bone loss is therefore a universal component of aging, but this process is now both preventable and treatable.

Osteoporosis in patients with rheumatic disease is of particular concern because bone loss may result from the disease process and from the medications used to control inflammation. Decreased bone mass, combined with an increased tendency of persons with musculoskeletal disease to fall, may also increase the risk of fracture. This chapter focuses (1) on the diagnosis and treatment of osteoporosis both in general and in patients with systemic rheumatic disorders and (2) on the skeletal effects of corticosteroids and other drugs used to treat rheumatic diseases.

## OSTEOPOROTIC RISK FACTORS AND SECONDARY CAUSES OF BONE LOSS AND OSTEOPOROSIS

Peak bone mass accumulation is achieved by the second to third decade, after which several factors influence the rate of bone loss. Risk factors for osteoporosis include a personal history of a fracture after age 40, first-degree relative with a history of fracture, white or Asian race, cigarette smoking, weight less than 127 pounds, height more than 5 feet 7 inches, advanced age, frailty, and dementia.[2] Secondary modifiable risk factors include inadequate intake of dietary calcium and vitamin D, low testosterone levels in men, premenopausal estrogen deficiency, excessive alcohol intake, impaired vision, neurologic disorders, lack of sunlight, and physical inactivity.[2] There is evidence that genetics are strong determinants of bone mass.[3] Collagen type $1\alpha1$ (COL1$\alpha$1) gene is associated with lower bone density and an increased risk of fracture.[4] There are racial differences in the prevalence of osteoporosis: 21% of postmenopausal American white women have osteoporosis, in comparison with 10% of African American women and 16% of Mexican American women.[5]

Although osteoporosis is a heterogeneous disorder, it develops as a consequence of a net increase in bone resorption with insufficient new bone formation. Secondary causes of osteoporosis may accelerate bone loss and increase the risk of osteoporosis with increasing age. Secondary causes include gonadal deficiencies (hypogonadism in men, premenopausal amenorrhea lasting more than 1 year, premature ovarian failure at less than 45 years of age, and menopause), decreased body mass index and decreased body fat, excessive alcohol intake, cigarette smoking, medical conditions altering bone turnover, and medications interfering with bone metabolism (Table 40–1). Hypercortisolism in Cushing's syndrome often produces osteoporosis, and administration of exogenous corticosteroids is the most common secondary cause of bone loss. Hyperthyroidism increases bone turnover; supraphysiologic doses of thyroid hormone (once the thyroid-stimulat-

## TABLE 40–1
## Causes of Osteoporosis/Osteopenia

*Primary osteoporosis:* Juvenile osteoporosis, idiopathic osteoporosis, postmenopausal osteoporosis, involutional osteoporosis
*Endocrine abnormalities:* Corticosteroid excess, thyrotoxicosis, hypogonadism (causes including anorexia nervosa and prolactinomas), primary hyperparathyroidism, hypercalciuria, vitamin D deficiency
*Process affecting the marrow:* Multiple myeloma, leukemia, lymphoma, anemias (sickle cell disease, thalassemia minor, Gaucher's disease, mastocytosis)
*Immobilization:* Bed rest, space flight
*Gastrointestinal diseases:* Postgastrectomy, celiac disease, primary biliary or alcoholic cirrhosis
*Drugs:* Anticonvulsants, heparin, methotrexate, corticosteroids, excess thyroid hormone, gonadotropin-releasing hormone agonist, cyclophosphamide, lithium, cyclosporine, aluminum, premenopausal tamoxifen, excessive alcohol
*Connective tissue disorders:* Osteogenesis imperfecta, scurvy, homocystinuria, Ehlers-Danlos syndrome
*Rheumatologic disorders:* Ankylosing spondylitis, rheumatoid arthritis, systemic lupus erythematosus

Modified from LeBoff MS, Fuleihan El-Hajj G, Brown E: Osteoporosis and Paget's disease of bone. *In* Branch WT (ed): Office Practice of Medicine. Philadelphia: WB Saunders, 1994:700.

ing hormone [TSH] level is suppressed) may cause bone loss,[6] even though concentrations of thyroid hormone may be within the normal range. Amenorrhea and hypogonadism may result from use of gonadotropin-releasing hormone (GnRH) agonists,[7] hyperprolactinemia, cytotoxic drugs, or anorexia nervosa,[8] and testosterone deficiency[9] in men may be associated with bone loss. Table 40–1 lists other secondary causes of osteopenia and osteoporosis.[10]

## BONE DENSITOMETRY

Bone density is the best single predictor of a future fracture risk. The advances in bone densitometry and the development of newer techniques such as dual energy x-ray absorptiometry (DEXA) make it possible to rapidly and precisely quantify the amount of bone in the relevant fracture sites of the spine, proximal femur, forearm, and total body with minimal radiation

k = 1.229  d0 = 110.1(1.000H)  6.461

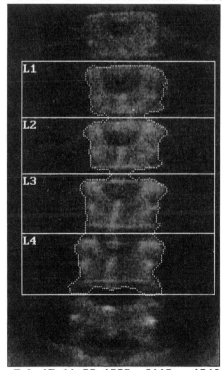

·Feb 17 11:00 1999  [113 x 134]
Hologic QDR-2000 (S/N 2413)
Array Spine Medium V4.66A:1

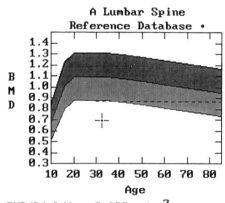

BMD(L1-L4) = 0.689 g/cm$^2$

| Region | BMD | T(30.0) | | Z | |
|--------|-----|---------|---|---|---|
| L1 | 0.660 | -3.16 | 65% | -3.16 | 65% |
| L2 | 0.710 | -3.49 | 65% | -3.49 | 65% |
| L3 | 0.698 | -3.68 | 63% | -3.68 | 63% |
| L4 | 0.688 | -4.15 | 60% | -4.15 | 60% |
| L1-L4 | 0.689 | -3.65 | 63% | -3.65 | 63% |

• Age and sex matched
T = peak BMD matched
Z = age matched          TK      11/04/91

FIGURE 40–1
Bone density of the lumbar spine (L1 to L4) in a 32-year-old man treated with corticosteroids, as measured by dual energy x-ray absorptiometry. Note the marked reduction in bone density, which is 3.65 standard deviations below peak bone mass (T score) and 3.65 standard deviations below age-matched controls (Z score).

exposure (e.g., 3 to 6 mrad each and 0.5 mrad for total body). The bone mineral density (BMD) in a patient is reported as a standard deviation in comparison with that of (1) young normal controls, to assess whether there is a decrease in BMD from peak bone mass (T score), and (2) age-matched controls, to determine whether the bone density is reduced relative to age-matched controls (Z score) (Fig. 40–1). Diagnostic criteria for BMD were established by the World Health Organization (WHO): normal BMD is represented by a T score of more than −1; osteopenia (low bone mass) is represented by a T score between −1 and −2.5; and established osteoporosis is represented by a T score of less than −2.5 and a previous history of a fragility fracture. Prospective studies show that in subjects over 60 years of age, a 1–standard deviation decrement in BMD in comparison with age-adjusted controls is associated with a 1.3 to 2.8 increase in relative risk of fracture.[11] A reduced bone density of the proximal femur is more predictive of increased risk of a fracture in the hip than at an alternative site.

The indications for bone densitometry measurements established by the Scientific Advisory Board of the National Osteoporosis Foundation are as follows: (1) estrogen deficiency or postmenopausal state in women less than 65 years old with one or more risk factors; (2) age over 65 years old for all women regardless of risk factors; (3) fractures in postmenopausal women; (4) monitoring efficacy of treatment in patients receiving prolonged estrogen replacement or other therapy for osteoporosis; (5) consideration of hormone therapy in women if a BMD would facilitate the decision. These indications are now incorporated into the Health Care Financing Administration policy, which also recommends BMD for (1) all patients with primary or secondary hyperparathyroidism, because a low bone mass identifies patients at risk for osteoporosis, is an indication for parathyroidectomy, or is an indication for therapeutic intervention, and (2) all corticosteroid-treated patients, to determine low bone mass and the need for therapy. In healthy premenopausal women, the use of bone densitometry for screening purposes is not cost effective.[5]

Therapeutic interventions are recommended for prevention of bone loss in patients with osteopenia and for treatment of patients with osteoporosis; these treatment options are discussed in later sections. Studies, however, suggest that changes in BMD may underestimate improvements in bone strength as seen when the mechanical force required to fracture a bone is calculated. Significantly different increases in BMD are seen with alendronate and calcitonin (6% per year vs. 2% to 3% per year) and yet both decrease fracture risk (48% vs. 37%, respectively). Future studies will increase our understanding of fracture prevention and how best to monitor therapy.

## OSTEOPOROSIS IN RHEUMATOID ARTHRITIS

Rheumatoid arthritis (RA) is associated with development of periarticular and generalized osteopenia and

increased incidence of fractures, which in turn may add substantially to the disability already associated with RA. Gough and associates[12] studied patients who had had RA for less than 2 years and compared them with healthy controls over a 2-year period, monitoring bone density and markers of bone turnover. Patients with early RA lost 3% of lumbar BMD and 5% of femoral neck BMD, in comparison with 1% losses in controls. This finding is in contrast with those of previous studies, which showed an increase in bone loss in the distal radius but failed to show accelerated spinal bone loss early in the course of the disease.[13] Investigations with bone densitometry in patients with long-standing RA showed significant decrements in BMD of the proximal femur, the lumbar spine, and the appendicular sites ranging from approximately 5% to 25%.[14, 15] Consistent with these findings is evidence of increased trabecular bone loss in iliac crest biopsies in women with RA.[16] Reported levels of circulating sex corticosteroids in women with RA are conflicting. Demir and colleagues studied patients with active and quiescent RA and found that basal and stimulated levels of cortisol, growth hormone, and adrenocorticotropic hormone (ACTH) were impaired by 65%, 85%, and 30%, respectively.[17] Other data showed reduced levels of the major adrenal androgen precursor to estrogen, dehydroepiandrosterone sulfate (DHEAS), in postmenopausal women with RA in comparison with control subjects. This may be a consequence of chronic illness and an alteration in the hypothalamic-pituitary-adrenal axis resulting from suppression of the immune system.[18] These low adrenal androgen levels are of potential importance because, in addition to being precursors of estrone, androgens are protective of bone. Sambrook and coworkers[19] showed a positive correlation between DHEAS levels and longitudinal changes in femoral neck bone density in postmenopausal women with RA.

Physical activity correlates with bone density measurements[3] and is an important determinant of osteoporosis in RA.[20] Patients with severe functional impairment have the lowest forearm bone density.[21] Other factors postulated to contribute to the decreased BMD and osteoporotic fractures in RA include enhanced inflammatory processes with elevated mediators of bone resorption; corticosteroid therapy; and other drug therapy.[3, 22]

## RHEUMATOID ARTHRITIS: POTENTIAL MEDIATORS OF BONE LOSS

The release of inflammatory cytokines or other local factors from the macrophages, fibroblasts, and T cells present in rheumatoid synovium may also contribute to the increased bone loss in RA.[23] Synovial biopsies from patients with RA, when cultured with 1,25(OH)$_2$ vitamin D, are capable of differentiating to osteoclasts.[24] The following are potential mediators of bone loss in RA: (1) interleukin (IL)–1, IL-6, IL-15, and IL-17; (2) tumor necrosis factor (TNF); (3) heparin;

(4) nitric oxide; and (5) prostaglandins. There are significant elevations of IL-1 in the blood and synovial fluid in patients with RA, which stimulates osteoclast formation, activation, and bone resorption.[23, 25] Elevations of TNF-$\alpha$ in the blood and synovial fluid[26] and high concentrations of IL-6 in the synovium,[25, 27] both of which can increase bone resorption and stimulate osteoclast formation, may also contribute to the development of osteoporosis in patients with RA. Studies have shown that IL-15 and IL-17 appear to induce osteoblasts to synthesize prostaglandins and promote osteoclastic maturation, which may be a crucial step in RA-induced bone resorption.[28, 29] In addition, release of mast cell heparin in patients with RA may accelerate bone loss. The mechanisms underlying the effects of heparin on skeletal metabolism have not been fully elucidated, although heparin promotes parathyroid hormone (PTH)–mediated bone loss and may increase bone collagen metabolism.[30] Nitric oxide and prostaglandins, regulated by cytokines such as IL-1 and TNF-$\alpha$, are produced in the rheumatoid synovium, and high concentrations of prostaglandins, particularly prostaglandin E$_2$ (PGE$_2$), enhance bone resorption.[31]

## BONE METABOLISM IN RHEUMATOID ARTHRITIS

To assess whether the skeletal changes in patients with RA represent more generalized abnormalities in mineral metabolism, investigators have examined indices of skeletal homeostasis. Normally, there is an inverse relationship between changes in calcium concentrations and PTH secretion, so that a small decrease in the ionized calcium concentration augments PTH release, with secondary renal conservation of calcium, mobilization of calcium from bone, and activation of 25-hydroxyvitamin D to 1,25-dihydroxyvitamin D, which in turn stimulates intestinal calcium absorption. The reduced serum calcium levels in patients with RA reported in early studies probably represent decreased calcium-binding proteins from chronic disease and not a reduction in ionized calcium concentrations, although the latter were not measured.[32] Moreover, in patients with RA, levels of PTH and vitamin D metabolites are generally similar to those in controls, thus indicating no abnormality in calcium metabolism.[33]

Studies of markers of bone turnover confirm the results of the in vivo and in vitro studies described earlier. Gough and associates[12] studied patients with RA for less than 2 years. In addition to the bone losses described earlier, the markers of bone formation, osteocalcin and alkaline phosphatase, are reduced in early disease but do not correlate well with disease activity or changes in bone density. Gough and associates found that urinary pyridinoline and deoxypyridinoline concentrations, the markers of bone resorption, are elevated in patients with active RA and closely correlated with changes in BMD. Levels of C-reactive protein correlated with markers of bone resorption and changes in bone density. This suggests that the degree

of systemic and local inflammation may control bone loss.

## RHEUMATOID ARTHRITIS AND CORTICOSTEROIDS

Early studies of patients with RA indicated accelerated bone loss caused by corticosteroid administration.[34] Corticosteroids are associated with an increased risk of osteoporosis. Consistent with these deleterious effects of corticosteroids on bone are the observations of Dykman and associates,[34] who showed that large cumulative doses of corticosteroids in patients with rheumatic diseases increased both trabecular bone loss in the forearm and the risk of skeletal fractures. Als and colleagues[35] observed decreased bone density in corticosteroid-treated premenopausal women with RA, which correlated with the duration of therapy and the cumulative dose. A randomized controlled trial by Laan and coworkers[36] showed early bone loss in the spine in a group of rheumatoid patients treated for up to 20 weeks with prednisone (mean dose, 7.5 mg/day), which was partially reversible with discontinuation of therapy. Reid and associates,[37] however, showed that although patients with RA who are treated with corticosteroids undergo an early reduction in bone density, patients receiving long-term corticosteroid therapy have less bone loss than do patients treated with calcium supplements or anti-inflammatory drugs, including nonsteroidal anti-inflammatory drugs (NSAIDs), penicillamine, and gold.

A large cross-sectional study of 195 patients with rheumatoid arthritis suggests that bone loss in patients with RA is more evident in the proximal femur than in the spine.[38] Both cumulative corticosteroid dose and disability correlate significantly with bone density. In patients who had discontinued corticosteroid therapy, however, bone densities were similar to those of patients who had never used corticosteroids. Other data indicate that postmenopausal women with RA who take long-term, low-dose corticosteroids or groups of premenopausal and postmenopausal women taking low doses of prednisone do not have an additional decrease in bone density in comparison with non–corticosteroid-treated subjects with RA.[13, 34, 35, 39] The lack of an adverse effect of low-dose corticosteroids on bone mass in postmenopausal women with RA probably results from suppression of the active inflammatory process and of cytokines and/or from improved function and increased physical activity.[21] Corticosteroids may therefore produce an early loss of bone, but this bone loss may be attenuated over time by better control of the disease process, increased ambulation, and physical activity.[40]

## CORTICOSTEROIDS AND OSTEOPOROSIS

Glucocorticoids have been known for many years to cause osteoporosis. Steroids are a necessary mainstay of therapy for many medical conditions, including RA, polymyalgia rheumatica, giant cell arteritis, connective tissue disease (systemic lupus erythematosus, mixed connective tissue disease, polymyositis, and overlap syndromes), and vasculitis. Osteoporotic fractures or osteonecrosis occurs in up to 50% of patients treated with long-term glucocorticoids. The risk of bone loss or associated fracture risk is determined by the cumulative corticosteroid dose, increasing age,[41] and/or menopausal status.[34]

Steroids primarily cause a decrease in bone formation.[42] The mechanism appears to be a decrease in osteoblast activity, resulting in a decrease in osteoblast function and premature apoptosis. Impaired osteoblast function is manifested as an initial induction of osteoblast differentiation, followed by decreased synthesis of both type I collagen and osteocalcin and decreased osteoblast replication.[43, 44] Corticosteroids reduce serum osteocalcin levels in a dose-dependent relationship, thereby indicating suppression of bone formation.[45, 46] These mechanisms contribute to incomplete repair of bone resorption cavities, thereby causing bone loss. The production of osteoclasts is also decreased, leading to a decrease in bone turnover. The result is a weakened bone matrix with thin, bony trabeculae that contributes to osteoporosis.[43]

Treatment of patients with more than 15 mg of prednisone per day impairs intestinal calcium absorption and increases urinary calcium excretion.[41, 45, 47, 48] These mechanisms appear to play an important role in the development of secondary hyperparathyroidism.[47, 49] Although in vitro studies have shown both stimulation and inhibition of bone resorption after corticosteroid exposure,[50, 51] parathyroidectomized rats exposed to corticosteroids do not display enhanced bone loss, which suggests that the bone resorption in this setting may be mediated by PTH.[52] PTH increases the resorption of bone directly and also increases the number of sites at which bone remodeling occurs. Lower doses of prednisone (range, 2.5 to 10 mg/day) in patients with RA do not affect PTH levels,[39] as measured by the immunoradiometric assay for intact hormone. Also, alternate-day glucocorticoid regimens may maintain intestinal calcium absorption and prevent elevations of PTH but do not prevent bone loss in adults.[53] Earlier studies indicated that corticosteroids interfere with the activation of vitamin D to 25-hydroxyvitamin D as well as to 1,25-dihydroxyvitamin D, but more recent data show that corticosteroids do not interfere with the metabolism of vitamin D.[42] Steroids may negatively influence calcium transport mechanisms in the bowel mucosa by reducing levels of vitamin D receptors and possibly inhibiting protein synthesis.[54]

Corticosteroid therapy causes hypogonadism, which may further contribute to bone loss. Corticosteroids inhibit pituitary secretion of gonadotropins and also directly decrease gonadal production of estrogen and testosterone. Steroid therapy[55, 56] reduces circulating free testosterone by as much as 50% in a dose-dependent manner. Reid and associates[55] showed that prednisone, more than 10 mg/day for an average of 7 years, caused a 33% reduction in total testosterone

and a 40% decrease in free testosterone. Steroids also reduce endogenous ACTH levels and adrenal androgen production of androstenedione and DHEAS.[18, 57] Decreases in sex hormones exacerbate the bone loss by increasing osteoclast-mediated bone resorption. Glucocorticoid-induced myopathy and muscle weakness also contribute to bone loss by removing the forces on bone produced by muscle contraction.

The phase of the most rapid glucocorticoid-induced bone loss occurs within the first 6 months of therapy, with losses of 3% to 15% in the lumbar spine at 1 year. In a meta-analysis of two randomized controlled trials in early RA, Verhoeven and Boers[40] showed that patients with RA treated with 1 to 10 mg of corticosteroid per day had no change in the lumbar spine and a 3.0% decrease in hip bone density; patients with RA not treated with steroids had a 0.6% decrease in bone density at the spine and a 0.7% decrease at the hip. However, Verhoeven and Boers also showed that patients without RA who took steroids had a 4.7% bone loss at the spine and 1.5% at the hip. Patients with nonrheumatologic diseases may lose up to 5% of bone mass per year; this loss occurs mostly in the first 6 months of therapy.

Corticosteroid use is associated with increased fractures of the predominantly trabecular bones, vertebrae, femoral head, distal radius, and ribs.[58] In postmenopausal women more than 65 years old, a decrease of bone density by 1 standard deviation doubles the risk of spinal fractures. However, glucocorticoid-treated patients appear to suffer fractures more easily with a higher bone density. The dosage of corticosteroid therapy influences the fracture risk. According to the preliminary data from Van Staa and colleagues,[59] an average daily prednisone dose of 2.5 to 7.5 mg is associated with a hip fracture risk of 1.77, and more than 7.5 mg/day, with a fracture risk of 2.27. The risk of vertebral fracture is also higher with prednisone: 2.5 mg/day is associated with a risk of 1.55; 2.5 to 7.5 mg/day, with a risk of 2.59; and more than 7.5 mg/day, with a risk of 5.18.[59] According to this study, the risk of fracture declined to baseline once steroid therapy was discontinued. Physicians are now more aware that glucocorticoids induce osteoporosis and increase the risk of fracture. Concern regarding bone loss remains a limiting factor in making treatment decisions regarding the dosage and duration of corticosteroid therapy. Corticosteroid-induced osteoporosis is therefore likely to continue to be a problem in the future.

## DRUG THERAPIES AND OSTEOPOROSIS

Other drugs used to treat RA may also have an effect on bone mineral metabolism. NSAIDs, gold, and penicillamine do not appear to prevent osteopenia in RA,[37] although the effects of nonsteroidal drugs on bone loss are conflicting. It is possible that some NSAIDs that inhibit prostaglandin synthesis may play a role in retarding the progressive bone loss in patients with high endogenous prostaglandin production, such as occurs in RA.[60] In vitro studies show that bovine osteoclast activity is inhibited by gold salts, and this may account for some of their beneficial effects in inhibiting disease activity in RA.[61] Methotrexate in high doses used to treat childhood leukemia is associated with osteoporotic fractures.[62] In vitro studies show that methotrexate inhibits osteoclast proliferation but not differentiation.[63] In a prospective, randomized, placebo-controlled study, low doses of methotrexate used for the treatment of RA did not reduce bone mass, although patients receiving more than 5 mg of prednisone per day lost an additional 8% bone at the lumbar spine over 3 years.[64] Data show that the immunosuppressant drug cyclosporine is effective in the treatment of RA. Cyclosporine produces time- and dose-dependent bone loss in rodent models, and therapy with both cyclosporine and prednisone is associated with osteoporosis in heart transplant recipients,[65, 66] which raises the possibility that use of this drug in patients with RA may accelerate the development of osteoporosis. Alternative agents, such as azathioprine or cyclophosphamide, do not produce osteoporosis, but these agents are associated with an increased risk of cancer. Cyclophosphamide may cause premature ovarian failure, resulting in a phase of rapid bone loss.[67]

Appropriate interventions for the treatment of rheumatologic diseases must have an effect on disease activity. Complications that result from therapy must be considered early, and alternative treatments or preventive strategies should be considered whenever possible.

## BONE LOSS IN SYSTEMIC LUPUS ERYTHEMATOSUS

The importance of bone loss in patients with systemic lupus erythematosus (SLE), as in RA, cannot be overemphasized. Disease activity is associated with elevated numbers of cytokines, such as interleukins and TNF, which directly affect bone metabolism, as discussed earlier. Young women are the people most susceptible to SLE, often have associated renal disease and/or premature ovarian failure as a result of immunosuppressive or alkylating therapy, and are frequently treated with high doses of prednisone for prolonged periods of time.[68] On the basis of studies of patients with cancer, daily oral cyclophosphamide for 6 to 48 months is associated with the development of amenorrhea in 50% to 70% of women treated. Regimens that involve pulse cyclophosphamide for shorter periods of time may minimize the risk of ovarian toxicity. Studies have shown that SLE is associated with a loss of trabecular bone. Teichmann and associates[69] showed that female patients with newly diagnosed SLE lose bone at the same rate as do women with long-standing SLE, and the reduction in BMD correlates with the excretion of urine hydroxyproline, with hypocalcemia, and with a decrease in osteocalcin. In a cohort of women with SLE,[70] 42% of the women had T scores of less than −1 at the spine and 44% at the hip; 13.4%

of the women had T scores of less than −2.5 at the spine and 6.3% at the hip. Previous use of steroids was strongly inversely related to BMD at the spine, but not as strongly at the hip.[70] There is a risk of lupus flares during pregnancy, and some investigators have therefore raised concerns about instituting hormone replacement therapy in postmenopausal women. The benefits of postmenopausal hormone replacement therapy are clear, and retrospective studies have suggested that hormone replacement therapy may be well tolerated in women with inactive or mild stable SLE.[71] A large, prospective, double-blind, placebo-controlled study, inclusive of all ethnic groups, the Safety of Estrogens in Lupus Erythematosus—National Assessment (SELENA) trial, should provide the basis for definitive recommendations in the near future.[72]

## BONE LOSS IN OSTEOARTHRITIS

Osteoarthritis (OA) is the most common musculoskeletal disorder treated by the rheumatologist. This primary disorder of chondrocyte function results in secondary changes in bone.[73] Bone biopsies from patients with severe OA show a significant increase in trabecular thickness and separation, with a decrease in trabecular number.[74] The osteophyte formation in OA may factitiously elevate bone density measurements of the spine without affecting the proximal femur sites; this makes it difficult to assess bone density in the lumbar spine.[75] Cautious interpretation of DEXA of the lumbar spine is essential to ensure that osteophytes do not falsely raise the spinal bone density reading. Osteophytes are seen in the lumbar spine in up to 75% of men and 61% of women over the age of 60 years, with 31% and 27%, respectively, at the hip.[75] Hannan and coworkers[76] demonstrated that proximal femur bone density was higher in women with mild OA of the knee than in subjects with no OA, although patients with advanced OA of the knee had bone density similar to that of control subjects. Moderate to severe OA is associated with increased appendicular and axial BMD. The association of increased body weight with OA may partly explain this higher bone mass. Degenerative arthritis of the axial skeleton and lower extremities results in decreased levels of function that may accelerate bone loss. Patients with OA may develop age-related bone loss, and the common co-occurrence of these two age-related disorders should be considered in managing these patients.[75, 76]

## BONE LOSS IN POLYMYALGIA RHEUMATICA

Osteopenia in patients with polymyalgia rheumatica (PMR) is not generally found to be a problem, although the bone loss has not been widely studied.[77] Persons with PMR are generally physically active soon after initiation of treatment. Although some patients with PMR may have associated low-grade peripheral synovitis, they lack significant joint involvement and are likely to participate in day-to-day weight-bearing activities. The initial dose of prednisone used to treat patients with PMR and the duration of therapy are widely variable. Clinicians frequently initiate therapy with NSAIDs before prednisone; this may facilitate a shorter duration of treatment with prednisone. Symptoms are occasionally controlled without corticosteroids. In some instances, prolonged intermediate doses of prednisone are required, and significant bone loss may be expected. Pearce and colleagues[78] studied 19 patients with PMR who took 2.5 to 10 mg of prednisone daily for a 14-month period. Markers of bone turnover showed a dose-related reduction in osteocalcin, which returned to normal at dosages of less than 5 mg/day; urine resorption markers were 57% higher than those of controls and decreased by 27% within 1 month of treatment; and muscle strength increased by 20% to 60%. Despite disease remission, bone density decreased by 2.6% at the spine and by 2.9% at the hip; in the first 6 months, spine BMD decreased by 1.7%, and after 6 months, BMD decreased by 8.5% at Ward's triangle and by 4.8% at the femoral neck. The decreases in BMD correlated with the cumulative dose of prednisone. Lower doses of prednisone may be bone sparing, but the underlying disease may not be controlled.[78]

## BONE LOSS IN ANKYLOSING SPONDYLITIS

Ankylosing spondylitis is also associated with the development of osteoporosis. Typically, patients with ankylosing spondylitis have symptoms, starting in the teenage years, that consist of persistent low back pain and morning stiffness. Eventually, the inflammatory symptoms and pain may subside, but patients have residual decreased range of motion in the axial skeleton and are less active. This disorder is often associated with peripheral arthritis, particularly of the large joints of the lower extremities, including the hips; therefore, there may be a further decrease in weight-bearing activity. Eventually, total joint arthroplasty may further limit physical activity and weight-bearing exercises.

Lee and associates[79] showed in men with ankylosing spondylitis that bone density is lower in the spine and hip and that this loss is more marked with later disease. No abnormal parameters of bone metabolism were identified, but bone biopsy revealed a reduced bone volume and trabecular width.[79] Evaluation of testicular function in 22 males with ankylosing spondylitis[80] showed increased luteinizing hormone levels and deficient testicular reserve, which may contribute to the development of osteoporosis. However, other investigators have shown no evidence of hypogonadism in males with ankylosing spondylitis.[81] An atypical osteomalacia diagnosed according to histologic criteria has also been documented in four men with ankylosing spondylitis who had no alterations in calcium or PTH levels.[82]

In patients with chronic ankylosing spondylitis, the most significant complication of concern is spinal fracture. The fracture potential increases in the cervical,

thoracic, and lumbar regions because of the ankylosed spine. Minor trauma is the most common cause of fracture in these persons. Serious complications include complete and incomplete spinal cord lesions and development of other associated neurologic deficits. Radiographic visualization of the fracture site may be difficult because of the extensive syndesmophyte formation. The use of a radionuclide bone scan or a computed tomographic (CT) scan may help visualize the fracture radiographically. The relationship between osteopenia and the risk of fracture is not fully understood. Donnelly and coworkers[83] examined the relationship between BMD and severity of disease in patients with ankylosing spondylitis. They found a significantly higher rate of fracture (10.3%) in the patients than in an age-matched control group, and they also found that there was no significant reduction in lumbar spine or hip BMD by DEXA in the patients with fracture. Patients with early disease had significantly lower spinal BMD, but BMD increased with advanced disease.[83] At the hip, BMD was lower in patients with more severe disease. Quantitative CT may be more useful than DEXA in determining the degree of osteopenia in late disease in these patients because of the extensive paravertebral syndesmophyte formation.[79] Nevertheless, active intervention with agents that reduce bone loss should be considered for these patients.

## EVALUATION OF A PATIENT WITH BONE LOSS OR OSTEOPOROSIS

The evaluation of a patient at risk for osteoporosis must include screening for secondary causes of bone loss, as outlined in Table 40–1. A complete history, physical examination, and laboratory evaluation are essential (Table 40–2). Laboratory tests include the

**TABLE 40–2**

**Screening and Follow-up Tests for Secondary Causes of Bone Loss in Steroid-Treated Patients**

**Screening Tests**

Complete blood cell count
Serum electrolytes, creatinine, calcium, phosphorus, liver enzymes, albumin, alkaline phosphatase measurements
Thyroid-stimulating hormone
Free testosterone in males/estradiol in premenopausal women
25(OH) vitamin D/1,25(OH)$_2$ vitamin D
24-hour urine calcium measurement
+/−Urine protein electrophoresis/serum protein electrophoresis
QCT or DEXA scan (bone density) lumbar spine and hip
+/−spinal radiograph to rule out fractures

**Annual Follow-up Testing**

Serum calcium
25(OH) vitamin D
24-hour urine calcium
Bone density lumbar spine and hip yearly (DEXA or QCT)

DEXA = dual energy x-ray absorptiometry; QCT = quantitative computed tomography.

measurement of serum electrolytes, calcium, phosphorus, and alkaline phosphatase levels; liver tests; a complete blood cell count; measurement of erythrocyte sedimentation rate; serum and possibly urinary protein electrophoresis; measurement of a sensitive TSH level and of 25(OH) vitamin D, urinary calcium, and creatinine levels; and, in some instances, tests of gonadal function and serum PTH concentrations. Markers of bone turnover, urinary N-telopeptides, may be helpful in determining whether this is a state of high or low bone turnover; these are measured in a second morning urine sample. Additional specific tests to rule out endocrinologic or neoplastic processes and a possible bone biopsy (after a double tetracycline label) should be considered in patients in whom there is a question of osteomalacia without biochemical changes to support the diagnosis. Candidates for a bone biopsy include patients with severe bone loss and those in whom primary osteoporosis is uncommon, such as children, premenopausal women, men less than 60 years of age, and black persons. All secondary causes of bone loss should be corrected before specific, therapeutic interventions for osteoporosis are considered, because substantial improvements in bone mass may be achieved.

## STRATEGIES FOR THE PREVENTION AND TREATMENT OF OSTEOPOROSIS

The goals of therapy for osteoporosis include the reduction of risk factors for bone loss, avoidance of prolonged immobilization, conservative management of pain, and an attempt to halt the disease progression by decreasing bone resorption and increasing bone formation. A regular weight-bearing program that includes endurance, resistance exercises, or both[84] may produce a modest increase in bone mass.

### Calcium

Adequate calcium intake is necessary for preventing calcium mobilization from the skeleton to maintain blood calcium levels. Studies have yielded widely varying results of the effect of calcium on bone turnover. Some data show that the benefit from calcium depends on the years since menopause, customary calcium intake, age, and vitamin D status. Prospective studies demonstrate that calcium supplementation is ineffective or minimally effective in preventing bone loss in women within 5 years of menopause, which is the period when estrogen deficiency has a predominant influence on bone loss.[85] Supplemental calcium is beneficial for late-postmenopausal women with low calcium intake (<400 mg/day) and vitamin D deficiency and may prevent up to 2.5% bone loss and decrease the risk of hip fracture by up to 30%. In prepubertal children, calcium intake of approximately 1600 mg/day increases bone density at different sites approximately 3% to 5%, which may ultimately confer an increased peak bone mass.[86]

The National Academy of Sciences[87] devised guidelines for adequate daily calcium intake for all ages in the population: To prevent a negative calcium balance, children require 500 to 800 mg; men and premenopausal women require 1000 mg; pregnant and lactating women require 1500 mg; and men over 50 years of age and postmenopausal women require 1200 mg of elemental calcium per day. These levels of calcium intake are generally safe, unless a patient has an underlying disorder of calcium homeostasis. Dairy products are the dietary sources that have the greatest amount of calcium. An 8-ounce glass of milk or calcium-supplemented orange juice contains approximately 300 mg of elemental calcium. Calcium carbonate, the most widely used calcium salt, contains 40% of elemental calcium. Each tablet of Tums E-X, for example, contains 300 mg of elemental calcium, and Os-Cal 500 and Tums 500 tablets each have 500 mg of elemental calcium. Calcium carbonate should be taken with food because patients with achlorhydria are unable to absorb this calcium salt well on an empty stomach.[88] Adverse effects of calcium carbonate include constipation. Calcium citrate contains 24% elemental calcium; this calcium salt is a more bioavailable calcium preparation than is calcium carbonate, and it may be taken during fasting.[89]

### Vitamin D: Maintenance and Therapy

Low dietary intake of vitamin D and inadequate sunlight exposure result in vitamin D deficiency, secondary hyperparathyroidism, and osteomalacia.[2] A study of patients with acute hip fractures showed that 50% of the patients had vitamin D deficiency.[90] Vitamin D (700 IU/day) and calcium carbonate (500 mg/day) reduce bone loss and decrease the incidence of nonvertebral fractures by 50%.[91] In elderly nursing home residents with low or low-normal vitamin D levels, vitamin D (800 IU/day) with calcium (1.2 g/day) decreased hip fractures by 43%.[92] Thus, in the elderly, treatment interventions may have a major impact in reducing fractures. Vitamin D deficiency is defined as 25(OH) vitamin D levels of less than 12 to 15 ng/mL; however, PTH levels rise at 25(OH) vitamin D levels ranging from less than 25 to 30 ng/mL. Replacement with vitamin D to this level may therefore prevent PTH-mediated bone loss. Vitamin D at 400 to 800 IU/day is usually adequate for replacement, but higher dose preparations are available, such as vitamin D, 50,000-IU tablet, or Drisdol Drops (vitamin D), 200 IU/drop.

Use of $1,25(OH)_2$ vitamin D may enhance calcium absorption and bone formation (at pharmacologic dosages; e.g., 0.5 $\mu$g/day). Although some studies show that administration of $1,25(OH)_2$ vitamin D for osteoporosis is ineffective in maintaining bone mass, high doses of $1,25(OH)_2$ vitamin D produced some increase in bone density.[93] A reduction in fractures in some studies with $1,25(OH)_2$ vitamin D therapy[94] may result from reversal of mild vitamin D deficiency. $1,25(OH)_2$ Vitamin D has a narrow margin of safety, with potential risks of hypercalcemia and hypercalciuria. In the absence of vitamin D insufficiency, however, most treatment regimens should ensure adequate intake with physiologic doses of vitamin D (400 to 800 IU/day).

## Estrogen

Estrogen therapy in postmenopausal women prevents bone loss and decreases the risk of fracture by 50%, possibly through direct interaction with estrogen receptors on bone cells[95] or through a reduction in cytokines that stimulate bone resorption (e.g., IL-1, IL-6).[96, 97] In women with no contraindications to its use, hormone replacement therapy is the treatment of choice for preventing and treating osteoporosis.[98] Estrogen decreases bone loss regardless of whether it is started at the onset of menopause or later in life when considerable bone loss has occurred. Estrogen replacement therapy should be continued for 10 years or more to reduce the risk of hip fractures in older women.[99, 100] Rapid bone loss does occur once estrogen is discontinued, and data show that even after 1 to 2 years of continuous estrogen therapy, bone loss may still occur.

According to data from several observational studies, estrogen therapy reduces the risk of cardiovascular disease, the leading cause of death in postmenopausal women, by approximately 50%. Improved lipoprotein profiles, a decrease in total and low-density lipoprotein (LDL) cholesterol and a rise in high-density lipoprotein (HDL) cholesterol, and other mechanisms, such as direct vascular and antioxidant effects, mediate the cardioprotective effect of estrogens. However, the Heart and Estrogen/Progestin Replacement Study[101] of the secondary prevention of heart disease in postmenopausal women showed an early increase in the risk of cardiac events, possibly as a result of increased thrombosis associated with oral estrogen therapy. Thus, this study showed no overall protective benefit conferred by the use of hormone replacement therapy in women with established heart disease.

Estrogen is administered in a sequential or continuous regimen with a progestin to diminish the risk of endometrial hyperplasia or carcinoma. Oral estrogen/progesterone regimens often used include (1) 0.625 mg of conjugated estrogen daily, with 10 mg of medroxyprogesterone added on days 1 to 14 of each month in a sequential regimen, and (2) 0.625 mg of conjugated estrogen daily, with 2.5 or 5 mg of medroxyprogesterone in a daily continuous hormone replacement regimen. Unlike the sequential hormone replacement regimen, which usually produces regular monthly withdrawal bleeding, daily continuous hormone replacement induces atrophy of the endometrium so that 80% or more of women are amenorrheic at 1 year. In the first 6 months of this latter regimen, 45% of women may experience irregular bleeding.[102] According to the guidelines of the American College of Obstetrics and Gynecology,[103] endometrial biopsies are not routinely necessary unless a woman has had irregular bleeding, is overweight before starting hormone replacement therapy, or experiences unexpected or severe vaginal bleeding while using hormone therapy. In women who have had a hysterectomy, estrogen is administered alone. Because of the possibility of a slight increase in the risk of breast cancer with estrogen use, regular breast examinations and annual mammography should be performed according to the guidelines of the American Cancer Society. Contraindications to estrogen therapy are breast or endometrial cancer and active thrombotic or liver disease (see other guidelines in reference 103). Transdermal estrogens, which, unlike oral estrogens, do not affect serum-binding proteins or clotting factors, also prevent bone loss but produce less beneficial effects on lipoproteins.

## Selective Estrogen Receptor Modulators

Selective estrogen receptor modulators (SERMs), a class of nonsteroidal drugs approved by the US Food and Drug Administration (FDA) for the prevention of osteoporosis, have been used in the treatment of breast cancer for many years; an example of these drugs is tamoxifen. They bind to estrogen-responsive tissues and act selectively as agonists or antagonists. Previous studies[104] in postmenopausal patients with breast cancer show that tamoxifen has estrogen agonist–like effects on clotting factors, on the endometrium, and on bone, preventing bone loss and reducing the risk of spinal fracture by up to 45%.[105] Raloxifene (Evista) is the FDA-approved SERM for the prevention of osteoporosis[106]; it has antagonistic effects to estrogen in the endometrium and breast, decreasing the risk of breast cancer by 76% in women treated for osteoporosis, and it has an estrogen-like effect on the lipid profile, decreasing LDL cholesterol 12% and increasing $HDL_2$ cholesterol 15%. Over 2 years in the Multiple Outcomes of Raloxifene trial,[106, 107] raloxifene, 60 mg/day, has been shown to increase bone density by 2% per year and to decrease vertebral fractures by 40% to 50%, without an effect on hip fractures. The side effects of raloxifene include an increase in deep venous thrombosis, hot flashes, leg cramps, and vaginal dryness. At present, raloxifene is approved for the prevention of osteoporosis in patients with osteopenia and is also approved for the treatment of osteoporosis.

## Calcitonin

Calcitonin is a 32–amino acid peptide produced by the parafollicular cells of the thyroid, which inhibits bone resorption through its direct effects on osteoclasts that have high-affinity calcitonin receptors. Intranasal calcitonin is approved by the FDA for the treatment of osteoporosis in a dosage of 200 IU/day and should be administered with calcium, 1 g/day, and vitamin D, 400 IU/day.[48, 108] Adverse effects of calcitonin include nausea in approximately 10% to 15% of patients, flushing, inflammation at the injection site, and rhinorrhea (nasal calcitonin). There may also be a beneficial analgesic effect in the presence of vertebral fractures. There may be a plateau to the effect on bone turnover after 18 to 26 months of therapy (tachyphylaxis), possibly a result of refilling in remodeling space and/or downregulation of calcitonin receptors. Studies in postmenopausal women with osteoporosis show that use of a calcitonin nasal spray (200 IU/day) for 12 months prevents bone loss in the spine and forearm.[109] The Prevention Recurrence of Osteoporotic Fractures (PROOF) study,[109a] a 3-year, randomized, placebo-controlled study of nasal calcitonin, 200 IU/day, versus placebo in postmenopausal women with established osteoporosis, demonstrated a 37% reduction in the risk of new vertebral fractures regardless of pretreatment characteristics.

## Bisphosphonates

Bisphosphonates are pyrophosphate analogs that are absorbed into the hydroxyapatite crystals of bone and inhibit bone resorption by interfering with osteoclast activity and inducing apoptosis, thereby reducing the depth of the osteoclast resorption cavity and preserving bone structure.[110] In addition, bisphosphonates cause osteoblasts to produce an osteoclastic inhibitory factor, also reducing bone resorption.[110] Bisphosphonates have a sustained effect because of their long half-life in bone. Etidronate, administered intermittently to older osteoporotic women over a period of 2 years, produced a 5% increase in spinal bone density and a 50% reduction in vertebral fractures[111] that was not sustained at 3 years. Etidronate is approved for the treatment of Paget's disease of bone but not for the treatment of osteoporosis.

Alendronate (Fosamax) is approved by the FDA for the prevention and treatment of osteoporosis. This is a more potent second-generation bisphosphonate. Prevention of bone loss in women with osteopenia who took alendronate, 5 mg/day for 2 years, increased bone density of the spine by 2.9% and hip by 1.3%.[112] In women with osteoporosis or a previous fracture, alendronate, 10 mg/day, increased bone density by 7% at the spine and 6% at the femoral neck.[113] The incidence of vertebral fractures was reduced by 50% in women with osteoporosis. However, the Fracture Intervention Study showed that patients with a T score higher than −2 and no previous fracture had no reduction in risk of fracture.[114] Bisphosphonates are poorly absorbed (<1%), and so they should be taken on an empty stomach with 8 ounces of water at least 30 minutes before meals. No calcium supplements should be taken within 2 to 4 hours of a dose, because calcium binds to alendronate and may impair absorption. Abdominal pain, constipation, diarrhea, flatulence, musculoskeletal pain, and headache may occur more frequently than experienced in the placebo group. Patients with esophageal abnormalities (stricture or achalasia), inability to stand upright for 30 minutes, or hypocalcemia are advised not to use this medication. Preexisting gastroesophageal reflux–type symptoms may be made worse by alendronate, and in rare cases, esophagitis, ulcerations, and erosions occur. To prevent the risk of reflux esophagitis, patients are advised to remain upright for at least 30 minutes after taking the medication.

Alendronate has been used to treat patients with osteoporosis in combination with estrogen replacement therapy, because these medications have different mechanisms of action. Combination therapy results in an additional 2.5% to 3% increase in bone density.[113]

More potent third-generation bisphosphonates are being studied in the treatment of osteoporosis. Risedronate (Actonel) is approved for the treatment of Paget's disease of bone and has recently been approved for the prevention and treatment of osteoporosis and the treatment of glucocorticoid-induced osteoporosis. Data[115, 116] have shown that 2 years of treatment with risedronate, 5 mg/day, in postmenopausal women with two or more spinal fractures increases spinal bone density by 7% and femoral neck bone density by 2.1%. Incident vertebral fractures are reduced by 40% to 50%, and nonvertebral fractures are reduced by 33% to 39%. Adverse effects were similar in both placebo and treatment groups and no increase in gastrointestinal symptoms was observed.

## Sodium Fluoride

Sodium fluoride stimulates bone formation and produces large increments in BMD. Adverse effects of fluoride occur in up to approximately 40% of subjects and include gastrointestinal irritation and a lower extremity pain syndrome with stress fractures. A slow-release fluoride preparation has fewer adverse effects.[117] In prospective, controlled studies of high doses of sodium fluoride for the treatment of osteoporosis (75 mg/day), there was no significant decrease in vertebral fractures, and nonvertebral fractures increased despite an increase in bone density.[118] Use of a slow-release fluoride preparation is associated with a 4% increase in spine bone density, a 2.3% increase in femoral neck bone density, a significant reduction in vertebral fractures, and fewer adverse effects. Meunier and colleagues[119] performed a 2-year multicenter, prospective, randomized, double-blind study of postmenopausal women with prevalent vertebral fractures. Subjects were treated with sodium fluoride, 50 mg/day; monofluorophosphate, 150 to 200 mg/day; or placebo (all patients received 1 g of calcium and 800 IU of vitamin D daily). Despite a 10.8% increase in spine bone density in all fluoride-treated subjects, in comparison with a 2.4% increase in subjects who received calcium and vitamin D alone, there was no prevention of new vertebral fractures.[119] At present, the use of fluoride therapy should be restricted to investigative protocols.

## Parathyroid Hormone

Low doses of parenteral PTH (PTH 1-34, the active amino terminus) given with calcitriol increased trabecular bone in the spine,[120] but it may cause small losses of cortical bone. Studies[121] have shown that postmenopausal women taking estrogen replacement therapy, calcium, and vitamin D, when treated with PTH 1-34 for 2 years, have a 13% increase in spinal bone density and an 8% increase of hip bone density with no significant decrease in forearm bone density. No fracture prevention data are available yet. PTH is not yet recommended for use beyond research protocols, particularly inasmuch as some studies have been stopped because of concerns of bone cancers that occur in animal models.

PTH-related protein is now being studied[122] as a potential anabolic agent in postmenopausal women, and results are promising, showing a decrease in markers of bone resorption and an increase in markers of bone formation, which suggest an increase in bone formation. Future directions in the treatment of osteoporosis may include use of anabolic growth factors or other approaches that may stimulate bone formation, but currently these are not yet available.

Because existing therapeutic interventions for established osteoporosis only partially reverse bone loss, preventive strategies to optimize skeletal mass—such as reduction of risk factors for bone loss, identification and treatment of patients at risk of bone loss (according to bone density criteria), adequate calcium and vitamin D nutrition, and a regular weight-bearing exercise program—are important. It is imperative to identify and treat underlying secondary causes of osteoporosis.

## Summary of the Treatment of Osteoporosis

Our approach to the treatment of postmenopausal women with osteoporosis is to use hormone replacement therapy as the first-line therapy because of the combined benefit of reducing the risk of cardiovascular disease and osteoporosis. The ongoing prospective randomized Women's Health Initiative will assess the effects of combined daily continuous estrogen and progesterone therapy on cardiovascular disease, fractures, and breast and uterine cancers. Physicians should therefore cautiously evaluate the risk/benefit ratio for hormone replacement therapy in individual patients. The rate of patient compliance with hormone replacement therapy is, however, only about 30%, and at present there is no widespread acceptance of this mode of therapy in postmenopausal women. Other strategies at present to prevent osteoporosis include use of alendronate, 5 mg/day, or raloxifene, 60 mg/day. FDA-approved therapeutic strategies to treat osteoporosis include the use of estrogen, with or without progesterone replacement therapy; intranasal calcitonin, 200 IU/day; and alendronate, 10 mg/day.

Because of the concerns about the long retention time of bisphosphonates in bone, we are cautious about administering these drugs to premenopausal women. We also withhold these agents from patients with vitamin D insufficiency until this is corrected. The availability of bone densitometry makes it feasible to ensure a therapeutic response to these treatment strategies. Patients who do not maintain or increase bone mass appropriately may require alternative therapeutic approaches. More potent future therapies may help prevent bone resorption and potentially promote bone formation, but further studies are awaited.

## STRATEGIES TO PREVENT OR TREAT CORTICOSTEROID-INDUCED BONE LOSS (Table 40–3)

Chronic corticosteroid use may cause about a 5% to 20% bone loss over 1 to 2 years, with osteoporosis as a well-documented sequela. Fracture risk is associated with the dosage of steroid therapy,[69] and discontinuation of steroids may reverse the bone loss in some instances. Strategies to prevent bone loss in all patients should therefore include use of the lowest steroid dosage possible and an evaluation for patients at risk of osteoporosis who may require prophylactic therapy.[123] Initial evaluation should identify the patient at risk for osteoporosis (see Table 40–1), as previously discussed. Additional risk factors include increased risk of fall as a result of steroid-induced myopathy and muscle wasting; cataracts; and altered mental status. Cooper and associates[124] showed that functional impairment increases the risk of hip fracture among patients with RA, independently of steroid use. Lifestyle modifications may be necessary, but they may not alter the rate of bone loss once corticosteroid treatment begins. An initial biochemical evaluation should include complete blood cell count; measurement of serum electrolytes, creatinine, calcium, alkaline phosphatase, phosphorus, albumin, liver enzymes, 25-hydroxyvitamin D, and TSH; possibly a measurement of free testosterone in males; and a 24-hour measurement of urine calcium[125] (see Table 40–2). Any secondary causes of bone loss should be identified and treated, as described earlier, to eliminate any treatable causes of bone loss and to recognize any factors that may increase the patient's risk of fracture.[2] Bone density should be determined at baseline by DEXA to establish risk of osteoporosis on the basis of WHO criteria.

Despite the severity of the bone loss in some patients with steroid use, there are few prospective, randomized, controlled investigations of therapeutic interventions in these patients. A prophylactic graduated exercise program, as is clinically feasible, may prevent the bone loss that results from immobilization and inactivity.[126] In patients who are taking corticosteroids, calcium, 1000 mg/day, inhibits bone resorption and de-

## TABLE 40–3
## Therapy for Corticosteroid-Induced Bone Loss or Osteoporosis

1. Reduce corticosteroid dose or discontinue therapy if feasible
2. Exercise against gravity
3. Maintain adequate calcium intake (1 g/day)
4. Hydrochlorothiazide (if urinary calcium ≥4 mg/kg/d)
5. Vitamin D or 25(OH) vitamin D therapy (monitoring serum and urinary calcium levels)
6. Estrogens/progesterone in postmenopausal women, testosterone when indicated in men
7. Calcitonin
8. Bisphosphonates (alendronate [Fosamax]*)

* Treatment approved by the US Food and Drug Administration.

creases bone loss.[89] Thus, patients should be advised to maintain adequate calcium intake, as discussed earlier for osteoporosis. Buckley and coworkers[127] showed that calcium, 1 g/day, with vitamin $D_3$, 500 IU/day, over 2 years in patients with RA taking more than 5 mg of prednisone daily, prevented bone loss at the spine and hip at rates of 2% and 0.9%, respectively, and increased bone density by 0.72% and 0.82%, respectively. Adachi and colleagues[128] randomly assigned 62 steroid-using patients to receive either 50,000 IU/week and 1 g of calcium or placebo, each for 36 months. Bone density decreased twice as fast in the steroid-treated patients; at 18 months, after the steroid dose was reduced to less than 7.5 mg/day, an increase in BMD was noted. Overall, the steroid users who took calcium and vitamin D had a 4.2% reduction in BMD, in comparison with a 9% decrease in the placebo recipients.

It was found that 1,25(OH)$_2$ vitamin D was ineffective in prevention of corticosteroid-induced osteoporosis.[49] However, as primary prevention, calcium and 1,25(OH)$_2$ vitamin D, with or without calcitonin, reduced vertebral bone loss in corticosteroid-treated subjects. Calcitonin therapy had a sustained effect during the second year when the other treatments were stopped.[129] Hahn and coworkers[130] showed in rheumatic patients taking corticosteroids that vitamin D (50,000 U two to three times weekly) and 25-hydroxyvitamin D (approximately 40 $\mu$g/day), each with 500 mg of elemental calcium daily, increased intestinal calcium absorption, suppressed PTH release, and had beneficial effects on bone density (approximately 8% and approximately 16% increments, respectively), although these were not long-term studies. Because of the negative calcium balance resulting from corticosteroid therapy, vitamin D supplementation raises the patient's 25-hydroxyvitamin D level to the upper range of normal and appears to offset the negative calcium balance. Careful monitoring of the serum and urinary calcium levels is necessary in order to minimize the risk of vitamin D intoxication.

In a corticosteroid-treated patient who has an elevated urinary calcium level ($\geq$4 mg/kg/day), possibly as a consequence of corticosteroid therapy or who develops hypercalciuria coincidentally with vitamin D treatment, hydrochlorothiazide therapy (25 to 50 mg two times daily) with a sodium-restricted diet is effective in reducing urinary calcium excretion.[123, 131] RA has been associated with a higher incidence of renal calculi and with hypercalciuria. In the absence of corticosteroid therapy, hydrochlorothiazide is associated with an 8% increase in BMD at the spine and a 3% increase at the hip per year,[132] higher bone density at multiple sites, and a reduction in the risk of hip fractures.[133]

Hypogonadism should be treated regardless of whether the patient is postmenopausal, as discussed earlier. In a randomized crossover trial, Reid and associates[134] studied men treated with long-term glucocorticoids for asthma and randomly assigned them to receive 250 mg of intramuscular testosterone monthly or placebo monthly for 1 year, and therapy was crossed over for the second year. All men had low free testosterone levels (330 to 380 pmol/L) before treatment, and testosterone therapy increased levels to the high normal range (1230 pmol/L). In the treatment group, bone density increased by 5% at the spine but not at the hip, and alkaline phosphatase and urinary hydroxyproline levels decreased significantly. There were no adverse effects on lipid profiles or prostate cancer risk, and an increase in lean body mass and decrease in total body fat were noted.[134] In men with testosterone deficiency resulting from corticosteroid therapy, treatment with parenteral testosterone (250 mg intramuscularly every 3 weeks) or a transdermal testosterone preparation (2.5 to 5 mg/day) may have beneficial effects on bone density in men with low pretreatment testosterone levels.[135] Dosage is determined by the free testosterone levels and should be monitored closely.

In a retrospective, case-control study, treatment with estrogen, 0.625 mg/day, and progesterone, 5 mg on days 15 to 25, prevented bone loss in corticosteroid-treated postmenopausal women receiving 5 to 15 mg of prednisone daily, resulting in a small but significant increase in spine BMD at 1 year.[136] In patients with RA not treated with corticosteroids, a prospective, placebo-controlled study showed that estrogen replacement increased bone density in both the spine and the proximal femur.[137] In a randomized controlled study, Hall and coworkers[138] treated patients with RA with transdermal estradiol, 50 $\mu$g/day; some of these patients were also treated with corticosteroids. Hormone replacement therapy increased BMD at the spine by 3.7%, whereas control groups (no estradiol) exhibited a 1% decrease; no change was seen at the hip.[19] Premenopausal women with amenorrhea or low estradiol levels should be treated with estrogen. A birth control pill containing a minimum of 50 $\mu$g of estradiol should be used unless there is a contraindication.[125] Further prospective, randomized, controlled studies of the effects of hormone replacement therapy on corticosteroid-induced bone loss are warranted.

The presence of enhanced bone resorption in corticosteroid-treated subjects has led investigators to examine the effects of calcitonin, an osteoclast inhibitor, on BMD in a variety of patients with rheumatic diseases. Adachi and colleagues[139] showed that patients with polymyalgia rheumatica who were treated with prednisone for 1 year had 3.7% less bone loss at the spine when treated with intranasal calcitonin, as opposed to placebo. A study of asthmatic patients[140] with glucocorticoid-induced osteoporosis who received steroids, calcium, and either intranasal calcitonin or placebo showed a 10.6% difference in spinal BMD at 2 years; BMD was higher in the calcitonin-treated group, but there was no significant protection against fracture. Ringe and Welzel[141] showed that parenteral calcitonin (100 units every other day) produced a small increase in bone density in the forearms of patients with rheumatic diseases, whereas bone density declined in the control group. A significant reduction in pain score was also noted. Kotaniemi and associates[142] showed that in patients with active RA taking low-dose steroids, treatment with intranasal calcitonin, 100 IU/day, versus placebo and calcium, 500 mg/day, for 1 year, resulted in an increase in femoral neck BMD but no significant change at the spine. Several studies, including preliminary data from a large multicenter placebo-controlled trial, have shown that calcitonin maintains bone mass or produces a small increment in bone in patients taking moderate doses of corticosteroids.[143] Low dosages of nasal calcitonin (200 IU/day for 1 month, then 100 IU/day) prevented bone loss at 1 year in patients with RA not treated with corticosteroids, although a 1.8% bone loss was noted in the second year of therapy; this loss, however, was significantly less than that in the control group.[144] Healey and co-workers[145] showed that patients treated with calcitonin injections maintained but had no increase in spinal BMD.

Unlike the antiresorptive drugs discussed earlier, fluoride stimulates bone formation. In a primary preventive study of patients without previous osteoporosis,[146] fluoride produced a nonsignificant 2% increase in BMD at the spine, in comparison with a 3% decrease in the placebo recipients. Monofluorophosphate plus calcium produced a 9.3% increase in spine BMD in patients treated with prednisone for 6 years.[147] Rickers and associates,[148] in a prospective randomized 24-week trial, were unable to demonstrate an effect of calcium, fluoride, and vitamin D in preventing corticosteroid-induced bone loss at a trabecular and cortical site in the forearm. Meunier and colleagues,[149] however, in a 2-year study, observed a 63% increment in trabecular bone on histomorphometric analysis of iliac crest biopsy specimens from corticosteroid-treated patients, which is consistent with an anabolic effect of fluoride on trabecular bone in this group of patients. Increases in BMD seen with fluoride therapy have not led to a decrease in the risk of fracture in patients with osteoporosis, but no fracture data are yet available for steroid-treated patients. Long-term, randomized, controlled studies demonstrating a beneficial effect of fluoride on the reduction of fractures would be necessary to establish a role for this therapy in the treatment of corticosteroid-induced bone loss.

Lane and coworkers[150] studied the role of PTH in the treatment of glucocorticoid-induced bone loss in postmenopausal women. All women were treated with 5 to 20 mg of prednisone daily and were receiving estrogen replacement therapy. Patients were randomly assigned to receive either PTH, 400 IU/day, or placebo, with calcium and vitamin D; after 1 year of the therapy, BMD increased by 9% at the lumbar spine. Markers of bone formation, osteocalcin and bone-specific alkaline phosphatase, increased within 1 month and bone resorption markers increased later[150]; fracture data are not yet available.

Increased osteoclastic activity is one of the mechanisms for increased bone resorption in RA. The use of bisphosphonates as antiresorptive therapy is proving to be beneficial in the treatment of corticosteroid-induced bone loss. In patients undergoing long-term corticosteroid therapy, a prospective placebo-controlled study of oral pamidronate (APD, or 3-amino-1-hydroxypropylidene-1, 1-bisphosphonate) and calcium produced an approximately 20% increment in lumbar spine bone density over 1 year,[151] with subsequent stable bone densities. However, oral pamidronate is not approved by the FDA for use in the United States. Cortet and associates[152] showed that in patients taking more than 7.5 mg of prednisone daily, etidronate, 400 mg/day, versus placebo, cycled every 76 days for 1 year with calcium, 500 mg/day, resulted in 0.3% increase in spinal BMD in etidronate recipients and a 2.79% decrease in placebo recipients. This overall 3% difference between groups is significant, but no changes were seen at the hip. Similarly, Adachi and colleagues[153] showed that intermittent cyclical therapy with etidronate significantly decreased bone loss in the lumbar spine by 3.23% and in the femoral trochanter by 4.14%. There was a trend toward fewer vertebral fractures in the etidronate-treated group. Side effects were mild, transient, and mostly gastrointestinal. A 1-year follow-up evaluation of these patients, after discontinuation of the study, showed no accelerated bone loss in the etidronate-treated group. A pooled data analysis from Roux and coworkers[154] showed that intermittent etidronate is effective at preventing corticosteroid-induced bone loss in subgroups defined by sex, menopausal status, and disease state (RA vs. polymyalgia rheumatica).

Intravenous pamidronate[54] was studied as a primary preventive therapy in patients commencing long-term prednisone treatment (<10 mg/day). Treatment involved 90 mg of pamidronate at the start of steroid therapy, followed by 30 mg every 3 months; at 1 year, 3.6% and 2.2% increases in BMD were noted in the spine and femoral neck, respectively, of the pamidronate recipients, whereas the control group had 5.3% and 5.3% reductions, respectively. A significant benefit is found when bisphosphonates are used at the outset of steroid therapy.

Saag and associates[155] pooled data from two randomized, double-blind trials, studying the effects of alendronate, 5 and 10 mg/day, and placebo on BMD in patients receiving more than 7.5 mg of prednisone per day for rheumatologic (54%) and other diseases. All patients received calcium, 800 to 1000 mg/day, and vitamin D, 250 to 500 IU/day. During the study, the median prednisone dosages decreased to 8.8 mg/day, 8.7 mg/day, and 9 mg/day, respectively, in each of the treatment groups. Over 48 weeks, the spinal BMD increased 2.1% and 2.9%, respectively, with a 0.4% decrease in the control group (significant). The femoral neck bone density increased by 1.2% and 1.0% in the alendronate groups, respectively, but decreased by 1.2% in the control group (significant). There was no significant reduction in the incidence of vertebral or nonvertebral fracture in either group. There was a slight increase in nonserious upper gastrointestinal symptoms in patients treated with 10 mg of alendronate, but there were no other significant adverse effects. A 24-month outcome analysis[155] of these patients, after a second year of therapy, revealed a 0.7% vertebral fracture rate in alendronate-treated patients, in contrast to 6.8% in control groups.

Risedronate, a bisphosphonate approved by the FDA for the treatment of Paget's disease of bone, has been studied in the treatment of steroid-induced osteoporosis. Cohen and colleagues,[156] in a double-blind, placebo-controlled trial of patients with primarily rheumatologic diseases who were starting long-term corticosteroid therapy, randomly assigned these patients to receive 500 mg of calcium for 1 year with risedronate, 2.5 mg; risedronate, 5 mg; or placebo. At 1 year, treatment with risedronate, 5 mg/day, decreased bone loss at the spine by 3.8% and at the femoral neck by 4.1%. Reid and associates[157] studied premenopausal women, postmenopausal women, and men with rheumatologic diseases; the patients were divided into two groups: those commencing steroid treatment, 7.5 mg for less than 3 months (to study prevention) and those taking long-term steroids, 7.5 mg for more than 6 months (to study treatment). All patients received 500 to 1000 mg of calcium plus 400 IU of vitamin D per day, with 2.5 mg or 5 mg of risedronate or placebo daily. The prevention study showed that risedronate, 5 mg/day, resulted in 0.5%, 0.8%, and 1.3% increases in BMD at the lumbar spine, femoral neck, and trochanter, respectively, but no increase in BMD with 2.5 mg of risedronate and a continued loss of up to 3% in the control group. The treatment study showed that risedronate, 5 mg, increased BMD by 2.8%, 1.9%, and 2% at the lumbar spine, femoral neck, and trochanter, respectively. The control group had no significant change in BMD. The vertebral fracture incidence was significantly lower in patients treated with risedronate, 5 mg, than in controls.[157] Risedronate was well tolerated, with no significant increase in gastrointestinal side effects. The American College of Rheumatologists[125] proposed the use of bisphosphonates in patients with corticosteroid-induced osteoporosis for whom hormone replacement therapy is contraindicated or refused or as an additional therapy if the BMD is low or continues to decrease despite hormone replacement therapy.

Studies show that the prednisolone derivative deflazacort appears to have fewer effects on bone metabolism than does prednisone.[158] At comparable anti-inflammatory dosages, deflazacort decreased BMD less than did prednisone (3% loss vs. 9.1% loss) at the spine, but no protection against bone loss was noted at the hip.[159] Use of this corticosteroid or other bone-sparing corticosteroid analogs may mitigate against the development or reduce the severity of corticosteroid-induced osteoporosis.

## AUTHORS' APPROACH TO MANAGEMENT

In corticosteroid-treated patients, an initial approach is to select the lowest corticosteroid dosage possible to treat the underlying disease process. Alternatives to corticosteroid therapy for the rheumatic process may be considered in patients whenever possible, particularly in patients with accelerated bone loss. Not all patients treated with corticosteroids develop osteoporosis, however; to identify those at risk, we obtain a bone density determination at baseline and repeat it at 1 year in patients starting long-term ($\geq 3$ months) corticosteroid therapy ($\geq 5$ to 7.5 mg/day). This allows us to correct any secondary causes of bone loss before steroid-induced changes occur and to institute therapy to protect the skeleton from steroid-induced osteoporosis when necessary. Bone densitometry results are monitored to assess the skeletal response to a treatment intervention so that modifications in therapy may be instituted appropriately.

At baseline in a patient with osteopenia or osteoporosis, other secondary causes of bone loss are vigorously sought and treated. All patients are advised to modify any lifestyle factors that increase the risk of osteoporosis: for example, smoking and excessive alcohol consumption. A physical activity program, including weight-bearing exercises for 30 to 60 minutes per day, is recommended.[20] Patients should be advised with regard to fall prevention strategies. To minimize the corticosteroid-induced negative calcium balance, we recommend adequate calcium intake (1000 mg for premenopausal women and 1500 mg for postmenopausal women). Vitamin D, 400 to 800 IU/day, or supraphysiologic dosages of vitamin D (e.g., 50,000 IU of vitamin D once weekly or bimonthly) may be necessary to maintain the 25-hydroxyvitamin D level in the upper normal range exceeding 25 ng/mL. Careful monitoring of the serum and urinary calcium concentrations is essential for preventing the development of hypercalcemia, hypercalciuria (24-hour urine calcium level, > 250 mg), and nephrolithiasis. Hydrochlorothiazide therapy (25 mg twice daily) may reduce the hypercalciuria associated with corticosteroid therapy or with concurrent calcium or vitamin D therapy, if necessary. Treatment of hypogonadism is essential; if there are no contraindications, as discussed earlier, we use gonadal steroid replacement in both the prevention and treatment of corticosteroid-induced bone loss in premenopausal women, postmenopausal women, and hypogonadal men.

Corticosteroid-treated patients may benefit from additional therapy to prevent or treat osteoporosis in patients with evidence of an increased risk of fracture, reduced bone mass, or previous fractures. Additional therapies are recommended for patients with a T score of less than $-1$. Patients with a normal BMD should have a follow-up BMD measurement at 6 to 12 months; if there has been more than a 5% loss, and if no secondary causes of bone loss that can be corrected are identified, additional therapy should be instituted. In patients with a previous fracture, pain relief may be an issue; calcitonin has been shown to have an analgesic effect in the treatment of vertebral fractures.[141] Premenopausal women should not be treated with bisphosphonates, although these agents appear to have the most potent effects in reducing bone loss both as a preventive and therapeutic intervention. They are not used in younger patients because of a theoretical concern regarding the long half-life of these drugs in the bone matrix. Intranasal calcitonin, 200 IU/day, alternating nostrils on alternate days to reduce nasal irritation and rhinorrhea, is well tolerated. Alendronate, 5 mg/day, may be used to prevent further bone loss in patients with osteopenia. Alendronate, 10 mg/day, has been approved by the FDA as a therapy for glucocorticoid-induced osteoporosis. Alendronate should be taken with care, as described earlier, to optimize absorption and to minimize side effects. Risedronate, 5 mg/day, has been approved by the FDA for the prevention and treatment of osteoporosis and glucocorticoid-induced osteoporosis. Intravenous pamidronate may be considered. When a patient treated with corticosteroids continues to lose bone or develops fractures while receiving a given intervention to protect bone mass, we reevaluate for concurrent secondary causes of bone loss and consider additional or alternative treatment options.

Glucocorticoids are essential in the treatment of many medical conditions, including pulmonary and several rheumatologic diseases. However, the disabilities resulting from glucocorticoid-induced osteoporosis and fractures are extensive. Information regarding the severity and prevalence of this disease is emerging from ongoing research, and physician awareness needs to be encouraged. Strategies for the management and prevention of steroid-induced bone loss are now available, as are therapeutic interventions. Early recognition of the risk of bone loss and prompt intervention are essential for optimizing care for patients who require glucocorticoid treatment.

### Acknowledgments

*We acknowledge our funding in part by National Institutes of Health grants RO1 AG 12271 and RO1 AG 13519 (Drs. LeBoff and Julie Glowacki) and the support by the National Institutes of Health (NIAMS) grant P60AR 36308 (Drs. LeBoff, Matthew Liang, and Julie Glowacki) for the Multi-Purpose Arthritis and Musculoskeletal Diseases Center, Brigham and Women's Hospital, Boston, Massachusetts.*

# REFERENCES

1. Riggs BL, Melton LJ III: The prevention and treatment of osteoporosis. N Engl J Med 1992; 327:620.
2. Delaney M, LeBoff MS: Metabolic bone disease. *In* Kelley WN, Harris ED, Ruddy S, et al (eds): Textbook of Rheumatology, 6th ed. Philadelphia: WB Saunders, in press.
3. Sambrook PN, Eisman JA, Champion GD, et al: Determinants of axial bone loss in rheumatoid arthritis. Arthritis Rheum 1987; 30:712.
4. Uitterlinden AG, Burger H, Huang Q, et al: Relation of alleles of the collagen type Iα1 gene to bone density and the risk of osteoporotic fractures in postmenopausal women. N Engl J Med 1998; 338:1016–1021.
5. Looker AC, Johnston CC Jr, Wahner HW, et al: Prevalence of low femoral bone density in older US women from NHANES III. J Bone Miner Res 1995; 10:769–802.
6. Ross DS, Neer RM, Ridgway EC: Subclinical hyperthyroidism and reduced bone density as a possible result of prolonged suppression of the pituitary-thyroid axis with L-thyroxine. Am J Med 1987; 82:1167.
7. Friedman AJ, Daly M, Juneau-Norcross M, et al: A prospective, randomized trial of gonadotropin-releasing hormone agonist plus estrogen-progestin add-back regimens for women with leiomyomata uteri. J Clin Endocrinol Metab 1993; 76:1439.
8. Rigotti NA, Neer RM, Skates SJ, et al: The clinical course of osteoporosis in anorexia nervosa: A longitudinal study of cortical bone mass. JAMA 1991; 265:1133.
9. Finkelstein JS, Klibanski A, Neer RM, et al: Osteoporosis in men with idiopathic hypogonadotropic hypogonadism. Ann Intern Med 1987; 106:354.
10. LeBoff MS, Fuleihan El-Hajj G, Brown E: Osteoporosis and Paget's disease of bone. *In* Branch WT (ed): Office Practice of Medicine. Philadelphia: WB Saunders, 1994:700.
11. Cummings SR, Black DM, Nevitt MC, et al: Bone density at various sites for prediction of hip fractures: The Study of Osteoporotic Fractures Research Group. Lancet 1993; 341(8837):72.
12. Gough A, Sambrook P, Devlin J, et al: Osteoclastic activation is the principal mechanism leading to secondary osteoporosis in rheumatoid arthritis. J Rheumatol 1998; 25(7):1282–1289.
13. Sambrook PN, Eisman JA, Yeates MG, et al: Osteoporosis in rheumatoid arthritis: Safety of low dose corticosteroids. Ann Rheum Dis 1986; 45:950.
14. Sambrook PN, Ansell BM, Foster S, et al: Bone turnover in early rheumatoid arthritis: 2. Longitudinal bone density studies. Ann Rheum Dis 1985; 44:580.
15. Hooyman JR, Melton LJ III, Nelson AM, et al: Fractures after rheumatoid arthritis. Arthritis Rheum 1984; 27:1353.
16. Mellish RWL, O'Sullivan MM, Garrahan NJ, et al: Iliac crest trabecular bone mass and structure in patients with non-steroid treated rheumatoid arthritis. Ann Rheum Dis 1987; 46:830.
17. Demir H, Kelestimur F, Tunc M, et al: Hypothalamo-pituitary-adrenal axis and growth hormone axis in patients with rheumatoid arthritis. Scand J Rheumatol 1999; 28(1):41–46.
18. Sambrook PN, Eisman JA, Champion GD, et al: Sex hormone status and osteoporosis in postmenopausal women with rheumatoid arthritis. Arthritis Rheum 1988; 31:973.
19. Sambrook P, Birmingham J, Champion GD, et al: Postmenopausal bone loss in rheumatoid arthritis: Effect of estrogens and androgens. J Rheumatol 1992; 19:357.
20. Laan RFJM, Buijs WCAM, Verbeek ALM, et al: Bone mineral density in patients with recent onset rheumatoid arthritis: Influence of disease activity and functional capacity. Ann Rheum Dis 1993; 52:21.
21. Hansen M, Florescu A, Stoltenberg M, et al: Bone loss in rheumatoid arthritis. Influence of disease activity, duration of the disease, functional capacity, and corticosteroid treatment. Scand J Rheumatol 1996; 25(6):367–376.
22. Avioli LV: Osteoporosis in rheumatoid arthritis [Editorial]. Arthritis Rheum 1987; 30:830.
23. Sambrook PN, Reeve J: Bone disease in rheumatoid arthritis [Editorial]. Clin Sci 1988; 74:225.
24. Takayanagi H, Oda H, Yamamoto S, et al: A new mechanism of bone destruction in rheumatoid arthritis: Synovial fibroblasts induce osteoclastogenesis. Biochem Biophys Res Commun 1997; 240(2):279–286.
25. Firestein GS, Alvaro-Garcia J, Maki R: Quantitative analysis of cytokine gene expression in rheumatoid arthritis. J Immunol 1990; 144:3347.
26. Saxne T, Palladino MA, Heinegard D, et al: Detection of tumor necrosis factor-alpha but not TNF-beta in rheumatoid arthritis synovial fluid and serum. Arthritis Rheum 1988; 31:1041.
27. Guerne PA, Zuraw BL, Vaughan JH, et al: Synovium as a source of interleukin-6 in vitro. J Clin Invest 1989; 83:585.
28. Ogata Y, Kukita A, Kukita T, et al: A novel role of IL-15 in the development of osteoclasts: Inability to replace its activity with IL-2. J Immunol 1999; 162(5):2754–2760.
29. Kokate S, Udagawa N, Takahashi N, et al: IL-17 in synovial fluids from patients with rheumatoid arthritis is a potent stimulator of osteoclastogenesis. J Clin Invest 1999; 103(9):1345–1352.
30. Goldhaber P: Heparin enhancement of factors stimulating bone resorption in tissue culture. Science 1965; 147:407.
31. Amin AR, Attur M, Abramson SB: Nitric oxide synthase and cyclooxygenases: Distribution, regulation, and intervention in arthritis. Curr Opin Rheumatol 1999; 11(3):202–209.
32. Scott DL, Farr M, Hawkins CF, et al: Serum calcium levels in rheumatoid arthritis. Ann Rheum Dis 1981; 40:580.
33. Weisman MH, Orth RW, Catherwood BD, et al: Measures of bone loss in rheumatoid arthritis. Arch Intern Med 1986; 146:701.
34. Dykman TR, Gluck OS, Murphy WA, et al: Evaluation of factors associated with glucocorticoid-induced osteopenia in patients with rheumatic diseases. Arthritis Rheum 1985; 28:361.

35. Als OS, Gotfredsen A, Christiansen C: The effect of glucocorticoids on bone mass in rheumatoid arthritis patients: Influence of menopausal state. Arthritis Rheum 1985; 28:369.
36. Laan RFJM, van Riel PLCM, van de Putte LBA, et al: Low-dose prednisone induces rapid reversible axial bone loss in patients with rheumatoid arthritis. Ann Intern Med 1993; 119:963.
37. Reid DM, Kennedy NSJ, Smith MA, et al: Bone loss in rheumatoid arthritis and primary generalized osteoarthrosis: Effects of corticosteroids, suppressive antirheumatic drugs and calcium supplements. Br J Rheumatol 1986; 25:253.
38. Hall GM, Spector ID, Griffin AJ, et al: The effect of rheumatoid arthritis and steroid therapy on bone density in postmenopausal women. Arthritis Rheum 1993; 36:1510.
39. LeBoff MS, Wade JP, Mackowiak S, et al: Low dose steroids do not have adverse effects on bone density or indices of mineral metabolism in postmenopausal women with rheumatoid arthritis. Clin Res 1989; 37:354A.
40. Verhoeven AC, Boers M: Limited bone loss due to corticosteroids: A systematic review of prospective studies in rheumatoid arthritis and other diseases. J Rheumatol 1997; 24(8):1495–1503.
41. Klein RG, Arnaud SB, Gallagher JC, et al: Intestinal calcium absorption in exogenous hypercortisolism: Role of 25-hydroxyvitamin D and corticosteroid dose. J Clin Invest 1977; 60:253.
42. Lane NE, Lukert B: The science and therapy of glucocorticoid-induced osteoporosis. Endocrinol Metab Clin North Am 1998; 27:465–483.
43. Canalis E: Mechanisms of glucocorticoid action in bone: Implications of glucocorticoid-induced osteoporosis. J Endocrinol Metab 1996; 81:3441–3447.
44. Weinstein RS, Jilka RL, Parfitt M, et al: Inhibition of osteoblastogenesis and promotion of apoptosis of osteoblasts and osteocytes by glucocorticoids. J Clin Invest 1999; 102:274–282.
45. Canalis E: Effect of glucocorticoids on type I collagen synthesis, alkaline phosphatase activity, and deoxyribonucleic acid content in cultured rat calvariae. Endocrinology 1983; 112:931.
46. Reid IR, Chapman GE, Fraser TR, et al: Low serum osteocalcin levels in glucocorticoid-treated asthmatics. J Clin Endocrinol Metab 1986; 62:379.
47. Dempster DW: Bone histomorphometry in glucocorticoid-induced osteoporosis. J Bone Miner Res 1989; 4:137.
48. Gennari C, Agnusdei D, Montagnani M, et al: An effective regimen of intranasal salmon calcitonin in early postmenopausal bone loss. Calcif Tissue Int 1992; 50:381.
49. Dykman TR, Haralson KM, Gluck OS, et al: Effect of oral 1,25-dihydroxyvitamin D and calcium on glucocorticoid-induced osteopenia in patients with rheumatic diseases. Arthritis Rheum 1984; 27:1336.
50. Reid IR, Katz JM, Ibbertson HK, et al: The effects of hydrocortisone, parathyroid hormone, and the bisphosphonate APD on bone resorption in neonatal mouse calvaria. Calcif Tissue Int 1986; 38:38.
51. Stern PH: Inhibition by steroids of parathyroid hormone-induced 45Ca release from embryonic rat bone in vitro. J Pharmacol Exp Ther 1969; 168:211.
52. Jee WSS, Park HZ, Roberts WE, et al: Corticosteroid and bone. Am J Anat 1970; 129:477.
53. Gluck OS, Murphy WA, Hahn TJ, et al: Bone loss in adults receiving alternate day glucocorticoid therapy. Arthritis Rheum 1981; 24:892.
54. Adachi J: Corticosteroid-induced osteoporosis. Am J Med Sci 1997; 313(1):41–49.
55. Reid IR, France JT, Pybus J, et al: Low plasma testosterone levels in glucocorticoid-treated male asthmatics. BMJ 1985; 291:574.
56. MacAdams MR, White RH, Chippus BE, et al: Reduction of serum testosterone levels during chronic glucocorticoid therapy. Ann Intern Med 1986; 104:648–651.
57. Rosen H, Jamed ML, Barkan AL: Dexamethasone suppresses gonadotropin-releasing hormone (GnRH) secretion and has direct pituitary effects in male rats: Differential regulation of GnRH receptor and gonadotropin responses to GnRH. Endocrinology 1988; 122:2873.
58. Adinoff AD, Hollister JR: Steroid-induced fractures and bone loss in patients with asthma. N Engl J Med 1983; 309:265.
59. Van Staa TP, Cooper C, Abenhaim L, et al: Use of oral corticosteroids and risk of fractures [Abstract 1222]. Bone 1998; 23(suppl):S202.
60. Morton DJ, Barrett-Connor EL, Schneider DL, et al: Nonsteroidal anti-inflammatory drugs and bone mineral density in older women: The Rancho Bernardo study. J Bone Miner Res 1998; 13(12):1924–1931.
61. Hall TJ, Jeker H, Nyugen H, et al: Gold salts inhibit osteoclastic bone resorption in vitro. Inflamm Res 1996; 45(5); 230–233.
62. Buckley LM, Leib ES, Cartularo KS, et al: Effects of low dose methotrexate on the bone mineral density of patients with rheumatoid arthritis. J Rheumatol 1997; 24(8):1489–1494.
63. Van Der Veen MJ, Scheven BA, Van Roy JL, et al: In vitro effects of methotrexate on human articular cartilage and bone-derived osteoblasts. Br J Rheumatol 1996; 35(4):342–349.
64. Katz JN, LeBoff MS, Wade JP, et al: Effect of methotrexate on bone density and calcium homeostasis in rheumatoid arthritis [Abstract]. Clin Res 1989; 37:509A.
65. Movsowitz C, Epstein S, Fallon M, et al: Cyclosporin A in vivo produces severe osteopenia in the rat: Effect of dose and duration of administration. Endocrinology 1988; 123:2571.
66. Rich GM, Mudge GH, Laffel GL, et al: Cyclosporine A and prednisone-associated osteoporosis in heart transplant recipients. J Heart Lung Transplant 1992; 11:950.
67. Saarto T, Blomquist C, Valimaki M, et al: Chemical castration induced by adjuvant cyclophosphamide, methotrexate, and fluorouracil causes rapid bone loss that is reduced by clodronate: A randomized study in premenopausal breast cancer patients. J Clin Oncol 1997; 15(4):1341–1347.
68. Boumpas DT, Austin HA III, Vaughan EM, et al: Risk for sustained amenorrhea in patients with systemic lupus erythematosus receiving intermittent pulse cyclophosphamide therapy. Ann Intern Med 1993; 119:366.
69. Teichmann J, Lange U, Stracke H, et al: Bone metabolism and bone mineral density of systemic lupus erythematosus at the time of diagnosis. Rheumatol Int 1999; 18(4):137–140.
70. Kipen Y, Buchbinder R, Forbes A, et al: Prevalence of reduced bone mineral density in systemic lupus erythematosus and the role of steroids. J Rheumatol 1997; 24:1922–1929.
71. Buyon JP: Hormone replacement therapy in postmenopausal women with systemic lupus erythematosus. J Am Med Womens Assoc 1998; 53(1):13–17.
72. Kim MY, Buyon JP, Petri M, et al: Equivalence trials in SLE research: Issues to consider. Lupus 1999; 8(8):620–626.
73. Dequecker J, Mokassa L, Aerssens J, et al: Bone density and local growth factors in generalized osteoarthritis. Microsc Res Tech 1997; 37(4):358–371.
74. Fazzalari NL, Parkinson IH: Femoral trabecular bone of osteoarthritic and normal subjects in an age and sex matched group. Osteoarthritis Cartilage 1998; 6(6):377–382.
75. Liu G, Peacock M, Eilam O, et al: Effect of osteoarthritis in the lumbar spine and hip on bone mineral density and diagnosis of osteoporosis in elderly men and women. Osteoporos Int 1997; 7(6):564–569.
76. Hannan MT, Anderson JJ, Zhang Y, et al: Bone mineral density and knee osteoarthritis in elderly men and women: The Framingham study. Arthritis Rheum 1993; 36:1671.
77. Reid DM, Nicoll JJ, Smith MA, et al: Corticosteroids and bone mass in asthma: Comparisons with rheumatoid arthritis and polymyalgia rheumatica. BMJ 1986; 293:1463.
78. Pearce G, Ryan PF, Delmas PD, et al: The deleterious effects of low-dose corticosteroids on bone density in patients with polymyalgia rheumatica. Br J Rheumatol 1998; 37(3):292–299.
79. Lee YS, Schlotzhauer T, Ott SM, et al: Skeletal status of men with early and late ankylosing spondylitis. Am J Med 1997; 103(3):233–241.
80. Tapia-Serrano R, Jiminez-Balderas FJ, Murrieta S, et al: Testicular function in active ankylosing spondylitis: Therapeutic response to human chorionic gonadotropin. J Rheumatol 1991; 18:841.
81. Bronson WD, Walker SE, Hillman LS, et al: Bone mineral density and biochemical markers of bone metabolism in ankylosing spondylitis. J Rheumatol 1998; 25(5):929–935.
82. Nelson AM, Riggs BL, Jowsey JO: Atypical axial osteomalacia. Arthritis Rheum 1978; 21:715.
83. Donnelly S, Doyle DV, Denton A, et al: Bone mineral density and vertebral compression fracture rates in ankylosing spondylitis. Ann Rheum Dis 1994; 53(2):117–121.

84. Dalsky GP, Stocke KS, Ehsani AA, et al: Weight-bearing exercise training and lumbar bone mineral content in postmenopausal women. Ann Intern Med 1988; 108:824.

85. Dawson-Hughes B, Dallal GE, Krall EA, et al: A controlled trial of the effect of calcium supplementation on bone density in postmenopausal women. N Engl J Med 1990; 323:878.

86. Johnston CC Jr, Miller JZ, Selmenda CW, et al: Calcium supplementation and increases in bone mineral density in children. N Engl J Med 1992; 327:82.

87. NIH Consensus Development Panel on Optimal Calcium Intake: Optimal calcium intake—NIH Consensus Conference. JAMA 1994; 272(24):1942–1948.

88. Recker RR: Calcium absorption and achlorhydria. N Engl J Med 1985; 313:70.

89. Reid IR, Ibbertson HK: Calcium supplements in the prevention of steroid-induced osteoporosis. Am J Clin Nutr 1986; 44:287.

90. LeBoff MS, Kohlmeier L, Hurwitz S, et al: Occult vitamin D deficiency in postmenopausal US women with acute hip fracture. JAMA 1999; 281(16):1505–1511.

91. Dawson-Hughes B, Harris SS, Krall EA, et al: Effect of calcium and vitamin D supplementation on bone density in men and women 65 years of age or older. N Engl J Med 1997; 337:670–676.

92. Chapuy MC, Arlot ME, Duboeuf F, et al: Vitamin $D_3$ and calcium to prevent hip fractures in elderly women. N Engl J Med 1992; 327:1637.

93. Gallagher JC, Goldgar O: Treatment of postmenopausal osteoporosis with high doses of synthetic calcitriol. Ann Intern Med 1990; 113:649.

94. Tilyard MW, Spears GF, Thompson J, et al: Treatment of postmenopausal osteoporosis with calcitriol or calcium. N Engl J Med 1992; 326(6):357–362.

95. Eriksen EF, Colvard DS, Berg NG, et al: Evidence of estrogen receptors in normal human osteoblast-like cells. Science 1988; 241:84.

96. Manolagas SC, Jilka RL: Cytokines, hematopoiesis, osteoclastogenesis, and estrogens [Editorial]. Calcif Tissue Int 1992; 50:199.

97. Pacifici R: Is there a causal role for IL-1 in postmenopausal bone loss? Calcif Tissue Int 1992; 50:295.

98. American College of Physicians: Guidelines for counseling postmenopausal women about preventative hormone therapy. Ann Intern Med 1992; 117:1038.

99. Felson DT, Zhang Y, Hannan MT, et al: The effect of postmenopausal estrogen therapy on bone density in elderly women. N Engl J Med 1993; 329:1141.

100. Lindsay R, Tohme JF: Estrogen treatment of patients with established postmenopausal osteoporosis. Obstet Gynecol 1990; 76:290.

101. Hulley S, Grady D, Bush T, et al: Randomized trial of estrogen plus progestin for secondary prevention of coronary heart disease in postmenopausal women. JAMA 1998; 280:605–613.

102. Weinstein L, Bewtra C, Gallagher JC: Evaluation of a continuous combined low-dose regimen of estrogen-progestin for treatment of the menopausal patient. Am J Obstet Gynecol 1990; 162:1534.

103. American College of Obstetrics and Gynecology: Hormone replacement therapy: A review of the recent guidelines of the American College of Obstetrics and Gynecology regarding hormone replacement therapy. ACOG Tech Bull 1992; 166:1.

104. Fisher B, Costantino JP, Wickerham DL, et al: Tamoxifen for prevention of breast cancer: Report of the National Surgical Adjuvant Breast and Bowel Project P-1 Study. J Natl Cancer Inst 1998; 90:1371–1388.

105. Love RR, Mazess RB, Barden HS, et al: Effects of tamoxifen on bone mineral density in postmenopausal women with breast cancer. N Engl J Med 1992; 326:852.

106. Delmas PD, Bjarnason NH, Mitlak BH, et al: Effects of raloxifene on bone mineral density, serum cholesterol concentrations, and uterine endometrium in postmenopausal women. N Engl J Med 1997; 337:1641–1647.

107. Cummings S, Eckert S, Krueger K, et al: The effect of raloxifene on risk of breast cancer in postmenopausal women. Results from the MORE randomized trial. JAMA 1999; 281:2189–2197.

108. Overgaard K, Riis BJ, Christiansen C, et al: Effect of calcitonin given intranasally on early postmenopausal bone loss. BMJ 1990; 299:477.

109. Overgaard K, Riis BJ, Christiansen C, et al: Nasal calcitonin for treatment of established osteoporosis. Clin Endocrinol 1989; 30:435.

109a. Silver S, Chestnut C, Andriano K, et al: Salmon calcitonin nasal spray reduces risk of vertebral fractures in established osteoporosis and has continuous efficacy with prolonged treatment: Accrued 5 year worldwide data of the PROOF study. [Abstract 1108]. Bone 1998; 23(suppl):S174.

110. Fleisch HA: Bisphosphonates: Preclinical aspects and use in osteoporosis. Ann Intern Med 1997; 29:55–62.

111. Watts NB, Harris ST, Genant HK, et al: Intermittent cyclical etidronate treatment of postmenopausal osteoporosis. N Engl J Med 1990; 323:73.

112. Black DM, Cummings SR, Karpf DB, et al: Randomized trial of effect of alendronate on risk of fracture in women with existing vertebral fractures. Fracture Intervention Trial Research Group. Lancet 1996; 348:1535–1541.

113. Liberman UA, Weiss SR, Broll J, et al: Effect of oral alendronate on bone mineral density and the incidence of fractures in postmenopausal osteoporosis. The Alendronate Phase III Osteoporosis Treatment Study Group. N Engl J Med 1998; 333:1437–1443.

114. Cummings SR, Black DM, Thompson DE, et al: Effect of alendronate on risk of fracture in women with low bone density but without vertebral fractures. JAMA 1998; 280:2077–2082.

115. Reginster J, Mirre HW, Sorensen OH, et al: Randomized trial of the effects of risedronate on vertebral fractures in women with established postmenopausal osteoporosis. Osteoporos Int 2000; 11(1):83–91.

116. Harris ST, Watts NB, Genont HK, et al: Effects of risedronate treatment on vertebral and nonvertebral fractures in women with postmenopausal osteoporosis: A randomized controlled trial. Vertebral Efficacy with Risedronate Therapy (VERT) Study Group. JAMA 1999; 282(14):1344–1352.

117. Pak CYC, Sakhaee K, Zerwekh JE, et al: Safe and effective treatment of osteoporosis with intermittent slow release sodium fluoride; Augmentation of vertebral bone mass and inhibition of fractures. J Clin Endocrinol Metab 1989; 68:150.

118. Riggs BL, Hodgson SF, O'Fallon WM: Effect of fluoride treatment on the fracture rate in postmenopausal women with osteoporosis. N Engl J Med 1990; 322:802.

119. Meunier PJ, Sebert JL, Reginster JY, et al: Fluoride salts are no better at preventing new vertebral fractures than calcium-vitamin D in postmenopausal osteoporosis: The FAVO Study. Osteoporos Int 1998;8(1):4–12.

120. Slovik DM, Rosenthal DI, Doppelt SH, et al: Restoration of spinal bone in osteoporotic men by treatment with human parathyroid hormone (1-34) and 1,25-dihydroxyvitamin D. J Bone Miner Res 1986; 4:377.

121. Lindsay R, Nieves J, Formica C, et al: Randomized controlled study of effect of parathyroid hormone on vertebral-bone mass and fracture incidence among postmenopausal women on oestrogen with osteoporosis. Lancet 1997; 350(9077):550–555.

122. Plotkin H, Gundberg C, Mitnick M, et al: Dissociation of bone formation from resorption during 2-week treatment with human parathyroid hormone-related peptide (1-36) in humans: Potential as an anabolic therapy for osteoporosis. J Clin Endocrinol Metab 1998; 83(8):2786–2791.

123. Hahn TJ: Steroid and drug induced osteopenia. In Favus MJ (ed): Primer of the Metabolic Diseases and Disorders of Mineral Metabolism. Philadelphia: Lippincott-Raven, 1993:250.

124. Cooper C, Coupland C, Mitchell M: Rheumatoid arthritis, corticosteroid therapy and hip fracture. Ann Rheum Dis 1995; 54:49–52.

125. American College of Rheumatology Task Force on Osteoporosis Guidelines: Recommendations for the prevention and treatment of glucocorticoid-induced osteoporosis. Arthritis Rheum 1996; 39:1792–1801.

126. Kotaniemi A, Savolainen A, Kroger H, et al: Weight-bearing physical activity, calcium intake, systemic glucocorticoids, chronic inflammation, and body constitution as determinants of lumbar and femoral bone mineral in juvenile chronic arthritis. Scand J Rheumatol 1999; 28(1):19–26.

127. Buckley LM, Leib ES, Cartularo KS, et al: Calcium and vitamin $D_3$ supplementation prevents bone loss in the spine secondary

to low-dose corticosteroids in patients with rheumatoid arthritis. A randomized, double-blind, placebo-controlled trial. Ann Intern Med 1996; 125:961–968.

128. Adachi JD, Bensen WG, Bianchi F, et al: Vitamin D and calcium in the prevention of corticosteroid-induced osteoporosis: A three-year follow-up. J Rheumatol 1996; 23:995–1000.

129. Sambrook P, Birmingham J, Kelly P, et al: Prevention of corticosteroid osteoporosis: A comparison of calcium, calcitriol, and calcitonin. N Engl J Med 1993; 328:1747.

130. Hahn TJ, Halstead LR, Teitelbaum SL, et al: Altered mineral metabolism in glucocorticoid-induced osteopenia: Effect of 25-hydroxyvitamin D administration. J Clin Invest 1979; 64:655.

131. Adams JS, Wahl TO, Lukert BP: Effects of hydrochlorothiazide and dietary sodium restriction on calcium metabolism in corticosteroid treated patients. Metabolism 1981; 30:217.

132. Adams JS, Song CF, Kantorovich V: Rapid recovery of bone mass in hypercalciuric, osteoporotic men treated with hydrochlorothiazide. Ann Intern Med 1999; 130:658–660.

133. Ray A, Downey W, Griffin MR, et al: Long-term use of thiazide diuretics and risk of hip fracture. Lancet 1989; 1:687.

134. Reid I, Wattie DJ, Evans MC, et al: Testosterone therapy in glucocorticoid-treated men. Arch Intern Med 1996; 156: 1173–1177.

135. Snyder PJ, Peachey H, Hannoush P, et al: Effect of testosterone treatment on bone mineral density in men over 65 years of age. J Clin Endocrinol Metab 1999; 84(6):1966–1972.

136. Luckert BP, Johnson BE, Robinson RG, et al: Estrogen and progesterone replacement therapy reduces glucocorticoid-induced bone loss. J Bone Miner Res 1992; 7:1063–1069.

137. Van den Brink HR, Lems WF, Ven Everdingen AA, et al: Adjuvant oestrogen treatment increases bone mineral density in postmenopausal women with rheumatoid arthritis. Ann Rheum Dis 1993; 52:302.

138. Hall GM, Daniels M, Doyle DV, et al: Effect of hormone replacement therapy on bone mass in rheumatoid arthritis patients with and without steroids. Arthritis Rheum 1994; 37:1499–1505.

139. Adachi JD, Bensen WG, Bell MJ, et al: Salmon calcitonin nasal spray in the prevention of corticosteroid-induced osteoporosis. Br J Rheumatol 1997; 36:255–259.

140. Luengo M, Pons F, Martinez de Osaba MJ, et al: Prevention of further bone mass loss by nasal calcitonin in patients on long-term glucocorticoid therapy for asthma: A two year follow up study. Thorax 1994; 49:1099–1102.

141. Ringe JD, Welzel D: Salmon calcitonin in the therapy of corticoid-induced osteoporosis. Eur J Clin Pharmacol 1987; 33:35.

142. Kotaniemi A, Piirainen H, Paimela L, et al: Is continuous intranasal salmon calcitonin effective in treating axial bone loss in patients with active rheumatoid arthritis receiving low dose glucocorticoid therapy? J Rheumatol 1996; 23(11):1875–1879.

143. Montemurro L, Schiraldi G, Fraioli P, et al: Prevention of corticosteroid-induced osteoporosis with salmon calcitonin in sarcoid patients. Calcif Tissue Int 1991; 49:71.

144. Sileghem A, Geusens P, Dequeker J: Intranasal calcitonin for the prevention of bone erosion and bone loss in rheumatoid arthritis. Ann Rheum Dis 1992; 51(6):761.

145. Healey JH, Paget S, Williams-Russo P, et al: A randomized controlled trial of salmon calcitonin to prevent bone loss in corticosteroid-treated temporal arteritis and polymyalgia rheumatica. Calcif Tissue Int 1996; 58(2):73–80.

146. Lems WF, Jacobs WG, Bijlsma JWJ, et al: Effect of sodium fluoride on the prevention of corticosteroid-induced osteoporosis. Osteoporos Int 1997; 7:575–582.

147. Guaydier-Souquieres G, Kotzki PO, Sabatier JP, et al: In corticosteroid-treated respiratory diseases, monofluorophosphate increases lumbar bone density: A double-masked randomized study. Osteoporos Int 1996; 6:171–177.

148. Rickers H, Deding A, Christiansen C, et al: Corticosteroid-induced osteopenia and vitamin D metabolism: Effect of vitamin $D_2$, calcium, phosphate, and sodium fluoride administration. Clin Endocrinol 1982; 16:490.

149. Meunier PJ, Briancon D, Chavassieu P, et al: Treatment with fluoride: Bone histomorphometric findings. *In* Christiansen C, Johansen JS, Riis BJ (eds): Osteoporosis. Viborg, Denmark: Norhaven AG, 1987:824.

150. Lane NE, Jenkins DK, Arnaud CD: Short-term increases in formation markers predict subsequent spine bone mineral density gains in women with glucocorticoid-induced osteoporosis treated with parathyroid hormone [Abstract 1042]. Bone 1998; 23(5, suppl):S159.

151. Reid IR, King AR, Alexander CJ, et al: Prevention of steroid-induced osteoporosis with (3-amino-1-hydroxypropylindene)-1, 1-bisphosphonate (APD). Lancet 1988; 1:143.

152. Cortet B, Hachulla E, Barton I, et al: Evaluation of the efficacy of etidronate therapy in preventing glucocorticoid-induced bone loss in patients with inflammatory rheumatic diseases. A randomized study. Rev Rhum Engl Ed 1999; 66(4):214–219.

153. Adachi JD, Bensen WG, Brown J: Intermittent etidronate therapy to prevent corticosteroid-induced osteoporosis. N Engl J Med 1997; 337:382–387.

154. Roux C, Adachi JD, Cooper C, et al: Pooled results from three randomized trials on the prevention of corticosteroid-induced osteoporosis with etidronate [Abstract W460]. Bone 1998; 23(suppl):S401.

155. Saag K, Emkey R, Schnitzer TJ, et al: Alendronate for the prevention and treatment of glucocorticoid-induced osteoporosis. N Engl J Med 1998; 339:292–299.

156. Cohen S, Levy RM, Keller M, et al: Risedronate therapy prevents corticosteroid-induced bone loss: A twelve-month, multicenter randomized, double-blind placebo-controlled parallel group study. Arthritis Rheum 1999; 42(11):2309–2318.

157. Reid D, Cohen S, Pack S, et al: Risedronate is an effective and well-tolerated therapy in both the treatment and prevention of corticosteroid-induced osteoporosis [Abstract]. Presented at the 81st Annual Meeting of the Endocrine Society, San Diego, June 1999.

158. Montecucco C, Caporali R, Caprotti P, et al: Sex hormones and bone metabolism in postmenopausal rheumatoid arthritis treated with two different glucocorticoids. J Rheumatol 1992; 19:1895.

159. Kurt L, Casez JP, Horber FF, et al: Effects of deflazacort versus prednisone on bone mass, body composition, and lipid profile: A randomized, double blind study in kidney transplant patients. J Clin Endocrinol Metab 1998; 83:3795–3802.

# INDEX

Note: Page numbers in *italics* refer to illustrations; page numbers followed by t refer to tables.

## A

Acetaminophen, in osteoarthritis, 464–465
Acetylcysteine, in dry eyes, 253
Achilles tendinitis, 66
  symptoms of, 67
  treatment of, 67–68
Achilles tendinosis, 66, 67
Achilles tendon, disorders of, 66–68
  insertional disorders of, 66, 67
  noninsertional disorders of, 66
Acid-suppression trial, in ulcers induced by nonsteroidal anti-inflammatory drugs, 470
Acrolein, side effects of, 330
Acupuncture, in fibromyalgia syndrome, 127
S-Adenosylmethionine, in fibromyalgia syndrome, 125
Adrenal suppression, corticosteroid-induced, 228–229
Adrenocorticotrophic hormone, in acute gout, 450–451
Alendronate, in osteoporosis, 537, 540, 541
  in Paget's disease, 498, 499
Alkylating agents, in amyloidosis in rheumatoid arthritis, 241
  in uveitis, 195
Allergic angiitis and granulomatosis. See *Churg-Strauss syndrome.*
Allopurinol, dose adjustment of, based on renal function, 454t
  in chronic gout, in organ transplant recipients, 115
  in gout, 36, 454–455
    hypersensitivity to, management of, 457
  toxicity of, 454–455
Alprazolam, in fibromyalgia syndrome, 124
Alveolitis, in scleroderma, management of, 371–372
American Medical Association, Current Procedural Terminology of, 132–133
Amitriptyline, in ankylosing spondylitis, 265–266
  in childhood fibromyalgia, 440–441
  in fibromyalgia syndrome, 42, 121–122, 123, 128

Amoxicillin, in Lyme disease, 519
  in Lyme disease prophylaxis, 523
  in Lyme disease-related carditis, 520
Amphotericin B, in fungal arthritis, 510–511, 512
Amyloidosis, 491–493
  AA (secondary), 493
  AL (primary), 492
  colchicine in, 492
  familial transthyretin, 493
  hemodialysis-associated, 493
  in familial Mediterranean fever, 494
  in rheumatoid arthritis, 241
  melphalan in, 492
  prednisone in, 492
  treatment of, 492, 492t
Analgesics, in complex regional pain syndrome-I, 105
  narcotic, in osteoarthritis, 34
  non-narcotic, in osteoarthritis, 34
Anaphylactoid purpura. See *Henoch-Schönlein purpura.*
Anemia, autoimmune hemolytic, in systemic lupus erythematosus, author's approach to, 202
  in rheumatoid arthritis, 198–200
    author's approach to, 199–200
    erythropoietin trials in, 198–199
    evaluation of, 198, *199*
    natural history of, 198
    treatment of, 198–199
  in systemic lupus erythematosus, 201–203, 281
  microangiopathic hemolytic, in systemic lupus erythematosus, 202–203
  of chronic disease, mechanism of, 198
    treatment of, 198
Anesthesia, and surgery, in Sjögren's syndrome, 259–260, 260t
Anesthetics, local, in fibromyalgia syndrome, 127–128
Angiitis, primary, of central nervous system. See *Central nervous system, primary angiitis of.*
Angiofibroblastic hyperplasia, 85
Angioplasty, percutaneous transluminal, in Takayasu's arteritis, 356
Ankle joint, pain in, 65–73
  range of motion of, 65–66

Ankylosing spondylitis, amitriptyline in, 265
  auranofin in, 266
  bone loss in, 534
  definition of, 263
  diagnosis of, 10–11, *11*
  disease modifying antirheumatic drugs in, 265–266
  management approach in, 266–267
  natural history of, 263
  neck pain in, 59
  nonarticular manifestations of, 264
  nonsteroidal anti-inflammatory drugs in, 264–265, 265t
  pamidronate in, 265
  patient education in, 264
  D-penicillamine in, 265–266
  physical therapy in, 264
  pulmonary manifestations of, 264
  radiotherapy in, 264, 266
  spinal disease in, 264
  sulfasalazine in, 266–267
  treatment of, 264–266
  uveitis in, 264
Antibiotics, in infectious arteritis, contraindications to, 508
  in infectious arthritis, 504–508, 505–506t, 506t, 507t
  in Lyme disease, 517–518, 521
  in Lyme disease prophylaxis, 523–524
  in Lyme disease–related carditis, 520
  in reactive arthritis, 267–268
  in rheumatoid arthritis, 226
Antibody tests, in Lyme disease, 516
Anticoagulation, in antiphospholipid syndrome in systemic lupus erythematosus, 282
  oral, in antiphospholipid syndrome, 293–294
Anticonvulsants, in complex regional pain syndrome-I, 106
Antidepressants, in fibromyalgia syndrome, 121–124
  tricyclic, in childhood fibromyalgia, 440–441
Antihistamines, in cutaneous vasculitis, 183
Anti-inflammatory agents, nonsteroidal. See *Nonsteroidal anti-inflammatory agents.*

Antilepromatous agents, in cutaneous lupus erythematosus, 177–178
Antimalarial agents, clinical pharmacology of, 284
　during pregnancy, 168
　in cutaneous lupus erythematosus, 176–177, *177*, 279–280
　in cutaneous vasculitis, 183
　in psoriatic arthritis, 270–271
　in rheumatoid arthritis, 224–225, 230
　in systemic lupus erythematosus, 274–275, 275t, 277, 278t
　in systemic lupus erythematosus in childhood, 425
　mechanism of action of, 284
　side effects of, 283
Antimetabolites, in uveitis, 195
Antiphospholipid syndrome, 289–296, 431–432
　clinical manifestations of, 290t
　definition of, 289
　diagnosis of, 291–292
　drug side effects and monitoring in, 293–294
　in systemic lupus erythematosus, 282
　investigational drugs in, 294
　long-term experience in, 291
　management of, 292–293, *293*
　　controlled clinical trials in, 290–291
　　open trials in, 290
　natural history of, 289–290
　oral anticoagulation in, 293–294
　pregnancy in, 289–290
　　management of, 292
　primary, 289
　University of Connecticut Health Center experience in, 291
　venous and arterial thromboses in, 289, 290t, 293
Antirheumatic drugs, disease-modifying, in ankylosing spondylitis, 265–266
　in Felty's syndrome, 242
　in rheumatoid arthritis, 221–226, 222t, 229
　in rheumatoid vasculitis, 244
　in pregnancy and lactation, and effects on fertility, 164–165t
　second-line, in psoriatic arthritis, 269–272
Antirheumatic therapies, toxicities of, during pregnancy, 167t
Antithymocyte globulin, in scleroderma, 369
Antiviral therapy, in hepatitis B virus–related polyarteritis nodosa, 326–327
　in type II mixed cryoglobulinemia, 336
Aortic root disease, inflammatory, in rheumatoid arthritis, 239
Apheresis, in polymyositis, 399
Aplasia, red cell, in rheumatoid arthritis, 200
Arachidonic acid metabolism, cyclooxygenase pathway for, *467*
Arnold-Chiari malformation, syringomyelia in, 61
Arteriography, in Takayasu's arteritis, 354
Arteritis, giant cell. See *Giant cell arteritis.*
　pulmonary, in rheumatoid arthritis, 238
　Takayasu's. See *Takayasu's arteritis.*
Arthritis, acute gouty. See *Gout, acute.*
　cognitive coping techniques in, 149
　costs of, 147
　family support of cognitive-behavioral management in, 150

Arthritis (*Continued*)
　group therapy intervention in, 149
　in elderly, comorbid conditions in, 31
　　economic impact of, 31
　　incidence of, 31
　infectious, 503–513
　　antibiotics in, 504–508, 505–506t, 506t, 507t
　　　contraindications to, 508
　　chronic, 510
　　detritus removal in, 509
　　diagnosis of, 503–504
　　fungal, 510–512, 511t
　　infections of prosthetic joints in, 509
　　joint rehabilitation in, 509–510
　　laboratory tests in, 503–504
　　mycobacterial infections in, 510
　　treatment of, clinical response to, 508, 508t
　inflammatory, in organ transplant recipients, 113–114
　interventions in perceived control in, 151–152
　Lyme disease-related, 520–521
　management of, cognitive-behavioral and psychoeducational interventions in, 147–161
　　cognitive-behavioral approach to, 148, 149t
　mixed, Arthritis Self-Management Program in, 154
　monarticular, hematologic disease presenting as, 3
　　in degenerative disease, 2
　　in neoplasm, 2
　　infection in, 1
　　inflammation in, 1
　　metabolic disease in, 1–2
　mutilans, 82
　outpatient group support in, 149–150
　pain in, and consequences of, management of, 148–150
　　comorbidity associated with, 147–148
　peripheral tuberculous, 510
　problem-solving interventions in, 151
　psoriatic. See *Psoriatic arthritis.*
　psychosocial management of, need for, 148
　reactive, 11–12, *12*
　　and human immunodeficiency virus disease, 267
　　antibiotics in, 267–268
　　definition of, 267
　　future directions in, 268
　　immunosuppressive drugs in, 267, 268
　　management approach in, 268
　　natural history of, 267
　　nonsteroidal anti-inflammatory drugs in, 267
　　sulfasalazine in, 267, 268
　　treatment of, 267–268
　rheumatoid. See *Rheumatoid arthritis.*
　self-management treatment strategies in, 152–158, 153t
　stress management interventions in, 150–151
　temperature biofeedback training in, 149
　with pyoderma gangrenosum, 187
Arthritis Foundation, Arthritis Self-Management Programs and, 153–154
Arthritis/periarthritis, in sarcoidosis, 489

Arthritis Self-Management Program(s), Arthritis Foundation and, 153–154
　clinical trials of, in mixed arthritis, 154
　　in rheumatoid arthritis, 155–156
　long-term follow-up studies of, 154
　self-efficacy and, 155
Arthrodesis, total wrist, in rheumatic disease, 78
　with arthroplasty, in shoulder pain, 47
Arthroplasty, in osteoarthritis, 475–476
　in shoulder pain, 47
　of metacarpophalangeal joint, arthroplasty of, 79–80
　of proximal interphalangeal joint, 80–81, *81*
　wrist, in rheumatic disease, 78
Arthroscopic débridement, in osteoarthritis, 35
Arthroscopy, in osteoarthritis, 475
Artificial tears, 253t
　evaluation of, 253
Aspirin, and Reye's syndrome, 404
　anti-inflammatory actions of, 465
　during pregnancy, 166
　in juvenile rheumatoid arthritis, 403–404
　　compliance rates for, 404
　　dosages of, 404
　　toxicity and monitoring of, 404
　in Kawasaki syndrome, 436
　in rheumatoid arthritis, 220, 221
　low-dose, in antiphospholipid syndrome, 292
Auranofin, in ankylosing spondylitis, 266
　in cutaneous lupus erythematosus, 178, *179*
　in juvenile rheumatoid arthritis, 412–413
　in rheumatoid arthritis, 223
Aurothioglucose, in rheumatoid arthritis, 223
Aurothiomalate, in rheumatoid arthritis, 223
Azathioprine, during pregnancy, 170
　in Behçet's disease, 491
　in childhood systemic lupus erythematosus, 429
　in Churg-Strauss syndrome, 328
　in cutaneous lupus erythematosus, 177, *178*
　in cutaneous vasculitis, 185, *185*
　in idiopathic inflammatory myopathies, 392, 393
　in inflammatory myopathies, 395
　in juvenile dermatomyositis, 434
　in juvenile rheumatoid arthritis, 415
　in lupus nephritis, 303, 306
　in polyarteritis nodosa, 328
　in psoriatic arthritis, 270, 272
　in rheumatoid arthritis, 38, 225–226, 230
　in rheumatoid vasculitis, 244, 245
　in scleroderma, 368–369
　in systemic lupus erythematosus, 276, 278, 279t
　in uveitis, 195
　side effects of, 397, 429
Azithromycin, in Lyme disease, 518–519
Azoles, in fungal arthritis, 511

**B**

Back pain, low. See *Low back pain.*
　postsurgical, 92
Bacterial endocarditis, subacute, in differential diagnosis of acute polyarthritis, 19–20
Bed rest, in lumbago, 93

Behçet's disease, azathioprine in, 491
  benzathine penicillin in, 491
  chlorambucil in, 491
  clinical features of, 490
  colchicine in, 490
  complications of, 490
  corticosteroids in, 491
  cyclophosphamide in, 491
  cyclosporine in, 490, 491
  epidemiology of, 490
  interferon-α in, 491
  methylprednisolone in, 491
  pentoxifylline in, 491
  prednisone in, 491
  sulfasalazine in, 491
  tetracycline in, 490
  thalidomide in, 490–491
  treatment of, 490–491
  triamcinolone in, 490
  uveitis in, 196
Bell's palsy, in Lyme disease, 520
Benzathine penicillin, in Behçet's disease, 491
  in Lyme disease-related arthritis, 521
Benzbromarone, in chronic gout, in organ transplant recipients, 115–116
  in crystal deposition disease, 458
Benzodiazepines, in fibromyalgia syndrome, 124
Benzylpenicillin, in Lyme disease–related arthritis, 521
  in Lyme disease–related carditis, 520
Betamethasone, during pregnancy, 166
Biologic agents, in juvenile rheumatoid arthritis, 415–416
Bisphosphonates, in complex regional pain syndrome-I, 106
  in osteoporosis, 537, 540, 541
  in Paget's disease, 498
Bladder, cyclophosphamide-induced injury to, 361
  cyclophosphamide toxicity to, 330
Blastomycosis, disseminated, 512
Bleeding abnormalities, in nonsteroidal anti-inflammatory drug usage, 471
Blood dyscrasias, in nonsteroidal anti-inflammatory drug usage, 471
Body composition, changes with aging, drug distribution and, 32–33
Bone, Paget's disease of. See *Paget's disease.*
Bone densitometry, in osteoporosis, *529,* 529–530
Bone loss, corticosteroid-induced, prevention and treatment of, 538t, 538–541
  corticosteroids and, 531–532
  tests for causes of, 534t
  evaluation in, 534t, 534–535
  in ankylosing spondylitis, 534
  in osteoarthritis, 533
  in polymyalgia rheumatica, 533–534
  in rheumatoid arthritis, 530–531
  in systemic lupus erythematosus, 533
  with aging, 528
Bone marrow suppression, azathioprine-induced, 397
  cyclophosphamide-induced, 428
Bone mineral density, bone densitometry to measure, *529,* 529–530
  in organ transplant recipients, 111
  measures to improve, in juvenile rheumatoid arthritis, 416
*Borrelia burdorferi,* biology of, 515–516
  transmission by ticks, 515

Boutonnière deformity, in rheumatic disease, 78–79, 80
Bowel, small, problems of, in scleroderma, 374–375
Bromhexine, in Sjögren's syndrome, 254
Bromocriptine, in systemic lupus erythematosus, 277
Bronchiectasis, in rheumatoid arthritis, 238
Bronchiolitis obliterans, in rheumatoid arthritis, 237, 238
Bronchiolitis obliterans–organizing pneumonia, in rheumatoid arthritis, 237–238
Brown's syndrome, in rheumatoid arthritis, 240
Budesonide, in sarcoidosis, 489
Bursitis, aseptic olecranon, 85–86
  causative factors in, 85
  septic olecranon, 86
  subdeltoid, treatment of, 46

## C

Calcinosis, in juvenile dermatomyositis, 180
Calcipotriene, in localized scleroderma, 182
Calcitonin, in complex regional pain syndrome-I, 106
  in osteoporosis, 536–537, 539–540, 541
  in Paget's disease, 497
Calcitriol, in localized scleroderma, 181–182
Calcium, in osteoporosis, 535, 539, 541
  metabolism of, prednisone and, 532
Calcium channel blockers, in benign angiopathy of central nervous system, 350
  in Raynaud's phenomenon, 384, 386t
Calcium phosphate crystal deposition, articular syndromes associated with, 458
Calcium pyrophosphate dihydrate deposition disease, 36–37, 457–458
  diagnosis of, *14,* 14–15, *15*
  pseudo-rheumatoid form of, 15, *15*
  treatment of, 37
Caplan's syndrome, 237
Capsaisin, in osteoarthritis, 464
Cardiac disease, in inflammatory myopathies, 397
  in rheumatoid arthritis, 238–239
Cardiopulmonary lupus erythematosus, 280–281
Cardiovascular disease, in scleroderma, management of, 378
Carditis, Lyme disease–induced, 520
Carpometacarpal joint, of thumb, in osteoarthritis, 84
Cartilage, in osteoarthritis, 461–462
  nonsteroidal anti-inflammatory drugs and, 465–466
Cauda equina syndrome, 96
Causalgia, 101
CD4 mAb, in rheumatoid arthritis, 212–213
CD40L, monoclonal antibody to, in lupus nephritis, 308
Cefotaxime, in Lyme disease meningitis, 519–520
Ceftriaxone, adverse affects of, 521
  in infectious arthritis, 504
  in Lyme disease in pregnancy, 521
  in Lyme disease meningitis, 519

Ceftriaxone (*Continued*)
  in Lyme disease–related arthritis, 521
  in Lyme disease–related carditis, 520
  in Lyme disease–related neuropathy, 520
Cefuroxime, in Lyme disease, 519
Cell-targeted therapies, in rheumatoid arthritis, 212–213
Central nervous system, benign angiopathy of, 346–347
  differential diagnosis and diagnostic tests in, 349t
  granulomatous angiitis of, 346
  and vasculitis after varicella-zoster virus infection, 350
  nonsteroidal anti-inflammatory drug usage and, 471–472
  primary angiitis of, 345
  criteria for diagnosis of, 345, 346t
  differential diagnosis of, 347, 349t
  historical perspective on, 345
  therapeutic approach in, 347, *348,* 349t
  treatment of, 347–350
  vasculitis of, 345–352
  in childhood Henoch-Schönlein purpura, 436
  infection-associated, 350–351
  secondary, 345
Cephalosporins, adverse effects of, 521
  in infectious arthritis, 504
  in Lyme disease meningitis, 519
Cervical medullary junction, surgical decompression of, 241
Cervical nerve roots, innervation of, 54t
Cervical spine. See *Spine, cervical.*
Cevimeline, in Sjögren's syndrome, 254
Charcot joint, classification of, 70
  diabetes with, 70
  symptoms of, 70
  treatment of, 70
Chemical sympathectomy, in complex regional pain syndrome-I, 104–105
Children, dermatomyositis in. See *Dermatomyositis, juvenile.*
  fibromyalgia in, 440–441
  nonsteroidal anti-inflammatory drugs in, adverse reactions to, 406–407
  polyarteritis nodosa in, 437
  recalcitrant myositis in, treatment of, 399–400
  reflex neurovascular dystrophy in. See *Reflex neurovascular dystrophy.*
  rheumatic diseases in, 423–445
  scleroderma in, 438
  systemic lupus erythematosus in. See *Systemic lupus erythematosus, in childhood.*
  vasculitic syndromes in, 435–438
  Wegener's granulomatosis in, 437–438
Chiropractic manipulation, in lumbago, 94–95
Chlorambucil, during pregnancy, 171–172
  in Behçet's disease, 491
  in juvenile dermatomyositis, 434
  in juvenile rheumatoid arthritis, 415
  in myositis, 397–398
  in rheumatoid vasculitis, 244, 245
  in scleroderma, 368–369
Chloramphenicol, in Lyme disease meningitis, 519
Chloroquine, in childhood systemic lupus erythematosus, 425
  in cutaneous lupus erythematosus, 176
  in sarcoidosis, 489
  side effects of, 425

Chondroitin sulfate, in osteoarthritis, 35
Chronic pain syndrome, 91–92
    chronic narcotic therapy in, 98
    chronic pain treatment centers and, 97
    facet injections in, 98
    spinal cord stimulation, 98–99
    spinal opiate administration in, 98
    transcutaneous electric nerve stimulation
        in, 98
Churg-Strauss syndrome, clinical features
        of, 324–325
    clinical pharmacology and drug
        interactions in, 329
    cyclophosphamide in, 326, 328
    glucocorticoids in, 325, 328
    laboratory studies in, 325
    natural history of, 325
    plasma exchange in, 326
    prednisone in, 326, 328
    prospective clinical trials in, 326–327
    treatment of, 327–329
        long-term experience with, 327
    treatment studies in, 325–326
Circinate balanitis, 12, 12
Clarithromycin, in Lyme disease, 519
Claw toe deformity, 71–72
Clodronate, in Paget's disease, 498
Clofazimine, in cutaneous lupus
        erythematosus, 178
Clonazepam, in Sjögren's syndrome, 257
Coccidioidomycosis, 511
Cogan's syndrome, clinical features of, 339
    management of, 340
    natural history of, 339
    treatment studies in, 339–340
Cognitive-behavioral interventions, in
        arthritis, 147–161
Cognitive-behavioral studies, in
        osteoarthritis, 150
Cognitive-behavioral treatment, in
        fibromyalgia syndrome, 128
Cognitive impairment, in neuropsychiatric
        systemic lupus erythematosus, 314
    treatment of, 320
Colchicine, in acute gout, 451–452
    in organ transplant recipients, 114–115
    in amyloidosis, 492, 493
    in Behçet's disease, 490
    in cutaneous vasculitis, 183
    in familial Mediterranean fever, 494, 495
    in gout, 36
    in hypersensitivity vasculitis, 339
    in psoriatic arthritis, 271
    in scleroderma, 367
    toxicity of, manifestations of, 452, 452t
        risk factors for, 451t, 452
        treatment of, 452
Cold response, reconditioning of, in
        Raynaud's phenomenon, 384
Colon, in scleroderma, 375
Complex regional pain syndrome-I,
        analgesics in, 105
    anticonvulsants and neurotropics in, 106
    anti-inflammatory agents in, 105–106
    bisphosphonates in, 106
    calcitonin in, 106
    chemical sympathectomy in, 104–105
    clinical features and natural history of,
        102
    diagnosis of, 103–104, 104t
    epidural and peripheral nerve blockade
        in, 106
    history and terminology in, 101
    neuroaugmentation in, 106–107
    oral sympathetic blockade in, 106

Complex regional pain syndrome-I
        (Continued)
    pathophysiology of, 102–103
    principles of management of, 101, 107
    staging system for, 102
    surgical sympathectomy in, 106
    treatment of, pharmacologic approaches
        to, 104–106
        physical modalities in, 106
        psychological interventions in, 107
        surgical approaches in, 106–107
    vasodilation in, 106
Complex regional pain syndrome-II,
        101
Computed tomography, in neck pain, 55
Computerized medical records, 134
Connective tissue disease(s), diagnosis of,
        15–17, 16, 17
    mixed, 17
    vasculitis of central nervous system in,
        351–352
Corrective surgery and amputation, in
        complex regional pain syndrome-I,
        106–107
Corticosteroids, adverse effects of, 39,
        228–229
    and immunosuppressive agents, in
        lupus nephritis, 304t
    and osteoporosis, 531–532
    bone loss associated with, 531–532
        prevention and treatment of, 538t,
            538–541
        tests for causes of, 534t
    clinical pharmacology of, 284–285
    drug interactions with, 285
    fractures associated with, 532
    in acute gout, 450–451
    in autoimmune hemolytic anemia in
        systemic lupus erythematosus, 202
    in Behçet's disease, 491
    in childhood systemic lupus
        erythematosus, 425–426
    in cutaneous lupus erythematosus, 175,
        177, 280
    in cutaneous vasculitis, 184
    in fibromyalgia syndrome, 124–125
    in gout, 36
    in hematologic lupus erythematosus, 281
    in inflammatory myopathies, 395, 396
    in juvenile dermatomyositis, 433
    in juvenile rheumatoid arthritis, 407–409
    in lupus nephritis, 302–303
    in musculoskeletal lupus erythematosus,
        280
    in neuropsychiatric systemic lupus
        erythematosus, 315–316
    in osteoarthritis, 473
    in pediatric spondyloarthropathies,
        407–409
    in polyarteritis nodosa in childhood,
        437
    in polymyalgia rheumatica, 40–41
    in psoriasis, 186
    in pyoderma gangrenosum, 187–188
    in relapsing polychondritis, 495, 496
    in rheumatoid arthritis, 39, 227–229, 531
    in sarcoidosis, 489
    in Sweet's syndrome, 188, 189
    in systemic lupus erythematosus,
        275–276, 276t
    in thrombocytopenia with systemic
        lupus erythematosus, 204
    in uveitis, 194–195
    injections of, in problems of hand and
        wrist, in rheumatoid arthritis, 75

Corticosteroids (Continued)
    intra-articular, in juvenile rheumatoid
        arthritis, 408–409
        protective effect of, 473
    intravenous pulse, in juvenile
        rheumatoid arthritis, 408
    pharmacologic effects of, 285
    side effects of, 41, 42, 228–229, 283, 316,
        397, 531–532
    toxicity of, monitoring of, 316
Cortisol, in rheumatoid arthritis, 227
Cranial neuropathies, in neuropsychiatric
        systemic lupus erythematosus,
        treatment of, 320
Cricoarytenoid ankylosis, in rheumatoid
        arthritis, 238
Crush injuries, of foot, 70–71
Cryoglobulinemia, mixed, in differential
        diagnosis of acute polyarthritis, 21, 22,
        24, 26, 27, 29
    type II mixed, antiviral therapy in, 336
        characteristics of, 334–335
        glomerulonephritis in, 335
        interferon-alpha in, 336, 337
        long-term experience with, 335
        lymphoproliferative disorders in, 335
        management of, 336–337
        natural history of, 335
        pathogenesis of, 335
        prospective trials in, 336
        skin lesions in, 335
        treatment studies in, 335–336
    with vasculitis. See Cryoglobulinemia, type
        II mixed.
Cryptococcal arthritis, 512
Crystal deposition diseases, 35–37,
        447–460
    diagnosis of, 13–17
    differential diagnosis of, 6
    investigational drugs and future
        directions in, 458
Current Procedural Terminology, of
        American Medical Association,
        132–133
Cutaneous lupus erythematosus. See Lupus
        erythematosus, cutaneous.
Cyclobenzaprine, in fibromyalgia
        syndrome, 42, 122–123
Cyclooxygenase, inducible, selective
        inhibitors of, 472
Cyclooxygenase-1 and -2 inhibitors,
        nonselective, in rheumatoid arthritis,
        220–221
Cyclooxygenase-2 inhibitors, selective, in
        rheumatoid arthritis, 219–220
Cyclooxygenase-2–specific inhibitors, in
        crystal deposition disease, 458
Cyclooxygenase inhibitors, nonselective,
        466t, 468–469
Cyclooxygenase pathway, for arachidonic
        acid metabolism, 467
Cyclophosphamide, clinical pharmacology
        of, and drug interactions, 329
    during pregnancy, 171
    in Behçet's disease, 491
    in childhood systemic lupus
        erythematosus, 427–428
        side effects of, 428
    in Churg-Strauss syndrome, 326,
        328–329
    in cutaneous vasculitis, 184
    in familial Mediterranean fever, 494–495
    in Henoch-Schönlein purpura, 338
    in juvenile rheumatoid arthritis, 415
    in lupus nephritis, 303–304, 305, 306

Cyclophosphamide (*Continued*)
  in myositis, 398
  in neuropsychiatric systemic lupus
    erythematosus, 316–317
  in polyarteritis nodosa, 326, 328–329
    in childhood, 437
  in primary angiitis of central nervous
    system, 347–350
  in rheumatoid vasculitis, 244, 245
  in systemic lupus erythematosus, 276,
    278
  in Takayasu's arteritis, 355
  in Wegener's granulomatosis, 332–333,
    333, 334
    in childhood, 438
  side effects of, 305, 317
    and monitoring in use of, 330, 331t
  toxicity of, monitoring of, 317
    and prevention of, 361
Cyclosporine, adverse effects of, 533
  and post-transplant hyperuricemia, 113
  during pregnancy, 169–170
  in Behçet's disease, 490, 491
  in childhood systemic lupus
    erythematosus, 430
  in cutaneous vasculitis, 185
  in dermatomyositis in children, 400
  in dry eyes, 253
  in juvenile dermatomyositis, 434
  in juvenile rheumatoid arthritis, 415
  in lupus nephritis, 307
  in myositis, 398
  in psoriasis, 186
  in psoriatic arthritis, 270
  in pyoderma gangrenosum, 188, *188*
  in rheumatoid arthritis, 38, 226, 229
  in systemic lupus erythematosus, 276
  in systemic vasculitis, 331
  in thrombocytopenia with systemic
    lupus erythematosus, 205
  side effects of, 398
  transplantation patients receiving,
    management of gout in, 456
Cystitis, hemorrhagic, cyclophosphamide-
    induced, 428
  in systemic lupus erythematosus, 281
Cytokine-targeted therapies, in rhuematoid
    arthritis, 208–212
Cytokine therapy, in cutaneous lupus
    erythematous, 178
Cytotoxic agents, in childhood systemic
    lupus erythematosus, 426–427
  in idiopathic inflammatory myopathies,
    393
  in ocular disease in rheumatoid arthritis,
    239–240
  in rheumatoid vasculitis, 245
Cytotoxic therapy, in Churg-Strass
    syndrome, 326, 327–328
  in cutaneous lupus erythematosus, 177,
    178
  in giant cell arteritis, 358
  in polyarteritis nodosa, 325, 327–328
  in polymyalgia rheumatica, 360
  in Takayasu's arteritis, 355–356

**D**

Danazol, in thrombocytopenia with
    systemic lupus erythematosus,
    204–205
Dapsone, in cutaneous lupus
    erythematosus, 177–178, 280
  in cutaneous vasculitis, 183
  in pyoderma gangrenosum, 187
  in relapsing polychondritis, 495, 496

de Quervain's tenosynovitis, 86
Deflazacort, bone metabolism and, 541
Dehydroepiandrosterone, in systemic
    lupus erythematosus, 277, 278–279
Delirium, in neuropsychiatric systemic
    lupus erythematosus, 313
  treatment of, 318
Dementia, in neuropsychiatric systemic
    lupus erythematosus, 313
  treatment of, 318
Depression, in fibromyalgia syndrome,
    41–42
  in neuropsychiatric systemic lupus
    erythematosus, 313
  in Sjögren's syndrome, 258
Dermatomyositis, cutaneous,
    hydroxychloroquine in, 179, *180*
  juvenile, calcinosis in, 180
  methotrexate in, 179–180, *181*
  treatment of, 179–180, *180, 181*
  immune globulins in, 398–399
  juvenile, azathioprine in, 434
    calcinosis in, 435
    chlorambucil in, 434
    clinical manifestations of, 433
    corticosteroids in, 433
    cyclosporine in, 434
    hydroxychloroquine in, 433
    intravenous immune globulin in, 434
    life-threatening, treatment of, 434–435
    methotrexate in, 433–434
    mild to moderate, treatment of,
      433–434
    morbidity in, 433
    rehabilitation in, 435
    severe, treatment of, 433–434
    supportive measures in, 435
    treatment of, 400
Dexamethasone, during pregnancy, 166
  in shoulder pain, 46
Diclofenac, in juvenile rheumatoid
    arthritis, 406
Dietary supplements, in psoriatic arthritis,
    271
Digital vasospasm, 16, *16*
Digits, deformities of, in psoriasis, 83
  in rheumatic disease, 80
  in systemic lupus erythematosus, 82
Dimethyl sulfoxide, in scleroderma, 368
Discectomy, in lumbar spine disease, 96
Documentation, medical, for rheumatology
    encounters. See *Medical documentation.*
Doxycycline, in Lyme disease, 518, 519
  in Lyme disease meningitis, 520
  in Lyme disease–related arthritis, 521
  in Lyme disease–related carditis, 520
  in Lyme disease–related neuropathy,
    520
  in osteoarthritis, 476
Drug surveillance, for elderly, 32
Drug therapy, controlled trials of, in
    fibromyalgia syndrome, 121–126
  in lumbago, 93
  in sciatica, 95
Drugs, adverse interactions of, with
    immunosuppressants, 116t, 117t
  antirheumatic. See *Antirheumatic drugs.*
  as disease-modifying agents in
    scleroderma, 366–370
  associated with dry eyes, 251, 251t
  interactions of, in fibromyalgia
    syndrome, clinical pharmacology of,
    129
  nonsteroidal anti-inflammatory. See
    *Nonsteroidal anti-inflammatory agents.*

Drugs (*Continued*)
  pharmacokinetics of, in elderly, 32–33
  side effects of, in antiphospholipid
    syndrome, 293–294
  in fibromyalgia syndrome, 129, 130t
  systemic, in Sjögren's syndrome,
    258–259
  trials of, in fibromyalgia syndrome,
    120–121, 121t
  vasculitis of central nervous system
    induced by, 351
Dysphagia, in scleroderma, 373

**E**

Elderly, pharmacokinetics of drugs in,
    32–33
  rheumatic disease in, 31–33
    epidemiology of, 31
    evaluation and treatment of, 31–32
Electroacupuncture, in fibromyalgia
    syndrome, 127
Electromyography, in neck pain, 55
Electromyography-biofeedback, in
    fibromyalgia syndrome, 126–127
Endocarditis, Libman-Sacks, 280
Enzymes, muscle, measurement of, in
    inflammatory myopathies, 394
Epicondylitis, lateral, 85
  medial, 85
Epidural and facet injections, in
    lumbago, 95
Epidural and peripheral nerve blockade, in
    complex regional pain syndrome-I,
    106
Epidural steroid injections, in lumbar
    spine disease, 97
  in sciatica, 95–96
Episcleritis, in rheumatoid arthritis, 239
Epoprostenol, in Raynaud's phenomenon,
    386
Erythema migrans, 515
  multiple, in Lyme disease, 519
Erythrocyte sedimentation rate, elevated,
    in organ transplant recipients, 117
Erythromycin, in Lyme disease, 518
Erythropoietin, in anemia in rheumatoid
    arthritis, 198–199
Esophagitis, in scleroderma, 373–374
Estrogen, in osteoporosis, 536, 539
Etanercept, during pregnancy, 172
  in juvenile rheumatoid arthritis, 416
  in rheumatoid arthritis, 39, 210, 226–227,
    230
Etidronate, in osteoporosis, 537
  in Paget's disease, 498
Exercise(s), in fibromyalgia syndrome,
    125–126
  in inflammatory myopathies, 395
  in lumbago, 93–94
  in osteoarthritis, 463
  rest and, in rheumatoid arthritis, 75
Extensor tendon rupture, in rheumatic
    disease of hand, *76*, 76–77
Extracorporeal photopheresis, in
    scleroderma, 369
Eye(s), diseases of, in rheumatoid arthritis,
    239–240
  dry, evaluation and treatment of,
    guidelines for, 252, 252t
    evaluation of patient with, 249, 250t,
      251–253
    topical therapy in, 253
  in sarcoidosis, 489
  inflammatory disease of, 192–197
    in Cogan's syndrome, 339

## F

Facet injections, in chronic pain
    syndrome, 98
  in lumbago, 95
Facial nerve paralysis, in Lyme disease,
    520
Failed back surgery syndrome, 92
Famciclovir, hepatitis B virus replication
    and, 327
Familial Mediterranean fever, amyloidosis
    in, 494
  colchicine in, 494, 495
  cyclophosphamide in, 494–495
  genetic defect in, 493–494
  manifestations of, 493
  prednisone in, 494–495
  treatment of, 494–495
Fatigue, in Sjögren's syndrome, 257–258
Felty's syndrome, 241–242
  author's approach to, 201
  clinical features of, 200
  disease-modifying antirheumatic drugs
    in, 242
  gold therapy in, 242
  granulocyte colony-stimulating factor in,
    201, 242
  granulocyte-macrophage colony-
    stimulating factor in, 201, 242
  in rheumatoid arthritis, 241–242
  methotrexate in, 201
  natural history of, 200
  neutropenia in, pathogenesis of, 200
    treatment of, 200–201
  splenectomy in, 200, 242
  treatment of, 242
Fertility, effects of antirheumatic drugs on,
    164–165t
Fever, in systemic lupus erythematosus,
    281
Fibromyalgia syndrome, 41–42, 120–131
  acupuncture in, 127
  S-adenosylmethionine in, 125
  affective spectrum disorders in, 120
  alpha-delta sleep in, 121
  alprazolam in, 124
  amitriptyline in, 121–122, 123, 128
  and rheumatoid arthritis, differential
    diagnosis of, 39
  antidepressants in, 121–124
  assessment of severity of, 128, 129
  benzodiazepines in, 124
  cognitive-behavioral treatment in, 128
  controlled trials of medication therapy
    in, 121–126
  corticosteroids in, 124–125
  cyclobenzaprine in, 42, 122–123
  depression in, 41–42
  diagnosis of, 41–42
  drug interactions in, clinical
    pharmacology of, 129
  drug side effects in, 129, 130t
  electroacupuncture in, 127
  electromyography-biofeedback in,
    126–127
  exercise therapy in, 125–126, 128
  fluoxetine in, 42, 123–124
  hormone therapy in, 125
  hypnotherapy in, 127
  ibuprofen in, 125
  in children, symptoms of, 440
    treatment of, 440–441
  incidence of, 41
  local anesthetics in, 127–128
  magnesium in, 126
  malic acid in, 126

Fibromyalgia syndrome (Continued)
  naproxen in, 121–122, 125
  neurohormonal function in, 120
  nonconventional therapy in, controlled
    trials of, 126–127
  nonmedication therapeutic trials in,
    125–126, 126t
  nonsteroidal anti-inflammatory drugs in,
    42, 124–125
  nortriptyline in, 42, 128
  pathologic mechanisms of, 120
  prednisone in, 124
  psychological distress in, 41
  psychotropic agents in, 121
  serotonin deficiency in, 121
  sleep disorders in, 41
  soma in, 125
  symptoms of, 41, 120
  temazepam in, 124
  tramadol in, 42
  transcutaneous electrical nerve
    stimulation in, 128
  trazodone in, 42
  treatment of, 42
  trials of medication in, 120–121, 121t
  tricyclic agents in, 42, 121–123, 128
  zolpidem in, 42
FK-506, in inflammatory myopathies,
    398
  in uveitis, 195
Flatfoot, acquired, differential diagnosis of,
    69–71
Flexor tendon rupture, in rheumatic
    disease of wrist, 77
Fluconazole, in fungal arthritis, 511
Flucytosine, in fungal arthritis, 511
Fluoxetine, in fibromyalgia syndrome, 42,
    123–124
Focal neurologic events, in
    neuropsychiatric systemic lupus
    erythematosus, treatment of, 318
Folic acid, in rheumatoid arthritis, 231
Foot, biomechanics of, 65–66
  crush injury of, 70–71
  evaluation of disorder of, 65
  pain in, 65–73
  plantigrade, 66
  posture of, 66
  valgus deformity of, 66
  varus deformity of, 66
Fractures, corticosteroid use and, 532
  in organ transplant recipients, 111,
    112
Functional status assessment, in rheumatic
    disease in elderly, 32
Fungal arthritis, 510–512, 511t

## G

Gastric emptying, delayed, in scleroderma,
    374
Gastritis, aspirin-induced, 404
Gastrointestinal bleeding, in childhood
    Henoch-Schönlein purpura, 436
Gastrointestinal lupus erythematosus, 281
Gastrointestinal reflux disease, in
    scleroderma, 374
Gastrointestinal tract, in scleroderma,
    management of, 373–375
  nonsteroidal anti-inflammatory drugs
    and, 469–470
  steroid effects on, 426
Gene therapy, in rheumatoid arthritis,
    214
Geriatric patient. See Elderly.
Geriatric rheumatology, 31–44

Giant cell arteritis, 353, 356–358
  cytotoxic therapy in, 358
  disease activity in, assessment of,
    356–357
  glucocorticoids in, 357–358
  in differential diagnosis of acute
    polyarthritis, 21, 22, 23–24, 26, 27,
    28–29
  methotrexate in, 358
  methylprednisolone in, 358
  natural history of, 356
  prednisolone in, 357–358
  prednisone in, 357–358
  treatment of, 355t, 357t, 357–358
  visual impairment in, 358
Glenohumeral osteoarthritis, shoulder pain
    in, 45
Glenoidectomy, with synovectomy, in
    shoulder pain, 47
Globulin, intravenous immune, during
    pregnancy, 172
Glomerulonephritis, in Henoch-Schönlein
    purpura, management of, 338
  in type II mixed cryoglobulinemia, 335
Glucocorticoids, as cause of osteoporosis,
    531–532
  biologic effects of, 473
  clinical pharmacology of, and drug
    interactions, 329
  during pregnancy, 166–168
  in Churg-Strauss syndrome, 326,
    327–328
  in giant cell arteritis, 357–358
  in Henoch-Schönlein purpura, 337,
    338
  in polyarteritis nodosa, 325, 327–328
  in polymyalgia rheumatica, 359–360
  in primary angiitis of central nervous
    system, 347–350
  in psoriatic arthritis, 269
  in rheumatoid arthritis, 228t, 236, 238
  in rheumatoid vasculitis, 243, 244
  in Takayasu's arteritis, 354–355, 355t
  in Wegener's granulomatosis, 332–333
  intra-articular, in osteoarthritis, 472–473,
    473t
  side effects of, and monitoring in use of,
    329–330
  toxic effects of, monitoring and
    prevention of, 360
Glucocorticosteroids, in ocular disease in
    rheumatoid arthritis, 239–240
  in rheumatoid pericarditis, 238–239
Glucosamine sulfate, in osteoarthritis, 35
Glycosaminoglycans, in osteoarthritis, 476
Gold therapy, during pregnancy, 168–169
  in Felty's syndrome, 242
  in psoriatic arthritis, 269
  in rheumatoid arthritis, 38–39, 223, 230
  injectable, administration of, 412
    background and efficacy of, 411–412
    in juvenile rheumatoid arthritis, 411
    in pediatric spondyloarthropathies,
      411–413
    mechanism of action of, 412
    toxicity and monitoring of, 412
  oral, in juvenile rheumatoid arthritis,
    412–413
  side effects of, 223
Golfer's elbow, 85
Gottron's papules, 17, 17
Gout, acute, in organ transplant recipients,
    diagnosis and treatment of,
    114–115
  management of, 448–452
  monarticular, treatment of, 36

Gout (*Continued*)
　　nonsteroidal anti-inflammatory drugs
　　　in, 449–450
　　therapeutic options in, 450t
　allopurinal hypersensitivity in,
　　management in, 457
　allopurinol in, 454t, 454–455
　chronic, in organ transplant recipients,
　　management of, 115–117
　classical, 447–448
　clinical presentation of, 35–36
　clinical spectrum of, 447
　colchicine in, 451t, 451–452, 452t
　complicated, management of, 456–457
　diagnosis of, 13–14, *14*, 36
　drug-related, 36
　hyperuricemia in, 447
　in transplantation patients receiving
　　cyclosporine, management of, 456
　incidence and prevalence of, 447
　intercritical, management of, 452–453
　　prophylaxis and follow-up of, 453,
　　　453t
　management of, 448
　oxypurinol in, 457
　polyarticular, 448
　post-transplantion, 113–114
　presentation of, 35–36
　probenecid in, 455
　refractory, management of, 456–457
　renal disease and/or edematous states
　　in, management in, 456
　risk for NSAID gastropathy in,
　　management in, 456–457
　salicylates in, 455–456
　sulfinpyrazone in, 455
　treatment of, 36
　untreated, 448
　uric acid defects in, 36
　uricosuric agents in, 455–456
Granulocyte colony-stimulating factor, in
　Felty's syndrome, 201, 242
Granulocyte-macrophage colony-
　stimulating factor, in Felty's
　syndrome, 201, 242
Growth, steroid effects on, 426
Growth hormone, in juvenile rheumatoid
　arthritis, 415–416
Gynecologic dryness, in Sjögren's
　syndrome, treatment of, 256–257

**H**

Haglund's deformity, 66
Hair, cyclophosphamide-induced loss of,
　428
Hammer toe, 66, 71
Hand, osteoarthritis of, *477*, 478–480, *480*
　rheumatic diseases of, 75–88
Headache, in neuropsychiatric systemic
　lupus erythematosus, 314
Hearing loss, in Cogan's syndrome, 339
　sensorineural, in neuropsychiatric
　　systemic lupus erythematosus,
　　treatment of, 320
Heart, in sarcoidosis, 489–490
Heart block, in rheumatoid arthritis, 239
Heart transplant recipients, hyperuricemia
　and gout in, 113
Heel pain syndrome, signs and symptoms
　of, 68
　structures involved in, 68
　treatment of, 68
Hematologic disease, 198–207
Hematologic lupus erythematosus, 281

Hemochromatosis, hereditary, diagnosis
　of, 496
　mode of inheritance of, 496
　prognosis in, 496
　symptoms of, 496
　treatment of, 496–497
Hemodialysis, amyloidosis associated
　with, 493
Henoch-Schönlein purpura, clinical
　features of, 337
　in childhood, 435–436
　management in, 338
　natural history of, 337
　treatment studies in, 337–338
Heparin, in antiphospholipid syndrome,
　292
　in systemic lupus erythematosus, 282
Hepatitis B, in differential diagnosis of
　acute polyarthritis, 19, 25
Hepatitis C, in differential diagnosis of
　acute polyarthritis, 19, 25
Herpesvirus infections, in organ transplant
　recipients, 117
Hindfoot, pain in, differential diagnosis of,
　66–69
Hip, arthroplasty of, 476
　osteoarthritis of, *478*, 480, *481*
Histoplasmosis arthritis, 511–512
Home care, in rheumatic disease in
　elderly, 32
Hormone therapy, in fibromyalgia
　syndrome, 125
Human immunodeficiency virus disease,
　reactive arthritis and, 267
Hyaluronan, in osteoarthritis, 473–474
Hydroxyapatite, 37
Hydroxychloroquine, in childhood
　systemic lupus erythematosus, 425
　in cutaneous dermatomyositis, 179, *180*
　in cutaneous lupus erythematosus, 176,
　　*177*
　in juvenile dermatomyositis, 433
　in juvenile rheumatoid arthritis, 413–414
　　background and efficacy of, 413–414
　　toxicity and monitoring of, 414
　in rheumatoid arthritis, 38, 224–225, 229,
　　230
　in sarcoidosis, 489
　in Sjögren's syndrome, 258–259
　in systemic lupus erythematosus, 282
　side effects of, 225, 283, 425
Hyperparathyroidism, corticosteroids and,
　532
Hypersensitivity reactions, to nonsteroidal
　anti-inflammatory drugs, 471
Hypersensitivity vasculitis, clinical
　features of, 338
　colchicine in, 339
　drug-related, 338
　management of, 339
　natural history of, 338
　treatment studies in, 338–339
Hypertension, in lupus nephritis,
　relationship to outcome, 308–309
　in Takayasu's arteritis, 356
Hyperuricemia, control of, drug therapy
　for, 453t
　indications for, 453–454
　in gout, 447
　patient evaluation in, *449*
　post-transplant, 113
Hypnotherapy, in fibromyalgia syndrome,
　127
Hypogonadism, corticosteroids and, 532,
　539

Hypomagnesemia, in heart transplant
　recipients, 112

**I**

Ibuprofen, in fibromyalgia syndrome, 125
　in juvenile rheumatoid arthritis, 405–406
　in osteoarthritis, 464–465
Iloprost, in Raynaud's phenomenon, 386
Immune globulin, in dermatomyositis in
　children, 400
　intravenous, in antiphospholipid
　　syndrome, 292
　in dermatomyositis, 398–399
　in inflammatory myopathies, 392–393,
　　398
　in juvenile dermatomyositis, 434
　in juvenile rheumatoid arthritis, 415
　in Kawasaki syndrome, 398, 436
　in systemic lupus erythematosus, 277
Immunochemical assessments, to predict
　disease activity in lupus nephritis, 301
Immunoglobulin(s), intravenous, in
　childhood systemic lupus
　erythematosus, 430
　in cutaneous lupus erythematosus,
　　177
　in lupus nephritis, 307
　in thrombocytopenia with systemic
　　lupus erythematosus, 204
　in uveitis, 195–196
Immunomodulatory therapy, in
　sarcoidosis, 488t
Immunosuppressive agents, adverse drug
　interactions with, 116t, 117t
　and steroids, in lupus nephritis, 304t,
　　308
　in cutaneous vasculitis, 184–185
　in inflammatory myopathies, 396
　in juvenile rheumatoid arthritis, 415
　in lupus nephritis, 303–305
　in primary angiitis of central nervous
　　system, 347
　in pyoderma gangrenosum, 188, *188*
　in reactive arthritis, 267, 268
　in relapsing polychondritis, 495, 496
　in sarcoidosis, 489
　in scleroderma, 368–369
　in uveitis, 192–193
　side effects of, 284
Immunosuppressive therapy, in
　sarcoidosis, 488t
　infection as complication of, 360
Indomethacin, in acute gout, 449–450, 450t
　in juvenile rheumatoid arthritis, 406
Infection, as cause of neck pain, 59–60
　as complication of immunosuppressive
　　therapy, 360
　in monarticular arthritis, 1
　vasculitis of central nervous sytem
　　associated with, 350–351
Infectious arthritis. See *Arthritis, infectious.*
Infertility, cyclophosphamide-induced, 361
Inflammation, in monarticular arthritis, 1
Inflammatory bowel disease, arthritis
　associated with, diagnosis of, 11, *11*
Inflammatory disease(s), idiopathic, of
　muscle, 390–402
　in Cogan's syndrome, 339
Inflammatory eye disease, 192–197
Infliximab, in rheumatoid arthritis, 227,
　230
　plus methotrexate, in rheumatoid
　　arthritis, 209–210
Injections, intra-articular, in
　osteoarthritis, 35

Intercellular adhesion molecule-1, in rheumatoid arthritis, 213–214
Interferon, in scleroderma, 368
Interferon-alpha, in Behçet's disease, 491
  in chronic hepatitis B, 327
  in Sjögren's syndrome, 255–256
  in uveitis, 196
  type II mixed cryoglobulinemia, 336, 337
Interferon-gamma, in psoriatic arthritis, 271
Interleukin-6, blockage of, in rheumatoid arthritis, 212
  in neuropsychiatric systemic lupus erythematosus, 315
Interleukin-10, in rheumatoid arthritis, 212
Interleukin-1 blockage, in rheumatoid arthritis, 211–212
Interphalangeal joint(s), distal, in osteoarthritis, 83–84
  in rheumatic disease, 82
  proximal, deformities of, arthroplasties for, 80–81, *81*
  in osteoarthritis, 84
Intestines, pseudo-obstruction of, in scleroderma, 375
Iron overload, in hereditary hemochromatosis, 496–497
Isoniazid, in spinal tuberculosis, 510
Isotretinoin, in cutaneous lupus erythematosus, 179, *180*
Itraconazole, in fungal arthritis, 511–512

**J**

Joint lavage, in osteoarthritis, 35, 474–475
Joint pain, in organ transplant recipients, 116
Joint prosthesis, in infectious arthritis, infections of, 509
Joint replacement, total, in osteoarthritis, 476
Juvenile rheumatoid arthritis, aspirin in, 403–404
  monitoring of use of, 404
  toxicity of, 404
  azathioprine in, 415
  biologic agents in, 415–416
  bone mineral density improvement in, 416
  chlorambucil in, 415
  conditioning and sports activities in, 418–419
  corticosteroids in, dosages of, 407–408
    general principles of, 407
    intra-articular, 408–409
    intravenous pulse, 408
    toxicity of, 408
  cyclosphosphamide in, 415
  cyclosporine in, 415
  diclofenac in, 406
  etanercept in, 415–416
  gold therapy in, injectable, 411–412
    oral, 412–413
  growth hormone in, 415
  hydroxychloroquine in, 413–414
  ibuprofen in, 405–406
  immunosuppresssive agents in, 415
  in 18-month-old girl, case illustrating, 416
  in 5-year-old boy, case illustrating, 417
  in 6-year-old girl, case illustrating, 416–417
  in 14-year-old girl, case illustrating, 417
  indomethacin in, 406
  intravenous immune globulin in, 415
  ketoprofen in, 406

Juvenile rheumatoid arthritis (*Continued*)
  management strategies in, cases illustrating, 416–418
  medications in, 418
  methotrexate in, 409–411
  morning stiffness in, measures to reduce, 418
  naproxen in, 406
  nonsteroidal anti-inflammatory drugs in, 404–407
  pain in, review of, 418
  patient-family education in, 418
  penicillamine in, 414–415
  piroxicam in, 406
  preparation for surgery, 419
  prognosis in, 403
  stem cell transplantation in, 415
  subsets of, 403
  sulfasalazine in, 413
  tolmetin in, 405
  treatment of, 403
    advances in, 419–420
    compliance with, 419
    when to stop, 419

**K**

Kawasaki syndrome, in children, aspirin in, 436
  epidemiology of, 436
  inflammatory manifestations of, 436
  intravenous immune globulin in, 436
  recommended treatment of, 436–437
Keratitis, peripheral ulcerative, in rheumatoid arthritis, 239–240
Keratoconjunctivitis sicca, in rheumatoid arthritis, 239, 240
Keratoderma blennorrhagicum, 12, *12*
Ketoprofen, in juvenile rheumatoid arthritis, 406
  in osteoarthritis, 464
Kidneys. See also *Renal* entries.
  disease of, in Henoch-Schönlein purpura, 337
    in childhood, 436
    in systemic lupus erythematosus, 297–312
    in sarcoidosis, 489
    in scleroderma, 375–376
  nonsteroidal anti-inflammatory drugs and, 470–471
Klippel-Feil deformity, 53, *54*, 61
Knee, arthroplasty of, 476
  arthroscopy of, 475
  osteoarthritis of, 475, *479*, 480–482, *482*
  osteotomy of, 476

**L**

β-Lactam antibiotics, in infectious arthritis, 504
Lactation, effects of antirheumatic drugs during, 164–165t
Laminectomy, decompressive, with medial facetectomy and spinal fusion, in lumbar spine disease, 97
Lamivudine, hepatitis B virus replication and, 327
Large granular lymphocyte syndrome, in rheumatoid arthritis, 241
Larynx, rheumatoid arthritis involving, 238
Leflunomide, during pregnancy, 172
  in rheumatoid arthritis, 39, 226, 230
Leg ulcers, in rheumatoid vasculitis, 245
Leprosy, lepromatous, 510

Leukapheresis, in idiopathic inflammatory myopathies, 392
Leukemia, large granular lymphocyte, and rheumatoid arthritis, treatment of, 201
Leukocytoclastic vasculitis, 182
Libman-Sacks endocarditis, 280
Limb pain, in organ transplant recipients, 116
Lisfranc joint arthrosis, 70
Liver, nonsteroidal anti-inflammatory drugs and, 471
Liver transplantation, osteoporosis and fracture following, 111
LJP394, in lupus nephritis, 308
Low back disorders, classification of, 89, 90t
Low back pain, acute, 93–97
  chronic, 91–92
    treatment of, 94t
  management of, general approach to, 92–93, 93t
Lumbago, alternative therapies in, 95
  bed rest in, 93
  chiropractic manipulations in, 94–95
  diagnostic features of, 89–90
  epidemiology of, 89
  epidural and facet injections in, 95
  exercises and modalities in, 93–94
  medications in, 93
  myofascial trigger point injection in, 94
  pathophysiology of, 89
  surgery in, 95
  therapies of, 93, 94t
Lumbar spine disease, 89–100
  discectomy in, 96
  neurogenic claudication in, 96–97
Lungs. See also *Pulmonary* entries.
  disease of, in rheumatoid arthritis, 236–238
    interstitial, in inflammatory myopathies, 396
    in systemic lupus erythematosus, 280
  in ankylosing spondylitis, 264
  in sarcoidosis, 489
  in scleroderma, management of, 370–373, *371*
Lupus erythematosus. See also *Systemic lupus erythematosus.*
  cardiopulmonary, 280–281
  cutaneous, antilepromatous agents in, 177–178
    antimalarial agents in, 176–177, *177*, 279–280
    auranofin in, 178, *179*
    azathioprine in, 177, *178*
    chloroquine in, 176
    clofazimine in, 178
    corticosteroids in, 175, *177*, 280
    cytokine therapy in, 178
    cytotoxic agents in, 177, *178*
    dapsone in, 177–178, 280
    hydroxychloroquine in, 176, *177*
    intravenous immunoglobulins in, 177–178
    isotretinoin in, 179, *180*
    management of, 279–280
    manifestations of, 175, *176*
    phenytoin in, 178
    retinoids in, 179, *180*
    standard therapy for, 175–177
    thalidomide in, 178
  gastrointestinal, 281
  hematologic, 281
  musculoskeletal, 280
  neonatal, 432–433

Lupus nephritis, alteration of immunologic function in, therapeutic agents for, clinical trials of, 308
  azathioprine in, 303, 306
  corticosteroids in, 302–303
  cyclophosphamide in, 303–304, 305, 306
  cyclosporine in, 307
  diffuse proliferative, 297, 298, 300
  disease activity in, immunologic predictors of, 300–302
  focal proliferative, 297, 298
  histologic classification of, 297–299
  histologic lesions of, clinical correlations and natural history of, 299, 299–300
  hypertension in, relationship to outcome, 308–309
  immunosuppressive agents in, 303–305, 308
    and steroids in, 304t
  in childhood, cyclophosphamide in, 427–428
  intravenous immunoglobulins in, 307
  lymphoid irradiation in, 307–308
  management of, monitoring of therapeutic efficacy in, 305–306
  membranous, 299, 299–300
  mesangial, 297, 298
  methylprednisolone in, 302–303, 306
  mycophenolate mofetil in, 307
  plasmapheresis in, 306–307
  prednisone in, 302, 306
  renal biopsy in, 302
Lyme disease, 515–527
  antibiotics in, 517–518
  antibody tests in, 516
  arthritis in, 520–521
  Bell's palsy in, 520
  carditis induced by, 520
  clinical manifestations of, 517–521
  diagnosis of, 516–517
  diagnostic work-up for, 522
  early, treatment of, 517–519
  early disseminated, treatment of, 519–521
  epidemiology of, 515
  in differential diagnosis of acute polyarthritis, 20, 25
  in pregnancy, 521
  in vitro and in vivo studies in, 517
  meningitis in, 519–520
  meningoencephalitis in, 519–520
  multiple erythema migrans in, 519
  peripheral neuropathy in, 520
  polymerase chain reaction in, 517
  post-Lyme syndrome and, 521
  prevention of, 522–524, 524t
  side effects of treatment of, 521–522
  treatment recommendations in, 517–521, 518t
  Western blot analysis in, 516–517
Lymphadenopathy, in systemic lupus erythematosus, 281
Lymphoid irradiation, in lupus nephritis, 307–308
Lymphoproliferative disorders, in type II mixed cryoglobulinemia, 335
  vasculitis of central nervous system in, 351

**M**

Magnesium, in fibromyalgia syndrome, 126
Magnetic resonance imaging, in neck pain, 55, 57
  in shoulder pain, 45

Malic acid, in fibromyalgia syndrome, 126
Mallet toe, 66, 71
Medical documentation, American Medical Association reporting conventions and, 132
  assessment section in, 138–139, 139
  computerized medical record for, 134
  medical record contents in, 132
  medical record design and, 133
  patient update and fact sheet of, 141–142, 145–146
  plan for future care in, 139–141, 140
  progress note in. See Progress note.
  template to record medical information and, 133–134
  third parties and, 132
Medications. See Drugs.
Mediterranean fever, familial. See Familial Mediterranean fever.
Melphalan, in amyloidosis, 492
Meningitis, chronic, differential diagnosis and basic evaluation in, 349t
  in Lyme disease, 519–520
Meningoencephalitis, in Lyme disease, 519–520
6-Mercaptopurine, during pregnancy, 170–171
  in psoriatic arthritis, 270
Metabolic disease, in monarticular arthritis, 1–2
Metacarpophalangeal joint(s), arthroplasty of, results of, 79–80
  in rheumatic disease, 79–80
Metastatic disease, neck pain in, 60–61
Metatarsalgia, 72
  causes of, 72
  treatment of, 72
Metatarsophalangeal joints, range of motion of, 66
Methotrexate, adverse effects of, 533
  clinical use of, 411
  during pregnancy, 171
  in childhood systemic lupus erythematosus, 429
  in cutaneous dermatomyositis, 179–180, 181
  in cutaneous vasculitis, 185
  in Felty's syndrome, 201
  in giant cell arteritis, 358
  in idiopathic inflammatory myopathies, 393
  in inflammatory myopathies, 395
  in juvenile dermatomyositis, 433–434
  in juvenile rheumatoid arthritis, 409–411
  in localized scleroderma, 182
  in myositis in children, 399–400
  in pediatric spondyloarthropathies, 409–411
  in psoriasis, 186
  in psoriatic arthritis, 269–270
  in relapsing polychondritis, 495, 496
  in rheumatoid arthritis, 37–38, 223–224, 229, 230
    background and efficacy of, 409
  in rheumatoid vasculitis, 244
  in sarcoidosis, 489
  in scleroderma in children, 438
  in systemic lupus erythematosus, 276, 277t, 278
  in Takayasu's arteritis, 355–356
  in uveitis, 195
  in Wegener's granulomatosis, 333, 334
    in childhood, 438
  kinetics of, 409–410
  mechanism of action of, 409

Methotrexate (Continued)
  plus infliximab, in rheumatoid arthritis, 209–210
  routes of administration of, 411
  side effects of, 270, 397
  toxicity of, 410–411
    monitoring and prevention of, 360–361
Methylprednisolone, in Behçet's disease, 491
  in Churg-Strauss syndrome, 328
  in cutaneous vasculitis, 184
  in giant cell arteritis, 358
  in Henoch-Schönlein purpura, 338
  in inflammatory myopathies, 395
  in lupus nephritis, 302–303, 306
  in polyarteritis nodosa, 328
  in polymyalgia rheumatica, 360
  in rheumatoid arthritis, 228, 230
  in rheumatoid vasculitis, 244
  in Wegener's granulomatosis, 333
  intravenous, in systemic lupus erythematosus, 277–278, 278t
  intravenous pulse, in childhood systemic lupus erythematosus, 426
    in polyarteritis nodosa in childhood, 437
    in systemic lupus erythematosus, 275–276, 276t
  side effects of, 283–284
Microdiskectomy, in lumbar spine disease, 96
Milwaukee shoulder, 33, 37
Misoprostol, in ulcers induced by nonsteroidal anti-inflammatory drugs, 469–470
Monoclonal antibodies, combination of, in systemic vasculitis, 331
Mouth, dry, evaluation of, 249, 250t
    and treatment of, guidelines for, 254t
Muscle(s), idiopathic inflammatory diseases of, 390–402
    lower extremity, weakness of, timed-stands test in, 393, 394
    strength of, evaluation of, in inflammatory myopathies, 394t
    weakness of, causes of, confused with polymyositis, 394t
Muscle enzymes, measurement of, in inflammatory myopathies, 394
Musculoskeletal system, in scleroderma, management of, 377–378
  infections of, in organ transplant recipients, 116
Mycobacterial infections, in infectious arthritis, 510
Mycobacterium leprae infections, 510
Mycobacterium tuberculosis infections, 510
Mycophenolate mofetil, in childhood systemic lupus erythematosus, 429–430
  in lupus nephritis, 307
  in psoriasis, 186
Myelitis, transverse, in neuropsychiatric systemic lupus erythematosus, 314
    treatment of, 318
Myelopathy, cervical, in rheumatoid arthritis, 240–241
Myocardial disease, with rheumatoid arthritis, 239
Myopathy(ies), inflammatory, azathioprine in, 395
    cardiac complications in, 397
    corticosteroids in, 395, 396

Myopathy(ies) (*Continued*)
   drug therapies in, 395–397
   exercise in, 395
   idiopathic, author's approach to,
      393–397
      classificaion of, *393*
      pretreatment decisions in, 393–395
      survival rates in, 391, *393*
   immunosuppressive agents in, 396
   interstitial lung disease in, 396
   investigational drugs in, 397–398
   methotrexate in, 395
   methylprednisolone in, 395
   natural history of, and long-term
      experience with, 390–391
   nonpharmacologic considerations in,
      395
   pulmonary complications in, 396–397
   treatment of, controlled clinical trials
      in, 392–393
   steroid-induced, 397
Myositis, autoantibodies associated with,
   390, *392*
   autoantibodies specific for, 390, *392*
   idiopathic, diagnostic criteria for, 390,
      391t
   inclusion body, diagnostic criteria for,
      390, 391t
      treatment of, 395, 399
   recalcitrant, in children, treatment of,
      399–400

## N

Naproxen, in fibromyalgia syndrome,
   121–122, 125
   in juvenile rheumatoid arthritis, 406
   in osteoarthritis, 465
Narcotic analgesics, in osteoarthritis, 34
Narcotic therapy, chronic, in chronic pain
   syndrome, 98
Neck, anatomy of, 51–52
   functional anatomy of, 51, *52*
   neuroanatomy and pain generators of,
      51–52, *52*
Neck pain, 51–64
   acute, approach to patient with, 62
   causes of, 56t, 56–62
   chronic, approach to patient with, 62
   congenital causes of, 61
   diagnostic evaluation in, 52–55
   diagnostic modalities in, 53–55
   epidemiology of, 52
   history taking in, 52–53
   in cervical degenerative disc disease,
      56, *57*
   in rheumatoid arthritis, 62
   infectious causes of, 59–60
   inflammatory causes of, 58–59, *59*
   laboratory studies in, 55
   neoplastic causes of, 60–61, *61*
   neurologic examination in, 53
   nonspinal causes of, 61
   physical examination in, 53, 62
   psychological causes of, 61–62
   traumatic causes of, 56–58
Neoplasms, neck pain in, 60–61
Nephritis, interstitial, in nonsteroidal anti-
   inflammatory drug usage, 470
   lupus. See *Lupus nephritis.*
Nerve blockade, epidural and peripheral,
   in complex regional pain syndrome-I,
   106
Nerve compression, in rheumatoid
   arthritis, 240
Nerve conduction studies, in neck pain, 55

Nerve stimulation, transcutaneous electric,
   in chronic pain syndrome, 98
   transcutaneous electrical, in fibromyalgia
      syndrome, 128
Neuroaugmentation, in complex regional
   pain syndrome-I, 106–107
Neurogenic claudication, diagnostic
   features of, 91
   epidemiology of, 91
   in lumbar spine disease, 96–97
   pathogenesis of, 91
Neurologic disease, in rheumatoid
   arthritis, 240–241
   in sarcoidosis, 490
Neuropathy(ies), peripheral, in Lyme
   disease, 520
   in neuropsychiatric systemic lupus
      erythematosus, 314
Neurotropics, in complex regional pain
   syndrome-I, 106
Neutropenia, chronic. See *Felty's syndrome.*
   in nonsteroidal anti-inflammatory drug
      usage, 471
   in rheumatoid arthritis, 241
Neutrophilic dermatosis, acute febrile. See
   *Sweet's syndrome.*
Newborns, lupus erythematosus in,
   432–433
Nifedipine, in Raynaud's phenomenon,
   385
Nitrates, topical, in Raynaud's
   phenomenon, 385
Nitrogen mustard, in childhood systemic
   lupus erythematosus, 129
Nonsteroidal anti-inflammatory agents,
   adverse reactions to, 451t
   in children, 407
   and cyclosporine, interaction of, in
      organ transplant recipients, 114
   anti-inflammatory actions of, 465, *467*
   anticoagulant effects of, 220
   cartilage metabolism and, 465–466
   central nervous system effects of,
      471–472
   clinical pharmacology of, 284
   common effects of, 406t
   cutaneous and hypersensitivity reactions
      to, 471
   drug interactions with, 284
   during pregnancy, 166
   gastrointestinal toxicity of, 469–470
   half-lives of, and molecular structures
      of, 468
   hepatic effects of, 471
   in acute gout, 449–450
   in ankylosing spondylitis, 264–265,
      265t
   in complex regional pain syndrome-I,
      105–106
   in cutaneous vasculitis, 183
   in fibromyalgia syndrome, 124–125
   in gout, 36
   in juvenile rheumatoid arthritis, 404–407
   in musculoskeletal lupus, 280
   in osteoarthritis, 34–35, 465–472
   in pediatric spondyloarthropathies,
      404–407
   in polymyalgia rheumatica, 360
   in pregnancy, 472
   in psoriatic arthritis, 269, 272
   in reactive arthritis, 267
   in rheumatoid arthritis, 37–38, *38,*
      218–219, 219t
   in serositis, 280

Nonsteroidal anti-inflammatory agents
   (*Continued*)
   in Sjögren's syndrome, 258
   in systemic lupus erythematosus, 274,
      275t, 277
      in childhood, 424
   in uveitis, 194
   mechanism of action of, 284
   metabolism of, 468–469
   monitoring for toxicity of, in children,
      405t
   pediatric dosages of, 405t
   peptic ulcer disease induced by,
      management of, 406t
   precautions in prescription of, 221
   renal toxicity of, 470–471
   side effects of, 283, 424, 469–472
   skin reactions to, 220
   toxicities associated with, 35, 42
      risk factors for, 450t
Nortriptyline, in fibromyalgia syndrome,
   42, 128
Nose, dryness of, in Sjögren's syndrome,
   treatment of, 256
Nystatin, in Sjögren's syndrome, 260

## O

Omeprazole, in ulcers induced by
   nonsteroidal anti-inflammatory drugs,
   470
Opiates, in osteoarthritis, 465
   spinal administration of, in chronic pain
      syndrome, 98
Oral sympathetic blockade, in complex
   regional pain syndrome-I, 106
Organ transplant recipients, acute gout in,
   114–115
   bone mineral density issues in, 111
   chronic gout in, 115–117
   elevated erythrocyte sedimentation rate
      in, 117
   fractures in, 111, 112
   hypomagnesemia in, 112
   inflammatory arthritis in, 113–114
   joint and limb pains in, 116
   musculoskeletal infections in, 116
   osteoporosis in, 111, 112
   rheumatologic consultations in, 111–119,
      112t
   vasculitis and pseudovasculitic
      syndromes in, 116–117
Organic brain syndrome, in
   neuropsychiatric systemic lupus
   erythematosus, 313
Osseous pain, 92
Osteitis deformans. See *Paget's disease.*
Osteoarthritis, 33–35, 461–486
   acetaminophen in, 464–465
   analgesics in, 464t, 464–465
   arthroplasty in, 475–476
   arthroscopy in, 475
   bone loss in, 533
   capsaicin in, 464
   cartilage degeneration in, 461–462
   clinical features of, 33–34, 83
   cognitive-behavioral studies in, 150
   corticosteroids in, 473
   destructive arthropathy in, 33
   diagnosis of, 15, *15*
      and treatment of, 462
   differential diagnosis of, 5–6
   doxycycline in, 476
   erosive, 33
   exercise in, 463
   functional impact of, 33

Osteoarthritis (*Continued*)
  glenohumeral, shoulder pain in, 45
  glycosaminoglycans in, 476
  hyaluronan in, 473–474
  ibuprofen in, 464–465
  incidence of, 33, 461
  intra-articular glucocorticoids in, 472–473, 473t
  intra-articular viscosupplementation in, 473–474
  invasive therapies in, 35
  investigational agents in, 476–477
  joint lavage in, 474–475
  joints involved in, 461
  ketoprofen in, 464
  management of, *477*, 477–482, *478–482*
  naproxen in, 465
  nonsteroidal anti-inflammatory drugs in, 465–472
    central nervous system effects of, 471–472
    cutaneous effects of, 471
    gastrointestinal toxicity of, 469–470
    hepatic side effects of, 471
    hypersensitivity reactions to, 471
    pregnancy and, 472
    renal toxicity of, 470–471
  of hand, *477*, 478–480, *480*
    classification criteria for, 462t
  of hip, *478*, 480, *481*
    classification criteria for, 462t
  of knee, 475, *479*, 480–482, *482*
    classification criteria for, 462t
  opiates in, 465
  osteotomy in, 476
  pathogenesis of, 461
  pathophysiology of, 461–462
  plaquenil, 477
  proteoglycans in, 476
  reduction of mechanical strain in, 463
  rehabilitation in, 463
  selective inhibitors of inducible cyclooxygenase in, 472
  specific deformities in, 83–84
  sulfasalazine in, 477
  symptoms of, 33–34
  tidal irrigation in, 475
  total joint replacement in, 476
  tramadol in, 465
  treatment of, nonpharmacologic, 34, 462–463
    pharmacologic, 34–35, 463–474
  vitamin C in, 476–477
  vitamin D in, 476
  vitamin E in, 476–477
  weight loss in, 463
Osteochondrosis, juvenile, 2
Osteodystrophy, renal, elements of, 111, 112t
Osteopenia, causes of, 529t
Osteoporosis, authors' approach to, 541
  bisphosphonates in, 537, 540, 541–542
  bone densitometry in, *529*, 529–530
  bone loss and, 528
  calcitonin in, 536–537, 539, 541
  calcium in, 535, 539, 541
  corticosteroids and, 531–532
  estrogen in, 536, 539
  evaluation in, 534t, 534–535
  fractures associated with, 528
  in organ transplant recipients, 111, 112
  in rheumatoid arthritis, 530
  parathyroid hormone in, 537–538, 540
  prevention of, and treatment of, 535–538
    before transplantation, 113t

Osteoporosis (*Continued*)
  risk factors for, 528
  secondary causes of, 528–529, 529t
  selective estrogen receptor modulators in, 536
  sodium fluoride in, 537, 540
  steroid-induced, 397
  treatment of, 535–538
  vitamin D in, 535–536, 539
Osteotomy, in osteoarthritis, 476
Oxypurinol, in gout, 457

**P**

Paget's disease, bisphosphonates in, 498–499
  calcitonin in, 497
  complications of, 497
  medications under investigation in, 499
  symptoms of, 497
  treatment of, indications for, 497
    medications in, 497–499, 498t
Pain, back, postsurgical, 92
  hindfoot, differential diagnosis of, 66–69
  in arthritis, and consequences of, management of, 148–150
    comorbidity associated with, 147–148
  neck. See *Neck pain.*
  of foot and ankle, 65–73
  osseous, 92
Pain syndrome, chronic. See *Chronic pain syndrome.*
  complex regional. See *Complex regional pain syndrome-I.*
Pamidronate, in ankylosing spondylitis, 265–266
  in Paget's disease, 498–499
  in steroid-induced osteoporosis, 540, 542
Panniculitis, four types of, 189
  treatment of, 189
Parathyroid hormone, in osteoporosis, 537–538, 540
Parathyroid hormone-related protein, 538
Parotid glands, swelling of, in Sjögren's syndrome, 259
Parvovirus, in differential diagnosis of acute polyarthritis, 20, 25
Penicillamine, adverse reactions to, 414–415
  during pregnancy, 169
  in juvenile rheumatoid arthritis, 414–415
  in rheumatoid arthritis, 38
    background and efficacy of, 414
    dosage and toxicity of, 414
D-Penicillamine, in ankylosing spondylitis, 265–266
  in psoriatic arthritis, 271
  in rheumatoid arthritis, 225, 230
  in rheumatoid vasculitis, 244
  in scleroderma, 366–367
  in scleroderma in children, 438
Penicillin(s), in infectious arthritis, 504
  in Lyme disease, 517–518
  in Lyme disease meningitis, 519–520
  in Lyme disease-related neuropathy, 520
Penicillin G, in Lyme disease in pregnancy, 521
Pentoxifylline, in Behçet's disease, 491
  in cutaneous vasculitis, 183
Peptic ulcer disease, NSAID-induced, management of, 406t
Percutaneous transluminal angioplasty, in Takayasu's arteritis, 356

Pericardiectomy, in rheumatoid arthritis, 238–239
Pericardiocentesis, in rheumatoid pericarditis, 238
Pericarditis, in rheumatoid arthritis, 238–239
Peripheral neuropathy, in Lyme disease, 520
  in neuropyschiatric systemic lupus erythematosus, 314
Periungual telangiectasia, 16, *16*
Phenytoin, in cutaneous lupus erythematous, 178
Photochemotherapy, in psoriatic arthritis, 271
Photopheresis, extracorporeal, in scleroderma, 369
Physical therapy, in ankylosing spondylitis, 264
  in osteoarthritis, 34
  in rheumatic disease in elderly, 32
Pilocarpine, in Sjögren's syndrome, 254
Piroxicam, in juvenile rheumatoid arthritis, 406
Plantigrade foot, 66
Plaquenil, in osteoarthritis, 477
  in rheumatoid arthritis, 231
Plasma exchange, in Churg-Strauss syndrome, 326
  in hepatitis B virus-related polyarteritis nodosa, 329
  in polyarteritis nodosa, 326
Plasmapheresis, in childhood systemic lupus erythematosus, 430
  in cutaneous vasculitis, 185
  in idiopathic inflammatory myopathies, 392
  in lupus nephritis, 306–307
  in neuropsychiatric systemic lupus erythematosus, 317–318
  in polymyositis, 399
  in systemic lupus erythematosus, 276
  side effects of, 317
Pneumoconiosis, in rheumatoid arthritis, 237
Pneumonia, bronchiolitis obliterans-organizing, in rheumatoid arthritis, 237–238
Polyangiitis, microscopic, 323
  laboratory studies in, 325
  natural history of, 325
  treatment studies in, 325–326
Polyarteritis, microscopic, 323
Polyarteritis nodosa, classic, definition of, 323–324
  clinical features of, 323
  clinical pharmacology and drug interactions in, 329
  cutaneous, treatment of, 328–329
  cyclophosphamide in, 326, 328
  glucorticoids in, 325, 328
  hepatitis B virus-related, treatment of, 325–326, 329
  in children, 437
    clinical manifestations of, 437
    treatment of, 437
  laboratory studies in, 325
  natural history of, 325
  plasma exchange in, 326
  prednisone in, 326, 328
  prospective clinical trials in, 326–327
  treatment of, 327–329
    long-term experience with, 327
  treatment studies in, 325–326

Polyarthritis, acute, case presentations of,
    18–29
    diagnosis of, 17–18
    differential diagnosis of, 18t, 18–29
    fever, rash, and arthritis in, 17
    incidence of, 17
  acute and chronic, differential diagnosis
    of, 4–29
  chronic, differential diagnosis of, rules
    for, 4–8
    extra-articular features of, 7
    in hand and foot, 7, 7
    joint involvement in, 6–7
    symptoms of, and physical findings
        in, 7–8
  nonsteroidal anti-inflammatory drugs in,
    280
Polychondritis, relapsing, complications of,
    495
    management of, 495–496
    symptoms of, 495
Polymerase chain reaction, in infectious
    arthritis, 503–504
  in Lyme disease, 517
Polymyalgia rheumatica, 40–41, 353,
    358–360
  and rheumatoid arthritis, differential
        diagnosis of, 39
  bone loss in, 533–534
  cytotoxic therapy in, 360
  diagnosis of, 40
  disease activity in, assessment of, 359
  drug toxicity in, monitoring and
        prevention of, 360–361
  glucocorticoids in, 359–360
  incidence of, 40
  infection and, 360
  methylprednisolone in, 360
  natural history of, 358–359
  nonsteroidal anti-inflammatory agents
        in, 360
  prednisolone in, 360
  prednisone in, 359–360
  treatment of, 40–41, 355t, 359t, 359–360
Polymyositis, causes of muscle weakness
        confused with, 394t
  plasmapheresis in, 399
  total body irradiation in, 399
Polymyositis-dermatomyositis, diagnostic
        criteria for, 390, 391t
Post-Lyme disease, 521
Potassium para-aminobenzoic acid, in
        scleroderma, 367–368
Pott's disease, 510
Prazosin, in Raynaud's phenomenon, 385
Prednisolone, during pregnancy, 166–168
  in giant cell arteritis, 357–358
  in polymyalgia rheumatica, 360
Prednisone, adverse effects of, 532
  calcium metabolism and, 532
  during pregnancy, 166, 168, 282
  in amyloidosis, 492
  in autoimmune hemolytic anemia in
        systemic lupus erythematosus, 202,
        202
  in Behçet's disease, 491
  in benign angiopathy of central nervous
        system, 350
  in Churg-Strauss syndrome, 326, 328
  in Cogan's syndrome, 339–340
  in cutaneous vasculitis, 184
  in familial Mediterranean fever, 494–495
  in fibromyalgia syndrome, 124
  in giant cell arteritis, 357–358
  in Henoch-Schönlein purpura, 338

Prednisone (Continued)
  in inflammatory myopathies, 392, 395
  in lupus nephritis, 302, 306
  in polyarteritis nodosa, 326, 328
  in polymyalgia rheumatica, 360
  in rheumatoid arthritis, 228, 237
  in rheumatoid pericarditis, 238–239
  in rheumatoid vasculitis, 245
  in Sweet's syndrome, 188, 189
  in systemic lupus erythematosus, 282
  in Takayasu's arteritis, 354–355, 356
  in thrombocytopenia with systemic
        lupus erythematosus, 204
  in uveitis, 194
Pregnancy, and lactation, effects of
        antirheumatic drugs in, 164–165t
  and rheumatoid arthritis, 163–166
    antimalarial agents during, 168
    azathioprine during, 170
    betamethasone during, 166
    chlorambucil during, 171–172
    cyclophosphamide during, 171–172
    cyclosporine during, 169–170
    dexamethasone during, 166
    etanercept during, 172
    glucocorticoids during, 166–168
    gold therapy during, 168–169
  in antiphospholipid syndrome, 289–290,
        292
  in systemic lupus erythematosus,
        281–282
    intravenous immune globulin during,
        172
    leflunomide during, 172
    Lyme disease in, 521
    medications during, 166–172
    6-mercaptopurine during, 170–171
    methotrexate during, 171
    nonsteroidal anti-inflammatory drugs in,
        472
    penicillamine during, 169
    prednisolone during, 166–168
    prednisone during, 166, 168
    progressive systemic sclerosis during,
        166
    sulfasalazine during, 169
    treatment of rheumatic diseases during,
        163–174
Probenecid, in chronic gout, in organ
        transplant recipients, 115
  in gout, 455
Progress note, 133, 134, 134–138, 143–144
    chief complaint on, 134, 135
    history of present illness on, 135, 136
    objective section of, 137, 137–138,
        138
    past medical, family, and social history
        on, 136, 136–137
    review of systems on, 135–136
    subjective section of, 135–137
Prolactin, in neuropsychiatric systemic
        lupus erythematosus, 315
Prostaglandins, in Raynaud's
        phenomenon, 385
Prosthetic joints, in infectious arthritis,
        infections of, 509
Proteoglycans, in osteoarthritis, 476
Proton pump inhibitor agents, in ulcers
        induced by nonsteroidal anti-
        inflammatory drugs, 470
Pseudogout. See Calcium pyrophosphate
        dihydrate deposition disease.
Pseudoosteoarthritis, 15, 15
Pseudovasculitic syndromes, in organ
        transplant recipients, 116–117

Psoriasis, 185–186
    corticosteroids in, 186
    cyclosporine in, 186
    diagnosis of, 186
    forms of, 186
    methotrexate in, 186
    mycophenolate mofetil in, 186
    retinoids in, 186
    treatment of, 186
    ultraviiolet B therapy in, 186
Psoriatic arthritis, 12–13, 13
    antimalarial agents in, 270–271
    antirheumatic drugs in, 269–272
    azathioprine in, 270, 272
    clinical features of, 83, 268
    colchicine in, 271
    cyclosporine in, 270
    definition of, 268
    dietary supplements in, 271
    digital deformities in, 83
    glucocorticoids in, 269
    gold therapy in, 269
    interferon gamma in, 271
    management approach in, 272
    6-mercaptopurine in, 270
    methotrexate in, 269–270
    natural history of, 268–269
    nonsteroidal anti-inflammatory drugs in,
        269, 272
    D-penicillamine in, 271
    photochemotherapy in, 271
    retinoids in, 271
    somatostatin in, 271
    specific deformities in, 83
    sulfasalazine in, 270
    thumb involvement in, 83
    treatment of, 269
    wrist involvement in, 83
Psychoeducational interventions, in
        arthritis, 147–161
Psychosis, in neuropsychiatric systemic
        lupus erythematosus, 313
    treatment of, 318
Psychosocial issues, in scleroderma,
        management of, 378–379
Psychotropic agents, in fibromyalgia
        syndrome, 121
Pulmonary. See also Lungs.
Pulmonary arteritis, in rheumatoid
        arthritis, 238
Pulmonary complications, in inflammatory
        myopathies, 396–397
Pulmonary fibrosis, in rheumatoid
        arthritis, treatment of, 237
Pulmonary hypertension, in scleroderma,
        management of, 372
  in systemic lupus erythematosus, 280
Pulmonary nodules, in rheumatoid
        arthritis, 237
Pulmonary vasoconstriction, hypoxic, in
        scleroderma, management of, 372–373
Purpura, anaphylactoid. See Henoch-
        Schönlein purpura.
    thrombotic thrombocytopenic, in
        systemic lupus erythematosus,
        203
Pyoderma gangrenosum, 186–188
    arthritis and, 186–187
    bowel disease and, 186–187
    corticosteroids in, 187–188
    cyclosporine in, 188, 188
    dapsone in, 187–188
    diagnosis of, 186–187
    immunosuppressive agents in, 188,
        188

Pyoderma gangrenosum (*Continued*)
  treatment of, 187–188
  ulcerations in, 186
Pyrazinamide, in spinal tuberculosis, 510

## Q

Quinolone, in infectious arthritis, 504

## R

Radiography, in neck pain, 53–55
  in shoulder pain, 45–46
Radiotherapy, in ankylosing spondylitis, 264, 266
  splenic, in thrombocytopenia with systemic lupus erythematosus, 204
Radioulnar joint, distal, in rheumatic disease, 78
Raloxifene, in osteoporosis, 536
Ranitidine, in ulcers induced by nonsteroidal anti-inflammatory drugs, 470
Raynaud's phenomenon, 16, *16*, 382–389
  calcium channel blockers in, 384, 386t
  critical ischemia in, approach to, 387
  definitions associated with, 382
  epoprostenol in, 386
  iloprost in, 386
  in scleroderma, management of, 376
  in systemic lupus erythematosus, 280
  nondrug management of, 383–384
  pharmacologic treatment of, 384–385
  prazosin in, 385
  primary, 382
  prostaglandins in, 385
  recommended evaluation in, 382–383, *383*
  reconditioning response to cold in, 384
  secondary, 382
  surgical treatment of, 387
  sympathectomy in, 387
  sympatholytic agents in, 385, 386t
  temperature biofeedback in, 383–384
  topical nitrates in, 385
  vasodilators in, 384–385, 386t
Reactive arthritis. See *Arthritis, reactive.*
Red cell aplasia, in rheumatoid arthritis, 200
Reflex neurovascular dystrophy, in children, management of, in rehabilitation center, 439–440
    therapeutic team members in, 439–440
  patient-parent education in, 439
  psychological factors in, 439
  symptoms of, 438–439
  treatment of, goal of, 439
Reflex sympathetic dystrophy. See *Complex regional pain syndrome-I; Reflex neurovascular dystrophy.*
Rehabilitation, in osteoarthritis, 463
Reiter's disease, 11–12, *12*
Relapsing polychondritis, complications of, 495
  management of, 495–496
  symptoms of, 495
Relaxin, in scleroderma, 368
Renal. See also *Kidneys.*
Renal allograft, survival of, in systemic lupus erythematosus, 309t, 309–310
Renal biopsy, in lupus nephritis, 302

Renal disease, end-stage, in systemic lupus erythematosus, management of, 309–310
  in systemic lupus erythematosus, 297–312
Renal toxicity, NSAID-related, 407
Rest, and exercise, in problems of hand and wrist, in rheumatoid arthritis, 75
  in rheumatoid arthritis, 218, 231
Retinoids, in cutaneous lupus erythematosus, 179, *180*
  in psoriasis, 186
  in psoriatic arthritis, 271
Reye's syndrome, aspirin and, 404
Rheumatic diseases, cutaneous disease associated with, treatment of, 175–191
  during pregnancy, treatment of, 163–174
  in childhood, 423–445
  in elderly, 31–33
    epidemiology of, 31
    evaluation and treatment of, 31–32
  of hand and wrist, 75–88
  uncommon, 487–502
Rheumatic fever, acute, in differential diagnosis of acute polyarthritis, 20, 25
Rheumatoid arthritis, 217–235
  age and, 38
  amyloidosis in, 241
  anemia in. See *Anemia, in rheumatoid arthritis.*
  antibiotics in, 226
  antimalarials in, 224–225, 230
  Arthritis Self-Management Program in, 155–156
  aspirin in, 220, 221
  azathioprine in, 38, 225–226, 230, 232
  bone loss in, 530–531
  bone mineral metabolism in, drugs affecting, 531–533
  bronchiectasis in, 238
  bronchiolitis obliterans in, 237, 238
  bronchiolitis obliterans-organizing pneumonia in, 237–238
  CD4 mAb in, 212–213
  cell-targeted therapies in, 212–214
  cervical spine in, 58–59, *59*
  chronic neutropenia in. See *Felty's syndrome.*
  clinical features of, 217
  corticosteroids in, 39, 227–229, 531
  cricoarytenoid ankylosis in, 238
  cyclosporine in, 38, 226, 229, 230
  cytokine-targeted therapies in, 208–212
  diagnosis of, *8*, 8–10, *9*, *10*, 37
  differential diagnosis of, 5, 37, 39–40
  disease-modifying antirheumatic drugs in, 221–226, 222t, 229, 231–232
  drug therapy in, 37
  during pregnancy, 163–166
  elderly-onset, shoulder in, 44
  etanercept in, 39, 210–211, 226–227, 230
  extra-articular manifestations of, 236–248
  flatfoot associated with, 71
  gene therapy in, 214
  glucocorticoids in, 228t, 236, 238
  gold therapy in, 38–39, 223, 230
  hydroxychloroquine in, 38, 224–225, 229, 230, 231
  immunologic mechanisms of, therapies targeted at, 209t
  in differential diagnosis of acute polyarthritis, 21, 22, 23, 26, 27, 28
  in elderly, diagnosis of, 37
    drug therapy in, 37–39

Rheumatoid arthritis (*Continued*)
  infliximab in, 211, 227, 230
    plus methotrexate, 209–210
  intercellular adhesion molecule-1 in, 213–214
  interleukin-1 blockage in, 211–212
  interleukin-6 blockage in, 212
  juvenile. See *Juvenile rheumatoid arthritis.*
  large granular leukemia and, treatment of, 201
  laryngeal involvement in, 238
  leflunomide in, 39, 226, 230
  management of, authors' approaches to, 231–232
  methotrexate in, 37–38, 223–224, 229, 230, 231, 232
    plus infliximab, 209–210
  methylprednisolone in, 228, 230
  morbid complications of, 217–218
  natural history of, 217–218
  neck pain in, 62
  nonselective cyclooxygenase-1 and -2 inhibitors in, 220–221
  nonsteroidal anti-inflammatory agents in, 37–38, 218–219, 219t
  novel therapies for, 208–216
  ocular disease in, 239–240
  osteoporosis in, 530
  outcomes in, 217
  penicillamine in, 38
  D-penicillamine in, 225, 230
  pneumoconiosis in, 237
  prednisone in, 228, 232, 237
  prevalence of, 37
  problems of hand and wrist in, nonsurgical treatment of, 75
    preventive and therapeutic surgery in, 75
  pulmonary arteritis in, 238
  pulmonary disease in, 236–238
  pulmonary fibrosis in, treatment of, 237
  red cell aplasia in, 200
  remissions in, 217
  rest in, 218, 231
  salicylates in, 221
  selective cyclooxygenase-2 inhibitors in, 219–220
  seropositivity for rheumatoid factor and, 218
  shoulder pain in, 44, 45
    treatment of, 46
  sulfasalazine in, 38, 224, 229, 230, 232, 413
  systemic inflammatory features of, management of, 236
  TNF inhibitors in, 226–227, 230
  treatment strategies for, 229–231
  tumor necrosis factor blockage in, 208–211
  younger-onset, shoulder in, 44
Rheumatoid disease, cardiac disease in, 238–239
Rheumatoid factor, 37–39
Rheumatoid vasculitis. See *Vasculitis(ides), rheumatoid.*
Rheumatology practice, medical documentation for. See *Medical documentation.*
Rifampin, in spinal tuberculosis, 510
Risedronate, in osteoporosis, 537, 540–541, 542
  in Paget's disease, 498, 499
Rose bengal staining, in dry eyes, 252
Rotator cuff disease, shoulder pain in, 45
  total shoulder prosthesis in, 47–48

RS3PE, and rheumatoid arthritis, differential diagnosis of, 39–40
Rubella, in differential diagnosis of acute polyarthritis, 19, 25

## S

Salicylates, advantages of, 221
adverse effects of, 220
in gout, 455–456
in rheumatoid arthritis, 221
in systemic lupus erythematosus in childhood, 424
side effects of, 424
Saliva substitutes, in Sjögren's syndrome, 255
Salivary flow, regulation of, 250, 251
Sarcoidosis, arthritis in, treatment of, 489
cardiovascular manifestations of, treatment of, 489–490
clinical spectrum of, 487
corticosteroids in, 489
dermatologic manifestations of, treatment of, 489
immunomodulatory therapy in, 488t
immunosuppressive therapy in, 488t
joint manifestations of, 487
natural history of, 487
neurologic manifestations of, treatment of, 490
ophthalmic manifestations of, treatment of, 489
prognostic signs in, 487
pulmonary manifestations of, treatment of, 489
remission of, 487
renal manifestations of, treatment of, 489
treatment of, 487–490
Schamberg's disease, in organ transplant recipients, 117
Schirmer I test, 252
Schirmer II test, 252
Sciatica, diagnostic features of, 90–91
epidemiology of, 90
epidural steroid injections in, 95–96
medications in, 95
observation in, 95
pathogenesis of, 90
Scleritis, 195
necrotizing, in rheumatoid arthritis, 239–240
Scleroderma, 365–381
antithymocyte globulin in, 369
as multisystem disease, 365
autologous stem cell transplantation in, 369
azathioprine in, 368–369
baseline evaluation in, 365, 366t
cardiovascular disease in, management of, 378
chlorambucil in, 368
colchicine in, 367
colonic involvement in, 375
cyclosporine in, 369
delayed gastric emptying in, 374
diffuse cutaneous, 365–366
dimethyl sulfoxide in, 368
disease-modifying agents in, drugs used as, 366–370
dysphagia in, 373
esophagitis in, 373–374
extracorporeal photopheresis in, 369
gastrointestinal reflux disease in, 374
gastrointestinal tract involvement in, management of, 373–375
immunosuppressive agents in, 368–369

Scleroderma (Continued)
in children, clinical manifestations of, 438
linear lesions in, 438
treatment of, 438
interferon in, 368
kidney involvement in, 375–376
limited, 365
localized, alternate therapies in, 182
calcipotriene in, 182
calcitriol in, 181–182
methotrexate in, 182
types of, 181, 181
ultraviolet A therapy in, 182
methotrexate in, 369
musculoskeletal system in, management of, 377–378
natural history of, 365–366
organ-specific treatment of, 370–379
potassium para-aminobenzoic acid in, 367–368
psychosocial issues in, management of, 378–379
pulmonary involvement in, management of, 370–373, 371
Raynaud's phenomenon in, management of, 376
relaxin in, 368
skin in, management of, 376–377
small bowel problems in, 374–375
therapeutic intervention in, authors' approach to, 370
future approaches to, 370
rationale for, 366
total lymphoid irradiation in, 369
Sclerosis, progressive systemic, during pregnancy, 166
Seizures, in neuropsychiatric systemic lupus erythematosus, 313–314
treatment of, 318
Selective estrogen receptor modulators, in osteoporosis, 536
Self-management treatment strategies, in arthritis, 152–158, 153t
Serositis, nonsteroidal anti-inflammatory drugs in, 280
Serpiginous choroiditis, 196
Shoulder pain, 44–49
clinical presentation of, 44
dexamethasone acetate in, 46
differential diagnosis of, 45–46
epidemiology of, 44–49
imaging in, 44–45
steroid injection in, 46
treatment of, conservative, 46
invasive, 46–48
Shoulder prosthesis, total, in rotator cuff disease, 47–48
Sinus disease, in Wegener's granulomatosis, 334
Sinusitis, in Sjögren's syndrome, treatment of, 256
Sjögren's syndrome, 10, 11
and rheumatoid arthritis, differential diagnosis of, 39
anesthesia and surgery in, 259–260, 260t
depression in, 258
diagnostic criteria in, controversy regarding, 249–250
disordered sleep in, 257–258
dry eyes in, evaluation of, 251–253
topical therapy of, 253
dry mouth in, evaluation and treatment of, 254–256
extraglandular manifestations of, 258t

Sjögren's syndrome (Continued)
fatigue in, 257–258
hydroxychloroquine in, 258–259
in differential diagnosis of acute polyarthritis, 21, 22, 24, 26, 27, 29
nasal dryness and sinusitis in, treatment of, 256
nonsteroidal anti-inflammatory agents in, 258
parotid gland swelling in, 259
primary, 249
routes of referral in, 249
schematic diagram of, 250–251, 251
secondary, 249
skin and gynecologic dryness in, treatment of, 256–257
symptoms in, pathogenesis of, 250–251
systemic medications in, 258–259
therapeutic considerations in, 259–260
treatment of, approaches to, 249–261
vasculitis of central nervous system in, 351–352
Skin, disease of, associated with rheumatic disease, treatment of, 175–191
dryness of, in Sjögren's syndrome, treatment of, 256–257
effects of nonsteroidal anti-inflammatory agents on, 220
in Henoch-Schönlein purpura, 337
in hypersensitivity vasculitis, 338
in scleroderma, management of, 376–377
in type II mixed cryoglobulinemia, 335
lesions of, in sarcoidosis, 489
nonsteroidal anti-inflammatory drug effects on, 471
Sleep, disordered, in Sjögren's syndrome, 257–258
Sodium fluoride, in osteoporosis, 537, 540
Soma, in fibromyalgia syndrome, 125
Somatostatin, in psoriatic arthritis, 271
Spinal cord, stimulation of, in chronic pain syndrome, 98–99
Spine, cervical, anatomy of, 51, 52
dislocations of, classification of, 58, 58
fracture(s) of, classification of, 58, 58
diagnosis of, 56–58
in rheumatoid arthritis, 58–59, 59
infections of, 59–60, 60
nerve plexus of, 51, 52
lumbar, disease of. See Lumbar spine disease.
mechanical disease of, in ankylosing spondylitis, 264
tuberculosis of, 510
Splenectomy, in Felty's syndrome, 200, 242
in thrombocytopenia with systemic lupus erythematosus, 204
Splinting, in problems of hand and wrist, in rheumatoid arthritis, 75
Spondyloarthropathies, diagnosis of, 10–13
differential diagnosis of, 6
pediatric, and adult-onset, compared, 403
aspirin in, 403–404
corticosteroids in, 407–409
methotrexate in, 409–411
nonsteroidal anti-inflammatory drugs in, 404–407
treatment of, 403

Spondyloarthropathies (*Continued*)
  seronegative, 263–273
    common features of, 263
    neck pain in, 59
*Sporothrix schenckii* arthritis, 512
Spurling's test, in neck pain, 53, *55*
Stem cell transplantation, autologous, in
    scleroderma, 369
  in juvenile rheumatoid arthritis, 415
  in systemic lupus erythematosus, 277
Sterility, cyclophosphamide-induced,
    428
"Steroid psychosis," 316
Steroids. See *Corticosteroids.*
Still's disease, adult-onset, in differential
    diagnosis of acute polyarthritis, 21, 22,
    24, 25, 27, 28
Stress management interventions, in
    arthritis, 150–151
Stroke syndromes, in neuropsychiatric
    systemic lupus erythematosus,
    313–314
Subtalar joint, pain in, 68
  range of motion of, 65–66
Sulfasalazine, clinical use of, 413
  during pregnancy, 169
  in ankylosing spondylitis, 266–267
  in Behçet's disease, 491
  in juvenile rheumatoid arthritis, 413
  in osteoarthritis, 477
  in psoriatic arthritis, 270
  in reactive arthritis, 267, 268
  in rheumatoid arthritis, 38, 224, 229,
    230
  monitoring of toxicity of, 413
Sulfinpyrazone, in chronic gout, in organ
    transplant recipients, 115
  in gout, 455
Sulindac, and renal toxicity in nonsteroidal
    anti-inflammatory drug usage,
    470–471
Swan-neck deformities, in rheumatic
    disease, 80
Sweet's syndrome, 188–189
  corticosteroids in, 188–189, *189*
  four types of, 188
  prednisone in, 188, *189*
Sympathectomy, chemical, in complex
    regional pain syndrome-I, 104–105
  in Raynaud's phenomenon, 387
  surgical, in complex regional pain
    syndrome-I, 106
Sympathetic blockade, oral, in complex
    regional pain syndrome-I, 106
Sympatholytic agents, in Raynaud's
    phenomenon, 385, 386t
Synovectomy, in rheumatic disease of
    hand and wrist, 77–78
  in shoulder pain, 46–47
Syringomyelia, 61
Systemic lupus erythematosus, and
    rheumatoid arthritis, differential
    diagnosis of, 39
  anemia in, 201–203, 281
  anticoagulation in, 282
  antimalarials in, 274–275, 275t, 277,
    278t
  antiphospholipid syndrome in, 282
  author's approach to, 279–282
  autoimmune hemolytic anemia in,
    author's approach to, 202
  azathioprine in, 276, 278, 279t, 282
  bone loss in, 533
  bromocriptine in, 277
  clinical features of, 82

Systemic lupus erythematosus (*Continued*)
  controlled clinical trials in, 277–279
  corticosteroids in, 275–276, 276t
  cyclophosphamide in, 276, 278, 281,
    282
  cyclosporine in, 276
  cystitis in, 281
  dehydroepiandrosterone in, 277, 278–279
  diagnosis of, 16, *16*, 17
  end-stage renal disease in, management
    of, 309–310
  fever in, 281
  hydroxychloroquine in, 282
  in childhood, antimalarial drugs in, 425
    antiphospholipid syndrome in,
      431–432
    azathioprine in, 429
    clinical manifestations of, 423
    cyclophosphamide in, 427–428
      side effects of, 428
    cyclosporine in, 430
    cytotoxic drugs in, 426–427
    immunoablation in, 430–431
    incidence of, 423
    intravenous immunoglobulin in,
      430
    methotrexate in, 429
    mycophenolate mofetil in, 429–430
    nitrogen mustard in, 429
    plasmapheresis in, 430
    salicylates and nonsteroidal anti-
      inflammatory drugs in, 424
    steroids in, 425–426
      indications for, 425
      low-dose, high-dose, and
        intravenous pulse, 425–426
      side effects of, 426
    treatment of, 431t, 432, *432*
      general measures in, 424
      goals of, 423–424
      pharmacologic therapy in, 424–432
  in differential diagnosis of acute
    polyarthritis, 21, 22, 23, 26, 27, 28
  intravenous immune globulin in, 277
  intravenous methylprednisolone in,
    277–278, 278t
  intravenous "pulse" methylprednisolone
    in, 275–276, 276t
  investigational drugs and future
    directions in, 285
  lymphadenopathy in, 281
  methotrexate in, 276, 277t, 278, 281
  microangiopathic hemolytic anemia in,
    202–203
  natural history of, 274
  neuropsychiatric, acute global
    dysfunction in, treatment of, 318
    central nervous system dysfunction in,
      causes of, 315
    clinical manifestations of, 313
    cognitive impairment in, treatment of,
      320
    corticosteroids in, 315–316
    cranial neuropathies in, treatment of,
      320
    cyclophosphamide in, 316–317
    differential diagnosis of, 315
    focal manifestations of, treatment of,
      318
    mortality associated with, 313
    neuropathologic studies in, 314–315
    plasmapheresis in, 317–318
    prolactin and interleukin-6 in, 315
    refractory, 317–318
    seizures in, treatment of, 318

Systemic lupus erythematosus (*Continued*)
  sensorineural hearing loss in,
    treatment of, 320
  specific manifestations of, treatment
    of, 318–320
  subacute global dysfunction in,
    treatment of, 318
  transverse myelitis in, treatment of,
    318
  treatment of, 313–322, 315–318, 319t
  vasculopathy in, 314
  nonsteroidal anti-inflammatory drugs in,
    274, 275t, 277, 282
  open-label trials in, 274–277
  plasmapheresis in, 276–277
  prednisone in, 282
  pregnancy in, 281–282
  prognosis in, 274
  pulmonary hypertension in, 280
  Raynaud's phenomenon in, 280
  renal allograft survival in, 309t,
    309–310
  renal disease in, 297–312
  specific deformities in, 82–83
  stem cell transplantation in, 277
  systemic thrombotic processes in,
    differential diagnosis/clinical
    manifestations of, 203t
  thrombocytopenia in, 203–205, 281
    author's approach to, 205
  thrombotic thrombocytopenic purpura
    in, 203
  vasculitis of central nervous system in,
    351

**T**

Takayasu's arteritis, 353–356
  active disease in, criteria for, 354t
  cyclophosphamide in, 355
  cytotoxic therapy in, 355–356
  disease activity in, assessment of,
    353–354
  glucocorticoids in, 354–355, 355t
  hypertension in, 356
  methotrexate in, 355–356
  natural history of, 353
  percutaneous transluminal angioplasty
    in, 356
  prednisone in, 354–355, 356
  surgery in, 356
  treatment of, 354–356, 355t
Tamoxifen, in osteoporosis, 536
Tarsal joint, transverse, pain in, 68–69
  range of motion of, 66
Tarsometatarsal joints, range of motion
  of, 66
Tears, artificial, 253t
  evaluation of, 253
  basal flow of, 252
  flow of, regulation of, 250, *251*
  volume of, measurement of, 252
Temazepam, in fibromyalgia syndrome,
  124
Temperature biofeedback, in Raynaud's
  phenomenon, 383–384
Temperature biofeedback training, in
  arthritis, 149
Temporal arteritis. See *Giant cell arteritis.*
Tennis elbow, 85
Tenosynovitis, de Quervain's, 86
  digital flexor, in rheumatic disease of
    hand, 77
  flexor, in rheumatic disease of hand, 76
  in rheumatic disease of hand, 75
  in rheumatoid arthritis, 240

Tenosynovitis (*Continued*)
  palmar (stenosing), in rheumatic disease of hand, 77
  wrist flexor, in rheumatic disease of hand, 76–77, *77*
Teratogenicity, cyclophosphamide-induced, 428
Tetracycline, in Behçet's disease, 490
  in Lyme disease, 517–518
Thalidomide, in Behçet's disease, 490–491
  in cutaneous lupus erythematosus, 178
Thrombocytopenia, in systemic lupus erythematosus, 203–205, 281
  author's approach to, 205
Thrombocytopenic purpura, thrombotic, in systemic lupus erythematosus, 203
Thromboses, in antiphospholipid syndrome, 289, 290t, 293
Thumb, arthritic involvement of, in psoriasis, 83
  carpometacarpal joint of, in osteoarthritis, 84
  deformities of, in systemic lupus erythematosus, 82–83
  in rheumatic disease, 78–79
    treatment of, 79, *79*
Tibial tendon, posterior, dysfunction of, natural history of, 69
  pathoanatomy of, 69
  symptoms of, 69
  treatment of, 69–70
  function of, 69
Tick bite control, for prevention of Lyme disease, 522–523
Tick bite prophylaxis, for prevention of Lyme disease, 523–524, 524t
Ticks, *Borrelia burdorferi* transmission by, in Lyme disease, 515
Tidal irrigation, in osteoarthritis, 475
Tiludronate, in Paget's disease, 498
Time-stands test, 393, *394*
Toes, lesser, problems of, 71–72
Tolmetin, in juvenile rheumatoid arthritis, 405
Topical agents, in osteoarthritis, 34
Total body irradiation, in polymyositis, 399
  side effects of, 399
Total lymphoid irradiation, in scleroderma, 369
Tramadol, in fibromyalgia syndrome, 42
  in osteoarthritis, 465
Transcutaneous electric nerve stimulation, in chronic pain syndrome, 98
  in fibromyalgia syndrome, 128
Transverse myelitis, in neuropsychiatric systemic lupus erythematosus, 314
  treatment of, 318
Transverse tarsal joint, pain in, 68–69
  range of motion of, 66
Trazodone, in fibromyalgia syndrome, 42
Triamcinolone, in acute gout, 450–451
  in Behçet's disease, 490
  in sarcoidosis, 489
Tricyclic agents, in fibromyalgia syndrome, 42, 121–123, 128
Trigger point injection, myofascial, in lumbago, 94
Trimethoprim-sulfamethoxazole, clinical trials of, in Wegener's granulomatosis, 333–334
Tuberculosis, spinal, 510

Tuberculous spondylitis, 59–60
Tumor(s), bone, neck pain in, 60–61
Tumor necrosis factor, blockage of, in rheumatoid arthritis, 208–211
Tumor necrosis factor-α inhibitors, in sarcoidosis, 490

## U

Ulcers, nonsteroidal anti-inflammatory drugs and, 469–470
Ulna, distal, in rheumatoid arthritis, 78
Ultraviolet A therapy, in localized scleroderma, 182
Ultraviolet B therapy, in psoriasis, 186
Urate oxidase, in crystal deposition disease, 458
Uricosuric agents, in gout, 455–456
Urothelial toxicity, of cyclophosphamide, 361
Uveitis, alkylators in, 195
  antimetabolites in, 195
  azathioprine in, 195
  complications of, 192
  corticosteroids in, 194–195
  cyclosporine in, 195
  diagnostic categorization of, 192, 193t
  during childhood, treatment of, 196
  FK-506 in, 195
  future approaches in, 195–196
  immunoglobulins in, 195–196
  immunosuppression in, 192–193
  in ankylosing spondylitis, 264
  in Vogt-Koyanagi-Harada syndrome, 196
  inferferon-alpha in, 196
  methotrexate in, 195
  nonsteroidal anti-inflammatory drugs in, 194
  periocular injections in, 194
  prednisone in, 194
  topical medications in, 194
  treatment of, 192
    guidelines for, 192–195
  types of, 192, *193*

## V

Vaccination, in Lyme disease prophylaxis, 524
Valvular disease, in rheumatoid arthritis, 239
Vancomycin, in infectious arthritis, 504
Varicella-zoster virus infection, vasculitis after, and granulomatous angiitis of central nervous system, 350
Vasculitis(ides), 323–344
  classification of, 323, 324t
  cryoglobulinemia with. See *Cryoglobulinemia, type II mixed*.
  cutaneous, antihistamines in, 183
    antimalarial agents in, 183
    azathioprine in, 185, *185*
    colchicine in, 183
    corticosteroids in, 184
    cyclophosphamide in, 184–185
    cyclosporine in, 185
    dapsone in, 183
    immunosuppressive agents in, 184
    methotrexate in, 185
    methylprednisolone in, 184
    nonsteroidal anti-inflammatory agents in, 183
    patient evaluation in, 182–183

Vasculitis(ides) (*Continued*)
    pentoxifylline in, 183
    prednisone in, 184
    syndromes displaying, 182
    treatment of, corticosteroids in, 183–184
      disease-specific considerations in, 183
      general, 183–185
      immunosuppressive agents in, 184–185
      nonimmunologic drug therapy in, 183
      plasmapheresis in, 185
  hypersensitivity. See *Hypersensitivity vasculitis*.
  in childhood, 435–438
  in Cogan's syndrome, 339, 340
  in organ transplant recipients, 116–117
  initial therapy of, guidelines for, 340t
  leukocytoclastic, 182
  of central nervous system, 345–352
    infection-associated, 350–351
  rheumatoid, azathioprine in, 244, 245
    chlorambucil in, 244, 245
    clinical features of, 242, 243
    cyclophosphamide in, 244, 245
    disease-modifying antirheumatic drugs in, 244
    in rheumatoid arthritis, 242–245
    inflammation in, 243
    leg ulcers in, 245
    methotrexate in, 244
    methylprednisolone in, 244
    myocardial disease in, 239
    organs involved in, 242
    prednisone in, 245
    relative survival in, 243t
    treatment of, 243–244, 244t
  systemic, investigational drugs and future directions in, 331
    necrotizing, glucocorticoid therapy without cytotoxic agents in, 328t
    secondary, treatment of, 350–352
    vasculitis of central nervous system in, 351
Vasodilation, in complex regional pain syndrome-I, 106
Vasodilators, in Raynaud's phenomenon, 384–385, 386t
Verapamil, in benign angiopathy of central nervous system, 350
Vertebrae, cervical, congenitally fused, *54*
Viscosupplementation, intra-articular, in osteoarthritis, 473–474
Vision, effects of hydroxychloroquine on, 425
  in giant cell arteritis, 358
Vitamin C, in osteoarthritis, 476–477
Vitamin D, corticosteroids and, 532
  in osteoarthritis, 476
  in osteoporosis, 535–536, 539
Vitamin E, in osteoarthritis, 476–477
Vitamin K antagonists, in antiphospholipid syndrome, 294
Vogt-Koyanagi-Harada syndrome, uveitis in, 196

## W

Warfarin, in venous thrombosis in systemic lupus erythematosus, 282
Wegener's granulomatosis, clinical features of, 331
  clinical trials in, 333–334
  cyclophosphamide in, 332–333, 334

Wegener's granulomatosis (*Continued*)
  diagnosis of, 332
  disease- and treatment-related morbidity
    in, 332
  generalized, 331
  glucocorticoids in, 332–333
  in children, clinical manifestations of,
    437–438
    treatment of, 438
  in differential diagnosis of acute
    polyarthritis, 21, 22, 23, 29
  investigational drugs and future
    therapies in, 334

Wegener's granulomatosis (*Continued*)
  limited, 331
  management of, 334
  methotrexate in, 333, 334
  methylprednisolone in, 333
  natural history of, 332
  sinus disease in, 334
  treatment studies and long-term
    experience with, 332–333
  trimethoprim-sulfamethoxazole in,
    333–334
Western blot analysis, in Lyme disease,
  516–517

Whiplash, treatment of, 56
Wrist, in osteoarthritis, 84
  in psoriasis, 83
  in systemic lupus erythematosus, 82
  rheumatic disease(s) of, 75–88
    patient evalution in, 75
    reconstructive and salvage surgery
      in, 78

**Z**
Zolpidem, in fibromyalgia syndrome, 42

ISBN 0-7216-8464-5

90038

9 780721 684642